Suki and Massry's THERAPY OF RENAL DISEASES AND RELATED DISORDERS,
THIRD EDITION

Suki and Massry's THERAPY OF RENAL DISEASES AND RELATED DISORDERS, THIRD EDITION

edited by

Wadi N. Suki, M.D.

Shaul G. Massry, M.D.

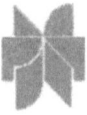

SPRINGER SCIENCE+BUSINESS MEDIA, LLC

Library of Congress Cataloging-in-Publication Data

Suki and Massry's therapy of renal diseases and related disorders.—3rd ed.
  p. cm.
 Rev. ed. of: Therapy of renal diseases and related disorders. 2nd ed. c1991.
 Includes bibliographical references and index.
  ISBN 978-1-4757-6634-9   ISBN 978-1-4757-6632-5 (eBook)
  DOI 10.1007/978-1-4757-6632-5

  1. Kidneys—Diseases—Treatment. 2. Urinary organs—Diseases—Treatment. I. Suki, Wadi N., 1934– .
 II. Massry, Shaul G.
  [DNLM: 1. Kidney Diseases—therapy.   WJ 300 S9475 1997]
 RC902. T49 1997
 616.6′106—dc21
 DNLM/DLC
 for Library of Congress   96-49630
                                                                                          CIP

Copyright © 1997 by Springer Science+Business Media New York
Originally published by Kluwer Academic Publishers in 1997
Softcover reprint of the hardcover 3rd edition 1997

Printed on acid-free paper.

CONTENTS

Foreword   ix
Preface to the First Edition   xi
Preface to the Second Edition   xiii
Preface to the Third Edition and Dedication   xv
List of Contributors   xvii

PART ONE: DISORDERS OF FLUID,
ELECTROLYTE, AND ACID–BASE BALANCE

1. Pathogenesis and treatment of hypoosmolar and hyperosmolar states   1
   J. CARLOS AYUS & ALLEN I. ARIEFF

2. Polyuric syndromes   21
   KIRBY GABRYS & MATTHEW D. BREYER

3. Edematous states   35
   JULES B. PUSCHETT & N. KEVIN KRANE

4. Disorders of potassium metabolism   53
   F. JOHN GENNARI

5. Disorders of calcium metabolism   85
   THERESA A. GUISE & GREGORY R. MUNDY

6. Disorders of magnesium homeostasis and magnesium in therapy   115
   JACK W. COBURN & BARTON S. LEVINE

7. Disorders of phosphate metabolism   143
   NORIMOTO YANAGAWA & MOUFID NEMEH

8. Nephrolithiasis and nephrocalcinosis   167
   JOAN H. PARKS & FREDRIC L. COE

9. Metabolic alkalosis: biochemical mechanisms, pathophysiology, and treatment   189
   SANDRA SABATINI & NEIL A. KURTZMAN

10. Therapy of lactic acidosis   211
    CHRISTINE P. BASTL, MICHAEL HEIFETS & LOUIS J. RILEY, JR.

11. Diabetic ketoacidosis and hyperosmolar nonketotic syndrome   233
    HORACIO J. ADROGUÉ

12. Metabolic acidosis   253
    MARTIN SCHREIBER, ROBERT M.A. RICHARDSON & MITCHELL L. HALPERIN

13. Renal tubular acidosis   275
    BRUCE KAPLAN & DANIEL BATLLE

14. Respiratory acid–base disorders   293
    HORACIO J. ADROGUÉ & NICOLAOS E. MADIAS

15. Mixed acid–base disorders   307
    NICOLAOS E. MADIAS & HORACIO J. ADROGUÉ

16. Fluid and electrolyte abnormalities in children   319
    CHARLES L. STEWART, FREDERICK J. KASKEL, & RICHARD N. FINE

17. Fluid and electrolyte disorders in the surgical patient   335
    KHALIL U. RAHMAN & WADI N. SUKI

18. Fluid and electrolyte disorders in the thermally injured   351
    CHARLES BAXTER & GEORGE J. KALOYANIDES

19. Acute renal failure   359
    GEORGE J. KALOYANIDES

PART TWO: INTRINSIC PARENCHYMAL DISEASE

A. GLOMERULAR

20. Acute glomerulonephritis   387
    FRANK G. BOINEAU & JOHN E. LEWY

21. Glomerulonephritis in bacterial endocarditis   395
DAVID S. BALDWIN &
JOEL NEUGARTEN

22. Goodpasture's syndrome   401
DAVID I. CHARNEY &
WAYNE A. BORDER ·

23. Nephrotic syndrome   413
PATRIZIA PASSERINI &
CLAUDIO PONTICELLI

24. Hematuria and IgA nephropathy   429
GIUSEPPE D'AMICO

B. TUBULOINTERSTITIAL

25. Infections of the urinary tract   435
NINA TOLKOFF-RUBIN &
ROBERT H. RUBIN

26. Vesicoureteral reflux and reflux nephropathy   441
ROBERT A. WEISS & ADRIAN SPITZER

27. Genitourinary tuberculosis   451
JAMES G. GOW

PART THREE: RENAL INVOLVEMENT IN
SYSTEMIC DISEASE

28. Systemic lupus erythematosus   459
STEPHEN MARK OLMSTEAD,
JOE VENZOR & DAVID P. HUSTON

29. Vasculitic diseases of the kidney   479
JAMES E. BALOW &
HOWARD A. AUSTIN III

30. Noninflammatory vascular disease of the
kidney   489
GARABED EKNOYAN

31. Thrombotic microangiopathy   513
PIERO RUGGENENTI &
GIUSEPPE REMUZZ

32. Multiple myeloma and plasma cell dyscrasias   529
PIETRO ZUCCHELLI &
SONIA PASQUALI

33. Hyperuricemic nephropathy   541
MOUFID N. NEMEH &
EDWARD J. WEINMAN

34. The effects of jaundice and cholemia on
kidney function and the cardiovascular system   547
JACOB GREEN & ORI S. BETTER

35. Renal complications of pregnancy   561
JOHN M. DAVISON, ADRIAN I. KATZ &
MARSHALL D. LINDHEIMER

36. Prevention and early treatment of diabetic
renal disease   605
CARL ERIK MOGENSEN

37. Renal complications of intravenous drug abuse
and human immunodeficiency virus infection   619
JACQUES J. BOURGOIGNIE

PART FOUR: HEREDITARY AND CONGENITAL
DISEASES

38. Renal cystic disease   639
R. DAVID GILE, BENJAMIN D. COWLEY,
JR. & JARED J. GRANTHAM

39. Therapy of the renal complications of sickle
cell hemoglobinopathy   663
CARLOS A. VAAMONDE &
JAMES R. OSTER

40. Inherited renal tubular disorders   671
DONALD L. BATISKY &
RUSSELL W. CHESNEY

41. Genetic diagnosis and counseling in inherited
renal diseases   685
JEAN-PIERRE GRÜNFELD,
GABRIEL CHOUKROUN &
BERTRAND KNEBELMANN

PART FIVE: NEOPLASIA

42. Cancers of the urinary tract   695
SETH P. LERNER & JAMES EASTHAM

PART SIX: CHEMICAL AND PHYSICAL INJURIES

43. Toxic nephropathy   723
WILLIAM M. BENNETT

44. Acute drug intoxications   747
JAMES F. WINCHESTER

PART SEVEN: CHRONIC RENAL FAILURE

A. MEDICAL THERAPY

45. Prevention of progression of renal disease   757
SAULO KLAHR

46. Renal insufficiency   767
FADI G. LAKKIS &
MANUEL MARTINEZ-MALDONADO

47. Anesthesia and surgery in the patient with
renal failure   777
DAVID R. BEVAN

48. Nutritional management of the uremic patient   783
AUGUST HEIDLAND, KATARINA
SÉBEKOVA & MARKUS TESCHNER

49. Treatment of hyperlipidemia in the nephrotic
syndrome   803
GEORGE A. KAYSEN

50. Cardiovascular complications in uremia and
    dialysis   817
    MIROSLAW SMOGORZEWSKI

51. Renal osteodystrophy: prevention and
    management   841
    ESTHER A. GONZALEZ &
    KEVIN J. MARTIN

52. Neurologic and psychiatric disorders in renal
    diseases   855
    ALBERTO ALBERTAZZI,
    MARIO BONOMINI & PAOLO CAPPELLI

53. Hematologic disorders in renal failure   875
    J. RADERMACHER &
    KARL M. KOCH

54. Hepatitis in the renal patient   893
    DAVID ROTH & GUIDO PEREZ

B. PERITONEAL DIALYSIS

55. Acute, intermittent, and cycled peritoneal
    dialysis   915
    JOSE A. DIAZ-BUXO

56. Continuous ambulatory peritoneal dialysis   935
    RAMESH KHANNA,
    ROBERT MACTIER & KARL D. NOLPH

57. Peritoneal catheter placement and
    management   953
    ZBYLUT J. TWARDOWSKI

58. Peritonitis and other complications   981
    CHARLES E. HALSTENSON &
    WILLIAM F. KEANE

C. HEMODIALYSIS

59. Dialysis access: temporary and permanent   989
    H. DAVID SHORT,
    WADE R. ROSENBERG &
    GEORGE P. NOON

60. Dialyzers, dialysates, and water treatment   1005
    NUHAD ISMAIL, BRYAN BECKER &
    RAYMOND M. HAKIM

61. Membrane biocompatibility   1021
    DANIEL F. WALTON &
    ALFRED K. CHEUNG

62. Hemodialysis, ultrafiltration, and
    hemofiltration   1043
    RAYMOND C. VANDERHOLDER,
    ANN A. VANLOO & SEVERIN M. RINGOIR

63. Use of drugs in uremia and dialysis   1065
    D. CRAIG BRATER

D. TRANSPLANTATION

64. Donor and recipient selection   1079
    STUART M. FLECHNER

65. Immunosuppression and treatment of
    rejection   1107
    M. ROY FIRST

66. Tubular and metabolic dysfunction following
    transplantation   1139
    LILIANA GRADOWSKA &
    LESZEK PĄCZEK

67. Transplantation in inherited systemic and
    metabolic diseases   1153
    ELEANOR D. LEDERER

68. Complications of renal transplantation   1169
    PETER J. MORRIS

PART EIGHT: HYPERTENSION

69. Essential hypertension   1183
    MICHAEL A. WEBER

70. Renal and renovascular hypertension   1195
    GEORGES MOURAD,
    JEAN-MICHEL HALIMI,
    JEAN RIBSTEIN & ALBERT MIMRAN

71. Posttransplant hypertension   1207
    DAVID A. LASKOW & JOHN J. CURTIS

PART NINE: UROLOGIC DISORDERS

72. The catheter   1219
    GRANNUM R. SANT &
    EDWIN M. MEARES, JR.

73. Nonsurgical management of vesicourethral
    dysfunction   1233
    J. KEITH LIGHT

Index   1241

Foreword[1]

"Where are all these kidney patients coming from? A few years ago we had never heard of kidney disease and now you are speaking of patients in the hundreds of thousands and indeed potentially millions." My reply, not meant to be grim, was "From the cemetery, Sir." This is a summary of some Congressional testimony I once gave on behalf of extending kidney disease under Medicare. Where indeed were all the patients with kidney disease in the United States before World War II? They were certainly not under the care of nephrologists! Nephrology was not listed in the questionnaires for any state or the American Medical Association as a subspecialty or even as a special interest. Indeed, even in the late 1960s, when I wrote the American Medical Association editor and asked why nephrology had not been included on a questionnaire to American physicians about their specialty interests, I received a "tongue in check" answer, "What's nephrology?" Indeed, for those of us who bridge back, it is often hard to realize the rapid evolution of our specialty. For uremia, we gave low-protein diets, adequate hydration, attention to fluid and electrolytes, comfort, and prayer. In my first two years at Georgetown, where every death in the hospital was reviewed, my nephrology division made death conference all but a few weeks out of the first two years. In a 1961 book on uremia[2] I wrote:

> The reversibility of uremic coma has received some attention but could use more. In a further effort to discourage pessimism we have therefore placed a capital 'R' following each of the potentially reversible types of renal disease. It is our sincere hope that the number of 'R's' will provide a pleasant surprise for the many physicians and medical students who want to think of the uremic syndrome as a terminal state during which little treatment can be instituted except that designed for the comfort of the patient.

This is not to say that the science underlying nephrology was inactive. Quite to the contrary, many cases of fruitful science relating to the kidney area not only existed but

flourished and had a profound impact on many young clinicians. Thomas Addis raised to a state of applied perfection the study of the urinary sediment, clinically practical kidney function tests, and the natural history of a number of kidney diseases including glomerulonephritis. William Goldring, Herbert Chasis, Dana Atchley, and others studied the effects of hypertension, endocarditis, and circulatory diseases on the kidney and spawned successive generations of alert clinical investigators, who began to chronicle the natural histories of a wide variety of kidney diseases. Quantitative studies of renal function flourished under a school headed by Homer Smith, and surprisingly precise techniques were developed for studying a whole range of explicit nephron functions. Imagine the joy with the advent of vascular catheterization to be able to apply extraction ratios and the Fick principle in a precise way to an organ such as the kidney by sampling arterial blood, venous blood, and the output of the urine! One had a quantitative handle on the entire function of a vital organ—perhaps for the first time in biologic history. One no longer looked only at the street side of the revolving door; one could find out, for example, that if ammonia did not go into the acid trap of the urine, it indeed might go back into the circulation via the renal vein.

The same story unfolded for a broad range of physiologic substances. In the metabolic school of nephrology, represented perhaps most brilliantly by Professor John Peters at Yale, a host of pioneer investigators applied the methods of quantitative clinical biochemistry to the elements of the blood whose homeostasis was so carefully regulated by the kidney. His deep interest in endocrinology and metabolism pointed our way to appreciate the endocrine role of the kidney in making or releasing a whole array of potent hormones affecting bodily function (e.g., erythropoietin, renin, aldosterone, etc.), and indeed the very survival of the human organism. The role of the kidney in controlling vitamin D metabolism, calcium absorption, parathyroid function, and the complex interrelationships comprising calcium/phosphorous homeostasis, bone growth, and bone repair were only mistily appreciated and became one of the great metabolic success

---

[1] Revised for the second edition.

[2] Schreiner GE Maher JF: Uremia, Chemistry and Pathogenesis & Treatment. Charles C. Thomas, Springfield, IL, p 24, 1961.

stories of postwar nephrology and metabolism. Postwar nephrology rushed to the fore and supplied nephrologists with such wonderful tools as the flamephotometer, electrophoresis, microchemistry, immunoassay, sonography, renal biopsy, immunofluorescence, electron microscopy, and unclear magnetic resonance, and permitted a total integration of form, histologic structure, and function. Clinical nephrology became indeed the real fusion of biochemistry, physiology, immunology, renal endocrinology, and the focus of newer imaging techniques.

With this precision in diagnosis, one could realistically hope for rational therapy, and one could be optimistic that some day the correct therapy would be correctly applied to the correct patient with the appropriately diagnosed disease.

With the evolution of such developments, an expert observer could indeed realistically hope that out of the myriad and mushrooming books of nephrology would come one with a message of constructive hope, focusing on the treatment of renal disease. Indeed, Dr. Suki and Dr. Massry have fulfilled that hope with this book, which is appropriately entitled, *The Therapy of Renal Disease and Related Disorders*. They have systematically taken the available scientific information and fused it into a practical text of therapy for the patient. The first section, entitled "Disorders of Fluid, Electrolyte and Acid-Base Balance," covers some of the more challenging general conditions, such as hyperosmolar and hypoosmolar states, polyuria, edema, and acute renal failure. The book then proceeds systematically to disorders of the ions, potassium, calcium, magnesium, phosphate, and the major quartet of acidbase balance, embracing alkalosis and acidosis in its clinically presentable forms. The book proceeds to the intrinsic parenchymal diseases, covering the major areas of glomerular and tubular interstitial disorders and what can be done about them. From there it launches into the vast sea of relationships with systemic diseases such as SLE, vasculitis, hyperuricemia, dysproteinemia, liver disease, pregnancy, and diabetes, among others. Adequate attention is paid to genetic and congenital disorders, including the genetic counseling of families beset by genetically determined disorders. Neoplasia, chemical and physical injuries, and a number of other unusual events are considered with practical insights. Then the book tackles the vast problem of uremia and newer experience with diet, dialysis, and transplantation.

Uremia is to the nephrologist what the baby is to the pediatrician, for it is the final common pathway of literally hundreds of disease processes that lead to scarring and destruction of nephrons.

We estimate that there are well in excess of 300,000 patients in the world living on the varied methodologies represented by the three basic forms of substituted kidney function—hemodialysis, peritoneal dialysis, and renal transplantation: over 100,000 persons in the United States alone, well over 110,000 in the countries compromising the EDTA Registry, and over 100,000 in the Pacific Rim. If we add on South America, Africa, and the lesser developed nations, the total could well be over 400,000 by the time this book is printed. These 400,000 plus persons and their families, who have intimate, repetitive personal experiences with uremia, serve as living withnesses of the medical progress of nephrology in the past three decades. They are witnesses of the fact that many of today's kidney patients have indeed, literally, "come from the cemetery."

But it is not enough to consider only the techniques of substitution therapy. For with living patients come not only the facets of uremia that are not yet handled by therapy, such as cardiovascular complications, renal osteodystrophy, anemia, disorders of immune surveillance, nutritional problems, etc., but there is also a necessity to know which particular patients fit which particular therapy best, and to choose the optimum time for applying one particular therapy to one particular patient. Indeed, the management of the uremic patients becomes essentially a life plan for that person, and the ills that kidney patients have live on with them, instead of going prematurely with them to the grave.

This is a book that is unique among many books available today. This is a book that presents material positively. This is a book that blends the analytical aspects of diagnosis with the hard realities of scientific and appropriate therapy. This is a book that will be enjoyed by young nephrologists and by physicians with a wide diversity of interests. Most of all, it is a book that will be deeply appreciated by their patients.

George E. Schreiner, M.D.
Distinguished Professor of Medicine
Former Director, Division of Nephrology
Georgetown University School of Medicine

Preface to the First Edition

In the last fifteen years, many books and monographs have been published which deal with different aspects of renal structure and function, and the various renal diseases. The number of published works reflects the explosion of scientific knowledge about the kidney and its diseases. Parallel with this increased knowledge have come major advances in the handling and management of patients suffering from disorders of the kidney. These advances, many of which are life-saving, in large measure have been responsible for the emergence of nephrology as a full-fledged medical specialty.

In spite of the progress made in the therapy of renal diseases and related disorders, there has not been a text devoted fully to this subject. The present text attempts to bring together in one ready reference what is known about renal therapeutics today thereby focusing attention on this vital aspect of nephrology and recording the present state-of-the-art.

The major strides forward in renal therapy shall be clear to the reader of this volume. Areas where advances or breakthroughs are still needed or where solid, objective proof of efficacy is still lacking shall be equally clear. The rapid pace of new research on renal therapy continued during the period that this text was in preparation, and this rapid pace attests to the vitality of nephrology as a discipline. We look forward to the preparation of new editions of this volume reflecting substantive advances which will continue to be made.

It is fitting, in closing, to acknowledge the generosity of each of the contributing authors who have given selflessly of their precious time to prepare their respective chapters, and the forbearance of our publisher, who has waited patiently as the process of assembling and editing this volume proceeded.

Wadi N. Suki
Shaul G. Massry

Preface to the Second Edition

It is said that a static science is a dead science, and to any observer of nephrology it is quite clear that there has been nothing static about this discipline. Even while the first edition was under preparation, newer treatments were being developed, the efficacy of new treatments was being tested, and the results of such trials were being published. It is impossible to capture in a book all the progress that is being made in a particular discipline that is changing rapidly, for to do so would be akin to capturing motion in a still picture. One can convey the impression of motion in a still picture, but it takes a video or a movie to capture motion. And so it is in nephrology, a field in which it should be clear to any one who takes more than a cursory look that major developments and important advances are being made steadily. We were almost prophetic, therefore, when we said in the preface to the first edition:

> The rapid pace of new research on renal therapy continued during the period that this text was in preparation, and this rapid pace attests to the vitality of nephrology as a discipline. We look forward to the preparation of new editions of this volume reflecting substantial advances which will continue to be made.

No sooner had the first edition come out in print than had a process of obsolescence already begun to set in as the wheels of progress kept on turning—hopefully leading us all forward. We were almost prophetic in predicting "the preparation of new editions." So now we come back with a new edition to report on some of the advances that were made since the first edition, and luckily for us all, and above all for our patients, advances have been made and continue to be made as we write these words. We have invited many of the past authors to update their chapters, while several new authors were invited to rewrite chapters on topics previously covered or to write new chapters on topics not previously covered. The task of writing a chapter is an onerous task and, having ourselves written many chapters for many texts, we are keenly aware of the time and effort that goes into the preparation of a chapter. In addition, it is all for very little reward, whether it is in terms of monetary returns to the author or in terms of the academic recognition that the author derives from writing a chapter, as compared with a scientific article in a peerreviewed journal reporting original scientific research. One can only conclude, therefore, that hundreds of authors undertake the task of writing a chapter propelled not by the motive of profit but by that of the noble commitment to convey to their fellow physicians the latest advances in their respective areas of expertise, with the aim of bettering the health of their patients and of raising the standards of the care they receive. It is fitting then to bear in mind that a text such as this is a tribute to each of the authors who contributed to it, and all of us who shall consult this text, as we tackle the complexities of managing our patients, are in their debt.

Wadi N. Suki
Shaul G. Massry

Preface to the Third Edition and Dedication

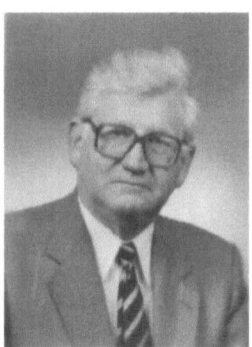

A discipline that stands still is lifeless. Anyone even peripherally involved in nephrology will know that this discipline is vigorous, vibrant, and very much alive. With vibrancy and life comes evolution, and one thing people who work in the field of nephrology will agree upon is that nephrology has been evolving and taking major strides forward. The revolution in the biological sciences has touched nephrology, just as it has other disciplines, and left an indelible mark. More importantly, it has energized this discipline and resulted in an outpouring of exciting new data and new concepts about renal disease and its therapy. These new concepts have already begun to have an impact on clinical nephrology practice and will do so even more in the years to come.

We began in 1984 to publish a treatise on the therapy of renal diseases and related disorders in order to catalogue for the student of nephrology what was known in this field. We subsequently published in 1991 another edition of this work to update it and to chronicle the changes that had come about in the interval. But since the discipline of nephrology has not stood still, it became necessary to follow up with yet another update, and it is our prediction that future updates will also become necessary as the old gives way to the new.

It is easy for one seeking information to reach to a shelf for a reference book such as this and leaf through the pages until one finds the information one seeks. Few people appreciate the time and effort that each author has put into each individual chapter. We as authors and editors have a deep appreciation for the arduousness of this task of writing and editing. No honorarium from the publisher can fully compensate an author for the effort that goes into preparing one of these chapters. One can only conclude then that each author is engaged in a selfless mission to share with, and to transmit to, others the knowledge that they have gained and the innovations in therapy that they have made. We hope that a word of very sincere thanks from the editors to each and every author will constitute sufficient recognition of the Herculean effort each has put into this final product.

The august group of contributors to this edition was to have been joined by Professor Henri Jahn[1]—a dear friend, an astute clinician, and a rigorous scientist who was also a master communicator. To those who knew him personally, Professor Jahn was a man who exuded warmth and friendliness. To those who knew him only as a physician scientist, he was a man with a keen intellect, whose excitement about a broad array of subjects was infectious. He was a serious student of human biology and made numerous contributions to nephrology as he journeyed through a career spanning more than a quarter of a century. His untimely death while this book was in preparation brought deep sadness to us. We would like to dedicate this volume to the memory of our warm, generous, and hospitable friend, Henri Jahn.

Wadi N. Suki
Shaul G. Massry

1. Professor Henri Jahn was until 1994 Professeur Titulaire and Chéf du Service de Néphrologie et Hémodialyse at the Faculté de Medecine et Hôpitaux de Strasbourg, France.

List of Contributors

Chapter 1
J. CARLOS AYUS, M.D., F.A.C.P.
Clinical Professor of Medicine
Baylor College of Medicine
Houston, TX 77024

ALLEN I. ARIEFF, M.D., F.A.C.P.
Chief, Geriatrics Research & Education
San Francisco V.A. Medical Center
Professor of Medicine
University of California School of Medicine
San Francisco, CA 94121

Chapter 2
KIRBY GABRYS, M.D.
Division of Nephrology
Vanderbilt University Medical Center
Nashville, TN 37232

MATTHEW D. BREYER, M.D.
Associate Professor
Departments of Medicine and Molecular Physiology and
 Biophysics
Vanderbilt University Medical Center
Nashville, TN 37232

Chapter 3
JULES B. PUSCHETT, M.D.
Professor and Chairman
Department of Medicine
Tulane University Medical Center
New Orleans, LA 70112-2699

N. KEVIN KRANE, M.D.
Associate Professor of Medicine
Chief, Clinical Nephrology
Section of Nephrology
Tulane University Medical Center
New Orleans, LA 70112-2699

Chapter 4
F. JOHN GENNARI, M.D.
Professor of Medicine
Director, Nephrology Unit
University of Vermont College of Medicine
Burlington, VT 05405

Chapter 5
THERESA A. GUISE, M.D.
Assistant Professor of Medicine
Division of Endocrinology
University of Texas Health Science Center at San
 Antonio
San Antonio, TX 78284

GREGORY R. MUNDY, M.D., F.R.A.C.P.
Professor and Head
Division of Endocrinology
Department of Medicine
University of Texas Health Science Center at San
 Antonio
San Antonio, TX 78284

Chapter 6
JACK W. COBURN, M.D.
Professor of Medicine
The Medical and Research Services
Veterans Affairs Medical Center, West Los Angeles
 (Wadsworth Division)
Department of Medicine
Nephrology Section (W111L)
UCLA School of Medicine
Los Angeles, CA 90073

BARTON S. LEVINE, M.D.
The Medical and Research Services
Veterans Affairs Medical Center, West Los Angeles
 (Wadsworth Division)
The Department of Medicine
Nephrology Section (W111L)
UCLA School of Medicine
Los Angeles, CA 90073

Chapter 7
NORIMOTO YANAGAWA, M.D.
Professor of Medicine
UCLA/San Fernando Valley Program
Nephrology Section, Sepulveda VAMC
Sepulveda, CA 91343

MOUFID NEMEH, M.D.
Assistant Professor of Medicine
UCLA/San Fernando Valley Program
Nephrology Section, Sepulveda VAMC
Sepulveda, CA 91343

Chapter 8
JOAN H. PARKS, M.B.A.
Program in Nephrology
Department of Medicine
The University of Chicago
Chicago, IL 60637

FREDRIC L. COE, M.D.
Professor of Medicine and Physiology
Director, Program in Nephrology
Department of Medicine
The University of Chicago
Chicago, IL 60637

Chapter 9
SANDRA SABATINI, Ph.D., M.D.
Chairman, Department of Physiology
Texas Tech University Health Sciences Center
Lubbock, TX 79430

NEIL A. KURTZMAN, M.D.
Chairman, Department of Medicine
Texas Tech University Health Sciences Center
Lubbock, TX 79430

Chapter 10
CHRISTINE P. BASTL, M.D.
Professor of Medicine
Chief of Nephrology
Temple University Health Sciences Center
Philadelphia, PA 19140

MICHAEL HEIFETS, M.D.
Associate Professor of Medicine
Division of Nephrology
Temple University Health Sciences Center
Philadelphia, PA 19140

LOUIS J. RILEY, JR., M.D.
Associate Professor of Medicine
Division of Nephrology
Temple University Health Sciences Center
Philadelphia, PA 19140

Chapter 11
HORACIO J. ADROGUÉ, M.D., F.A.C.P.
Professor of Medicine
Baylor College of Medicine
Chief, Renal Section
Department of Veterans Affairs Medical Center
Houston, TX 77030

Chapter 12
MARTIN SCHREIBER, M.D.
Renal Division
St. Michael's Hospital and The Toronto Hospital
University of Toronto
Toronto, CANADA M5B 1A6

ROBERT M.A. RICHARDSON, M.D.
Renal Division
St. Michael's Hospital and The Toronto Hospital
University of Toronto
Toronto, CANADA M5B 1A6

MITCHELL L. HALPERIN, M.D., F.R.C.P.(C)
Professor of Medicine
Division of Nephrology
St. Michael's Hospital and The Toronto Hospital
University of Toronto
Toronto, CANADA M5B 1A6

Chapter 13
BRUCE KAPLAN, M.D.
The University, Fexas Health Science Centr & Housth
    Division of Benal Disease and Hypertension
6431 Faxnin M5B 4.148.
Housth TX 77030

DANIEL BATLLE, M.D.
Division of Nephrology and Hypertension
Northwestern University Medical School
Chicago, IL 60611

Chapter 14
HORACIO J. ADROGUÉ, M.D.
Professor of Medicine
Baylor College of Medicine
Chief, Renal Section
Department of Veterans Affairs Medical Center
Houston, TX 77030

NICOLAOS E. MADIAS, M.D.
Professor of Medicine
Tufts University School of Medicine
Chief, Division of Nephrology
New England Medical Center
Boston, MA 02111

Chapter 15
NICOLAOS E. MADIAS, M.D.
Professor of Medicine
Tufts University School of Medicine
Chief, Division of Nephrology
New England Medical Center
Boston, MA 02111

HORACIO J. ADROGUÉ, M.D.
Professor of Medicine
Baylor College of Medicine
Chief, Renal Section
Department of Veterans Affairs Medical Center
Houston, TX 77030

Chapter 16
CHARLES L. STEWART, M.D.
Department of Pediatrics
University Medical Center at Stony Brook
Stony Brook, NY 11794-8111

FREDERICK J. KASKEL, M.D., Ph.D.
Department of Pediatrics
University Medical Center at Stony Brook
Stony Brook, NY 11794-8111

RICHARD N. FINE, M.D.
Professor and Chairman
Department of Pediatrics
University Medical Center at Stony Brook
Stony Brook, NY 11794-8111

Chapter 17
KHALIL U. RAHMAN, M.D.
Nephrology Assoc
Department, KY 40503

WADI N. SUKI, M.D.
Professor of Medicine and of Molecular Physiology and
    Biophysics
Department of Medicine
Chief, Renal Section
Baylor College of Medicine
Houston, TX 77030

Chapter 18
CHARLES BAXTER, M.D.
Professor of Surgery
Department of Surgery
University of Texas Health Sciences Center at Dallas
Dallas, TX 75235

Chapter 19
GEORGE J. KALOYANIDES, M.D.
Professor of Medicine
Division of Nephrology and Hypertension
Health Scinences Center, CST15-020
State University of New York at Stony Brook
Stony Brook, NY 11794-8152

Chapter 20
FRANK G. BOINEAU, M.D.
Professor of Pediatrics
Chief, Section of Pediatric Nephrology
Tulane University Medical Center
New Orleans, LA 70112-2699

JOHN E. LEWY, M.D.
Reily Professor and Chairman
Department of Pediatrics
Tulane University Medical Center
New Orleans, LA 70112-2699

Chapter 21
DAVID S. BALDWIN, M.D.
Professor of Medicine
New York University School of Medicine
Co-Director, Renal Section
New York University and Bellevue Medical Centers
New York, NY 10016

JOEL NEUGARTEN, M.D., J.D.
Associate Professor of Medicine
Albert Einstein College of Medicine
Associate Director, Renal and Hypertension Division
Montefiore Medical Center
Bronx, NY 10467

Chapter 22
DAVID I. CHARNEY, M.D.
Assistant Professor of Medicine
Division of Nephrology
Department of Medicine
University of Utah School of Medicine
Salt Lake City, UT 84132

WAYNE A. BORDER, M.D.
Professor of Medicine
Chief, Division of Nephrology
University of Utah School of Medicine
Salt Lake City, UT 84132

Chapter 23
PATRIZIA PASSERINI, M.D.
Ospedale Maggiore di Milano
Instituto di Ricovero e Cura a Carattere Scientifico
Divisione di Nefrologia e Dialisi—Pad. Croff
20122 Milano
ITALY

CLAUDIO PONTICELLI, M.D.
Ospedale Maggiore di Milano
Instituto di Ricovero e Cura a Carattere Scientifico
Divisione di Nefrologia e Dialisi—Pad. Croff
20122 Milano
ITALY

Chapter 24
GIUSEPPE D'AMICO, M.D.
Divisione di Nefrologia
Ospedale San Carlo Borromeo—Milano
20153 Milano
ITALY

Chapter 25
NINA TOLKOFF-RUBIN, M.D., F.A.C.P.
Director, End-Stage Renal Disease Program
Chief, Hemodialysis and CAPD Units
Massachusetts General Hospital
Associate Professor of Medicine
Harvard Medical School
Boston, MA 02114

ROBERT H. RUBIN, M.D., F.A.C.P.
Director, Center for Experimental Pharmacology and
    Therapeutics
Harvard–M.I.T. Division of Health Sciences and
    Technology
Chief, Transplantation Infectious Disease
Massachusetts General Hospital
Associate Professor of Medicine
Harvard Medical School
Boston, MA 02114

Chapter 26
ROBERT A. WEISS, M.D.
Associate Professor of Pediatrics
New York Medical College
Valhalla, NY 10595

ADRIAN SPITZER, M.D.
Professor of Pediatrics
Director, Division of Pediatric Nephrology
Albert Einstein College of Medicine
Bronx, NY 10461

Chapter 27
JAMES G. GOW, M.D.
"Ingerthorpe"
25 Merrilocks Road
Liverpool L23 6UL
ENGLAND

Chapter 28
STEPHEN MARK OLMSTEAD, D.O.
760 N. Shiloh
Garland, TX 75042
JOE VENZOR, M.D.
Immunology Section
Department of Medicine
Baylor College of Medicine
Houston, TX 77030

DAVID P. HUSTON, M.D.
Associate Professor of Medicine and Microbiology and
    Immunology
Chief, Immunology Section
Department of Medicine
Baylor College of Medicine
Houston, TX 77030

Chapter 29
JAMES E. BALOW, M.D.
Clinical Director
Kidney Disease Section
National Institute of Diabetes and Digestive and Kidney
    Disease
National Institutes of Health
Bethesda, MD 20892-1818

HOWARD A. AUSTIN III, M.D.
Kidney Disease Section
National Institute of Diabetes and Digestive and Kidney
    Disease
National Institutes of Health
Bethesda, MD 20892-1818

Chapter 30
GARABED EKNOYAN, M.D.
Professor of Medicine
Department of Medicine
Baylor College of Medicine
Houston, TX 77030

Chapter 31
PIERO RUGGENENTI, M.D.
Mario Negri Institute for Pharmacological Research
Division of Nephrology and Dialysis
Ospedali Riuniti de Bergamo
24125 Bergamo, ITALY

GIUSEPPE REMUZZI, M.D.
Mario Negri Institute for Pharmacological Research
Division of Nephrology and Dialysis
Ospedali Riuniti de Bergamo
24125 Bergamo, ITALY

Chapter 32
PIETRO ZUCCHELLI, M.D.
Malpighi Department of Nephrology
Policlinico S. Orsola-Malpighi
Bologna, ITALY

SONIA PASQUALI, M.D.
Malpighi Department of Nephrology
Policlinico S. Orsola-Malpighi
Bologna, ITALY

Chapter 33
MOUFID N. NEMEH, M.D.
Assistant Clinical Professor
Department of Medicine
UCLA/San Fernando Valley Program
VA Medical Center
Sepulveda, CA 91343

EDWARD J. WEINMAN, M.D.
Professor and Chair
Department of Medicine
UCLA/San Fernando Valley Program
VA Medical Center
Sepulveda, CA 91343

Chapter 34
JACOB GREEN, M.D.
Department of Nephrology
Rambam Medical Center
Haifa, ISRAEL 31096

ORI S. BETTER, M.D.
Department of Nephrology
Rambam Medical Center
The B. Rappaport Faculty of Medicine
Technion, Israel Institute of Technology
Bat Galim
Haifa, ISRAEL 31096

Chapter 35
JOHN M. DAVISON, M.D.
Department of Obstetrics and Gynaecology
University of Newcastle
Royal Victoria Infirmary
Newcastle upon Tyne NE1 4LP
ENGLAND

ADRIAN I. KATZ, M.D.
The University of Chicago
Departments of Obstetrics and of Gynecology and
  Medicine
Sections of Nephrology and of Maternal Fetal Medicine
Chicago, IL 60637

MARSHALL D. LINDHEIMER, M.D.
Professor of Medicine and of Obstetrics and Gynecology
The University of Chicago
Departments of Obstetrics and of Gynecology and
  Medicine
Sections of Nephrology and of Maternal Fetal Medicine
Chicago, IL 60637

Chapter 36
CARL ERIK MOGENSEN, M.D.
Professor of Medicine
Medical Department M
(Diabetes and Endocrinology)
Kommunehospitalet, University Hospital in Aarhus
DL-8000 Aarhus C, DENMARK

Chapter 37
JACQUES J. BOURGOIGNIE, M.D.
Professor of Medicine
Chief, Division of Nephrology (R-126)
University of Miami School of Medicine
Miami, FL 33101

Chapter 38
R. DAVID GILE, M.D.
Wichita Nephrology Group
Wichita, KS 67214-3766

BENJAMIN D. COWLEY, JR., M.D.
Division of Nephrology and Hypertension
Department of Medicine
Kansas University Medical Center
Kansas City, KS 66106

JARED J. GRANTHAM, M.D.
Division of Nephrology and Hypertension
Department of Medicine
Kansas University Medical Center
Kansas City, KS 66106

Chapter 39
CARLOS A. VAAMONDE, M.D.
Professor of Medicine
Chief, Nephrology Section
Nephrology Section and Research Services
Veterans Affairs Medical Center
Department of Medicine
University of Miami School of Medicine
Miami, FL 33125

JAMES R. OSTER, M.D.
Nephrology Section and Research Services
Veterans Affairs Medical Center
Department of Medicine
University of Miami School of Medicine
Miami, FL 33125

Chapter 40
DONALD L. BATISKY, M.D.
Division of Pediatric Nephrology
Department of Pediatrics
The University of Tennessee, Memphis
LeBonheur Children's Medical Center
Memphis, TN 38103

RUSSELL W. CHESNEY, M.D.
Division of Pediatric Nephrology
Department of Pediatrics
The University of Tennessee, Memphis
LeBonheur Children's Medical Center
Memphis, TN 38103

Chapter 41
JEAN-PIERRE GRÜNFELD, M.D.
Université René Descartes—Paris V
Service de Néphrologie
Hôpital Necker
75015 Paris, FRANCE

GABRIEL CHOUKROUN, M.D.
Université René Descartes—Paris V
Service de Néphrologie
Hôpital Necker
75015 Paris, FRANCE

BERTRAND KNEBELMANN, M.D.
Université René Descartes—Paris V
Service de Néphrologie
Hôpital Necker
75015 Paris, FRANCE

Chapter 42
SETH P. LERNER, M.D.
Assistant Professor of Medicine
Scott Department of Urology
Baylor College of Medicine
Houston, TX 77030

JAMES EASTHAM, M.D.
Scott Department of Urology
Baylor College of Medicine
Houston, TX 77030

Chapter 43
WILLIAM M. BENNETT, M.D.
Professor of Medicine and Pharmacology
Division of Nephrology, Hypertension, and Clinical
  Pharmacology
Oregon Health Sciences University
Portland, OR 97201

Chapter 44
JAMES F. WINCHESTER, M.D.
Professor of Medicine
Georgetown University Medical Center
PHC 6003
Washington, DC 20007

Chapter 45
SAULO KLAHR, M.D.
Simon Professor of Medicine and Co-Chairman
Department of Medicine
Washington University School of Medicine
Physician-in-Chief
The Jewish Hospital of St. Louis
St. Louis, MO 63110

Chapter 46
FADI G. LAKKIS, M.D.
Nephrology Division
Department of Medicine
Emory University School of Medicine and The Medical
  and Research Services
Atlanta Department of Veterans Affairs Medical Center
Decatur, GA 30033

MANUEL MARTINEZ-MALDONADO, M.D.
Professor and Vice Chairman
Emory University School of Medicine and The Medical
  and Research Services
Chief, Medical Service
Atlanta Department of Veterans Affairs Medical Center
Decatur, GA 30033

Chapter 47
DAVID R. BEVAN, M.D., M.R.C.P., F.R.C.A.
Professor and Head
Department of Anaesthesia
University of British Columbia
Vancouver General Hospital
Vancouver, B.C.
CANADA V5Z 4E3

Chapter 48
AUGUST HEIDLAND, M.D.
Professor of Medicine
Kuratorium für Dialyse und Nierentransplantation
97080 Würzburg
GERMANY

KATARINA SÉBEKOVA, M.D.
Kuratorium für Dialyse und Nierentransplantation
97080 Würzburg
GERMANY

MARKUS TESCHNER, M.D.
Kuratorium für Dialyse und Nierentransplantation
97080 Würzburg
GERMANY

Chapter 49
GEORGE A. KAYSEN, M.D., Ph.D.
Professor of Medicine
Chief, Division of Nephrology
University of California, Davis School of Medicine
Department of Veterans Affairs Northern California
  System of Clinics
Sacramento, CA 95817

Chapter 50
MIROSLAW SMOGORZEWSKI, M.D.
Assistant Professor of Medicine
Division of Nephrology
University of Southern California
School of Medicine
Los Angeles, CA 90033

Chapter 51
ESTHER A. GONZALEZ, M.D.
Division of Nephrology
Department of Internal Medicine
St. Louis University Health Sciences Center
St. Louis, MO 63110

KEVIN J. MARTIN, M.D.
Professor of Medicine
Director, Division of Nephrology
Department of Internal Medicine
St. Louis University Health Scineces Center
St. Louis, MO 63110

Chapter 52
ALBERTO ALBERTAZZI, M.D.
Professor of Medicine and Nephrology
Chief, Department of Nephrology and Dialysis
G. D'Annunzio University
Institute of Nephrology
University of Chieti
S. Camillo De Lellis Hospital
66100 Chieti, ITALY

MARIO BONOMINI, M.D.
Institute of Nephrology
University of Chieti
S. Camillo De Lellis Hospital
66100 Chieti, ITALY

PAOLO CAPPELLI, M.D.
Institute of Nephrology
University of Chieti
S. Camillo De Lellis Hospital
66100 Chieti, ITALY

Chapter 53
J. RADERMACHER, M.D.
Medizinische Hochschule Hannover
Abteilung Nephrologie
Zentrum Innere Medizin und Dermatologie
W-3000 Hannover 61
GERMANY

KARL M. KOCH. M.D.
Medizinische Hochschule Hannover
Abteilung Nephrologie
Zentrum Innere Medizin und Dermatologie
W-3000 Hannover 61
GERMANY

Chapter 54
DAVID ROTH, M.D.
Professor of Medicine
University of Miami School of Medicine
The Veterans Administration Medical Center
Division of Nephrology (R-126)
Miami, FL 33101

GUIDO PEREZ, M.D.
Professor of Medicine
University of Miami School of Medicine
The Veterans Administration Medical Center
Division of Nephrology (R-126)
Miami, FL 33101

Chapter 55
JOSE A. DIAZ-BUXO, M.D., F.A.C.P.
Director Home Dialysis, Metrolina Kidney Center
Charlotte, NC 28204

Chapter 56
RAMESH KHANNA, M.D.
Professor of Medicine
Division of Nephrology
School of Medicine
University of Missouri–Columbia
Columbia, MO 65212

ROBERT MACTIER, M.D.
Division of Nephrology
School of Medicine
University of Missouri–Columbia
Columbia, MO 65212

KARL D. NOLPH, M.D.
Professor of Medicine
Director, Division of Nephrology
School of Medicine
University of Missouri–Columbia
Columbia, MO 65212

Chapter 57
ZBYLUT J. TWARDOWSKI, M.D.
Division of Nephrology
Department of Medicine
University of Missouri
Harry S. Truman Veterans Administration Hospital
Dalton Research Center
MA 436 Health Sciences Center
Columbia, MO 65212

Chapter 58
CHARLES E. HALSTENSON, Pharm.D., F.C.P.,
   F.C.C.P.
Professor of Pharmacy
University of Minnesota College of Pharmacy
Co-director, The Drug Evaluation Unit
Hennepin County Medical Center
Minneapolis, MN 55415

WILLIAM F. KEANE, M.D., F.A.C.P.
Professor of Medicine
University of Minnesota Medical School
Co-Director, The Drug Evaluation Unit
Chairman, Department of Medicine
Hennepin County Medical Center
Minneapolis, MN 55415

Chapter 59
H. DAVID SHORT, M.D.
Assistant Professor of Surgery
Department of Surgery
Baylor College of Medicine
Houston, TX 77030

WADE R. ROSENBERG, M.D.
Assistant Professor of Surgery
Department of Surgery
Baylor College of Medicine
Houston, TX 77030

GEORGE P. NOON, M.D.
Professor of Surgery
Department of Surgery
Baylor College of Medicine
Houston, TX 77030

Chapter 60
NUHAD ISMAIL, M.D., F.A.C.P.
Assistant Professor of Medicine
Division of Nephrology
Vanderbilt University Medical Center
Nashville, TN 37232-2372

BRYAN BECKER, M.D.
Division of Nephrology
Vanderbilt University Medical Center
Nashville, TN 37232-2372

RAYMOND M. HAKIM, M.D., PH.D.
Professor of Medicine
Division of Nephrology
Vanderbilt University Medical Center
Nashville, TN 37232-2372

Chapter 61
DANIEL F. WALTON, D.O.
Division of Nephrology and Hypertension
Oceania Kidney Disease of Hypertension Center
Phoenix, AZ 85006

ALFRED K. CHEUNG, M.D.
Associate Professor of Medicine
Division of Nephrology and Hypertension
University of Utah School of Medicine and
Veterans Affairs Medical Center
Salt Lake City, UT 84148

Chapter 62
RAYMOND C. VANHOLDER, M.D.
Professor of Medicine
Nephrology Department
University Hospital
De Pintelaan, 185
B9000 Ghent, BELGIUM

ANN A. VAN LOO, M.D.
Nephrology Department
University Hospital
De Pintelaan, 185
B9000 Ghent, BELGIUM

SEVERIN M. RINGOIR, M.D.
Professor of Medicine
Director, Nephrology Department
University Hospital
De Pintelaan, 185
B9000 Ghent, BELGIUM

Chapter 63
D. CRAIG BRATER, M.D.
Chairman, Department of Medicine
Professor of Medicine and of Pharmacology and
    Toxicology
Indiana University School of Medicine
WOP 316, Wishard Memorial Hospital
Indianapolis, IN 46202

Chapter 64
STUART M. FLECHNER, M.D.
Department of Urology/A100
Section of Renal Transplantation
Cleveland, Clinic Foundation
Cleveland, OH 44195

Chapter 65
M. ROY FIRST, M.D.
Professor of Medicine
University of Cincinnati Medical Center
Division of Nephrology and Hypertension
Cincinnati, OH 45267-0585

Chapter 66
LILIANA GRADOWSKA, M.D.
Professor of Medicine
Chief, Department of Immunotherapy
The Transplantation Institute
School of Medicine
02006 Warsaw
Nowogrodzka 59, POLAND

LESZEK PACZEK, M.D.
Associate Professor of Medicine
The Transplantation Institute
School of Medicine
02006 Warsaw
Nowogrodzka 59, POLAND

Chapter 67
ELEANOR D. LEDERER, M.D.
Assistant Professor of Medicine
Kidney Disease Program
University of Louisville
Louisville, KY 40292

Chapter 68
PETER J. MORRIS, M.D., Ph.D., F.R.C.S., F.R.A.C.S.,
    F.A.C.S. (hon), F.R.S.
Nuffield Professor of Surgery
Chairman, Nuffield Department of Surgery
University of Oxford
Oxford Radcliffe Hospital
The John Radcliffe
Headington, Oxford OX3 9DU
UNITED KINGDOM

Chapter 69
MICHAEL A. WEBER, M.D.
Professor of Medicine
Hypertension Center—W130
Veterans Affairs Medical Center, Long Beach and the
    University of California, Irvine
Long Beach, CA 90822

Chapter 70
GEORGES MOURAD, M.D.
Medecine Interne et Hypertension Artérielle
Centre Hospitalier Universitaire
Hôpital Lapeyronie
34295 Montpellier Cedex 5, FRANCE

JEAN-MICHEL HALIMI, M.D.
Medecine Interne et Hypertension Artérielle
Centre Hospitalier Universitaire
Hôpital Lapeyronie
34295 Montpellier Cedex 5, FRANCE

JEAN RIBSTEIN, M.D.
Professor of Medicine
Medecine Interne et Hypertension Artérielle
Centre Hospitalier Universitaire
Hôpital Lapeyronie
34295 Montpellier Cedex 5, FRANCE

ALBERT MIMRAN, M.D.
Professor of Medicine
Medecine Interne et Hypertension Artérielle
Centre Hospitalier Universitatire
Hôpital Lapeyronie
34295 Montpellier Cedex 5, FRANCE

Chapter 71
DAVID A. LASKOW, M.D.
Department of Surgery
University of Alabama–Birmingham
Birmingham, AL 35294-0006

JOHN J. CURTIS, M.D.
Department of Medicine
University of Alabama–Birmingham
Birmingham, AL 35294-0006

Chapter 72
GRANNUM R. SANT, M.D.
Professor and Vice-Chairman
Associate Urologist in Chief
Tufts University School of Medicine and
New England Medical Center Hospitals
Boston, MA 02111

EDWIN M. MEARES, JR., M.D.
Charles M. Whitney Professor and Chairman
Tufts University School of Medicine and
New England Medical Center Hospitals
Boston, MA 02111

Chapter 73
J. KEITH LIGHT, M.D.
Professor and Chairman
Department of Urology
State University of New York
Health Science Center–Syracuse
College of Medicine
Syracuse, NY 13210

CHAPTER 45

Prevention of Progression of Renal Disease

SAULO KLAHR

INTRODUCTION

In most forms of chronic renal disease, glomerular filtration rate (GFR) tends to decrease inexorably once a certain threshold of nephron destruction has occurred. The progressive decrease in GFR is accompanied histologically by increasing glomerulosclerosis and interstitial fibrosis, in which specialized segments of the nephron are progressively replaced by extracellular matrix (1). Renal diseases of diverse etiology culminate in nephrosclerosis, the hallmark of the end-stage diseased kidney. This suggests that a heterogenous array of initial insults can induce pathologic responses that converge upon a common avenue in which normal renal tissue is replaced by nonfunctional elements.

The mechanisms underlying the progression of renal disease are complex and very likely multifactorial (2). Histologic similarities between glomerulosclerosis and atherosclerosis are striking and have led to the suggestion that both lesions share a common pathogenesis (3,4). Factors that may participate in the development of atherogenesis include endothelial cell injury, lipid deposition, macrophage infiltration, cellular proliferation, and connective tissue deposition (5,6). Similar factors may account for the development of glomerulosclerosis. In addition, it should be remembered that mesangial cells closely resemble vascular smooth muscle cells (7).

The progression of chronic renal disease is most likely mediated by several risk factors acting alone or in combination. Potential risk factors that may contribute to the progression of chronic renal failure include systemic hypertension, proteinuria, hyperlipidemia, high protein or phosphorus intake, and probably conditions that promote glomerular hypertrophy. Therapeutic maneuvers designed to minimize the potential contributions of one or more of these risk factors may halt or ameliorate the loss of renal function (Table 1).

ASSESSING THE PROGRESSION OF RENAL DISEASE

The progression of chronic renal failure is best assessed by sequential measurements of GFR using exogenous markers, such as inulin. This determination, however, requires the intravenous infusion of inulin and at least three precisely timed urine collections; this procedure often requires water loading the patient to increase urine flow. To avoid water loading and timed urine collections, the plasma disappearance of radioactive compounds such as ^{125}I-iothalamate, ^{99}Tc DTPA, or ^{51}Cr EDTA (8) has been used to measure GFR. Plasma levels of the marker must be relatively constant and urine flow adequate. Several blood samples must be collected following the intravenous injection of the radiolabeled compound. The timing of blood sampling is critical to determine the rate (slope) of disappearance of the radiolabeled compound. Clinically, the use of exogenous markers is not practical. Instead, the clearance of endogenous creatinine has been used to assess GFR (9).

Creatinine clearance

Creatinine, an endogenous metabolic product of creatine, is not an ideal filtration marker in humans (10). It is excreted in the urine as a result of both glomerular filtration and tubular secretion. Consequently, the creatinine clearance generally exceeds the inulin clearance (or GFR), and this difference increases as renal disease progresses due to an elevation of serum creatinine and a greater contribution of tubular secretion of creatinine to the total amount of creatinine excreted in the urine. To avoid this problem, several groups have used the average of urea and creatinine clearances and shown that this corresponds closely to inulin clearance in both adults and children with renal insufficiency (11–14).

Serum creatinine

The serum creatinine concentration remains the most widely used measure of renal function. However, a single value of serum creatinine is a crude estimate of GFR or creatinine clearance because the serum levels of creatinine are influenced not only by the level of GFR but also by creatinine production (muscle mass) or ingestion (dietary intake of meats) (10). The sensitivity of serum creatinine for detection of mild renal insufficiency (inulin clearances

Suki, WN and Massry SG (eds), Suki and Massry's Therapy of Renal Diseases and Related Disorders, Third Edition. ISBN 978-1-4757-6634-9.
©1998, Kluwer Academic Publishers, Boston/Dordrecht/London. All rights reserved.

Table 1. Therapeutic interventions druing the course of chronic renal failure

Stage of chronic renal impairment (GFR)	Blood pressure	Dietary protein (g/kg/day)	Calcium supplement- ation (mg/day)	Phosphorus restriction (mg/day)	Hyperlipidemia	Proteinuria
Early (50–80 mL/min)	Requires treatment throught course of disease[a]	1.0–1.2	500–1000	≤900	Aim to reduce serum cholesterol by diet and drug therapy if ≥6.5 mmol/L	Aim to reduce if in excess of 1 g/24 hr
Moderate (25–5-0 mL/min)		0.8–1.0	1000–1200	700–900 with mealtime calcium carbonate		
Advanced (5–25 mL/min)		0.6 (high- biological- value protein)	1200–1500	≤700 with 1200 mg mealtime calcium carbonate		
Dialysis		1.2–1.4	1200–1800	As for advanced impairment, although higher doses of phosphate binders may be required		—

[a] In patients with proteinuria in excess of 1 g/day, the level of blood pressure should be kept below 92 mmHg (mean arterial pressure). Protein restriction at GFR values below 25 mL/min is indicated to improve metabolic acidosis and to decrease phosphorus intake. From Klahr (19); used with permission.

of 50–90 mL/min/1.73 m^2) is not very high. Normal upper values for serum creatinine depend on the specific methodology used. The values of serum creatinine rise from 0.6 mg/dL at age 5 to 1.2–1.3 mg/dL at age 40. Little change in serum creatinine (in the absence of renal disease) is seen after age 40, despite the fall in GFR with aging due to a simultaneous reduction in creatinine generation. Serum creatinine is typically 10% higher in men than in women.

Reciprocal of serum creatinine

Some investigators have proposed (15,16) that in a particular patient, regardless of the etiology of the renal disease, a plot of the reciprocal of the serum creatinine concentration (1/serum creatinine) versus time is a linear function and that a change in the slope of this relationship indicates a change in the rate of progression of the renal disease. Another suggestion is that if a linear decline in 1/serum creatinine is valid for all patients with a variety of renal diseases, then patients can serve as their own controls and there is no need to compare different patient groups (17). Although the 1/serum creatinine versus time plots have been used to assess the progression of renal disease and the effect of therapeutic interventions, there are several problems with this approach. In many of the published studies, the beneficial effects reported may have

been due to factors not considered, such as loss of muscle mass, changes in creatinine intake, spontaneous stabilization of renal function, and particularly the effects of frequent follow-up visits and blood pressure control measures (18).

Urea

The blood urea nitrogen (BUN) should probably never be used by itself to evaluate renal function, but in conjunction with serum creatinine levels it has additive value. Urea is filtered and reabsorbed by the renal tubules to a variable degree. Tubular reabsorption of urea is affected by volume status, urine flow, and protein intake. Tubular reabsorption of urea is increased when tubular flow is decreased (congestive heart failure, volume depletion, etc.). In this setting, the BUN can rise in the absence of intrinsic renal disease (prerenal azotemia). Increased generation of urea also contributes to the BUN elevation observed in patients with congestive heart failure. The ratio of BUN to serum creatinine concentration may be considered an indirect estimate of renal function and of the patient's volume status. BUN levels are markedly affected by changes in protein intake, higher BUN levels being observed when protein intake increases. Low levels of BUN can be found in patients with liver disease or malnutrition or in those eating a low protein diet.

RISK FACTORS

As mentioned above, progression of chronic renal disease may be modified by several risk factors that operate alone or in combination (19). These risk factors include systemic hypertension, proteinuria, hyperlipidemia, high protein or phosphorus intake, and conditions that promote clotting or infiltration of the renal parenchyma by immune cells.

Systemic hypertension

Systemic hypertension, whether primary or secondary, may cause renal disease or may accelerate the loss of function in kidneys with established parenchymal disease (20).

Hypertension may damage the kidney by increasing arteriolar wall thickness, thereby leading to ischemia and subsequent glomerulosclerosis, or it may damage the glomeruli directly through increased intraglomerular pressure (20). Although careful documentation of the effects of control of blood pressure on the progression of renal disease in humans is limited, most of the evidence suggests an important role of hypertension in the progression of chronic renal failure.

ANGIOTENSIN CONVERTING ENZYME INHIBITORS

Hypertension in patients with chronic renal disease is correlated with the decrease in renal function (21). Several antihypertensive agents may slow the progression of renal disease. Inhibitors of the angiotensin-converting enzyme (ACE) have a more specific benefit in reducing renal injury, although definitive clinical evidence supporting a differential effect is lacking. ACE inhibitors have been reported to influence favorably the course of a variety of renal diseases in man, including primary glomerulopathies, diabetic nephropathy, the nephropathy of systemic lupus erythematosus, hypertensive renal disease, polycystic kidney disease, and chronic pyelonephritis (22–25). In most cases, converting enzyme inhibition was associated with a reduction in proteinuria (26,27), and in some cases with a slowing in the rate of progression of renal disease. However, most studies have not examined an optimal control population to differentiate between the effects of blood pressure reduction and a more specific effect of ACE inhibitors on renal function.

Several studies have compared the effect of ACE inhibitors and other agents on the progression of renal disease. Ruilope et al. (28) examined the rate of progression of renal disease in 10 patients treated for 12 months with captopril and compared this rate to the patients' previous rate of progression while they were receiving an antihypertensive regimen consisting of propranolol, hydralazine, and furosemide. These investigators found a decrease in the rate of progression of the renal disease with ACE inhibitors. The use of the patients' previous rate of progression complicates the interpretation of the result of

this study, since unidentified "time" effects may be associated with slowing of progression (29). Heeg et al. (30,31) also compared the antiproteinuric effects of the ACE inhibitor lisinopril with those arising from prior therapy with methyldopa and other conventional agents; there was a more consistent reduction in proteinuria after ACE inhibition.

In patients with essential hypertension, treatment with an ACE inhibitor (captopril) reduced microalbuminuria, whereas no change in albumin excretion occurred in a separate group of patients treated with β-blockers and diuretics (32). Comparison of different agents in normotensive diabetic patients with microalbuminuria has yielded somewhat conflicting results: some studies have demonstrated a beneficial effect unique to ACE inhibitors, but other studies have not (33,34). The issue is further clouded by the significant slowing of the progression of diabetic kidney disease observed when patients follow regimens without ACE inhibitors and by the reduced proteinuria associated with these regimens (29,35,36). Therefore, the question of whether there are differential effects of antihypertensives on renal injury is not completely answered, although ACE inhibitors appear to have a therapeutic advantage.

BLOOD PRESSURE LEVELS AND PROGRESSION OF RENAL DISEASE

Bergström et al. (29) found a significant correlation between the degree of reduction in mean arterial blood pressure and the decrement in the rate of loss of renal function (29). Similarly, Kajiwara et al. found that successful treatment of hypertension with propranolol slowed the rate of progression in patients with glomerulonephritis (37), and Brazy et al. (38) found that patients successfully treated for hypertension had a slower rate of progression of renal disease. Yet none of these observations fully resolves the nature of the association between hypertension and rapid progression; that is, the blood pressure improvement might be the consequence of and not the cause of a slower progression of the underlying renal disease. It appears, therefore, that in diabetic and nondiabetic nephropathies, treatment with ACE inhibitors controls systemic hypertension, reduces proteinuria, and slows the progression of the underlying renal failure (22–26). It has been suggested that the effect of ACE inhibitors on the progression of diabetic nephropathy is unrelated to its hypotensive effect. This notion is difficult to validate without prospective randomized studies comparing ACE inhibitors to other antihypertensive agents. Animal studies have suggested that reduction of glomerular capillary pressures may protect residual renal function and that ACE inhibitors and calcium channel blockers may be particularly effective in reducing the progression of kidney disease through such a mechanism (2).

Several studies suggest that reduction of diastolic blood pressure to levels below 90 mmHg should be the goal of antihypertensive therapy in patients with established hypertension. All these trials were conducted in patients with essential hypertension. In a recent study (39), however, renal disease progressed even with "good control" of blood pressure. At least two explanations may account for this observation: 1) other factors besides elevated blood pressure had a role in the progression of renal disease in these patients: and 2) lowering blood pressure to levels of 140/90 mmHg or less may not prevent the untoward effect of hypertension on the kidney. In the pilot phase of the multicenter Modification of Diet in Renal Disease (MDRD) Study (40), there was a significant correlation between blood pressure levels and the decrease in GFR. The decrease in GFR was greater in patients with higher blood pressure. This correlation persisted even in patients whose blood pressure was lower than 140/90 mmHg. This observation suggests that it may be necessary to reduce blood pressure below this widely accepted target level to preserve renal function in patients with chronic renal disease. In such patients, the capacity of the afferent arteriole to vasoconstrict in response to elevations in blood pressure may be abnormal, and transmission of pressure to glomerular capillaries may cause "damage" even at levels of blood pressure considered adequate. Therefore, the "target" level for adequate control of blood pressure in patients with chronic renal failure needs to be defined.

In the full-scale MDRD study (41), the effect of two levels of blood pressure control on the progression of renal disease were also examined. In Study 1, 585 patients with GFR levels of 25–55 mL/min were randomly assigned to groups in which mean arterial pressure was regulated to conform to usual or low levels (107 or 92 mmHg). In Study 2, 255 patients with GFR levels of 13–24 mL/min were similarly randomized to a usual or low blood pressure group. In Study 1, patients assigned to the low blood pressure group had a greater decline in GFR during the first four months after randomization as compared to the usual blood pressure group. However, after that the decline in GFR was slower in the patients randomized to the low blood pressure group, and this trend continued to the end of the study period. Patients in Study 2 randomized to the low blood pressure group did not demonstrate a greater decrease in GFR in the first four months of follow-up or a significantly slower decline in GFR thereafter. The difference in mean blood pressure between the usual- and low-blood-pressure groups during the follow-up period was 4.7 mmHg (p < 0.001) in both Study 1 and Study 2. The percent of patients taking antihypertensive (including diuretic) drugs for more than half of the follow-up period was 80% and 90%, respectively, in the usual- and low-blood-pressure groups in Study 1 and was 85% and 98%, respectively, in Study 2. The percent of patients taking ACE inhibitors alone or in combination for more than half the follow-up period in Study 1 was, respectively, 34% and 54% in the usual- and low-blood-pressure groups. In Study 2, the percent of patients taking ACE inhibitors was, respectively, 27% and 43% in the usual- and low-blood-pressure groups.

PROTEINURIA, RACE, AND THE EFFECTS OF BLOOD PRESSURE CONTROL

The MDRD Study (41) also found a significant interaction between the prescribed blood pressure, the magnitude of proteinuria during the baseline period, and the rate of decline in GFR beginning at 4 months into follow-up (p = 0.006), as well as the projected decline in GFR from baseline to 3 years (p = 0.02). The beneficial effect of the low-blood-pressure intervention was greatest in 54 patients in Study 1 whose urinary protein excretion was greater than 3 g/day at baseline. It was intermediate in the 104 patients in Study 1 in whom proteinuria was 1–3 g/day, and it was absent in the 420 patients in Study 1 in whom proteinuria was less than 1 g/day. A similar trend, although less pronounced, was observed in patients in Study 2. We also found that 53 blacks in Study 1 had a more rapid projected decline in GFR (19 mL/min/3 years) than 525 other patients (11 mL/min/3 years, p = 0.02). Blacks assigned to the low-blood-pressure group had a projected loss of GFR approximately half (14 mL/min/3 years) that of blacks in the usual-blood-pressure group (25 mL/min/3 years, p = 0.11). The lack of a significant effect may be related to the small number of black patients enrolled in the study. The results of blood pressure control in patients with proteinuria in the multicenter study suggest that the levels of blood pressure should be kept about 92 mmHg (mean arterial pressure). This is equivalent to a blood pressure of 125/75 mmHg.

DIABETIC NEPHROPATHY

In specific diseases, particularly diabetic nephropathy, substantial evidence indicates that blood pressure reduction prevents the progression of renal failure. Mogensen (42) reported initially in 1982 that treatment of hypertension in six patients with diabetic nephropathy led to a 60% reduction in their rate of loss of GFR. These observations were confirmed by Parving et al. (43) and Bjorck et al. (25). Each of these studies included only a small number of patients, and in each case the investigator used the patients' rate of GFR loss prior to entry into the study as a control. Subsequent studies (44) demonstrated in a randomized placebo-controlled trial that administration of the ACE inhibitor enalapril significantly reduced blood pressure and proteinuria and increased GFR in normotensive patients with diabetic nephropathy. No such improvement was observed in the placebo-controlled patients. Although none of these patients had progressive renal insufficiency, the results of the study call into question the generally accepted blood pressure goal of 140/90 mmHg for patients with diabetic (or other forms of) nephropathy and suggests that there may be a special role for angiotensin–converting enzyme (ACE) inhibitors in the treatment of these patients.

The results of a randomized clinical trial of the effects of treatment with captopril, an angiotensin-converting enzyme inhibitor, in patients with insulin-dependent diabetes mellitus (IDDM) and diabetic nephropathy have also been published (45,46). This study was designed to determine whether treatment of patients with IDDM and established diabetic nephropathy with an ACE inhibitor is associated with a reduction in the rate of progression of their renal disease. In contrast to previous studies, this trial was prospective, randomized, and double-masked; a large number, 409, of relatively homogeneous patients with IDDM were studied, with sufficient follow-up time for assessing the progression of renal insufficiency. Participants were randomized to receive either captopril, 25 mg orally three times a day, or placebo. In all participants, diastolic blood pressure was controlled at levels below 90 mmHg, and systolic blood pressure was lowered appropriately according to baseline blood pressure values obtained. Blood pressure control during the follow-up period was achieved using a variety of antihypertensives that excluded other ACE inhibitors or calcium channel blockers. The primary outcome of the study was the documentation of the time required for doubling of the baseline serum creatinine to at least 2 mg/dL. Secondary outcomes included a profile of urinary protein excretion and measurement of the time preceding end-stage renal disease or death. During the scheduled follow-up visits, there were no reported differences between the captopril-treated and placebo-treated groups in either blood sugar control as measured by glycosylated hemoglobin, or in protein intake as measured by 24-hour urinary urea excretion. As mentioned above, the primary outcome for this trial was documentation of the time required for doubling of the serum creatinine. During the period of follow-up, 25 of the participants receiving captopril reached the doubling of serum creati-

nine stop point, while 43 of those participants in the placebo-treated group reached that stop point. This difference between the captopril- and placebo-treated groups was significant. The time required for creatinine doubling for the captopril-treated participants was longer than that in the placebo-treated participants. The overall percent risk reduction conferred by captopril was 48.5% based on the proportion of hazard regression model (see Figure 1).

An important secondary outcome was the time interval before death, dialysis, or transplantation. In the captopril-treated group, there were 23 combined endpoints of death, dialysis or transplantation, while in the placebo group there were 43 endpoints reached, with a percent risk reduction of 50.5% in those participants receiving captopril. Mean arterial pressure was approximately 4 mmHg lower during follow-up in the participants in the captopril group versus the placebo. The lower blood pressure in the captopril-treated group contributed only minimally to the more promising results in this group when data were analyzed by a proportional hazards regression model with blood pressure as a time-dependent covariate. However, it cannot be completely ruled out that lower blood pressure influenced the outcome of the study and had a role in the benefit provided. This study represents the largest group of patients with diabetic nephropathy in whom a beneficial effect of captopril on preserving renal function was demonstrated. These results suggest that ACE inhibitors have an effect beyond that of blood pressure reduction as compared to other antihypertensives. On the other hand, the difference of 4 mmHg in blood pressure may itself be responsible for differences in results obtained in the two groups. The authors also found that the medium protein excretion during follow-up decreased in the captopril-treated participants compared to the placebo-treated group. This is consistent with previous studies using meta-regression analysis (47). The effect of captopril was influenced by the patients' serum creatinine level at entry, since participants with worse renal insufficiency had a greater demonstrable benefit. This finding in part reflects fewer doublings of serum creatinine events in participants with lower serum creatinines at baseline and a longer time of observation required for doubling of serum creatinine in patients with higher GFRs.

In summary, angiotensin-converting enzyme inhibition with captopril significantly slowed the rate of decline of renal function in the patients with diabetic nephropathy. Several questions remain unanswered by this study. The possible interaction between the use of ACE inhibitors and other interventions such as low protein diets, calcium channel blockers, and tight blood sugar control were not addressed. This study was done using captopril as the ACE inhibitor, and whether or not the results can be attributed to the ACE inhibitor effect of this agent or generalized to other ACE inhibitors is not known. It is possible that captopril could be exerting effects through mechanisms other than ACE inhibition. The free sulfhydryl group of

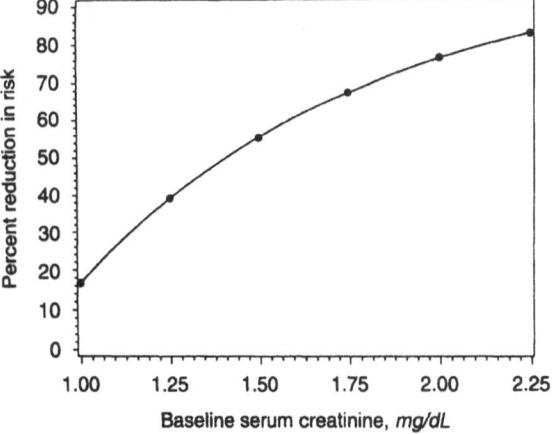

Figure 1. Percent reduction in risk with captopril as a function of baseline serum creatinine. From Breyer et al. (46); used with permission.

captopril is a unique chemical feature of this ACE inhibitor. It has been reported to be responsible for scavenging free oxygen radicals and attenuating reperfusion-induced myocardial injury (48).

OTHER EFFECTS OF ANGIOTENSIN II THAT MAY AFFECT THE PROGRESSION OF RENAL DISEASES

Other effects of angiotensin II may affect the course of chronic renal disease. Angiotensin II promotes growth of a number of cells and tissues, including vascular smooth muscle, adrenal cortex, heart, and kidney (49–52). Renal growth, particularly glomerular enlargement, may predispose to injury (53). In the kidney, angiotensin II induces hypertrophy of proximal tubular cells and potentiates the mitogenic response of these cells to epidermal growth factor (52,54). In mesangial cells, angiotensin II increases ^{3}H-thymidine incorporation, induces hypertrophy, and stimulates collagen and actin synthesis (55–57). In vivo, intrarenal infusion of angiotensin II increases the expression of several early growth response genes, an effect associated with cellular growth in other tissues (58). Besides its direct effects, angiotensin II promotes renal growth through its ability to stimulate ammoniagenesis in renal tubular cells (59). Ammonia stimulates renal tubular hypertrophy (60). Furthermore, increased concentrations of ammonia in the renal cortex can induce tubulointerstitial disease by interacting with the C3 component of complement, resulting in activation of the complement cascade (61). Angiotensin II also effects mesangial trafficking, leading to increased uptake of macromolecules in the mesangium, which may predispose to eventual glomerular sclerosis (62). Thus, angiotensin II could contribute to the progression of renal disease through both its hemodynamic and nonhemodynamic actions.

Dietary protein

The past decade has seen renewed interest in the use of low-protein diets in the treatment of progressive renal insufficiency, due mainly to the suggestive evidence that a low protein intake may slow or even halt the progression of renal failure (63). Several reported trials support the concept that protein restriction may modify the course of progressive renal disease. However, because most of the published studies (64) were uncontrolled, the results are difficult to evaluate.

Two different protein-restricted diets have been used in patients with progressive renal disease: 1) a diet containing 0.6 g/kg/day of protein and 2) a more restricted diet containing 0.3 g/kg/day of protein predominantly of "high biological value" (i.e., proteins containing a high proportion of essential amino acids) supplemented with either essential amino acids or a mixture of essential amino acids and ketoanalogues of essential amino acids.

The protein requirement of normal subjects, about 0.6 g of protein/kg of ideal body weight/day, is the same for patients with chronic renal disease. However, neutral nitrogen balance and, hence, maintenance of protein stores are possible only if the following conditions are met: 1) a high proportion of the protein (>60%) must be of high biologic value; 2) caloric intake must be adequate (about 35 kcal/kg/day) (65); 3) there is a daily supplement of vitamins B and C (66); and (4) there is no coexisting catabolic condition (e.g., metabolic acidosis (67)). A skilled dietitian is critical to ensure that a nutritionally adequate regimen is provided and that each patient's food preferences are included when recipes are planned. Compliance can be achieved with these diets during long-term therapy.

CLINICAL ASSESSMENT OF THE PATIENT ON A PROTEIN-RESTRICTED DIET

Since some of the diets utilized provide amounts of protein below the recommended standard for adequate nutrition, patients following such diets should be closely monitored for early signs of protein depletion. They also need to be assessed for adherence to the diet.

Adherence to the diet is best assessed by determining the excretion of urea in the urine. It is known that urea is the major component of urine nitrogen to vary with protein intake. Thus, it is important to measure the rate of urea production when evaluating protein intake. This is best done by collecting 24-hour urine specimens and measuring urea in such specimens. It is important at the same time to determine whether or not blood urea concentrations are relatively constant. If these levels are changing, urinary excretion of urea may be affected and consequently may not be an accurate reflection of protein intake. Urea balance can be calculated from changes in the urea pool, which can be ascertained by multiplying the concentration of serum urea nitrogen in grams per liter by approximately 60% of body weight in kilograms, which is approximately the total body water. Once the size of the urea pool is calculated, the net production of urea, which is referred to as *urea appearance rate*, can be calculated as the sum of urinary urea nitrogen excretion plus accumulation (positive or negative) of urea nitrogen. If serum urea nitrogen and weight are stable, urea appearance rate equals excretion rate. Body weight, serum albumin levels, and serum transferrin levels, as well as anthropometric measurements (skin fold thickness, midarm circumference, etc.) should be determined at regular intervals to assess any untoward effects of the protein-restricted diet and hence the development of malnutrition.

The current recommendations for dietary protein intake in patients with chronic renal failure are based on 1) the degree of renal insufficiency, 2) the presence of progressive renal failure, 3) the level of proteinuria, 4) the presence of a concomitant coexistent catabolic illness, and 5) whether glucocorticoids are prescribed. It should be appreciated that phosphorus restriction is an essential component of dietary therapy for two reasons: 1) phosphorus restriction is the initial step in the management of secondary hyperparathyroidism, and 2) studies in both animals and humans have suggested that low phosphorus diets may retard the progression of renal failure independent of the level of protein intake (68–71).

DIETARY PROTEIN RESTRICTION AT DIFFERENT LEVELS OF RENAL FUNCTION

There is no clear evidence to indicate whether dietary protein restriction is of benefit in patients with mild renal insufficiency (GFR > 60 mL/min). These individuals typically have serum creatinine levels below 2 mg/dL and in the absence of coexistent systemic disease are for the most part asymptomatic. These patients should be informed that, at this level of renal function, no clear benefit of dietary protein restriction has been established, and low-protein diets are not typically recommended in such patients unless there is evidence of progressive renal disease. Most of the effort in these patients should be directed towards control of hypertension and other coexistent problems such as edema and hyperlipidemia.

In patients with moderate chronic renal failure (GFR 25–60 mL/min), some degree of protein restriction may be indicated. Although the evidence is not clearly established that protein restriction at this level of GFR benefits or affects the progression of chronic renal disease, there are other reasons why some degree of protein restriction should be recommended. Protein restriction will decrease the ingestion of phosphorus and decrease the generation of acid, hence forestalling the development of mild metabolic acidosis, and will diminish the need for administering phosphate-binding drugs to decrease the serum levels of phosphorus. Depending on the level of renal function in this group, diets could be restricted to contain between 0.8 and 0.6 g of protein/kg body weight. Approximately two thirds of this diet should be of high biological value (i.e., meat, fish, eggs). This ensures that the daily requirement for essential amino acids is achieved. Although dietary protein restriction to this level requires considerable commitment, an advantage is that the patient's protein needs can be achieved with the use of traditional foods.

In patients with advanced renal insufficiency (GFR 5–25 mL/min), protein restriction is required to decrease the levels of phosphorus ingestion and hence hyperphosphatemia, to prevent further decreases in the serum levels of bicarbonate (metabolic acidosis), and to decrease uremic symptoms related to accumulation of products derived from protein catabolism. Two diets have been recommended for patients with renal function at this level: 1) a diet containing approximately 0.6 g of protein/kg body weight, with most of the protein of high biological quality, or 2) a more restricted diet of 0.3 g of protein/kg body weight of high biological protein, supplemented with a mixture of amino acids and keto acid analogues. Although protein-restricted regimens are designed to forestall some of the complications of uremia, some evidence exists that they may also affect the rate of progression of renal disease

(see below). It is important, again, to assure that appropriate nutrition is being provided, since clear evidence has emerged that patients reaching end-stage renal disease and undergoing dialysis have an increased mortality if malnutrition is present, as reflected by lower levels of serum albumin.

EFFECTS OF PROTEIN RESTRICTION ON THE PROGRESSION OF CHRONIC RENAL DISEASES

Clinical evidence generated during the last two decades has suggested a potential role for dietary protein restriction in slowing the progression of chronic renal failure (63). It should be pointed out that chronic renal failure is caused by entities with different etiologic characteristics and with unique responses to dietary protein restriction. Diabetic nephropathy is the major cause of end-stage renal failure in the United States. Very few trials of the effects of dietary protein restriction on the progression of renal disease in this setting have been conducted. In two reports, short-term protein restriction reduced proteinuria in diabetic patients with microalbuminuria (72,73). In one of these studies, Walker et al. (72) examined the pathologic course of 19 insulin-dependent diabetic patients who had persistent proteinuria and ate an unrestricted diet containing an average of 1.13 g protein/kg/day. When they were switched to a diet averaging 0.67 g protein/kg/day, the rate of decline in GFR slowed significantly, from 0.61 to 0.4 mL/min/ month. This slowing of progression was significant, even after the results were adjusted for differences in blood pressure, energy intake, and levels of glycosylated hemoglobin. Albumin excretion and its fractional clearance also fell when the low-protein diet was instituted.

The most convincing evidence for a response to a low-protein diet in diabetic patients was reported by Zeller et al. (73). In this study, two groups of patients were randomly assigned to a diet containing 1 g protein/kg/day (35 patients) or to a diet containing 0.6 g protein/kg/day (33 patients). Changes in renal function were evaluated by measuring the renal clearances of creatinine and ^{125}I-iothalamate. Albuminuria was also measured. Reasonable compliance with the protein restriction was achieved, since only 2 of the 33 patients in the protein-restricted diet persistently ate more than 0.8 g protein/kg/day. However, the difference in protein intake between the two groups was not large, about 0.3 g/kg/day. There was no loss of body weight or muscle mass and no decrease in serum albumin in the protein-restricted group. Thus, no evidence of malnutrition was evident over the $1\frac{1}{2}$–2-year duration of the study. The average decline in GFR and creatinine clearance was significantly slower in the protein-restricted group. The mean rate of loss of GFR was 1.01 mL/min/ month in the control group and only 0.36 mL/min/month in the protein-restricted group. The loss of creatinine clearance was 0.81 mL/min/month in the group ingesting 1 g of protein as compared to 0.33 mL/min/month in the group ingesting 0.6 g of protein. It should be emphasized that in this study some of the patients eating the unrestricted diet had stable values of GFR during the duration of the study. Although this makes the positive results more startling, it also indicates the difficulty in carrying out a trial in which progressive renal failure is being analyzed. It is important to try to enroll in such trials patients who demonstrate progression of their renal disease. In this study, the authors also analyzed factors other than dietary protein restriction and found that the apparent beneficial effect of the dietary manipulation could not be attributed to differences between the two groups in blood pressure or glycemic control or to differences in the frequency of examination. The conclusion was that protein restriction accounted for the slower progression of renal disease.

The Modification of Diet in Renal Disease (MDRD) Study, as mentioned above, was a multicenter, randomized trial in the United States involving 840 patients with various renal diseases. It examined the effects of blood pressure control (see above) and protein restriction on the progression of chronic renal failure (41). In Study 1, 585 patients with GFR values of 25–55 mL/min were randomly assigned to a usual- or a low-protein diet (1.3 or 0.58 g/kg body weight/day). In Study 2, patients with GFR levels of 13–24 mL/min were randomly assigned to a low- or a very-low- (0.28 g/kg body weight/day) protein diet, supplemented with keto amino acids. The average follow-up of these patients was 2.2 years. Compared to the usual protein diet group, patients assigned to the low-protein diet group in Study 1 had a greater decline in GFR during the first 4 months after randomization and a lesser decline thereafter. However, the total mean decline in GFR projected to 36 months did not differ between the two dietary groups. In Study 2, the very-low-protein diet had a marginal ($p = 0.007$) effect on the decline in GFR projected to 3 years when compared with the low-protein diet. If one assumes that the initial decline in GFR in the patients assigned to the low-protein diet in Study 1 is related to the hemodynamic effects of decreasing protein intake, and if one examines the subsequent change in GFR (slope) during the time period from the follow-up visit at 4 months after randomization to the end of the study, there is a 29% decrease in the rate of GFR loss in the patients ingesting the low-protein diet as compared to those ingesting the usual protein diet. Adherence results revealed that the patients assigned to the usual-protein diet ingested an average of 1.12 g protein/kg body weight as compared to approximately 0.7 g/kg body weight in those randomized to the low-protein diet. It appears, therefore, that in most instances when protein restrictions to 0.6 or to 0.4 g protein are prescribed as a target, the adherence rates are closer to 0.7 g protein/kg body weight. In this multicenter study, there was no evidence for the development of malnutrition or signs of protein depletion in the patients randomized to the low-protein diets. Although there is no clear definitive evidence that protein restriction ameliorates the progression of renal disease in humans, the overwhelming majority of data suggest a beneficial effect. Some degree of protein restriction should be recommended in patients with progressive renal failure, but the protein restriction should not be so severe as to require major modification in the eating patterns of patients.

EFFECTS OF PHOSPHORUS RESTRICTION

Several reports suggest an adverse effect of high phosphorus intake on renal function in both normal laboratory animals and those with reduced renal function, and it has been assumed that tissue injury in hyperphosphatemia results from calcium-phosphate deposition (74). A low-protein diet may affect progression of renal disease by decreasing the amount of phosphate in the diet. Whether the effects of dietary phosphate and protein are synergistic in slowing the progression of renal disease remains to be confirmed. Since phosphate restriction is required to prevent hyperparathyroidism and bone disease in patients with chronic renal failure, this maneuver is often recommended for patients with chronic renal disease, especially those with GFR values below 30 mL/min. Hyperphosphatemia is best treated by protein restriction and administration of phosphate-binding agents such as a calcium carbonate or calcium acetate.

INTERCURRENT EVENTS AFFECTING THE PROGRESSION OF RENAL DISEASE

During the course of chronic renal disease, several intercurrent events (Table 2) may accelerate the rate of loss of renal function. These intercurrent events should be considered when a sudden decrement in GFR occurs and, if present, should be corrected to slow the progression of renal failure. These events may cause a transient or a permanent loss of renal function. Treatment should address the major underlying disorder, e.g., correction of extracellular fluid volume, adequate treatment of infection, reversal of congestive heart failure, and discontinuation of

Table 2. Events that may accelerate rate of loss of renal function in patients with chronic renal failure

Extracellular fluid volume depletion—e.g., diarrhea and vomiting
Infection—e.g., systemic or of the urinary tract
Congestive heart failure
Nephrotoxic drugs—e.g., nonsteroidal anti-inflammatory drugs, antibiotics, anesthetic agents, cytotoxic drugs, radiographic contrast media
Urinary tract obstruction
Severe hypertension
Pregnancy
Hypotension—e.g., volume depletion or drug-induced
Metabolic derangements—e.g., hypercalcemia, hyperuricemia

Adapted from Klahr (19); used with permission.

nephrotoxic drugs. Urinary tract obstruction should be considered and, if present, should be corrected. Metabolic derangements such as hypercalcemia and hyperuricemia should also be treated.

ACKNOWLEDGMENTS

Supported by Program Project Grant DK-09976, from the NIDDK, National Institutes of Health (U.S.A.). The author acknowledges with thanks the editorial assistance of Mr. James Havranek.

REFERENCES

1. Border WA, Okuda S, Nakamura T: Extracellular matrix and glomerular disease. *Semin Nephrol* 9:307–317, 1989.
2. Klahr S, Schreiner G, Ichikawa I: The progression of renal disease. *N Engl J Med* 318:1657–1666, 1988.
3. Schmitz PG, Kasiske BL, O'Donnell MP, Keane WF: Lipids and progressive renal injury. *Semin Nephrol* 9:354–369, 1989.
4. Diamond FR, Karnovsky MJ: Focal and segmental glomerulosclerosis: analogies to atherosclerosis. *Kidney Int* 33:917–924, 1988.
5. Ross R: The pathogenesis of atherosclerosis—an update. *N Engl J Med* 314:488–500, 1986.
6. Steinberg D: Lipoproteins and the pathogenesis of atherosclerosis. *Circulation* 76:508–514, 1987.
7. Schlondorff D: The glomerular mesangial cell: an expanding role for a specialized pericyte. *FASEB J* 1:272–281, 1987.
8. Levey AS: Measurement of renal function in chronic renal disease. *Kidney Int* 38:167–184, 1990.
9. Bauer JH, Brooks CS, Burch RN: Clinical appraisal of creatinine clearance as a measurement of glomerular filtration rate. *Am J Kidney Dis* 3:337–346, 1982.
10. Levey AS, Perrone RD, Madias NE: Serum creatinine and renal function. *Annu Rev Med* 39:465–490, 1988.
11. Lavender S, Hilton PJ, Jones NF: The measurement of glomerular filtration rate in renal disease. *Lancet* 2:1216–1218, 1969.
12. Lubowitz H, Slatopolsky E, Shankel S, Rieselbach RE, Bricker NS: Glomerular filtration rate: determination in patients with chronic renal disease. *JAMA* 199:252–256, 1967.
13. Manz F, Alatas H, Kochen W, Lutz P, Rebien W, Scharer K: Determination of glomerular function in advanced renal failure. *Arch Dis Child* 52:721–724, 1977.
14. Milutnovic J, Cutler RE, Hoover P, Meijsen B, Scribner BH: Measurement of residual glomerular filtration rate in the patient receiving repetitive hemodialysis. *Kidney Int* 8:185–190, 1975.
15. Mitch WE, Walser M, Buffington GA, Lemann J: A simple method of estimating progression of chronic renal failure. *Lancet* 2:1326–1328, 1976.
16. Rutherford WE, Blondin J, Miller JP, Greenwalt AS, Vavra JD: Chronic progressive renal disease: rate of change of serum creatinine concentration. *Kidney Int* 11:62–70, 1977.
17. Mitch WE: The influence of the diet on the progression of renal insufficiency. *Annu Rev Med* 35:246–264, 1984.
18. El Nahas AM, Coles GA: Dietary treatment of chronic renal failure: ten unanswered questions. *Lancet* 1:597–600, 1986.
19. Klahr S: Chronic renal failure: management. *Lancet* 338:423–427, 1991.
20. Klahr S: The kidney in hypertension—villain and victim. *N Engl J Med* 320:731–733, 1989.
21. Lindeman RD, Tobin JD, Shock NW: Association between blood pressure and the rate of decline in renal function with age. *Kidney Int* 26:861–868, 1984.
22. Keane WF, Anderson S, Aurell M, de Zeeuw D, Narins RG, Povar G: Angiotensin converting enzyme inhibitors and progressive renal insufficiency. Current experience and future directions. *Ann Intern Med* 111:503–516, 1989.
23. Herlitz H, Edeno C, Mulec H, Westberg G, Aurell M: Captopril treatment of hypertension and renal failure in systemic lupus erythematosus. *Nephron* 38:253–256, 1984.
24. Hommel E, Parving H-H, Mathiesen E, Edsberg B, Damkjaer Nielsen M, Giese J: Effect of captopril on kidney function in insulin-dependent diabetic patients with nephropathy. *Br Med J [Clin Res]* 293:467–470, 1986.
25. Bjorck S, Nyberg G, Mulec H, Granerus G, Herlitz H, Aurell M: Beneficial effects of angiotensin converting enzyme inhibition on renal function in patients with diabetic nephropathy. *Br J Med [Clin Res]* 293:471–474, 1986.
26. Bakris GL: Effects of diltiazem or lisinopril on massive proteinuria associated with diabetes mellitus. *Ann Intern Med* 112:707–708, 1990.
27. Rosenberg ME, Hostetter TH: Comparative effects of antihypertensives on proteinuria: angiotensin-converting enzyme inhibitor vs. α1-antagonist. *Am J Kidney Dis* 18:472–482, 1991.
28. Ruilope LM, Miranda B, Morales JM, Rodicio JL, Romero JC, Ray L: Converting enzyme inhibition in chronic renal failure. *Am J Kidney Dis* 13:120–126, 1989.
29. Bergström J, Alvestrand A, Bucht H, Gutierrez A: Progression of chronic renal failure in man is retarded with more frequent clinical follow-ups and better blood pressure control. *Clin Nephrol* 25:1–6, 1986.
30. Heeg JE, de Jong PE, Van Der Hem GK, De Zeeuw D: Efficacy and variability of the antiproteinuric effect of ACE inhibition by lisinopril. *Kidney Int* 36:272–279, 1989.
31. Heeg JE, de Jong PE, Van der Hem GK, De Zeeuw D: Reduction of proteinuria by angiotensin converting enzyme inhibition. *Kidney Int* 32:78–93, 1987.
32. DeVenuto G, Andreotti C, Mattarei M, Pegoretti G: Prolonged treatment of essential hypertension and renal function: comparison of captopril and beta blockers considering microproteinuria values. *Curr Ther Res* 38:710–718, 1985.
33. Insua A, Ribstein J, Mimran A: Comparative effect of captopril and nifedipine in normotensive patients with incipient diabetic nephropathy. *Postgrad Med J* 64 (Suppl 3):59–62, 1988.
34. Baba T, Murabayashi S, Takebe K: Comparison of the renal effects of angiotensin converting enzyme inhibitor and calcium antagonist in hypertensive type 2 (non-insulin dependent) diabetic patients with microalbuminuria: a randomised controlled trial. *Diabetologia* 32:40–44, 1989.
35. Parving HH, Andersen AR, Smidt UM, Hommell E, Mathiesen ER: Effect of antihypertensive treatment on kidney function in diabetic nephropathy. *Br Med J* 294:1443–1447, 1987.
36. Christensen CK, Mogensen CE: Effect of antihypertensive treatment on progression of incipient diabetic nephropathy. *Hypertension* 7 (Suppl II):109–113, 1985.

37. Kajiwara N: Therapy and prognosis of hypertension in chronic nephritis. *Jpn Circ J* 39:779–786, 1975.

38. Brazy PC, Stead WW, Fitzwilliam JF: Progression of renal insufficiency: role of blood pressure. *Kidney Int* 35:670–674, 1989.

39. Rostand SG, Brown C, Kirk KA, Rutsky EA, Dustan HP: Renal insufficiency in treated essential hypertension. *N Engl J Med* 320:684–688, 1989.

40. Klahr S: The modification of diet in renal disease study. *N Engl J Med* 320:864–866, 1989.

41. Klahr S, Levey AS, Beck GJ, Caggiula AW, Hunsicker L, Kusek JW, Striker G, and the Modification of Diet in Renal Disease (MDRD) Study Group: The effects of dietary protein restriction and blood pressure control on the progression of chronic renal disease. *N Engl J Med*, in press.

42. Mogensen CE: Long-term antihypertensive treatment inhibiting progression of diabetic nephropathy. *Br Med J [Clin Res]* 285:685–688, 1982.

43. Parving H-H, Andersen AR, Smidt UM, Svendsen PA: Early aggressive antihypertensive treatment reduces rate of decline in kidney function in diabetic nephropathy. *Lancet* 1:1175–1179, 1983.

44. Marre M, Leblanc H, Suarez L, Guyenne T-T, Menard J, Passa A: Converting enzyme inhibition and kidney function in normotensive diabetic patients with persistent microalbuminuria. *Br Med J [Clin Res]* 294:1448–1452, 1987.

45. Lewis EJ, Hunsicker LG, Bain RP, Rohde RD, for the Collaborative Study Group: The effect of angiotensin-converting enzyme inhibition on diabetic nephropathy. *N Engl J Med* 329:1456–1462, 1993.

46. Breyer JA, Hunsicker LG, Bain RP, Lewis EJ, the Collaborative Study Group: Angiotensin converting enzyme inhibition in diabetic nephropathy. *Kidney Int* 45 (Suppl 45):S-156–S-160, 1994.

47. Kasiske BL, Kalil RSN, Ma JZ, Liao M, Keane WF: Effect of antihypertensive therapy on the kidney in patients with diabetes: a meta-regression analysis. *Ann Intern Med* 118:129–138, 1993.

48. Westlin W, Mullane K: Does captopril attenuate reperfusion-induced myocardial dysfunction by scavenging free radicals? *Circulation* 77 (Suppl 1):I-30–I-39, 1988.

49. Campbell-Boswell M, Robertson AL Jr: Effects of angiotensin II and vasopressin on human smooth muscle cells in vitro. *Exp Mol Pathol* 35:265–276, 1981.

50. Simonian MH, Gill GN: Regulation of deoxyribonucleic acid synthesis in bovine adrenocortical cells in culture. *Endocrinology* 104:588–595, 1979.

51. Aceto JF, Baker KM: [Sar¹] angiotensin II receptor-mediated stimulation of protein synthesis in chick heart cells. *Am J Physiol* 258:H806–H813, 1990.

52. Wolf G, Neilson EG: Angiotensin II induces cellular hypertrophy in cultured murine proximal tubular cells. *Am J Physiol* 259:F768–F777, 1990.

53. Daniels BS, Hostetter TH: Adverse effects of growth in the glomerular circulation. *Am J Physiol* 258:F1409–F1416, 1990.

54. Norman J, Badie-Dezfooly B, Nord EP, Kurtz I, Schlosser J, Chaudhari A, Fine LG: EGF-induced mitogenesis in proximal tubular cells: potentiation by angiotensin II. *Am J Physiol* 253:F299–F309, 1987.

55. Ray PE, Aguilera G, Kopp JB, Horikoshi S, Klotman PE: Angiotensin II stimulates proliferation of human fetal mesangial cells by a receptor-mediated mechanism (abstract). *J Am Soc Nephrol* 1:424, 1990.

56. Homma T, Hoover RL, Ichikawa I, Harris RC: Angiotensin II (A II) induces hypertrophy and stimulates collagen production in cultured rat glomerular mesangial cell (abstract). *Clin Res* 38:358A, 1990.

57. Singhal PC, Franki N, Hays RM: Angiotensin II induces actin synthesis in cultured mesangial cell (abstract). *Clin Res* 38:401A, 1990.

58. Rosenberg ME, Hostetter TH: The effect of angiotensin II on early growth response genes in the rat kidney (abstract). *J Am Soc Nephrol* 1:426, 1990.

59. Chobanian MC, Julin CM: Angiotensin II stimulates ammoniagenesis in canine renal proximal tubule segments. *Am J Physiol* 260:F19–F26, 1991.

60. Golchini K, Norman J, Bohman R, Kurtz I: Induction of hypertrophy in cultured proximal tubule cells by extracellular NH₄Cl. *J Clin Invest* 84:1767–1779, 1989.

61. Nath KA, Hostetter MK, Hostetter TH: Pathophysiology of chronic tubulointerstitial disease in rats: interaction of dietary acid load, ammonia, and complement component C3. *J Clin Invest* 76:667–675, 1985.

62. Keane WF, Raij L: Relationship among altered glomerular barrier permselectivity, angiotensin II, and mesangial uptake of macromolecules. *Lab Invest* 52:599–604, 1985.

63. Klahr S: Effects of protein intake on the progression of renal disease. In: *Annual Review of Nutrition*, vol. 9. Annual Reviews, Palo Alto, CA, pp 87–108, 1989.

64. Hunsicker LG: Studies of therapy of progressive renal failure in humans. *Semin Nephrol* 9:380–394, 1989.

65. Kopple JD, Monteon FJ, Shaib JK: Effect of energy intake on nitrogen metabolism in nondialyzed patients with chronic renal failure. *Kidney Int* 29:734–742, 1986.

66. Hirschberg RR, Kopple JD: Requirements for protein, calories, and fat in the predialysis patient. In: WE Mitch, S Klahr, eds, *Nutrition and the Kidney*. Little, Brown, Boston, pp 131–153, 1988.

67. Mitch WE: Uremia and the control of protein metabolism. *Nephron* 49:89–93, 1988.

68. Barsotti G, Giannoni A, Morelli E, Lazeri M, Vlamis I, Baldi R, Giovanetti S: The decline of renal function slowed by very low phosphorus intake in chronic renal patients following a low nitrogen diet. *Clin Nephrol* 21:54–59, 1984.

69. Gimenez L, Walker WG, Tew WP, Hermann JA: Prevention of phosphate-induced progression of uremia in rats by 3-phosphocitric acid. *Kidney Int* 22:36–41, 1982.

70. Lau K: Phosphate excess and progressive renal failure: the precipitation–calcification hypothesis. *Kidney Int* 36:918–937, 1989.

71. Lumlertgul D, Burke TJ, Gilum DM, Alfrey AC, Harris DC, Hammond WS, Schrier RW: Phosphate depletion arrests progression of chronic renal failure independent of protein intake. *Kidney Int* 29:658–666, 1986.

72. Walker JD, Bending JJ, Dodds RA, Mattock MB, Murrells TJ, Keen H, Viberti GC: Restriction of dietary protein and progression of renal failure in diabetic nephropathy. *Lancet* 2:1411–1415, 1989.

73. Zeller K, Whittaker E, Sullivan L, Raskin P, Jacobson H: Effect of restricting dietary protein on the progression of renal failure in patients with insulin-dependent diabetes mellitus. *N Engl J Med* 324:78–84, 1991.

74. Gimenez LF, Solez K, Walker WG: Relation between renal calcium content and renal impairment in 246 human renal biopsies. *Kidney Int* 31:93–99, 1987.

CHAPTER 46

Renal Insufficiency

FADI G. LAKKIS & MANUEL MARTINEZ-MALDONADO

INTRODUCTION

Regardless of the primary etiology of renal disease, the progressive decline in renal function eventually leads to uremia. In most patients with chronic renal insufficiency the signs and symptoms of uremia manifest when glomerular filtration rate (GFR) decreases to less than 15–20 mL/min. When GFR reaches a level lower than 5 mL/min, end-stage renal disease sets in and replacement therapy in the form of dialysis or transplantation becomes unavoidable. This chapter focuses on the conservative management of patients with chronic renal insufficiency who do not yet require renal replacement therapy.

Caring for patients with chronic renal failure encompasses four basic strategies (Table 1). First is the attempt to control the rate of progression of renal disease. Second is the prevention of further damage to the kidneys. Third is the management of individual aspects of the uremic syndrome and its complications. Finally, patients with chronic renal insufficiency should be educated about renal replacement therapies and prepared for the appropriate treatment modality when necessary.

CONTROLLING THE RATE OF PROGRESSION OF RENAL DISEASE

The natural history of established chronic renal insufficiency is that of relentless progression to end-stage renal disease. Most chronic renal failure patients lose residual GFR in a predictable fashion, even when the primary insult that initiated renal injury is no longer present (1). Based on both animal and clinical studies, several potential inducers of glomerulosclerosis and progression of renal disease have been identified. These include systemic and glomerular hypertension, dietary protein and phosphate, proteinuria, hyperlipidemia, and several growth factors and cytokines (2,3). Therapeutic interventions designed to minimize the impact of these factors are warranted; however, definite proof of the efficacy of some of these interventions awaits the completion of prospective clinical trials.

Treatment of hypertension

Approximately 85% of patients with chronic renal failure are hypertensive. Sodium retention and increased activity of the renin–angiotensin system are important etiologic factors. There is ample evidence indicating that uncontrolled hypertension superimposed on renal disease accelerates the decline in GFR. Several clinical studies suggest that treatment of hypertension slows the progression of renal disease (4,5). Antihypertensive therapy exerts its salutary effects on the kidney by ameliorating arteriolar nephrosclerosis and, more importantly, by reducing intraglomerular hypertension, which in experimental animals has been shown to lead to glomerulosclerosis (5–7).

The first step in the treatment of hypertension in chronic renal failure is dietary sodium restriction. The majority of patients, however, will require additional pharmacological therapy. Both angiotensin-converting enzyme (ACE) inhibitors and calcium channel blockers are effective first-line therapy. ACE inhibitors lower intraglomerular pressure by controlling systemic hypertension and by preferentially vasodilating the efferent arterioles (7). The intrarenal hemodynamic effects of ACE inhibitors translate into a decreased rate of decline in renal function, especially in diabetic patients (8). The beneficial effect of ACE inhibitors seems to be independent of treatment of systemic hypertension and is probably related to modification of intrarenal hemodynamics and/or reduction of proteinuria in diabetics (see below) (8,9). Although generally well tolerated, a few adverse side effects of ACE inhibitors are observed in patients with impaired renal function (7). These include hyperkalemia and an acute decline in GFR; the latter may occur in the presence of severe congestive heart failure, volume depletion, or significant bilateral renovascular disease. Cautious initiation of therapy using smaller doses of a short-acting ACE inhibitor and close follow-up of serum potassium and creatinine are recommended. Excessive doses of a sulfhydryl group containing ACE inhibitor can result in neutropenia in patients with advanced renal insufficiency and should be avoided. Calcium channel blockers are safe and effective

Suki, WN and Massry SG (eds), Suki and Massry's Therapy of Renal Diseases and Related Disorders, Third Edition. ISBN 978-1-4757-6634-9.

Table 1. Management of the patient with chronic renal failure

I. Attempt to control the rate of progression of renal disease
    1. Treatment of hypertension
    2. Dietary protein and phosphate restriction
    3. Reduction of proteinuria
    4. Management of hyperlipidemia
II. Avoid further damage to the kidneys (*non nocere*)
III. Manage the individual complications of uremia
    1. Fluid and electrolyte disorders
    2. Secondary hyperparathyroidism
    3. Other endocrine disorders
    4. Reproductive and sexual dysfunction
    5. Hematologic abnormalities
    6. Immunological impairment
    7. Neurological disorders
    8. Gastrointestinal complications
    9. Cardiac dysfunction and uremic pericarditis
    10. Pruritus
IV. Prepare the patient for renal replacement therapy

monotherapeutic agents that may retard the rate of decline in GFR. Whether calcium channel blockers confer specific renoprotective effects as observed with ACE inhibitors remains uncertain (5). The diuretic class of antihypertensives is generally ineffective as monotherapy in the case of moderate to severe renal insufficiency (10). However, diuretics potentiate the antihypertensive effect of ACE inhibitors when used in combination therapy. This is especially beneficial in African-American patients, who are generally less responsive to ACE inhibitors than Caucasians. Beta blockers exert their antihypertensive action partly by inhibiting renin release in the kidney and are effective in the patient with chronic renal failure. Their renoprotective effect, however, seems to be less pronounced than that of ACE inhibitors. In patients with uremic symptoms, beta blockers can exacerbate central nervous system depression and sexual dysfunction. The utility of central alpha-2-adrenergic agonists and peripheral alpha-1-adrenergic antagonists is often limited by their side effects, which include orthostatic hypotension and fluid retention. Neither group has been shown to reduce glomerular hypertension in a specific manner.

The degree of reduction in blood pressure required to slow the decline in GFR has not been clearly determined. Data generated by the Modification of Diet in Renal Disease (MDRD) study demonstrated that reduction in blood pressure below a mean arterial pressure (MAP) of 95 mmHg significantly decreased the rate of progression of renal insufficiency only in patients with pronounced proteinuria (>1 g/24 hr) (11). A trend towards slower decline in GFR was also observed in African-American individuals. No significant increase in adverse side effects of "aggressive" antihypertensive treatment was noted in this study.

Dietary protein and phosphate restriction

High protein intake in experimental animals leads to glomerular hyperfiltration and progressive glomerulosclerosis. Restriction of dietary protein, on the other hand, favorably alters the natural course of experimental renal disease. Several clinical studies have demonstrated that protein restriction may slow the decline in GFR in patients with chronic renal disease (12). The conclusions, however, are indefinite due to deficiencies in study design and the influence of confounding variables. The most rigorous study to date is the modification of Diet in Renal Disease (MDRD) study, which evaluated the effect of dietary protein restriction on the progressive decline of GFR over a 3-year period in 840 patients with various chronic renal diseases (11). The results of this study suggest that progression of renal disease in humans is minimally retarded by dietary protein restriction. Even a highly restricted diet providing 0.3 g of high-biological-value protein per kg body weight per day (supplemented with ketoacid analogues of essential amino acids) provided a marginal reduction in the rate of progression of renal disease. Dietary protein restriction seems to be more effective in retarding the progression of diabetic nephropathy.

Pending further data on the role of protein restriction in the progression of renal disease, it seems prudent to prescribe diets containing 0.4–0.6 g high-biological-value protein/kg body weight/day to patients with chronic renal insufficiency. Adequate caloric intake (approximately 35 kcal/kg/day) is necessary for efficient utilization of dietary protein. Diets containing less than 0.4 g protein/kg body weight/day should be supplemented with a keto acid–amino acid preparation to prevent malnutrition.

Several reports suggest an adverse effect of phosphorus intake on renal function and on the progression of renal disease (13). Because this causal relationship remains uncertain, the main purpose of restricting dietary phosphate in chronic renal failure should be the prevention of renal osteodystrophy, as discussed later in the chapter.

Reduction of proteinuria

Several studies suggest a direct correlation between the magnitude of proteinuria and rate of decline of renal function in patients with chronic glomerular disease (14). Maneuvers that diminish proteinuria would be expected to be beneficial. A large collaborative study demonstrated that treatment of diabetic patients with captopril significantly reduces the rate of decline in GFR independent of control of systemic hypertension (8). Because captopril also decreases 24-hour urinary protein excretion in these patients, it is postulated that the salutary effect of ACE inhibitors on diabetic nephropathy is at least partially mediated by reduction of proteinuria.

In many forms of glomerulonephritis, the control of proteinuria depends on specific immunosuppression, but ACE inhibitors may be helpful in nontreatable forms of the nephrotic syndrome (15). Although nonsteroidal anti-inflammatory drugs (NSAIDs) diminish proteinuria of glomerular disease, their renal side effects preclude long-term use.

Management of hyperlipidemia

The most common dyslipidemia of chronic renal failure is hypertriglyceridemia which occurs in 30%–70% of the patients (16). Hypercholesterolemia, on the other hand, is present in the majority of nephrotics and in only 20% of nonnephrotic subjects. Both groups of patients have a decreased ratio of high-density lipoprotein (HDL) to low-density lipoprotein (LDL) and manifest accelerated atherosclerosis. Data derived from animal models of renal disease suggest a causal relationship between hypercholesterolemia and glomerulosclerosis, but clinical evidence in support of this hypothesis is not available (17). The main goal of treatment of hyperlipidemia in chronic renal failure, therefore, is the prevention of atherosclerosis.

Dietary modification and exercise should be recommended to all patients with hyperlipidemia. Pharmacological intervention is not warranted in the patient with mild to moderate elevation of serum triglycerides due to the lack of association between hypertriglyceridemia and atherosclerotic disease. Moreover, effective triglyceride-lowering drugs (fibric acids) are cleared by the kidney and result in higher incidence of side effects in patients with renal insufficiency. Their use should be reserved for patients with severe hypertriglyceridemia in whom the risk of pancreatitis is significantly increased. Persistently elevated cholesterol levels can be treated with HMG-CoA reductase inhibitors such as lovastatin. Since less than 10% of an administered dose of lovastatin is eliminated by the kidneys, dose adjustment is not required when renal function is impaired. Probucol is an effective cholesterol-lowering agent, but its long-term protective effect is debatable, since it also decreases blood HDL levels. Moreover, probucol reduces levels of oxidized LDL and may prove to be beneficial in slowing the progression of renal failure, because preliminary evidence suggests a pathogenetic role for oxidized LDL in glomerulosclerosis (17).

Experimental therapies

Several growth factors, cytokines, and biologically active lipids have been found to play a role in the pathogenesis of glomerulosclerosis. Of note is the TGF-β family of proteins, which induces synthesis of extracellular matrix proteins and promotes glomerular destruction (18). Administration of monoclonal antibodies to TGF-β_1 has been shown to suppress glomerular matrix accumulation in experimental glomerulonephritis (19). Similar results were obtained with the use of decorin, a naturally occurring inhibitor of TGF-β (20). The use of an interleukin-1 receptor antagonist, IL-1RA, has also generated promising data in experimental models of glomerulonephritis (21). More recently, taxol, a microtubule-specific agent, has been shown to inhibit formation of renal cysts in an animal model of congenital polycystic kidney disease (22). Although it will be several years before these targeted therapeutic agents reach clinical utility, their use may eventually enhance our ability to alter the natural course of renal disease.

AVOIDING FURTHER DAMAGE TO THE KIDNEYS (NON NOCERE)

The list of causes of acute renal failure in the normal population also applies to the patient with chronic renal insufficiency (Table 2). In many respects, patients with preexisting kidney disease are more sensitive to these insults. Diligent care should be exercised in avoiding nephrotoxic agents and in recognizing reversible acute renal failure in these patients.

Drugs

The list of nephrotoxic drugs is ever growing. In the hospitalized patient, aminoglycoside antibiotics are the most common offenders (23). Although acute renal failure caused by aminoglycosides is usually reversible, residual damage is not uncommon. Patients who are advanced in age and those with underlying chronic renal insufficiency or volume depletion are at an increased risk. The cumulative amount administered and the duration of exposure to an aminoglycoside during the dosing interval (i.e., frequency of dosing) correlate better with the incidence of nephrotoxicity than the measured peak and trough of serum levels of antibiotic. Increasing individual doses while prolonging the dosing interval has been advocated to re-

Table 2. Potentially reversible causes of acute renal failure in patients with chronic renal disease

---

Intravascular volume depletion
Low cardiac output state
Sepsis
Malignant or accelerated hypertension
Drug toxicity
Acute interstitial nephritis
Urinary tract infection
Obstructive uropathy
Radiocontrast nephrotoxicity
Atheroembolic renal disease
Endogenous nephrotoxic substances
  Rhabdomyolysis
  Hyperuricemia
  Hypercalcemia
Acute glomerulonephritis
Exacerbation of preexisting glomerulonephritis
Renal vein thrombosis
Pregnancy-related complications

---

duce nephrotoxicity (24). Furthermore, dosage should be meticulously adjusted according to GFR in order to avoid both renal and auditory toxicities. Nonsteroidal anti-inflammatory drugs (NSAIDs) inhibit the production of vasodilatory prostaglandins in the kidney and can further compromise GFR in patients with chronic renal insufficiency (25). Even over-the-counter doses of an NSAID such as ibuprofen are sufficient to cause adverse renal effects (26). Although sulindac has been reported to cause fewer renal side effects than other NSAIDs, its long half-life can lead to toxic accumulation in patients with liver and renal disease (25). In addition to their hemodynamic effects, NSAIDs are an important etiology of interstitial nephritis (27). Other medications that commonly cause acute interstitial nephritis include β-lactam antibiotics, sulfonamides, rifampin, diuretics (thiazides, furosemide and butenamide), cimetidine, captopril, and diphenylhydantoin. Acute interstitial nephritis should be recognized promptly and the offending agent withdrawn (28). In some cases, a short course of corticosteroids may hasten recovery and limit the extent of renal damage from interstitial nephritis (29).

Medications normally excreted by the kidney can accumulate to dangerous levels in the presence of reduced GFR and can lead to both renal and nonrenal side effects. Several references and handbooks that guide medication dosing in patients with chronic renal failure are available and should be consulted (30).

Radiographic contrast agents

The nephrotoxicity of contrast agents is well recognized and occurs following intra-arterial, intravenous, or oral administration. Patients with preexisting renal insufficiency (diabetic nephropathy, in particular), volume depletion, or low cardiac output are at increased risk (31). Ionic and nonionic radiocontrast agents are equally nephrotoxic, although the latter causes less cardiovascular complications (32). The administration of a large volume of radiocontrast or repeated injections over the period of a few days is associated with a higher incidence of nephrotoxicity and should be avoided. One retrospective study provides a formula that estimates the maximum "safe" volume of radiocontrast that could be administered during a procedure (33):

Maximum contrast (mL) = *5 mL contrast/kg body weight (not to exceed 300 mL)* divided by *serum creatinine (mg/dL)*.

Adherence to the numbers derived from this formula does not guarantee prevention of nephrotoxicity, and the numbers should be used as rough guidelines only. Contrast studies are best avoided in patients at risk. If the use of radiocontrast is necessary, adequate hydration of the patient before and during the procedure is imperative. The prophylactic value of mannitol or loop diuretics in reducing the incidence of nephrotoxicity is still uncertain due to the lack of controlled prospective studies.

Atheroembolic renal disease

Arterial catheterization can result in another renal complication unrelated to the administration of radiocontrast. Atheroembolic renal disease, also referred to as *cholesterol emboli*, usually occurs in patients with peripheral vascular disease following angiography or aortic surgery (34). It manifests as either acute oliguric renal failure or insidious, gradual decline in renal function. Unlike radiocontrast nephropathy, atheroembolic disease is usually irreversible and in many cases culminates in end-stage kidney disease. The decision to perform arterial catheterization in the patient with chronic renal insufficiency should take into consideration the risk of renal injury.

Pregnancy

Whether pregnancy is contraindicated in the patient with chronic renal insufficiency is a matter of debate. A conservative approach is to advise women of child-bearing age of the risks associated with pregnancy in the presence of renal insufficiency: accelerated decline in GFR, worsening of hypertension, higher incidence of preeclampsia, intrauterine fetal growth retardation, and preterm delivery (35,36). Women with serum creatinine greater than 1.5 mg/dL and, more importantly, uncontrolled hypertension are at a higher risk of developing the above complications, and it is prudent to advise against pregnancy when the serum creatinine level is above 3.0 mg/dL. Certain nephropathies such as lupus nephritis and perhaps membranoproliferative glomerulonephritis are more sensitive to intercurrent gestation (36). The presence of both proteinuria and hypertension in women with chronic glomerulonephritis constitutes an additional risk factor for developing preeclampsia. Women with moderate renal insufficiency who elect to become pregnant should receive close prenatal surveillance with serial blood pressure and creatinine clearance measurements. If GFR declines during gestation in the absence of an obvious reversible cause, and especially when accompanied by uncontrolled hypertension, termination of pregnancy should be considered. Other renal complications associated with pregnancy include urinary tract infections, cortical necrosis, and (less commonly) renal failure associated with acute fatty liver of pregnancy.

MANAGEMENT OF UREMIA AND ITS COMPLICATIONS

The uremic syndrome is the end result of progressive glomerulosclerosis irrespective of the primary etiology of renal disease. The multiorgan derangements of uremia are generally incapacitating and often life-threatening. The remainder of this chapter focuses on the management of the individual manifestations of the uremic syndrome.

Fluid and electrolyte disorders

Patients with advanced renal failure have increased extracellular fluid volume due to sodium and water retention. The increase in intravascular volume contributes to hypertension, while expansion of the interstitial spaces manifests as edema. Treatment of hypertension is imperative for the prevention of cardiovascular catastrophes. The different antihypertensive agents discussed earlier in relation to controlling the progression of renal disease are also effective in more advanced renal failure. The spectrum of edema in uremic patients ranges from pretibial swelling to anasarca and pulmonary edema. The mainstay treatment of edema is dietary sodium restriction; diets containing less than 4 g of sodium, and often less than 2 g, are necessary. If symptomatic edema persists despite salt restriction, diuretics can be prescribed (37). Loop diuretics are the agents of choice due to their potent natriuretic effect. Since the actions of furosemide and bumetanide depend on their active secretion in the proximal tubule, advanced renal failure necessitates the use of higher doses. Very high doses (greater than 300–500 mg of furosemide or 6–10 mg of bumetanide bolus), however, are associated with increased incidence of ototoxicity. Ethacrynic acid should be avoided in patients with advanced renal insufficiency due to significant ototoxicity as well. Recent data suggest that slow, continuous infusion of a loop diuretic may be safer and more natriuretic than an equivalent dose administered in repeated boluses. Thiazides, given alone, are ineffective when GFR is less than 20–30 mL/min, with the exception of metolazone. Metolazone inhibits sodium transport in both the distal and proximal tubules and remains effective in advanced renal failure when given in larger doses (10–25 mg/day). More importantly, thiazide diuretics given in combination with a loop agent are helpful in the treatment of the diuretic-resistant patient. Osmotic diuretics, such as mannitol, are cleared exclusively by the kidneys and should not be used in the uremic patient due to the risk of elevation of extracellular fluid osmolality leading to pulmonary edema, hyponatremia, and hyperkalemia. Potassium-sparing diuretics can lead to serious hyperkalemia and are also contraindicated. Carbonic anhydrase inhibitors are generally ineffective in the presence of a very low GFR and may worsen metabolic acidosis.

Hyponatremia is a common disturbance of plasma composition in patients approaching end-stage renal disease, and results from reduced water clearance by the kidneys. Free water restriction to less than 1 L/day, and occasionally to less than 500 mL, may be necessary. If hypoosmolar intravenous fluids are to be administered, the physician must pay attention not only to the total amount of sodium the patient is going to receive but also to the volume of free water. For example, compared to normal saline, administration of half-normal saline solutions carries the additional risk of inducing hyponatremia in the patient with advanced renal insufficiency.

Decreased ammoniagenesis in the chronically diseased kidneys leads to metabolic acidosis, which usually becomes manifest when GFR drops below 25 mL/min (38). The acidosis in turn contributes to renal osteodystrophy and myocardial depression. Reducing dietary intake of protein to 0.4–0.6 g/kg body weight/day is the first line of treatment. If the serum bicarbonate level falls below 15–17 mEq/L despite dietary adjustment, oral alkali supplementation should be instituted. Either sodium bicarbonate or a sodium citrate/citric acid solution (Shohl's solution) can be prescribed to provide 0.5–1 mEq bicarbonate/kg/day. A 650-mg tablet of sodium bicarbonate delivers 8 mEq bicarbonate while 1 mL of either sodium bicarbonate or Shohl's solution provides 1 mEq. Since the conversion of citrate to bicarbonate occurs in the liver, citrate-containing solutions should not be administered in the presence of severe hepatic dysfunction. Moreover, the sodium load that accompanies either bicarbonate or citrate therapy should be taken into account in the patient with edema. Calcium carbonate frequently prescribed for the management of hyperphosphatemia and hypocalcemia in uremics is an alkali and may obviate the need for additional bicarbonate supplements. In patients with renal failure secondary to diabetes, hypertension- or interstitial nephritis-decreased renin secretion leading to reduced aldosterone production can contribute to the pathogenesis of acidosis. Hyperkalemia is commonly present in these patients and further suppresses renal ammoniagenesis. A small dose of a synthetic mineralocorticoid (fludrocortisone) is sometimes required for the treatment of hyporeninemic hypoaldosteronism.

Like acidosis, hyperkalemia manifests when the GFR drops below 20% of normal (39), and dietary potassium restriction becomes essential. Exogenous sources of potassium (oral potassium supplements and certain salt substitutes) and medications that can cause hyperkalemia (potassium-sparing diuretics, ACE inhibitors, β-blockers, NSAIDs, and occasionally heparin) should be avoided or discontinued. Endogenous causes of hyperkalemia such as hemolysis, gastrointestinal bleeding, hematomas, rhabdomyolysis, acidosis, and hyporeninemic hypoaldosteronism should be diagnosed promptly and corrected when possible. If hyperkalemia persists despite dietary restriction, potassium-binding resins (Kayexalate) can be prescribed. Loop diuretics and metolazone result in significant kaliuresis and are beneficial to the patient with both hyperkalemia and edema.

Secondary hyperparathyroidism

Essential for the prevention and treatment of uremic secondary hyperparathyroidism is the control of serum phosphorus levels (40,41). Reduced urinary excretion of phosphate occurs early in the course of renal insufficiency and results in compensatory hyperparathyroidism that maintains serum phosphate levels in the normal range. In order to correct the hyperparathyroidism, dietary restriction of phosphate intake is essential when GFR decreases below 50–60 mL/min. Meat and dairy products are the major sources of phosphate in the average diet. As GFR reaches a level below 30 mL/min, the renal capacity to excrete phosphate is overwhelmed, and serum levels begin to rise. At this stage, oral phosphate binders must be prescribed. Aluminum-containing antacids such as aluminum hydroxide and aluminum carbonate are potent phosphate binders. The systemic absorption and accumulation of aluminum in the presence of renal insufficiency may result in serious complications such as dementia, osteomalacia, microcytic anemia, and proximal myopathy. Although magnesium-containing antacids are effective phosphate binders, the risk of hypermagnesemia precludes their use. Calcium salts are currently the phosphate binders of choice. Calcium carbonate and calcium acetate have been shown to control hyperphosphatemia when administered during or immediately after meals. Their most common side effects are constipation and gastric discomfort, both of which can be managed symptomatically.

In addition to hyperphosphatemia, decreased calcium absorption in advanced renal insufficiency contributes to the pathogenesis of secondary hyperparathyroidism. Calcium salts prescribed as phosphate binders also serve as calcium supplements. Patients who have normal serum phosphorus but low calcium levels should receive additional doses of a calcium salt between meals. Vitamin D supplements are usually required to compensate for the decreased renal production of 1,25-dihydroxyvitamin D_3 and to enhance absorption of calcium from the gastrointestinal tract. The administration of 1,25-dihydroxyvitamin D_3 may directly suppress the secretion of parathyroid hormone as well. Because all forms of vitamin D therapy can cause hypercalcemia, close follow-up of serum calcium is recommended. Moreover, hyperphosphatemia should be corrected before vitamin D supplements are initiated to avoid extraskeletal deposition of calcium phosphate.

Other endocrine disorders

Multiple hormonal systems are affected by chronic renal failure. The extent to which endocrine derangements other than hyperparathyroidism contribute to the uremic syndrome is unclear. End-organ resistance to insulin and glucose intolerance are universally present in uremics (42). Fasting hyperglycemia, however, rarely occurs in the nondiabetic subject. Uremic patients also demonstrate decreased levels of tri-iodothyronine (T_3) due to decreased peripheral conversion of thyroxine (T_4) to T_3, as seen in the euthyroid-sick syndrome (43). The majority of these patients are clinically euthyroid. Treatment is not required for either the insulin resistance or the thyroid hormone abnormality.

Reproductive and sexual dysfunction (44)

Most premenopausal women with uremia are anovulatory and have abnormal menstrual cycles. Decreased libido and have abnormal menstrual cycles. Decreased libido and diminished ability to reach orgasm are commonly reported. Low serum estrogen levels and mildly elevated prolactin levels are observed in these patients, but neither estrogen replacement nor treatment with a dopaminergic agonist (bromocryptine) has significant clinical benefits. Psychological factors contributing to sexual dysfunction should be investigated and treated. Pregnancy is not recommended in patients with moderate to severe renal failure, as discussed earlier in this chapter.

Erectile impotence and decreased libido are commonly reported by male uremic patients. The major pathogenetic factors include psychological, vascular, and hormonal abnormalities. Diminished spermatogenesis is also observed and may lead to infertility. Although testosterone levels are uniformly low in these patients, testosterone therapy does not offer significant benefit. Dopaminergic agonists (bromocryptine, lisuride, and parlodel) decrease prolactin levels and may partially restore sexual function in men with advanced renal failure. The correction of anemia with erythropoeitin has also been shown to improve sexual function in these patients.

Hematologic abnormalities

The three major hematological manifestations of uremia are anemia, bleeding diathesis, and mild hemolysis (45). The management of anemia of chronic renal failure has radically changed with the advent of recombinant human erythropoeitin. The efficacy of erythropoeitin in the dialysis patient is well documented. Correction of anemia results in improved cardiac function, exercise tolerance, central nervous system symptoms, appetite, and sexual function (46). The utility of erythropoeitin in the predialysis patient has been demonstrated in clinical studies (47,48). The usual dose of erythropoeitin in the patient with chronic renal failure is 50–150 U/kg administered subcutaneously 2–3 times per week. The target hematocrit ranges between 30% and 35%. Higher hematocrits may worsen hypertension and are in rare cases associated with seizures. In addition to monitoring blood pressure, it is necessary to measure serum iron, iron-binding capacity, and ferritin levels prior to and during erythropoeitin therapy. Iron supplements are often necessary to maintain an adequate response to erythropoeitin. Unlike data derived from animal experiments, correction of anemia with erythropoeitin does not adversely affect the progression of renal disease in human studies (47,48).

The hallmark of the hemostatic abnormality of uremia is a prolonged bleeding time secondary to abnormalities of platelet aggregation and platelet-vascular wall interactions. Correction of the bleeding tendency in uremic patients is often required prior to surgical procedures and is imperative during active bleeding. Several therapeutic measures are effective (Table 3) (45). First, correction of anemia with either erythropoeitin or transfusions shortens the bleeding time in most patients. Second, 1–deamino-8-D-arginine vasopressin (DDAVP) administered intrave-

Table 3. Treatment of bleeding diathesis in uremia

Therapy	Dose	Peak action	Duration of action
DDAVP	0.3 µg/kg I.V.	1–4 hours	≤8 hours
Cryoprecipitate	10 units I.V.	4–12 hours	12–18 hours
Estrogen	0.6 mg/kg daily for 5 days	5–7 days	10–14 days

nously (0.3 mg/kg) or intranasally (3 mg/kg) restores hemostasis within 1–4 hours, and its effect lasts up to 8 hours (49). Tachyphylaxis develops rapidly with repeated doses of DDAVP. Third, cryoprecipitate has a rapid onset of action and may be administered to the actively bleeding patient. The effect of cryoprecipitate lasts 12–18 hours, but repeated use is hindered by expense, volume overload, and risk of transmission of viral infections. Fourth, conjugated estrogens (emopremarin, for example) correct hemostasis in uremics for up to 14 days when given daily for 5 days (0.6 mg/kg). The onset of action of estrogens is usually within 24 hours. The above treatments should be considered complementary rather than mutually exclusive.

Immunological impairment

Immunological defects in uremia include abnormalities in granulocyte and lymphocyte function. Uremic patients are more prone to infections and may have an increased incidence of bacteremia. Adherence to sterile techniques when performing invasive procedures, as well as early recognition and treatment of bacteremia, is necessary. Although antibody responses in uremics are depressed, immunoglobulin titers achieved following vaccination are protective in most patients. Pneumococcal and hepatitis B vaccines are therefore recommended. Follow-up antibody titers help determine the need for booster vaccination. In general, immunocompromised patients should not receive live-attenuated-virus or live-bacteria vaccines due to the increased risk of complications (50). Strict control of secondary hyperparathyroidism and zinc repletion may correct some of the immunological impairments in uremia.

Neurological disorders

The central nervous system manifestations of uremia include sleep abnormalities, decreased mentation, lethargy, asterixis, and myoclonus. When central nervous system impairment is severe, dialysis becomes a necessity. Because none of these signs and symptoms is specific to uremia, other etiologies should be ruled out before initiating dialysis. The differential diagnosis includes metabolic causes (hyponatremia, hypernatremia, hypoglycemia, hyperglycemia, and severe hypophosphatemia), accumulation of a medication that has central nervous system side effects, hepatic encephalopathy, hypertensive encephalo-

pathy, strokes, subdural hematoma, and central nervous system infections. Many of these etiologies are reversible and should be diagnosed promptly.

The peripheral neuropathy of chronic renal disease is usually distal and symmetric and can affect both sensory and motor nerves. It manifests with paresthesias, muscle weakness, and muscle twitching (restless leg syndrome). Quinine sulfate and benzodiazepines effectively control the latter disorder. It is important to note that the progression of peripheral neuropathy in uremic patients can be controlled with dialysis and that clinical remission may occur following renal transplantation (51).

Gastrointestinal complications

Nausea and anorexia are common complaints among uremic patients. Treatment with a drug such as metoclopromide can control the nausea and enhance gastric emptying. Because uremia predisposes patients to gastrointestinal bleeding, ulcerogenic medications (steroids and NSAIDs) should be avoided when possible. The management of gastrointestinal bleeding in chronic renal failure is similar to that in nonuremic subjects except for the need to adjust the doses of H_2-blockers and to correct the bleeding time when necessary. High dietary fiber intake and nonmagnesium laxatives are recommended for patients with constipation resulting from oral calcium supplements.

Cardiac dysfunction and uremic pericarditis

Left ventricular dysfunction is commonly observed in uremic patients, and improvement has been reported following either hemodialysis or renal transplantation (52). In the patient with chronic renal insufficiency who is not on renal replacement therapy, adequate control of hypertension and hypervolumia is required to ameliorate cardiac dysfunction. The occurrence of uremic pericarditis is an indication for acute and intensive dialysis. In fact, the incidence of uremic pericarditis has declined sharply with the use of early or prophylactic dialysis. Large pericardial effusions and tamponade are infrequent complications. If they do occur, pericardiocentesis or pericardiectomy may become necessary. NSAIDs and steroids are ineffective for the treatment of uremic pericarditis.

Pruritus (53)

The management of pruritus in patients approaching end-stage renal disease begins with excluding etiologies other than uremia. These include dermatological disorders, liver disease, and occult malignancy. The next step is the correction of serum phosphorus levels. Strict control of secondary hyperparathyroidism may alleviate itching in some patients. The most commonly used pharmacological therapy are the antihistaminics (H_1-blockers). H_1-blockers are effective for mild pruritus; in more severe cases, ultraviolet phototherapy (UVB) may be helpful.

PREPARING THE PATIENT FOR RENAL REPLACEMENT THERAPY

Despite conservative management, patients with uremia will eventually progress to end-stage renal disease and may become candidates for renal replacement therapy. One should not assume that every patient with end-stage renal disease is suitable for replacement therapy. The presence of serious and chronic comorbidities such as terminal cancer, multiple strokes, and dementia should be taken into consideration. Patients and their families should be actively involved in making the decision whether or not to initiate renal replacement therapy.

Dialysis is the most commonly utilized form of treatment for end-stage renal disease. The patient who is a hemodialysis candidate should have an arteriovenous fistula created 6–8 weeks before the anticipated date of initiating therapy to allow for adequate maturation of the vessels. The decision to begin dialysis depends on the severity of uremic signs and symptoms in the individual patient rather than on the blood urea nitrogen and creatinine levels. Table 4 summarizes the indications for initiation of dialysis in the patient with chronic renal failure. Many nephrologists, however, advocate early initiation of dialysis to avert the more serious complications of uremia, such as pericarditis, pulmonary edema, motor neuropathy, and encephalopathy.

Table 4. Indications for initiation of chronic hemodialysis

Uncontrolled fluid and electrolyte abnormalities
  Hyperkalemia
  Metabolic acidosis
  Fluid overload (pulmonary edema)

Uncontrolled uremic symptoms or signs
  Nausea, vomiting, anorexia
  Malaise
  Uremic pericarditis
  Uremic encephalopathy
  Peripheral motor neuropathy (wrist or foot drop)
  Worsening peripheral sensory neuropathy

The option of peritoneal dialysis should not be overlooked. With the advent of new surgical techniques, peritoneal dialysis can be initiated as early as 1–2 days following the placement of a peritoneal catheter. Occasionally, patients with an appropriate living related kidney donor may bypass the need for dialysis. In the latter case, potential family donors should be sought and adequately screened (54). Most transplant candidates, however, receive dialysis therapy in preparation for surgery or while waiting for a cadaver kidney.

REFERENCES

1. Hebert LA, Bay WH: On the natural tendency to progressive loss of remaining kidney function in patients with impaired renal function. *Med Clin North Am* 74:1011–1024, 1990.
2. Martinez-Maldonado M, Benabe JE, Cordova HR: Chronic clinical intrinsic renal failure. In: DW Seldin, G Giebisch, eds, *The Kidney: Physiology and Pathophysiology*, 2nd ed. Raven Press, New York, 1992.
3. Jacobson H: Chronic renal failure: pathophysiology. *Lancet* 338:419–423, 1991.
4. Kasiske BL, Kalil RSN, Ma JZ, Liao M, Keane WF: Effect of antihypertensive therapy on the kidney in patients with diabetes: a meta-regression analysis. *Ann Intern Med* 118:129–138, 1993.
5. Tolins JP, Raij L: Antihypertensive therapy and the progression of chronic renal disease. Are there renoprotective drugs? *Semin Nephrol* 11:538–548, 1991.
6. Hostetter TH, Rennke HG, Brenner BM: The case for intrarenal hypertension in the initiation and progression of diabetic and other glomerulopathies. *Am J Med* 72:375–380, 1982.
7. Keane WF, Anderson S, Aurell M, de Zeeuw D, Narins RG, Povar G: Angiotensin converting enzyme inhibitors and progressive renal insufficiency. Current experience and future directions. *Ann Intern Med* 111:503–516, 1989.
8. Lewis EJ, Hunsicker LG, Bain RP, Rohde RD, for the Collaborative Study Group: The effect of angiotensin-converting enzyme inhibition on diabetic nephropathy. *N Engl J Med* 329:1456–1462, 1993.
9. Ravid M, Savin H, Jutrin I, Bental T, Katz B, Lishner M: Long-term stabilizing effect of angiotensin-converting enzyme inhibition on plasma creatinine and on proteinuria in mormotensive type II diabetic patients. *Ann Intern Med* 118:577–581, 1993.
10. Kaplan NM: Renal parenchymal hypertension. In: *Clinical Hypertension*, 5th ed. Williams & Wilkins, Baltimore, 1990.
11. Klahr S, Levey AS, Beck GJ, Caggiula AW, Hunsicker L, Kusek JW, Striker G, for the Modification of Diet in Renal Disease study group: The effects of dietary protein restriction and blood-pressure control on the progression of chronic renal disease. *N Engl J Med* 330:877–884, 1994.
12. Mitch WE: Dietary protein restriction in patients with chronic renal failure. *Kidney Int* 40:326–341, 1991.
13. Lau K: Phosphate excess and progressive renal failure: the precipitation–calcification hypothesis. *Kidney Int* 36:918–937, 1989.
14. Remuzzi G, Bertani T: Is glomerulosclerosis a consequence of altered glomerular permeability to macromolecules? *Kidney Int* 38:384–394, 1990.

15. Praga M, Hernandez E, Montoyo C, Andres A, Ruilope LM, Rodicio JL: Long-term beneficial effects of angiotensin-converting enzyme inhibition in patients with nephrotic proteinuria. *Am J Kidney Dis* 20:240–248, 1992.
16. Grundy SM: Management of hyperlipidemia of kidney disease. *Kidney Int* 37:847–853, 1990.
17. Keane WF, Mulcahy WS, Kasiske BL, Kim Y, O'Donnell MP: Hyperlipidemia and progressive renal disease. *Kidney Int* 39:S41–48, 1991.
18. Isaka Y, Fujiwara Y, Ueda N, Kaneda Y, Kamada T, Imai E: Glomerulosclerosis induced by in vivo transfection of transforming growth factor β or platelet-derived growth factor gene into the rat kidney. *J Clin Invest* 92:2597–2601, 1993.
19. Border WA, Okuda S, Languino LR, Sporn MB, Ruoslahti E: Suppression of experimental glomerulonephritis by antiserum against transforming growth factor β1. *Nature* 346:371–374, 1990.
20. Border WA, Noble NA, Yamamoto T, Harper JR, Yamaguchi Y, Pierschbacher MD, Ruoslahti E: Natural inhibitor of transforming growth factor β protects against scarring in experimental kidney disease. *Nature* 360:361–364, 1992.
21. Tang WW, Feng L, Vannice JL, Wilson CB: Interleukin-1 receptor antagonist ameliorates experimental anti-glomerular basement membrane antibody-associated glomerulonephritis. *J Clin Invest* 93:273–279, 1994.
22. Woo DDL, Miao SYP, Pelayo JC, Woolf AS: Taxol inhibits progression of congenital polycystic kidney disease. *Nature* 368:750–753, 1994.
23. Kaloyanides GJ: Aminoglycoside nephrotoxicity. In: RW Schrier, CW Gottschalk, eds, *Diseases of the Kidney*, vol 2, 5th ed. Little, Brown, Boston, 1993.
24. Levison ME: New dosing regimens for aminoglycoside antibiotics. *Ann Intern Med* 117:693–694, 1992.
25. Schlondorff D: Renal complications of nonsteroidal antiinflammatory drugs. *Kidney Int* 44:643–653, 1993.
26. Whelton A, Stout RL, Spilman PS, Klassen DK: Renal effects of ibuprofen, piroxicam, and sulindac in patients with asymptomatic renal failure. *Ann Intern Med* 112:568–576.
27. Clive DM, Stoff JS: Renal syndromes associated with nonsteroidal antiinflammatory drugs. *N Engl J Med* 310:563–572, 1984.
28. Ten RM, Torres VE, Milliner DS, Schwab TR, Holley KE, Gleich GJ: Acute interstitial nephritis: immunologic and clinical aspects. *Mayo Clin Proc* 63:921–930, 1988.
29. Galpin JE, Shinaberger JH, Stanley TM, Blumenkrantz MJ, Bayer AS, Friedman GS, Montgomerie JZ, Guze LB, Coburn JW, Glassock RJ: Acute interstitial nephritis due to methicillin. *Am J Med* 65:756–765, 1978.
30. Bennet WM, Aronoff GR, Golper TA, Morrison G, Singer I, Brater DC: *Drug Prescribing in Renal Failure. Dosing Guidelines for Adults*, 2nd ed. American College of Physicians, Philadelphia, 1991.
31. Berns AS: Nephrotoxicity of contrast media. *Kidney Int* 36:730–740, 1989.
32. Schwab SJ, Hlatky MA, Pieper KS, Davidson CJ, Morris KG, Skelton TN, Bashore TM: Contrast nephrotoxicity: a randomized controlled trial of a nonionic and an ionic radiographic contrast agent. *N Engl J Med* 320:149–153, 1989.
33. Cigarroa RG, Lange RA, Williams RH, Hillis LD: Dosing of contrast material to prevent contrast nephropathy in patients with renal disease. *Am J Med* 86:649–652, 1989.
34. Coburn JW, Agre KL: Renal thromboembolism, atheroembolism, and other acute diseases of the renal arteries. In: RW Schrier, CW Gottschalk, eds, *Diseases of the Kidney*, vol 2, 5th ed. Little, Brown, Boston, 1993.
35. Hou SH, Grossman SD, Madias NE: Pregnancy in women with renal disease and moderate renal insufficiency. *Am J Med* 78:185–194, 1985.
36. Surian M, Imbasciati E, Cosci P, et al.: Glomerular disease and pregnancy. A study of 123 pregnancies in patients with primary and secondary glomerular diseases. *Nephron* 36:101–105, 1984.
37. Rose BD: Diuretics. *Kidney Int* 39:336–352, 1991.
38. Warnock DG: Uremic acidosis. *Kidney Int* 34:278–287, 1988.
39. Ypersele De Strihou CVY: Potassium homeostasis in renal failure. *Kidney Int* 11:491–504, 1977.
40. Delmez JA, Slatopolsky E: Recent advances in the pathogenesis and therapy of uremic secondary hyperparathyroidism. *J Clin Endocrinol Metab* 72:735–739, 1991.
41. Malluche H, Faugere MC: Renal bone disease 1990: an unmet challenge for the nephrologist. *Kidney Int* 38:193–211, 1990.
42. De Fronzo RA, Tobin JD, Rowe JW, et al.: Glucose intolerance in uremia. Quantification of pancreatic beta cell sensitivity to glucose and tissue sensitivity to insulin. *J Clin Invest* 62:425–435, 1978.
43. Kaptein EM, Quion-Verde H, Choolzian CJ, et al.: The thyroid in end-stage renal disease. *Medicine (Baltimore)* 67:187–197, 1988.
44. Schaefer F, Ritz E, Kokot F, Massry SG: Metabolic and endocrine dysfunctions in uremia. In: RW Schrier, CW Gottschalk, eds, *Diseases of the Kidney*, vol 3, 5th ed. Little, Brown, Boston, 1993.
45. Paganini EP, Rothmann SA, Paul P, Meagher RC: Hematologic abnormalities. In: JT Daugirdas, TS Ing, eds, *Handbook of Dialysis*, 1st ed. Little, Brown, Boston, 1988.
46. Lundin AP: Recombinant erythropoietin and chronic renal failure. *Hosp Pract* 26(4):61–69, 1991.
47. Abels R: Rate of progression of chronic renal failure in predialysis patients treated with erythropoietin. *Semin Nephrol* 10 (Suppl 1):20–25, 1990.
48. Lim VS, DeGowin RL, Zavala D, Kirchner PT, Abels R, Perry P, Fangman J: Recombinant human erythropoietin treatment in pre-dialysis patients. A double-blind placebo-controlled trial. *Ann Intern Med* 110:108–114, 1989.
49. Mannucci PM, Remuzzi G, Pusineri F, Lombardi R, Valsecchi C, Mecca G, Zimmerman TS: Deamino-8-D-arginine vasopressin shortens the bleeding time in uremia. *N Engl J Med* 308:8–12, 1983.
50. Centers for Disease Control: General recommendations on immunization. Guidelines from the immunization practices advisory committee. *Ann Intern Med* 111:133–142, 1989.
51. Bolton CF, Baltzan MA, Baltzan RB: Effects of renal transplantation on uremic neuropathy. *N Engl J Med* 284:1170, 1971.
52. Burt RK, Gupta-Burt S, Suki WN, Barcenas CG, Ferguson JJ, Van Buren CT: Reversal of left ventricular dysfunction after renal transplantation. *Ann Intern Med* 111:635–640, 1989.
53. Balaskas EV, Oreopoulos DG: Uremic pruritus. *Dial Transplant* 21:278–284, 1992.
54. Bay WH, Hebert LA: The living donor in kidney transplantation. *Ann Intern Med* 106:719–727, 1987.

CHAPTER 47

Anesthesia and Surgery in the Patient with Renal Failure

DAVID R. BEVAN

INTRODUCTION

Most patients with chronic renal failure (CRF) will receive anesthesia for vascular access before hemodialysis, for renal transplantation, or for surgery unrelated to their renal disease. CRF is associated with systemic disease, which increases the problems of anesthesia. The purpose of this chapter is to review the major obstacles to safe anesthesia, to describe the changes induced by renal failure, in the activity of drugs used during anesthesia, and to recommend safe approaches to anesthesia in CRF. Most patients are now well controlled by dialysis and, before renal transplantation, will usually have received hemodialysis within 48 hours of the procedure, so severe cardiovascular and biochemical disturbances are seldom observed at the time of surgery.

SYSTEMIC DISEASE

Cardiovascular disturbances

ANEMIA

The most common abnormality affecting the cardiovascular system in CRF is severe anemia. The causes are discussed elsewhere in this book but include decreased erythropoiesis, hemolysis, bleeding, and iatrogenic blood sampling. In most studies (1–4), the mean hemoglobin concentration at the time of renal transplantation is 6–8 g/ 100 mL. Despite the more frequent use of blood transfusion (5), the hemoglobin concentration before surgery seldom exceeds 10 g/100mL, although this may be correctable with recombinant human erythropoietin (6). This level of hemoglobin in normal patients is below that at which anesthesiologists used to advise postponement of surgery (7,8). The chronic anemia is compensated for by an increase in cardiac output and a shift to the right of the oxyhemoglobin dissociation curve by stimulation of 2:3 DPG synthesis. Thus, the off-loading of oxygen at the tissues is increased, and there is no indication for preoperative blood transfu-

sion to correct the anemia. Nevertheless, oxygen delivery (O_2 delivery = cardiac output × arterial oxygen content) is threatened and may be severely reduced in the presence of cardiac or respiratory disease. In addition, the increase in cardiac output predisposes to the development of congestive failure. Consequently, particular care is taken during and after anesthesia to preserve oxygen delivery with respect to blood loss replacement, oxygen therapy, and cardiovascular support. Most general anesthetic agents are associated with some myocardial depression and impairment of pulmonary oxygen transfer, which exacerbate the problem.

HYPERTENSION

The majority of CRF patients are hypertensive. Arrhythmias and myocardial ischemia during anesthesia are common in the untreated hypertensive patient, particularly at the time of laryngoscopy and tracheal intubation (9). If time allows, attempts should be made to gain control of the blood pressure before anesthesia. More frequently, particularly in the renal transplant patient, urgent control is undertaken before induction of anesthesia using the ultra-short-acting cardioselective beta$_1$-sympathetic blocking drug esmolol, 2µg/kg I.V. (10), or the combined alpha$_1$- and beta-sympathetic blocking drug labetalol, 5mg bolus I.V. (11). The risk of uncontrolled hypertension far exceeds that of impaired cardiovascular responsiveness during surgery.

CONGESTIVE FAILURE

Preoperative fluid-volume status will be determined by local hemodialysis practices. Nevertheless, a tendency to fluid overload persists. Some authors have found surprisingly high right- and left-sided filling pressures at the time of transplantation, even in the apparently well-controlled patient (13,14). Thus, the theoretical advantages of "loading" the transplanted kidney to encourage early function (14,15) may be hazardous, but should encourage greater use of central venous pressure measurement. Uremic

Suki, WN and Massry SG (eds), Suki and Massry's Therapy of Renal Diseases and Related Disorders, Third Edition. ISBN 978-1-4757-6634-9.
©1998, Kluwer Academic Publishers, Boston/Dordrecht/London. All rights reserved.

pericarditis is a rare complication of CRF but may, theoretically, contribute to hemodynamic complications.

Respiratory disturbances

Good hemodialysis treatment ensures that pulmonary edema is uncommon. Nevertheless, the CRF patient usually has a PaO_2 that is lower than expected for his or her age. Several predisposing factors may be involved, particularly infection and, rarely, uremic lung disease. Consequently, attention should be paid to oxygen therapy in the perioperative period, particularly since O_2 delivery is already compromised. Hypoxemia during hemodialysis is common, although the cause is not understood clearly (16).

Electrolytes and hydrogen ion

Severe disturbances of electrolytes and hydrogen ion are uncommon, but mild hyponatremia and metabolic acidosis are not. The latter may induce hyperventilation and a compensatory respiratory alkalosis, and unless this is appreciated, positive-pressure ventilation without hyperventilation will encourage hyperkalemia (17).

Hyperkalemia is unusual, but if above 6 mEq/L should be treated with calcium and with glucose and insulin. Hyperkalemia poses a particular danger during anesthesia, because the muscle relaxant succinylcholine usually increases serum potassium concentration by a further 0.5 mEq/L (18), again predisposing to arrhythmia after the induction of anesthesia. However, it seems that this risk has been exaggerated, and a much greater increase in potassium concentration during transplantation occurs if the preserving fluid, with its high K^+ concentration, is not drained from the kidney before anastomotic connections are made (19).

Disordered calcium metabolism and the risk of pathological fractures necessitate that the unconscious patient be moved carefully.

Alimentary tract

Renal transplantation is performed as an emergency procedure, so it must be assumed that recipients will have full stomachs and be prone to the dangers of regurgitation and pulmonary aspiration if adequate precautions are not taken. In addition, the CRF patient is at greater risk due to delayed gastric emptying (20). Consequently, an H_2 receptor blocker, such as ranitidine, 150 mg P.O., 1 hour before the induction of anesthesia is useful prophylaxis. However, the routine precautions of pre-oxygenation, cricoid pressure, and rapid tracheal intubation will usually avoid problems The use of an antacid such as magnesium trisilicate is not recommended because it may lead to hypermagnesemia.

Associated disease

Many CRF patients have widespread disease. Diabetes mellitus is common and may add vascular and neurologic complications, which will introduce further fluid imbalance if plasma glucose concentrations are uncontrolled. Autonomic failure may predispose to hemodynamic instability and peripheral neuropathy.

Concomitant drug therapy is common. Those receiving corticosteroids for immunologic control may require additional supplements to maintain hemodynamic stability, but this is not always necessary, and supplements can be administered as required (21). Immunologic suppression increases the risk of infection, and antibiotic therapy, particularly with the aminoglycosides, tetracyline, vancomycin, and clindamycin, may potentiate nondepolarizing muscle relaxants (22).

ANESTHETIC PROBLEMS

General anesthesia

Anesthetic agents are fat-soluble compounds and consequently are normally reabsorbed by the kidney. Their termination of action depends upon redistribution, metabolism, and, for inhalational agents, excretion by the lungs. Thus, their action is unaffected in patients with CRF unless the disease modifies organ sensitivity or unless cardiovascular effects are produced.

The CRF patient must be handled gently to avoid damage to brittle bones and to shunts and fistulae. For example, I.V. and arterial cannula and blood pressure cuffs should not be placed on limbs used for hemodialysis access. The danger of sepsis exists, so all anesthetic instruments, laryngoscopes, suction apparatus, etc. should be sterilized before use. The immunologically impaired CRF patient may also be a carrier of viral disease, so medical staff should take appropriate precautions for their own safety.

The aim of anesthesia in the CRF patient is to provide comfort for the patient, to allow access for the surgeon, and to avoid further compromise to the kidney by the direct or indirect effects of anesthesia. It should be remembered that these goals can be achieved by several techniques and that the success of transplantation depends upon immunologic techniques, ischemic time, and operative technique.

FLUID THERAPY

The principles of fluid therapy in the CRF patient are no different from normal. Fluid will be required for maintenance and to replace losses. Maintenance fluids, approximately 20 mL/kg/day, can be provided by D5W solution. The choice of other fluid will depend upon the composition of the fluid lost. Blood should be replaced with blood, and if the preoperative hemoglobin concentration is less than 10 g/dL, attempts should be made to ensure that it does not decrease further during surgery. Third-space losses during intra-abdominal surgery can be replaced with either 0.9% saline or Ringer's lactate at 5–10 mL/kg/hr. The risks of fluid overload during surgery in CRF have been exaggerated, to the detriment of the maintenance of hemodynamic integrity. Intraoperative fluid loading or the addition of mannitol or frusemide do not help to preserve renal function in the patient with renal insufficiency.

PREMEDICATION

Several years of hemodialysis do not make repeated venepunctures any more comfortable. CRF patients realize the importance of a successful transplant. Understandably, they will be anxious before surgery and will often require premedication, usually with oral diazepam 10–20 mg, to control psychological and cardiovascular states. Opioids are better avoided as premedication because their duration of action may be prolonged (23).

MONITORING

International standards now mandate that, during anesthesia, the following monitors are required in all patients: pulse oximeter, plethysmograph, stethoscope, ECG, capnograph, and temperature measurement; in addition, the lighting should be adequate to see the patients's color (24). The requirements for additional monitoring depend both on the severity and control of the renal failure and on the extent of the intended surgery. In the well-controlled patient, hemodynamic monitoring may be restricted to blood pressure and ECG. However, the unstable patient, in whom considerable fluid and blood shifts are anticipated, will require central venous and probably pulmonary and systemic artery monitoring. The latter should be embarked upon judiciously due to the possible need for peripheral vessels for future hemodialysis.

INDUCTION OF ANESTHESIA

Induction of general anesthesia is usually achieved with the intravenous barbiturate thiopental, 2.5–5 mg/kg. Its duration of action may be prolonged in the uremic patient as a result of decreased plasma protein binding (24), altered cerebral metabolism (25), or increased permeability of the blood–brain barrier (26). However, the duration of action in the recently dialysed patient is not changed. Other induction agents, such as methohexital (9) or ketamine (27), produce more problems in the hypertensive patient. The recently introduced, and expensive, short-acting agent propofol has no particular advantage in CRF patients undergoing prolonged surgery.

MAINTENANCE OF ANESTHESIA

Anesthesia is maintained in CRF patients with N_2O/O_2 together with low concentrations of inhalational agents, usually in combination with small doses of opioids.

Inhalation anesthesia

Isoflurane is the most common inhalational vapor used in the maintenance of anesthesia. It is only minimally metabolized (29) and thus avoids the theoretic hepatic toxicity of halothane and the fluoride nephrotoxicity induced by inorganic fluoride from the metabolism of methoxyflurane. Anesthetic agents have little direct effect upon kidney function as long as severe hypotension is avoided. The low blood and tissue solubility of isoflurane ensures that its elimination is more rapid and that emergence, particularly after prolonged exposure, occurs more quickly than after halothane or enflurane (30).

Opioids

There remains some controversy in the use of opioids in patients with renal failure. Opioids are fat-soluble compounds and are not normally excreted by the kidney. However, there are reports of prolonged respiratory depression and sedation following the use of morphine (31) and demerol (32). Renal failure does not does not alter the elimination of these drugs, but it is likely that accumulation of their metabolites occurs (23), which is probably responsible for their prolonged effects. Renal failure may also decrease protein binding and hence increase the amount of free basic drugs such as the opioids. However, studies with fentanyl, sufentanil, and alfentanil suggest that plasma clearance, and hence duration of action, are unaffected in CRF (33,34). Consequently, one of these drugs, usually fentanyl (1–3 µg/kg/hr), is chosen to supply perioperative analgesia.

MUSCLE RELAXATION

Neuromuscular blocking drugs are necessary to facilitate tracheal intubation and to allow relaxation for intra-abdominal procedures. Abnormal effects can be anticipated with almost all of these drugs in the CRF patient.

Depolarizing relaxants

Succinylcholine is associated with many complications (Table 1), yet it remains the only relaxant with a very rapid onset (1 min) and duration (5–8 min) of action and continues to be popular to facilitate tracheal intubation, particularly in the emergency patient. The most frequent and severe complication is *hyperkalemia.* In normal and renal-failure patients, an increase of plasma concentration of 0.5 mEq/L can be expected (18), and succinylcholine is therefore avoided if the plasma concentration is higher than 6 mEq/L. Greater increases are seen in burns, trauma, neurological disease, and muscular dystrophy when succinylcholine is contraindicated (35). Gradually, the use of succinylcholine is declining due to the availability of the intermediate-duration nondepolarizing relaxants *atracurium* and *vecuronium.*

The duration of action of succinylcholine may be prolonged in renal failure because plasma cholinesterase concentrations are decreased by hemodialysis (36) and after transplantation (37). The latter decrease is accentuated because azathioprine potentiates succinylcholine by inhibi-

Table 1. Complications associated with succinylcholine

Common	Rare
Fasciculations	Malignant hyperthermia
Hyperkalemia	Anaphylaxis
Muscle pains	Prolonged apnea
Myoglobinemia	Pulmonary edema
Cardiac bradyarrhythmias	Severe hyperkalemia
Catecholamine release	
Increased intraocular pressure	
Increased intragastric pressure	

Table 2. Median values for volume of distribution (Vd_{ss} l/kg), plasma clearance (Cp mL/kg/min), and terminal half-lives ($t\frac{1}{2}\beta$) or mean residence times (MRT) from several pharmacokinetic studies in normal patients (N) and patients with renal failure (RF) (39,42,43,56)

		Vd_{ss}	Cp	$t\frac{1}{2}\beta$
Atracurium	N	0.16	5.5	20
	RF	0.17	6.3	24
Mivacurium	N	0.11	70.4	1.5 (MRT)
	RF	0.15	76.6	1.9 (MRT)
Pancuronium	N	0.23	1.9	145
	RF	0.25	0.67	534
Rocuronium	N	0.21	2.89	71
	RF	0.26	2.89	97
Tubocurarine	N	0.39	1.9	239
	RF	—	—	—
Vecuronium	N	0.26		62
	RF	0.24		97

tion of phosphodiesterase, which leads to increased acetylcholine release (38).

Nondepolarizing relaxants

The kidney is the predominant route of excretion for most of the nondepolarizing relaxants. It is the only route for *gallamine* (whose use is thus contraindicated), but for others the proportion excreted through the kidney will depend upon alternative routes of excretion or metabolism. *Pancuronium, d-tubocurarine, doxacurium,* and *pipecuronium* are long-acting relaxants for whom the kidney is the major excretory route. *Vecuronium* is mainly excreted via the liver (39), *atracurium* is metabolized both by a spontaneous process—Hoffman elimination (40)—and by hydrolysis by non-specific esterases (41), and *mivacurium* is a recently introduced short-duration agent that is metabolized (42), like *succinylcholine,* by plasma cholinesterase. Experience with *rocuronium,* which has pharmacokinetic and pharmacodynamic behavior similar to *vecuronium,* is very limited (43). Currently, there is some emphasis throughout anesthesia to replace the long-acting by the intermediate-acting relaxants to ensure full recovery of neuromuscular function after the end of anesthesia. This is particularly important in the CRF patient. Thus, *atracurium* is very widely used (0.4–0.5 mg/kg to facilitate intubation, and maintenance by small boluses 0.1–0.2 mg/kg or by infusion) in these patients due to the absence of organ-based excretion. The introduction of *mivacurium* has occurred too recently for its place to be assessed (44). However, the rapid rate of recovery make it an attractive option.

Sensitivity to the nondepolarizing relaxants is not altered in CRF, nor is the volume of distribution of these agents; however, the clearance and elimination of all except atracurium and mivacurium are modified (Table 2). The keys to the safe use of muscle relaxants in these patients is to provide doses just sufficient to maintain neuromuscular blockade, as assessed by a nerve stimulator, preferably with *atracurium* (45), and to reverse the block at the end of surgery.

Reversal of neuromuscular blockade

The drugs used to reverse muscle relaxants—anticholinergic and anticholinesterases—are also water-soluble, ionized compounds normally excreted by the kidney (46,47). The reduction of plasma clearance of the anticholinesterases is greater than can be explained by a reduction in GFR, so they are probably actively secreted into the tubular lumen (48). The choice and dose of anticholinesterase is determined from the extent of the block—neostigmine (0.035–0.07 mg/kg) for deep block and edrophonium (0.5–1.0 mg/kg) for less intense paralysis (49). Once adequate recovery has been established, reparalysis will not occur (50).

POSTOPERATIVE ANALGESIA

Most major hospitals now undertake more careful control of pain after surgery with the help of an Acute Pain Service. CRF patients undergoing major surgery will require the same attention to pain relief. Systemic opioids administered by either the epidural or intravenous route (patient-controlled analgesia) should be given with care in consideration of the pharmacological behavior of opioids in CRF.

Regional anesthesia

Several surgical procedures in the CRF patient are suitable for regional analgesia. Brachial plexus block, by the axillary or interscalene routes, is ideal to allow the creation of vascular access for hemodialysis in the arm and produces the highest fistula flows with less hemodynamic change than inhalational anesthesia with halothane or isoflurane (51). Some (52), but not all (53), investigators have noticed that the duration of action of the local anesthetics may be reduced in CRF. Regional anesthesia is more difficult when several sites are involved. Bilateral axillary block is inadvisable due to the risk of pneumothorax.

Spinal analgesia and epidural analgesia have both been recommended for renal transplantation (54) because they cause autonomic block. However, most transplant patients prefer to be asleep. Some authors consider epidural analgesia contraindicated in the patient with a hemorrhagic tendency (55), but there are no reports of epidural hematoma in the CRF patient.

PROTECTING THE KIDNEY

Major surgery in CRF patients is often followed by deterioration in renal function. Several regimens have been suggested to preserve urine flow with mannitol or loop diuretics (57), renal perfusion with low-dose, 1–3 µg/kg, or "renal" dopamine (58), or to maintain intravascular volume with fluid loading (59). Given in an uncontrolled fashion, such regimens have been disappointing. At the present time, renal function seems to be best preserved by maintaining cardiovascular stability and cardiac output arterial blood pressure, thus ensuring the maintenance of renal perfusion. There is some experimental work suggesting that the combination of atrial natriuretic factor with mannitol (60) may have some beneficial role. Also, administration of nonsteroidal anti-inflammatory agents seems to worsen renal function (61), probably by decreasing the production of vasodilating prostaglandins. Thus, there is mounting evidence that renal function is best preserved by maintaining renal perfusion. As yet, there is no conclusive evidence to support the use of specific "renal" therapy.

REFERENCES

1. Bastron RD, Bailey G, Deutsch S, Vandam LD: Anesthesia for patients with chronic renal failure for renal homotransplantation. *Anesthesiology* 30:335–336, 1969.
2. Samuel JR, Powell D: Renal transplantation. Anaesthetic experience of 100 cases. *Anaesthesia* 25:165–176, 1970.
3. Monks PS, Lumley J: Anaesthetic aspects of renal transplantation. *Ann R Coll Surg Engl* 50:354–366, 1972.
4. Logan DA, Howie HB, Crawford J: Anaesthesia for renal transplantation: an analysis of fifty-six cases. *Br J Anaesth* 46:69–72, 1974.
5. Uldall PR, Wilkinson R, Dewar PJ, et al.: Factors affecting the outcome of cadaver renal transplantation in Newcastle upon Tyne. *Lancet* 2:316–319, 1977.
6. Jindal HH, Hirsch DJ, Belitsky P, Whalen MA: Low-dose subcutaneous erythropoietin corrects the anaemia of renal transplant faailure. *Nephrol Dial Transplant* 7:143–146, 1992.
7. Haljamae H, Rosenberg PH: Present and future concepts in transfusion practice. *Acta Anaesthesiol Scand* 32 (Suppl 89):1–3, 1988.
8. Gillies IDS: Anaemia and anaesthesia. *Br J Anaesth* 46:589–602, 1974.
9. Prys-Roberts C: Anaesthesia and hypertension. *Br J Anaesth* 56:711–724, 1984.
10. Miller DR, Martineau RJ, Wynands JE: Bolus administration of esmolol for controlling the haemodynamic response to tracheal intubation: the Canadian multicentre trial. *Can J Anaesth* 38:849–858, 1991.
11. Singh PP, Dimich I, Sampson I, Sonnenklar N: A comparison of esmolol and labetalol for the treatment of perioperative hypertension in geriatric ambulatory surgical patients. *Can J Anaesth* 39:559–562, 1992.
12. Goldman L, Caldera DL: Risks of general anesthesia and elective operation in the hypertensive patient. *Anesthesiology* 50:285–292, 1979.
13. Cronnelly R, Kremer PF, Beaupre P, Cahalan MK, Salvatierra O, Feduska N: Hemodynamic response to fluid challenge in anesthetized patients with end-stage renal disease. *Anesthesiology* 59:A49, 1983.
14. Carlier M, Squifflet J-P, Pirson Y, Gribomont B, Alexandre GPJ: Maximal hydration during anesthesia increases pulmonary artery pressures and improves early function of human renal transplants. *Transplantation* 34:201–204, 1982.
15. Tasker PRW, MacGregor GA, de Wardener HE: Prophylactic use of intravenous saline in patients with chronic renal failure undergoing major surgery. *Lancet* 2:911–912, 1974.
16. Eiser AR: Pulmonary gas exchange during hemodialysis and peritoneal dialysis: interaction between respiration and metabolism. *Am J Kidney Dis* 6:131–142, 1985.
17. Goggin MJ, Joekes AM: Gas exchange in renal failure. I. Dangers of hyperkalaemia during anaesthesia. *Br Med J* 2:244–147, 1971.
18. Koide M, Waud BE: Serum potassium concentrations after succinylcholine in patients with renal failure. *Anesthesiology* 36:142–144, 1972.
19. Soulillou JP, Fillaudeau F, Keribin JP, Guenel J: Acute hyperkalemia risks in recipients of kidney graft cooled with Collins' solution. *Nephron* 19:301–304, 1977.
20. McNamee PT, Moore GW, McGeown MG, Doherty CC, Collins BJ: Gastric emptying in chronic renal failure. *Br Med J* 291:310–11, 1985.
21. Symreng T, Karlberg BR, Kagedal B, Schildt B: Physiological cortisol substitution of long-term steroid-treated patients undergoing major surgery. *Br J Anaesth* 53:949–954, 1981.
22. Sokoll MD, Gergis SD: Antibiotics and neuromuscular function. *Anesthesiology* 55:148–159, 1981.
23. Chauvin M, Sandouk P, Scherrmann JM, Farinotti, Strumza P, Duvaldestin P: Morphine pharmacokinetics in renal failure. *Anesthesiology* 66:327–331, 1987.
24. Guidelines to the practice of anaesthesia as recommended by the Canadian Anaesthetists' Society. *Can J Anaesth* 41 (Suppl 3):1–16, 1994.
25. Ghonheim MM, Pandya H: Plasma protein binding of thiopental in patients with impaired renal or hepatic function. *Anesthesiology* 42:545–549, 1975.
26. Richet G, de Novales EL, Verroust P: Drug intoxication and neurological episodes in chronic renal failure. *Br Med J* 2:394–395, 1970.
27. Freeman RB, Sheff MF, Maher JF, Schreiner GE: The blood cerebrospinal fluid barrier in uremia. *Ann Intern Med* 56:233–240.
28. Hobika GH, Evers JL, Mostert JW, Trudnowski RJ, Moore RH, Murphy GP: Comparison of hemodynamic effects of glucagon and ketamine in patients with chronic renal failure. *Anesthesiology* 37:654–658, 1972.

29. Holaday DA, Fiserova-Bergerova V, Latto IP, Zumbiel MA: Resistance of isoflurane to biotransformation in man. *Anesthesiology* 43:325–332.

30. Eger EI II: Recovery from anesthesia. In: Eger EI II, ed, *Anesthetic Uptake and Action*. Baltimore: Williams & Wilkins, p. 228, 1974.

31. Osborne RJ, Joel SP, Slevin ML: Morphine intoxication in renal failure: the role of morphine-6-glucuronide. *Br Med J* 292:1548–1549, 1986.

32. Szeto, HH, Inturrisi CE, Houde R, Saal S, Cheigh J, Redenberg MM: Accumulation of normeperidine, an active metabolite of meperidine, in patients with renal failure or cancer. *Ann Intern Med* 86:738–741, 1977.

33. Chauvin M, Lebrault C, Levron JC, Duvaldestin P: Pharmacokinetics of alfentanil in chronic renal failure. *Anesth Analg* 66:53–56, 1987.

34. Sear JW: Sufentanil disposition in patients undergoing renal transplantation: influence of choice of kinetic model. *Br J Anaesth* 63:60–67, 1989.

35. Martyn JAJ, White DA, Gronert GA, Jaffe RS, Ward JM: Up-and-down regulation of skeletal muscle acetylcholine receptors. *Anesthesiology* 76:822–843, 1992.

36. Holmes JH, Makamoto S, Sawyer KC: Changes in blood composition before and after dialysis with the Kolff twin coil kidney. *Trans Am Soc Artific Intern Organs* 4:16–18, 1958.

37. Ryan DW: Postoperative serum cholinesterase activity following successful renal transplantation. *Br J Anaesth* 51:881–884, 1979.

38. Dretchen KL, Morgenroth VH, Standaert FG, Walts LF: Azathioprine: effects on neuromuscular transmission. *Anesthesiology* 45:604–609, 1976.

39. Fahey MR, Morris RB, Miller RD, Nguyen T-L, Upton RA: Pharmacokinetics of ORG NC45 (Norcuron) in patients with and without renal failure. *Br J Anaesth* 55:6–11, 1981.

40. Stenlake JB, Waugh RD, Dewar GH, Hughes R, Chapple DJ, Coker GG: Biodegradable neuromuscular blocking agents. Part 4. Atracurium besylate and related polyalkylene diesters. *Eur J Med Chem* 16:515–524, 1981.

41. Nigrovic V, Pandya JB, Auen M, Wajskol A: Inactivation of atracurium in human and rat plasma. *Anesth Analg* 64:1047–1052, 1985.

42. Cook DR, Freeman JA, Lai AA, et al.: Pharmacokinetics of mivacurium in normal patients and in those with hepatic or renal failure. *Br J Anaesth* 69:580–585, 1992.

43. Szenohradszky J, Fisher DM, Segredo V, et al.: Pharmacokinetic of rocuronium bromide (ORG 9426) in patients with normal renal function or patients undergoing renal transplantation. *Anesthesiology* 77:899–904, 1992.

44. Phillips BJ, Hunter JM: Use of mivacurium chloride by constant infusion in the anephric patient. *Br J Anaesth* 68:492–498, 1992.

45. Hunter JM, Jones RS, Utting JE: Use of atracurium in patients with no renal function. *Br J Anaesth* 54:1251–1258, 1982.

46. Cronnelly R, Stanski DR, Miller RD, Sheiner LB, Soh YJ: Renal function and the pharmacokinetics of neostigmine in anesthetized man. *Anesthesiology* 51:222–226, 1979.

47. Morris RB, Cronnelly R, Miller RD, Stanski DR, Fahey MR: Pharmacokinetics of edrophonium in anephric and renal transplant patients. *Br J Anaesth* 53:1311–1314, 1981.

48. Rennick BR: Renal tubule transport of organic cations. *Am J Physiol* 9:F83–F89, 1981.

49. Bevan DR, Donati F, Kopman A: Reversal of neuromuscular blockade. *Anesthesiology* 77:785–805.

50. Bevan DR, Archer DP, Donati F, Ferguson A, Higgs BD: Reversal of pancuronium in renal failure: no recurarization. *Br J Anaesth* 54:63–68, 1982.

51. Mouquet C, Bitker MO, Bailliart O, et al.: Anesthesia for creation of a forearm fistula in patients with endstage renal failure. *Anesthesiology* 70:909–914, 1989.

52. Bromage PR, Gertel M: Brachial plexus block in chronic renal failure. *Anesthesiology* 36:488–493, ••.

53. Beauregard L, Martin R, Tetrault J-P: Brachial plexus block and chronic renal failure. *Can J Anaesth* 34:S118, 1987.

54. Wyant GM: The anaesthetist looks at tissue transplantation: three years experience with kidney transplantation. *Can Anaesth Soc J* 14:225–234, 1967.

55. Lofstrom B: Anaesthetic problems in renal transplantation. *J Urol Nephrol* 1:161–169, 1967.

56. Shanks CA: Pharmacokinetics of the non-depolarizing neuromuscular relaxants applied to calculation of bolus and infusion dose regimens. *Anesthesiology* 64:72–86, 1986.

57. Levinsky NG, Bernard DB: Mannitol and loop diuretics in acute renal failure. In: JM Brenner, JM Lazarus, eds, *Acute Renal Failure*, 2nd ed. Churchill Livingstone, New York, pp 841–856, 1988.

58. Myles PS, Buckland MR, Schenk NJ, et al.: Effect of "renal-dose" dopamine on renal function following cardiac surgery. *Anaesth Intensive Care* 21:56–61, 1993.

59. Luciani J, Franz P, Thibault P, Ghesquiere F, Conseiller C, Cousin M-T, Glaser P, LeGrain M, Viars P, Kuss R: Early anuria prevention in human kidney transplantation. Advantages of fluid loading under pulmonary artery pressure monitoring during the surgical period. *Transplantation* 28:308–312, 1979.

60. Lieberthal W, Sheridan AM, Valeri CR: Protective effect of atrial natriuretic factor and mannitol following renal ischemia. *Am J Physiol* 258:F1266–F1272, 1990.

61. Power I, Cumming AD, Pugh GC: Effect of diclofenac on renal function and prostacyclin after surgery. *Br J Anaesth* 69:451–456, 1992.

CHAPTER 48

Nutritional Management of the Uremic Patient

AUGUST HEIDLAND, KATARINA SÉBEKOVA, & MARKUS TESCHNER

INTRODUCTION

Dietary treatment of patients with chronic renal failure (CRF) has many components. These include appropriate protein intake, adequate calories, vitamins, and trace elements. The clinical impact of the dietary management of CRF patients is enormous, since uremia is characterized by a state of protein–calorie malnutrition with consequent high morbidity and mortality.

GUIDELINES FOR ASSESSING PATIENTS' COMPLIANCE WITH PROTEIN INTAKE AND NUTRITIONAL STATUS IN CHRONIC RENAL FAILURE (Table 1)

Recognition of nutritional deficiencies, in particular before clinical evidence, is of increasing importance to prevent malnutrition-associated morbidity and mortality by an optimal dietary therapy. There are a number of possibilities for evaluating both adherence to dietary prescription and nutritional status: assessment of dietary intake, anthropometry, biochemical parameters, immune function, and body composition.

Assessment of dietary intake

Adequacy of protein and energy intake may be assessed retrospectively by 24-hour recalls or prospectively by food diaries. A 4-day dietary history is considered to correlate well with the true dietary intake (1), although some data indicate that diet histories tend to underestimate protein intake (2).

Assessment of dietary compliance

A reliable quantitative method to assess dietary compliance is the measurement of urea nitrogen appearance (UNA). It approximates dietary protein intake (DPI) if the patient is in a steady state. UNA can be calculated from the sum of urea excretion and its accumulation (positive or negative) in the body pool (3). Urea space corresponds to body water and averages about 60% of body weight. In hemodialysis (HD) patients, UNA can be calculated from the sum of urea dialyzed and excreted plus its accumulation in the body pool. UNA is calculated from the following equation:

$$UNA(gN/day) = \text{urinary urea } N(g/day) + (SUN_f - SUN_i)$$
$$\times 0.6BW + (Bw_f - Bw_i) \times SUN_f,$$

where i and f are the initial and final values for the period of measurement. Due to a lack of equilibrium of urea between extracellular and intracellular urea at the end of dialysis, the measurement should be performed 30 minutes after completion of the treatment (4). To convert the nitrogen intake to protein equivalence (5), the protein catabolic rate (PCR) can be calculated from the sum of UNA and the excretion of nonurea nitrogen (PCR averages 31 mg/kg/day of nitrogen) by multiplication by a factor of 6.25. PCR may also be calculated from total urea removal and predialysis and postdialysis BUN. The normalized protein catabolic rate (NPCR) is obtained by dividing PCR by "dry" body weight. The role of NPCR as a marker of nutritional intake stems from the demonstration that PCR is linearly related to urea generation rate and thus dietary protein intake when the patient is in a steady state. PCR values of about 1.3 to 1.4 g/kg/day are needed to maintain lean body mass (LBM) in maintenance hemodialysis (MHD) (6). Catabolic events, leading to muscle proteolysis, increase PCR falsely.

Nitrogen balance techniques

Determination of nitrogen balance is still regarded as the gold standard in the evaluation of protein requirements. It might roughly be estimated as the difference between nitrogen intake and UNA minus the average nonurea nitrogen excretion. The shortcomings of this measurement are the influence of previous dietary intake and nutritional status of the patient. Malnourished patients may attain nitrogen equilibrium with less protein intake than well-

Suki, WN and Massry SG (eds), Suki and Massry's Therapy of Renal Diseases and Related Disorders, Third Edition. ISBN 978-1-4757-6634-9.

Table 1. Diagnostic parameters for nutritional intake and malnutrition in patients with chronic renal failure

---

Nutritional intake
  Dietary interviews (retrospective)
  Dietary diaries (prospective)
Protein intake
  Urinary urea excretion
  Urea nitrogen appearance (UNA)
  Urea generation rate (UGR)
  Protein catabolic rate (PCR)
  Serum urea/serum creatinine ratio
Anthropometric measurement
  Height, "dry weight"
  Body mass index (BMI)
  % weight loss (from usual body weight)
  % of ideal body weight
  Triceps and subscapular skinfold thickness
  Midarm muscle circumference (MAMC)
Body composition[a]
  Bioelectrical impedance (BEI)
Biochemical measurements
  Predialysis urea, creatinine, potassium
  Cholesterol (<150 mg/dL)
  Albumin (<4.0 g/dL)
  Prealbumin (<30 mg/dL)
  Transferrin (<200 mg/dL)
  Cholinesterase, pseudocholinesterase
  Plasma amino acid profile
  IGF-1 (<300 μg/L)
Immunological parameters
  Total lymphocyte count
  Delayed hypersensitivity skin testing
  Complement proteins (except C_4)

---

[a] In addition to the mentioned routine techniques of body composition assessment, additional methods may be of use in the near future (e.g., total body electrical conductance, dual-energy x-ray absorptiometry, nuclear magnetic resonance imaging) or may have importance in research (e.g., total body water measurement employing deuterium, tritium, or bromide isotope dilution, neutron activation analysis employing nitrogen, exchangeable Na/exchangeable K ratio, infrared impedance, ultrasound, densitometry, computerized tomography).

nourished ones. Furthermore, results of short-term studies inadequately reflect the disturbances of long-term conditions (7).

Body composition in uremic patients

Components of body composition include lean body mass, adipose tissue, bone, and water. In uremic patients, in contrast to healthy adults, not only water balance and adipose tissue but also lean body mass can change over a short time period.

WEIGHT

Longitudinal measurements of weight loss and gains are critical. Attention must be paid to dry weight in MHD patients and in patients with edema. The choice of standards is still disputed. The relative body weight (defined as the patient's weight compared with the weight of normal persons of the same age, sex, and weight) or premorbid weight give important clues to the nutritional state. Body mass index (BMI) has the advantage of avoiding standardized tables of height and weight (8).

HEIGHT

Serial measures are important in adults for monitoring a potential shrinkage of the patient.

BODY FAT

Since body fat closely correlates with subcutaneous fat, measurement of skin-fold thickness from at least three different locations gives reproducible information, particularly in lean individuals. Although errors of repeated measurements are seldom below 7%, edema must be excluded (9).

LEAN BODY MASS

Skeletal mucle mass forms the major store of protein and is estimated from measurement of midarm muscle circumference (MAMC). It can be calculated by subtraction of triceps skin-fold thickness from midarm circumference according to the following equation:

$$MAMC = \text{midarm circumference (cm)} - 0.314 \times \text{triceps skin-fold thickness.}$$

Only gross changes can be distinguished, and results are influenced by overhydration. The reproducibility of this measurement depends upon the skill of the observer (8). New standards for weight and body composition by frame size and height for assessment of nutritional status were derived from a cross-sectional study in 21,752 subjects (10).

Measurement of *total body protein* can be performed by neutron activation (11). This very accurate method was successfully employed in MHD patients. Furthermore, total body potassium (TBP) can be used to determine total body protein. In chronic renal failure, however, potassium homeostasis is markedly disturbed (12), rendering TBK less useful for the assessment of nitrogen stores. Estimation of lean body mass by measurement of total body water (TBW) with deuterinized water (D_2O) is not accurate in CRF due to fluid balance disorders.

PROTEINS

Measurement of the 3-methylhistidine (3-MEH): creatinine ratio in urine or in plasma is an index of myofibrillar protein degradation. 3-MEH forms an integral component of both actin and myosin in the myofibrils of skeletal muscle (13). During muscle proteolysis, this amino acid is released into the circulation and cannot be reutilized for protein synthesis. A dietary source of 3-MEH has to be eliminated.

Leucine turnover techniques provide information of whole-body protein metabolism (protein synthesis, protein degradation, and amino acid oxidation) (14).

TOTAL BODY COMPOSITION

Bioelectric impedance (BEI) measurement estimates the body composition indirectly in a noninvasive, rapid, and accurate fashion. Results of BEI analysis have correlated with anthropometry for the proportion of lean body mass, fat mass, and malnutrition index. Its reproducibility is best when performed post-HD. BEI was successfully applied during long-term studies in MHD patients (15,16).

A useful tool for the evaluation of the principal components of the body is dual-energy X-ray absorptiometry (DXA). It is simple to perform, of high precision and accuracy, and convenient for the patients (17).

Biochemical measurements

Transport proteins have been widely used in the assessment of protein malnutrition in both uremic and nonuremic patients (18). However, these parameters are also influenced by the renal disease itself.

ALBUMIN

The most convincing link between malnutrition and morbidity has been provided by albumin measurements. However, apart from dietary factors, plasma albumin concentration is lowered by many other factors such as extracorporal losses (nephrotic rage proteinuria, hemo- and peritoneal dialysis), fluid retention, increased vascular permeability, enhanced catabolism, and decreased synthesis as a "negative acute phase protein". Moreover, due to its long half-life (20 days), albumin is a late parameter of malnutrition. Its validity as a nutritional indicator is questionable in patients receiving albumin infusions.

SHORT HALF LIFE PROTEINS

Serum proteins with a short half-life, such as prealbumin (PA, $t\frac{1}{2}$ = 2 days) and retinol-binding protein (RBP, $t\frac{1}{2}$ = 10 hours), are early indices of malnutrition in nonrenal patients. In end-stage renal failure, however, the concentrations of these low-molecular-weight plasma proteins may be elevated due to their decreased glomerular filtration (8). Furthermore, PA is a negative acute-phase reactant. In spite of these shortcomings, plasma levels of PA less than 0.29 g/L are considered to be a sensitive and specific index of malnutrition in MHD patients (19).

PLASMA TRANSFERRIN

Plasma transferrin (TF) ($t\frac{1}{2}$ = 9 days) has a smaller extravascular pool than albumin and is not influenced by renal function. Values of less than 0.2 g/L are a sign of protein deficiency (20). A shortcoming of this measurement is its dependence upon iron status: TF concentration is increased when iron stores are depleted and diminished in iron overload (for instance due to repeated blood transfusions). Furthermore, in patients with malignant tumors, infections, or rheumatoid arthritis, decreases of TF-concentration may occur.

Insulin-like growth factor 1 (IGF-1) is low in cases of malnutrition. Levels less than 300 µg/L indicate an advanced stage (21).

OTHER PARAMETERS

Plasma creatinine levels reflect muscle mass in a rough fashion (8). Low concentrations in relation to GFR indicate malnutrition. Also, low predialysis concentrations of BUN, potassium (K^+), or inorganic phosphate (if no phosphate binders are administered) may indicate malnutrition. Finally, low cholesterol levels (<150 mg/dL) are an index of undernutrition (22).

AMINO ACIDS (AAS)

Plasma amino acid profiles demonstrate marked abnormalities (decreases of most essential amino acids and some nonessential amino acids) in CRF that are related to the nutritional state, severity of uremia, and altered renal metabolism (synthesis and uptake of amino acids). Distribution of intracellular amino acids differs from that of plasma levels (23,24).

IMMUNE FUNCTION

Malnutrition also impairs immunocompetence. For evaluation of cell-mediated immunity, skin reaction after application of multiple antigens is a useful tool (25). Other indicators are total lymphocyte count (26) and various complement proteins (C_3, C_{3a}, C_{1q}) except C_4 (27).

SUBJECTIVE GLOBAL ASSESSMENT (SGA)

SGA combines the evaluation of protein intake and clinical judgment of the nutritional state (28) and is widely used.

Summary

No single parameter provides reliable information about the overall nutritional state. Combined evaluation of dietary history as well as serial anthropometric and biochemical measurements offer the best approach to the assessment of nutritional status. Another useful tool seems to be the recently suggested *malnutrition index*, which is based on anthropometric (bioelectrical impedance), laboratory, and clinical parameters (29).

NUTRITION IN THE PRE DIALYSIS STAGE OF CHRONIC RENAL FAILURE (CRF)

CRF is a state of protein intolerance (30); as a consequence, the waste products of protein metabolism accumulate in proportion to the loss of functional renal mass and protein intake, finally resulting in uremic intoxication. The fact that protein restriction ameliorates many clinical symptoms of uremia has been known for more than 100 years. Low-protein diet (LPD) not only decreases serum urea levels but also reduces accumulation of hydrogen ions, inorganic phosphate, and numerous organic acids and amines, all of which contribute to uremic toxicity. In the past, the beneficial effects of LPD frequently were hampered by the development of severe protein calorie malnutrition. Thus, the goals of nutritional therapy in CRF are both 1) reduction of uremic toxicity and 2) maintenance of a good nutritional state. Furthermore, LPD may retard the progression of many renal diseases. Two approaches to protein restriction have been developed: 1) the conventional low-protein diet (0.6 g protein/kg/day) and 2) the very-low-protein diet (VLPD) (0.28 g protein/kg/day), supplemented with either a mixture of essential amino acids (EAAs) or a mixture of EAAs and their ketoanalogues.

Conventional low-protein diet (LPD)

Patients with CRF require at least 0.6 g protein/kg/day (31), two thirds of which should be of high biological value (eggs, lean meat) in order to secure an adequate intake of essential amino acids. This protein intake corresponds to the requirement in normal individuals ((32), page 31). In a small number of patients, neutral nitrogen balance was demonstrated (32); however, other investigators reported development of undernutrition (33).

Very-low-protein diet (VLPD) supplemented with essential amino acids

This diet should provide 0.30 g protein/kg/day and is supplemented with the nine essential amino acids (0.25 g/kg/day). Since the protein is of mixed biological value, the diet is much more variable and palatable as compared to the conventional LPD (35,35). Initially, the composition of the supplemented EAA mixtures corresponded to the proportion for normal individuals as recommended by Rose. To adapt the mixture to the disturbed amino acid pattern in CRF, a number of qualitative and quantitative changes in amino acids were performed. In particular, the semi-essential amino acids histidine, arginine, and tyrosine were included. These amino-acid-supplemented VLPDs have been shown to be highly effective in controlling the symptoms of CRF and may postpone the need of dialysis for many months. Even during long-term treatment, nitrogen balance can be maintained (36). The VLPD is particularly indicated in patients with advanced renal failure (GFR less than 10 mL/min).

Very-low-protein diet supplemented with keto acids

This VLPD (0.28 g protein/kg/day) is supplemented with the nitrogen-free keto acids or hydroxy acid analogues of leucine, isoleucine, valine, methionine, and phenylalanine. In addition, four crystalline essential amino acids (histidine, lysine, threonine, and tryptophan) are provided: their transamination to the corresponding EAA decreases the formation of urea and other nitrogenous metabolites (40). In addition, the keto acid of leucine may exert a nitrogen-sparing effect (41). There are two main keto acid formulations: the calcium salts of keto acids and hydroxy acids as well as the keto acid formulation EE, which provides the branched chain amino acids as salts of the basic amino acids ornithine, lysine, and histidine, as well as tyrosine, threonine, and the hydroxyanalogue of methionine (42). As compared to the EAA-supplemented VLPD, the keto acid formulation contains about 15% less nitrogen, resulting in an additional decrease in urea nitrogen appearance.

Apart from improvement of nitrogen metabolism, the keto acid-based dietary regimen exerts a number of favorable hormonal effects. Thus, an improvement of secondary hyperparathyroidism has been evidenced by a decrease of parathyroid hormone levels and alkaline phosphatase as well as amelioration of renal osteodystrophy (43). These effects are mediated at least in part by reduction of dietary phosphorus intake as well as by suppression of intestinal phosphate absorption due to Ca binding (44). Furthermore, amelioration of metabolic acidosis due to less hydrogen ion generation may be involved.

The keto acid VLPD regimen also improves the uremia-induced impairment of glucose metabolism. Thus, a decrease of fasting hyperglycemia and plasma insulin levels (45,46), an increased insulin sensitivity (in the euglycemic insulin clamp technique), and an improved metabolic clearance rate of insulin (47) have been reported and are explained by the decline of circulating uremic toxins.

Meanwhile, the mixture of keto acid and EAAs has been successfully used in a multitude of clinical studies in CRF patients (48–52). However, it must be stressed that both the EAA- and the keto acid-supplemented diet exert their beneficial effects only in combination with VLPD. At a higher protein intake, both supplements are presumably oxidized (53).

Despite the beneficial actions upon uremic symptoms and nutritional status of a VLPD with EAA or keto acid supplements, maintenance dialysis treatment should be started at the latest if the GFR is 5 mL/min. A further postponing of dialysis therapy runs the risk of loss of lean body mass and physical fitness.

Energy requirements in chronic renal failure

Energy intake in patients with CRF (GFR < 25 mL/min) is substantially decreased and averaged about 23 kcal/kg/day (54). According to metabolic studies, CRF patients should ingest about 35 kcal/kg/day to ensure a neutral or positive nitrogen balance. In obesity (body weight >120%) and in elderly patients (>65 years), energy intake should be reduced (55,56).

Effects of nutritional therapy on progressive renal insufficiency

The metaanalysis and the Modification of Diet in Renal Disease (MDRD) study "strongly suggest that the dietary protein restriction delays the progression of renal disease" (56a,b,c).

REASONS FOR WASTING IN CHRONIC RENAL FAILURE

The pathogenesis of protein–caloric malnutrition in chronic renal failure is multifactorial. Poor dietary intake and enhanced needs due to catabolism, unresolved uremia, intercurrent illnesses, comorbid conditions (diabetes), and metabolic acidosis are involved. Furthermore, metabolic and endocrine disorders as well as elevated cytokine levels play a contributory role (Table 2).

Poor protein energy intake

Poor protein energy intake from anorexia is related to uremic toxicity, drug therapy, emotional depression, unpalatable diets, or intercurrent illnesses. In addition, production of toxic compounds (such as dimethylamines and trimethylamines as well as nitrosodimethylamine) in the small bowel due to bacterial overgrowth (57,58) may inter-

Table 2. Factors involved in protein calorie malnutrition in CRF

Poor protein-energy intake (anorexia)
  Uremic toxicity
  Toxic components from small bowel
  Emotional depression
  Unpalatable diets
  Intercurrent illness
  Drug therapy
Inability to adapt the metabolism to dietary protein restriction
  Hormonal disturbances (insulin and 76F-l resistance, cortisol
    PTH and glucagon excess)
  Altered amino acid, protein, and carbohydrate metabolism
Decreased protein synthesis and/or enhanced protein
    degradation due to
  Metabolic acidosis
  Uremic toxins
  Enhanced cytokin levels (TNFα, IL-1)
  Physical inactivity
  Superimposed illnesses

fere with both caloric intake through poor appetite and intestinal absorptive mechanisms.

Metabolic and endocrine disorders

Animal studies suggest that chronic uremia may promote mild catabolism and protein wasting (59). In starved uremic rats, protein synthesis is reduced and breakdown is increased. In fed uremic rats, protein synthesis is either decreased or normal (59,60). Ultrafiltrates of uremic patients have been shown to reduce protein synthesis in vitro (61). Recent evidence suggest that plasma cytokine (tumor necrosis factor α TNFα) and interleukin (IL-1) are enhanced in endstage renal failure and mediate some of the metabolic dysfunctions (61a). Apart from uremic toxicity endocrine disorders and metabolic acidosis are involved in protein wasting. Target organs are resistant to the anabolic effect of insulin (62,63). Also, glucagon and parathyroid hormone have been suggested to play a role in uremic catabolism (64–66). The most important stimulus for protein catabolism is cortisol. Even a rise in the physiological range increases body protein degradation (67).

Metabolic acidosis (MA) represents an independent mediator of protein breakdown, amino acid oxidation, and urea production (68,69). The adaptation to LPD is impaired. Muscle protein turnover measurements (forearm phenylalanine kinetics) in men showed a direct relationship between proteolysis and severity of MA (70). In addition, a direct relationship between proteolysis and plasma cortisol, which is increased in rats with MA (71), was found (70). MA enhances skeletal branched chain keto acid (BCKA) decarboxylation (valine, leucine, and isoleucine) by stimulating BCKA dehydrogenase activity (72). Correspondingly, in MHD patients, intracellular muscle levels of valine are reduced in direct correlation to arterial $[HCO_3^-]$ (73). Recently, it was demonstrated that the proteolysis of MA involves an ATP-dependent nonlysosomal pathway. In line with these investigations, a stimulation of gene transcription for enzymes that degrade proteins was found. Thus, the mRNA for ubiquitin and for several subunits of proteasome, a multisubunit enzyme complex for protein degradation, was sharply enhanced in MA (74).

In subtotal nephrectomized rats, MA is associated with insulin resistance and defective glucose utilization (75). Also, a resistance to the anabolic actions of recombinant human growth hormone (rHuGH) concerning growth, food efficacy, protein synthesis, and formation of IGF-1 was reported (76). The sensitivity of parathyroid glands to calcium is impaired (77).

Correction of MA in CRF patients improves nitrogen balance (78) and reduces the 3-methylhistidine, creatinine ratio in urine due to decreased skeletal muscle protein degradation (79).

Superimposed illnesses such as infections and septicemia promote muscle protein catabolism. In massive proteolysis ("autocannibalism"), both increased protein degradation and impaired protein synthesis (80) are involved. The principal metabolic event is probably the enhanced formation

Table 3. Additional factors involved in wasting in MHD patients

Underdialysis
　$K_t/V < 1.0$ and complicated course of dialysis
Bioincompatible membranes (cuprophane)
Transmembrane losses of:
　Amino acids, peptides and H
　proteins after multiple reuses of the dialyzer
　Calories with no-glucose dialysates
Blood losses
Effects of endotoxins (interleukin-1 TNFα and other cytokines)
　Use of acetate dialysis fluid
　Contaminated dialysate

of interleukin-1 and tumor necrosis factor α (TNFα), which stimulate proteolysis via prostaglandin E_2 (80–82). This effect is enhanced during fever (83,84). According to a recent concept promoted by Wilmore (85), repeated complicating events (injuries, insults, infections) lead to a continuous depletion of body protein stores and ultimately result in death.

ADDITIONAL CATABOLIC FACTORS OF HEMODIALYSIS TREATMENT (Table 3)

An important catabolic factor of hemodialysis treatment is underdialysis, as documented by a urea reduction ratio of less than 60% or a K_t/V_{urea} less than 1 (86). Furthermore, high BUN levels trigger a feedback mechanism that results in poor nutritional intake. A direct correlation between the dose of dialysis (K_t/V) and protein catabolic rate (PCR) has been demonstrated in a randomized prospective study in patients with a K_t/V less than 1.3 (85). According to preliminary data, this relationship was also dependent on the dialysis membrane (87). Thus, a higher PCR was found when using the more biocompatible high-flux membrane, as compared to cuprophane. However, since both K_t/V and PCR are calculated from urea kinetics, a direct relationship of these parameters was postulated (88).

Apart from underdialysis, many patients experience a complicated dialysis course, with hypotension, headache, and vomiting during and even several hours after the treatment procedure, leading to a poor food intake. The incidence and extent of poor food intake is especially pronounced in diabetic patients due to both hemodynamic instability and the gastroparesis diabeticorum.

HD treatment is a catabolic event in itself, as indicated by a negative nitrogen balance and an increased nitrogen appearance on the dialysis days (89,90). The catabolic stimulus results from the blood membrane interaction. In normal individuals with sham HD without dialysate flow, the blood contact with the dialyzer (cuprophane membrane) induced a marked release of amino acids from muscle, corresponding to a protein breakdown of about 15–20 g (91). Since the catabolic response was abolished by pretreatment with indomethacin, the effect seems to be

mediated by prostaglandines. It is of note that the increased release of amino acids was not observed when the more biocompatible synthetic membranes were used (92). Correspondingly, in MHD patients, dialysis with cuprophane membranes is associated with a massive activation of granulocytes and monocytes as well as the alternative complement pathway (93,94). In particular, the release of cytokines (interleukin-1, TNFα) enhances protein breakdown partly via prostaglandin E_2 liberation (95,96). In contrast to these findings, no enhanced protein degradation during cuprophane hemodialysis in MHD patients was found in a leucine kinetic study. Nevertheless, protein synthesis was reduced (97).

Dialysis fluid may also contribute to muscle protein catabolism when sodium acetate is used or when endotoxin fragments pass from the dialysate through the membrane. Interleukin-1 formation is enhanced in both cases (98,99).

Dialysis-induced wasting may also be promoted by removing nutrients. When cellulosic dialyzers are used, there are losses of approximately 4–9 g of free amino acids in the fasting state and approximately 8–12 g when the patients eat (100). Use of high-flux membranes may increase these losses. However, when the amino acid losses were adjusted to surface area and blood flow, no difference between various dialyzers (cellulosic and high-flux polysulfone membranes) was found (101). It is of note that the losses of total amino acids and proteins are exacerbated during multiple reuses. After the sixth reuse of a dialyzer, amino acid losses are increased by 50% compared to first use. Albumin is also lost into the dialysate with increasing reuses (101). With 25 reuses, protein losses of about 20 g/HD were reported (102). The losses of amino acids and proteins after reuses are probably caused by the reprocessing of the dialysis membranes with bleach and formaldehyde, which enlarges the pores. The massive protein losses after reuses may abolish the potential benefits of increasing the dialysis dose on the nutritional state.

Apart from amino acids, peptides, and protein, glucose is also lost into the dialysate when glucose-free dialysate is used. In normoglycemic individuals, approximately 15–25 g of glucose may be removed, which could contribute to a negative energy balance and enhanced protein catabolism via gluconeogenesis (103). Wasting of the MHD patient is further intensified by blood losses related to blood drawings, occult or profound gastrointestinal bleeding, and sequestration of blood in the dialyzers (104). In a patient on regular MHD, the total amount of blood loss per year is about 6–8 L.

PREVALENCE AND CLINICAL OUTCOME OF MALNUTRITION IN MAINTENANCE HEMODIALYSIS (MHD)

Malnutrition is a frequent finding in patients on MHD, as indicated by decreases of subcutaneous fat, skeletal muscle mass, total body nitrogen, low concentrations of visceral proteins, and abnormal plasma and intracellular amino acid profiles. An impaired nutritional intake was documented in a number of studies. In the National Cooperative Dialysis Study (NCDS), caloric intake averaged only 24 kcal/kg/day (105); a protein intake of less than 0.8 g/kg/day at entry of the study was found in 23%. Jakob et al. (21) reported a protein intake of less than 1 g/kg/day in 45% of 61 MHD patients and Bergström et al. (106) in 25% of 117 MHD patients.

Morbidity and mortality in malnourished MHD patients

Poor nutritional intake, as assessed by low predialysis urea as well as by low cholesterol and triglyceride levels, was associated with an increased overall mortality in the French Diaphane Collaborative Study of 1453 MHD patients (107). Similarily, Acchiardo et al. (108) reported that morbid events occurred more commonly in malnourished MHD patients. In a subgroup with a PCR less than 0.65 g/kg/day, the days of hospitalizations and the mortality rate was substantially higher than in patients with a PCR of 1.2 g/kg/day and more. In a longitudinal study from Finland, 17% of the MHD patients were malnourished and died within 3 years (19). Lowrie and Lew (109) analyzed the relationship between various nutritional parameters and survival in more than 12,000 MHD patients, monitored over the course of 1 year. Low serum albumin was an independent and strong predictor of mortality. In patients with an albumin concentration of less than 30 g/L, the annual death rate was seven times higher than in those with an albumin level of more than 40 g/L. Even a mild decline of serum albumin (35–40 g/L) was associated with a doubling of death rate. The strong relationship between plasma albumin and the risk of death was underlined in a further study of Lowrie et al. in 17,185 MHD patients (110). In a Canadian multicenter study including 486 MHD patients, low albumin levels (<30 g/L) were associated with

a dramatic rise in infections (in particular pneumonia and septicemia) and an increased mortality rate (111). The predictive value of low albumin was also supported by the U.S. Renal Data Service (USRDS) study in 3349 MHD patients (112) and by a recent retrospective analysis in 13,473 MHD patients (113).

How can the enhanced morbidity and mortality in malnourished MHD patients be explained?

In a subgroup of the MHD patients, malnutrition is caused by severe concomitant cardiovascular (particular in diabetics), liver, and gastrointestinal diseases, which per se have an unfavorable prognosis. In these patients, malnutrition may only be an indicator of the bad outcome. In many other patients, malnutrition favors the development of infections and septicemia due to impaired immunocompetence (114,115). Furthermore, poor nutritional state may promote cardiovascular complications due to its frequent association with overhydration, which favors the development of hypertension and congestive heart failure. According to a hypothesis of Ritz et al. (116), malnutrition may exert a number of additional adverse effects by influencing the L-arginine nitric oxide (NO) pathway. In renal failure, NO formation is impaired due to low plasma and tissue levels of L-arginine (117) (in the presence of decreased renal synthesis of L-arginine (118)) as well as the accumulation of the endogenous inhibitor of NO-synthase, asymmetric dimethyl-L-arginine (ADMA) (119). Reduced dietary protein intake may result in a further decline of the arginine and NO levels in plasma and tissues. As a consequence of decreased NO-formation vasoconstriction (120) as well as hypertension, platelet aggregation, proliferation of vascular smooth muscle cells, and atherosclerosis may develop, which ultimately predisposes to cardiac death. Furthermore, NO also is involved in antibacterial defence and bacterial killing.

Table 4. Prevention and treatment of malnutrition in maintenance hemodialysis (124)

Protein	To maintain protein stores: 1.0–1.2 g/kg/day (approximately 50% of high biological value)
	To regain the lost protein stores: up to 1.4 g/kg/day
Energy	Approximately 35 kcal/kg/day—unless patient's relative body weight is >120%
	Approximately 30 kcal/kg/day for patients older than 60 years
Fat	30% of total energy intake
	Polyunsaturated : saturated fatty acids ratio × 1.0 : 1.0—if serum triglyceride levels are enhanced, fat may be increased to approximately 40% of total calories
Carbohydrates	Rest of nonprotein calories
	Primarily complexed carbohydrates
Total fiber intake	20–25 g/day

Increase of dialysis dose: $K_t/V > 1.35$
Use of biocompatible membranes
Correction of metabolic acidosis: $HCO_3^- > 22$ mmol/L
Intradialytic parenteral nutrition in severe and resistant malnutrition
Administration of anabolic hormones: (rHuGH, IGF_1)?

PREVENTION AND TREATMENT OF MALNUTRITION IN MHD PATIENTS (Table 4)

Protein and energy intake

In healthy adults, the mean protein requirement is approximately 0.6 g/kg/day, and the safe level of protein intake, corresponding to a plus of two standard deviations, is 0.75 g/kg/day (32). MHD patients require a higher intake due to the catabolic effect of HD treatment. The recommended daily protein intake is about 1.2 g/kg. Proteins of high biological value should be preferred (>50%) (121–124).

Energy requirements in MHD patients are not generally different from those in normal subjects (125). Since a low-energy intake reduces the utilization of protein and high-energy intake exerts a protein-saving effect, the daily energy intake is recommended to be 35 kcal/kg, unless the patient is not obese (body weight >120%) or older than 65 years (124).

Malnourished patients should be educated to increase their protein and energy intake. They should be encouraged to supplement their diets with high-energy foods or with carbohydrate polymers or high-caloric milk shakes. In some individuals, it will be inevitable to reduce the dietary restrictions concerning the risk of hyperkalemia and hyperphosphatemia.

An important prerequisite for successful nutritional therapy is an adequate blood purification; enhancing the dose of dialysis may improve the appetite with a subsequent increase of protein and caloric intake. An optimal dialysis requires a K_t/V of about 1.3–1.4, corresponding to a urea reduction ratio higher than 65% (84).

Dialytic-induced losses of amino acids may be compensated for to a certain extent by allowing a normal food intake during HD. However, gastric emptying is impaired even during uneventful hemodialysis (126). Enteral food supplementation via nasogastric tubes in general is badly tolerated. However, in diabetic patients with severe gastroparesis, jejunostomy tubes have been used successfully.

Intradialytic parenteral nutrition (IDPN)

In malnourished patients who are unable to increase their oral nutrient intake, infusions of amino acids and calories during HD treatment is of potential value. To avoid the induction of amino acid imbalances, solutions should be adapted to the metabolic alterations of uremia. Besides essential amino acids, some nonessential amino acids (histidine, arginine, serine and tyrosine), which become indispensible in renal failure, must also be included (127). Moreover, the altered pharmacokinetic behavior of individual amino acids in uremia has to be taken into consideration (128). Infusion therapy can be performed throughout the whole dialysis procedure, since less than 10% of the infused amino acids are lost into the dialysate due to their high endogenous clearance (129). In a few but not all stud-

ies, an improvement of plasma proteins, dry weight, and cellular immunity was reported; however, a minimum of 4 months was required to influence the nutritional parameters (128,130–132). Potential effects of IDPN on mortality rate were analyzed in a retrospective study in 81 malnourished MHD patients receiving a mixture of glucose, amino acids, and lipids with about 700 kcal/HD. After a treatment time of 9 months, mortality rate was significantly reduced, in association with a rise in body weight and serum albumin as compared to patients who did not receive IDPN (133). Although these data are promising at the present time, the extremely expensive IDPN cannot be generally recommended in malnourished MHD patients, since its benefit is still not proven (134) and the optimal composition of the nutrition still remains to be defined (128). Nevertheless, IDPN is justified in severely malnourished patients.

Drug intervention

EPO therapy exerts some anabolic actions, as shown by urea kinetics (135), a small weight gain, and an increase in triceps skin-fold thickness (136). An improvement of abnormal circulating amino acids was reported (137) but not observed by others (138). Probably the anabolic EPO effects are limited to patients with severe malnutrition. EPO seems to exert no specific action on appetite improvement.

Growth hormone (GH)

Administration of recombinant human growth hormone (rHuGH) is a potential strategy for enhancing protein anabolism in malnourished renal failure patients (83). In uremic rats and in children with CRF, an improvement of BUN, nitrogen balance, and UNA, as well as food utilization and growth velocity, was shown (139–142). Preliminary data also demonstrate an anabolic action in MHD patients. A decrease of predialysis BUN levels, urea generation rate, and PCR have been found, which may be potentiated by IDPN (143–145). Since many of the anabolic and metabolic actions of rHuGH are mediated through insulin-like growth factor 1 (IGF-1), and since rHuGH treatment may fail to increase the synthesis of IGF-1 in sepsis and in severe malnutrition, administration of IGF-1 seems to be a promising strategy in protein catabolism (146). However, there is a need for further studies of the potential beneficial and adverse effects of both GH and IGF-1.

NUTRITIONAL MANAGEMENT DURING CONTINUOUS AMBULATORY PERITONEAL DIALYSIS (CAPD)

Prevalence and outcome of malnutrition in CAPD

A high incidence of malnutrition in CAPD patients has been demonstrated (147,148). Data from a cross-sectional multicenter study involving 224 CAPD patients in Europe and North America showed an incidence of about 40%; 8% were classified as severely malnourished (149). Malnutrition was more pronounced in diabetic CAPD patients (149). The prevalence of protein malnutrition seems to be higher in CAPD as compared to MDH patients (42% vs. 30%), as demonstrated in a large-scale cross-sectional study involving 265 MHD and 224 CAPD patients (150). In contrast, fat stores, as evaluated by skin-fold thickness, were higher in CAPD.

In line with the numerous data in MHD patients, undernutrition in CAPD also is associated with a bad clinical outcome. Low serum albumin was shown to be a strong and independent predictor of morbidity (days of hospitalization) and deaths in a 5-year retrospective study in 51 CAPD patients (151) and in a prospective study in 80 CAPD patients (152). Rocco et al. (153) studied 45 CAPD patients for at least 1 year and found that a low serum albumin initially, as well as after 12 months, strongly predicted both hospitalizations and mortality. Blake et al. (154) monitored 76 new CAPD patients over 222 6-month periods and found that low serum albumin correlated with hospital days, fatique index, impairment of nerve conduction, and technical failure of the CAPD procedure. Mean serum albumin was lower in diabetics and in patients older than 65 years. In contrast to these investigations, Fine and Cox (155) demonstrated in a prospective study that moderately decreased serum albumin levels (25–30 g/L) persisting for 12 months did not lead to apparent clinical consequences. However, the significance of this study is limited due to its relative short duration (15 months) and the small number of patients.

Additional causes of malnutrition in CAPD patients

Apart from the common reasons of protein energy malnutrition in CRF, various additional factors are involved in CAPD patients. These include suppressed appetite due to the constant glucose absorption from dialysate as well as abdominal distention. An important factor seems to be underdialysis. Up to 94% of the severely malnourished patients had no residual renal function (156). Since in many

of them the daily dialysate volume was not adjusted to the loss of renal function, control of the uremic state was inadequate, with consequent anorexia. In addition, the dialysis procedure itself contributes to the wasting. Losses of free amino acids into the dialysate vary between 1.2–3.4 g/24 hr and that of proteins (albumin, transferrin, immunoglobulins, complement factors) between 5–15 g/24 hr (157,158). With mild peritonitis, the protein losses increase by 50%–100%; much higher losses are observed with severe peritonitis (159). In addition, the inflammation itself represents a strong catabolic factor due to enhanced formation of interleukin-1 and other mediators of protein catabolism that also suppress appetite (160).

Recommendations for prevention of protein energy malnutrition in CAPD patients (Table 5)

Protein requirements in CAPD patients are greater than the recommended dietary allowances for normal adults or MHD patients, but the energy requirements for CAPD patients do not differ from those of normal subjects. Due to substantial absorption of glucose from peritoneal dialysate (161), energy needs are satisfied in most patients.

The recommended nutritional intakes for CAPD patients, based on recent reviews (159,162), are summarized in Table 5. To achieve serum albumin levels greater 38 g/L, approximately 1.2–1.3 g/kg protein/day (50% of high biological value) are prescribed. In malnourished patients, up to 1.5 g protein/kg/day may be given.

Since residual renal function has an important influence on appetite as well as on dialysis efficiency, an increase of the dialysis dose is needed if renal function declines (29). In addition, several studies have demonstrated that dietary protein intake (assessed by PNA) increases when the dialysis dose (as assessed by K_t/V) is enhanced. According to Twardowski and Nolph (163), a total creatinine clearance of at least $50 \, L/week/1.73 \, m^2$ body surface area and a weekly K_t/V_{urea} of 1.7 must be achieved.

Prevention of malnutrition in CAPD patients includes the flexible correction of even slight MA (oral administration of alkaline agents or altering the dialysate buffer concentration).

Table 5. Recommended dietary nutritional intake for patients undergoing CAPD (154,162)

Protein	To maintain protein stores: 1.2–1.5 g/kg/day (approximately 50% of high biological value) To regain lost protein stores: up to 1.5 g/kg/day for malnourished patients
Energy	Approximately 35 kcal/kg/day, including glucose absorption from dialysate[a]—unless patient's relative body weight is >120% Approximately 30 kcal/kg/day for patients older than 60 years
Fat	See Table 4
Carbohydrates	See Table 4
Total fiber intake	See Table 4

[a] Peritoneal glucose absorption can be roughly estimated by multiplying the 24-hour glucose load by 0.6 (in CAPD patients with a normal peritoneal transport characteristic).

Supplementation of amino acids to dialysate is indicated in malnourished patients who are unable to ingest additional proteins (>1 g/kg/day), in hypercatabolic illnesses, and in those who require reduction of glucose load. It has been demonstrated that the preponderance of amino acids are absorbed (80% after 4 hours, on average). Thus, intraperitoneal amino acid (IPAA) solution becomes an important source of protein formation (159,164). A combination of essential and nonessential amino acids is probably most conductive to the achievement of a positive nitrogen balance. Amino acid solutions should be administered during the postprandial state. The dosage should be calculated to increase patients' daily protein plus amino acid intake to about 1.2–1.3 g/kg/day (165,166). Benefits derived from amino acid-containing dialysis solutions include improvement of nitrogen balance, hypoalbuminemia, amino acid levels, and hypertriglyceridemia.

The ultrafiltration patterns of 1% and 2% amino acid solutions are similar to those of 2.5% and 4.25% conventional dialysis solutions (167). The major limitation of amino acids as osmotic agents is the generation of nitrogenous waste products, with a consequent rise of blood urea nitrogen.

A potential side effect of IPAA administration is MA, which develops due to the acid load delivered by salts of basic amino acids and/or from the degradation of sulfuric amino acids, which generates protons. Complicating nausea can be controlled by reducing the dose of amino acids. Fewer side effects are observed with the use of only one amino acid dialysis exchange, with an amino acid concentration lower than 1.5%.

Recently, the effectiveness of rHuGH (5 mg/day s.c.) was prospectively studied in CAPD patients. Short-term administration resulted in a potent anabolic effect, with decrease of BUN, PCR, and dialysate urea nitrogen (DUN) and a rise of IGF 1 without any side effects (168).

NUTRITIONAL SUPPORT IN ACUTE RENAL FAILURE (ARF)

Metabolic abnormalities in ARF

Metabolic alterations in ARF result from the combined effects of uremia and the underlying disease (trauma, septicemia, circulatory shock) and include changes in the metabolism of amino acids, proteins, carbohydrates, and lipids.

AMINO ACID AND PROTEIN METABOLISM

ARF is characterized by protein hypercatabolism with a negative nitrogen balance. In severe ARF (particularly in multiple organ failure), BUN may increase by more than 30 mg/dL/day and UNA up to 40 g/day (169,170). There is an enhanced release of amino acids from skeletal muscle

(171,172). However, instead of their utilization for protein synthesis, the amino acids are preferentially used for gluconeogenesis and ureagenesis as well as synthesis of acute-phase proteins (173). Although the endogenous clearance of most amino acids is increased, that of phenylalanine, proline, and valine is suppressed (174). Insulin resistance contributes to accelerated protein breakdown and to decreased protein synthesis (175–177). Defects in protein and glucose metabolism are interrelated: insufficient intracellular energy metabolism stimulates protein breakdown and disrupts protein turnover (178). Furthermore, MA, secondary hyperparathyroidism, and glucagon excess play a contributory role. Of particular importance are elevated glucocorticoid levels, which markedly enhance protein degradation, hepatic gluconeogenesis, and ureagenesis (179). These effects can be reversed in vitro and in vivo by the antiglucocorticoid RU 38486 (180,181). Protein catabolism is stimulated by increased levels of proteinases, interleukin-1, and tumor necrosis factor α (182–184). In addition, renal failure itself contributes to altered amino acid and protein metabolism: thus, renal synthesis of cysteine, tyrosine, arginine, and serine is impaired (185,186).

CARBOHYDRATE METABOLISM

A main feature of ARF is insulin resistance due to a defect at the postreceptor level. In spite of hyperinsulinemia, glucose uptake of skeletal muscle is decreased, contributing to hyperglycemia (187).

LIPID METABOLISM

Impaired lipolysis due to the decreased activites of lipoprotein lipase and hepatic glyceride lipase increases triglycerides (particularly VLDL and LDL) levels, whereas total cholesterol and apoprotein A I and A II levels are decreased. In contrast to chronic renal failure, plasma carnitine is elevated due to release from skeletal muscle and enhanced synthesis in the liver (188,189).

ENERGY METABOLISM

Oxygen consumption and energy expenditure in complicated ARF are increased (190,191). In contrast, in uncomplicated ARF, energy metabolism may even tend towards a decreased expenditure. Due to insulin resistance and depressed hepatic glycogen stores, oxydation of fat increases while that of carbohydrates decreases.

ELECTROLYTES

Catabolism in ARF is generally associated with hyperkalemia and hyperphosphatemia; however, parenteral nutrition may cause reactive hypokalemia and hypophosphatemia (192).

Nutritional approach in acute renal failure

Energy requirements in ARF are determined by the under-lying and concomitant disease(s). Overnutrition exceeding the actual energy needs can cause adverse effects. Energy requirements can be estimated by calculating the basic energy expenditure (BEE) and by correcting for stress factors. BEE is approximately 25 kcal/kg/day and can be calculated by employing the Harris Benedict formula (178):

Males: $66.47 + (13.75 \times BE) + (5 \times height) - (6.76 \times age)$;

Females: $66.51 + (9.56 \times BW) + (1.85 \times height) - (4.67 \times age)$.

Energy requirements for hypercatabolism are calculated by multiplication with the following factors: 1.1–1.3 for peritonitis or sepsis; 1.2–1.4 for severe infection, multiple trauma, and multiple organ failure; and 1.2–2.0 for burns (190).

In patients with *mild protein catabolism* (UNA < 6 g/day above nitrogen intake), the prognosis of ARF is good, and oral feeding usually is sufficient. *Moderate hypercatabolism* (UNA 6–12 g/day) points to a complicated course of ARF. Tube feeding or intravenous nutritional support is usually required. In severe hypercatabolism (UNA > 12 g/day) due to trauma, infection, or burns, a complex treatment should be provided to ameliorate the massive protein degradation.

ORAL OR ENTERAL FEEDING

Oral or enteral feeding should be used in all cases when possible. Digestion of food helps to maintain the gastrointestinal barrier and prevents the translocation of bacteria and systemic infection (193). Initially, a simple carbohydrate diet with 0.6 g/kg/day of high-quality proteins is recommended. Protein intake might be gradually increased up to 0.8 g/kg/day, if BUN levels are below 100 mg/dL. To counteract the catabolic effects of hemodialysis treatment, the protein intake should be adjusted to 1.2 g/kg/day in HD and 1.4 g/kg/day in peritoneal dialysis (178).

PARENTERAL NUTRITION

Glucose infusion

Glucose is the major energy substrate. Due to impaired glucose tolerance, addition of insulin is obviously necessary to maintain normoglycemia. The infusion speed should not exceed 5 g/kg/day to prevent enhanced lipogenesis. If the energy needs cannot be covered solely by glucose, lipid emulsions (1 g/kg/day) can be administered. Contraindications of fat emulsions are hyperlipidemia (>350 mg/dL), intravascular coagulation, MA, impaired circulation, or hypoxemia.

Amino acid infusion

Apart from EAAs, the nonessential amino acids histidine, arginine, tyrosine, serine, and cysteine also become indispensable in ARF (194). Therefore, infusion of conventional solutions of EAAs according to the Rose profile can aggravate the preexisting imbalance of circulating amino acids and may even induce ammonia intoxication (195). Requirement for protein or amino acids in ARF is determined by the underlying illness, degree of hypercatabolism, and the frequency of required hemodialysis. If there is no enhanced catabolism, the protein or amino acid intake should be slightly greater than 0.6 g/kg/day. In the case of severe catabolism, protein intake might be increased up to 1.5 g/kg/day (196). Further increases only promote formation of nitrogenous waste products.

It is recommended to start the infusion at a rate providing about 50% of nutrients over the first 24 hours and to increase it gradually over 3 days to meet the patient's need (178).

Nutritional support in ARF should not be initiated during the acute phase (within the first 48 hours after injury), since infusions of large quantities of glucose and amino acids during the "ebb phase" might even aggravate the tubular damage and the loss of renal function (197).

Complications of parenteral nutrition include disturbances of mineral and electrolyte metabolism, acid–base disorders, volume overload, and lipid disturbances. Hypokalemia is frequently observed, in particular due to insulin administration; furthermore, enhanced phosphorylation after refeeding, favors development of phosphate deficiency. MA results from the metabolism of certain amino acids, such as histidine, arginine, and lysine, with consequent enhanced hydrogen ion production (192).

The effectiveness of parenteral nutrition in ARF patients for survival, rate of renal recovery, and nitrogen balance was critically analyzed recently from nine studies (196). According to these data, the combined administration of glucose + EAAs as compared to glucose alone enhanced survival in four studies. In four other prospective studies, no difference was observed with the additional use of amino acid therapy. In two studies (198,199) in which nitrogen balance data were reported, only 10% of the 40 patients achieved a positive balance, and this improvement was limited only to those patients who were less catabolic and had a better renal function. In contrast, in patients with severe hypercatabolism, no positive nitrogen balance was achieved, although the magnitude of negative nitrogen balance may have been diminished. Therefore, it was concluded that aggressive parenteral nutrition with amino acids does not convincingly affect recovery from complicated ARF. However, it is conceivable that the prognosis may be improved by application of anticatabolic hormones such as GH and IGF-1 or glucocorticoid antagonists (139,145).

NUTRITION IN THE RENAL TRANSPLANT PATIENT

Protein metabolism in transplant recipients is influenced by many factors, such as kind and dose of immunosuppression, time point of transplantation, function of the allograft, rejection episodes, and intercurrent illnesses.

In the immediate posttransplantation period, protein catabolism is frequently accelerated due to the combined effects of large doses of steroids, the stress of surgery, persistence of the uremic state (due to delayed onset of the graft function), need of frequent dialysis procedures, and complicating bleedings or infections (200). In particular, glucocorticoids promote protein catabolism in a dose-dependent manner. Interestingly, an increase in dietary protein was shown to improve nitrogen balance to neutral or even positive values without a rise in protein catabolic rate (201,202). Therefore, when higher doses of steroids are given, the daily protein intake should be 1.3–1.5 g/kg. An increased protein intake is also recommended if the clinical course is complicated by delayed graft function or if a pulse steroid therapy for rejection episodes is performed. However, there are no data as to whether an enhanced protein intake may exert adverse effects on graft function. Concerning energy intake, 30–35 kcal/kg/day seems to be adequate.

Recommendations for the long-term nutritional treatment of transplanted patients are less well established. One argument for the continued increase of protein intake is the observation of wasting of striated muscle, even when low doses of corticosteroids are administered (204). This atrophy involves all three types of muscle fibers (205). In particular, transplanted diabetics are prone to reduced muscle mass (206). Whether a rise of protein intake above 1 g/kg/day minimizes muscle wasting is unknown but conceivable. In contrast to the decreased muscle mass, there is an overcorrection of cutaneous fat during long-term corticoid therapy. There is also evidence that prednisone-induced myopathy is reversed by physical training (204).

Feehally et al. (207) suggested that the progressive loss of renal function during chronic transplant rejection may be mediated at least in part by glomerular capillary hypertension. Accordingly, induction of low-protein diet (0.6 g/kg/day) has been conducted in a small number of patients. In one study, 4 of 5 patients demonstrated a distinct change in the slope of reciprocal serum creatinine within a follow-up of 6 months on average (207). However, a decrement of creatinine intake as well as muscle wasting could have contributed to the stabilization of serum creatinine. The diet has been well tolerated by the patients, whose weight remained stable after a small initial drop; also, midarm muscle circumference did not change. Similarly, in two other short-term studies with low-protein diet, nitrogen balance was maintained when the energy intake exceeded 25 kcal/kg/day (208,209). There is, of course, the need for additional studies to assess the long-term effects of a low-protein diet on both nutritional state and renal function before a low-protein diet can be generally recommended.

TRACE ELEMENTS AND VITAMINS

Data on trace elements metabolism in renal disease are limited. Alterations in both directions, toxicity and deficiency, are reported. In deficiency states, inadequate nutrition (protein-restricted diets and/or anorexia), impaired gastrointestinal absorption, increased urinary excretion, and losses into dialysate may play a role. Accumulation of trace elements in chronic renal failure (such as Al or Cu) may result from a contaminated dialysate or dialysis equipment and reduced excretory renal function.

Iron

The incidence of iron deficiency is already high in conservatively treated CRF patients. Low iron intake during LPD and/or gastrointestinal bleeding are of importance (104). In nephrotic-range proteinuria, urinary losses of iron and transferrin might be of significance (210). In MHD patients, blood losses related to the dialysis procedure aggravate iron deficiency (104). On the other hand, blood transfusions and the reduced half-life of red blood cells may cause iron overload (211).

Regular determination of serum iron, transferrin, and ferritin is necessary for the assessment of iron status. Iron supplementation should be considered if serum ferritin levels are below normal limits and throughout certain periods of erythropoietin treatment. An oral route of administration is preferred; intravenous administration of iron endangers the patient with iron overload, and, very rarely, anaphylactoid reaction.

Selen

Selenium (Se) is a coenzyme of glutathione peroxidase, one of the enzymes scavenging toxic peroxides and lipid hydroperoxides. Decrease in glutathione peroxidase activity parallels the degree of Se deficiency. Se concentration decreases with age.

Both normal and low levels of Se were reported in CRF patients (212,213). Se deficiency was found regardless of the type of treatment. Dialysis procedure does not influence Se concentration in plasma, since Se is bound to high-molecular-weight proteins. In CRF patients with cardiovascular complications, Se levels are even more suppressed as compared to patients without complication (213).

Low Se concentration in CRF may be due to a protein-restricted diet: a correlation between whole-blood Se level and nutritional parameters (serum albumin) was found (214,215). Disturbed gastrointestinal absorption of Se (216) or a deficit of Se carriers (plasma proteins and red blood cells) may contribute to Se deficiency (217). Therefore, restoration of normal concentrations of Se carriers instead of Se supplementation has been advocated.

Se deficiency is associated with cardiovascular diseases, atherosclerosis, myopathy, impaired immune function, and cancer (218,219).

In clinical praxis, determination of glutathione peroxidase activity in blood cells (platelets, red blood cells, or granulocytes) instead of Se concentration itself is favored in order to assess the Se status. If supplements of Se are to be added, the levels of Se should be carefully monitored to avoid toxicity, since Se has a narrow therapeutic window.

Zinc

Data concering the zinc (Zn) status of CRF are conflicting. Plasma Zn levels are low, normal, or even elevated (220–222). Since plasma Zn levels represent only 0.5% of total body Zn, its plasma concentration is an unreliable indicator of the total body zinc stores. An altered distribution of body Zn (plasma versus tissue, or among the tissues) was proposed (223). It is still not clear whether absolute or relative (due to translocation) Zn deficiency occurs in uremia.

Zn deficiency seems to mediate some uremic symptoms, such as impaired gustatory and olfactory acuity, anorexia, delayed wound healing, impaired chemotaxis of leukocytes, and sexual dysfunction (220,223,225).

Decreased intestinal absorption, disturbance of tubular transport, urinary losses of Zn (nephrotic range proteinuria) (226), and a decrease in circulating Zn-binding proteins may contribute to Zn deficiency. Moreover, plasma Zn levels are influenced by stress even in healthy subjects.

Zn supplementation is indicated in the presence of symptoms assumed to be caused by Zn deficiency. Supplementation might be achieved by the intake of Zn-rich animal protein, by administration of Zn acetate, or via dialysate enrichment.

Copper

Hypercupremia occurs in CRF regardless of the type of treatment (226,227). In addition, in patients hemodialyzed with cuprammonium-based cellulose, membrane elution of copper from the membrane may occur. Since plasma coeruloplasmin levels are normal in renal failure, free copper must accumulate. Impairment in hepatic handling of copper, as well Zn deficiency (which potentiates intestinal copper absorption), may contribute. Urinary losses of copper, and hypocupremia may be associated with nephrotic-range proteinuria (210). No clinical symptoms of uremia attributed to hypercupremia have been described.

Pyridoxine (B₆) (Table 6)

Pyridoxalphosphate (the phosphorylated form of pyridoxine) is essential for the metabolism of amino acids. Despite normal plasma levels of pyridoxine, functional tests (erythrocyte glutamic pyruvic transaminase, or aspartate aminotransferase tests) indicate deficiency of pyridoxine in CRF patients regardless of the treatment (237,238). However, neither extreme dialysate losses nor markedly reduced intake of this vitamin has been found. Prevalence of pyridoxine deficiency increases with time. It is suggested that accumulation of uremic toxins inhibit the conversion of pyridoxine to its active form. Therefore, uremic patients have higher requirements for this vitamin than do healthy individuals (237).

Pyridoxine deficiency induces symptoms similar to those of uremia (depression, anemia, peripheral neuropathy, depressed immune function, and oxalosis) (228,238).

Supplementation of pyridoxine in a dose of 5 mg/day is recommended in conservatively treated patients. MHD and CAPD patients should receive 10 mg/day. If vitamin B₆ antagonists (e.g., hydralazine) are coadministered, the dose should be adequately increased (236).

Cyanocobalamin (B₁₂)

Vitamin B₁₂ acts as a coenzyme of isomerase and methyltransferase reactions. Although its deficiency causes megaloblastic anemia, in the clinical picture the neurological symptoms often dominate. B₁₂ is largely protein bound, and therefore its intradialysate losses are smaller compared to those of other water-soluble vitamins. CRF patients, regardless of the type of treatment, show B₁₂ levels in the normal range without supplementation (236).

Ascorbic acid (vitamin C)

Ascorbic acid is a substrate in many oxidation-reduction reactions. Its deficiency causes scurvy. Restriction of proteins and potassium in the diet goes hand in hand with ascorbic acid deficiency. Moreover, ascorbic acid is easily dialyzed. In 50% of CRF patients, plasma ascorbate levels were decreased (228). However, normal values were reported in a longitudinal follow-up of 15 MHD patients without vitamin supplementation (239). In renal failure, daily supplementation of ascorbic acid in a dose of 100 mg/day is recommended (230). Higher doses (0.5–1.0 g/day) endanger the patient by oxalosis, which may contribute to vascular disease (240).

Table 6. Vitamins (recommended supplementation) (228,234–236)

Thiamin (B₁)	2 mg/day (not routinely)
Riboflavin (B₂)	Conservatively treated CRF patients on protein-restricted diet: 1.6–2.0 mg/day
Pyridoxine (B₆)	5 mg/day in conservatively treated patients 10 mg/day in MHD and CAPD patients
Cobalamin (B₁₂)	None
Ascorbic acid	100 mg/day
Folic acid	1 mg/day
Vitamin A	None
Vitamin K	None
Vitamin D	Individualized supplementation

Folic acid

Folate requirements are about 100 μg daily. Low plasma levels of folic acid has been reported in about 10% of chronically uremic patients (228). This deficiency is supposed to be caused by inadequate dietary intake and by dialysis losses of about 32 μg/dialysis (229). Red blood cell folate levels, however, have commonly been shown to be normal in these patients (230). A daily supplementation of 1 mg of folate in MHD patients is supposed to be adequate. However, higher folate doses ameliorate the hyperhomocysteinemia in uremic patients (231,232), which is an independent risk factor for arteriosclerosis (233).

Tocopherol (vitamin E)

Tocopherol acts as an antioxidant and is a scavenger of free-oxygen radicals. Its intake is independent from that of protein. Data on tocopherol levels in CRF patients are contradictory: in conservatively treated patients on a protein-restricted diet, high levels were reported, whereas those on an unrestricted protein diet showed normal tocopherol levels (235). In HD patients, high, normal, and even low levels were reported (236).

Retinol (vitamin A)

Retinol is obviously necessary to maintain the integrity of epithelial membranes and for the formation of the visual pigment rhodopsin. Patients with CRF have hypervitaminosis A regardless of the treatment (240,241). No differences due to dietary regimen were observed. Dialysis clears retinol poorly. Although retinol-binding protein levels are markedly increased in CRF, no abnormal tissue concentration of vitamin A was found (241). Correspondingly, toxicity is rare, since most of the vitamin is present in the inactive form, bound to its transport protein (243).

REFERENCES

1. El Nahas AM, Coles GA: Dietary treatment of chronic renal failure: Ten unanswered questions. *Lancet* 2:597–600, 1986.
2. Schoenfeld PY, Henry RR, Laird NM, Roxe DM: Assessment of nutritional status of the national cooperative dialysis study population. *Kidney Int* 23(13):80–88, 1983.
3. Grodstein G, Kopple JD: Urea nitrogen appearance, a simple and practical indicator of total nitrogen output (abstract). *Kidney Int* 16:953, 1979.
4. Gotch FA: Kinetic modelling in hemodialysis. In: AR Nissensen, DE Gentile, RN Fine, eds, *Clinical Dialysis*, vol 2. Appleton & Lange, Norwalk, CT, pp 130–132, 1990.
5. Maroni BJ, Steinman TI, Mitch WE: A method for estimating nitrogen intake of patients with chronic renal failure. *Kidney Int* 27:58–65, 1985.
6. Hakim RM, Levin N: Malnutrition in hemodialysis patients. *Am J Kidney Dis* 21(2):125–137, 1993.
7. Guarnieri G, Toigo G, Situlin R, Crapesi L, Del Bianco MA, Zanettovich A, Faccini L, Lucchesi A, Oldrizzi L, Rugiu C, Maschio G: Nutritional assessment in patients with early renal insufficiency on long-term low protein diet. *Contr Nephrol* 53:40–50, 1986.
8. Blumenkrantz MJ, Kopple JD, Gutman RA, et al.: Methods for assessing nutritional status of patients with renal failure. *Am J Clin Nutr* 33:1567–1585, 1980.
9. Womersly J, Durmin JVGA: An experimental study on variability of measurements of skin-fold thickness in young adults. *Hum Biol* 45:281–292, 1973.
10. Frisancho AR: New standards of weight and body composition by frame size and height for assessment of nutritional status of adults and the elderly. *Am J Clin Nutr* 40:808–819, 1984.
11. Cohn SH, Brennan BL, Yasamara S, Vartsky D, Vaswar AN, Ellis KJ: Evaluation of body composition and nitrogen content of renal patients on chronic dialysis as determined by total body nitrogen activation. *Am J Clin Nutr* 38:52–58, 1983.
12. Letteri JM, Ellis KJ, Asad SN, Cohn SH: Serial measurement of total body potassium in chronic renal disease. *Am J Clin Nutr* 31:1937–1944, 1978.
13. Munro HN, Young VR: Urinary excretion of 3-methylhistidine: a tool to study metabolic responses in relation to nutrient and hormonal status in health and disease of man. *Am J Clin Nutr* 31:1608–1614, 1978.
14. Berkelhammer CH, Baker JP, Leiter LA, Uldall PR, Whittall R, Wolman SL: Whole-body protein turnover in adult hemodialysis patients as measured by ^{13}C-leucine. *Am J Clin Nutr* 46:778–783, 1987.
15. Kurtin PS, Shapiro AC, Tomita H, Raizman D: Volume status and body composition of chronic dialysis patients: utility of bioelectric impedance plethysmography. *Am J Nephrol* 10:363–367, 1990.
16. Dumler F, Schmidt R, Kilates C, Faber M, Lubkowski T, Frinak S: Use of bioelectrical impedance for the nutritional assessment of chronic hemodialysis patients. *Miner Electrolyte Metab* 18:284–287, 1992.
17. Stenver DI, Gotfredsen A, Hilsted J, Nielsen B: Body composition in hemodialysis patients measured by dual-energy X-ray absorptiometry. *Am J Nephrol* 25:105–110, 1995.
18. Golden M: Transport proteins as indices of protein status. *Am J Clin Nutr* 35:1159–1165, 1982.
19. Oksa H, Ahonen K, Pasternack A, Marnela KM: Malnutrition in hemodialysis patients. *Scand J Urol Nephrol* 25:157–161, 1991.
20. Kluthe R, Baumann G, Bischoff V, Quirin H: Serumtransferrin und Eiweißernährung bei chronisch intermittierender Hämodialyse. *Med Ernährung* 12:73–77, 1971.
21. Jacob V, LeCarpentier JE, Salzano S, Naylor V, Wild G, Brown CB, El Nahas AM: IGF-1, a marker of undernutrition in hemodialysis patients. *Am J Clin Nutr* 52:39–44, 1990.
22. Degoulet P, Legrain M, Reach I, Aime F, Devries C, Rojas P, Jacobs C: Mortality risk factors in patients treated by chronic hemodialysis. *Nephron* 31:103–110, 1982.
23. Kopple JD, Swenseid MD: Nitrogen balance and plasma amino acid levels in uremic patients fed an essential amino acid diet. *Am J Clin Nutr* 27:806, 1974.
24. Alvestrand A, Furst P, Bergström J: Plasma and muscle free amino acids in uremia: influence of nutrition with amino acids. *Clin Nephrol* 18:297, 1982.

25. Bansal VK, Popli S, Pickering J, Ing TS, Vertuno LL, Hano JE: Protein-caloric malnutrition and cutaneous energy in hemodialysis maintained patients. *Am J Clin Nutr* 33:1608–1611, 1980.

26. Wolfson M, Strong CJ, Minturn D, Gray DK, Kopple JD: Nutritional status and lymphocyte function in maintenance hemodialysis patients. *Am J Clin Nutr* 37:547–555, 1984.

27. Kult J, Richter U, Scheitza E, Hennemann H, Heidland A: Störungen im Komplementsystem bei Niereninsuffizienz und ihre Beeinflussung durch Aminosäurensubstitution. *Dtsch Med Wochenschr* 99:339–343, 1974.

28. Detsky AS, McLaughlin JH, Jeejeelkoy KN: What is subjective global assessment of nutritional status? *J Parenter Enter Nutr* 11:8–13, 1987.

29. Madore F, Wuest M, Ethier JH: Nutritional evaluation of hemodialysis patients using an impedance index. *Clin Nephrol* 41(6):377–382, 1994.

30. Mitch WE, Walser M: Nutritional therapy of the uremic patient. In: BM Brenner, FC Rector, eds, *The Kidney*, 4th ed. WB Saunders, Philadelphia, pp 2186–2222, 1991.

31. Kluthe R, Oechslen D, Quirin H, Jesdinsky HJ: Six years experience with a special low-protein diet. In: R Kluthe, G Berlyne, B Burton, eds, Uremia. Thieme, Stuttgart, pp 250–256, 1972.

32. FAO/WHO/UNU: *Energy and Protein Requirements*. In: Technical Report Series 724, World Health Organization, Geneva, pp 1–110, 1985.

33. Kopple JD, Coburn JW: Metabolic studies of low protein diets in uremia: I. Nitrogen and potassium. *Medicine (Baltimore)* 52:583–595, 1973.

34. Goodship THJ, Mitch WE, Hoerr RA, Wagner DA, Steinmann TI, Young VR: Adaptation to low protein diets in renal failure: leucine turnover and nitrogen balance. *J Am Soc Nephrol* 1:66–75, 1990.

35. Bergström K, Fürst P, Norée L-O: Treatment of chronic uremic patients with protein-poor diet and oral supply of essential amino acids. I. Nitrogen balance studies. *Clin Nephrol* 3:187–194, 1975.

36. Attmann PO, Ewald J, Isaksson B: Body composition during long-term treatment of uremia with amino acid supplemented low-protein diets. *Am J Clin Nutr* 33:801–806, 1980.

37. Röckel A, Roller F, Kult J, Heidland A: Comparative studies of potato–egg diet and mixed low-protein diet combined with essential amino acids in patients with endstage renal failure. In: A Heidland, ed, *Renal Insufficiency*. Georg Thieme Verlag, Stuttgart, pp 163–168, 1976.

38. Kopple JD, Swendseid M: Evidence that histidine is an essential amino acid in normal and chronically uremic man. *J Clin Invest* 55:881–890, 1975.

39. Alvestrand A, Ahlberg M, Fürst P, Bergström J: Clinical results of long-term treatment with a low protein diet and a new amino acid preparation in patients with chronic uremia. *Clin Nephrol* 19:69–74, 1983.

40. Walser M: Ketoacids in the treatment of uremia. *Clin Nephrol* 3:180–186, 1975.

41. Mitch WE, Walser M, Sapir DG: Nitrogen sparing induced by leucine compared with that induced by its keto analogue, alpha-ketoisocaproate in fasting obese man. *J Clin Invest* 67:553–560, 1981.

42. Mitch WE, Walter M, Steinman TI, Hill S, Zeger S, Tungasanga K: The effect of a ketoacid/amino acid supplement to a restricted diet on the progression of chronic renal failure. *N Engl J Med* 311:623–629, 1984.

43. Fröhling PT, Kokot F, Vetter K, et al.: Influence of keto acid treatment on hormonal disorders in chronic renal failure. *Contrib Nephrol* 65:95–99, 1988.

44. Schaefer K, von Herrath D, Asmus G, Umlauf E: The beneficial effect of ketoacids on serum phosphate and parathyroid hormone in patients with chronic uremia. *Clin Nephrol* 30:93–98, 1988.

45. Heidland A, Kult J, Röckel A, Heidbreder E: Evaluation of essential amino acids and keto acids in uremic patients on low-protein diet. *Am J Clin Nutr* 31:1784–1792, 1978.

46. Aparicio M, Gin H, Potaux L, et al.: Effect of a ketoacid diet on glucose tolerance and tissue insulin sensitivity. *Kidney Int* 36 (Suppl 27):231, 1989.

47. Gin H, Combe C, Rigalleau V, Delafaye C, Aparicio M, Aubertin J: Effects of a low-protein, low-phosphorus diet on metabolic insulin clearance in patients with chronic renal failure. *Am J Clin Nutr* 59(3):663–666, 1994.

48. Kampf D, Fischer HC, Kessel M: Efficacy of an unselected protein diet (25 g) with minor oral supply of essential amino acids and keto analogues compared with a selective protein diet (40 g) in chronic renal failure. *Am J Clin Nutr* 33:1673–1678, 1980.

49. Barsotti G, Guiducci A, Ciardella F, Giovannetti S: Effects on renal function of a low-nitrogen diet supplemented with essential amino acids and ketoanalogues and of hemodialysis and free protein supply in patients with chronic renal failure. *Nephron* 27:113, 1981.

50. Ciardella F, Morelli E, Niosi F, et al.: Effects of a low phosphorus, low nitrogen diet supplemented with essential amino acids with ketoanalogues on serum triglycerides of chronic uremic patients. *Nephron* 42:196, 1986.

51. Walser M, LaFrance ND, Ward L, Van Duyn MA: Progression of chronic renal failure in patients given ketoacids following amino acids. *Kidney Int* 32:123–128, 1987.

52. Masud T, Young VR, Maroni BJ: Metabolic responses to protein restriction: the first comparison of ketoacids to essential amino acids. *J Am Soc Nephrol* 3:286, 1992.

53. Burns J, Crosswell J, Ell S, et al.: Comparison of the effects of keto acid analogues and essential amino acids on nitrogen homeostasis in uremic patients on moderately protein-restricted diets. *Am J Clin Nutr* 31:1767, 1978.

54. Modification of Diet in Renal Disease (MDRD) Study Group, prepared by Kopple J, Berg R, Houser H, Steinman T, Teschan P: Nutritional status of patients with different levels of chronic renal insufficiency. *Kindey Int* 36(27):184–194, 1989.

55. Kopple JD, Monteon FJ, Shaib JK: Effect of energy intake on nitrogen metabolism in nondialyzed patients with chronic renal failure. *Kidney Int* 29:734, 1986.

56. Hirschberg RR, Kopple JD: Requirements for protein, calories and fat in the pre-dialysis patient. In: WE Mitch, S Klahr, eds, *Nutrition and the Kidney*. Little, Brown, Boston, pp 131–153, 1988.

56a. Pedrini MT, Levey AS, Lasu J, Chalmers TC, Wang PH: The effects of dietary protein restriction on the progression of diabetic and non diabetic renal disease: A meta-analysis. *Ann Intern Med* 124:627–632, 1996.

56b. Fouque D, Laville M, Boissel R, Labeeuw M, Zech PY: Controlled low protein diets in chronic renal insufficiency: meta-analysis. *BMJ* 304:216–220, 1992.

56c. Klahr S: Role of dietary protein and blood pressure in the progression of renal disease. *Kidney Int* 49:1783–86, 1996.

57. Simenhoff ML, Burke JF, Sankkonen JJ, et al.: Amine metabolism and the small bowel in uremia. *Lancet* 2:818–822, 1976.

58. Lele PS, Dunn SR, Simenhoff ML: Nutritional and metabolic modulation of the carcinogen, nitrosodimethylamine, in chronic renal failure. *Kidney Int* 32 (Suppl 22):159–161, 1987.

59. Li JB, Wassner SJ: Protein synthesis and degradation in skeletal muscle of chronically uremic rats. *Kidney Int* 29:1136–1143, 1986.

60. Garber AJ: Skeletal muscle protein and amino acid metabolism in experimental chronic uremia in the rat. Accelerated alanine and glutamine formation and release. *J Clin Invest* 62:L623–L632, 1978.

61. Cernacek P, Spustova V, Dzurik R: Inhibitors of protein synthesis in uremic serum and urine. Partial purification and relationship to amino acid transport. *Biochem Med* 27:305–310, 1982.

61a. Pereira BJG, Shapiro L, King AJ, Falagas ME, Strom JA, Dinarello CA: Plasma levels of IL-1β, TNF-α and their specific inhibitors in undialyzed chronic renal failure, CAPD and hemodialysis patients. *Kidney Int* 45:890–896, 1994.

62. Maloff BL, McCaleb ML, Lockwood DH: Cellular basis of insulin resistance in chronic uremia. *Am J Physiol* 245:E178, 1983.

63. Castellino P, Solini A, Luzi L, Barr JG, Smith DJ, Petrides A, Giordano M, Carroll C, DeFronzo RA: Glucose and amino acid metabolism in chronic renal failure: effect of insulin and amino acids. *Am J Physiol* 262:F168–F176, 1992.

64. Bilbrey GL, Faloona GR, White MG, Knochel JP: Hyperglucagonemia of renal failure. *J Clin Invest* 53:841, 1974.

65. Garber AJ: Effect of parathyroid hormone on selected muscle protein and amino acid metabolism in the rat. *J Clin Invest* 71:1806, 1983.

66. Akmal M, Massry SG, Goldstein DA, Fanti P, Weisz A, DeFronzo RA: Role of parathyroid hormone in the glucose intolerance of chronic renal failure. *J Clin Invest* 75:1037–1044, 1985.

67. Darmaun D, Matthews DE, Bier DM: Physiological hypercortisolemia increases proteolysis, glutamine, and alanine production. *Am J Physiol* 255:E366–E373, 1988.

68. Reaich D, Channon SM, Scrimgeour CM, Goodship TH: Ammonium chloride-induced acidosis increases protein breakdown and amino acid oxidation in humans. *Am J Physiol* 263:E735–E739, 1992.

69. May RC, Masud T, Logue B, Bailey J, England B: Chronic metabolic acidosis accelerates whole body proteolysis and oxidation in awake rats. *Kidney Int* 41:1535–1542, 1992.

70. Garibotto G, Russo R, Sofia A, Sala MR, Robaudo C, Moscatelli P, Deferrari G, Tizianello A: Skeletal muscle protein synthesis and degradation in patients with chronic renal failure. *Kidney Int* 45:1432–1439, 1994.

71. May RC, Kelly RA, Mitch WE: Metabolic acidosis stimulates protein degradation in rat muscle by a glucocorticoid-dependent mechanism. *J Clin Invest* 77:614–621, 1986.

72. May RC, Hara Y, Kelly RA, Block KP, Buse M, Mitch WE: Branched-chain amino acid metabolism in rat muscle: abnormal regulation in acidosis. *Am J Physiol* 252:E712–E718, 1987.

73. Bergström J, Alvestrand A, Fürst P: Plasma and muscle free amino acids in maintenance hemodialysis patients without protein malnutrition. *Kidney Int* 38:108–114, 1990.

74. Mitch WE, Medina R, Greiber S, et al.: Accelerated muscle proteolysis in acidosis involves increased mRNA for ubiquitin and subunits of the proteosome (multicatalytic proteinase). *FASEB J* 5:3210, 1991.

75. DeFronzo RA, Alvestrand A, Smith D, Hendler R, Hendler E, Wahren J: Insulin resistance in uremia. *J Clin Invest* 67:563–568, 1981.

76. Maniar S, Laouari D, Motel V, Déchaux M, Kleinknecht C: Growth hormone (GH) resistance induced by chronic metabolic acidosis (CMA) in uremic rats (abstract 102). *7th International Congress on Nutrition and Metabolism in Renal Disease*, Stockholm, May 29–June 1, 1994.

77. Graham KA, Goodship THJ: Correction of acidosis in hemodialysis patients (HD) suppresses parathyroid hormone secretion (abstract 196). *7th International Congress on Nutrition and Metabolism in Renal Disease*, Stockholm, May 29–June 1, 1994.

78. Papadoyannikis NJ, Stefanidis CS, McGeown M: The effect of the correction of metabolic acidosis on nitrogen and potassium balance of patients with chronic renal failure. *Am J Clin Nutr* 40:623–627, 1984.

79. Williams B, Hattersley J, Layward E, Walls J: Metabolic acidosis and skeletal muscle adaption to low protein diets in chronic uremia. *Kidney Int* 40:779–786, 1991.

80. Goldberg AL, Baracos VE, Rodemann P, Waxmann L, Dinarello CA: Control of protein degradation in muscle by prostaglandins, Ca^{2+}, and leukocytic pyrogen (interleukin I). *Fed Proc*: 1301–1306, 1984.

81. Baracos V, Rodemann P, Dinarello CA, Goldberg AL: Stimulation of muscle protein degradation and prostaglandin E_2 release by leukocytic pyrogen (Interleukin 1). *N Engl J Med* 308:553–558, 1983.

82. Dinarello CA, Wolff SM: Molecular basis of fever in humans. *Am J Med* 72:799–819, 1982.

83. Wilmore DW: Catabolic illness: strategies for enhancing recovery. *N Engl J Med* 325:695–702, 1991.

84. Jindal KK, Manuel A, Goldstein MB: Percent reduction in blood urea concentration during hemodialysis (PRU). A simple and accurate method to estimate K_t/V (urea). *ASAIO Trans* 33:286–288, 1987.

85. Lindsay RM, Spanner E: A hypothesis: the protein catabolic rate is dependent upon the type and amount of treatment in dialyzed uremic patients. *Am Kidney Dis* 13:382–389, 1989.

86. Lindsay RM, Spanner E, Heidenheim AP, Lefebvre JMJ, Hodsman A, Baird J, Allison MEM: Which comes first, K_t/V or PCR—Chicken or egg? *Kidney Int* 42(38):S32–S36, 1992.

87. Lindsay RM, Spanner E, Heidenheim AP, Burton H, Lindsay S, Lefebvre JMJ: A multicentre study of short hour dialysis using AN69S—Preliminary results. *ASAIO Trans* 37(3):M465–M467, 1991.

88. Venning MC, Faragher EB, Harty JC, Hartley G, Goldsmith DJA, Tapson JS, Gokal R: The relationship between K_t/V and NPCR in haemodialysis patients in cross-sectional studies is mathematical coupling (abstract). *J Am Soc Nephrol* 4:393, 1993.

89. Borah MF, Schönfeld PY, Gotch FA, Sargent JA, Wolfson M, Humphreys MH: Nitrogen balance during intermittent dialysis therapy of uremia. *Kidney Int* 14:491–500, 1978.

90. Lim VS, Flanigan MJ: The effect of interdialytic interval on protein metabolism: evidence suggesting dialysis-induced catabolism. *Am J Kidney Dis* 14:96–101, 1989.

91. Gutierrez A, Alvestrand A, Wahren J, Bergström J: Effect of in vivo contact between blood and dialysis membranes on protein catabolism in humans. *Kidney Int* 38:487–494, 1990.

92. Gutierrez A, Bergström J, Alvestrand A: Protein catabolism in sham hemodialysis: the effect of different membranes

on protein catabolism in humans. *Kidney Int* 38:20–29, 1992.

93. Heidland A, Hörl W, Heller N, Heine H, Neumann S, Heidbreder E: Proteolytic enzymes and catabolism: enhanced release of granulocyte proteinases in uremic intoxication and during hemodialysis. *Kidney Int* 24 (Suppl 16):S27–S36, 1983.

94. Hörl W, Jochum M, Heidland A, Fritz H: Release of granulocyte proteinases during hemodialysis. *Am J Nephrol* 3:213–217, 1983.

95. Betz M, Hänsch GM, Rauterberg EW, Bommer J, Ritz E: Cuprammonium membranes stimulates interleukin-1 release and arachidonic acid metabolism in monocytes in the absence of complement. *Kidney Int* 34:67–73, 1988.

96. Herbelin A, Nguyen AT, Zingraff J, Urena P, Descamps-Latscha B: Influence of uremia and hemodialysis on circulating interleukin-1 and tumor necrosis factor alpha. *Kidney Int* 37:116–125, 1990.

97. Lim VS, Bier DM, Flanigan MJ, Sum-Ping ST: The effect of hemodialysis on protein metabolism. A leucine kinetic study. *J Clin Invest* 91:2429–2436, 1993.

98. Lonnemann G, Bingel M, Floege J, Koch KM, Shaldon S, Dinarello CA: Detection of endotoxin-like interleukin-1-inducing activity during in-vitro dialysis. *Kidney Int* 33:29–35, 1988.

99. Bingel M, Lonnemann G, Koch KM, Dinarello CA, Shaldon S: Enhancement of in-vitro human interleukin-1 production by sodium acetate. *Lancet* 1:14–16, 1987.

100. Kopple JD, Swendseid ME, Shinaberger JH, Umezawa CY: The free and bound amino acids removed by hemodialysis. *Trans Am Soc Artif Intern Organs* 19:309–313, 1973.

101. Ikizler TA, Flakoll PJ, Parker RA, Hakim RM: Amino acid and albumin losses during hemodialysis. *Kidney Int* 46:830–837, 1994.

102. Graeber W, Halley SE, Lapkin RA, Graeber CA, Kaplan AA: Protein losses with reused dialyzers (abstract). *J Am Soc Nephrol* 4:349, 1993.

103. Wathen RL, Keshaviah P, Hommeyer P, Cadwell K, Comty CM: The metabolic effects of hemodialysis with and without glucose in the dialysate. *Am J Clin Nutr* 31:1870–1875, 1978.

104. Koch KM, Bechstein PB, Fassbinder W, Kaltwasser P, Schoeppe W, Werner E: Occult blood loss and iron balance in chronic renal failure. *Proc Eur Dial Transplant Assoc* 12:362–369, 1975.

105. Laird NM, Berkey CS, Lowrie EG: Modeling success or failure of dialysis therapy: the National Cooperative Dialysis Study. *Kidney Int* 23 (Suppl 13):101–106, 1983.

106. Bergström J: Nutrition and adequacy of dialysis in hemodialysis patients. *Kidney Int* 43 (Suppl 41):261–267, 1993.

107. Degoulet P, Legrain M, Reach I, et al.: Mortality risk factors in patients treated by chronic hemodialysis: Report of the Daiphane Collaborative Study. *Nephron* 31:103–110, 1982.

108. Acchiardo SR, Moore LE, Latour PA: Malnutrition as the main factor in morbidity and mortality of hemodialysis patients. *Kidney Int* 24 (Suppl 16):199–203, 1983.

109. Lowrie EG, Lew LN: Death risk in hemodialysis patients: the predictive value of commonly measured variables and an evaluation of death rate differences between facilities. *Am J Kidney Dis* 5:458–482, 1990.

110. Lowrie EG, Lew NL, Huang WH: Race and diabetes as death risk predictors in hemodialysis patients. *Kidney Int* 42(38):S22–S31, 1992.

111. Churchill DN, Taylor DW, Cook RJ, LaPlante P, Barre P, Cartier P, Fay WP, Goldstein MB, Jindal K, Mandin H, McKenzie JK, Muirhead N, Parfrey PS, Posen GA, Slaughter D, Ulah RA, Werb R: Canadian hemodialysis morbidity study. *Am J Kidney Dis* 3:214–234, 1992.

112. Held PJ, Port FK, Gaylin DS, Wolfe RA, Levin NW, Blagg CR, Garcia J, Agodoa L: Hemodialysis prescription and delivery in the US: results from USRDS case mix study (abstract). *J Am Soc Nephrol* 2:328, 1991.

113. Owen WF, Lew NL, Liu Y, Lowrie EG, Lazarus JM: The urea reduction ratio and serum albumin concentrations as predictors of mortality in patients undergoing hemodialysis. *N Engl J Med* 329:1001–1006, 1993.

114. Mattern WD, Hak LJ, Lamanna RW, et al.: Malnutrition, altered immune function, and the risk of infection in maintenance hemodialysis patients. *Am J Kidney Dis* 1:206–218, 1982.

115. Haag-Weber M, Dumann H, Hörl WH: Effect of malnutrition and uremia on impaired cellular host defence. *Miner Electrolyte Metab* 18:174–185, 1992.

116. Ritz E, Vallance P, Nowicki M: The effect of malnutrition on cardiovascular mortality in dialysis patients: is L-arginine the answer? *Nephrol Dial Transplant* 9:129–130, 1994.

117. Bergström J, Alvestrand A, Fürst P: Plasma and muscle free amino acids in maintenance hemodialysis patients without protein malnutrition. *Kidney Int* 38:108–114, 1990.

118. Jones MR, Kopple JD, Swendseid ME: Phenylalanine metabolism in uremic and normal man. *Kidney Int* 14:169–179, 1978.

119. Vallance P, Leone A, Calver A, Collier J, Moncada S: Accumulation of an endogenous inhibitor of nitric oxide synthesis in chronic renal failure. *Lancet* 339:572–575, 1992.

120. Vallance P, Collier J, Moncada S: Effects of endothelium-derived nitric oxide on peripheral arteriolar tone in man. *Lancet* 2:997–1000, 1989.

121. Kluthe R, Lüttgen FM, Capetianu T, Heinze U, Katz N, Südhoff A: Protein requirements in maintenance hemodialysis. *Am J Clin Nutr* 31:1812–1820, 1978.

122. Kopple JD: Dietary considerations in patients with advanced chronic renal failure, acute renal failure, and transplantation. In: RW Schrier, CW Gottschalk, eds, *Diseases of the Kidney*, 5th ed. Little, Brown, Boston, pp 3167–3210, 1992.

123. Mitch W, Klahr S, eds: *Nutrition and the Kidney*, 2nd ed. Little, Brown, Boston, 1993.

124. Kopple JD: Effect of malnutrition on morbidity and mortality in maintenance hemodialysis patients. *Am J Kidney Dis* 24(6):1002–1009, 1994.

125. Slomowitz LA, Monteon FJ, Grosvenor M, Laidlaw SA, Kopple JD: Effect of energy intake on nutritional status in maintenance hemodialysis patients. *Kidney Int* 35:704–711, 1989.

126. Grodstein G, Harrison A, Roberts C, Ippoliti A, Kopple J: Impaired gastric emptying in hemodialysis patients (abstract). *Kidney Int* 16:952, 1979.

127. Druml W, Lochs H, Roth E, Hübl W, Balcke P, Lenz K: Utilisation of dipeptides and acetyl-tyrosine in normal and uremic humans. *Am J Physiol* 260:E280–E285, 1991.

128. Smolle KH, Kaufmann P, Holzer H, Druml W: Intradialytic parenteral nutrition in malnourished patients on chronic hemodialysis therapy. *Nephrol Dial Transplant*, 10, 14, 11–16, 1995.

129. Wolfson M, Jones MR, Kopple JD: Amino acid losses during hemodialysis with infusion of amino acids and glucose. *Kidney Int* 21:500–506, 1982.

130. Heidland A, Kult J: Long-term effects of essential amino

acids supplementation in patients on regular dialysis treatment. *Clin Nephrol* 3:234–239, 1975.

131. Cano N, Labastie-Coeyrehourq J, Lacombe P, Stroumza P, diConstanzo-Dufetel J, Durbec J-P, Coudray-Lucas C, Cynober L: Peridialytic parenteral nutrition with lipids and amino acids in malnourished hemodialysis patients. *Am J Clin Nutr* 52:726–730, 1990.

132. Matthys DA, Vanholder RC, Ringoir SM: Benefit of intravenous essential amino-acids parenteral nutrition in the malnourished hemodialysis patient. *J Renal Nutr* 1:23–33, 1991.

133. Capelli JP, Kushner H, Camiscioli TC, Chen S-M, Torres MA: Effect of intradialytic parenteral nutrition on mortality rates in end-stage renal disease care. *Am J Kidney Dis* 23:808–816, 1994.

134. Wolfson M: Intradialytic parenteral nutrition (IDPN) is of no proven benefit in hemodialysis patients. *Semin Dial* 6:170–173, 1993.

135. Canaud B, Bouloux C, Rivory JP, Taib J, Garred LJ, Florence P, Mion C: Erythropoietin-induced changes in protein nutrition: quantitative assessment by urea kinetic modeling analysis. *Blood Purif* 8:301–308, 1990.

136. Barany P, Pettersson E, Ahlberg M, Hultman E, Bergström J: Nutritional assessment in anemic hemodialysis patients treated with recombinant human erythropoietin. *Clin Nephrol* 35:270–279, 1991.

137. Riedel E, Hampl H, Scigalla P, Nündel M, Kessel M: Correction of amino acid metabolism by recombinant EPO in hemodialysis patients. *Kidney Int* 36(27):S216–S221, 1989.

138. Garibotto G, Gurreri G, Robaudo C, Saffioti S, Magnasco A, Sofia A, Marchelli M, Sala MR: Erythropoietin treatment and amino acid metabolism in hemodialysis. *Nephron* 65(4):533–536, 1993.

139. Heidland A, Schaefer RM, Teschner M, Huang S: New approaches in the control of hypercatabolism in experimental uremia. *Acta Med Pol* 3:1–4, 1990.

140. Mehls O, Ritz E, Hunziker EB, Eggli P, Heinrich U, Zapf J: Improvement of growth and food utilization by human recombinant growth hormone in uremia. *Kidney Int* 33:45–52, 1988.

141. Fine RN, Pyke-Grimm K, Nelson PA, et al.: Recombinant human growth hormone treatment of children with chronic renal failure: long-term (1 to 3 year) outcome. *Pediatr Nephrol* 5:477–481, 1991.

142. Mehls O, Tönshoff B, Tönshoff C, Haffner D: The therapeutic value of rhGH in children with chronic renal failure. *Miner Electrolyte Metab* 18:320–324, 1992.

143. Kopple JD, Brunori G, Leiserowitz M, Mattimore C, Hirschberg R: Growth hormone treatment for patients with renal failure. *Jpn J Nephrol* 33:468–474, 1991.

144. Ziegler TR, Lazarus JM, Young LS, Hakim R, Wilmore DW: Effects of recombinant human growth hormone in adults receiving maintenance hemodialysis. *J Am Soc Nephrol* 2:1130–1135, 1991.

145. Schulman G, Wingard RL, Hutchison RL, Lawrence P, Hakim RM: The effects of recombinant human growth hormone and intradialytic parenteral nutrition in malnourished hemodialysis patients. *Am J Kidney Dis* 21:527–534, 1993.

146. Kopple JD: The rationale for the use of growth hormone or insulin-like growth factor I in adult patients with renal failure. *Miner Electrolyte Metab* 18:269–275, 1992.

147. Marckmann P: Nutritional status of patients on hemodialysis and peritoneal dialysis. *Clin Nephrol* 29:75–78, 1988.

148. Mejia JL, Gamba G, Correa-Rotter R, Saldivar S, Pena JC: Early clinical and laboratory predictors of death risk in CAPD patients. *J Am Soc Nephrol* 3:415, 1992.

149. Young GA, Kopple J, Lindholm B, et al.: Nutritional assessment of continuous ambulatory peritoneal dialysis patients. An international study. *Am J Kidney Dis* 17:462–471, 1991.

150. Cianciaruso B, Brunori G, Traverso G, Panarello G, Enia G, Strippoli P, DeVecchi A, Querques M, Viglino G, Vonesh E, Kopple JD, Maiorca R: Cross-sectional comparison of malnutrition in continuous ambulatory peritoneal dialysis (CAPD) and hemodialysis (MHD) patients (pts) (abstract 73). *7th International Congress on Nutrition and Metabolism in Renal Disease*, Stockholm, May 29–June 1, 1994.

151. Teehan BP, Schleifer CR, Brown JM, Sigler MH, Raimondo J: Urea kinetic analysis and clinical outcome on CAPD. A five year longitudinal study. *Adv Peritoneal Dial* 6:181–185, 1990.

152. Avram MM, Goldwasser P, Erroa M, Fein PA: Predictors of survival in continuous ambulatory peritoneal dialysis patients: the importance of prealbumin and other nutritional and metabolic markers. *Am J Kidney Dis* 233(1):91–98, 1994.

153. Rocco MV, Jordan JR, Burkart JM: The efficacy number as a predictor of morbidity and mortality in peritoneal dialysis patients. *J Am Soc Nephrol* 4:1184–1191, 1993.

154. Blake PG, Flowerdew G, Blake RM, Oreopoulos PG: Serum albumin in patients on continuous ambulatory peritoneal dialysis—predictors and correlations with outcomes. *J Am Soc Nephrol* 3:1501–1507, 1993.

155. Fine A, Cox D: Modest reduction of serum albumin in continuous ambulatory peritoneal dialysis patients is common and of no apparent clinical consequence. *Am J Kidney Dis* 20:50, 1992.

156. Jones MR: Etiology of severe malnutrition: results of an international cross-sectional study in continuous ambulatory peritoneal dialysis patients. *Am J Kidney Dis* 23:412–420, 1994.

157. Giordano C, DeSanto NG, Capodicasa G: Amino acid losses during CAPD. *Clin Nephrol* 14:230–232, 1980.

158. Kopple JD, Blumenkrantz MJ, Jones MR, Moran JK, Coburn JW: Plasma amino acid levels and amino acid losses during continuous ambulatory peritoneal dialysis. *Am J Clin Nutr* 36:395–402, 1982.

159. Kopple JD, Hirschberg R: Nutrition and peritoneal dialysis. In: WE Mitch, S Klahr, eds, *Nutrition and the Kidney*, 2nd ed. Little, Brown, Boston, pp 290–313, 1993.

160. Grimbl RF: Cytokines: their relevance for nutrition. *Eur J Clin Nutr* 43:217–230, 1989.

161. Grodstein GP, Blumenkrantz MJ, Kopple JD, Moran JK, Coburn JW: Glucose absorption during continuous ambulatory peritoneal dialysis. *Kidney Int* 19:564–567, 1981.

162. Heimburger O, Bergström J, Lindholm B: Maintenance of optimal nutrition in CAPD. *Kidney Int* 584:S39–S46, 1994.

163. Twardowski ZJ, Nolph KD: Opinion: Peritoneal dialysis—how much is enough? *Semin Dial* 1:75–76, 1988.

164. Schilling H, Wu G, Pettit J, Mitwalli A, Anderson HG, Ogilve R, Oreopoulos DG: Use of amino acid containing solutions in continuous ambulatory peritoneal dialysis patients after peritonitis. Results of a prospective controlled trial. *Proc EDTA-ERA* 22:421–425, 1985.

165. Jones RJ, Martis L, Algrim CE, Bernard D, Swartz R, Messana J, Bergström J, Lindholm B, Lim V, Serkes KD, Vonesh E, Kopple JD: Amino acid solutions for CAPD: rationale and clinical experience. *Miner Electrolyte Metab* 18:309–315, 1992.

166. Young GA, et al.: The use of an amino-acid-based CAPD fluid over 12 weeks. *Nephrol Dial Transplant* 4:285, 1989.
167. Goodship THJ, Lloyd S, McKenzie PW, et al.: Short-term studies on the use of amino acids as an osmotic agent in continuous ambulatory peritoneal dialysis. *Clin Sci* 73:471, 1987.
168. Hakim RM, Ikizler A, Wingard R, Breyer JA, Schulman G: Short-term effects of recombinant human growth hormone (rhGH) therapy in CAPD patients (abstract 7). *7th International Congress on Nutrition and Metabolism in Renal Disease,* Stockholm, May 29–June 1, 1994.
169. Kopple JD, Jones M, Fukuda S, Swendseid ME: Amino acid and protein metabolism in renal failure. *Am J Clin Nutr* 31:1532–1540, 1978.
170. Giordano C, DeSanto NG, Senatore R: Effects of catabolic stress in acute and chronic renal failure. *Am J Clin Nutr* 31:1561–1571, 1978.
171. Bondy PK, Engle F, Farror B: The metabolism of amino acids and protein in the adrenalectomized-nephrectomized rat. *Endocrinology* 44:476, 1949.
172. Fürst P, Alvestrand A, Bergström J: Effects of nutrition and catabolic stress on intracellular amino acids pools in uremia. *Am J Clin Nutr* 33:1387–1395, 1980.
173. Maier KP, Hoppe-Seyler G, Talke H, Fröhlich J, Schollmeyer P, Gerok W: Enzymatic and metabolic studies on carbohydrate and amino acid metabolism in rat liver during acute uremia. *Eur J Clin Invest* 3:201–207, 1971.
174. Druml W, Fischer M, Liebisch B, Lenz K, Roth E: Elimination of amino acids in renal failure. *Am J Clin Nutr* 60:418–423, 1994.
175. Arnold WE, Holliday MA: Tissue resistance to insulin stimulation of amino acid uptake in acutely uremic rats. *Kidney Int* 16:124, 1979.
176. Maroni BJ, Haesemeyer RW, Kutner MH, Mitch E: Kinetics of system A amino acid uptake by muscle: effects of insulin and acute uremia. *Am J Physiol* 258:F1304, 1990.
177. May RC, Clark AS, Goheer A, Mitch WE: Specific defects in insulin-mediated muscle metabolism in acute uremia. *Kidney Int* 28:490, 1985.
178. Druml W: Nutritional support in acute renal failure. In: WE Mitch, S Klahr, eds, *Nutrition and the Kidney.* Little, Brown, Boston, pp 314–345, 1993.
179. Heidland A, Schaefer RM, Weipert J, Heidbreder E, Teschner M, Peter G, Hörl WH: Catabolism in acute renal failure: importance of glucocorticoids and lysosomal enzymes. *Adv Exp Med Biol* 212:41–55, 1987.
180. Schaefer RM, Teschner M, Kulzer P, Leibold J, Peter G, Heidland A: Evidence for reduced catabolism by the antiglucocorticoid RU 38486 in acutely uremic rats. *Am J Nephrol* 7:127–131, 1987.
181. Schaefer RM, Riegel W, Stephan E, Keller H, Hörl WH, Heidland A: Normalization of enhanced hepatic gluconeogenesis by the antiglucocorticoid RU 38486 in acutely uremic rats. *Eur J Clin Invest* 20:35, 1990.
182. Hörl W, Heidland A: Enhanced proteolytic activity—cause of protein catabolism in acute renal failure. *Am J Clin Nutr* 33:1423–1427, 1980.
183. Heidland A, Schaefer RM, Heidbreder E, Hörl WH: Catabolic factors in renal failure: therapeutic approaches. *Nephrol Dial Transplant* 3:8–16, 1988.
184. Hörl WH, Wanner C, Thaiss F, Schollmeyer P: Detection of a metalloproteinase in patients with acute and chronic renal failure. *Am J Nephrol* 6:6–13, 1986.

185. Tizianello A, Deferrari G, Garibotto G, Gurreri G, Robaudo C: Renal metabolism of amino acids and ammonia in subjects with normal renal function and in patients with chronic renal insufficiency. *J Clin Invest* 65:1162–1173, 1980.
186. Mitch WE, Chesney RW: Amino acid metabolism by the kidney. *Miner Electrolyte Metab* 9:190, 1983.
187. May RC, Clark AS, Goheer MA, Mitch WE: Specific defects in insulin-mediated muscle metabolism in acute uremia. *Kidney Int* 28:490–497, 1985.
188. Druml W: Lipid metabolism and amino acid metabolism in acute renal failure (in German). *Klin Ernähr* 28:1, 1987.
189. Wanner C, Riegel W, Schaefer RM, Hörl WH: Carnitine and carnitine esters in acute renal failure. *Nephrol Dial Transplant* 4:951, 1989.
190. Soop M, Forsberg E, Thörne A, Alvestrand A: Energy expenditure in postoperative multiple organ failure with acute renal failure. *Clin Nephrol* 31:139, 1989.
191. Om P, Hohenegger M: Energy metabolism in acute uremic rats. *Nephron* 25:249, 1980.
192. Knochel J: Complications of total parenteral nutrition. *Kidney Int* 27:489–496, 1985.
193. Deitch EA, Winterton J, Berg R: The gut as a portal of entry for bacteremia. Role of protein malnutrition. *Ann Surg* 205:681, 1987.
194. Druml W: Nutritional importance of non-essential amino acids. *J Clin Nutr Gastroenterol* 4:71, 1989.
195. Grazer RE, Sutton JM, Friedstrom S, McBarron FD: Hyperammoniemic encephalopathy due to essential amino acid hyperalimentation. *Arch Intern Med* 144:2278, 1984.
196. Sponsel H, Conger D: Is parenteral nutrition therapy of value in acute renal failure patients? *Am J Kidney Dis* 25(1):96–102, 1995.
197. Imai E, Yamamoto S, Isaka Y, Fukuhara Y, Fujii Y, Kikuchi T, Tanaka T, Kamada T, Ueda N: Delay of recovery from renal ischemic injury by administration of glutamine (Gln). *J Am Soc Nephrol* 2:648A, 1991.
198. Abel R, Beck C, Abbott W, Ryan J, Barnett G, Fischer J: Improved survival from acute renal failure after treatment with intravenous essential α-amino acids and glucose. *N Engl J Med* 288:695–699, 1973.
199. Feinstein EI, Blumenkrantz M, Healy M, Koffler A, Silberman H, Massry S, Kopple J: Clinical and metabolic responses to parenteral nutrition in acute renal failure. *Medicine (Baltimore)* 60:124–137, 1981.
200. Hoy WE, Sargent JA, Hall D, McKenna BA, Byer BM: Protein catabolism during the postoperative course after renal transplantation. *Am J Kidney Dis* 5:186, 1985.
201. Whittier FC, Evans DH, Datton S, Ross G, More H: Nutrition in renal transplantation. *Am J Kidney Dis* 6:405, 1985.
202. Prachno CH J, Hunsicker LG: Nutritional requirements of renal transplant patients. In: W Mitch, S Klahr, eds, *Nutrition and the Kidney.* Little, Brown, Boston, pp 346–364, 1993.
203. Cogan MG, Sargent JA, Yarbrough SG, Vincenti F, Amend WJ: Prevention of prednisone-induced negative nitrogen balance: effect of dietary modification on urea generation rate in patients on hemodialysis receiving high-dose glucocorticoids. *Ann Intern Med* 95:158, 1981.
204. Horber FF, Scheidegger JR, Grüning BE, Frey FJ: Evidence that prednisone-induced myopathy is reversed by physical training. *J Clin Endocrinol Metab* 61:83, 1985.
205. Horber FF, Huppeler H, Herren D, Claasen H, Howald H, Gerber Ch, Frey FJ: Altered skeletal muscle ultrastructure in

renal transplant paitents on prednisone. *Kidney Int* 30:411, 1986.

206. Miller DG, Levine SE, D'Elia JA, Bistrian BR: Nutritional status of diabetic and non-diabetic patients after renal transplantation. *Am J Clin Nutr* 44:66, 1986.

207. Feehally J, Binnett SE, Morris KPG, Walls J: Is chronic renal transplant rejection a non-immunological phenomenon? *Lancet* 2:486, 1986.

208. Windus DW, Lacson S, Delmez JA: The short-term effects of a low-protein diet in stable renal transplant recipients. *Am J Kidney Dis* 17:693, 1991.

209. Salahudeen AK, Hostetter Th, Raatz SK, Rosenberg ME: Effects of dietary protein in patients with chronic renal transplant rejection. *Kidney Int* 41:183, 1992.

210. Brown EA, Markanda ND, Sagnella GA, Jones BER, MacGreger GA: Urinary iron loss in the nephrotic syndrome—unusual cause of iron deficiency with a note on urinary copper losses. *Postgrad Med J* 60:125, 1984.

211. Van de Vyrer FL, Vanheule AO, Verbueken AH, Haese PD, Visser WJ, Bekaert AB, van Grieken RE, Buyssens N, de Broe ME: Pattern of iron storage in patients with severe renal failure. *Contr Nephrol* 38:153–166, 1984.

212. Milly K, Wit L, Diskin C, Tulley R: Selenium in renal failure patients. *Nephron* 61:139–144, 1992.

213. Kallistratos G, Evangelou A, Seferiadis K, Vezyraki P, Barboutis K: Selenium and hemodialysis: serum selenium levels in healthy persons, non-cancer and cancer patients with chronic renal failure. *Nephron* 41:217–222, 1985.

214. Dworkin B, Weseley S, Rosenthal WS, Schwartz EM, Weiss L: Diminished blood selenium levels in renal failure patients on dialysis: correlations with nutritional status. *Am J Med Sci* 293:6–12, 1987.

215. Girelli D, Olivieri O, Stanzial AM, Azzini M, Lupo A, Bernich P, Menini C, Gammaro L, Corrocher R: Low platelet glutathione peroxidase activity and serum selenium concentration in patients with chronic renal failure: relations to dialysis treatments, diet and cardiovascular complications. *Clin Sci* 84:611–617, 1993.

216. Leung A, Henderson I, Fell G, Hall D, Kennedy AC: Selenium deficiency in chronic uraemia and dialysis. *Proc Eur Dial Transplant Soc Eur Renal Assoc* 22:1134–1138, 1985.

217. Diskin CJ: Selenium deficiency? *Trans Am Soc Artif Intern Organs* 32:665–669, 1986.

218. Salonen JT, Alfthen F, Hattunen JK, Puska P: Association between cardiovascular death and myocardial function and serum selenium in a matched-pair longitudinal study. *Lancet* 1:175–177, 1982.

219. Serfass RE, Ganther HE: Defective microbicidal activity in glutathione peroxidase-deficient neutrophils of selenium-deficient rats. *Nature* 255:640, 1975.

220. Atkin-Thor E, Goddard B, O'Nion J, Stephen RL, Kolff WJ: Hypogeusia and zinc depletion in chronic dialysis patients. *Am J Clin Nutr* 31:1948–1951, 1978.

221. Mansouri K, Halsted JA, Gombos EA: Zinc, copper, magnesium, and calcium in dialyzed and non-dialyzed uremic patients. *Arch Intern Med* 125:88, 1970.

222. Bogden JD, Oleske JM, Weiner B, Smith LG, Najem GR: Elevated plasma zinc concentrations in renal dialysis patients. *Am J Clin Nutr* 33:1088, 1980.

223. Mahajan SK, Prasad AS, Lambujo J, et al.: Improvement of uremic hypogeusia by zinc: a double-blind study. *Am J Clin Nutr* 33:1517, 1980.

224. Tsukamoto Y, Iwanami S, Marumo F: Disturbances of trace element concentrations in plasma of patients with chronic

renal failure. *Nephron* 26:174, 1980.

225. Sprenger KBG, Bandscha D, Lewis K, Spohn B, Schmitz J, Franz H: Improvement of uremic neuropathy and hypogeusia by dialysate zinc supplementation. A double blind study. *Kidney Int* 24 (Suppl 16):315, 1983.

226. Stec J, Podsacka L, Pavkovcekava O, Kollar M: Zinc and copper metabolism in nephrotic syndrome. *Nephron* 56:186, 1990.

227. Sondheimer JH, Mahajan SK, Rye DL, et al.: Elevated plasma copper in chronic renal failure. *Am J Clin Nutr* 47:896, 1988.

228. Stein G, Schön S, Sperschneider H, Richter R, Fünfstück R, Günther K: Vitamin status in patients with chronic renal failure. *Contrib Nephrol* 65:33, 1988.

229. Hemmelhoff-Andersen KE: Folic acid status of patient with chronic renal failure maintained by dialysis. *Clin Nephrol* 8:510–513, 1977.

230. Swainson CP: Do dialysis patients need extrafolate? *Lancet* 1:239, 1983.

231. Janssen MJFM, van Guldener C, De Jong GMTh, van den Berg M, Stehouwer CDA, Donker AJM: Folic acid treatment of hyperhomocysteinemia in dialysis patients. *Miner Electrolyte Metab* 22:110–114, 1996.

232. Wilcken DEL, Dudman NPB, Tyrrell PA, Robertson MR: Folic acid lowers elevated plasma homocysteine in chronic renal insufficiency: Possible implications for prevention of vascular disease. *Metabolism* 37:697–••, 1988.

233. Clarke R, Daly R, Robinson K, Naughten E, Cahalane S, Fowler B, Graham I: Hyperhomo-cysteinemia: An independent risk factor for vascular disease. *N Engl J Med* 324:1149–1155, 1991.

234. Boeschoten EW, Schrijver J, Krediet RT, Schreurs WHP, Arisz L: Deficiencies of vitamins in CAPD patients: the effect of supplementation. *Nephrol Dial Transplant* 2:187, 1988.

235. Gentile MG, Manna BM, D'Amico, et al.: Vitamin nutrition in patients with chronic renal failure and dietary manipulation. *Contrib Nephrol* 65:43, 1988.

236. Gilmour ER, Hartley GH, Goodschip THJ: Trace elements and vitamins in renal disease. In: WE Mitch, S Klahr, eds, *Nutrition and the Kidney*. Little, Brown, Boston, pp 114–131, 1993.

237. Kopple JD, Mercurio K, Blumenkrantz MJ, Jones MR, Roberts C, Card B, Saltzman R, Casciato DA, Swenseid MA: Daily requirement for pyridoxine supplement in chronic renal failure. *Kidney Int* 19:694–704, 1981.

238. Dobbelstein HW, Körner WF, Mempel W, Grosse-Wilde H, Edel HH: Vitamin B_6 deficiency in uremia and its implications for the depression of immune responses. *Kidney Int* 5:233–237, 1974.

239. Ramirez G, Chen M, Boyce HW, Fuller SM, Ganguly R, Brüggemeyer CD, Butcher DE: Longitudinal follow-up of chronic hemodialysis patients without vitamin supplementation. *Kidney Int* 30:99–106, 1986.

240. Pru C, Eaton J, Kjellstrand C: Vitamin C intoxication and hyperoxalemia in chronic hemodialysis patients. *Nephron* 39.112–116, 1985.

241. Gentile M, Fellin G, Manna GM, D'Amico, et al.: Vitamin A and retinol binding protein in chronic renal insufficiency. *Int J Artif Organs* 11:403, 1988.

242. Stein G, Schone S, Geinitz D, et al.: No tissue level abnormality of vitamin A concentration despite elevated serum vitamin A of uremic patients. *Clin Nephrol* 25:87, 1986.

243. Muth I: Implications of hypervitaminosis A in chronic renal failure. *J Renal Nutr* 1:2, 1991.

CHAPTER 49

Treatment of Hyperlipidemia in the Nephrotic Syndrome

GEORGE A. KAYSEN

INTRODUCTION

The nephrotic syndrome is defined by urinary protein excretion of more than 3.5 g/day (1) and is generally accompanied by hypoalbuminemia and increased blood lipid levels (2). Both plasma cholesterol and triglyceride concentration are usually inversely related to plasma cholesterol concentration (3) or to a marker of glomerular permselectivity, the renal clearance of albumin (4). Cholesterol generally bears a negative first-order correlation with serum albumin concentration, while triglyceride levels increase asymptotically as plasma albumin concentration declines (3,4).

Hyperlipidemia is found in nearly all nephrotic patients with an albumin concentration below 20 mg/mL (5,6). Cholesterol and phospholipids correlate closely with one another, but cholesterol and triglycerides do not (6), indicating that multiple disturbances in lipid metabolism may exist in nephrotic patients. Although changes in plasma concentrations of apolipoproteins A-I (apo A-I) and A-II (apo A-II) are variable (7,8), apolipoprotein B (apo B) is increased consistently (7,8).

DISLIPIDEMIA IN THE NEPHROTIC SYNDROME

Plasma lipoproteins are abnormally rich in lipids and poor in apolipoproteins (8). The abnormal composition of lipoproteins affects virtually every lipoprotein class (6,8). Total high-density lipoprotein (HDL) cholesterol is either unchanged (9) or decreased in patients with the nephrotic syndrome (8,10), although HDL concentration is markedly elevated in experimental models of the nephrotic syndrome in the rat (11–13). Within the HDL lipoproteins, the lower-molecular-weight (200-kDa) HDL_3 variety remains unaffected (14), while the larger (400-kDa) HDL_2 is decreased (15). This change is important because it is felt that HDL_2 rather than HDL_3 is the negative cardiovascular risk factor.

Both low-density lipoprotein (LDL) and intermediate-density lipoprotein (IDL) are increased (16), as is the LDL:HDL ratio. Both LDL and IDL are atherogenic.

Lipoprotein (a) (Lp(a)) has recently been identified as a prominent risk factor in atherogenesis (17,18). Generally, the quantity of this lipoprotein in plasma is genetically determined and is not affected by diet (19). The size of the apolipoprotein moiety in Lp(a), apo(a), is heterogeneously distributed in the population (20). Those individuals having the largest apo(a) subtypes have the lowest concentration of Lp(a) in plasma (16). It has become recently apparent that Lp(a) levels are increased in patients with a variety of renal diseases, including the nephrotic syndrome (21–23) and in CRF (24). Lp(a) levels decrease during remission from the nephrotic syndrome (25), even if that remission is brought about by loss of renal function resulting in end-stage renal disease. Thus, increased Lp(a) in nephrotic patients represents an acquired disorder in lipid levels resulting from the nephrotic state and is not a consequence of a "nephrotogenic" effect of an inherited increase in Lp(a) levels.

Unlike inherited increases in plasma Lp(a) levels, acquired increases in Lp(a) are not associated with decreased size of apo(a). Whether an acquired increase in Lp(a) has the same implications for the development of cardiovascular disease is unknown.

Potential deleterious role of lipid disorders

There are two potential adverse effects of the lipid disorders in the nephrotic syndrome. The first is the potential risk of atherosclerotic disease. The second is the recently proposed hypothesis that hyperlipidemia may play a contributory role in the progression of renal injury. While evidence is building that both processes are of significance in humans, neither hypothesis is as yet completely accepted as true.

CARDIOVASCULAR RISKS OF THE NEPHROTIC SYNDROME

The changes that occur in blood lipoprotein composition in the nephrotic syndrome (8,14), namely, reduced HDL_2 cholesterol, a relative increase in HDL_3 cholesterol, and the massive increase in total cholesterol, mostly found in the LDL, IDL, and VLDL fractions, should be expected to cause increased risk of atherosclerotic disease. Indeed, accelerated atherosclerosis has been reported in patients with proteinuria and hyperlipidemia and in some studies has been associated with a sharply increased incidence of cardiovascular disease and stroke (26). One study reported an 85-fold increase in the incidence of ischemic heart disease in such patients (27). In another recent retrospective analysis of 142 patients with proteinuria greater than 3.5 g/day, the relative risk of myocardial infarction was found to be 5.5 and the risk of cardiac death 2.8 compared to age-matched, sex-matched controls (28). It is not clear from this study, however, whether hyperlipidemia or instead some other manifestation of the nephrotic syndrome was responsible for the increased prevalence of coronary artery disease. The failure to identify the nephrotic syndrome as a risk factor for atherosclerotic disease in some studies may be due to the transient nature of proteinuria or to its short duration in some subjects (29). It is generally difficult to find comparable groups—patients who have the same level of renal function, blood pressure, and proteinuria with consistently different lipid levels for prolonged periods of time—in order to independently analyze the effect of hyperlipidemia alone on the development of atherosclerotic vascular disease.

Hyperlipidemia of the nephrotic syndrome may be severe and is characterized by a high LDL:HDL cholesterol ratio. This pattern is associated with accelerated atherosclerosis in other clinical situations, and there is no reason to believe that hyperlipidemia of the nephrotic syndrome would not have similar consequences should this metabolic disorder persist. These abnormalities are further complicated by the increase in plasma Lp(a) levels, increased platelet aggregability (30), increased plasma viscosity, increased concentration of highly atherogenic remnants of VLDL, and chylomicron catabolism in plasma. It would be surprising indeed if hyperlipidemic patients with the nephrotic syndrome did not have considerable risk for development of serious atherosclerotic disease. For this reason, there is no rationale for leaving pronounced hyperlipidemia untreated for prolonged periods of time in a patient with the nephrotic syndrome. Appropriate therapy will be discussed subsequently in this chapter.

PROGRESSIVE NATURE OF RENAL DISEASE

It has been proposed, based primarily upon observations in several models of renal disease in the rat, that hyperlipidemia per se may accelerate the progression of renal disease and increase urinary protein excretion (31–34). In studies on rats, LDL cholesterol was found to be taken up by the mesangium of the glomerulus, increasing renal vascular resistance by enhancing thromboxane generation (35) and causing progression of renal failure (36,37). The human glomerulus also takes up apo-B- and apo-E-rich lipoproteins by specific receptor-mediated pathways (38), so the potential for the same

pathophysiologic changes that occur in rat are present in man. Al Shabeb et al. (34) found that feeding a high-cholesterol diet to guinea pigs for 70 days induced proteinuria and hematuria as well as significant glomerular abnormalities, mainly focal glomerular sclerosis. Feeding a high-cholesterol diet to rats (31,39) induces significant albuminuria, accelerates focal glomerulosclerosis, and increases glomerular capillary pressure. The hemodynamic effects may be mediated by generation of thromboxane A_2 and may also require oxidation of circulating lipoproteins (35). Furthermore, a high-cholesterol diet increases cholesterol esters and linoleic acid and decreases the content of arachidonic acid in the renal cortex (31). These changes correlate with glomerular injury. In the obese Zucker rat with endogenous hyperlipidemia, proteinuria and progressive glomerulosclerosis occur commonly and can be attenuated by cholesterol-lowering agents (31,40). Interestingly, in this model, glomerular capillary pressure and SNGFR are within normal range, suggesting that hyperfiltration is not the mediator of glomerular injury induced by hyperlipidemia (31,40).

Diamond et al. (41) found that rats with nephrotic syndrome induced by puromycin aminonucleoside (PAN) had more proteinuria and lower inulin clearance when fed a high-cholesterol diet than did nephrotic rats eating a regular diet. The glomeruli in the high-cholesterol group were more sclerotic and had mesangial cell proliferation and foam cells. Lowering serum cholesterol by administration of cholestyramine resin attenuated both acute and chronic proteinuria in rats with PAN nephrosis (31,42). Grond et al. (43) found that the severity of glomerular changes was much greater in PAN-induced nephrotic syndrome than in that caused by adriamycin, although the severity of hyperlipidemia was comparable. Therefore, the effect of lipids on proteinuria may be dependent upon both the model of disease and the species studied.

High-cholesterol diets cause increased proteinuria and glomerulosclerosis in the Dahl salt-sensitive rat, but not in the Dahl salt-resistant rats (44), suggesting that under certain circumstances increased blood lipid levels may not in and of themselves cause renal disease, but may act to increase disease severity in the presence of other pathologic processes, such as glomerular injury, diabetes, or hypertension.

THE EFFECT OF HYPERLIPIDEMIA ON PROGRESSION OF RENAL DISEASE IN PATIENTS

In all likelihood, hyperlipidemia per se could only rarely be implicated as the primary cause of glomerular disease in man, e.g., in the condition of congenital lecithin cholesterol acyltransferase deficiency (45). Support for a hypothesis that hyperlipidemia is an independent risk factor for progression of renal disease in humans is still scant, but evidence is accumulating that lipids may indeed contribute to the progressive nature of renal disease in humans, especially those with diabetes mellitus (46). In a relatively small study analyzing the effect of a variety of variables on progression of renal disease in diabetic patients, defined as the loss of GFR using the Cockcroft and Gault formula, Dillon (47) reported that serum cholesterol concentration independently correlated with loss of renal function. Hypertriglyceridemia and decreased HDL cholesterol are also found with greater prevalence in diabetic patients with microalbuminuria compared with those without urinary abnormalities (48). Of course, it is difficult to distinguish cause and effect in these findings. Mulec et al. (49), in a prospective study of 30 patients with Type 1 diabetes, reported that hypercholesterolemia, hypertriglyceridemia, and increased apo-B levels correlated with a more rapid deterioration in kidney function. A single case of a diabetic patient with Type III familial hyperlipoproteinemia showed remission of renal biopsy abnormalities characterized by a massive cluster of foam cells containing apolipoprotein B and E in the mesangial region following with intensive therapy that included plasmapheresis using a dextran sulfate-cellulose column (46).

These findings suggest that in humans, unlike rats, hyperlipidemia by itself is unlikely to cause renal disease. However, at least in the case of diabetes mellitus, increased cholesterol levels may indeed shorten renal survival. Whether this is because the injured glomerulus is more likely to take up lipoproteins than is the normal glomerulus or whether this apparent nephrotoxicity of cholesterol in the presence of diabetes is peculiar to diabetic nephropathy is unknown at this time. Renal disease might modify the glomerulus or induce local growth factors, or alternatively, glucose might modify lipoproteins by the now well-characterized pathway leading to advanced glycosylation end products added to LDL, easing their access to cells within the glomerulus.

Mechanism of acquired disorders in blood lipids

Hyperlipidemia in the nephrotic syndrome is a consequence both of increased synthesis (50) and decreased catabolism of lipoproteins. The clearance of chylomicrons (CMs) (51) and very-low-density lipoproteins (VLDLs) (52) is reduced. The precise cause and relative contribution of increased lipogenesis and decreased lipid catabolism to hyperlipidemia, as well as their relationship to urinary protein loss, hypoalbuminemia, and reduced serum oncotic pressure (π), remain controversial.

INCREASED SYNTHESIS

It has been well established that hepatic synthesis (53,54) and secretion of lipoproteins (50,55–57) are increased in nephrotic syndrome in the rat both by direct measurement of lipoprotein synthesis and secretion and by kinetic analysis of the turnover rate of ^{125}I-labeled apolipoproteins (57). Apolipoprotein synthesis and secretion is also increased (55,58). Of these, the gene encoding apo A-I is regulated at the transcriptional level (11–13), while apo E and apo B are

posttranscriptionally regulated in the nephrotic syndrome. Similar changes both in apolipoprotein levels and in hepatic gene expression occur in the condition of hereditary analbuminemia in the rat, suggesting that reduced plasma albumin concentration or π in some is responsible not only for establishing the increased concentration of these apolipoprotiens in plasma but also for altering hepatic gene expression (13).

Conflicting data on lipoprotein synthesis in patients with the nephrotic syndrome have been reported. Triglyceride synthesis was reported to be increased in patients with the nephrotic syndrome (59,60). However, Vega and Grundy (61) reported that the synthesis of VLDL was not increased in the four nephrotic patients that they studied. Warwick (62) found that the synthesis of apo B was increased in nephrotic subjects and correlated with proteinuria in those patients in whom urinary protein loss exceeded 9 g/day. Apo B synthesis was not increased in patients with less proteinuria.

MECHANISM OF INCREASED HEPATIC SYNTHESIS OF LIPOPROTEINS IN THE NEPHROTIC SYNDROME; EFFECT OF PLASMA ONCOTIC PRESSURE

The specific mechanism causing increased lipogenesis has not been elucidated. Most evidence suggests that the principal organ responsible for increased synthesis both of lipids and of apolipoproteins in the nephrotic syndrome is the liver. Furthermore, evidence suggests that reduced extracellular albumin concentration (63) and/or reduced extracellular π (64) in some way regulates apolipoprotein synthesis and lipogenesis by the hepatocyte.

Marsh and Drabkin suggested that lipoprotein synthesis was increased in parallel with that of albumin in the nephrotic syndrome, since all share a common secretory pathway (56). This hypothesis was supported in part by the previous studies of Soothill and Kark (65), who showed that infusion of albumin partially corrected nephrotic hyperlipidemia. Davis reported that apolipoprotein secretion (apo B) by hepatocytes in culture could be reduced by increasing π in the culture medium, but albumin synthesis could not (66). Although these observations would sever the link between apolipoprotein synthesis and that of albumin, they do support the hypothesis that extracellular π regulates apo B synthesis.

Pullinger (63) and Moberly (67) report that albumin specifically regulates secretion of apo B by HepG2 cells by binding oleic acid and other free fatty acids. However, it has not been established that this is the mechanism whereby hypoalbuminemia stimulates lipogenesis in vivo, and this mechanism cannot explain the effect of nonalbumin macromolecules (dextran and polyvinyl pyrrolodone) on hyperlipidemia or the effect of nonprotein solutes on lipoprotein secretions by cultured hepatocytes. Therefore, although changing albumin concentration might modulate synthesis of some apolipoproteins by binding substances in the plasma that can affect lipid metabolism, this outcome cannot be the entire effect of albumin on blood lipid levels.

THE EFFECT OF CHANGES IN THE ACTIVITIES OF LIPOREGULATORY ENZYMES

HDL arises initially as a cholesterol, phospholipid bilayer called nascent HDL (68). Nascent HDL may be secreted by the liver, is also found in intestinal lymph, and can arise in the peripheral circulation from detritus of chylomicrons and VLDL catabolism on the vascular endothelium. The cholesterol on the surface of this bilayer is esterified by the action of lecithin cholesterol ester transferase (LCAT), forming lysolecithin and cholesterol esters (68). The latter sink into the core of the nascent HDL, forming a spherical particle, HDL_3. Further action of this same enzyme ma-

tures HDL_3 to the larger HDL_2, a particle whose core is now rich with cholesterol esters. Cholesterol ester transfer protein (CETP) catalyzes the transfer of this cholesterol-ester-rich core of HDL_2 to VLDL remnant particles, creating LDL (Figure 1) and increasing plasma LDL cholesterol at the expense of HDL cholesterol. CETP is increased in the plasma of nephrotic patients and correlates positively with VLDL cholesterol and negatively with HDL cholesterol (16). CETP levels decrease significantly following reduction of proteinuria after treatment with an angiotensin-converting enzyme inhibitor (69) in conjunction with a reduction in VLDL and LDL. CETP plays a significant role in the enrichment of VLDL with cholesterol esters, and may also contribute to increased concentrations of apo-B lipoproteins and decreased HDL cholesterol in some nephrotic patients. The mechanism

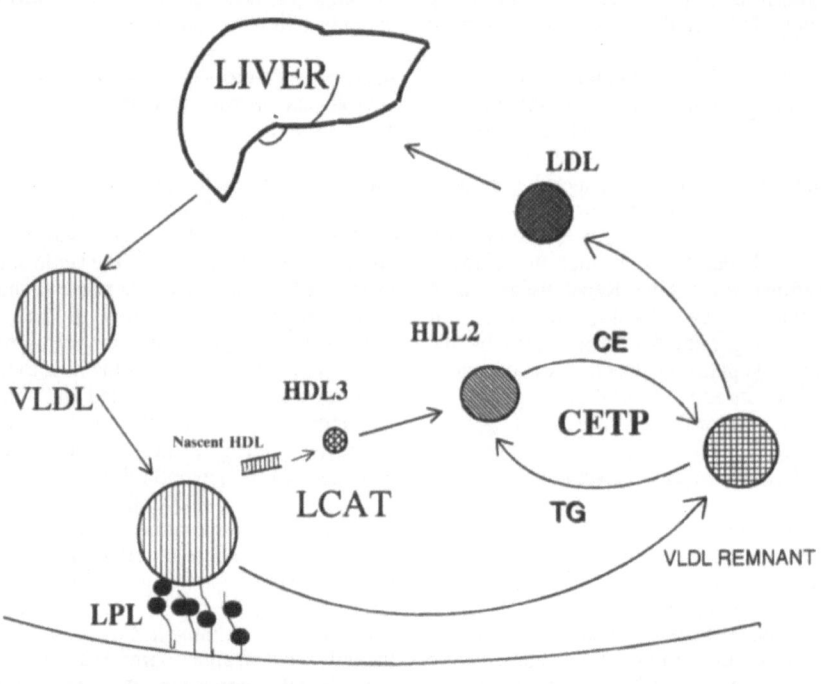

Figure 1. **Metabolism of VLDL.** Very-low-density lipoprotein (VLDL) is secreted by the liver and is hydrolyzed on the vascular endothelium by lipoprotein lipase (LPL). LPL (small, filled circles) is bound electrostatically to heparin sulfate and, in the presence of apo C-II, hydrolyzes triglycerides (TG), thereby releasing free fatty acids, monoglycerides, and diglycerides for cellular uptake. Other surface constituents of VLDL, free cholesterol, and phospholipids participate in the formation of nascent HDL. The free cholesterol on the surface of nascent HDL is esterified by the action of lecithin cholesterol ester transferase (LCAT) to produce cholesterol esters. These sink into the core as nascent HDL is metabolized to the small, dense HDL_3, and finally into the cholesterol ester-(CE-) rich HDL_2. The relatively TG-depleted VLDL remnant particle is released from the endothelial surface and then either is taken up by the liver directly via the remnant receptor or interacts with CE-rich HDL_2. In that interaction, catalyzed by cholesterol ester transfer protein (CETP), the CE-rich core of HDL_2 is exchanged for the TG-rich core of the VLDL remnant, yielding a TG-rich HDL molecule (not shown) and LDL. The latter is then taken up by the liver through the LDL receptor, and the former is processed by lipases to HDL_3 to continue the cycle.

responsible for increased plasma CETP levels in nephrotic patients is unknown.

Plasma LCAT activity has been found to be increased in the plasma of patients with the nephrotic syndrome when measured in assays using excess exogenous substrate (69). HDL free-cholesterol content was inversely related to LCAT activity. ACE inhibition resulted in a 40% reduction of proteinuria, a partial normalization of LCAT activity, and a decrease in VLDL and LDL cholesterol. LCAT activity is also increased in the rat when similar assay conditions are used (70). These findings are opposite to those of Sestack et al. (71). Differences may be explained by the different assay conditions used, but the physiologic consequences of these studies depend upon the specific reaction catalyzed by LCAT in vivo. The protein LCAT catalyzes two separate reactions: the transfer of an acyl group, usually arachidonic acid, to free cholesterol, increasing the cholesterol ester content of HDL, and the lysolecitin acyltransferase (LAT) reaction, which takes place on LDL. Sestack et al. found that while esterified cholesterol correlated positively with LCAT activity in normal rats, it correlated negatively in nephrotic animals, suggesting that increases of the enzyme in vivo may increase the LAT rather than the LCAT reaction (71).

The observation that HDL_3 is preserved in plasma in nephrotic patients at the apparent expense of HDL_2 suggests that the LCAT reaction is reduced in nephrotic patients. However, this pattern of HDL distribution could also be explained by increased activity of CETP rapidly cycling the core of HDL_2 to VLDL remnant particles, thus increasing the flux of cholesterol from the surface of nascent HDL into the core of LDL by increased activities of both enzymes (Figure 1). This model would also clarify the HDL pattern in rats with the nephrotic syndrome characterized by increased HDL_2 and also the HDL pattern of an even larger variety, HDL_1, found in humans to only a limited extent. Rats lack CETP, and thus the cycle would be interrupted. Against this explanation is the observation by Warwick that the transition of apo B from VLDL to LDL is impeded in nephotic humans (72). At this time, it is unclear whether the LCAT reaction is indeed increased in the forward direction in the nephrotic syndrome.

Decreased lipoprotein catabolism

Chylomicrons are synthesized in the gut and VLDLs in the liver. Both are catabolized on the vascular endothelium by LPL. The nascent chylomicrons and VLDLs are decorated with a series of apolipoproteins by interacting with HDL, specifically with HDL_2. Of these apolipoproteins, apo C-II is a necessary cofactor for LPL activity, and apo C-III is a competitive inhibitor (73). Thus, the interaction between properly functioning HDL and both chylomicrons and VLDL and the relative amounts of apo C-II and apo C-III are critically important determinants of the rate of lipolysis of these lipoproteins on the vascular endothelium in the presence of LPL.

Once the action of LPL is completed, remnant particles enriched in cholesterol and apolipoproteins are released. The chylomicron remnant particles are immediately catabolized by the liver (74). This process is impaired in the livers of nephrotic rats (75), although the mechanism has not been clarified. VLDL remnants may also be taken up immediately, and may also be further processed to LDL by the enzymatic action of CETP through interaction with HDL. These processes also are impaired in the nephrotic syndrome (72).

The rate of catabolism of triglyceride-laden lipoproteins, CMs and VLDLs, is greatly reduced in the nephrotic syndrome (76). The clearance of CM and VLDL is delayed in nephrotic rats (76,77). Garber et al. (52) found that LPL activity was reduced in nephrotic rats and suggested that reduction in LPL activity was responsible for incomplete conversion of VLDL to IDL and LDL and reduced transfer of lipids to HDL. Uptake of triglycerides is reduced to about 30% of normal in all organs (75), even in the heart, reported to have normal levels of LPL activity (77). We found that while catabolism of CM by hearts isolated from nephrotic rats is decreased in vitro, the LPL pool bound to the vascular endothelium was reduced by approximately 90%, while LPL activity not bound to the vascular endothelium, and hence unable to interact with large lipoproteins, was normal (75). Thus, specific reduction of LPL attached to the vascular endothelium may play a role in the reduced catabolism of VLDL and CM in the nephrotic syndrome (78).

The relationship between reduced endothelial-bound LPL activity and reduced catabolism of CM and VLDL is by no means an open-and-shut story. Furukawa found that HDL isolated from normal animals corrects defective catabolism of VLDL isolated from nephrotic rats by LPL in vitro (79), while HDL isolated from nephrotic rats did not. Davies reported that VLDL and CM catabolism by analbuminemic rats was normal, despite a marked reduction in heparin-releasable LPL activity (76). Thus, multiple separate defects in the peripheral catabolism of triglyceride-rich lipoproteins may be responsible for delayed clearance of these particles from the circulation.

Studies in patients with the nephrotic syndrome have not been as detailed as in the rat. However, when comparable studies are evaluated, both species exhibit similar disturbances in lipid metabolism. The fractional turnover rate of triglycerides is reduced in nephrotic subjects compared to controls and the $t\frac{1}{2}$ of triglyceride is prolonged from 4 to 11 hours in VLDL (59). Not only is VLDL catabolism decreased but also the disappearance curve has an unusual shape, presumed to result from a delay in the conversion of VLDL to IDL (80).

The delay in lipolysis in humans, as in rats, is proposed to be due to a decrease in LPL activity. Evidence supporting this hypothesis is that LPL activity is reduced in children with the nephrotic syndrome and increases after remission. Furthermore, there is a tight inverse correlation between LPL and the concentration of triglycerides in the VLDL fraction (81). It should be noted that not all investigators find a decrease in LPL activity in nephrotic patients (82). These same investigators (72), however, find a decrease in the rate of apo-B transfer from VLDL$_1$ to VLDL$_2$ and subsequently to IDL and conclude that decreased peripheral catabolism and hepatic removal of apo-B-rich lipoproteins is as important as their increased synthesis in establishing their increased levels in plasma of nephrotic patients.

Although total plasma apo C-II is raised in nephrotic patients, the amount of this LPL cofactor per unit of VLDL is reduced by more than 50%, since the total amount of VLDL is increased more than is total apo C-II (83). These findings are similar to those described in rats (58). Chylomicron metabolism has not been studied in human nephrotic syndrome. However, the fractional rate of disappearance of Intralipid, a surrogate for CMs administered intravenously, is lower in nephrotic patients than in healthy controls (84).

Although the delayed catabolism of triglycerides and the triglyceride-rich lipoproteins has been very well established, much less is known about the catabolism of cholesterol and cholesterol-rich lipoproteins. LDL catabolism has been reported to be either normal or reduced (60) in patients with the nephrotic syndrome and only marginally reduced in nephrotic rats (57). LDL is not the principal cholesterol-bearing lipoprotein in rats, however. That function is carried out by HDL. The catabolism of the protein moieties, apo A-I and apo C, is reduced in HDL by 50% in nephrotic rats (85) irrespective of whether the HDL is derived from normal or from nephrotic rats. Nothing, however, is known about the fate of cholesterol in HDL in the nephrotic syndrome.

TREATMENT OF HYPERLIPIDEMIA

Treatment of the nephrotic syndrome should primarily be directed at 1) treating the primary renal disease, if possible, and 2) using nonspecific treatments to reduce proteinuria. If the primary mechanism causing the nephrotic syndrome can be directly treated—with the use of glucocorticoids for the treatment of minimal-change nephrotic syndrome, for example—then treatment of hyperlipidemia is of limited clinical utility. If the primary disease process causing the nephrotic syndrome is untreatable, and proteinuria is anticipated to be prolonged, specific therapy should be directed at reducing markedly elevated blood lipid levels.

Proteinuria predicts a bad renal outcome in a variety of diseases that cause the nephrotic syndrome. Microalbuminuria predicts progression of renal disease in diabetic patients (86), and the combination of microalbuminuria and hypercholesterolemia predicts the development of atherosclerosis (87). While treatment of microalbuminuria would not be anticipated to alter blood lipid levels, if a component of the dyslipidemia of the nephrotic syndrome is a consequence either of a liporegulatory substance lost in the urine or of the synthesis of an inhibitor of lipid metabolism by the proteinuric kidney, then a significant reduction in urinary protein excretion should result in decreased blood lipid levels. Indeed, this is the case.

Treatment of nephrotic patients with either ACE inhibitors (88) or cyclooxygenase inhibitors (89,90) results in a decline in both proteinuria and blood lipid levels (69) even if plasma albumin concentration does not increase (91) or increases only slightly (92). The decline in blood lipid levels includes a decrease in total cholesterol, Lp(a) (92), a decrease in VLDL and LDL cholesterol, and a decrease in the activities of CETP and LCAT (69). The effect of ACE inhibitors is a class effect and appears to be shared by all drugs within this class.

ACE inhibitors have been shown to reduce the rate of progression of renal disease in animals with a variety of renal lesions (93) and, more significantly, in patients with diabetic renal disease (94,95). This effect is greater than can be accounted for by their antihypertensive action alone and is due to either their inhibition of generation of angiotensin-II or their effect on the kinin system or both. For this reason alone, treatment with an ACE inhibitor is preferred to treatment with a cyclooxygenase inhibitor in the effort to control proteinuria.

As with ACE inhibitors, treatment with cyclooxygenase inhibitors may cause hyperkalemia (96), especially in patients with diabetic renal disease and patients with underlying hyperkalemia. The decrease in GFR caused by these agents may also limit their utility. Unlike ACE inhibitors, cyclooxygenase inhibitors are likely to increase renal sodium retention, potentially worsening edema formation or increasing the need for diuretic therapy (97). Treatment of nephrotic patients with an ACE inhibitor and a cyclooxygenase inhibitor simultaneously may be clinically hazardous, resulting in a marked decrease in GFR and in hyperkalemia. Other potential risks of cyclooxygenase inhibition include acute renal failure and interstitial nephritis, in addition to gastrointestinal disturbances. Furthermore, cyclooxygenase inhibitors will accentuate renal sodium retention and can produce gastrointestinal bleeding. For this reason, cyclooxygenase inhibitors are not the agent of choice.

ACE inhibitors should be started with a low dose (6.25–12.5 mg of captopril or 2.5–5 mg of enalapril, for example). Blood pressure should be checked within 24 hours to make certain that the decline in pressure is not clinically unacceptable, as might occur with renal artery stenosis. Renal function and serum potassium should be evaluated within a week of initiation of therapy, and blood count (white blood cells) should be checked within a month. If renal function remains stable, the ACE inhibitor should be increased until mean arterial pressure decreases by 10 mmHg.

Urinary protein excretion declines gradually, even if the

fall in blood pressure is abrupt. Urinary protein excretion should be checked at the end of the first month of therapy. If urinary protein excretion has not decreased, or if there has been no effect on blood pressure, an effect may be elicited by either further restricting dietary sodium or adding a diuretic. If there is no effect of high doses of an ACE inhibitor on either blood pressure or on proteinuria, even after sodium restriction and/or the use of loop diuretics, the ACE inhibitor should be discontinued.

Dietary treatment

DIETARY PROTEIN

High-protein diets should not be prescribed for adult patients with the nephrotic syndrome in an attempt to repair depleted albumin stores (98). Since dietary protein augmentation causes an increase in urinary albumin excretion (99,100) and albumin synthesis rate, a high-protein diet may actually cause a decrease in serum albumin concentration (4). Therefore, diets that provide more than the recommended daily allowance for protein of 0.8 g/kg are probably contraindicated. The composition of the diet—specifically, the type of protein provided by the diet—may also be of significance. The ability of high-protein diets to increase urinary albumin excretion in the rat is a consequence of only a few of the amino acids. The branch chain amino acids (101)—arginine, proline, aspartate, and glutamate, for example—affect on urinary albumin excretion (102). Several laboratories have shown that diets composed essentially of vegetable proteins cause a reduction in urinary protein excretion when compared to isonitrogenous diets composed of a mixture of foods including animal protein (103–106). Patients receiving the soy protein diet also exhibited a decrease in total serum cholesterol, LDL-cholesterol, and apo B. It is not clear whether the reduction in blood lipids was a consequence of a reduction in dietary lipid intake or instead a consequence of reduced urinary protein excretion.

DIETARY FAT

It is probably prudent to restrict dietary cholesterol and saturated lipids in patients with the nephrotic syndrome. It is indeed possible that the changes in lipoprotein levels that follow consumption of a soy protein diet are a consequence of the lipid composition of the diet, rather than of the amino acid composition. It is unlikely however, that changes in urinary protein excretion are a consequence of changes in plasma lipoprotein levels. Indeed, with the exception of one study without contemporaneous time controls (107), reduction in blood lipid levels in patients with the nephrotic syndrome is without effect in urinary protein losses. The decrease in blood lipid levels reported by D'Amico and coworkers is also beyond that generally encountered by consumption of a low fat diet alone (108),

and perhaps is a consequence of the type of lipids provided in the vegetarian diet.

FISH OILS

Glomerular blood flow, and as a consequence hydraulic pressure, is regulated in part by the interplay between locally produced vasoconstrictors and vasodilators. Prostaglandins are among the more important of these autocoids. Both the vasodilatory PGE_2 and $PGF_2\alpha$ and the vasoconstrictor thromboxane A_2 (TxA_2) are products of metabolism of arachadonic acid, an omega-6 polyunsaturated fatty acid (PUFA).

Lipids derived from marine sources are enriched with omega-3 PUFA (e.g., eicosapentaenoic acid (EPA)), while those derived from vegetable oils are enriched with omega-6 PUFA (e.g., arachidonic acids (AAs)) (109). The effect of dietary supplementation with PUFA, particularly fish oil, has been studied in a variety of experimental models of renal disease, including the nephrotic syndrome (110–113). EPA competes with AA as a substrate for cyclooxygenase and lipooxygenase. Cyclooxygenase converts AA and EPA to the diene (e.g, PGI_2, TXA_2) and triene (e.g, PGI_3, TXA_3) metabolites, respectively (114,115). Lipooxygenase converts AA and EPA to the four and five series of leukotrienes, respectively (116,117). TXA_2, an AA metabolite, is a potent vasoconstrictor, while TXA_3, a metabolite of EPA, is biologically inert (118). In contrast, the vasodilators PGI_2 and PGI_3 are equipotent (115). Thus, substitution of EPA for AA in the diet may result in alterations in tissue fatty acid composition and possibly may alter expression of renal injury inasmuch as the balance between vasoconstricting and vasodilating eicosanoids is altered (119,120).

In adriamycin-induced nephrosis in the rat, Ito et al. (121) found that plasma levels of cholesterol and triglycerides, proteinuria, and serum creatinine were significantly lower in rats fed fish oil than in rats fed beef tallow. Glomerular hyalinosis and endothelial swelling were also less in the rats fed fish oil, and these changes correlated with the changes in plasma concentration of triglyceride and cholesterol.

In a subsequent study (122) utilizing the same model, these investigators found that dietary fish oil supplementation induced a dose-dependent reduction in glomerular synthesis of the dienoic eicasanoids, PGE_2, 6-keto-$PGF_1\alpha$ (a stable metabolite of PGI_2), and TXB_2. Fish oil also decreased the generation of TXB_2 from platelets. In further studies in rats with nephrotic syndrome induced by low-dose adriamycin, Barcelli et al. (123) reported that dietary supplementation with fish oil as a source of omega-3 PUFA, evening primrose oil as a source of omega-6 PUFA, or a mixture of both reduced plasma triglyceride and cholesterol levels compared to those in rats fed beef tallow. The fatty acid composition of the kidney was also different in each dietary group of rats. However, in this study, neither the magnitude of proteinuria nor the changes in plasma creatinine concentration were affected by dietary fish oil. These studies suggest that alterations in the type of dietary PUFA may alter some manifestation of the nephrotic state; however, these effects are very dependent upon the disease model investigated. For example, fish oil actually accelerates renal damage when fed to rats following partial renal ablation (124).

The effect of fish oil on either renal disease or on the lipid disorders of the nephrotic syndrome are less clear-cut than are the data from experimental animals. While fish oil supplementation lowered serum triglycerides and VLDL cholesterol (125) in patients with systemic lupus, there was no effect on proteinuria or GFR. The addition of fish oil to a soy protein diet had no further effect on proteinuria or on serum triglycerides (104) The long-term effects of dietary supplementation with fish oil in the nephrotic syndrome are as yet unknown; therefore, this diet cannot be recommended for treatment of the nephrotic syndrome except within the context of a controlled investigative trial.

Lipid-lowering agents

If specific therapy for the disease causing the nephrotic syndrome is not available and if hyperlipidemia does not remit after dietary intervention and reduction in proteinuria with an ACE inhibitor, then increased lipid levels can be treated with specific lipid-lowering agents. A variety of lipid-lowering agents have proved useful in treatment of hyperlipidemia in the nephrotic syndrome.

The 3-hydroxy-3-methylglutaryl coenzyme A reductase (HMG CoA reductase) inhibitors have proved especially useful. Treatment with pravastatin caused an approximately 28% reduction in cholesterol and a 31% reduction in triglycerides in a group of 11 severely hyperlipidemic patients with the nephrotic syndrome (126). The decrease in cholesterol was essentially entirely due to a decrease in LDL cholesterol, resulting in a decrease in the HDL:LDL cholesterol ratio.

Similar results have been obtained with simvastatin (127) and lovastatin (108,128,129). The use of these agents may engender some morbidity (such as rhabdomyolysis with lovastatin (130), especially in combination with gemfibrozil (131)). Serum lipid levels should be monitored, and patients should also be followed for evidence of rhabdomyolysis.

Although HMG CoA reductase inhibitors lower serum cholesterol, this reduction may not be the mechanism whereby these agents reduce the progression of renal disease in experimental animals. 3-Hydroxy-3-methylglutaryl coenzyme A reductase is the rate-limiting enzyme necessary for the synthesis of mevalonic acid. Mevalonic acid, in turn, is necessary for the growth of eukaryotic cells. Mevalonate is necessary not only for the synthesis of cholesterol but also for the synthesis of a group of nonsteroid compounds, including farnesyl. O'Donnell and

coworkers found that while lovastatin inhibited the growth of cultured mesangial cells, this effect could be overcome with either mevalonate or farnesyl but not with LDL or cholesterol, suggesting that this class of drugs may have a direct antiproliferative effect on glomerular cells independent of their ability to lower serum cholesterol levels (132,133).

ANTIOXIDANTS

Antioxidants such as probucol (134,135) have proved useful in lowering serum cholesterol and ameliorating the progression of renal diseases in the rat. Probucol reduced both LDL and total serum cholesterol in nephrotic patients (136–139) and also tends to lower HDL cholesterol. Its effects in ameliorating disease in animal models may be due to its antioxidant effects (140). LDL cholesterol is taken up both through the regulated LDL receptor-mediated pathway and, in its oxidized form, through a scavenger pathway. The latter pathway is not downregulated by increased intracellular cholesterol. Thus, oxidized LDL presents a much more significant danger to cells, since excessive cholesterol may be endocytosed, resulting in cell damage or death.

Reduction in cholesterol level is less than that reported with HMG CoA reductase inhibitors (138,141).

FIBRIC ACID DERIVATIVES

Fibric acids, such as gemfibrozil (142) have been reported to reduce triglycerides by as much as 50% when used in conjunction with colestipol. Although the fibric acids will lower triglyceride levels in nephrotic patients, they are not effective in lowering cholesterol levels (143). When used in combination with other lipid-lowering agents, these drugs have also been associated with myositis (131). Use of these drugs in the presence of renal failure may also predispose to muscle damage (144).

BILE ACID-BINDING RESINS

The bile acid sequestrants colestipol and cholestyramine bind bile acids in the gut and deplete the hepatic cholesterol pool, thus inducing LDL hepatocyte receptors. Recent studies showed a reduction of total cholesterol of 8%–20% and a reduction of LDL cholesterol of 19%–31% without significant changes in HDL cholesterol.

SUMMARY

Hyperlipidemia in the nephrotic syndrome is a consequence of increased synthesis and decreased catabolism of lipoproteins. LDL, IDL, atherogenic remnants of chylomicrons, and VLDL catabolism increase in plasma. The LDL:HDL ratio is increased. Platelet aggregability is also increased, as is the concentration of the especially atherogenic lipoprotein Lp(a). Changes in lipoprotein concentration and composition should put patients at increased risk of atherosclerotic disease, and this effect most likely is the case. In addition, hyperlipidemia may play a role in the progression of renal disease. For these reasons, it would be unwise not to treat hyperlipidemia if it persists in a patient with the nephrotic syndrome.

Most of the lipid disorders improve when urinary protein excretion is reduced. This reduction can most easily be accomplished with an ACE inhibitor. Although restriction in dietary fat is the first line of therapy for patients with hyperlipidemia of other causes, there is as yet no agreement on the nutritional management of hyperlipidemia in nephrotic patients. Unlike the situation with other hyperlipidemic patients, attention must be paid to dietary protein intake in nephrotic patients due to the potential deleterious effect of dietary protein on the course of progressive renal disease. Vegetarian soy diets have been found useful in reducing both blood lipid levels and proteinuria. The most prudent suggestion for dietary manipulation at this time is to avoid dietary protein supplementation, to choose a protein intake of approximately 0.8 g/kg, and to reduce dietary cholesterol and saturated fatty acids.

If hyperlipidemia persists despite dietary management and treatment with an ACE inhibitor, a group of lipid-lowering agents are useful. Of these, the HMG CoA reductase inhibitors have proved to be most effective, although significant reduction in blood lipid levels has been reported with all classes of lipid-lowering agents.

ACKNOWLEDGMENT

This work was supported in part by the research service of the United States Department of Veterans Affairs and in part by a grant from the National Institutes of Health RO1 DK 42297.

REFERENCES

1. Earley LE, Farland M: Nephrotic syndrome. In: MB Strauss, LG Welt, eds, *Diseases of the Kidney*, 3rd ed. Little, Brown, Boston, pp 765–813, 1979.
2. Earley LE, Havel RJ, Hopper J, Graus H: Nephrotic syndrome. *Calif Med* 115:23–41, 1971.
3. Thomas EM, Rosenblum AH, Lander HB, Fisher R: Relationship between blood lipid and blood protein levels in the nephrotic syndrome. *Am J Dis Child* 81:207–214, 1951.
4. Kaysen GA, Gambertoglio J, Felts J, Hutchison FN: Albumin synthesis, albuminuria and hyperlipidemia in nephrotic patients. *Kidney Int* 31:1368–1376, 1987.
5. Conwill DE, Granger DN, Cook BH, Johnson BB, Taylor AE: The effect of serum oncotic pressure on serum cholesterol levels: a study in "normal" and nephrotic subjects. *South Med J* 70:456–458, 1977.
6. Baxter JH, Goodman HC, Havel RJ: Serum lipid and lipoprotein alterations in nephrosis. *J Clin Invest* 39:455–498, 1960.

7. Nayak SS, Bhaskaranand N, Kamath KS, Baliga M, Venkatesh A, Aroor AR: Serum apolipoproteins A and B, lecithin:cholesterol acyl transferase activities and urinary cholesterol levels in nephrotic syndrome patients before and during steroid treatment. *Nephron* 54:234–239, 1990.
8. Gherardi E, Rota E, Calandra S, Genova R, Tamborino A: Relationship among the concentrations of serum lipoproteins and changes in their chemical composition in patients with untreated nephrotic syndrome. *Eur J Clin Invest* 7:563–570, 1977.
9. Joven J, Villabona C, Vilella E, Masana L, Albertí R, Vallés M: Abnormalities of lipoprotein metabolism in patients with the nephrotic syndrome. *N Engl J Med* 323:579–584, 1990.
10. Antikainen M, Holmberg C, Taskinen MR: Growth, serum lipoproteins and apoproteins in infants with congenital nephrosis. *Clin Nephrol* 38:254–263, 1992.
11. Marshall JF, Apostolopoulos JJ, Brack CM, Howlett GJ: Regulation of apolipoprotein gene expression and plasma high-density lipoprotein composition in experimental nephrosis. *Biochim Biophys Acta* 1042:271–279, 1990.
12. Tarugi P, Calandra S, Chan L: Changes in apolipoprotein A-I mRNA level in the liver of rats with experimental nephrotic syndrome. *Biochim Biophys Acta* 868:51–61, 1986.
13. Sun X, Jones H Jr, Joles JA, Van Tol A, Kaysen GA: Apolipoprotein gene expression in analbuminemic rats and in rats with Heymann nephritis. *Am J Physiol* 262 (*Renal Fluid Electrolyte Physiol* 31):F755–F761, 1992.
14. Muls E, Rosseneu M, Daneels R, Schurgers M, Boelaert J: Lipoprotein distribution and composition in the human nephrotic syndrome. *Atherosclerosis* 54:225–237, 1985.
15. Keane WF, St. Peter JV, Kasiske BL: Is the aggressive management of hyperlipidemia in nephrotic syndrome mandatory? *Kidney Int Suppl* 38:S134–S141, 1992.
16. Moulin P, Appel GB, Ginsberg HN, Tall AR: Increased concentration of plasma cholesteryl ester transfer protein in nephrotic syndrome: role in dyslipidemia. *J Lipid Res* 33:1817–1822, 1992.
17. Kostner GM, Avogaro P, Cazzolato G, Marth E, Bittolo-Bon G, Quinci GB: Lipoprotein Lp(a) and the risk for myocardial infarction. *Atherosclerosis* 38:51–61, 1981.
18. Utermann G: The mysteries of lipoprotein(a). *Science* 246:904–910, 1989.
19. Boerwinkle E, Menzel HJ, Kraft HG, Utermann G: Genetics of the quantitative Lp(a) lipoprotein trait. III. Contribution of Lp(a) glycoprotein phenotypes to normal lipid variation. *Hum Genet* 82:73–78, 1989.
20. Gavish D, Azrolan N, Breslow J: Plasma Lp(a) concentration is inversely correlated with the ratio of kringle IV/kringle V encoding domains in the apo(a) gene. *J Clin Invest* 84:2021–2027, 1989.
21. Karádi I, Romics, L, Pálos G, Doman J, Kaszas I, Hesz A, Kostner GM: Lp(a) lipoprotein concentration in serum of patients with heavy proteinuria of different origin. *Clin Chem* 35:2121–2123, 1989.
22. Short CD, Durrington PN, Mallick NP, Bhatnagar D, Hunt LP, MBewu A: Serum lipoprotein (a) in men with proteinuria due to idiopathic membranous nephropathy. *Nephrol Dial Transplant* 7 (Suppl 1):109–113, 1992.
23. Thomas ME, Freestone A, Varghese Z, Persaud JW, Moorhead JF: Lipoprotein(a) in patients with proteinuria. *Nephrol Dial Transplant* 7:597–601, 1992.
24. Guillausseau P-J, Peynet J, Chanson P, Legrand A, Altman J-J, Poupon J, N'Guyen M, Rousselet F, Lubetzki J: Lipopro-

tein (a) in diabetic patients with and without chronic renal failure. *Diabetes Care* 15:976–979, 1992.

25. Wanner C, Rader D, Bartens W, Kramer J, Brewer HB, Schollmeyer P, Wieland H: Elevated plasma lipoprotein(a) in patients with the nephrotic syndrome. *Ann Intern Med* 119:263–269, 1993.

26. Mallick NP, Short CD: The nephrotic syndrome and ischaemic heart disease. *Nephron* 27:54–57, 1981.

27. Berlyne GM, Mallick NP: Ischemic heart disease as a complication of nephrotic syndrome. *Lancet* 2:399–400, 1969.

28. Ordonez JD, Hiatt RA, Killebrew EJ, Fireman BH: The increased risk of coronary heart disease associated with nephrotic syndrome. *Kidney Int* 44:638–642, 1993.

29. Wass V, Cameron JS: Cardiovascular disease and the nephrotic syndrome: the other side of the coin. *Nephron* 27:58–61, 1981.

30. Zwaginga JJ, Koomans HA, Sixma JJ, Rabelink TJ: Thrombus formation and platelet-vessel wall interaction in the nephrotic syndrome under flow conditions. *J Clin Invest* 93:204–211, 1994.

31. Schmitz PG, Kasiske BL, O'Donnell MP, Keane WF: Lipids and progressive renal injury. *Semin Nephrol* 9:354–369, 1989.

32. Wellman KF, Volk BW: Renal changes in experimental hyper-cholesterolemia in normal and subdiabetic rabbits: I. Short term studies. *Lab Invest* 22:36–48, 1970.

33. Drevon CA, Hoving T: The effects of cholesterol/fat feeding on lipid levels and morphological structures in liver, kidney and spleen in guinea pigs. *Acta Pathol Microb Immunol Scand* 85:1–18, 1977.

34. Al-Shebeb T, Frohlich J, Magil AB: Glomerular disease in hypercholesterolemic guinea pigs: a pathogenetic study. *Kidney Int* 33:498–507, 1988.

35. Kaplan R, Aynedjian HS, Bank N, Schlondorff D: Cholesterol feeding causes renal vasoconstriction via oxidized lipoprotein activation of thromboxane. *Kidney Int* 37:371A, 1990.

36. Moorhead JF, Wheeler DC, Varghese Z: Glomerular structures and lipids in progressive renal disease. *Am J Med* 87:12–20N, 1989.

37. Keane WF, Kasiske BL, O'Donnell MP: Lipids and progressive glomerulosclerosis: a model analogous to atherosclerosis. *Am J Nephrol* 8:261–271, 1988.

38. Grone HJ, Walli AK, Grone E, Kramer A, Clemens MR, Seidel D: Receptor mediated uptake of apo B and apo E rich lipoproteins by human glomerular epithelial cells. *Kidney Int* 37:1449–1459, 1990.

39. Schmitz PG, O'Donnell MP, Kasiske BL, Keane WF: Dietary induced hypercholesterolemia elevates glomerular capillary pressure. *Kidney Int* 35:473A, 1989.

40. Kasiske BL, O'Donnell MP, Cleary MP, Keane WF: Treatment of hyperlipidemia reduces glomerular injury in obese zucker rats. *Kidney Int* 33:667–672, 1988.

41. Diamond JR, Karnovsky MJ: Exacerbation of chronic aminonucleoside nephrosis by dietary cholesterol supplementation. *Kidney Int* 31:671–677, 1987.

42. Hanchak NA, Karnovsky MJ, Diamond JR: Cholestyramine lowers acute and recurrent proteinuria in chronic puromycin aminonucleoside nephrosis. *Kidney Int* 33:376A, 1988.

43. Grond J, Weening JJ, Elema JD: Glomerular sclerosis in nephrotic rat. *Lab Invest* 51:277–285, 1984.

44. Tolins JP, Stone BG, Raij L: Interactions of hyper-cholesterolemia and hypertension in initiation of glomerular injury. *Kidney Int* 41:1254–1261, 1992.

45. Lager DJ, Rosenberg BF, Shapiro H, Bernstein J: Lecithin cholesterol acyltransferase deficiency: ultrastructural examination of sequential renal biopsies. *Mod Pathol* 4:331–335, 1991.

46. Suzaki K, Kobori S, Ueno S, Uehara M, Kayashima T, Takeda H, Fukuda S, Takahashi K, Nakamura N, Uzawa H: Effects of plasmapheresis on familial type III hyperlipoproteinemia associated with glomerular lipidosis, nephrotic syndrome and diabetes mellitus. *Atherosclerosis* 80:181–189, 1990.

47. Dillon JJ: The quantitative relationship between treated blood pressure and progression of diabetic renal disease. *Am J Kidney Dis* 22:798–802, 1993.

48. Haffner SM, Gonzales C, Valdez RA, Mykkanen L, Hazuda HP, Mitchell BD, Monterrosa A, Stern MP: Is microalbuminuria part of the prediabetic state? The Mexico City Diabetes Study. *Diabetologia* 36:1002–1006, 1993.

49. Mulec H, Johnsen SA, Wiklund O, Bjorck S: Cholesterol: a renal risk factor in diabetic nephropathy? *Am J Kidney Dis* 22:196–201, 1993.

50. Marsh JB: Lipoprotein metabolism in experimental nephrosis. *J Lipid Res* 25:1619–1623, 1984.

51. Staprans I, Felts JM, Couser WG: Glycosaminoglycans and chylomicron metabolism in control and nephrotic rats. *Metabolism* 36:496–501, 1987.

52. Garber DW, Gottlieb BA, Marsh JB, Sparks CE: Catabolism of very low density lipo-proteins in experimental nephrosis. *J Clin Invest* 74:1375–1383, 1984.

53. Shafrir E, Brenner T: Lipoprotein lipid and protein synthesis in experimental nephrosis and plasmaphoresis. I. Studies in rat in vivo. *Lipids* 14:695–702, 1979.

54. Brenner T, Shafrir E: Lipoprotein lipid and protein synthesis in experimental nephrosis and plasmapheresis. II. Perfused rat liver. *Lipids* 15:637–643, 1980.

55. Calandra S, Gherardi F, Fainaru M, Guaitani A, Bartosek I: Secretion of lipoproteins, apolipoprotein A-I and apolipoprotein E by isolated and perfused liver of rat with experimental nephrotic syndrome. *Biochim Biophys Acta* 665:331–338, 1981.

56. Marsh JB, Drabkin DL: Experimental reconstruction of metabolic pattern of lipid nephrosis: key role of hepatic protein synthesis in hyperlipemia. *Metabolism* 9:946–955, 1960.

57. Joven J, Masana L, Villabona C, Vilella E, Bargallo T, Trias M, Figueras M, Turner PR: Low density lipoprotein metabolism in rats with puromycin aminonucleoside-induced nephrotic syndrome. *Metabolism* 38:491–495, 1989.

58. Marsh JB, Sparks CE: Hepatic secretion of lipoproteins in the rat and the effect of experimental nephrosis. *J Clin Invest* 64:1229–1237, 1979.

59. Kekki M, Nikkilä EA: Plasma triglyceride metabolism in the adult nephrotic syndrome. *Eur J Clin Invest* 1:345–351, 1971.

60. McKenzie IFC, Nestel PJ: Studies on the turnover of triglyceride and esterified cholesterol in subjects with the nephrotic syndrome. *J Clin Invest* 47:1685–1695, 1968.

61. Vega GL, Grundy SM: Lovastatin therapy in nephrotic hyperlipidemia: effects on lipoprotein metabolism. *Kidney Int* 33:1160–1168, 1988.

62. Warwick GL, Caslake MJ, Boulton-Jones JM, Dagen M, Packard CJ, Shepherd J: Low-density lipoprotein metabolism in the nephrotic syndrome. *Metabolism* 39:187–192, 1990.

63. Pullinger CR, North JD, Teng BB, Rifici VA, Ronhild de Brito AE, Scott J: The apolipoprotein B gene is constitutively expressed in HepG2 cells: regulation of secretion by oleic

acid, albumin, and insulin, and measurement of the mRNA half-life. *J Lipid Res* 30:1065–1977, 1989.

64. Yamauchi A, Yamamoto S, Fukuhara Y, Orita Y, Kamada T, Nogouchi T, Tanaka T: Oncotic pressure regulates the levels of albumin (Alb) mRNA and apolipoprotein B (ApoB) mRNA in cultured rat hepatoma cells (H4IIE) (abstract). *Kidney Int* 35:441A, 1989.

65. Soothill JA, Kark RM: The effects of infusions of salt-poor human serum albumin on serum cholesterol cholinesterase, and albumin levels in healthy subjects and in patients ill with the nephrotic syndrome. *Clin Res Proc* 4:140–141, 1956.

66. Davis RA, Engelhorn SC, Weinstein DB, Steinberg D: Very low density lipoprotein secretion by cultured rat hepatocytes: inhibition by albumin and other macromolecules. *J Biol Chem* 255:2039–2045, 1980.

67. Moberly JB, Cole TG, Alpers DH, Schonfeld G: Oleic acid stimulation of apolipoprotein B secretion from HepG2 and Caco-2 cells occurs post-transcriptionally. *Biochim Biophys Acta* 1042:70–80, 1990.

68. Eisenberg E: High density lipoprotein metabolism. *J Lipid Res* 25:1017–1058, 1984.

69. Dullaart RP, Gansevoort RT, Dikkeschei BD, de Zeeuw D, de Jong PE, Van Tol A: Role of elevated lecithin: cholesterol acyltransferase and cholesteryl ester transfer protein activities in abnormal lipoproteins from proteinuric patients. *Kidney Int* 44:91–7, 1993.

70. Agbedana ED, Yamamoto T, Moriwaki Y, Suda M, Takahashi S, Higashino K: Studies on abnormal lipid metabolism in experimental nephrotic syndrome. *Nephron* 64:256–61, 1993.

71. Sestak TL, Alavi N, Subbaiah PV: Plasma lipids and acyltransferase activities in experimental nephrotic syndrome. *Kidney Int* 36:240–248, 1989.

72. Warwick GL, Packard CJ, Demant T, Bedford DK, Boulton-Jones JM, Shepherd J: Metabolism of apolipoprotein B-containing lipoproteins in subjects with nephrotic-range proteinuria. *Kidney Int* 40:129–138, 1991.

73. Brown WV, Baginsky ML: Inhibition of lipoprotein lipase by an apoprotein of human very low density lipoprotein. *Biochem Biophys Res Commun* 46:375–382, 1972.

74. Felts JM, Itakura H, Crane RT: The mechanism of assimilation of constituents of chylomicrons, very low density lipoproteins and remnants—a new theory. *Biochem Biophys Res Commun* 6:1467–1475, 1975.

75. Kaysen GA, Mehendru L, Pan XM, Staprans I: Both peripheral chylomicron catabolism and hepatic uptake of remnants are defective in nephrosis. *Am J Physiol* 263:F335–F341, 1992.

76. Davies RW, Staprans I, Hutchison FN, Kaysen GA: Proteinuria, not altered albumin metabolism, effects hyperlipidemia in the nephrotic rat. *J Clin Invest* 86:600–605, 1990.

77. Levy E, Ziv E, Bar-On H, Shafrir E: Experimental nephrotic syndrome: removal and tissue distribution of chylomicrons and very-low-density lipoproteins of normal and nephrotic origin. *Biochim Biophys Acta* 1043:259–266, 1990.

78. Kaysen GA, Pan XM, Couser WG, Staprans I: Defective lipolysis persists in hearts of rats with Heymann nephritis in the absence of nephrotic plasma. *Am J Kidney Dis* 22:128–134, 1993.

79. Furukawa S, Hirano T, Mamo JCL, Nagano S, Takahashi T: Catabolic defect of triglyceride is associated with abnormal very-low-density lipoprotein in experimental nephrosis. *Metabolism* 39:101–107, 1990.

80. Vega GL, Grundy SM: Lovastatin therapy in nephrotic hyperlipidemia: effects on lipoprotein metabolism. *Kidney Int* 33:1160–1168, 1988.

81. Yamada M, Matsuda I: Lipoprotein lipase in clinical and experimental nephrosis. *Clin Chim Acta* 30:787–794, 1970.

82. Warwick GL, Packard CJ, Stewart JP, Watson TD, Burns L, Boulton-Jones JM, Shepherd J: Post-prandial lipoprotein metabolism in nephrotic syndrome. *Eur J Clin Invest* 22:813–820, 1992.

83. Kashyap ML, Srivastava LS, Hynd BA, Brady D, Perisutti F, Glueck CJ, Gartside PS: Apolipoprotein CII and lipoprotein lipase in human nephrotic syndrome. *Atherosclerosis* 35:29–40, 1980.

84. Chan MK, Persaud JW, Ramdial L, Varghese Z, Seveny P, Moorhead JF: Hyperlipidemia in untreated nephrotic syndrome, increased production or decreased removal? *Clin Chem Acta* 117:317–323, 1981.

85. Sparks CE, Tennenberg SD, Marsh JB: Catabolism of the apolipoproteins of HDL in control and nephrotic rats. *Biochim Biophys Acta* 665:8–12, 1981.

86. Mogensen CE, Christiansen CE: Predicting diabetic nephropathy in insulin-dependent patients. *N Engl J Med*, 311:89–93, 1984.

87. Tkac I, Molcanyiova A, Tkacova R, Takac M: Levels of cardiovascular risk factors in type 2 diabetes mellitus are dependent on the stage of proteinuria. *J Intern Med* 231(2):109–113, 1992.

88. Don BR, Kaysen GA, Hutchison FN, Schambelan M: The effect of angiotensin-converting enzyme inhibition and dietary protein restriction in the treatment of proteinuria. *Am J Kidney Dis* 17:10–17, 1991.

89. Goldbetz H, Black V, Shemesh O, Myers BD: Mechanism of the antiproteinuric effect of indomethacin in nephrotic humans. *Am J Physiol* 256 (*Renal Fluid Electrolyte Physiol* 25):F44–F51, 1989.

90. Gansevoort RT, Heeg JE, Vriesendorp R, de Zeeuw D, de Jong PE: Antiproteinuric drugs in patients with idiopathic membranous glomerulopathy. *Nephrol Dial Transplant* 7 (Suppl 1):91–96, 1992.

91. Kaysen GA, Don B, Schambelan M: Proteinuria, albumin synthesis and hyperlipidaemia in the nephrotic syndrome. *Nephrol Dial Transplant* 6:141–149, 1991.

92. Keilani T, Schlueter WA, Levin ML, Batlle DC: Improvement of lipid abnormalities associated with proteinuria using fosinopril, an angiotensin-converting enzyme inhibitor. *Ann Intern Med* 118:246–254, 1993.

93. Zatz R, Dunn RB, Meyer TW, Anderson S, Rennke HG, Brenner BM: Prevention of diabetic glomerulopathy by pharmacological amelioration of glomerular capillary hypertension. *J Clin Invest* 77:1925–1930, 1986.

94. Bain R, Rohde R, Hunsicker LG, McGill J, Kobrin S, Lewis EJ: A controlled clinical trial of angiotensin-converting enzyme inhibition in type I diabetic nephropathy: study design and patient characteristics. The Collaborative Study Group. *J Am Soc Nephrol* 3 (Suppl):S97–S103, 1992.

95. Lewis EJ, Hunsicker LG, Bain RP, Rohde RD: The effect of angiotensin-converting-enzyme inhibition on diabetic nephropathy. *N Engl J Med* 329:1456–1462, 1993.

96. Tan SY, Shapiro R, Franco R, Stockard H, Mulrow PJ: Indomethacin-induced prostaglandin inhibition with hyperkalemia. *Ann Intern Med* 90:783–785, 1979.

97. Tiggeler RGWL, Koene RAP, Wijdeveld PGAB: Inhibition of furosemide-induced natriuresis by indomethacin in pa-

tients with the nephrotic syndrome. *Clin Sci Mol Med* 52:149–152, 1977.

98. Kaysen GA, Gambertoglio J, Jiminez I, Jones H, Hutchison FN: Effect of dietary protein intake on albumin homeostasis in nephrotic patients. *Kidney Int* 29:572–577, 1986.

99. Keutmann EH, Bassett SH: Dietary protein in hemorrhagic Bright's disease. II. The effect of diet on serum proteins, proteinuria and tissue proteins. *J Clin Invest* 14:871–888, 1935.

100. Peters JP, Bulger HA: The relation of albuminuria to protein requirement in nephritis. *Arch Intern Med* 37:153–185, 1926.

101. Kaysen GA, al-Bander H, Martin VI, Jones H Jr, Hutchison FN: Branched-chain amino acids augment neither albuminuria nor albumin synthesis in nephrotic rats. *Am J Physiol* 260:R177–R184, 1991.

102. Kaysen GA, Martin VI, Jones H Jr: Arginine augments neither albuminuria nor albumin synthesis caused by high-protein diets in nephrosis. *Am J Physiol* 263:F907–914, 1992.

103. Barsotti G, Morelli E, Cupisti A, Bertoncini P, Giovannetti S: A special, supplemented "vegan" diet for nephrotic patients. *Am J Nephrol* 11:380–385, 1991.

104. D'Amico G, Gentile MG: Influence of diet on lipid abnormalities in human renal disease. *Am J Kidney Dis* 22:151–157, 1993.

105. D'Amico G, Gentile MG: Effect of dietary manipulation on the lipid abnormalities and urinary protein loss in nephrotic patients. *Miner Electrolyte Metab* 18:203–206, 1992.

106. D'Amico G, Gentile MG, Manna G, Fellin G, Ciceri R, Cofano F, Petrini C, Lavarda F, Perolini S, Porrini M: Effect of vegetarian soy diet on hyperlipidaemia in nephrotic syndrome. *Lancet* 339(8802):1131–1134, 1992.

107. Rabelink AJ, Hene RJ, Erkelens DW, Joles JA, Koomans HA: Partial remission of nephrotic syndrome in patients on long-term simvastatin. *Lancet* 335:1045–1046, 1990.

108. Kasiske BL, Velosa JA, Halstenson CE, La Belle P, Langendorfer A, Keane WF: The effects of lovastatin in hyperlipidemic patients with the nephrotic syndrome. *Am J Kidney Dis* 15:8–15, 1990.

109. Moncada S, Flower R, Vane JR: Prostaglandins, prostacyclin, thromboxane A2 and leukotrienes. In: AG Gilman, LS Goodman, TW Rall, F Murad, eds, *The Pharmacological Basis of Therapeutics*. McMillan, New York, pp 660–673, 1985.

110. Sinclair HM: Essential fatty acids in perspective. *Hum Nutr Clin Nutr* 38:245–260, 1984.

111. Klahr S, Buerkert J, Purkerson ML: Role of dietary factors in the progression of chronic renal disease. *Kidney Int* 24:579–587, 1983.

112. Prickett JD, Robinson DR, Steinberg AD: Dietary enrichment with the polyunsaturated fatty acids eicosapentaenoic acid prevents proteinuria and prolongs survival in NZBxNZWf1 mice. *J Clin Invest* 68:556–559, 1981.

113. Scharschmidt LA, Gibbons NB, McGarry L, Berger P, Axelord M, Janis R, Ko YH: Effects of dietary fish oil on renal insufficiency in rats with subtotal nephrectomy. *Kidney Int* 32:700–709, 1987.

114. Zoja C, Benigni A, Verroust P, Ronco P, Bertani T, Remuzzi G: Indomethacin reduces proteinuria in passive heymann nephritis in rats. *Kidney Int* 31:1335–1343, 1987.

115. Culp BR, Titus BG, Lands WEM: Inhibition of prostaglandin biosynthesis by eicosapentaenoic acid. *Prostaglandin Med* 3:269–278, 1979.

116. Remuzzi G, Imberti L, Rossini M, Morelli C, Carminati C,

117. Cattaneo GM, Bertani T: Increased glomerular thromboxane synthesis as a possible cause of proteinuria in experimental nephrosis. *J Clin Invest* 75:94–101, 1985.

117. Spector AA, Kaduce TL, Figard PH, Norton KC, Hoak JC, Czervionke RL: Eicosapentaenoic acid and prostaglandin production by cultured human endothelial cells. *J Lipid Res* 24:1595–1604, 1983.

118. Needleman P, Raz A, Minkes MS, Ferrendelli JA, Sprecher H: Triene prostaglandins: prostacyclin and thromboxane biosynthesis and unique biological properties. *Proc Natl Acad Sci USA* 76:944–948, 1979.

119. von Schaky C, Fischer S, Weber PC: Long-term effects of dietary marine -3 fatty acids upon plasma and cellular lipids, platelet function, and eicosanoid formation in humans. *J Clin Invest* 76:1626–1631, 1985.

120. Higgs GA: The effects of dietary intake of essential fatty acids on prostaglandin and leukotriene synthesis. *Proc Nutr Soc* 44:181–187, 1985.

121. Ito Y, Yamashita W, Barcelli U, Pollak V: Dietary fat in experimental nephrotic syndrome: beneficial effects of fish oil on serum lipids and, indirectly, on the kidney. *Life Sci* 40:2317–2324, 1987.

122. Ito Y, Barcelli U, Yamashita W, Weiss W, Glas-Greenwalt P, Pollak V: Fish oil has beneficial effects on lipids and renal disease of nephrotic rats. *Metabolism* 37:352–357, 1988.

123. Barcelli UO, Beach DC, Thompson M, Weiss M, Pollak VE: A diet containing n-3 and n-6 fatty acids favorably alters the renal phospholipids, eicosanoid synthesis and plasma lipids in nephrotic rats. *Lipids* 23:1059–1063, 1988.

124. Logan JL, Michael UF, Benson B: Dietary fish oil interferes with renal arachidonic acid metabolism in rats: correlations with renal physiology. *Metabolism* 41:382–389, 1992.

125. Clark WF, Parbtani A, Naylor CD, Levinton CM, Muirhead N, Spanner E, Huff MW, Philbrick DJ, Holub BJ: Fish oil in lupus nephritis: clinical findings and methodological implications. *Kidney Int* 44:75–86, 1993.

126. Tokoo M, Oguchi H, Terashima M, Tokunaga S, Miyasaka M, Hora K, Higuchi M, Yoshie T, Furuta S: Effects of pravastatin on serum lipids and apolipoproteins in hyperlipidemia of the nephrotic syndrome. *Nippon Jinzo Gakkai Shi* 34:397–403, 1992.

127. Thomas ME, Harris KP, Ramaswamy C, Hattersley JM, Wheeler DC, Varghese Z, Williams JD, Walls J, Moorhead JF: Simvastatin therapy for hypercholesterolemic patients with nephrotic syndrome or significant proteinuria. *Kidney Int* 44:1124–1129, 1993.

128. Chan PC, Robinson JD, Yeung WC, Cheng IK, Yeung HW, Tsang MT: Lovastatin in glomerulonephritis patients with hyperlipidaemia and heavy proteinuria. *Nephrol Dial Transplant* 7:93–99, 1992.

129. Golper TA, Illingworth DR, Morris CD, Bennett WM: Lovastatin in the treatment of multifactorial hyperlipidemia associated with proteinuria. *Am J Kidney Dis* 13:312–320, 1989.

130. McCorpier CL, Jones PH, Suki WN, Lederer ED, Quinones MA, Schmidt SW, Young JB: Rhabdomyolysis and renal injury with lovastatin use. Report of two cases in cardiac transplant recipients. *JAMA* 260:239–241, 1988.

131. Marais GE, Larson KK: Rhabdomyolysis and acute renal failure induced by combination lovastatin and gemfibrozil therapy. *Ann Intern Med* 112:228–230, 1990.

132. O'Donnell MP, Kasiske BL, Kim Y, Atluru D, Keane WF:

Lovastatin inhibits proliferation of rat mesangial cells. *J Clin Invest* 91:83–87, 1993.

133. O'Donnell MP, Kasiske BL, Kim Y, Atluru D, Keane WF: The mevalonate pathway: importance in mesangial cell biology and glomerular disease. *Miner Electrolyte Metab* 19:173–179, 1993.

134. Modi KS, Schreiner GF, Purkerson ML, Klahr S: Effects of probucol in renal function and structure in rats with subtotal kidney ablation. *J Lab Clin Med* 120:310–317, 1992.

135. Hirano T, Mamo JC, Nagano S, Sugisaki T: The lowering effect of probucol on plasma lipoprotein and proteinuria in puromycin aminonucleoside-induced nephrotic rats. *Nephron* 58:95–100, 1991.

136. Appel GB, Appel AS: Lipid-lowering agents in proteinuric diseases. *Am J Nephrol* 10 (Suppl 1):110–115, 1990.

137. Buckley MM, Goa KL, Price AH, Brogden RN: Probucol. A reappraisal of its pharmacological properties and therapeutic use in hypercholesterolaemia. *Drugs* 37:761–800, 1989.

138. Iida H, Izumino K, Asaka M, Fujita M, Nishino A, Sasayma S: Effect of probucol on hyperlipidemia in patients with nephrotic syndrome. *Nephron* 47:280–283, 1987.

139. Valeri A, Gelfand J, Blum C, Appel GB: Treatment of the hyperlipidemia of the nephrotic syndrome: a controlled trial. *Am J Kidney Dis* 8:388–96, 1986.

140. Carew TE, Schwenke DC, Steinberg D: Antiatherogenic effect of probucol unrelated to its hypocholesterolemic effect: evidence that antioxidants in vivo can selectively inhibit low density lipoprotein degradation in macrophage-rich fatty streaks and slow the progression of atherosclerosis in the Watanabe heritable hyperlipidemic rabbit. *Proc Nat Acad Sci USA* 84:7725–7729, 1987.

141. Kesaniemi YA, Grundy SM: Influence of probucol on cholesterol and lipoprotein metabolism in man. *J Lipid Res* 25:780–790, 1984.

142. Groggel GC, Cheung AK, Ellis-Benigni K, Wilson DE: Treatment of nephrotic hyperlipoproteinemia with gemfibrozil. *Kidney Int* 36:266–271, 1989.

143. Grundy SM, Vega GL: Rationale and management of hyperlipidemia of the nephrotic syndrome. *Am J Med* 87(5N):3N–11N, 1989.

144. Pierides AM, Alvarez-Ude F, Kerr DN: Clofibrate-induced muscle damage in patients with chronic renal failure. *Lancet* 2(7948):1279–1282, 1975.

CHAPTER 50

Cardiovascular Complications in Uremia and Dialysis

MIROSLAW SMOGORZEWSKI

INTRODUCTION

Cardiovascular complications occur frequently in patients with renal disease and are the leading cause of death in patients with end-stage renal disease (ESRD). Cardiac disease accounted for 39% of all deaths in dialysis patients between 1988 and 1990 in the U.S. (1), 37.8% of deaths in Canada (2), and up to 30% in Europe (3). U.S. Renal Data Systems (USRDS) classifies cardiac diseases as a cause of death into three categories: myocardial infarction, pericarditis, and other cardiac causes, with a death rate of 19.9, 1, and 42.4 per 1000 patients per year, respectively, during the period 1988–1990. The category *other cardiac causes* includes congestive heart failure, subacute and chronic ischemic heart disease, cardiomyopathy, arrhythmias, and valvular disease. For all patients between 45 and 65 years of age on dialysis, the death rate from cardiovascular disease was approximately 3.5 times the age-specific rate for the normal population (4).

The presence of cardiac failure, dysrhythmia requiring therapy, and coronary artery disease increased the risk of death within 6 months from the start of maintenance dialysis by a factor of 2.5 (5).

The high incidence of cardiovascular complications can result from cardiac alterations present before ESRD develops and can be linked to primary disease that causes ESRD, as well as to uremia and metabolic disturbance or therapeutic modalities used for its treatment. Diabetic patients with ESRD had a cardiovascular mortality rate two times that of nondiabetic patients (1), and diabetes mellitus is an independent factor for the development of heart failure and coronary artery disease (CAD) in population epidemiological studies (6). Significant CAD was present in 21%–50% of diabetic patients with ESRD, and a high percentage (35%) of those patients had no clinical presentation of the disease (7,8). On the other hand, some diabetic patients with ESRD developed diabetic cardiomyopathy with impaired left ventricular function despite their normal coronary arteries (9).

The factors that contribute to the high cardiovascular morbidity and mortality in uremia patients are summarized in Table 1. Hypertension, either as a primary event or secondary to renal disease and renal failure, accelerates the development of atherosclerosis within coronary vessels and induces hypertrophy of the myocardium. These responses may result in an imbalance between the myocardial oxygen supply and its demand and lead to heart ischemia and complications such as congestive heart failure, arrhythmias, and sudden death (10). Data from the Framingham Study show that the incidence of cardiac endpoints, including coronary heart disease, increases progressively with rising systolic or diastolic pressure or both (11). Mac Mohon et al. reached similar conclusions in their meta-analysis of nine major prospective studies and found that persistent diastolic blood pressure of 5 mmHg is associated with at least a 21% increase in coronary heart disease (12).

Hypertension in patients with ESRD is also strongly associated with increased mortality from cardiac disease (13). The control of blood pressure correlates with the improvement of left ventricular systolic function in patients on chronic dialysis (14).

The pathogenesis of hypertension in chronic renal failure is multifactorial and difficult to define, given the heterogenicity of the patient population (15). There is clearly a relationship between patients' volume status and their blood pressure. In a majority of patients, avoidance of fluid overload will control blood pressure. Furthermore, increased peripheral vascular resistance with or without high output state (14,16), sympathetic overactivity (17), and enhanced reactivity to the pressor mediators such as angiotensin have been noted, as well as derangements in intracellular electrolytes. Multiple other factors also contribute to cardiovascular disease in uremia patients. Correction of anemia by blood transfusion (16) or by treatment with erythropoietin (18–21) reduces cardiac output and improves left ventricular function but can increase peripheral vascular resistance, thereby increasing blood pressure and compromising heart function. Approximately 30% of patients who receive erythropoietin therapy will develop hypertension or will require an increased dose of hypertensive medication.

Chronic excess of intravascular fluid between hemodialysis treatments and inadequate volume removal during

Suki, WN and Massry SG (eds), Suki and Massry's Therapy of Renal Diseases and Related Disorders, Third Edition. ISBN 978-1-4757-6634-9.

Table 1. Factors contributing to the increased incidence of cardiovascular disease in uremia

1. Demographic characteristics of patients with ESRD: age, race, and gender
2. Diseases that cause ESRD: diabetes, essential hypertension, glomerulonephritis, nephrotic syndrome, vasculitis, amyloidosis
3. Uremic syndrome: volume overload, anemia, electrolyte and acid–base alterations, hyperparathyroidism, glucose intolerance and insulin resistance, aluminum toxicity, hyperlipidemia, coagulopathy
4. Dialysis-related factors: hypotension, hypoxemia, hypokalemia and arrhythmia, arteriovenous fistula, dialysis solution component membrane biocompatibility, β_2-microglobulinemia, iron overload
5. Treatment before or during dialysis therapy: steroids, erythropoietin
6. Left ventricular hypertrophy, pericarditis, endocarditis

dialysis increase preload and cardiac work requirements and may contribute to heart hypertrophy.

The introduction of high-flux dialysis with rapid ultrafiltration can lead to hypotension before the dry weight of the patient is achieved due to the delay rate in movement of the fluid from the interstitial and intracellular compartments into the vascular space, compare to rate of fluid rennoval.

Alterations in lipid and carbohydrate metabolism in chronic renal failure may accelerate atherosclerosis (22,23), although clear evidence for accelerated atherosclerosis in ESRD patients is lacking.

Recent analysis (24) supports previous findings (25) that males and whites on dialysis had a higher risk of death due to acute myocardial infarction and other cardiac causes than females and blacks.

Several clinical studies concluded that secondary hyperparathyroidism of chronic renal failure contribute to left ventricular abnormalities (26). Low cardiac output, as well as inadequate left ventricular hypertrophy, correlates with a degree of secondary hyperparathyroidism (27,28) in dialysis patients, and parathyroidectomy was followed by a significant improvement in cardiac function (29). Experimental animal studies in vivo and in vitro, as well as studies with isolated cardiac myocytes, indicate that the heart is a target organ for PTH (26,30). An excess of PTH in chronic renal failure adversely affects myocardial metabolism and function (26). This action of PTH is mediated by a sustained rise in cytosolic calcium of cardiac myocytes both through excess entry of calcium into the cell and through decreased extrusion (31), despite the significant downregulation of the PTH–PTHrP receptor of the heart in uremia (32). The entry of calcium into the myocardium can be prevented by calcium channel blockers. These agents also reduced the metabolic derangements of the heart, despite high circulating PTH (33). Additionally, there is evidence that PTH plays a permissive role in the induction of interstitial fibrosis of the heart with collagen fiber deposition (34). This finding is common in uremia (35), which can be responsible for diastolic dysfunction of the left ventricle.

PERICARDITIS

Pericarditis is the result of inflammation processes of various etiologies of the pericardium. Both parietal pericar-

dium (the fibrous outer coat, covered inside by a serosal layer) and visceral pericardium (the serosal membrane and epicardial surface of the heart) can be involved. The pericardial cavity between the two serosal membranes contains 15–50 mL of the fluid under normal physiological conditions. The stiffness of the parietal pericardium is the limiting factor for the amount of fluid that can be accommodated in the pericardial cavity, especially in the short term, without the compromise of heart function. There is a steep rise in pericardial pressure when the fluid volume acutely exceeds approximately 200 mL. In response to chronic enlargement of the heart or slow accumulation of fluid, the pericardium undergoes hypertrophy and becomes more compliant (36).

Incidence

The incidence of symptomatic pericarditis in the early stages of dialysis therapy was 40%–60% prior to the initiation of dialysis (37,38) and significantly decreased to approximately 10% with the availability of an earlier initiation of dialysis (39–44). The likelihood that a patient on chronic dialysis will develop pericarditis is still around 8%–12% (43,44). This means that pericarditis remains one of the most frequent and potentially life-threatening complications in ESRD patients. It causes death in at least 1% of the dialysis population studied (1) and in up to 10% in some reports (43). Autopsies performed on 106 patients with ESRD who had received dialysis for a mean of 36 months found the frequency of pericarditis to be 33% (45). The incidence of asymptomatic pericardial effusion discovered by echocardiography in uremic patients who are about to initiate dialysis is between 15% and 40%, while in chronically dialyzed patients it is approximately 30% (37,39,42,44).

Pathology and pathogenesis

Table 2 depicts the pathologic features of pericarditis associated with renal failure.

There are some differences between the pathologies of acute pericarditis occurring prior to the initiation of dialysis. Generally, the pericardial fluid tends to be hemorrhagic in dialyzed patients, and hemorrhage in patients with uremic pericarditis is commonly serous but may contain blood. The final evolution of the disease may lead to con-

Table 2. Pathologic findings in uremic pericarditis

Type of pericarditis	Findings
Acute fibrinous or dry pericarditis	Fibrinous deposits with characteristic bread-and-butter appearance
	Thickening of pericardial walls
	Acute inflammation
Acute pericarditis with pericardial effusion	As above plus pericardial effusion: serous, serosanguinous, or hemorrhagic
Subacute constrictive pericarditis	Fibrinous deposits
	Active inflammation
	Vascularization of pericardial walls
	Fibrosis
Chronic constrictive pericarditis	Fibrosis and adhesions of epicardium and pericardial sac

Table 3. Factors contributing to the development of pericarditis in patients with renal failure

1. Late start of dialysis, inadequate dialysis, "uremic toxins"
2. Underlying systemic disorders such as SLE, vasculitis, dermatomyositis, scleroderma
3. Infections: viral, bacterial, fungal, tuberculosis, etc.
4. Electrolyte and fluid disturbances: volume overload, calcium and phosphorous, uric acid
5. Coagulation defects: platelet dysfunction, anticoagulants
6. Drugs: minoxidil, procainamide, hydralazine

strictive pericarditis, with predominant findings of fibrosis and adhesion of both layers of pericardium (46).

A large number of etiologic factors have been postulated in the pathogenesis of uremic pericarditis (Table 3). In uremic patients, pericarditis usually appears when the glomerular filtration rate has dropped below 5 mL/min. In most instances (80%–90%), pericarditis will resolve after initiation of dialysis and infrequently (3%) will progress to cardiac tamponade (43,46). These observations suggest that factors removable by hemodialysis play a role in the pathogenesis of pericarditis. In contrast, when pericarditis appears more than 2 weeks after initiation of chronic dialysis, resolution occurs only in 53% and tamponade in 20% of the patients, despite intensive dialysis therapy, suggesting that nondialyzable factors also contribute to the genesis of pericarditis (43). The incidence of pericarditis is lower in patients on peritoneal dialysis than in those on hemodialysis (47). This finding suggests that factors such as "middle molecules," for which the better clearance is achieved by peritoneal dialysis, may be important in the pathogenesis of pericarditis. Volume overload contributes to pericardial effusion both in predialysis- and dialysis-associated pericarditis; therefore, correction of this abnormality is an essential element of the therapy (39,46,48,49).

The possibility of infectious causes must always be kept in mind when evaluating uremic patients with pericarditis. Uremic patients are immune compromised; they have increased frequency of infection, and their response to systemic or local infection can be abrogated. Fever in excess of 38.5°C and revoked leukocytosis with a shift toward the left should alert the physician to the possibility of either a purulent pericarditis or an infection elsewhere in the body that precipitated the pericarditis. Viral infections such as influenza virus A, Coxsackie virus B, or CMV virus have also been reported in dialysis patients (50,51) and in the early period after kidney transplantation (52). These etiologies should be suspected especially if the pericarditis episodes appear in a cluster (51). Immunological factors have been postulated in two studies (53,54), but it is not clear whether the antibodies of the IgM and IgG classes against sarcolemma were the cause of pericarditis or the consequence of the disease.

Clinical presentation

The major signs and symptoms of uremic pericarditis are summarized in Table 4. Chest pleuropericardial pain is a common (40%–70%) presenting complaint (39,40,55). It is aggravated by breathing or by recumbent position and is relieved by sitting up or by leaning forward. Pericardial friction rub was present in over 75% of patients at the time of admittance and in more than 90% during hospitalization with uremic pericarditis (39,40,55). It indicates pericardial inflammation and usually does not disappear with the accumulation of pericardial fluid. A low-grade fever associated with leukocytosis frequently proceeds pericarditis and was found in 75%–95% of cases. Mental confusion, lethargy, and disorientation have been reported in patients with large pericardial effusion and probably reflects low-cardiac-output syndrome (40). Unexplained increases in heart size, especially in the absence of pulmonary edema, could be a sign of progressive enlarging pericardial effusion. Pericardial effusion without clinical evidence of pericarditis was found in 36% of 50 uremic patients before initiation of dialysis and in approximately 25% of patients during maintenance dialysis (42). Therefore, tests that demonstrate pericardial effusion are consistent with the diagnosis of pericarditis if other clinical features are also present at any time during the disease. The most specific and sensitive test for pericardial effusion is echocardiography (56), which should be performed whenever there is reasonable suspicion of a pericardial disease. Pericardial fluid appears as an echo-free space on the M-mode echocardiogram. A small amount of fluid is usually

Table 4. Clinical features of pericarditis in patients with end-stage renal failure

Timing	Features

1. Prior to the initiation of dialysis	Symptoms
	   Chest pain without exertion, with or without radiation:
	      dyspnea, cough, mental confusion
	Signs
	   Pericardial friction rub
	   Fever
	   Cardiomegaly
	   Pulsus paradoxus
	   Hypotension
	   Jugular vein distension
	   Anasarca, edema, ascites
	   Cardiac arrhythmias
	Laboratory findings
	   Pericardial effusion by echocardiography, changes in
	      EKG (abnormalities in ST–T segment, low voltage)

2. During chronic dialysis	Symptoms and signs can be very similar to the above. Intolerance to ultrafiltration hypotension on dialysis, rapid weight gain

located behind the left ventricular posterior wall, but a larger effusion is associated with an echo-free space in front of the right ventricle. This latter finding is associated with hemodynamic compromise of the heart (43). Two-dimensional echocardiography can further quantitate the amount of fluid, demonstrating fibrinous adhesions and the thickened pericardium (57). Echocardiography of patients with pericardial effusion allows assessment of the size of the cardiac chamber, wall motion, and diastolic filling—findings that are useful in determining whether heart failure or cardiac tamponade is present (57,58). In patients with tamponade, right ventricular collapse and slight atrial diastolic collapse occur in 81% and 88%, respectively. Other findings include abnormal respiratory flow velocities at the mitral valves and tricuspid valves, changes in ventricular dimensions (58), and changes in left atrial and ventricular compression (59). These echocardiographic signs are highly sensitive and specific (56), and they appear when cardiac tamponade is hemodynamically significant and before the pulsus paradoxus or profound hypertension is noticed (60). Computerized tomography and magnetic resonance imaging can even better indicate the presence of chronic pericarditis by identifying the thickened pericardial membrane, adhesions, or calcium deposits in the constrictive pericarditis.

Electrocardiographic changes of acute pericarditis evolve through ST-segment elevation with subsequent return toward isoelectrical status with inverted T waves (61). These changes can be noticed in 10%–40% of patients with uremic pericarditis, reflecting a relative sparing of the epicardium; however, other less specific abnormalities can affect up to 80% of the patients (43,49,55). A decrease in the voltage of the QRS complex in all leads is typical for effusion or pericardial membrane thickening.

Chest x-ray in uremic pericarditis is almost always abnormal, with cardiomegaly present in 90% of the cases. The sudden onset of cardiomegaly is suggestive of pericardial effusion.

Pericardioscopy, a new diagnostic tool, has not been used as yet in patients with uremic pericarditis.

Complications

Table 5 depicts complications that may occur in uremic patients with pericarditis.

Acute pericardial tamponade secondary to pericardial effusion is a life-threatening event. It was reported in approximately 20% of the patients with uremic pericarditis (43).

Diagnosis of tamponade is made by clinical examination that shows elevated systemic venous pressure due to right heart failure, tachycardia, dyspnea, low systemic blood pressure, or the rapid fall of blood pressure with pulsus paradoxus during dialysis. The latter is defined as a systolic blood pressure decline of more than 10 mmHg with inspiration. Frequently, cardiac tamponade occurs immediately after hemodialysis, when fluid removal from the intravascular compartment decrease diastolic filling of the ventricles.

The diagnosis is supported by the echocardiographic changes described above. Rapid increase in heart size on the x-ray in the presence of clear lungs in the clinical setting also suggest tamponade. Cardiac catheterization can be used in questionable cases and will show diastolic equilibration of the intracardiac pressure.

Myocarditis may accompany uremic pericarditis (39,46) and may play a role in the hypotension and cardiac arrhythmias occurring in patients with pericarditis.

Supraventricular arrhythmia has been reported in 27% of ESRD patients with pericarditis, including atrial fibrillation or flutter in 18% and supraventricular tachycardia in 7% (44). Arrhythmia was also common in other studies (39,46,47). The rapid change in the electrolyte composition during hemodialysis and the high incidence of heart diseases other than pericarditis can further contribute to the genesis of arrhythmias.

Constrictive pericarditis may follow pericardial inflammation and should be suspected in dialysis patients who have had pericardial disease, have developed refractory right heart failure, or have difficulties tolerating volume removal during hemodialysis. In chronic cases, the pericardium may be calcified. Cardiac catheterization and angiography can be done to evaluate the severity of constriction, to determine cardiac function and the underlining diseases, and to differentiate these from restrictive cardiomyopathy.

Management

The discussion of treatment of pericarditis will be limited to the uremic causes, since it is obvious that if standard diagnostic evaluation establishes, for example, a specific infectious cause, then the appropriate therapy for that condition must be instituted. The best treatment for uremic

Table 5. Complications of pericarditis in patients with end-stage renal failure

Timing	Complications
Acute	Pericardial tamponade
	Cardiac arrhythmias
	Myocarditis
Chronic	Constriction

pericarditis is prevention. This can be achieved by starting dialysis treatment at the appropriate time during the course of chronic renal failure and by delivery of adequate therapy. Figure 1 depicts the therapeutic approaches to uremic pericarditis. The appearance of pericarditis in patients with ESRD is a clear indication for the initiation of dialysis. These patients generally show an excellent response to dialytic treatment, with approximately 80%–90% showing regression of symptoms (41,43) with daily therapy. In some other studies, however, this response rate was only 50% (42). Dialysis-associated pericarditis or recurrent pericarditis is much more refractory to intensive dialysis. Rutsky and Rostand found that 56% of 123 episodes of dialysis-associated pericarditis did resolve without invasive intervention (43). A course of intensive daily dialysis for 10–14 days is usually used before other steps of therapy are undertaken. Close monitoring during and following dialysis is extremely important, as is careful removal of fluid during each dialysis, since a deterioration of heart hemodynamic and cardiac tamponade may occur with rapid ultrafiltration. The presence of a large pericardial effusion may indicate that intensive dialysis may not be successful.

Tight heparinization and regional heparinization or regional citrate anticoagulation can be used to minimize the chances of intrapericardial bleeding (63,64). If the patient fails to respond within a period of 10–14 days, or if pericardial effusion increases or the patient becomes hemodynamically unstable, then surgical intervention procedures must be undertaken.

There is controversy in the literature as to whether an invasive procedure should be used concomitantly with intensive dialysis for the treatment of pericardial effusion or whether such procedures should be reserved for conditions where the 10–14 days of intensive therapy is not effective. It is also not clear what type of invasive intervention, e.g.,

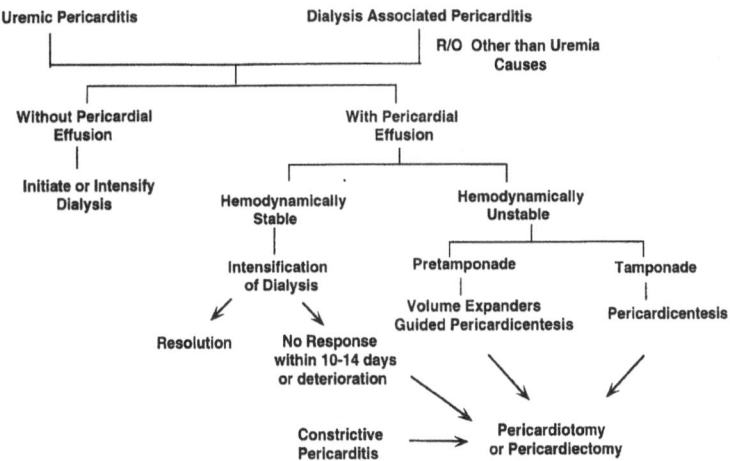

Figure 1. The therapeutic approach to pericarditis in patients with end-stage renal disease.

pericardiocentesis with or without steroid installation (47,66,67,70) or pericardiectomy (68,69,71), is the procedure of choice, since most of these studies are retrospective and lack proper randomization of the patients (43,46,70). The approach presented in Figure 1 is based on the most current experience and seems to be most effective and safe.

Pericardiocentesis is a life-saving procedure if cardiac tamponade occurs but is seldom used alone for treatment of pericardial effusion, since it has a high rate of complications (43,46) and up to a 70% recurrence rate (46). It is recommended to perform pericardiocentesis in the cardiac catheterization laboratory under echocardiographic guidance (72). The combination of pericardiocentesis and catheter installation for drainage or periodic instillation of steroids has been used successfully by some centers (66,67,70) but discouraged by others (73) due to infection complications.

Surgical drainage is performed either by a pericardiotomy through the subxiphoid route or by a pericardiectomy. Pericardiectomy, either parietal for effusion pericarditis only or visceral for those patients with constrictive pericarditis, is the definitive procedure, with a recurrence rate and a mortality rate less than 1% (43). The procedure led to substantial morbidity, however, with pulmonary complications in 19 of 41 patients, cardiac arrhythmias in 8, and hypotension in 8 (43). Pericardiotomy is a less extensive procedure which generates the pericardial window and drains the pericardium. It has a low complication rate and a high success rate (40,43,49), but incomplete drainage and effusion recurrence may require a pericardiectomy.

Nonsteroidal anti-inflammatory agents have been used successfully to relieve the symptoms and to reduce the need for invasive intervention (74), but a better-controlled study showed that except for fever, other pathologies were not affected by indomethacin (75).

Acute pericardial tamponade

The first step in the management of cardiac tamponade is a rapid expansion of the intravascular volume by normal saline, plasma expanders, or blood. If this maneuver establishes hemodynamic stability, then drainage of the effusion can be performed in the optimal conditions of the cardiac catherization laboratory under echocardiographic guidance. Otherwise, pericardiocentesis can be safely performed at the bedside by experienced personnel, especially in patients with massive pericardial effusion (76). Subsequently, one must proceed with a pericardiectomy as a definitive therapy, since otherwise the effusion is very likely to recur and further complicate the patient status.

Pericardiectomy is also the procedure of choice for chronic constrictive pericarditis. Although pericardiectomy provides immediate relief, it is a major procedure with a higher rate of immediate complications, and recent studies also show late complications such as increase in the left ventricular mass and tricuspid regurgitation. For these reasons, subtotal pericardiectomy has been recommended (77).

UREMIC CARDIOMYOPATHY AND HEART FAILURE

Cardiac failure is due to systolic and/or diastolic dysfunction in most cases. The majority of patients with chronic renal failure will have elements of both systolic and diastolic dysfunction. Systolic dysfunction is determined by the contractile state of the myocardium, the preload (described by end-diastolic volume and the length of the myocardial fiber prior to onset of the contraction), the afterload applied to the ventricles, and the heart rate. The diastolic dysfunction is caused by the stiff noncompliance of the left or right ventricle. Both types of dysfunction can result in low cardiac output, high ventricular filling pressure, and eventually congestive failure.

Figure 2 depicts the systolic dysfunction represented by dilating cardiopathy (right panel) and diastolic dysfunction represented by hypertrophic cardiopathy (central panel). The upper set of curves describes the compliance expressed as a relationship between end-diastolic pressure and end-diastolic volume, and the lower set presents the Starling relationship of the stroke work to end-diastolic pressure. Under normal conditions, cardiac work increases as filling volume increases, and the normal compliance curve is such that the filling pressure does not reach "pulmonary edema" level. Pathological hypertrophy or other processes that increase the stiffness of the wall do not change the Starling curve, but an increase in filling volume necessary to increase cardiac work may disproportionately elevate the end-diastolic pressure, since the compliance curve is steeper than in normal subjects. During heat dialation, the starling curve is flat and cardiac work does not increase properly in response to volume (78).

Finally, cardiac function may be above normal but inadequate for the metabolic demands or requirements for blood flow in conditions such as anemia or an arteriovenous fistula.

Incidence

The current prospective study (79) of 433 dialysis patients who have been followed for a mean of 41 months demonstrates that 133 (31%) of the patients had congestive heart failure at the initiation of dialysis and another 25% developed de novo heart failure during dialysis. Seventy-five of the 133 patients with CHF at baseline had recurrent episodes; and during follow-up echocardiographic examination showed systolic dysfunction (left ventricular (LV) ejection fraction ≤ 40% or fractional shortening ≤ 25%) in 33% and LV dyskinesia in 47%. In patients without CHF, only 6.7% had systolic dysfunction, and 11% had LV

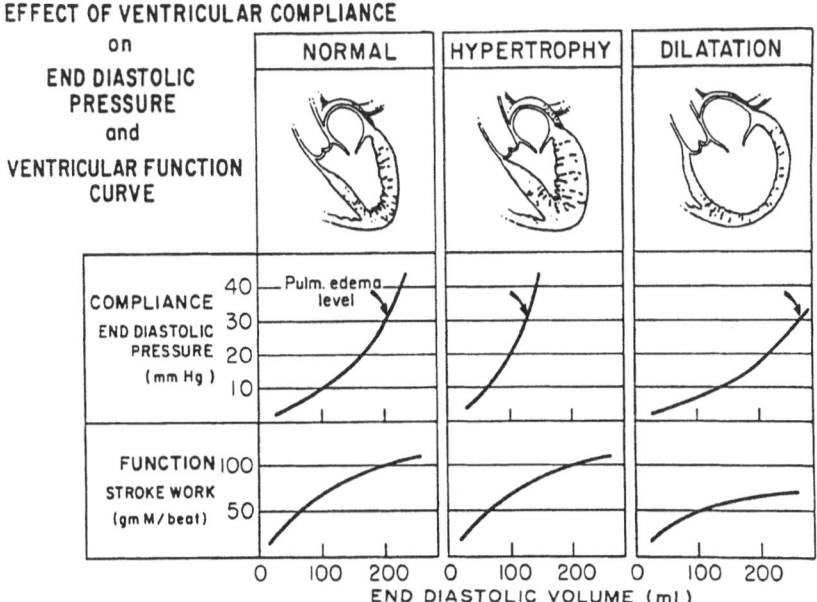

Figure 2. The relationship of end-diastolic filling pressure and end-diastolic volume (upper set of curves) and the Starling relationship (lower set of curves) in normal heart (left panel), heart hypertrophy (center panel), and dilated cardiopathy (right panel). From (78).

dyskinesia. These data are similar to those from smaller studies previously published (80–82).

Etiology

The various factors that contribute to the development of heart failure in uremic patients are depicted in Figure 3. Patients with ESRD develop salt and water retention, which can be controlled by dialysis and diet. Frequently, such control is inadequate, and volume expansion may precipitate CHF (83). Chronic increase in preload due to chronic volume expansion in patients with normal heart increases stroke volume and causes compensatory ventricular dilatation and hypertrophy. Also, in patients on dialysis, LV volume correlates with the blood volume, and ultrafiltration reduces LV size (84,85). Rapid volume expansion, even in patients with normal LV function, may produce pulmonary edema. This outcome is more likely to occur when LV compliance is decreased, as it is in many patients with uremia. In these patients, a small increase in volume may cause a rise in ventricular diastolic pressure and precipitate pulmonary edema.

Volume expansion can also induce hypertension (86); and two of many consequences of hypertension are an increase in coronary artheosclerosis (87,88) and an increase in afterload.

Arteriovenous fistula is an additional burden to the heart, especially in patients with borderline LV performance and high blood flow through the shunt (89–92). An acute effect of occlusion of the fistula resulted in a decrease in the cardiac index and in a mean velocity of fiber shortening (90). In the long term, a decrease in the diameter of the left ventricle was observed (92), as well as an improvement in its contractility after closure of the fistula.

Anemia causes hyperkinetic circulation and contributes to the development of LV hypertrophy (93) and LV enlargement in normotensive patients on hemodialysis (28). Improvement of the anemia by erythropoietin treatment (hematocrit approximately 34%–36%) also decreased elevated cardiac output, cardiac index, and heart rate and increased total peripheral vascular resistance (94,95). Echocardiographic studies performed 24 months after initiation of erythropoetin therapy showed a decrease in LV mass and LV index and improvement in diastolic myocardial function (95). The potential role of secondary hyperparathyroidism has been discussed previously. Diffuse calcification of the myocardium (96–98) and of the mitral or aortic valve (98–100) is related to secondary hyperparathyroidism and a high calcium phosphate product (99,100). These valvular diseases are underrecognized complications of chronic uremia. Recent cross-sectional studies (101) showed by echocardiography that 40 of 62 patients had structural alterations of aortic or mitral valves, with aortic stenosis hemodynamically relevant in 8 patients.

Myocardial calcification and calcified valve lesions may impair LV function (96–98) and induce arrhythmia and heart block.

Carnitine deficiency induced by hemodialysis can con-

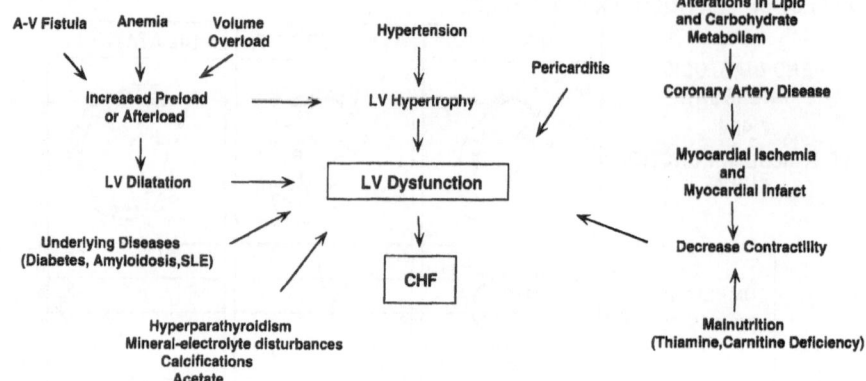

Figure 3. A schematic representation of the major factors in heart failure in patients with chronic renal failure.

tribute to myopathy. Supplementation of carnitine in patients with chronic renal failure produces improvement in LV performance (102).

Left ventricular morphology

In patients on dialysis, left ventricular hypertrophy (LVH) and dilated cardiomyopathy are independent predictors of recurrent or persistent heart failure (81) and long-term survival (103). It is apparent that the assessment of heart morphology is an important part of the diagnostic workup and has an impact on the management of this heart dysfunction. Echocardiography and cardiac Doppler evaluations are most frequently used, since they are easy to obtain, are safe, and provide both anatomical and hemodynamic data. The use of other methods such as radionuclide left ventriculography, MRI, and CT may provide even more accurate information (104). Data from the echocardiographic study of the Framingham population define, in general, four patterns of LVH (105): disproportionate septal asymmetric LVH, concentric LVH, eccentric dilated LVH, and eccentric nondilated LVH. The LVH was classified into concentric and eccentric types by using a relative wall thickness of 45% or more to indicate concentric and less than 45% to define eccentric LVH. Three of these patterns are presented in Figure 4. Since relative wall thickness was found to be inadequate for differentiating various types of LV enlargement, it was proposed to use LV mass and volume indexed to body surface to classify LV geometry (106). The prevalence of LVH using the Framingham echocardiographic criteria was 20% of all adults over the age of 39 years and 17%–42% of those with hypertension (107,108).

The prevalence of LVH is about 60% in ESRD patients (109,110). In a study of 275 dialysis patients by Parfrey et al., mild hypertrophy was present in 33%, severe hypertrophy in 22%, and dilated cardiomyopathy in 9%; only 28% had a normal echocardiogram (111).

Concentric and eccentric hypertrophy are part of the early and late adaptive mechanisms to volume overload and hypertension. The genesis of septal hypertrophy is not well defined. Concentric hypertrophy and septal hypertrophy are the most frequent variants of LVH and were found in 11% (81) and 18% (103) of patients, respectively.

Dilated left ventricles and dilated cardiopathy responsible for systolic dysfunction are less frequently found in the dialysis population (8% and 9%, respectively) (113), but half the patients who presented with CHF had this echocardiographic presentation, indicating its clinical importance.

London et al. introduced the term *inadequate LVH* based on the observation that, in dialysis patients without history of cardiovascular diseases, the ventricular mass: volume ratio was lower than expected (28), i.e., the left ventricles had adapted inappropriately to the volume load. This condition is associated with hypertension and secondary hyperparathyroidism (112) and can predispose to dilated cardiomyopathy. In the most recent study by Foley et al. (114), LVH was present in 74% and LV dilatation in 32% of 433 patients starting dialysis. Only 16% of those patients had a normal heart.

Management (Table 6)

The basic principles of the prevention and treatment of heart failure in patients with chronic renal failure are similar to those applied in other populations, with certain modifications. The reversible causes of CHF, such as valvular heart disease, coronary artery disease, and pericardial effusion, may need interventional correction.

Prevention of CHF can be achieved by controlling the extracellular fluid volume, treating hypertension, and controlling the risk factors for coronary diseases. The removal of excess fluid in patients with GFR below 10 mL/min usually requires dialysis with ultrafiltration or hemofiltration.

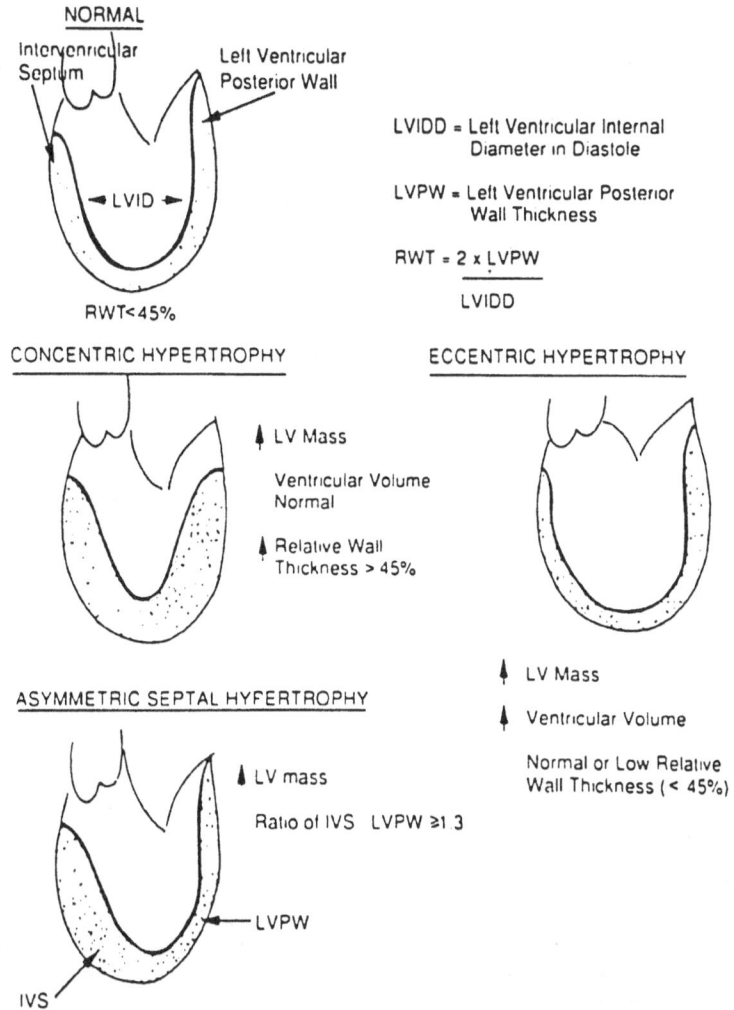

Figure 4. The three patterns of left ventricular hypertrophy commonly recognized by echocardiography. LVID, left ventricular internal diameter; RWT, relative wall thickness; LV, left ventricular; IVS, intraventricular septum. From Foley RN, Parfrey PS, Harnett JD: Left ventricular hypertrophy in dialysis patients. *Semin Dial* 5:34–41, 1992.

The use of high-dose loop diuretics, especially in ESRD patients who presented with pulmonary edema, may not be effective, carries the risk of side effects, may delay dialysis, and as such may endanger the lives of patients. Hemodialysis with sequential ultrafiltration or hemofiltration not only corrects some of the metabolic derangements of uremia but also allows for the removal of excess volume, even in unstable cardiovascular patients.

Correction of the volume by ultrafiltration in a group of ESRD patients with normal LV function will relieve the symptoms of CHF without changing the LV ejection fraction (115). In patients with impaired LV function (an ejection fraction ≤ 50%), the acute effect of hemodialysis with or without (85) volume losses improves ejection fraction

(83,114) and myocardial contractility (85,116). The pure ultrafiltration lowers the ejection fraction without change in contractility (85). This acute net improvement in myocardial function was related to an increase in ionized calcium (117,118) and to the correction of metabolic acidosis, with greater improvement in LV performance with bicarbonate than acetate dialysis solution (119).

The impact of long-term hemodialysis on LV function is more complicated and unclear (120). There are studies suggesting that LV function may improve, deteriorate, or remain unchanged during long-term dialysis, depending on the baseline status of the LV structure, its function, and underlying cardiovascular disease.

Compared to hemodialysis, CAPD possesses some ad-

Table 6. Management of left ventricular dysfunction in patients with chronic renal failure

Principle	Methods of attainment
1. Control of extracellular volume	a. Dietary sodium restriction to 2 g/day
	b. Restriction of fluid intake (1 L/day + visible fluid losses)
	c. Adequate ultrafiltration during hemodialysis or peritoneal dialysis
2. Control of blood pressure	a. Reduction of excess of extracellular volume to achieve "dry" weight
	b. Antihypertensive medication
3. Correction of anemia	a. Erythropoetin therapy (Ht 34%–36%)
	b. Replacement of iron stores
4. Improvement of systolic dysfunction	a. Correction of coronary artery disease
	b. Digitalis, inotropic agents in selected patients
5. Improvement of diastolic dysfunction	a. ACE inhibitor
	b. Calcium-channel blockers
	c. β-blockers
6. Decrease high-output state	a. Reduction or closure of the arteriovenous fistula in selected cases
7. Correction of calcium/phosphate metabolism	a. Calcitriol therapy
	b. Parathyroidectomy when indicated

vantages for heart hemodynamics (121). LV function in patients on CAPD was similar to performance in patients immediately following hemodialysis (122) and did not change during the follow-up (123). However, the deterioration of the LV systolic function may occur in CAPD patients with LV hypertrophy and decreased compliance when patients use more than 2 L of dialysis solution for a single exchange (124). These patients are sensitive to decreased LV preload resulting from a reduction in venous return due to inferior vena cava compression and increased intrathoracic pressure. The long-term positive effect of CAPD on the heart can be jeopardized by hyperlipidemia and hyperinsulinemia, which may increase the risk of atherosclerosis.

The correction of anemia reverses the hyperkinetic state of circulation, i.e., decreases the cardiac index and increases peripheral vascular resistance. In addition, a controlled, randomized study of 38 patients (95) with a normal ejection fraction before the treatment showed improvement of diastolic dysfunction and partial regression of LV hypertrophy after 2 years of erythropoietin therapy. Myocardial contractility has been reported to improve (125,126), not change (18) or decrease (21). The decrease in contractility without altering LV systolic load decreases myocardial energy demand (21). Erythropoietin therapy is then an important step in the prevention of the functional and morphological changes in the heart that can lead to CHF.

Hypertension is another factor that must be controlled. The first step is to achieve the *dry weight*, defined as the weight below which a normoalbuminemic patient on dialysis becomes hypotensive with fluid removal and above which the same patient will be either hypertensive or show signs of fluid expansion (127). Achieving the dry weight will control blood pressure in more than 50% of patients with ESRD enrolled for dialysis and can be obtained by

conventional dialysis with ultrafiltration. Patients who, despite expanded volume and hypertension before the dialysis session, become hypotensive during attempts to remove fluid may benefit either from sequential dialysis or sodium modeling during dialysis. CAPD seems to offer more effective control of blood pressure than hemodialysis, but 25% of the patients on CAPD still have uncontrolled hypertension. There are no specific guidelines concerning the optimal blood pressure level to aim for in ESRD patients. For both systolic and diastolic blood pressure, a goal similar to that for the nonrenal population is generally advised (129). The choice of hypertensive medication for dialysis patients is also not clear, since there is a lack of controlled trials assessing the efficacy of various hypertensive medication in this population. These issues are discussed in detail in Chapter 10. One aspect of hypertensive therapy relates to the prevention of LVH. Dahlof et al. (130) performed a meta-analysis of echocardiographically demonstrable regression of LVH for 109 treatment studies involving 2357 patients with essential hypertension. These authors concluded that angiotensin-converting enzyme (ACE) inhibitors were associated with a 16% regression of LV mass and calcium channel antagonists with an 8% regression. If this effect is also found in patients with ESRD, these drugs should be preferentially used in patients on dialysis.

The goal of drug therapy of CHF in chronic uremia is to provide symptomatic relief, to increase exercise capacity, to avoid hospitalization, to prevent progression of LV dysfunction, and to prolong life. Treatment should be based on the carefully performed medical history, physical examination with a chest x-ray, and electrocardiogram. An echocardiogram for the assessment of LV morphology and function should be used to evaluate whether the main dysfunction is systolic or diastolic in nature. Systolic dysfunction may be improved by digoxin or other inotropic agents, while diastolic dysfunction may benefit from ACE inhibitors, calcium channel blockers, or vasodilators. Although this principle seems reasonable, neither of the large studies in CHF patients used these criteria to allocate patients for specific medication.

The conclusions from the Cooperative North Scandinavian Enalapril Survival Study (CONSENSUS) (131), Studies of Left Ventricular Dysfunction (SOLVD) (132,133), and the Veterans' Administration Heart Failure Trial II (134) are that ACE inhibitor therapy can improve survival and prevent the progression of disease in a broad spectrum of patients without advanced renal failure, whether or not overt manifestation of CHF is present (135).

Two other studies (136,137) show that digoxin treatment of CHF patients receiving diuretics and ACE inhibitors increases the ejection fraction, enhances exercise capacity, and reduces clinical events due to the worsening of CHF. The β-blockers have been shown to improve the cardiac status of patients with dilated cardiomyopathy (138) and are frequently used in postinfarction mild heart failure. Calcium antagonists of the first generation (nifedipine, diltiazem, and verapamil) have shown a short-term positive effect in patients with heart failure, but the long-term studies show hemodynamic and clinical deterioration. This outcome may differ for the second generation of calcium antagonists with less negative inotropy (139). In fact, the recent, study with amlodipine show improvement in LV function in patients with CHF without myocardial infarction. The results of all these studies cannot be directly applied to patients with ESRD. But since many of the pathophysiological mechanisms of CHF are similar in patients with and without uremia, one may also conclude that these studies support the use of ACE inhibitors, digoxin, and possibly calcium channel blockers for the treatment of dialysis patients with New York Heart Association functional Class II–Class IV heart failure. The use of nitrates if ACE inhibitors are contraindicated or not tolerated also seems reasonable. Digoxin is also indicated for the treatment of supraventricular tachyarrhythmias. The use of these medications requires detailed knowledge of their kinetics in patients with impaired renal function and of their potential side effects, some of which may appear only in the dialysis population. The prevention of digoxin-induced arrhythmia requires adjusting the dialysate potassium concentration to avoid postdialytic hypokalemia. The measurement of digoxin levels in dialysis patients may be useful.

Recent clinical observations (140–142) have shown an association between anaphylactoid reaction during dialysis in patients receiving ACE inhibitors and the use of polyacrylonitrile high-flux dialyzers. This reaction is mediated by a bradykinin release during the early period of dialysis (142). Although no fatalities have been reported, patients who experience this reaction should be given either a different class of medication or a different type of membrane.

Other measures are also important for correction of cardiac failure in uremia. Correction of the serum calcium phosphate product by appropriate diet control, administration of nonaluminum-containing phosphate binders, and parathyroidectomy, when indicated, may prevent calcification of the myocardium. Improvement of cardiac index and cardiac contractility, as well as an increase in LV ejection fraction, was observed after parathyroidectomy (29,143). Also, treatment with vitamin D analogues and suppression of parathyroid hormone secretion were followed by improvement of LV function (144).

Renal transplantation may result in improvement of LV performance in uremic patients with dilated cardiomyopathy (145). In addition, significant regression of LVH after kidney transplantation has been reported in several studies (146,147) but not in others (148). On the other hand, cardiovascular complications are the major cause of graft losses, especially in those patients that are diabetic and older than 55 years of age. Screening of diabetic transplant candidates older than 35 years of age should include stress thallium imaging and/or coronary angiography. Nondiabetic asymptomatic patients older than 55 should also undergo noninvasive cardiac evaluation. For those with positive stress tests, cardiac catheterization and correction of underlying disease should be actively pursued (149).

CORONARY HEART DISEASE

Patients with ESRD are at high risk for ischemic heart disease and its consequences. Myocardial infarction was responsible for 12% of deaths of all dialysis patients in 1988–1990 in the U.S. (1). Dialysis patients have a high prevalence of well-known coronary risk factors such as hypertension, altered lipid metabolism, and LVH. In addition, 34% of patients accepted for dialysis had diabetes mellitus, and 43% were older than 65 years (1). Additionally, the hearts of these patients are exposed to a multitude of metabolic and hemodynamic derangements associated with uremia and dialysis that can precipitate the cardiac events. The increased myocardial oxygen demand and altered coronary microcirculation have been postulated as a cause of ischemic heart disease in these patients. Indeed, a decrease in capillary density in the myocardium in uremia has been reported (150).

Thirty to 60 percent of patients on dialysis will present with the clinical symptoms of ischemic heart disease (151,152). Rostand and Rutsky (153,154) found that 24% of 110 symptomatic patients did not show significant occlusion of the coronary artery when assessed by angiography. This finding is much higher than in general population where only 10%–20% of patients undergoing cardiac catheterization for angina-like chest pain had no significant occlusion. White males older than 50 years had a greater risk for atherosclerotic lesions, as did those with elevated serum levels of cholesterol and segmental LV dyskinesia. Patients with myocardial ischemia without stenosis were younger, more likely to be black, and more likely to develop LVH (155). Two studies suggest that women on dialysis are 50% more likely to have symptomatic coronary disease than those the same age in the general population (152,154).

The clinical diagnosis of coronary artery disease is difficult in patients with ESRD, since some of them will have significant coronary arteriosclerosis without angina pectoris, while others may have symptoms of ischemia without the narrowing of the major coronary artery. Nevertheless, the majority of the patients will present either with stable angina, unstable angina, or myocardial infarction.

The noninvasive exercise stress testing normally used as a first step for diagnosis of ischemic heart disease is not very useful in the dialysis population, especially in patient without ischemic symptoms (156). Thirty to 80 percent of patients cannot reach the target heart rate (154,156). In 103 patients with ESRD without clinical symptoms of ischemia, the thallium stress test had a sensitivity of 88%, a specificity of 70%, and predictive value for development of cardiovascular events during 4-year follow up of 73% (157). The accuracy of the pharmacological stress tests using vasodilators such as dipyridamole or adenosine combined with ^{201}Thallium scan high in the general population is unknown for dialysis patients. Dobutamine stress echocardiography and analysis of wall motion were 90% accurate in detecting coronary artery disease and very successfully identified patients with low risk for cardiovascular events (158).

Coronary angiographies should be limited to patients who have positive noninvasive tests, unstable angina, or failed intensive medical therapy and who are, at the same time, acceptable candidates for interventional procedures such as coronary artery bypass grafting (CABG) or percutaneous transluminal coronary angioplasty (PTCA).

Treatment of ischemic heart disease

The management of coronary heart disease includes an aggressive modification of risk factors, correction of anemia, pharmacological therapy, and revascularization in a selected group of patients.

Increased physical activity and weight reduction may lower plasma triglyceride (159). The use of lipid-lowering agents is problematic, since none has been proven to be effective in reducing cardiovascular events in the ESRD population. Lidpid-lowering agents are also potentially toxic in patients with chronic renal failure (160). HMG-CoA reductase inhibitors can be added in the smallest working dose if patients present with significant hypercholesterolemia. Careful monitoring of CPK, liver function, and hematological parameters is necessary until the dose is established. Prevention of the development of LVH through early blood pressure control and correction of anemia is highly desirable.

Pharmacological therapy in patients with angina includes the use of nitrates, β-blockers, and calcium channel antagonists either as monotherapy or in combination (161). The choice of specific agents must be tailored to the indi-

vidual patient, keeping in mind their side effects and the fact that chronic renal failure may modify metabolism and excretion.

Table 7 summarizes the retrospective analysis of CABG surgery and PTCA in chronic dialysis patients, with an early mortality for CABG ranging from 3.3% to 20% and for PTCA from 4.2% to 14% (162–167). The severity of the complications and late mortality as well as the 2-year survival were worse in the CABG surgery group than in those reported for the same procedure in the general population (166). The potential causes for these findings include biological aging of the dialysis population, high prevalence of diabetes, congestive heart failure, and arrhythmia (155). The results of PTCA seems even less favorable due to the similar rate of early mortality as compared to CABG surgery, with a high chance of restenosis and a need for subsequent surgical intervention (167). CABG surgery effectively relieves symptoms of angina and may improve the quality of life, but it creates significant risks and may or may not improve overall survival. With this limited experience and no control trial, it is difficult to define indications for a revascularization procedure. PTCA seems to be ineffective, but new developments and modifications of the procedure may change this conclusion. CABG surgery can be considered in patients with three-vessel disease or significant left main artery stenosis, those who failed medical therapy, or those with unstable angina and moderately impaired LV function (ejection fraction ≥ 35% < 50%) (155). This last recommendation is based on the observation made in the general population that patients with well-preserved LV function have good prognoses.

CARDIAC ARRHYTHMIAS

A high incidence of both atrial and ventricular arrhythmias was found in cross-sectional studies of patients with ESRD. The prevalence of atrial arrhythmia was between 68% and 88%; ventricular arrhythmias were present in 56%–76% of patients, and premature ventricular complexes (PVCs) were found in 14%–21% (168–170). Older age, preexisting heart disease, LVH, and use of digitalis therapy were associated with higher prevalence and greater severity of cardiac arrhythmias (171). There are conflicting data about the effect of dialysis, various dialysate compositions, and dialysis protocols on the occurrence of rhythm disturbances, with some studies showing higher incidence of PVCs during dialysis or in the immediate postdialysis period (169,170), whereas in others no differences could be observed (168). Most of the atrial arrhythmias are of low clinical and hemodynamic significance, except the bradyarrhythmias and atrial tachyarrhythmias. The majority of PVCs are unifocal and below 30 per hour, but high-grade ventricular arrhythmias (multiple PVCs, ventricular couplets, and ventricular tachycardia) were found in 27% of 92 patients with 24-hour Holter monitoring (172). The finding of high-grade ventricular arrhythmias in the pres-

Table 7. Results of coronary artery bypass graft (CABG) and percutaneous transluminal coronary angioplasty (PTCA) in chronic dialysis patients

Reference	Procedure	Patients (n)	Age (mean)	% of 3 vessels or main left artery disease	Ejection fraction	Early mortality	Restenosis within 6 months (%)	2-year survival	Comments
Rineharl et al. (162)	CABG	60	62.1	85%	16 patients ≤ 40%	2 (3.3%)	—	66%	
	PTCA	24	63.6	29%	7 patients ≤ 40%	1 (4.2%)	At least 47%	51%	CABG is preferable for patients with multivessel disease
Rostand and Rutsky (154,163)	CABG	42	51.6	81%	45.6%	8 (19.1%)	—	—	Higher risk for older patients
Batiuk et al. (164)	CABG	25	56.7	68%	45%	5 (20%)	—	77%	Higher early mortality in patients with previous myocardial infarction
Kahan et al. (165)	PTCA	17	60	70%	6 patients ≤ 40%	1 (6%)	81%	—	High rate of restenosis; CABG may be preferred therapy
Deutsch et al. (166)	CABG	16	62	81%	55%	1 (6.3%)	—	—	Increased morbidity compared to controls matched for severity of disease
Ahmed et al. (167)	PTCA	21	59	48%	—	3 (14%)	—	—	High rate of acute complications, poor long-term prognosis; other strategies should be considered

ence of coronary artery disease was associated with increased risk of cardiac mortality and sudden death (173,174).

Asymptomatic nonsustained supraventricular arrhythmias and unifocal PVCs that are not associated with symptoms or hemodynamic compromise usually do not require therapy. If the same rhythm disturbances are present in a setting of coronary heart disease, pericarditis, or severe cardiomyopathy, treatment may be indicated. Some patients will require only short-term treatment during or immediately after dialysis, and the approach is very similar to that used for nonuremic patients, with proper adjustment of the dose of medication (175).

Emergency treatment of symptomatic supraventricular tachyarrhythmias includes cardioversion and/or digoxin and verapamil (for younger patients with good LV function) followed by quinidine. Sustained ventricular tachycardia should be treated urgently with lidocaine followed by quinidine or mexiletene, and ventricular fibrillation with defibrillation followed by lidocaine. Bradyarrhythmias may require permanent placement of a pacemaker in patients with syncope caused by sinus node dysfunction, sick sinus syndrome, high-degree AV block, and carotid sinus hypersensitivity.

Treatment of underlying cardiac disorders and correction of precipitable factors are of primary importance in the prevention of cardiac arrhythmias. These treatments include correction of anemia, adjustment of potassium in the dialysate solution (especially in patients treated with digoxin to prevent hypokalemia), and prevention of severe

hyperpotassemia before dialysis, as well as prevention of hypomagnesamia and hypercalcemia. Some patients may benefit after switching from hemodialysis to CAPD.

HYPOTENSION AND HEMODYNAMIC STABILITY

Hypotension episodes occur during 25%–50% of hemodialysis treatment (176). The etiology of such events is multifactorial and not fully understood (177). The major contributing factors are presented in Table 8. A recent study in which sympathetic nerve activity was measured directly by intraneural microelectrode in a group of patients without diabetes or other conditions known to impair autonomic reflexes showed that hemodialysis-induced hypotension was caused by paradoxical withdrawal of sympathetic vasoconstrictive drive. This paradoxical reaction produced the vasodepressor syncope (178). The baroreceptor function in these patients was normal, in contrast to previous studies (179,180). The nature of the inappropriate sympathetic discharge is not known.

The first step in the management of hemodynamic instability during dialysis requires recognition of cardiac problems that may precipitate a hypotensive reaction, such as pericarditis, significant LV dysfunction, and arrhythmias. Rapid and in access volume removal should be avoided, especially in older patients. The use of sodium modeling and bicarbonate dialysate may be beneficial (181,182). A decrease in the frequency of intradialytic hypotension due

Table 8. Factors contributing to development of hypotension during hemodialysis

1. Reduction of intravascular volume
2. Decreased plasma osmolality
3. Left ventricular dysfunction and decreased cardiac reserve
4. Autonomic nervous system dysfunction
5. Antihypertensive medication

to increased LV contractility (183) and peripheral vasoconstriction (184) was observed by lowering the dialysate temperature from 37°C to 35°C (185,186). This simple maneuver can be use in patients with chronic hypotension problems if they tolerate cooler temperatures well.

INFECTIVE ENDOCARDITIS IN END-STAGE RENAL DISEASE

The overall incidence of endocarditis seems to be below the previously reported 5% (187–189) in end-stage renal disease, given that the number of reported cases has decreased. But outbreaks of bacteremia with drug-resistant bacteria, an older dialysis population, and frequent treatment of patients with immunosuppressive medications before dialysis may significantly increase the prevalence of endocarditis in the future. Bacteremia may also occur in patients on peritoneal dialysis, most commonly due to exit infection and peritonitis.

Infections are a frequent complication of uremia (190) and account for approximately 13% of deaths in the dialysis population and 80% of deaths due to septicemia (1). The causes of infection are multifactorial and include impaired cellular and humoral immune response by T and B cells (191) and phagocytic dysfunction of polymorphonuclear leukocytes and macrophages (192,193) in a context of high exposure to infective pathogens before and during dialysis, as experienced by uremic patients. Infections of the primary arteriovenous fistula occur in 1%–5% of the dialysis population with a frequency of 0.15 episodes per patient per year, but prosthetic grafts are infected at a rate of 10%–15% with a frequency of one to three episodes per patient per dialysis per year (194). Central venous access catheter infection with septicemia was observed in 22% of 118 catheters over a period of 3.5 years (195). Arteriovenous fistulas are not, surprisingly, the major source of bacteremia and metastatic infections that can involve both pathologically changed and normal heart valves. In a 1966 in a paper on the use of internal fistula for dialysis, Brescia et al. have already reported bacterial endocarditis complicating hemodialysis in a patient with rheumatic fever (196).

Etiology

Although almost any bacteria can produce endocarditis, staphylococci, streptococci, and enterococci are the most

Table 9. Presenting clinical features of infective endocarditis in the general population

Clinical feature	% Present
CHF	25–65
Malaise, myalgias, arthralgias	25–45
Fever	80–90
Chills	40
Weight loss, anorexia	25
Heart murmurs	60–85
Changing murmur	5–10
Neurological deficits	33
Skin manifestitation	
Osler nodes	0–10
Petechiae	30–60
Splinter hemorrhages	15
Janeway lesions	<10
Splenomegaly	20–57
Clubbing	12–52
Anemia	40–50
Leukocytosis	25–50

Data from (197).

common pathogens. In earlier studies, *Staphylococcus aureus* accounted for approximately 50% of infective endocarditis followed by *Streptococcus viridans* and enterococci (187–189). This figure is probably still true today, since the major source of bacteremia in patients on dialysis is vascular access, and *Staphylococcus aureus* accounts for 40%–70% of the infections of vascular accesses, followed by *Staphylococcus epidermidis* (10%–15%) and gramnegative rods, including *Pseudomonas aeruginosa* and enterobacter species (194). *Streptococcus viridans* is a normal inhabitant of the oropharynx, and since these streptococci are easy to eradicate by prophylactic use of penicillin before dental procedures—an approach common for dialysis patients—they may be less frequently seen as a cause of endocarditis in the future.

Clinical presentation

Table 9 presents clinical findings associated with infective endocarditis in the general population (197). Patients with ESRD will also demonstrate these features, with some variability.

The criteria for diagnosis of endocarditis have, lately been extensively discussed (198). The new criteria proposed by Durack et al. (Duke criteria, Table 10) retain in slightly modified form the pathologic criteria of Von Reyn et al. (199) but add the echocardiographic entities for the detection of intracardiac vegetation. Positive transesophageal echocardiogram for vegetation has a specificity of more than 90%. A negative study does not rule out endocarditis, but it has a negative predictive accuracy of almost 90% (200). A definite diagnosis of infective endocarditis requires the demonstration of two major findings, such as positive blood cultures and positive

Table 10. Proposed new criteria for diagnosis of infective endocarditis and definitions of terminology

A. Proposed new criteria

Definite infective endocarditis
Pathologic criteria
   Microorganisms: demonstrated by culture or histology in a vegetation, or in a vegetation that has embolized, or in an intracardiac
     abscess
   Pathologic lesions: vegetation or intracardiac abscess present, confirmed by histology showing active endocarditis
Clinical criteria, using specific definitions listed in part B
   2 major criteria
   1 major and 3 minor criteria
   5 minor criteria

Possible infective endocarditis
Findings consistent with infective endocarditis that fall short of "Definite," but not "rejected"

Rejected
Firm alternate diagnosis for manifestations of endocarditis
Resolution of manifestations of endocarditis, with antibiotic therapy for 4 days or less
No pathologic evidence of infective endocarditis at surgery or autopsy, after antibiotic therapy for 4 days or less

B. Definitions of terminology used in the proposed new criteria

Major criteria
Positive blood culture for infective endocarditis
   Typical microorganism for infective endocarditis from two separate blood cultures
Viridans streptococci, *Streptococcus bovis*, HACEK group[a], or
Community-acquired *Staphyloccus aureus* or enterococci, in the absence of a primary focus, or
Persistently positive blood culture, defined as recovery of a microorganism consistent with infective endocarditis from:
   1. Blood cultures drawn more than 12 hours apart, or
   2. All of three or a majority of four or more separate blood cultures, with first and last drawn at least 1 hour apart
Evidence of endocardial involvement
   Positive echocardiogram for infective endocarditis
     1. Oscillating intracardiac mass, on valve or supporting structures, or in the path of regurgitant jets, or on implanted material, in
       the absence of an alternative anatomic explanation, or
     2. Abscess, or
     3. New partial dehiscence of prosthetic valve, or
   New valvular regurgitation (increase or change in preexisting murmur not sufficient)

Minor criteria
Predisposition: predisposing heart condition or intravenous drug use
Fever: ≥38.0°C (100.4°F)
Vascular phenomena: major arterial emboli, septic pulmonary infarcts, mycotic aneurysm, intracranial hemorrhage, conjunctival
   hemorrhages, Janeway lesions
Immunologic phenomena: glomerulonephritis, Osler's nodes, Roth spots, rheumatoid factor
Microbiologic evidence: positive blood culture but not meeting major criterion as noted previously[b] or serologic evidence of active
   infection with organism consistent with infective endocarditis
Echocardiogram: consistent with infective endocarditis but not meeting major criterion as noted previously

---

[a] Including nutritional variant strains.
[b] Excluding single positive cultures for coagulase-negative staphylococci and organisms that do not cause endocarditis.
HACK HACEK = *Haemophilus spp.*, *Actinobacillus actinomycetemcomitans*, *Cardiobacterium hominis*, *Eikenella spp.*, and *Kingella*
kingae.
From (198).

echocardiogram; or one of the major findings and at least three minor criteria; or five minor criteria. A positive diagnosis must be followed by appropriate antimicrobial therapy and surgical intervention. The category of possible endocarditis does not imply that antimicrobial therapy should or should not be given, but clinicians must draw their own conclusion—i.e., the likelihood of endocarditis and the need for empirical therapy in each case (198).

In patients with normal renal function and streptococcal endocarditis, the cure rate is about 90%, but there is a

40% mortality rate in those with *Staphylococcus aureus* endocarditis. It is not surprising that of 30 patients on dialysis reviewed by Cross et al. (187), where a clinical outcome was noted, 16 patients died (53%), since the majority had endocarditis due to staphyloccocus infection. Other factors associated with the significant mortality within this group include multivalvular involvement, enterococcal infections, previous steroid therapy, and a patient age greater than 46.

Management

The prophylaxis of infective endocarditis with antimicrobial agents is recommended for hemodialysis patients for some dental and surgical procedure (Table 11) due to the

Table 11. Dental and surgical procedures indicated for antimicrobial prophylaxis[a]

Dental procedures known to induce gingival or mucosal
 bleeding
Tonsillectomy and/or adenoidectomy
Surgical operations that involve intestinal or respiratory mucosa
Bronchoscopy with a rigid bronchoscope
Sclerotherapy for esophageal varices
Esophageal dilatation
Gallbladder surgery
Cystoscopy
Urethral dilatation
Urinary tract surgery if urinary tract infection is present
Prostatic surgery
Incision and drainage of infected tissue
Vaginal hysterectomy
Vaginal delivery in the presence of infection

[a]This table lists selected procedures but is not meant to be all-inclusive.

abnormal vascular communication (fistula) present. However, there is no definite proof of the efficacy of the prophylaxis either in cardiac conditions or in dialysis patients. The current regimen, presented in Table 12, is the one recommended by the American Heart Association (201) and modified for hemodialysis population.

Patients on hemodialysis have a high carriage of *Staphylococcus aureus* as compared to patients with chronic renal failure (60% versus 20%), and generally the same organisms were cultured from infection of vascular access as from the nose, throat, and skin (202,203). The effort to eradicate this carriage has been successful only in a short follow-up, but recolonization with resistant bacteria occurred after 2–3 months, and more studies are needed before any recommendations can be made.

In dialysis patients with a temporarily placed central venous catheter, fever, and no clear source of infections, a blood culture must be obtained, catheter removed and a single dose of vancomycin 1 g I.V. may be given. The tip of the catheter should be cultured. A new catheter can be inserted on the opposite side after 48 hours as long as the blood cultures are negative. Infection of the permanent vascular access (native fistula or prosthetic graft) requires appropriate antibiotic therapy for 2–4 weeks based on blood culture and sensitivity. Whenever prompt clinical response is not achieved, bacteremia continues despite therapy, or there is local abscess formation, the shunt should be either partially or totally removed (204).

Infective endocarditis in patients with ESRD is difficult to eradicate and frequently requires valve replacement to prevent recurrent systemic emboli, as well as for treatment of severe valvular destruction, persistent infection, and congestive heart failure. Proper choice of antibiotic therapy must be based on blood cultures and sensitivity data. Three sets of blood cultures obtained a few hours apart during the first day of hospitalization yield the caus-

Table 12. Antibiotic regimens for endocarditis prophylaxis in adults (modified for patients on dialysis)

Dental, oral, and upper respiratory tract procedures	
Standard regimen	Amoxicillin 3 g P.O. 1 hr before procedure and 1.5 g 6 hr after initial dose
Allergy to penicillin	Erythromycin ethylsuccinate 800 mg or erythromycin stearate 1 g P.O. 2 hr before procedure; then half the dose 6 hr after initial dose OR clindamycin 300 mg P.O. 1 hr before procedure and 150 mg 6 hr after intitial dose
For patients unable to take oral medications	Ampicillin 2 g I.V. 30 min before procedure; then 1 g I.V. 6 hr after initial dose
Patients at high risk and allergic to penicillin	Vancomycin 1 g I.V. over 1 hr, starting 1 hr before procedure; no repeat dose necessary
Regimens for GU/GI procedures	
Standard regimen	Ampicillin 2 g I.V. or I.M. plus gentamicin 1.5 mg/kg (not to exceed 80 mg) 30 min before procedure; then amoxicillin 1.5 g P.O. 6 hr after initial dose or repeat parenteral dose of ampicillin 2 g
Alternate regimen for low-risk patients	Amoxicillin 3 g p.o. 1 hr before procedure, then 1.5 g P.O. 6 hr after initial dose
Allergy to penicillin and high-risk patients	Vancomycin 1 g I.V. over 1 hr plus gentamicin 1.5 mg/kg (not to exceed 80 mg) 1 hr before procedure

Modified from Dajansias AS, Bisno AL, Chung KJ, et al.: Prevention of bacterial endocarditis: recommendations of the American Heart Association. *JAMA* 264:2919–2922, 1992.

Table 13. Therapy of infective endocarditis in adult patients with end-stage renal disease

Organism	Therapy of choice	Effect of dialysis	Duration of treatment	Comments
Streptococcus				
1. Penicillin sensitive (e.g., *S. viridans*, *S. bovis*, β-hemolityc streptococci (MIC < 0.1 ug/mL)	Penicillin G 2 million units I.V., then 1 million units I.V. q 8 hr or	Supplement maintenance dose after HD	4 weeks	1.7 mEg potassium per 10 million units; maximum 6 million units/day
	Vancomycin 15 mg/kg I.V. q 7–10 days or		4 weeks	If history of anaphylaxis to penicillin Vancomycin peak serum concentration 30–40 μg/mL; trough, 5–10 μg/mL
	Cefazolin 1 g I.V. q 24 hr, or	Supplement maintenance dose after HD (1 g I.V.)		
	Ceftriaxone 1 g I.V. g 12 hr		4 weeks	If history of rash to penicillin
2. Penicillin-resistant streptococci (e.g., enterococci other streptococci) (MIC > 0.1 μg/mL)	Penicillin G loading dose 2 million units I.V., then 2 million units I.V. g 8 hr, Gentamicin 1.5 mg/kg I.V., then 1 mg/kg after dialysis or	2/3 of normal dose after HD	4–6 weeks	Gentamicin can be used only for 2 weeks if 0.1 > MIC ≥ 0.5
	Ampicillin 2 g I.V., then 2 g I.V. q 12–16 hrs. Gentamicin 1.5 mg/kg I.V. then 1 mg/kg I.V. after dialysis 7–10 days or	Maintenance dose after HD	4–6 weeks	Daily dialysis Gentamicin 0.5–0.75 mg/kg after dialysis, peak 5 μg/mL, trough ≤ 2 μg/mL
	Vancomycin 15 mg/kg I.V. q and Gentamicin as above			
Staphylococcus aureus				
1. Penicillin sensitive	Penicillin G 2 million units I.V., then 2 million units q 8 hr or		4–6 weeks	
	Vancomycin 15 mg/kg I.V. q 7–10 days			
2. Penicillin resistant, methicillin sensitive	Nafcillin or oxacillin 2 g I.V. q 4–6 hr or	Negligible removal by HD	4–6 weeks	No need for dose adjustmen
	Cefazolin 1 g I.V. q 24 hr or	Negligible removal by HD		
	Vancomycin 15 mg/kg I.V. q 7–10 days		4–6 weeks	
3. Meticillin resistant	Vancomycin 15 mg/kg I.V. q 7–10 days		4–6 weeks	
Staphylococcus epidermidis				
1. Meticillin sensitive	Same as meticillin sensitive S. aureus		4–6 weeks	
2. Meticillin resistant	Vancomycin 15 mg/kg I.V. g 7–10 days plus rifampin 300 mg p.o. q 8 hr		4–6 weeks	
Gram-negative organisms				
1. HACEK group (penicillin sensitive)	Ampicillin 2 g I.V. then 2 g I.V. q 12–16 hr plus gentamicin 1.5 mg/kg I.V then 1 mg/kg after dialysis		4–6 weeks	Peak and trough levels as above
2. HACEK group (pencillin resistant)	Cefotaxime 2 g I.V. q 24 hr Imipenem 1 g I.V., then 0.25 g q 6 hr	Add 1 g after HD Add dose after HD	4–6 weeks	
3. Enterobacteriaceae	Cefotaxime 2 g I.V. q 24 hr or Imipenem 1 g I.V. then 0.25 g q 6 hrs or Aztreonam and gentamicin		6 weeks	Alternatives to cefotaxime can also be used
4. *Pseudomonas aeruginosa*	Pipracillin 3 g q 8 hr or	Additional dose of 3 g after HD	6 weeks	
	Ceftazidime 2 g q 48 hr or	Additional dose of 1 g after HD		
	Imipenem 1 g I.V. then 0.25 g I.V. q 6 hr plus Tobramycin 1.7 mg/kg I.V. then 0.5 mg/kg q 48 hr	Add dose after HD 2/3 of normal dose after HD		
5. *Fungi candida spp*	Amphotercin B 1.0 mg/kg I.V. every 36 hr. Start with 0.25 mg/kg and increase by 0.25 mg/kg/day upto maximum dose, then lower the dose to achieve total dose of 30–40 mg/kg after 6–8 weeks plus	Dose not modified by HD	6–8 weeks	Flucytosine level keep at 50–100 μg/mL
	Flucytosine 150 mg/kg P.O. q 24–36 hr	Add dose after HD		Flucytosine level keet at 50–100 μg/mL
6. *Aspergillus spp*	Amphotericin B as above		6–8 weeks	

Adopted from: Bisno AL, et al.: Antimicrobial treatment of infective endocarditis due to viridans streptococci, enterococci and staphylococci. *JAMA* 261: 1471–1477, 1989; Durack DT: Infective endocarditis. In: PD Hoeprich, MC Jordan, AR Bonald, eds, *Infectious Disease*. JB Lippincott, Phililedphia, pp 1233–1248, 1994; Bennett WM, et al.: *Drug Prescribing in Renal Failure*, 3rd ed. American College of Physicians, Phililedphia, 1994; Matthews SJ: Aminoglycosides. In: GE Schumacher, ed, *Therapeutic Drug Monitoring*. Appleton and Lange, Norwalk, Conn pp 237–294, 1995.

ative bacteria in 98% of all cases unless the patient has been treated during the previous 2 weeks (205). The minimum inhibitory and bactericidal concentrations (MIC and MBC) should be determined and compared with the bactericidal activity of the patient's serum during antibiotic therapy. A serum bactericidal titer of 1:8 or greater is thus desirable. Repeated blood culture should be drawn 2 and 5 days after initiation of the therapy and 1 and 3 weeks after completion of the therapy. Patients with acute fulminant infective endocarditis must be treated with an empirical regimen as soon as three sets of blood culture have been obtained at 15-minute intervals. Early cardiovascular consultation should be obtained for all patients with aortic valve endocarditis or with valvular prosthesis even if they are hemodynamically stable. Table 13 lists the drugs of choice, dosage, administration route, and treatment duration for infective endocarditis as adopted by the American Heart Association (206,207) and modified for patients with end-stage renal failure. The details of dose adjustment and specific problems related to the use of these drugs in chronic renal failure will not be discussed here, since they are reviewed elsewhere in this book.

REFERENCES

1. U.S. Renal Data Systems: *USRDS 1993 Annual Data Report.* The National Institute of Health, National Institute of Diabetes and Digestive and Kidney Disease, Bethesda, MD, pp 49–54, 1993.
2. Canadian Organ Replacement Register: *1991 Annual Report.* Hospital Medical Records Institute, Don Mills, Ontario, Canada, April 1993.
3. European Dialysis and Transplant Association: *Annual Report on Regular Dialysis and Transplantation in Europe XXII*, 1991.
4. Greaves SC, Sharpe DN: Cardiovascular disease in patients with end-stage renal failure. *Aust NZ J Med* 22:153–159, 1992.
5. Foley RN, Parfrey PS, Hefferton D, Singh I, Simons A, Brendan J, Barrett MB: Advance prediction of early death in patients starting maintenance dialysis. *Am J Kidney Dis* 23:836–845, 1994.
6. Kennel WB, McGee DL: Diabetes and cardiovascular disease: the Framingham Study. *JAMA* 241:2035–2038, 1979.
7. Braun WE, Phillips DF, Vidt DG, et al.: Coronary artery disease in 100 diabetics with end-stage renal failure. *Transplant Proc* 16:603–607, 1984.
8. Philipson JD, Carpenter BJ, Itzkoff J, et al.: Evaluation of cardiovascular risk for renal transplantation in diabetic patients. *Am J Med* 81:630–634, 1986.
9. Bennett WM, Kloster F, Rosch J, Barry J, Porter CA: Natural history of asymptomatic coronary angiographic lesions in diabetic patients with end-stage renal disease. *Am J Med* 65:779, 1978.
10. Massie BM, Tubau TF, Szlachcic J, et al.: Hypertensive heart disease: the critical role of left ventricular hypertrophy. *J Cardiovasc Pharmacol* 13 (Suppl 1):S18–S24, 1989.
11. Kannel WB: Role of blood pressure in cardiovascular disease: The Framingham Study. *Angiology* 26:1–14, 1975.
12. Mac Mahon S, Peto R, Cutler J, Collins R, Sorlie P, Neaton J, Abbot FR, Godwin J, Dyer A, Stamler J: Blood pressure, stroke and coronary heart disease. *Lancet* 335:765–774, 1990.
13. Haire HM, Sherrand DJ, Scandapane D, et al.: Smoking, hypertension and mortality in a maintenance dialysis population. *Cardiovasc Med* 3:1163–1168, 1978.
14. Ayus JC, Frommer P, Olivero JJ, et al.: Effect of long-term dialysis on left ventricular ejection fraction in end-stage renal disease. *Kidney Int* 19:142A, 1981.
15. de-Leeuw PW: Pathophysiology of hypertension in patients on renal replacement therapy. *Blood Purif* 12:245–251, 1994.
16. Neff MS, Kim KE, Persoff M, Onesti G, Swartz C: Hemodynamics of uremic anemia. *Circulation* 63:876–883, 1971.
17. Converse RL Jr, Jacobsen TN, Toto RD, Jost CM, Cosentino F, Fouad-Tarazi F, Victor RG: Sympathetic overactivity in patients with chronic renal failure. *N Engl J Med* 327:1912–1918, 1992.
18. London GM, Zins B, Pannier B, Naret C, Berthelot M, Jacquot C, Safar M, Drueke TB: Vascular changes in hemodialysis patients in response to recombinant human erythropoietin. *Kidney Int* 36:878–882, 1989.
19. Satoh K, Masuda T, Ikeda Y, Kurokawa S, Kamata K, Kikawada R, Takamoto T, Marumo F: Hemodynamic changes by recombinant erythropoietin therapy in hemodialyzed patients. *Hypertension* 15:262–266, 1990.
20. Martinez-Vea A, Bardaji A, Garcia C, Ridao C, Richart C, Oliver JA: Long-term myocardial effects of correction of anemia with recombinant human erythropoietin in aged patients on hemodialysis. *Am J Kidney Dis* 19:353–357, 1992.
21. Fellner SK, Lang RM, Neumann A, Korcarz C, Borow KM: Cardiovascular consequences of correction of the anemia of renal failure with erythropoietin. *Kidney Int* 44:1309–1315, 1993.
22. Lindner A, Charra B, Sherrard DJ, Scribner BH: Accelerated atherosclerosis is prolonged maintenance hemodialysis. *N Engl J Med* 290:697–701, 1974.
23. Attman PO, Alaupovic P: Lipid abnormalities in chronic renal insufficiency. *Kidney Int* 39:516–523, 1991.
24. Bloembergen WE, Port FK, Mauger EA, Wolfe RA: Causes of death in dialysis patients: racial and gender differences. *J Am Soc Nephrol* 5:1231–1242, 1994.
25. Silins J, Fortier L, Mao Y, et al.: Mortality rates among patients with end-stage renal disease in Canada, 1981–1986. *Can Med Assoc J* 141:677–682, 1989.
26. Massry SG, Smogorzewski M, Perne AF: Parathyroid hormone and myocardiopathy of chronic renal failure. In PS Parfrey, JD Harnett, eds, *Cardiac Dysfunction in Chronic Uremia.* Kluwer Academic Publishers, Boston, pp 139–160, 1992.
27. Parfrey PS, Harnett JD, Griffiths S, Gualt MH, Barre PE, Guttman RD: Low-output left ventricular failure in end-stage renal disease. *Am J Nephrol* 7:184–191, 1987.
28. London GM, Fabiani F, Marchais SJ, De Vernejoul M Ch, Guerin A, Safar ME, Metivier F, Llach F: Uremic cardiomyopathy: an inadequate left ventricular hypertrophy. *Kidney Int* 31:973–980, 1987.
29. Drueke T, Fauchet M, Fleury J, Lesourd P, Toure V, Le-Pailleur C, de-Vernejoul P, Crosnier J: Effect of parathyroidectomy on left ventricular function in haemodialysis patients. *Lancet* 1:112–114, 1980.
30. Smogorzewski M, Zayed M, Zhang Y-B, Roe J, Massry SG: Parathyroid hormone increases cytosolic calcium concentra-

tion in adult rat cardiac myocytes. *Am J Physiol* 264:H1998–H2006, 1993.

31. Zhang Y-B, Smogorzewski M, Ni Z, Massry SG: Altered cytosolic calcium Homeostasis in rat cardiac myocytes in CRF. *Kidney Int* 45:1113–1119, 1994.

32. Smogorzewski M, Tian J, Massry SG: Downregulation of PTH-PTHrP receptor of the heart in CRF: role of [Ca²⁺]i. *Kidney Int* 47:1182–1186, 1995.

33. Perna AF, Smogorzewski M, Massry SG: Effect of verapamil on the abnormalities in fatty acid oxidation of myocardium. *Kidney Int* 36:453–457, 1989.

34. Amann K, Ritz E, Wiest G, Klaus G, Mall G: A role of parathroid hormone for the activation of cardiac fibroblasts in uremia. *J Am Soc Nephrol* 4:1814–1819, 1994.

35. Mall G, Huther W, Schneider J, Lundin P, Ritz E: Diffuse intermyocytic fibrosis in uremic patients. *Nephrol Dial Transplant* 5:39–44, 1990.

36. Freeman GL, LeWinter MM: Pericardial adaptations during cardiac dilatation in dogs. *Circ Res* 54:294–300, 1984.

37. Wacker W, Merill JP: Uremic pericarditis in acute and chronic renal failure. *JAMA* 156:764–765, 1954.

38. Bailey GL, Hampers CL, Hager EB, Merrill JP: Uremic pericarditis: clinical features and management. *Circulation* 38:582–591, 1968.

39. Compty CM, Cohen SL, Shapiro FL: Pericarditis in chronic uremia and its sequels. *Ann Intern Med* 75:173–183, 1971.

40. Ribot S, Frankel JH, Gielchincky I, et al.: Treatment of uremic pericarditis. *Clin Nephrol* 2:127–130, 1974.

41. Wray TM, Stone WJ: Uremic pericarditis: a prospective echocardiographic and clinical study. *Clin Nephrol* 6:295–302, 1976.

42. Frommer JP, Young JB, Ayus JC: Asymptomatic pericardial effusion in uremic patients: effect of long-term dialysis. *Nephron* 39:296–301, 1985.

43. Rutsky EA, Rostand SG: Treatment of uremic pericarditis and pericardial effusion. *Am J Kidney Dis* 10:2–8, 1987.

44. Rostand SG, Rutsky EA: Pericarditis in end-stage renal disease. *Cardiol Clin* 8:701–707, 1990.

45. Ansari A, Kaupke CJ, Vaziri ND, Miller R, Barbari A: Cardiac pathology in patients with end-stage renal disease maintained on hemodialysis. *Int J Artif Organs* 16:31–36, 1993.

46. Renfrew RM, Buselmeier TJ, Kjellstrand CM: Pericarditis and renal failure. *Annu Rev Med* 31:345–360, 1980.

47. Silverberg S, Oreopoulos DG, Wise DJ, et al.: Pericarditis in patients undergoing long-term hemodialysis and peritoneal dialysis. Incidence, complications and management. *Am J Med* 63:874–880, 1977.

48. Young JB, Frommer P, Ayus JC, Alexander JK, Miller RR: Effect of dialysis on pericardial effusion: a prospective echocardiographic study in end-stage renal failure patients. *Circulation* 62:111–186, 1980.

49. Drueke T, LePailleur C, Zingraff J, Jungers P: Uremic cardiomyopathy and pericarditis. *Adv Nephrol Necker Hosp* 9:33–70, 1980.

50. Osanloo E, Shalhoub RJ, Cioffi RF, Parker RH: Viral pericarditis in patients receiving hemodialysis. *Arch Intern Med* 139:301–303, 1979.

51. Joffe P, Johannessen AC: Uremic pericarditis, an epidemic disease. *Danish Med Bull* 34:117–118, 1987.

52. Sever MS, Steinmuller DR, Hayes JM, Steem SB, Novick AC: Pericarditis following renal transplantation. *Transplantation* 51:1229–1232, 1991.

53. Twardowski ZJ, Alpert MA, Gupta RC, Nolph KD, Madsen

BT: Circulating immune complexes: possible toxins responsible for serositis (pericarditis, pleuritis, and peritonitis) in renal failure. *Nephron* 35:190–195, 1983.

54. Maisch B, Kochsiek K: Humoral immune reactions in uremic pericarditis. *Am J Nephrol* 3:264–271, 1983.

55. De Pace NL, Nestico PF, Schwartz AB, et al.: Predicting success of intensive dialysis in the treatment of uremic patients. *Am J Med* 76:38–46, 1984.

56. Engel PJ: Echocardiographic findings in pericardial disease. In: NO Fowler, ed, *The Pericardium in Health and Disease.* Futura, mount kisco N.Y. pp 99–151, 1985.

57. Martin RP, Bowden R, Filly K, Popp RL: Intrapericardial abnormalities in patients with pericardial effusion. Findings by two dimensional echocardiography. *Circulation* 61:568–572, 1980.

58. Burstow DJ, Oh JK, Bailey KR, et al.: Cardiac tamponade: characteristic Doppler observations. *Mayo Clin Proc* 64:312–324, 1989.

59. Fowler NO: Cardiac tamponade: a clinical or an echocardiographic diagnosis? *Circulation* 87:1738–1741, 1993.

60. Klopfenstein HS, Schuchard GH, Wann LS, Palmer TE, Hartz AJ, Gross CM, et al.: The relative merits of pulsus parodoxus and right ventricular diastolic collapse in the early detection of cardiac tamponade: an experimental echocardiographic study. *Circulation* 71:829–833, 1985.

61. Spodick DH: The electrocardiogram in acute pericarditis: distributions of morphological and axial changes by stage. *Am J Cardiol* 33:470–474, 1974.

62. Singhal MJ, Jha R, Agarwal SK, et al.: Uremic pericarditis—prevention of complications. *J Nephrol* 8:113–117, 1995.

63. Sanders PW, Taylor Z, Curtis JJ: Hemodialysis without anticoagulation. *Am J Kidney Dis* 5:32–35, 1985.

64. Von Brecht JH, Flanigan MY, Freeman RM, Lim VS: Regional anticoagulation: hemodialysis with hypertonic trisodium citrate. *Am J Kidney Dis* 8:196–201, 1986.

65. Luft FC, Gilman JK, Weyman DE: Pericarditis in the patient with uremia: clinical and echocardiographic evaluation. *Nephron* 25:160–166, 1980.

66. Buselmeier TJ, Simmons RL, Najarian JS, Mauer SM, Matas AJ, Kjellstrand CM: Uremic pericardial effusion. Treatment by catheter drainage and local nonabsorbable steroid administration. *Nephron* 16:271–280, 1976.

67. Fuller TJ, Knochel JP, Brennan JP, Fetner CD, White MG: Reversal of intractable uremic pericarditis by triamcinolone hexacetonide. *Arch Intern Med* 136:979–982, 1976.

68. Connors JP, Kleiger RE, Shaw RC, et al.: The indication for pericardiectomy in the uremic pericardial effusion. *Surgery* 80:689–694, 1976.

69. Ghavamin M, Gutch CF, Hughes RK, et al.: Pericardial tamponade in chronic hemodialysis patients. Treatment by pericardiectomy. *Arch Intern Med* 131:249–253, 1973.

70. Gafter U, Chachkes M, Zevin D, Levi J: Therapeutic approach to pericarditis in uremia. *Isr J Med Sci* 26:107–109, 1990.

71. Morin JE, Mulder DS, Long R: Pericardiectomy for uremic tamponade. *Can J Surg* 19:109–112, 1976.

72. Shabetai R: Pericardial disease: etiology, pathophysiology, clinical recognition and treatment. In: JT Willerson, JN Cohn, eds, *Cardiovascular Medicine.* Churchill Livingston, New York, pp 1011–1040, 1995.

73. Feinroth MV, Goldstein EJC, Josephson A, Friedman EA: Infection complicating intrapericardial steroid instillation in uremic pericarditis. *Clin Nephrol* 15:331–333, 1981.

74. Minuth ANW, Nottebohm GA, Eknoyan G, Suki WN: Indomethacin treatment of pericarditis in chronic hemodialysis patients. *Arch Intern Med* 135:807–810, 1975.

75. Spector D, Alfred H, Siedlecki M, Briefel G: A controlled study of the effect of indomethacin in uremic pericarditis. *Kidney Int* 24:663–669, 1983.

76. Miller JI: Surgical management of pericardial disease. In: RC Schlant, W Alexander, eds, *Hurst's The Heart Arteries and Veins*, 8th ed, pp 1675–1680, 1994. Mc Graw-Hill N.Y.

77. Nataf P, Cacoub P, Dorent R, Jault F, Pavie A, Cabrol C, Gandjbakhch I: Results of subtotal pericardiotomy for constrictive pericarditis. *Eur J Cardiothorac Surg* 7:252–256, 1993.

78. Gorlin R, Hoseupud JD, Greenberg BH: Evolution of concepts of myocardial function in the treatment of congestive heart failure. In: JD Hoseupud, BH Greenberg, eds, *Congestive Heart Failure*. N. York Springer-Verlag, pp 3–8, 1994.

79. Harnett JD, Foley RN, Kent GM, Barre PE, Murray D, Parfrey PS: Congestive heart failure in dialysis patients. Prevalence, incidence, prognosis and risk factors. *Kidney Int* 47:884–890, 1995.

80. Cruz IA, Bhatt GR, Cohen HC, et al.: Echocardiographic detection of cardiac involvement in patients with chronic renal failure. *Arch Intern Med* 138:720–724, 1978.

81. Parfrey PS, Harnett JD, Griffiths SM, Gault MH, Barre PE: Congestive heart failure in dialysis patients. *Arch Intern Med* 148:1519–1525, 1988.

82. Lai KN, Ng J, Whitford J, Buttfield I, Fassett RG, Mathew TH: Left ventricular function in uremia: echocardiographic and radionuclide assessment in patients on maintenance hemodialysis. *Clin Nephrol* 23:125–133, 1985.

83. Wizemann V, Kramer W, Thormann J, Kindler M: Exercise-induced ventricular dysfunction: reversible by hemodialysis. *Trans Am Soc Artif Intern Organs* 30:567–570, 1984.

84. Chaignon M, Chen WT, Tarazi RC, Bravo EL, Nakamato S: Effect of hemodialysis on blood volume distribution and cardiac output. *Hypertension* 3:327–332, 1981.

85. Nixon JV, Mitchell JH, McPhaul JJ, Henrich WL: Effect of hemodialysis on left ventricular function. *J Clin Invest* 71:377–384, 1983.

86. Kim KE, Onesti G, Del Guercio ET, et al.: Sequential hemodynamic changes in end-stage renal disease and the anephric state during volume expansion. *Hypertension* 2:102–110, 1980.

87. Vincenti F, Amend JW, Abele J, et al.: The role of hypertension in hemodialysis-associated atherosclerosis. *Am J Med* 68:363–369, 1980.

88. Rostand SG, Kirk KA, Rutsky EA: Relationship of coronary risk factors to hemodialysis-associated ischemic heart disease. *Kidney Int* 22:304–308, 1982.

89. Ahearm DH, Maher JF: Heart failure as a complication of a hemodialysis arteriovenous fistula. *Ann Intern Med* 77:201–204, 1972.

90. Timmis AD, Mc Gonigle RJ, Weston MJ, Mc Leod AA, Jackson G, Jewitt DE, Parsons V: The influence of hemodialysis fistulas on circulatory dynamics and left ventricular function. *Int J Artif Organs* 5:101–104, 1982.

91. Payne RM, Sodeblom RE, Lobstein PH, et al.: Exercise-induced hemodynamic effects of arterio-venous fistulas used for hemodialysis. *Kidney Int* 2:344–348, 1972.

92. Cohn SJ, Chandraratna PAN, Winer RL, Shah GM, Aronow WS: Echocardiographic assessment of the hemodynamic effects of arteriovenous fistulas in patients with chronic renal failure. *J Cardiovasc Ultrasonogr* 2:5, 1983.

93. Silberberg JS, Rahel DP, Patton DR, et al.: Role of anemia in the pathogenesis of left ventricular hypertrophy in end-stage renal disease. *Am J Cardiol* 64:222–224, 1989.

94. Fellner SK, Lang RM, Neuman A, Korcarz C, Borow KM: Cardiovascular consequences of correction of the anemia of renal failure with erythropoietin. *Kidney Int* 14:1309–1315, 1993.

95. Sikole A, Polenakovic M, Spirovska V, Polenakovic B, Masin G: Analysis of heart morphology and function following erythropoietin treatment of anemic dialysis patients. *Artif Organs* 17:977–984, 1993.

96. Terman DS, Alfrey AC, Hammond WS, et al.: Cardiac calcification in uremia. A clinical, biochemical and pathologic study. *Am J Med* 50:744, 1971.

97. Rostand SG, Sanders C, Kirk KA, Rustky EA, Fraser RG: Myocardial calcification and cardiac dysfunction in chronic renal failure. *Am J Med* 85:651–657, 1988

98. Abrahams C, D'Cruz I, Kathpalia S: Anormalities in the mitral valve apparatus in patients undergoing long-term hemodialysis. Autopsy and echocardiographic correlation. *Arch Intern Med* 142:1796–1800, 1982.

99. Nestico PF, DePace NL, Kotler MN, et al.: Calcium phosphorus metabolism in dialysis patients with and without mitral anular calcium. Analysis of 30 patients. *Am J Cardiol* 51:497–500, 1983.

100. Maher ER, Young G, Smyth-Walsh B, Pugh S, Curtis JR: Aortic and mitral valve calcification in patients with end-stage renal disease. *Lancet* 2:875–877, 1987.

101. Straumann E, Meyer B, Misteli M, Blumberg A, Jenzer HR: Aortic and mitral valve disease in patients with end stage renal failure on long term haemodialysis. *Br Heart J* 67:236–239, 1992.

102. Khoss AE, Steger H, Legenstein E, Proll E, Salzer-Muhar M, Schlemmer M, Balzar E, Wimmer M: L-carnitine therapy and myocardial function in children treated with chronic hemodialysis. *Wien Klin Wochenschr* 101:17–20, 1989.

103. Silberberg JS, Barre PE, Prichard SS, Sniderman AD: Impact of left ventricular hypertrophy on survival in end-stage renal disease. *Kidney Int* 36:286–290, 1989.

104. Alpert MA, Wizeman V, Huting J, Massey CV: Nominvassive assessment of left ventricular structure and function in patients with end-stage renal disease. In: M Timino, V Wizemann, eds, *Contribution to Nephrology*, vol 106. S Karger, AG Basel, pp 13–25, 1994.

105. Savage DD, Garrison RJ, Kannel WB, Levy D, Anderson SJ, Stokes J III, Feinleib M, Castelli WP: The spectrum of left ventricular hypertrophy in a general population sample: The Framingham Study. *Circulation* 75 (Suppl I):I-26–I-33, 1987.

106. Huwez FV, Pringle SD, Macfarlane PW: A new classification on left ventricular geometry in patients with cardiac disease based on M-mode echocardiography. *Am J Cardiol* 70:681–688, 1992.

107. Devereux RB, Pickering TG, Alderman MH, et al.: Left ventricular hypertrophy in hypertension: prevalence and relation to pathophysiologic variables. *Hypertension* 9:1153–1160, 1987.

108. Hammond IN, Devereux RB, Alderman MH, Lutas EM, Spitzer MC, Crowley JS, Laragh JH: The prevalence and correlation of echocardiographic left ventricular hypertrophy among employed patients with uncomplicated hypertension. *J Med Coll Cardiol* 7:639–650, 1986.

109. Cohen MV, Diaz P, Scheuer J: Echocardiographic assessment of left ventricular function in patients with chronic uremia. *Clin Nephrol* 12:156–162, 1979.

110. Ikram H, Lynn KL, Bailey RR, Little PJ: Carvascular changes in chronic hemodialysis patients. *Kidney Int* 24:371–376, 1983.

111. Harnett JD, Parfrey PS, Griffiths SM, Gault MH, Barre P, Guttman RD: Left ventricular hypertrophy in end stage renal disease. *Nephron* 48:107–115, 1988.

112. London GM, de Vernejoul MC, Fabiani F, et al.: Secondary hyperparathyroidism and cardiac hypertrophy in hemodialysis patients. *Kidney Int* 32:900–907, 1987.

113. Parfrey PS, Harnett JD: Long-term cardiac morbidity and mortality during dialysis therapy. *Adv Nephrol Necker Hosp* 23:311–330, 1994.

114. Foley RN, Parfrey PS, Harnett JD, Kent GM, Martin CJ, Murray DC, Barre PE: Clinical and echocardiographic disease in patients starting end-stage renal disease therapy. *Kidney Int* 47:186–192, 1995.

115. Hung J, Harris PJ, Uren RF et al.: Uremic cardiomyopathy-effect of hemodialysis on left ventricular function in end stage renal failure. *N Engl J Med* 302:547–557, 1980.

116. Madsen BR, Alpert MA, Whiting RB, Van Stone J, Ahmad M, Kelly DL: Effect of hemodialysis on left ventricular performance. *Am J Nephrol* 4:86–91, 1984.

117. Chaignon M, Chen WT, Tarazi RC, Nakamoto S, Salcedo: Acute effects of hemodialysis on echographic-determined cardiac performance: improved contractility resulting from serum-increased calcium with reduced potassium despite hypovolemic-reduced cardiac output. *Am Heart J* 103:374–378, 1982.

118. Henrich WL, Hung J, Nixon JV: Increased ionized calcium and left ventricular contractility during hemodialysis. *N Engl J Med* 310, 1984.

119. Ruder MA, Alpert MA, Van Stone J et al.: Comparative effects of acetate and bicarbonate hemodialysis on left ventricular function. *Kidney Int* 27:768–773, 1985.

120. Huting J, Kramer W, Schutterle, Wizemann V: Analysis of left-ventricular changes associated with chronic hemodialysis. A noninvasive follow-up study. *Nephron* 49:284–290, 1989.

121. Rottenbourg JB: CAPD is more advantageous than hemodialysis. *Semin Dial* 5:212–214, 1992.

122. Alpert MA, Van Stone J, Twardowski ZJ, Nolph KD: Comparative cardiac effects of hemodialysis and continuous ambulatory pertoneal dialysis. *Clin Cardiol* 9:52–58, 1986.

123. Tabacchi GC, Castiglioni A, Giongranole A, et al.: Echocardiographic evaluation of left ventricular function in patients in CAPD. *Peritoneal Dial Bull* 7:578–581, 1987.

124. Franklin JA, Alpert MA, Twardowski ZJ: Effect of increasing intrabdominal pressure and volume on left ventricular function in CAPD. *Am J Kidney Dis* 12:291–298, 1988.

125. Low I, Grutzmacher P, Bergmann M, Schoeppe W: Echocardiographic findings in patients on maintenance hemodialysis substituted with recombinant human erythropoietin. *Clin Nephrol* 31:26–30, 1989.

126. Low-Friedrich I, Grutzmacher P, Marz W, Bergmann M, Schoeppe W: Therapy with recombinant human erythropoietin reduces cardiac size and improves heart function in chronic hemodialysis patients. *Am J Nephrol* 11:54–60, 1991.

127. Paganini EP, Fouad FM, Tarazi RC: Systemic hypertension in chronic renal failure. In: RA O'Rourke, BM Brenner, JH Stein, eds, *The Heart and Renal Disease*. Churchill Livingstone, New York, p 127, 1984.

128. Stablen DM, Hamburger RJ, Lindgloid AS, Nolph KD, Novak JW: The effect of CAPD on hypertension control: a report of the national CAPD registry. *Peritoneal Dial Int* 8:141–144, 1988.

129. Roy LF, Leehen FHH: Therapy of hypertension in end-stage renal disease. In: P Parfrey, JD Harnett, eds, *Cardiac Dysfunction in Chronic Uremia*. Kluwer Academic Publishers, Boston, pp 245–266, 1992.

130. Dahlof B, Pennert K, Hansson L: Reversal of LVH in hypertensive patients. A metaanalysis of 109 treatment studies. *Am J Hypertens* 5:95–110, 1992.

131. The CONSENSUS Trial Study Group: Effect of enalapril on mortality in severe congestive heart failure. Results of the Cooperative North Scandinavian Enalapril Survival Study (CONSENSUS). *N Engl J Med* 316:1429–1435, 1987.

132. The SOLVD Inestigators: Effect of enalapril on survival in patients with reduced left ventricular ejection fraction on congestive heart failure. *N Engl J Med* 325:293–302, 1991.

133. The SOLVD Investigators: Effect of enalapril on mortality and the development of heart failure in asymptomatic patients with reduced left ventricular ejection fraction. *N Engl J Med* 325:303–310, 1991.

134. Cohn JN, Johnson G, Ziesche S, et al.: A comparison of enalapril with hydralazine-isosorbide dinitrate in the treatment of chronic congestive heart failure. *N Engl J Med* 325:303–310, 1991.

135. Greenber BH: The medical managment of chronic congestive heart failure. In: JD Hosenpud, BH Greenberg, eds, *Congestive Heart Failure: Pathophysiology, Diagnosis and Comprehensive Approach to Management*. Springer-Verlag, New York, pp 628–644, 1994.

136. Packer M, Gheorghiade M, Young JB, Constantini PJ, Adams KF, Cody RJ, Smith LK, Van Voorhees L, Gourely LA, Jolly MK, for the RADIANCE Study: Withdrawal of digoxin from patients with chronic heart failure treated with angiotensin-converting-enzyme inhibitors: RADIANCE study. *N Engl J Med* 329:1–7, 1993.

137. Uretsky BF, Young JB, Shahidi FD, Yellen LG, Harrison MC, Jolly MK, on behalf of the PROVED Investigative Group: Randomized study assessing the effect of digoxin withdrawal in patients with mild to moderate chronic congestive heart failure: results of the PROVED trial. *J Am Coll Cardiol* 22:955–962, 1993.

138. Waagstein F, Bristow MR, Swedberg K, Camerini F, Fowler MD, Silver MA, Gilbert EM, Johnson MR, Goss FG, Hjalmarson A, for the Metoprolol in Dilated Cardiomyopathy (MDC) Trial Study Group: Beneficial effect of metoprolol in idiopathic dilated cardiomyopathy. *Lancet* 342:1441–2446, 1993.

139. Ferrari R: Calcium antagonists and left ventricular dysfunction. *Am J Cardiol* 75:71E–76E, 1995.

140. Verresen L, Waer M, Vanrenterghem Y, Michielsen P: Angiotensin converting-enzyme inhibitors and anphilactoid reactions to high-flux membranes. *Lancet* 336:1360–1362, 1990.

141. Pegues DA, Beck-Sague CM, Woollen SW, Greenspan B, Burns SM, Bland LA, Arduino MJ, Favero MS, Mackow RC, Jarvis WR: Anaphylactoid reactions associated with reuse of hollow-fiber hemodialyzers and ACE inhibitors. *Kidney Int* 42:1232–1237, 1992.

142. Verrsen L, Fink E, Lenske H-D, Vanrenterghem Y: Bradykinin is a mediator of anphylactoid reactions during hemodialysis with AN 69 membranes. *Kidney Int* 45:1497–1503, 1994.

143. Hara S, Ubara Y, Arizono K, Ikeguchi H, Katori H, Yamada A, Ogura Y, Murata H, Mimura N: Relation between parathyroid hormone and cardiac function in long-term

hemodialysis patients. *Miner Electrolyte Metab* 21:72–76, 1995.

144. McGonigle RJS, Fowler MB, Timmis AB, Weston MJ, Parsons V: Uremic cardiomyopathy: potential role of parathyroid hormone. *Nephron* 36:94–100, 1984.

145. Burt RK, Gupta-Burk S, Suki WN, et al.: Reversal of left ventricular dysfunction after kidney transplantation. *Ann Intern Med* 111:635–640, 1989.

146. Cueto-Garcia L, Herrera J, Arriaga J, Laredo C, Meaney E: Echocardiographic changes after successful renal transplantation in young nondiabetic patients. *Chest* 83:56–62, 1983.

147. Larsson O, Attman PO, Beckman-Suurkula M, Wallentin I, Wikstrand J: Left ventricular function before and after kidney transplantation. A prospective study in patients with juvenile-onset diabetes mellitus. *Eur Heart J* 7:779–791, 1986.

148. Huting J: Course of left ventricular hypertrophy and function in end-stage renal disease after transplantation. *Am J Cardiol* 70:1481–1484, 1992.

149. Smogorzewski M: Renal transplantation in specific disease. In: SG Massry, RJ Glassock, eds, *Massry's and Glassock Textbook of Nephrology*. Williams & Wilkins, Baltimore, pp 1707–1717, 1994.

150. Amann K, Wiest G, Zimmer G, Gretz N, Ritz F, Mall G: Reduced capillary density in the myocardium of uremic rats—a stereological study. *Kidney Int* 42:1079–1085, 1992.

151. Rostand SG, Kirk KA, Rutsky EA: The epidemiology of coronary artery disease in patients on maintenance hemodialysis: implications for management. *Contrib Nephrol* 52:34–41, 1985.

152. Simon P, Autuly V, Ang KS, et al.: Epidemiologic data on ischemic heart disease (IHD) in a dialyzed population (abstract). *J Am Soc Nephrol* 3:395, 1992.

153. Rostand SG, Kirk KA, Rutsky EA: Dialysis-associated ischemic heart disease: Insights from coronary antiography. *Kidney Int* 25:653–659, 1984.

154. Rostand SG, Rutsky EA: Coronary artery disease in end-stage renal disease. In: WL Henrich ed, *Principles and Practice of Dialysis*. Williams & Wilkins, Baltimore, pp 181–195, 1994.

155. Rostand SG, Kirk KA, Rutsky EA: Relationship of coronary risk factors to hemodialysis-associated ischemic heart disease. *Kidney Int* 22:304–308, 1982.

156. Holley JL, Fenton RA, Arthur RS: Thallium stress testing does not predict cardovascular risk in diabetic patients with end-stage renal disease undergoing cadaveric renal transplantation. *Am J Med* 90:503–570, 1991.

157. Brown JH, Vites NP, Testa HH, Prescott MC, Hunt LP, Gokol R, Mallick NP: Value of thallium myocardial imaging in the prediction of future cardiovascular events in patients with end-stage renal failure. *Nephrol Dial Transplant* 8:433–437, 1993.

158. Reis G, Marcovitz PA, Leichtman AB, Merion RM, Fay WP, Wernes SW, Armstrong WF: Usefuness of dobutamine stress echocardiography in detecting coronary artery disease in end-stage renal disease. *Am J Cardiol* 75:707–710, 1995.

159. Goldberg AP, Hagberg JM, Delmez JA, et al.: Metabolic effects of exercise training in hemodialysis patients. *Kidney Int* 18:754–761, 1980.

160. Grundy SM: Management of hyperlipdemia of kidney disease. *Kidney Int* 37:847–853, 1990.

161. Boudaulas H: Cardiovascular drug therapy in patients with renal disease. In: CV Leier, H Boudoulas, eds, *Cardiorenal Disorders and Diseases*. Futura, Mount Kisco, NY, pp 275–315, 1992.

162. Rinehart AL, Herzog CA, Collins AJ, Fack JM, Jennie Z, Ma MS, Opsahl JA: A comparison of coronary angioplasty and coronary artery bypass grafting outcomes in chronic dialysis patients. *Am J Kidney Dis* 25:281–290, 1995.

163. Rostand SG, Kirk KA, Rutsky EA, Pacifico AD: Results of coronary artery bypass grafing in end-stage renal disease. *Am J Kidney Dis* 12:266–270, 1988.

164. Batiuk T, Kurtz SB, Oh JK, Orszulak TA: Coronary artery bypass operation in dialysis patients. *Mayo Clin Proc* 66:45–53, 1991.

165. Kahn JK, Rutherford BD, McConahay DR, et al.: Short- and long-term outcome of percutaneous transluminal coronary angioplasty in chronic dialysis patients. *Am Heart J* 119:484–489, 1990.

166. Deutsch E, Bernstein RC, Addonizio P, Kussmaul WG III: Coronary artery bypass surgery in patients on chronic hemodialysis. *Ann Intern Med* 110:369–372, 1989.

167. Ahmed WH, Shubrooks SJ, Gibson MC, Bain DS, Bittl JA: Complications and long-term outcome after percutaneous coronary angioplasty in chronic hemodialysis patients. *Am Heart J* 128:252–255, 1994.

168. Wizemann V, Kramer W, Thormann J, Kindler M, Schutterle G: Cardiac arrhythmias in patients on maintenance hemodialysis: causes and management. *Contrib Nephrol* 52:42–53, 1986.

169. Kimura K, Tabei K, Asano Y, Hosoda S: Cardiac arrhythmias in hemodialysis patients. A study of incidence and contributory factors. *Nephron* 53:201–207, 1989.

170. Redaelli B, Cavalli A, Catini R, et al.: (Gruppo emodialisi e patologie cardiovasculari): Multicentre, cross-sectional study of ventricular arrhythmias in chronically hemodialyzed patients. *Lancet* 2:305–308, 1988.

171. Wizemann V, Kramer W: Cardiac arrhythmias in end-stage renal disease: prevalence, risk factors, and management. In: PS Parfrey, JD Harnett, eds, *Cardiac Dysfunction in Chronic Uremia*. Kluwer Academic Publishers, Boston, pp 67–81, 1992.

172. Niwa A, Taniguchi K, Ito H, Nakagawa S, Takeuchi J, Sasaoka T, Kanayama M: Echocardiographic and Holter findings in 321 uremic patients on maintenance hemodialysis. *Jpn Heart J* 26:403–411, 1985.

173. D'Elia J, Weinrauch L, Gleason R, et al.: Application of the ambulatory 24-hour electrocardiogram in the prediction of cardiac death in dialysis patients. *Arch Intern Med* 148:2381–2385, 1988.

174. Sforzini S, Latini R, Mingadi G, Vincent A, Redaelli B: Ventricular arrhythmias and four-year mortality in hemodialysis patients. Gruppo Ernodialisi e Patologie Cardiovasculari. *Lancet* 339:212–213, 1992.

175. Rutsky EA: Arrhythmias in hemodialysis patients. In: AR Nissenson, RN Fine, eds, *Dialysis Therapy*, 2nd ed. Hanley and Belfus, Philadelphia, pp 116–123, 1992.

176. Abuelo JG, Shemin D, Chazan JA: Acute symptoms produced by hemodialysis: a review of their causes and association. *Semin Dial* 6:59–69, 1993.

177. Victor RG, Henrich WL: Autonomic neuropathy and hemodynamic stability in end-stage renal disease patients. In: WL Henrich, ed, *Principles and Practice of Dialysis*. Williams & Wilkins, Baltimore, pp 196–208, 1994.

178. Converse RL, Jacobsen TN, Jost CM, Toto RD, Grayburn PA, Obregon TM, Fouad-Tarazi F, Victor RG: Paradoxical withdrawal of reflex vasoconstriction as a cause of hemodialysis-induced hypotension. *J Clin Invest* 90:1657–1665, 1992.

179. Lilley JJ, Golden J, Stone RA: Adrenergic regulation of blood pressure in chronic renal failure. *J Clin Invest* 57:1190–1200, 1976.
180. Campese VM, Romoff MS, Levitan D, Lane K, Massry SG: Mechanisms of autonomic nervous system dysfunction in uremia. *Kidney Int* 20:246–253, 1981.
181. Velez RL, Woodard TD, Henrich WL: Acetate and bicarbonate hemodialysis in patients with and without autonomic dysfunction. *Kidney Int* 26:59–65, 1984.
182. Schilling Lehman H, Hampl H: Studies on circulatory stability during bicarbonate hemodialysis with constant dialysate sodium versus acetate hemodialysis with sequential dialysate sodium. *Artif Organs* 9:17–21, 1985.
183. Levy FL, Grayburn PA, Foulks CJ, Brickner ME, Henrich WL: Improved left ventricular contractility with cool temperature hemodialysis. *Kidney Int* 41:961–965, 1992.
184. Jost CM, Agarwal R, Khair-el-Din T, Graybourn PA, Victor RG, Henrich WL: Effect of cooler temperature dialysate on hemodynamic stability in "problem" dialysis patients. *Kidney Int* 44:606–612, 1993.
185. Maggiore Q, Pizzarelli F, Sisca S, Zocalli C, Parlongo S, Nicolo F, Creazzo G: Blood temperature and vascular stability during hemodialysis and hemofiltration. *Trans Am Soc Artif Intern Organs* 28:523–527, 1982.
186. Sherman RA, Faustino EF, Bernholc AS, Eisinger RP: Effect in variations in dialysate temperature on blood pressure during hemodialysis. *Am J Kidney Dis* 4:66–68, 1984.
187. Cross AS, Steigbigel RT: Infective endocarditis and access site infections in patients on hemodialysis. *Medicine (Baltimore)* 55:453–466, 1976.
188. Nichols A, Edward N, Cutto G: Staphylococcal septicemia, endocarditis and osteomyelitis in dialysis and renal transplant patients. *Postgrad Med J* 56:642–648, 1980.
189. Leonard A, Roy L, Shapiro FL: Bacterial endocarditis in regularly dialyzed patients. *Kidney Int* 4:407–422, 1973.
190. Birkeland SA: Uremia as a state of immune deficinecy. *Scand J Immunol* 5:107–1115, 1976.
191. Descamps-Latscha B, Herbelin L: Long-term dialysis and cellular immunity: a critical survey. *Kidney Int* 43 (Suppl 4):S135–S142, 1993.
192. Ruiz P, Gomez F, Schreiber AD: Impaired function macrophage F_c gamma receptors in end-stage renal disease. *N Engl J Med* 322:717–722, 1990.
193. Alexiewicz JM, Smogorzewski M, Fadda GZ, Massry SG: Impaired phagocytosis in dialysis patients. Studies on mechanisms. *Am J Nephrol* 11:102–111, 1992.
194. Albers FJ: Causes of hemodialysis access failure. *Adv Renal Replacement Ther* 1:107–118, 1994.
195. Swartz RD, Messana JM, Boyer CJ, Lunde NM, Weitzel WF, Hartman TL: Successful use of cuffed central venous hemodialysis catheters inserted percutaneously. *J Am Soc Nephrol* 4:1719–1725, 1994.
196. Brecia MJ, Cimino JE, Appel K, Hurwitz BJ: Chronic hemodialysis using venipuncture and a surgically created arteriovenous fistula. *N Engl J Med* 275:1089–1092, 1966.
197. Scheld WM, Sande MA: Endocarditis and intravascular infections. In: GL Mandell, JE Bennett, R Dolin, eds, *Mandell, Douglas and Bennett's Principles of Infectious Diseases.* Churchill Livingstone, New York, pp 740–783, 1995.
198. Durack DT, Lukes AS, Bright DK: New criteria for diagnosis of infective endocarditis: utilization of specific echocardiographic findings. *Am J Med* 96:200–203, 1994.
199. Von Reyn CF, Levy BS, Arbeit RD, Friedlander G, Crumpacker CS: Infective endocarditis: an analysis based on strict case definitions. *Ann Intern Med* 94:505–517, 1981.
200. Stewart WJ, Shank: The diagnosis of prosthetic valve endocarditis by echocardiography. *Semin Thorac Cardiovasc Surg* 7:7–12, 1995.
201. Dajan AS, Bisno AL, Chung KJ, et al.: Prevention of bacterial endocarditis: recommendations of the American Heart Association. *JAMA* 264:2919–2922, 1992.
202. Yu VL, Goetz A, Wagener M, Smith PB, Rihs JD, Hanchett J, Zuravleff JJ: Staphylococcus aureus nasal carriage and infection in patients on hemodialysis. *N Engl J Med* 315:91–96, 1986.
203. Chow JW, Yu VL: Staphylococcus aureus nasal carriage in hemodialysis patients. Its role in infection and approaches to prophylaxis. *Arch Intern Med* 49:1258–1262, 1989.
204. Padberg FT Jr, Lee BC, Curl GR: Hemoaccess site infection. *Surg Gynecol Obstet* 174:103–108, 1992.
205. Durack DT: Infective endocarditis. In: PD Hoeprich, MC Jordan, AR Ronald, eds, *Infectious Diseases.* JB Lippincott, Philadelphia, pp 1233–1248, 1994.
206. Bisno AL, Dismukes WE, Durack DT, et al.: Antimicrobial treatment of infective endocarditis due to viridans streptococci, enterococci and staphylococci. *JAMA* 261:1471–1477, 1989.
207. Kaul TK, Fields BL, Reddy MA, Kahn DR: Cardiac operations in patients with end-stage renal disease. *Ann Thorac Surg* 57:691–696, 1994.

CHAPTER 51

Renal Osteodystrophy: Prevention and Management

ESTHER A. GONZALEZ & KEVIN J. MARTIN

INTRODUCTION

Renal osteodystrophy is the term used to describe the complex abnormalities of bone that may occur, to variable extents, in many patients with renal disease. The spectrum of disorders of the skeleton in these patients is broad and extends from states of accelerated bone turnover with increased bone resorption due to excessive levels of parathyroid hormone (PTH) (osteitis fibrosa) to disorders of bone mineralization (osteomalacia) and other states of decreased bone turnover (adynamic bone). In addition, osteosclerosis, bone cysts, loss of bone mineral, and skeletal fractures may occur. The pathogenesis of these abnormalities has been the subject of intense investigation for the past two decades; the consequences of decreased renal function that give rise to these disorders of bone have been characterized and serve as the basis for a rational approach to the prevention and therapy of the skeletal abnormalities of renal dysfunction.

With the recognition of the need for prevention and therapy of renal osteodystrophy and with advances in dialysis techniques, the prevalence of the various types of bone abnormalities in patients with advanced renal failure has changed. A recent breakdown of the types of bone abnormalities from a single center of patients with end-stage renal disease is shown in Figure 1. The data have been divided according to the modality of dialysis (1). The most prevalent bone abnormalities in patients on hemodialysis are osteitis fibrosa and the adynamic pattern of bone histology, while in patients on peritoneal dialysis the adynamic pattern predominates. The following sections will deal with the prevention and management of renal osteodystrophy based upon pathophysiologic considerations, which are shown in diagrammatic format in Figure 2. Several factors related to chronic renal insufficiency are responsible for the pathogenesis of uremic osteodystrophy. Phosphorus retention, calcitriol deficiency, and abnormal function of the parathyroid glands are the principal consequences of chronic renal failure that

contribute to the development of hyperparathyroid bone disease. Attempts to prevent and treat secondary hyperparathyroidism may result in low-bone-turnover osteodystrophy. Even hemodialysis itself may contribute to renal osteodystrophy with the accumulation of β-2-microglobulin or from impurities in the water supply.

The essentials of the diagnostic assessment of patients with renal osteodystrophy include regular measurements of serum biochemistries such as BUN, creatinine, calcium, phosphorus, and bicarbonate together with measurements of PTH and aluminum. Other parameters of bone metabolism such as alkaline phosphatase, osteocalcin, tartrate-resistant acid phosphatase, and products of collagen metabolism may be useful in selected circumstances. Currently, assays of intact PTH using two-site immunoradiometric (IRMA) or immunochemiluminescent (ICMA) techniques are the most widely used and are replacing the previously used region-specific radioimmunoassays such as midregion or C-terminal PTH radioimmunoassays. The assay of intact PTH has a well-defined normal range and allows comparison of results between different laboratories so that uniform guidelines may be derived. While the precise values for intact PTH required for normal bone turnover have not been established for all levels of renal function, it appears that values of 100–150 pg/mL, which is above the upper limit of normal of 65 pg/mL, are associated with normal bone turnover in patients with end-stage renal disease (2).

While bone biopsy and examination of undecalcified sections after tetracycline labeling is clearly the 'gold standard' for the diagnosis of renal osteodystrophy, this invasive test is usually reserved for selected circumstances. Indications for biopsy include
— Evaluation of bone pain and fractures
— Evaluation of positive noninvasive aluminum testing, particularly prior to parathyroidectomy
— Evaluation of hypercalcemia, either spontaneous or on therapy with low doses of calcium and/or calcitriol, particularly if the levels of PTH are low

Suki, WN and Massry SG (eds), Suki and Massry's Therapy of Renal Diseases and Related Disorders, Third Edition. ISBN 978-1-4757-6634-9.
©1998, Kluwer Academic Publishers, Boston/Dordrecht/London. All rights reserved.

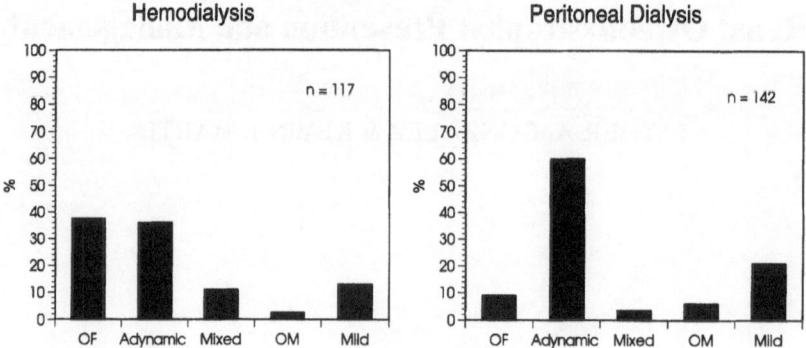

Figure 1. Incidence of the various histologic patterns of renal osteodystrophy in patients on chronic hemodialysis and CAPD. OF: osteitis fibrosa, OM: osteomalacia (Modified from reference 1 with permission).

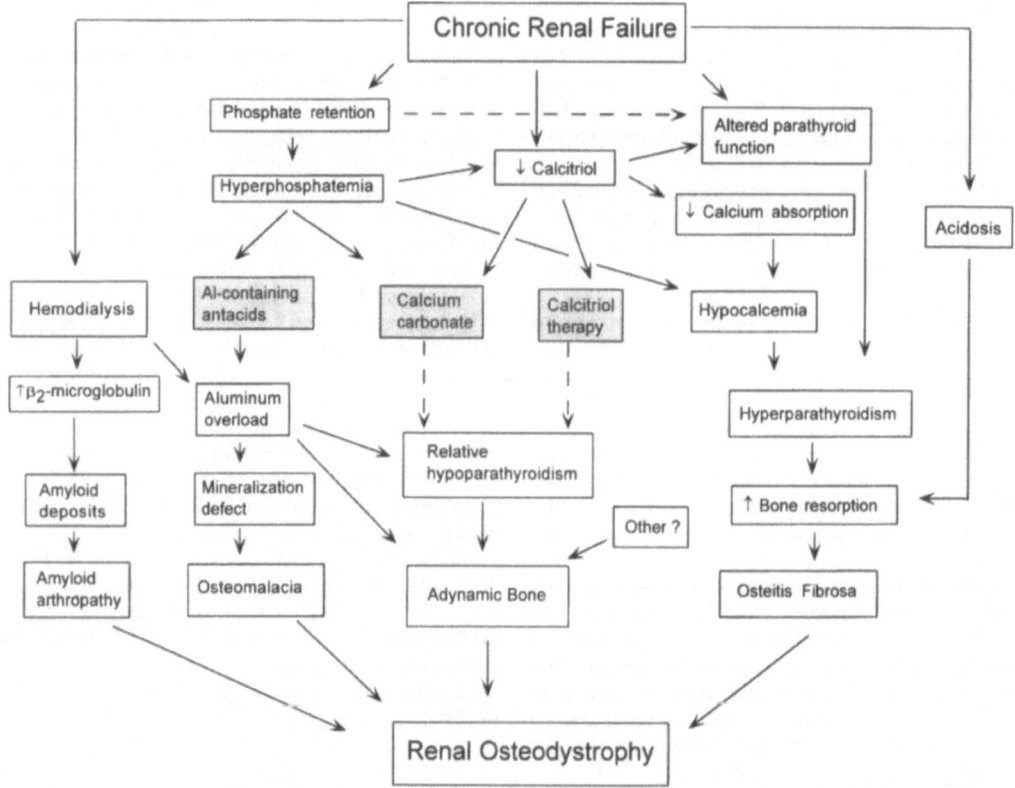

Figure 2. Schematic representation of the factors involved in the pathogenesis of renal osteodystrophy. Solid lines indicate mechanisms that are well established. Dashed lines indicate mechanisms which have not yet been definitively established. Shaded boxes denote therapeutic interventions in the management of osteitis fibrosa.

OSTEITIS FIBROSA

Osteitis fibrosa results from high levels of circulating PTH. The main factors involved in the development of hyperparathyroidism in chronic renal failure include 1) retention of phosphorus, 2) decreased levels of calcitriol, and 3) abnormal function of the parathyroid glands.

Phosphorus retention

The role of phosphorus retention in the genesis of secondary hyperparathyroidism has been clearly demonstrated (3,4). Due to impaired phosphorus excretion by the failing kidney, there is an increase in serum phosphorus that results in decreased levels of ionized calcium, which in turn leads to stimulation of PTH secretion. In addition, hyperphosphatemia may inhibit the synthesis of 1–25 dihydroxyvitamin D (calcitriol) (5), resulting in decreased intestinal calcium absorption and hypocalcemia, thereby contributing to the increased secretion of PTH. Even though hyperparathyroidism can be triggered by phosphorus-induced hypocalcemia and by low levels of calcitriol, there is evidence that other factors may be involved, since it has been shown that lowering dietary phosphorus results in decreased levels of PTH even in the absence of changes in the levels of ionized calcium or calcitriol (6,7). In addition to lowering PTH secretion, dietary phosphorus restriction has also been shown to prevent proliferation of parathyroid cells in rats with mild chronic renal failure (8). These data indicate that phosphorus restriction per se is of paramount importance in the management of secondary hyperparathyroidism.

Prevention and management of hyperphosphatemia

Dietary restriction of phosphorus should be initiated early in the course of renal insufficiency (8). This may be achieved by avoiding foods rich in phosphorus (9). A list of the phosphorus content of selected foods is presented in Table 1. In general, there is a good correlation between the phosphorus and protein contents of most foods; thus, whereas a normal diet provides 1–1.5 g of phosphorus per day, a diet restricting daily protein intake to 0.6 g/kg provides approximately 650 mg of phosphorus (10). Subsequently, attempts to restrict phosphorus intake below 700–900 mg/day should be avoided lest protein–calorie malnutrition develops. As renal function deteriorates, it becomes increasingly difficult to control hyperphosphatemia by dietary restriction alone, and even when hemodialysis is instituted, only about 900 mg of phosphorus can be removed during a standard treatment—an amount lower than that absorbed from the intestine with a diet providing adequate protein intake. Therefore, it is necessary to limit the absorption of phosphorus through the use of compounds that bind ingested phosphorus in the intestine and thus prevent its absorption. Aluminum salts are potent phosphate binders; however, their use is limited in

Table 1. Phosphorus content of selected foods (mg per serving)

Egg	90
Peanuts	100
Sunflower seeds	330
Milk	125
Meats	200
Cheese	150
Cream cheese	30
Whole wheat bread	65
Pasta/noodles	25
Oatmeal	130
Cream of wheat	32
Beans	130
Vegetables	30–50
Beverages	
Coffee	2
Cola	30
Root beer	0
Fruit	10–25

patients with chronic renal failure, since these compounds can be absorbed (11) and contribute to the development of dementia and osteomalacia (12). If the use of aluminum hydroxide is necessary, the dose should be restricted to no more than 40–45 mg/kg/day (13) in order to minimize the risk of aluminum toxicity.

Calcium salts, taken with meals, have been shown to be effective in binding phosphorus in the intestine (14,15), and their use is now preferred over that of aluminum-containing antacids in view of the undesirable side-effect profile of the latter. When administered to patients with chronic renal failure, calcium carbonate has been shown to be an effective phosphate binder in 60%–70% of the cases (15). The dose required to prevent hyperphosphatemia ranges from 4 to 12 g daily. Hypercalcemia is a well-known side effect of calcium carbonate treatment that may be minimized by the use of dialysate with a low calcium content (2.5 mEq/L) (16). When compared to calcium carbonate, calcium acetate has been found to be more effective as a phosphate binder (17). A lower dose, ranging from 1.5 to 9 g daily, is required, and no significant difference has been found in the incidence of hypercalcemia; however, somewhat lower tolerance has been reported with calcium acetate (18). In addition, calcium acetate has been shown to reduce intestinal absorption of zinc (19), thus contributing to the development of zinc deficiency, which may be responsible for abnormal taste or smell as well as sexual dysfunction. Calcium citrate has the same phosphate-binding effect as calcium carbonate (20); however, its use should be avoided in the setting of chronic renal failure, since citrate may increase aluminum absorption by increasing its solubility and opening cellular tight junctions (21).

Magnesium salts have also been used as phosphate binders (22); however, they should be used cautiously, since high magnesium levels may have serious effects on nerve conduction and myocardial conductivity. At low doses (2 g daily), magnesium hydroxide in combination with calcium carbonate has been shown to be safe in dialysis patients, provided that the magnesium concentration in the dialysate is lowered to 0.2–0.3 mmol/L. Furthermore, although hypermagnesemia may result in impaired bone mineralization, mildly elevated serum magnesium levels (between 1 and 1.5 mmol/L) have not been associated with defective mineralization (23–25).

Thus, the management of hyperphosphatemia includes dietary restriction of phosphorus to 700–900 mg daily and the use of calcium salts with meals. The daily dose of calcium salts should be distributed according to the phosphorus content of each meal, and the risk of hypercalcemia may be reduced by lowering the dialysate calcium concentration to 2.5 mEq/L. Although aluminum intake should be avoided in chronic renal failure, the use of calcium salts may be limited in some cases due to hypercalcemia. Under those circumstances, it may become necessary to use aluminum-containing phosphate binders in combination with calcium salts in order to prevent an elevated calcium–phosphorus product and subsequent risk for metastatic calcification.

Calcitriol deficiency

Progression of renal insufficiency is accompanied by low levels of calcitriol, since its synthesis takes place in the kidney by the actions of the enzyme 1-alpha-hydroxylase (26,27). Calcitriol deficiency may contribute to the development of secondary hyperparathyroidism by several mechanisms (Figure 3), including impaired intestinal calcium absorption leading to hypocalcemia, abnormal func-

tion of the parathyroid glands, and skeletal resistance to the actions of PTH. Studies have shown that hyperplastic parathyroid glands have an increased set-point for calcium (the concentration of calcium required to decrease PTH release by 50%) and that this abnormality in parathyroid gland function can potentially be reversed by the administration of calcitriol (28,29). Low levels of calcitriol may also result in abnormal parathyroid gland function by increasing PTH gene transcription and parathyroid cell growth and by decreasing the number of vitamin D receptors on the parathyroid glands (30–32). It has been demonstrated that in renal failure, the skeleton is resistant to the calcemic action of PTH and that this defect can be partially corrected with calcitriol treatment (33,34). Thus, it appears that calcitriol deficiency plays a central role in the pathogenesis of secondary hyperparathyroidism. Therefore, the prevention and management of osteitis fibrosa should include supplementation with vitamin D metabolites in addition to the control of serum phosphorus.

Supplementation with vitamin D metabolites

Several vitamin D metabolites have been used for the treatment of renal osteodystrophy (35–38); however, with the exception of 1-alpha-hydroxycholecalciferol, calcitriol has largely replaced their use. Calcitriol has been shown to be effective in lowering PTH levels and improving bone histology (39,40). Early in the course of renal failure, oral calcitriol at a dose of 0.5 ug or less per day has been found to minimize hyperparathyroidism (41,42). Despite such findings, concern exists about the use of calcitriol in this setting due to the potential adverse effects on renal function. Calcitriol has been reported to decrease renal func-

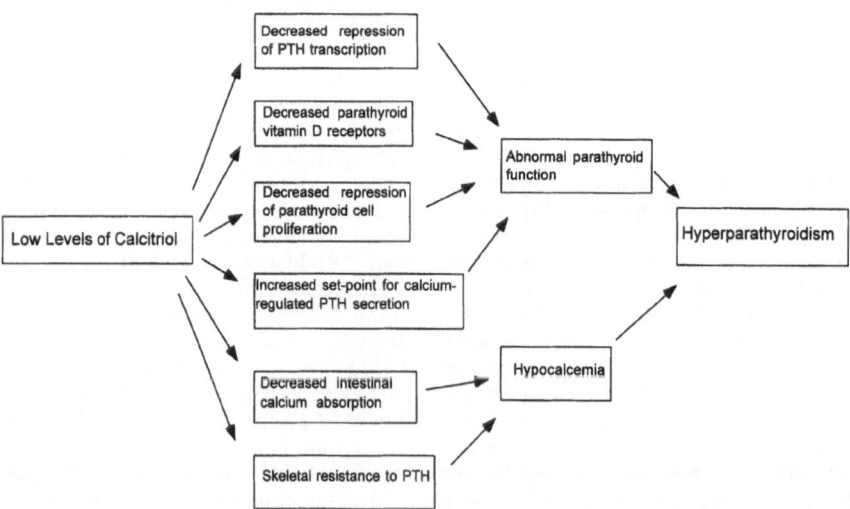

Figure 3. Mechanisms by which calcitriol deficiency contributes to secondary hyperparathyroidism.

tion, an effect that may be due to hypercalcemia or to a direct effect of the drug (43); other studies, however have not detected impairment in renal function during calcitriol treatment, provided that the dose used remained below 0.5 ug/day (44,45). Moreover, calcitriol may reduce the renal tubular excretion of creatinine, since decreases in creatinine clearance in patients treated with 0.5 ug of calcitriol per day have been detected in the absence of changes in inulin clearance (46). Thus, even though the development of hypercalcemia may accelerate the progression of renal failure during calcitriol treatment, such risk appears to be small when low doses are used and therapy is adequately monitored.

Calcitriol has also been found to be beneficial in the treatment of hyperparathyroid bone disease in advanced renal failure (47). Intermittent high doses of calcitriol given intravenously (1–3 ug) with each dialysis have been shown to suppress hyperparathyroidism in hemodialysis patients (48). In addition, patients with severe secondary hyperparathyroidism and hypercalcemia refractory to treatment with oral calcitriol have been shown to respond to intravenous calcitriol (49). "Pulse" administration has also been effective in the oral form (2–5 ug twice per week) in both hemodialysis and peritoneal dialysis patients (50–52). The pathogenetic background for the superior action of intermittent high doses of calcitriol, whether given by the intravenous or oral route, is unclear. It may be that when given in this manner, higher plasma concentrations of calcitriol are achieved, resulting in increased delivery of the drug to the parathyroid glands (53). As previously discussed, calcitriol receptors in the parathyroid glands are downregulated in chronic renal failure, and calcitriol may increase the number of such receptors in hyperplastic parathyroid glands. Thus, calcitriol, when present at high levels, may upregulate its own receptors and improve its effect on the parathyroid glands. In cases of severe hyperparathyroidism, the parathyroid tissue may become resistant to the actions of calcitriol. The recent demonstration of the relative lack of calcitriol receptors in nodular hyperplastic parathyroid tissue may provide the explanation for such observations (54).

To summarize, the use of calcitriol varies with the degree of renal insufficiency and hyperparathyroidism. In early renal failure, oral calcitriol at a dose of 0.25–0.5 ug/day can be used with careful monitoring of serum calcium and renal function. Pulse therapy with calcitriol, whether oral or intravenous, may provide effective suppression of hyperparathyroidism in patients receiving dialysis. The occasional patient with severe secondary hyperparathyroidism resistant to calcitriol should be considered for parathyroidectomy. In addition to increasing intestinal absorption of calcium, calcitriol increases intestinal phosphorus absorption (55); therefore, hyperphosphatemia should be adequately corrected prior to initiating therapy with calcitriol, and serum calcium and phosphorus levels need to be monitored closely during therapy, since hypercalcemia and metastatic calcification are potential compli-

cations. If hypercalcemia develops, it may be necessary to reduce the dose or stop treatment with calcium-containing phosphate binders as well as treatment with calcitriol. Lowering the dialysate calcium to 2.5 mEq/L may also be considered. The occurrence of hypercalcemia shortly after initiating therapy suggests that the diagnosis be reevaluated to ensure that aluminum or other low-turnover bone disease has been excluded and that the levels of intact PTH are indeed elevated above the desirable range of 100–150 pg/mL. On the other hand, the development of hypercalcemia late during the course of therapy may occur as a result of healing of osteitis fibrosa (56,57). In the future, noncalcemic vitamin D analogues may prove valuable in the management of osteitis fibrosa, while decreasing the risk of hypercalcemia (58). In addition to calcium and phosphorus, PTH levels should also be monitored closely, not only to assess the effectiveness of therapy but also to avoid excessive suppression of parathyroid hormone secretion.

Calcium supplementation

Hypocalcemia is not uncommon during the course of renal failure, due to decreased intestinal calcium absorption and decreased dietary calcium intake (59,60). Although emphasis has been placed on controlling hyperphosphatemia, and replacing calcitriol, it is important to avoid hypocalcemia, since the effects of calcitriol on PTH secretion are minimized in the presence of hypocalcemia, which is a powerful stimulus for PTH secretion. The minimum requirement is 1.5 g of elemental calcium per day, and this can be easily achieved with the use of calcium salts as phosphate binders.

Role of parathyroidectomy

While in many cases the strategies for the prevention and treatment of osteitis fibrosa discussed above can be effective, there are a number of circumstances in which these efforts fail or are associated with significant complications such that surgical removal of parathyroid tissue must be considered. The indications for parathyroidectomy are summarized in Table 2. Surgical parathyroidectomy should be considered in patients who are noncomplaint with dietary phosphorus restriction and with the ingestion of phosphate binders, and in whom persistent hyperphosphatemia develops with steadily increasing levels of intact PTH to very high values (>1000 pg/mL). In these circumstances, severe hyperparathyroid bone disease may develop, and medical treatment with calcium supplementation and calcitriol cannot be considered due to the risk of inducing severe hypercalcemia and an elevated calcium–phosphorus product, which might lead to metastatic calcification. The use of calcitriol may indeed aggravate the hyperphosphatemia (55). Some patients with severe hyperparathyroidism may become hypercalcemic without calcitriol therapy, reflecting increased bone resorption by

Table 2. Indications for parathyroidectomy

1. Severe hyperparathyroidism and persistent hyperphosphatemia
2. Severe hyperparathyroidism with hypercalcemia
3. Severe hyperparathyroidism in transplant candidate for living related donor
4. Severe hyperparathyroidism unresponsive to vitamin D and calcium
5. Persistently elevated calcium phosphorus product leading to metastatic calcification
6. Calciphylaxis
7. Severe pruritus?

PTH, and this outcome too may limit efforts to begin or continue treatment with calcium and calcitriol. In such cases, it is necessary to be certain that the hypercalcemia is due to hyperparathyroidism and not to associated aluminum-induced osteomalacia. Thus, it should be documented that PTH levels are very high (>1000 pg/mL) and that aluminum accumulation has been directly excluded (vide infra). A potential indication for parathyroidectomy is a patient who will receive a living related kidney transplant within the near future. In such cases, if hyperparathyroidism is severe, parathyroidectomy should be considered prior to transplant in order to prevent posttransplant hyperparathyroidism, which might require intervention later. No firm guidelines have been established for this clinical situation, but circumstances such as PTH level persistently greater than 1500 pg/mL, young age, and female sex might be important considerations. Parathyroidectomy should also be considered in patients with high levels of intact PTH and with a persistently elevated calcium–phosphorus product, particularly if there is any demonstrable evidence of metastatic calcification. The indication for parathyroidectomy would become more urgent if calciphylaxis develops.

If parathyroidectomy is considered, it is important to exclude coexisting aluminum accumulation in bone, since the syndrome of aluminum-induced osteomalacia may become worse postparathyroidectomy (61). It is therefore appropriate to specifically screen for aluminum accumulation prior to parathyroidectomy by measurements of serum aluminum, Deferroxamine (DFO) testing, and bone biopsy if necessary (vide infra).

SURGICAL PROCEDURE

Several procedures for parathyroidectomy are currently being practiced. These include 1) subtotal parathyroidectomy with reimplantation of parathyroid tissue in the forearm, 2) subtotal parathyroidectomy, and 3) total parathyroidectomy (62,63). Although the most prevalent procedure is subtotal parathyroidectomy with or without re-implantation of parathyroid tissue in the arm, recent evidence has been presented to indicate that total parathyroidectomy may be safely performed in selected patients. While further data are needed to evaluate the safety and efficacy of total parathyroidectomy, the procedure probably should not be considered in patients who are destined to have renal transplant in the future.

The efficacy of parathyroidectomy is reasonably well established; however, if residual parathyroid tissue remains and the patient continues to be noncomplaint, recurrence can be seen in approximately 10% of cases. The advantage of reimplantation of parathyroid tissue in the forearm is that excess parathyroid tissue can again be removed should recurrence be encountered. Malignant transformation of parathyroid implants is a serious complication associated with this procedure (64,65).

NONSURGICAL PARATHYROID GLAND ABLATION

There have been several reports of successful ablation of the parathyroid glands by injection of ethanol using computerized tomography or ultrasound guidance (66–68). This procedure may be considered in selected patients who are at high risk for surgery. Further experience is required to fully evaluate the indications and efficacy of this approach.

PERIOPERATIVE MANAGEMENT

In order to minimize severe hypocalcemia postoperatively, it is advisable to start calcitriol preoperatively. Thus, if patients are not already receiving calcitriol therapy, they should be started on calcitriol with each dialysis at a dose of 2–3 ug for 1–2 weeks prior to parathyroidectomy. Following the surgical procedure, hypocalcemia may be anticipated, and it is imperative to measure serum calcium frequently postoperatively and to begin a calcium infusion before severe hypocalcemia develops. A dosage of 2 mg/kg/hr is a reasonable starting point and may be adjusted according to the measurements of serum calcium. When the patient is able to ingest medications, large amounts of calcium carbonate should be administered orally and increased as tolerated. In many instances, doses in excess of 12 g of elemental calcium per day are required. This oral calcium therapy should be supplemented with oral calcitriol at a dose of 1–2 ug twice a day in the early stages. Frequent physical examinations should also be performed to monitor the appearance of Chvostek's or Trousseau's signs or the appearance of tetany. Serum alkaline phosphatase may increase in the days to weeks postoperatively, indicating increased osteoblastic activity; when alkaline phosphatase begins to fall, caution should be exercised with regard to the dosage of calcium and calcitriol, since hypercalcemia may occur shortly thereafter.

OSTEOMALACIA AND OTHER LOW-BONE-TURNOVER STATES

There are two syndromes of low-bone-turnover uremic osteodystrophy that are best classified histologically. The first is osteomalacia, that is, excess osteoid with decreased rate of mineralization, which is often due to aluminum accumulation. This disorder is becoming less common and now accounts for 4% of cases of renal osteodystrophy. The second low-bone-turnover state is termed *adynamic* or *aplastic bone* and is characterized by decreased bone formation without osteoid accumulation. This histologic pattern now accounts for 60% of cases of renal osteodystrophy in patients on CAPD and 36% of cases on hemodialysis (Figure 1).

Aluminum-related bone disease

Aluminum is known to be a major risk factor for the development of low-bone-turnover osteodystrophy. Aluminum accumulation is most often associated with osteomalacia; however, it may also give rise to the adynamic pattern. The pathogenetic role of aluminum in this syndrome is supported by the positive correlation of aluminum in the dialysate water with the development of osteomalacia (12). Furthermore, aluminum administration can result in osteomalacia and increased bone aluminum, and its discontinuation improves the osteomalacia (69,70). The mechanisms by which aluminum accumulation results in low-bone-turnover osteodystrophy are not clear. There is evidence to support that aluminum has effects on mineralization as well as on bone formation (71,72). In addition, calcitriol production and PTH secretion can both be decreased by aluminum (73,74). However, other factors must also be involved in the pathogenesis of this disorder, since not all patients exposed to aluminum develop bone disease. The existing level of bone turnover at the time of aluminum accumulation may determine the effects of aluminum on bone so that the lower the bone turnover, the more likely aluminum is to localize at the mineralization front. This would explain the finding of worsening aluminum-associated osteomalacia after decreased bone turnover is produced by parathyroidectomy (61).

PREVENTION OF ALUMINUM ACCUMULATION

Aluminum overload may be prevented and even reversed by removing all sources of aluminum. It has been demonstrated that improvement in water purification for dialysis decreases the incidence of aluminum-related osteodystrophy (12). Adequate water purification and close monitoring of aluminum in the dialysis fluids should be performed routinely in order to maintain aluminum levels below 10 ug/L (75). The avoidance of aluminum-containing phosphate binders has been shown to be effective in lowering plasma aluminum levels, as illustrated in Figure 4 (76); thus, the latter compounds should be restricted if at all possible. As previously discussed, citrate increases intestinal aluminum absorption (77); therefore, an effort should be made to avoid citrate-containing compounds such as Shohl's solution. Another factor that contributes to enhanced aluminum absorption is iron deficiency (78), which can be easily avoided by routine assessment of iron status and prompt institution of iron supplementation when necessary.

REMOVAL OF ALUMINUM

If serum aluminum is elevated, further aluminum exposure must be avoided and efforts made to assess aluminum burden. Bone biopsy remains the gold standard for identifying aluminum accumulation in bone; however, because this procedure is invasive and not widely available to all dialysis patients, emphasis has been placed on assessing aluminum accumulation by noninvasive means. Since serum aluminum levels are not of definitive value in identifying patients with aluminum-related bone disease (79), the Deferroxamine (DFO) test is used as a diagnostic tool in this setting. The test is performed by administering DFO (5 mg/kg) intravenously during the last 60 minutes of hemodialysis and obtaining serum aluminum levels prior to that hemodialysis session and again before the next ses-

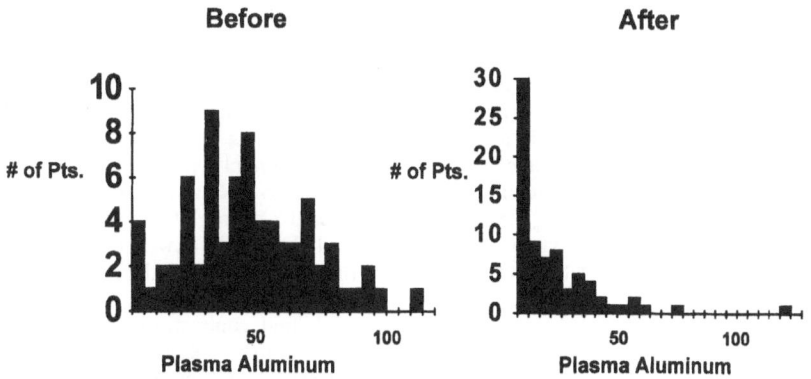

Figure 4. Levels of plasma aluminum in 75 patients on maintenance hemodialysis before and 18 months after the discontinuation of aluminum-containing phosphate binders (Redrawn from reference 76 with permission).

sion. An increment in serum aluminum by 150 ug/L or greater constitutes a positive test. The diagnostic efficacy of this test can be improved by combining the results with measurements of intact PTH. Thus, if serum aluminum increases by 150 ug/L or more during the DFO test and intact PTH is less than 200 pg/mL, the positive predictive value for aluminum bone disease is greater than 95% (80).

In order to remove aluminum by dialysis, it is necessary to use long-term intermittent treatment with DFO, since 80%–90% of aluminum is protein bound (81) and therefore not available for removal by dialysis. DFO chelates aluminum and forms complexes small enough to cross the dialysis membranes (82). Treatment with DFO is indicated in all patients with symptoms of aluminum overload and should be considered in asymptomatic patients in whom the serum aluminum level is consistently greater than 60 ug/L, the result of the DFO test is positive, and especially if bone histology is consistent with aluminum bone disease. Recent recommendations are to use low-dose DFO (5 mg/kg) intravenously once weekly. If after 3 months of therapy, followed by a washout period of 4 weeks, two successive DFO tests 1 month apart fail to demonstrate an increment in serum aluminum greater than 75 ug/L, no further treatment is recommended (83).

Several adverse side effects of DFO have been reported in dialysis patients. Some of the minor complications described include hypotension, ocular and auditory disturbances, gastrointestinal symptoms, and neuromuscular irritability (84,85). Thus, baseline auditory and ophthalmological evaluations are indicated. In addition, the patients should be monitored closely for the development of iron deficiency. Among the most serious complications associated with DFO therapy are the development of encephalopathy (84) and systemic mucormycosis (86). The encephalopathy has been attributed to DFO-induced increased levels of aluminum in the blood, which may subsequently accumulate in the brain (87,88). The potential for *Rhizopus* infection is of great concern, since it follows a fatal course in most cases. In order to minimize these potential complications of DFO, low doses should be given, and high-performance extraction procedures are recommended for hemodialysis as a means of promoting removal of the aluminum–DFO complexes in selected patients (81). Polysulfone dialyzers have been shown to be more effective in promoting removal of DFO–aluminum complexes when compared to cuprophane dialyzers (89). In addition, charcoal hemoperfusion and the combination of hemodialysis and hemoperfusion are superior to hemodialysis alone in achieving aluminum removal following the administration of DFO (90,91). Such procedures may be considered during the early phases of treatment, when the highest aluminum levels are achieved, and in patients with symptoms of aluminum overload.

Idiopathic adynamic bone disease

With the avoidance of aluminum sources by adequate water purification and decreased use of aluminum-containing phosphate binders, aluminum-related bone disease is becoming less of a problem; however, there has been an increase in the incidence of adynamic bone disease in the absence of aluminum accumulation (1,92). This lesion has been associated with old age, diabetes, CAPD, parathyroidectomy, the use of vitamin D metabolites, and (less commonly) with iron and fluoride intoxication (93–96). Although the pathogenesis of the adynamic bone disorder remains unclear, it has been suggested that a relative hypoparathyroid state, such as that associated with diabetes and with the increased use of calcium salts and vitamin D metabolites, is partially responsible for the development of this lesion (94,97). Furthermore, the higher incidence of adynamic bone in CAPD when compared to hemodialysis may be related to the more sustained and higher calcium levels obtained with the former dialysis modality (98), resulting in more effective suppression of PTH secretion. The significance of the adynamic bone lesion is not clear, and its designation as a disease may be premature at the present time. Usually the patients are asymptomatic, and it has been suggested that due to the absence of osteopenia, the risk of fractures should not be increased (1,94); however, this entity is associated with bone aging due to stunted bone remodeling, which may in turn result in inadequate repair of physiologic microdamages, thus leading to mechanical incompetence and a higher risk for fractures (93). Long-term follow-up of patients with adynamic bone is necessary in order to adequately assess the prognosis of this condition.

The increasing incidence of idiopathic adynamic bone disease poses a new therapeutic challenge, since its pathogenesis remains an enigma. Fortunately, most patients are asymptomatic, with the major difficulty being a predisposition to hypercalcemia. This can be managed by reducing oral calcium intake and/or dialysate calcium concentration. Furthermore, excessive suppression of PTH secretion should be avoided by adjusting the dose of vitamin D metabolites so that intact PTH levels are not allowed to fall much below 100 pg/mL.

BETA-2-MICROGLOBULIN AMYLOIDOSIS

Recently, a new syndrome has been described in patients on long-term dialysis; it is characterized by juxta-articular radiolucent cysts in the bone, destructive arthropathies, and carpal tunnel syndrome. There is evidence to suggest that the pathogenesis of this disorder is related to the deposition of β-2-microglobulin in the tissues in the form of amyloid fibrils (99); however, the mechanisms responsible for the production and deposition of amyloid in dialysis patients are not clear. Neither the blood levels nor the synovial fluid concentrations of β-2-microglobulin have been shown to correlate with the presence of amyloid deposits (100,101). Other factors such as glycosaminoglycans, collagen, and serum amyloid protein, as well as aluminum and iron deposits, have also been implicated in the pathogenesis of dialysis amyloidosis (102–105). Recent evidence suggests a relationship between the type of dialysis membrane used and the incidence of amyloidosis. A lower incidence of carpal tunnel syndrome and cystic radiolucencies has been reported with the use of polyacrylonitrile (PAN) as compared to cuprophane membranes (106,107). It is possible that due to its greater biocompatibility, the PAN membrane produces less inflammation and lesser generation of acute-phase reactive proteins that may be involved in the generation of amyloid.

Removal of β-2-microglobulin

At present, there is no effective treatment for dialysis amyloidosis. Since removal of β-2-microglobulin may be important in delaying symptomatic disease, it seems worthwhile to remove as much of it from the blood as possible. High-flux dialysis membranes can remove β-2-microglobulin (108); however, it is not clear if this promotes the mobilization of β-2-microglobulin from the tissues into the circulation. Recently, the use of specific adsorbents of β-2-microglobulin has also been proposed (109). Once the factors contributing to the pathogenesis of β-2-microglobulin-associated skeletal disease are better understood, this complication of long-term dialysis should become easier to manage.

INTEGRATION OF THERAPEUTIC STRATEGIES

Since the pathophysiological abnormalities that give rise to renal osteodystrophy begin early in the course of renal failure, it is highly desirable to start preventive treatment early and to modify the therapeutic strategy as renal disease progresses. A summary of the various approaches to the management of renal osteodystrophy according to the severity of renal insufficiency is presented in Table 3. The main goals of therapy are

— Control of hyperparathyroidism (target values for intact PTH: 100–150 pg/mL)
— Absence of metastatic calcification
— Absence of skeletal symptoms
— Prevention of aluminum accumulation

In the early stages of renal insufficiency, it is desirable to begin mild dietary phosphorus restriction and to begin calcium supplementation. Even at this stage, the levels of intact PTH should be measured. As renal disease progresses, additional measures should be considered, such as the correction of acidosis. Acidosis may lead to loss of bone mineral, since hydrogen ions are buffered by bone, and may exaggerate the effects of PTH in the skeleton (110). If PTH remains elevated in spite of phosphorus restriction and calcium supplementation, the administration of calcitriol should be considered. Hypercalcemia must be avoided lest the decline in renal function be accelerated. When renal insufficiency becomes severe, the above measures should be intensified, and increasing doses of phosphate binders may be required. Calcitriol therapy should be monitored closely, and the dosage should be guided by

Table 3. Guidelines for Prevention and Treatment of Renal Osteodystrophy

Stage of Renal Insufficiency	

Mild
c_{cr} 50–80 ml/min
	1. Dietary Pi restriction
	2. Pi binders
	    Calcium carbonate or acetate
	    0.5–1 gram of calcium with meals
	3. Monitor PTH

Moderate
c_{cr} 25–50 ml/min
	1. Dietary Pi restriction
	2. Pi binders
	    Calcium carbonate or acetate
	    0.5–1 gram of calcium with meals
	3. Monitor PTH
	4. Treat acidosis
	5. Consider calcitriol p.o.

Severe and ESRD
c_{cr} < 25 ml/min
	1. Dietary Pi restriction
	2. Pi binders
	    Calcium carbonate or acetate
	    0.5–3 grams of calcium with meals
	    Aluminum salts — if Pi >7.5 mg/dl
	    minimize duration of Tx
	3. Monitor calcium phosphorus, PTH
	4. Treat acidosis
	    sodium bicarbonate
	
	Consider the following:
	5. Calcitriol p.o.
	    0.5–1 µg daily
	    2–4 µg twice per week
	6. Calcitriol i.v.
	    0.5–3 µg i.v. post dialysis
	7. Evaluate dialysate calcium
	8. Choice of dialyzer
	9. Indications for parathyroidectomy
	10. Indications for bone biopsy

measurements of intact PTH, calcium, and phosphorus. Desirable values for intact PTH are 100–150 pg/mL; suppression of PTH to values much less than 100 pg/mL should probably be avoided lest low bone turnover (adynamic bone) be induced. If aluminum salts are used, therapy should be short term in order to avoid aluminum intoxication. When end-stage renal disease occurs, additional options become available, such as the intravenous administration of calcitriol to patients on hemodialysis. Similar intermittent dosing with oral calcitriol may be used in patients on peritoneal dialysis. The control of hyperphosphatemia must be monitored closely during calcitriol therapy, and consideration should be given to the choice of dialysate calcium so that hypercalcemia may be minimized and metastatic calcification prevented. Parathyroidectomy may become necessary for refractory hyperparathyroidism. Whether increased use of biocompatible dialyzers and improved techniques for the removal of β-2-microglobulin will lead to decreased incidence of β-2 amyloidosis remains to be determined.

In summary, measures for the prevention of renal osteodystrophy should be initiated as early as possible in the course of renal insufficiency. Patients must be monitored closely and therapy begun according to the above guidelines. It is anticipated that if these therapeutic measures can be effectively instituted, the complications of renal osteodystrophy should be preventible.

REFERENCES

1. Sherrard DJ, Hercz G, Pei Y, Maloney NA, Greenwood Celia, Manuel A, Saiphoo C, Fenton SS, Segre G: The spectrum of bone disease in end-stage renal failure—an evolving disorder. *Kidney Int* 43:436–442, 1993.
2. Quarles LD, Lobaugh B, Murphy G: Intact parathyroid hormone overestimates the presence and severity of parathyroid mediated osseus abnormalities in uremia. *J Clin Endocrinol Metab* 75:145–150, 1992.
3. Slatopolsky E, Caglar S, Pennell JP, Taggart J, Canterbury J, Reiss E, Bricker NS: On the pathogenesis of hyperparathyroidism in chronic experimental insufficiency in the dog. *J Clin Invest* 50:492–499, 1971.
4. Slatopolsky E, Caglar S, Gradowska L, Canterbury J, Reiss E, Bricker NS: On the prevention of secondary hyperparathyroidism in experimental chronic renal disease using "proportional reduction" of dietary phosphorus intake. *Kidney Int* 2:147–151, 1972.
5. Tanaka Y, DeLuca HF: The control of 25-hydroxyvitamin D metabolism by inorganic phosphorus. *Arch Biochem Biophys* 159:566–574, 1973.
6. Lopez-Hilker S, Dusso AS, Rapp NS, Martin KJ, Slatopolsky E: Phosphorus restriction reverses hyperparathyroidism in uremia independent of changes in calcium and calcitriol. *Am J Physiol* 259:F432–F437, 1990.
7. Aparicio M, Combe C, Lafage MH, De Precigout V, Potaux L, Bouchet JA: In advanced renal failure, dietary phosphorus restriction reverses hyperparathyroidism independent of changes in the levels of calcitriol. *Nephron* 63:122–123, 1992.
8. Fugakawa M, Kurokawa K: Mild dietary phosphorus restriction directly prevents enhanced parathyroid hormone secretion and synthesis and proliferation of parathyroid cells in chronic renal failure in rats. *J Am Soc Nephrol* 3:703, 1992.
9. Delmez JA, Slatopolsky E: Hyperphosphatemia: its consequences and treatment in patients with chronic renal disease. *Am J Kidney Dis* 19:303–317, 1992.
10. Portale AM, Booth BE, Halloran BP, Morris RC: Effect of dietary phosphorus on circulating concentration of $1,25(OH)_2D_3$ and immunoreactive parathyroid hormone in children with moderate renal insufficiency. *J Clin Invest* 73:1580–1589, 1984.
11. Kaehny W, Hegg A, Alfrey A: Gastrointestinal absorption of aluminum from aluminum-containing antacids. *N Engl J Med* 296:1389–1390, 1977.
12. Platts MM, Goode GC, Hislop JS: Composition of the domestic water supply and the incidence of fractures and encephalopathy in patients on home dialysis. *Br Med J* 2:657–660, 1977.
13. Winney RJ, Cowie JF, Robson JS: Role of plasma aluminum in the detection and prevention of aluminum toxicity. *Kidney Int* 18:S-91–S-95, 1986.
14. Sheikh MS, Maquire JA, Emmett M, Santa Ana CA, Nicar MJ, Schiller LR, Fordtran JS: Reduction of dietary phosphorus absorption by phosphorus binders. *J Clin Invest* 83:66–73, 1989.
15. Slatopolsky E, Weerts C, Lopez-Hilker S, Norwood K, Zink M, Windus D, Delmez J: Calcium carbonate is an effective phosphate binder in dialysis patients. *N Engl J Med* 315:157–161, 1986.
16. Slatopolsky E, Weerts C, Norwood K, Giles K, Fryer P, Finch J, Windus D, Delmez J: Long term effects of calcium carbonate and 2,5 meq/liter calcium dialysate on mineral metabolism. *Kidney Int* 36:897–903, 1989.
17. Delmez JA, Tindira CA, Windus DW, Norwood KY, Giles KS, Nighswander TL, Slatopolsky EL: Calcium acetate as phosphorus binder in hemodialysis patients. *J Am Soc Nephrol* 3:96–102, 1992.
18. Caravaca F, Santos I, Cuberoj J, Esparragp JF, Arrobas M, Pizarro JL, Robles R, Sanches-Casado E: Calcium acetate versus calcium carbonate as phosphate binders in hemodialysis patients. *Nephron* 60:423–427, 1992.
19. Hwang S-J, Lai Y-H, Chen H-C, Tsai J-H: Comparison of the effects of calcium carbonate and calcium acetate on zinc tolerance test in hemodialysis patients. *Am J Kidney Dis* 19:57–60, 1992.
20. Mai L, Emmett M, Sheikh MS, Santa Ana CA, Schiller LR, Fordtran JS: Calcium acetate an effective phosphorus binder in patients with renal failure. *Kidney Int* 36:690–695, 1989.
21. Froment DP, Molitoris Ba, Buddington B, Miller N, Alfrey AC: Site and mechanism of enhanced gastrointestinal absorption of aluminum by citrate. *Kidney Int* 36:978–984, 1989.
22. O'Donovan R, Baldwin D, Hammer M, Moniz C, Parsons V: Substitution of aluminum salts by magnesium salts in control of dialysis hyperphosphatemia. *Lancet* 1:880–882, 1986.
23. Moriniere PH, Fournier A, Leflon A, Herve M, Sebert JL, Gregoire I, Bataille P, Fueris J: Comparison of 1-α OH vitamin D_3 and high doses of calcium carbonate for the control of hyperparathyroidism and hyperaluminemia in patients on maintenance dialysis. *Nephron* 39:309–315, 1985.
24. Moriniere PH, Boudailliez N, Hocine CH, Belbrik S, Renaud H, Westeel PF, Cohen Solal ME, Fournier A: Prevention of osteitis fibrosa, aluminum bone disease and soft tissues calcification in dialysis patients: a long term comparison of moderate doses of oral calcium ± $Mg(OH)_2$ versus $Al(OH)_3$ ± 1α OH vitamin D_3. *Nephrol Dial Transplant* 4:1045–1053, 1989.
25. Moriniere PH, Vinatier I, Westeel PF, Cohen Solal ME, Belbrik S, Abdulmassih Z, Leflon P, Roche D, Fournier A: Magnesium hydroxide as a complementary aluminum free phosphate binder to high doses of oral calcium in uremic patients on chronic hemodialysis: lack of deleterious effect on bone mineralization. *Nephrol Dial Transplant* 3:651–656, 1988.
26. Wilson L, Felsenfeld A, Drezner MK, Llach F: Altered divalent ion metabolism in early renal failure: role of $1,25(OH)_2D$. *Kidney Int* 27:565, 1985.
27. Gray R, Boyle I, DeLuca HF: 1971. Vitamin D metabolism: the role of kidney tissue. *Science* 172:1232–1234, 1971.
28. Brown EM, Wilkson RE, Eastman RC, Pallotta J, Marynick SP: Abnormal regulation of parathyroid hormone release by calcium in secondary hyperparathyroidism due to chronic renal failure. *J Clin Endocrinol Metab* 54:172–179, 1982.
29. Delmez AJ, Tindira C, Grooms P, Dusso A, Windus DW, Slatopolsky E: Parathyroid hormone suppression by intrave-

nous 1,25-dihydroxyvitamin D: a role for increased sensitivity to calcium. *J Clin Invest* 83:1349–1355, 1989.

30. Okazaki T, Igarashi T, Kronenberg HM: 5'-Flanking region of the parathyroid hormone gene mediates negative regulation by 1,25(OH)$_2$D$_3$. *J Biol Chem* 263:2203–2208, 1988.

31. Kremer R, Bolivar I, Goltzman D, Hendy GN: Influence of calcium and 1,25-dihydroxycholecalciferol on proliferation and proto-oncogene expression in primary cultures of bovine parathyroid cells. *Endocrinology* 125:935–941, 1989.

32. Korkor AB: Reduced binding of [^{3}H] 1,25-dihydroxyvitamin D$_3$ in the parathyroid glands of patients with, renal failure. *N Engl J Med* 316:1573–1577, 1987.

33. Somerville PJ, Kaye M: Resistance to parathyroid hormone in renal failure: role of vitamin D metabolites. *Kidney Int* 14:245–254, 1978.

34. Massry SG, Stein R, Garty J, Aruff AI, Coburn JW, Norman AW, Friedler RM: Skeletal resistance to the calcemic action of parathyroid hormone in uremia: role of 1,25(OH)$_2$D$_3$. *Kidney Int* 9:467–474, 1976.

35. Kaye M, Chatterjee G, Cohen GF, Borra S, Sarar S: Arrest of hyperparathyroid bone disease with dihydrotachysterol in patients undergoing chronic hemodialysis. *Ann Intern Med* 73:225–233, 1970.

36. Kaye M, Sagar S: Effect of dihydrotachysterol on calcium absorption in uremia. *Metabolism* 21:815–824, 1972.

37. Witmer G, Margolis A, Fontaine O, Fritsch J, Lenoir G, Broyer M, Balsan S: Effects of 25-hydroxycholecalciferol on bone lesions of children with terminal renal failure. *Kidney Int* 10:395–408, 1976.

38. Recker R, Schoenfeld P, Letten J, Slatopolsky E, Goldsmith R, Brickman A: The efficacy of calcifediol in renal osteodystrophy. *Arch Intern Med* 138:857–863, 1978.

39. Brickman AS, Sherrard DJ, Jowsey J, Singer FR, Baylink DJ, Maloney N, Massry SG, Norman AW, Coburn JW: 1,25-dihydroxycholecalciferol: effect on skeletal lesions and plasma parathyroid hormone in uremic osteodystrophy. *Arch Intern Med* 134:883–888, 1974.

40. Silverberg DS, Bettcher KB, Dossetor JB, Overton TR, Holick MR, DeLuca HF: Effect of 1,25-dihydroxycholecalciferol in renal osteodystrophy. *Can Med Assoc J* 112:190–195, 1975.

41. Baker LRI, Abrams SML, Roe CJ, Faugere MC, Fanti P, Subayti Y, Malluche HH: 1,25(OH)$_2$D$_3$ administration in moderate renal failure: a prospective double-blind trial. *Kidney Int* 35:661-669, 1989.

42. Nordal KP, Dahl E: Low dose calcitriol versus placebo in patients with pre-dialysis chronic renal failure. *J Clin Endocrinol Metab* 67:661–669, 1988.

43. Christiansen CL, Rodbro P, Christiansen MS, Hartnack B, Transbol I: Deterioration of renal function during treatment of chronic renal failure with 1,25-dihydroxycholecalciferal in chronic renal failure. *Lancet* 2:700–703, 1978.

44. Coen G, Mazzaferro S, Bonucci E, Ballanti P, Massimetti C, Donato G, Landi A, Smacchi A, Della Rocca C, Cinotti GA: Treatment of secondary hyperparathyroidism of predialysis chronic renal failure with low doses of 1,25(OH)$_2$D$_3$: humoral and histomorphometric results. *Miner Electrolyte Metab* 12:375–382, 1986.

45. Baker LRI, Abrams SML, Roe CJ, Faugere M-C, Fanti P, Subayti Y, Malluche HH: Early therapy of renal bone disease with calcitriol: a prospective double-blind study. *Kidney Int* 36(S27):S140–S142, 1989.

46. Bertoli M, Luisetto G, Ruffatti A, Urso M, Romagnoli G:

Renal function during calcitriol therapy in chronic renal failure. *Clin Nephrol* 33:98–102, 1990.

47. Massry SG, Goldstein DA, Malluche HH: Current status of the use of 1,25(OH)$_2$D$_3$ in the management of renal osteodystrophy. *Kidney Int* 19:409–418, 1980.

48. Slatopolsky E, Weerts C, Thielan J, Horst R, Harter H, Martin KJ: Marked suppression of secondary hyperparathyroidism by intravenous administration of 1,25-dihydroxycholecalciferol in uremic patients. *J Clin Invest* 74:2136–2143, 1984.

49. Andress DL, Norris KC, Coburn JW, Slatopolsky EA, Sherrard DJ: Intravenous calcitriol in treatment of refractory osteitis fibrosa of chronic renal failure. *N Engl J Med* 321:274–279, 1989.

50. Tsukamoto Y, Nomura M, Maurno F: Pharmacological parathyroidectomy by oral 1,25(oh)$_2$D$_3$ pulse therapy. *Nephron* 51:130–131, 1989.

51. Tsukamoto Y, Nomura M, Takahashi Y, Takagi Y, Yoshida A, Nagaoka T, Togashi K, Kikawada R, Marumo F: The "oral 1,25(OH)$_2$D$_3$ pulse therapy" in hemodialysis patients with severe secondary hyperparathyroidism. *Nephron* 57:23–28, 1991.

52. Martin KJ, Ballal HS, Domoto DT, Blalock S, Weindel M: Pulse oral calcitriol for the treatment of hyperparathyroidism in patients on continuous ambulatory peritoneal dialysis: preliminary observations. *Am J Kidney Dis* 19:540–545, 1992.

53. Reichel H, Szabo A, Uhl J, Resian S, Schmitz A, Schmidt-Gayk H, Ritz E: Intermittent versus continuous administration of 1,25-dihydroxyvitamin D$_3$ in experimental renal hyperparathyroidism. *Kidney Int* 44:1259–1265, 1993.

54. Fukada N, Tanaka H, Tominaga Y, Fukagawa M, Kurokawa K, Seino Y: Decreased 1,25-dihydroxyvitamin D$_3$ receptor density is associated with a more severe form of parathyroid hyperplasia in chronic uremic patients. *J Clin Invest* 92:1436–1443, 1993.

55. Walling MW: Intestinal Ca and phosphate transport: differential responses of vitamin D$_3$ metabolites. *Am J Physiol* 233:E488–E494, 1977.

56. Ott SM, Maloney NA, Coburn JW, Alrey AC, Sherrard DJ: The prevalence of bone aluminum deposition in renal osteodystrophy and its relation to the response to calcitriol therapy. *N Engl J Med* 307:709–713, 1982.

57. Malluche HH, Faugere MC: Effects of 1,25(OH)$_2$D$_3$ administration on bone in patients with renal failure. *Kidney Int* 28 (Suppl 29):S48–S53, 1990.

58. Brown AJ, Ritter CR, Finch JL, Morrissey J, Martin KJ, Murayama E, Nishii Y, Slatopolsky E: The noncalcemic analogue of vitamin D, 22-oxacalcitriol, suppresses parathyroid hormone synthesis and secretion. *J Clin Invest* 84:728–732, 1989.

59. Kopple JD, Coburn JW: Metabolic studies of low protein diets in uremia. II. Calcium, phosphorus and magnesium. *Medicine (Baltimore)* 52:597–607, 1973.

60. Clarkson EM, Eastwood JB, Koutsaimanis KG, de Wardener HE: Net intestinal absorption of calcium in patients with chronic renal failure. *Kidney Int* 3:258–263, 1973.

61. Andress D, Otts S, Maloney N, Sherrard D: Effect of parathyroidectomy on bone aluminum accumulation in chronic renal failure. *N Engl J Med* 31:468–473, 1985.

62. Kaye M, D'Amour P, Henderson J: Elective total parathyroidectomy without transplantation in end stage renal disease. *Kidney Int* 35:1390–1399, 1989.

63. Takagi H, Tominaga Y, Uchida K, Yamada N, Kawai M,

Kano T, Morimoto T: Subtotal versus total para-thyroidectomy with forearm autograft for secondary hyper-parathyroidism in chronic renal failure. *Ann Surg* 200:18–23, 1984.

64. White JV, LoGerfo P, Fiend C. Weber C: Autologous par-athyroid transplantation. *Lancet* 2:461, 1983.

65. Ellis HA: Fate of long-term parathyroid autografts in patients with chronic renal failure treated by parathy-roidectomy: a histopathological study of autografts, parathy-roid glands and bone. *Histopathology* 13:289–309, 1988.

66. Giangrande A, Castiglioni A, Solbiati L, Allaria P: Ultrasound-guided percutaneous fine-needle ethanol injec-tion into parathyroid glands in secondary hyper-parathyroidism. *Nephrol Dial Transplant* 7:412–421, 1992.

67. Page B, Zingraff J, Souberbielle JC, Coutris G, Sarfati E, Drueke T, Moreau JF: Correction of severe secondary hyperparathyroidism in two dialysis patients: surgical re-moval versus percutaneous ethanol injection. *Am J Kidney Dis* 19:378–381, 1992.

68. Takeda S, Michigishi T, Takakura E: Successful ultrasoni-cally guided percutaneous ethanol injection for secondary hyperparathyroidism. *Nephrology* 62:100–103, 1992.

69. Ellis HA, McCarthy JH, Herrington J: Bone aluminum in haemodialysed patients and in rats injected with aluminum chloride: relationship to impaired bone mineralization. *J Clin Pathol* 32:832–844, 1979.

70. Finch JF, Bergfeld M, Martin KJ, Chan YL, Teitelbaum S, Slatopolsky E: The effects of discontinuation of aluminum exposure on aluminum-induced osteomalacia. *Kidney Int* 30:318–324, 1986.

71. Posner AS, Blumenthal NC, Boskey AL: Model of aluminum induced osteomalacia: inhibition of apatite formation and growth. *Kidney Int* 29:S17–S19, 1986.

72. Lieberherr M, Grosse B, Cournot-Witmer G, Hermann-Erlee MPM, Balsan S: Aluminum action on mouse bone cell metabolism and response to PTH and 1,25(OH)$_2$D$_3$. *Kidney Int* 31:737–743, 1987.

73. Goodman WG, Henry DA, Horst R, Nudelman RK, Alfrey AC, Coburn, JW: Parenteral aluminum administration in the dog: II. Induction of osteomalacia and effect on vitamin D metabolism. *Kidney Int* 25:370–375, 1984.

74. Morrissey J, Slatopolsky E: Effect of aluminum on parathy-roid hormone secretion. *Kidney Int* 29:S-41–S-44, 1986.

75. Alfrey A: Aluminum metabolism. *Kidney Int* 29:S8–S11, 1986.

76. Gonzalez EA, Martin KJ: Aluminum and renal osteo-dystrophy: a diminishing clinical problem. *Trends Endocrinol Metab* 3:371–375, 1992.

77. Molitoris BA, Froment DH, MacKenzie TA, Huffer WH, Alfrey AC: Citrate: a major factor in the toxicity of orally administered aluminum compounds. *Kidney Int* 36:949–953, 1989.

78. Cannatta JB, Fernandez-Soto I, Fernandez MMJ, Brock JH, Fernandez MJL, Halls D: The role of iron metabolism in absorption and cellular uptake of aluminum. *Kidney Int* 39:799–803, 1991.

79. Nebeker HG, Andress DL, Milliner DS, Ott SM, Alrey AC, Slatopolsky EA, Sherrard DJ, Coburn JW: Indirect methods for the diagnosis of aluminim bone disease: plasma alumi-num, the desferrioxamine infusion test, and serum iPTH. *Kidney Int* 29 (Suppl 18):S96–S99, 1986.

80. Pei Y, Hercz G, Greenwood C, Sherrard D, Segre G, Manuel A, Saiphoo C, Fenton S: Non-invasive prediction of alumi-num bone disease in hemo and peritoneal dialysis patients. *Kidney Int* 41:1374–1382, 1992.

81. Kaehny WD, Alfrey AC, Holman RE, Shorr WJ: Aluminum transfer during hemodialysis. *Kidney Int* 12:361–365, 1977.

82. Milliner DS, Hercz G, Milliner JH, Shinaberger JH, Nissenson A, Coburn JW: Clearance of aluminum in hemodialysis: effect of desferrioxamine. *Kidney Int* 29:S-100–S-103, 1986.

83. CONSENSUS conference: Diagnosis and treatment of alu-minum overload in end stage renal failure patients. *Nephrol Dial Transplant Suppl* 1:1–4, 1993.

84. Swartz RD: Deferoxamine and aluminum removal. *Am J Kidney Dis* 6:358–364, 1985.

85. Olivieri NF, Buncic JR, Chew E, Gallant Tsvi, Harrison RV, Keenan N, Logan W, Mitchell D, Ricci G, Skarf B, Taylor M, Freedman MH: Visual and auditory neurotoxicity in patients receiving subcutaneous deferoxamine infusions. *N Engl J Med* 314:869–873, 1986.

86. Windus DW, Stokes TJ, Julian BA, et al.: Rhizopus infec-tions in hemodialysis patients receiving deferoxamine. *Ann Intern Med* 107:678–680, 1987.

87. Sherrard DJ, Andress DL: Aluminum-related osteo-dystrophy. *Adv Intern Med* 34:307–324, 1989.

88. Malluche HH, Monier-Faugere MC: Uremic bone disease: current knowledge, controversial issues, and new horizons. *Miner Electrolyte Metab* 17:281–296, 1991.

89. Molitoris BA, Alfrey AC, Alfrey PS, Miller NL: Rapid re-moval of DFO-chelated aluminum during hemodialysis using polysulfone dialyzers. *Kidney Int* 34:98–101, 1988.

90. Delmez J, Weerts C, Lewis-Finch J, Windus D, Slatopolsky E: Accelerated removal of deferoxamine Mesylate-chelated aluminum by charcoal hemoperfusion in hemodialysis pa-tients. *Am J Kidney Dis* 13:308–311, 1989.

91. Weiss LG, Danielson BG, Fellstrom B, Wikstrom B: Alumi-num removal with hemodialysis, hemofiltration and hemo-perfusion in uremic patients after desferrioxamine infusion. *Nephron* 51:325–329, 1989.

92. Morniere P, Cohen-Solal M, Belbrik S, Boudailliez B, Marie A, Westeel PF, Renaud H, Fievet P, Lalau JD, Sebert JL, Fournier A: Disappearance of aluminic bone disease in a long term asymptomatic dialysis population restricting Al(OH)3 intake: emergence of an idiopathic adynamic bone disease not related to aluminum. *Nephron* 53:93–101, 1989.

93. Malluche HH, Monier-Faugere MC: Risk of adynamic bone disease in dialyzed patients. *Kidney Int* 42(38):S-62–S-67, 1992.

94. Cohen-Solal ME, Sebert JL, Boudailliez B, Westeel PF, Moriniere PH, Marie A, Garabedian M, Fournier A: Non-aluminic adynamic bone disease in non-dialyzed uremic pa-tients: a new type of osteopathy due to overtreatment? *Bone* 13:1–5, 1992.

95. De Vernejoul MC, Girot R, Gueris J, Cancela L, Bang S, Bielakoff J, Mautalen C, Goldberg D, Miravet L: Calcium phosphate metabolism and bone disease in patients with ho-mozygous thalassemia. *J Clin Endocrinol Metab* 54:276–281, 1982.

96. Boivin G, Chapuy MC, Baud C, Meunier PJ: Fluoride con-tent in human iliac bone. Results in controls, patients with fluorosis, and osteoporotics treated with fluoride. *J Bone Miner Res* 3:497–502, 1988.

97. Vincenti F, Arnaud SB, Recker R, Genant H, Amend W, Feduska N, Salvatierra O: Parathyroid and bone response of the diabetic patient to uremia. *Kidney Int* 25:677–682, 1984.

98. Morton AR, Hercz G: Hypercalcemia in dialysis patients: 1991. Comparison of diagnostic methods. *Dial Transplant* 20:661–694, 1991.

99. Geyko F, Yamada T, Odani S, Nakagawa Y, Arakawa M, Kunitomo T, Kataoka H, Suzuki M, Hirasswa Y, Shirahama T, Cohen AS, Schmid K: A new form of amyloid protein associated with chronic hemodialysis was identified as β-2 microglobulin. *Biochem Biophys Res Commun* 129:701–706, 1985.

100. Geyko F, Homma N, Suzuki Y, Arakawa M: Serum levels of β-2 microglobulin as a new form of amyloid protein in patients undergoing long-term hemodialysis. *N Engl J Med* 314:585–586, 1986.

101. Sethi D, Grower PE: Synovial fluid β-2 microglobulin levels in dialysis arthropathy. *N Engl J Med* 315:1419–1420, 1986.

102. Linker A, Carney HC: Presence and role of glycosaminoglycans in amyloidosis. *Lab Invest* 57:297–305, 1987.

103. Saito A, Ogawa H, Chung TG, Ohkubo I: Accumulation of serum amyloid P and its deposition in the carpal tunnel region of long-term hemodialysis patients. *Trans Am Soc Artif Intern Organs* 33:512–513, 1987.

104. Netter P, Kessler M, Burnel D, Hutin MF, Delones S, Benoit J, Gaucher A: Aluminum in the joint tissues of chronic renal failure patients treated with regular hemodialysis and aluminum compounds. *J Rheumatol* 11:66–70, 1984.

105. Cary NRB, Sethi D, Brown EA, Erhardt CC, Woodrow DF, Gower PE: Dialysis arthropathy. Amyloid or iron? *Br Med J* 293:1392–1394, 1986.

106. Van Ypersele De Strihou C, Jadoul M, Malghem J, Maldague B, Jamart J: Effect of dialysis-related amyloidosis. *Kidney Int* 39:1012–1019, 1991.

107. Miura Y, Ishiyama T, Inomata A, Takeda T, Senma S, Okuyama K, Suzuki Y: Radiolucent bone cysts and type of dialysis membrane used in patients undergoing long-term hemodialysis. *Nephron* 60:268–273, 1992.

108. Acchiardo S, Kraus AP, Jennings BR: β-2-microglobulin levels in patients with renal insufficiency. *Am J Kidney Dis* 13:70–74, 1989.

109. Gejyo F, Homma N, Arakawa M: Long-term complications of dialysis: pathogenetic factors with special reference to amyloidosis. *Kidney Int* 43(41): S-78–S-82, 1993.

110. Lefebvre A, deVernejoul MC, Gueris J, Goldfarb B, Graulet AM, Morieux C: Optimal correction of acidosis changes progression of dialysis osteodystrophy. *Kidney Int* 36:1112–1118, 1989.

CHAPTER 52

Neurological and Psychiatric Disorders in Renal Diseases

ALBERTO ALBERTAZZI, MARIO BONOMINI, & PAOLO CAPPELLI

INTRODUCTION

Neurological abnormalities specifically related to uremia constantly occur in patients with end-stage renal disease (ESRD), although they only become clinically well defined in severe acute renal failure (ARF) or late in the course of chronic renal failure (CRF) and sometimes in connection with metabolic acidosis and/or electrolyte disturbances secondary to renal disease (1–5).

These abnormalities can affect the central (encephalopathy) or peripheral (polyneuropathy) nervous system or both. The autonomic nervous system may be involved as well.

After the institution of adequate maintenance dialysis therapy, the symptoms generally subside, although many patients may continue to have more subtle kinds of nervous system dysfunction; only successful kidney transplantation is followed by a full clinical recovery in most cases. Dialysis itself is associated with distinct disorders of the central nervous system, including dialysis disequilibrium syndrome, dialytic encephalopathy, some kinds of mononeuropathy such as carpal tunnel syndrome, intracranial hemorrhage, and Wernicke's encephalopathy.

In addition, psychological and psychiatric disturbances, not necessarily related to uremic toxicity or to the type of substitutive treatment, may cause specific disorders.

Finally, it is worth remembering that in some diseases both the nervous system and the kidney may be affected independently of each other and that the nervous system may suffer from renal hypertension (6,7) and side effects of drugs used in the treatment of renal disease (6).

UREMIC ENCEPHALOPATHY

Uremic encephalopathy has been defined as a constellation of potentially or actually disabling neurobehavioral symptoms that may occur abruptly in ARF or progressively in CRF. They are readily reversible by various modalities of dialysis treatment (3).

Clinical features

Clinical features of uremic encephalopathy correlate not so much with specific biochemical abnormalities or the degree of uremia, except in a very general fashion, as with the rate of progression of renal failure. In ARF, these features are more abrupt in onset, are more fulminant, and occur at lower BUN or serum creatinine levels (8). In progressive CRF, cyclic intervals of well-being merge with an otherwise downhill course of the symptomatology. This process may reflect the capacity of the brain to adapt more readily to slowly developing than to acute systemic biochemical alterations (3).

The neurological changes mainly involved in uremia, when renal function declines below 10% of normal, are those concerning complex mental functions and the level of consciousness on the one hand and motor disturbances on the other (1).

The initial neuropsychological changes consist in a decrease in alertness and attention span, and an inability to sustain attention and to concentrate on tasks. Patients are apathetic and irritable and complain of fatigue. When the renal function deteriorates further, the sensorium becomes clouded, and a delirious condition may supervene. Eventually, the untreated patient becomes stuporous and then comatose (9).

The initial motor abnormality is tremulousness, only apparent during limb movements. Then follows asterixis and so-called *flapping tremor*. Myoclonus can be observed in a late phase of uremic encephalopathy; it occurs irregularly and asymmetrically in the limbs, trunk, and head (2).

Generalized tonic and clonic convulsions are a manifestation of acute or late chronic uremia and sometimes precede sudden death.

Electrophysiological findings

New neurophysiological techniques have recently been employed to detect and record conduction abnormalities in central and peripheral pathways even when clinical appearances are normal (10–12). Electroencephalographic (EEG) changes include disorganization, slowing and loss of alpha frequency, diffuse slow wave bursts, and specific paroxysmal discharges.

EEG with Berg's analysis has shown an increase in the percentages of frequencies lower than 7 Hz, 7–10 Hz, and 10–13 Hz, and a reduction in the 13–20-Hz band. These abnormalities are directly related to serum creatinine concentration (13). After at least 8 months of efficient maintenance hemodialysis (MHD), the EEG frequency is usually near normal (14).

In the uremic patient, the latency of the P100 wave of visual evoked potentials (VEPs) rises in the predialysis period. It falls, although not significantly, after the first months of MHD and increases again after long-term treatment. Latency only returns to the normal range after successful renal transplantation (15–17).

Acoustic evoked potentials (AEPs), exploring the polysynaptic auditory pathway, are abnormal in the end stages only. Recordings taken after the end of the first hemodialytic session show increased latencies, attributed to disequilibrium, but regular treatment brings response latencies down towards normal within 4–6 weeks (18,19). Prolonged MHD, lasting more than 5 years, is associated with significant alteration in the morphology of the tracing.

Results with somatosensitive evoked potentials (SEPs) indicate that, while a significant loss in velocity of peripheral nerve conduction is present, intracranial propagation along the short nervous fibers remains near normal (20).

Morphology

Morphological study of the uremic brain by computerized tomography (CT) shows different patterns of cerebral atrophy: global (36.8%), cortical (31.5%), and focal (36.3%). Clear calcifications at various levels, as an epiphenomenon of vascular damage, are present in nearly all patients. A correlation seems to exist between cortical atrophy and the duration of uremia before substitutive treatment. In patients undergoing MHD, the periodic variations in cerebral water content are manifest. Postdialytic density values decrease compared to predialytic ones owing to lower water content in nervous parenchyma. At the end of dialysis, the densitometric values reported are very similar to those of controls. These densitometric changes do not involve CAPD patients who show a trend similar to that of controls (21).

Nuclear magnetic resonance imaging (MRI), a rapidly developing technique, has replaced CT as the first-choice examination in most neurological conditions. Our preliminary experience in MHD and CAPD patients, however, indicates that MRI yields no better information than CT for differential diagnosis between uremic lesions and aspecific abnormalities due to aging, vascular pathology, or atrophy, frequently present in patients older than 60 (personal communication).

Concerning light microscopy examination, the classic study by Olsen (22) did not detect any specific structural changes within the brain. Necrosis of the granular layer of the cerebral cortex, small intracerebral hemorrhages, and necrotic foci have been seen.

Pathophysiology

Although multiple factors may contribute to causing uremic encephalopathy, the most obvious observation is that its symptomatology is rapidly reversible after substitutive treatment has begun, and connects with the overall uremic retention products. A long list of neurotropic uremic "toxins" resulting from protein metabolism has already been drawnup (23). These compounds may affect enzyme activity, like Na^+-K^+-ATPase, and oxygen use, thus reducing the energy available for brain metabolism. They may also interfere with synaptic transmission and in this context could explain the increase in latency of visual and acoustic pathways.

In addition, hyperparathyroidism, a common occurrence in chronic uremia, probably exerts an important neurotoxic action, and its catabolic effect may also contribute to the increasing accumulation of toxic metabolites (24,25).

As a third causal fact, it should be remembered that a wasting syndrome is frequently present in uremia. During MHD and CAPD, removal of glucose and losses of amino acid and protein are additional factors, together with discontinuous and partial detoxification. These factors may well account for the long-term treatment abnormalities in the electrophysiological tracings, such as the morphology of AEPs after more than 5 years of MHD, when most patients present nutritional defects (26).

Treatment

Nowadays one rarely observes any significant manifestation of uremic encephalopathy where dialysis treatment starts promptly, whether in ARF or in CRF. The rapid abatement of even severe clinical features after institution of effective dialytic therapies that remove low-molecular-weight retained substances remains one of the strongest arguments for uremic toxins being involved in the pathogenesis of encephalopathy.

On the other hand, a correct diet schedule during chronic progressive renal disease may enable onset of encephalopathic symptomatology to be postponed.

DIETARY TREATMENT

Only very few studies (27,28) have specifically investigated whether dietary treatment might prevent, stabilize, or improve uremic neuropathy. The studies in which nutritional treatment is most precisely defined have concluded that it may exert a beneficial effect. In particular, a very-low-nitrogen diet (0.3 g/kg/day of unselected proteins) supplemented with a mixture of essential amino acids and ketoanalogues, with 35–40 kcal/kg/day and 400–500 mg/day of phosphorus, the so-called *supplemented diet* (SD), allows stable central nervous conduction to be preserved (28). Complete normality of the acoustic pathway in this group of patients might reflect reduced generation of the toxic compounds believed to interfere with synaptic transmission. With reference to the possible role of hyperparathyroidism, it is recognized that PTH rises as renal function declines in patients on conventional low-nitrogen diet (CLND), whereas it may fall in those on SD (29).

In conclusion, a correct dietary treatment with a very-low-nitrogen content, supplemented with essential amino acids and ketoanalogues, not only prevents protein–calorie malnutrition but reduces the retention of potentially toxic metabolites and achieves a partial reversal of hyperparathyroidism, i.e., it exerts a positive effect on the various factors that are regarded as the pathogenetic causes of uremic neuropathy (30).

MHD AND CAPD

When renal failure is clearly running its relentless progressive course, despite patient compliance with a correct dietary regimen, the prevention of uremic encephalopathy is best achieved by starting MHD or CAPD before the patient becomes severely uremic. On the other hand, even when the clinical manifestations are severe, the whole syndrome clears up within days or weeks after the onset of adequate dialysis treatment (1–4).

Following the rapid subsiding of major clinical features, less severe symptoms, like sluggishness, memory disturbances, fatigue, and sleep disturbances may persist to blight the quality of life of uremic patients. Although it was initially suggested that peritoneal dialysis was associated with a reduced prevalence of neuropathy, a well-defined difference between MHD and CAPD has never been demonstrated, at least from the clinical point of view (21,31). In addition, no clear evidence for an optimum regimen of dialysis or type of dialysis membrane has been forthcoming.

The best way to follow the natural course of encephalopathy during substitutive treatment is by electrophysiological tests (11–21). EEG activities recorded prior to CAPD and 3 months afterwards undergo a similar modification to those occurring in MHD and mentioned above. These consist in a significant reduction of the 10–13 Hz band and an increase of the 13–20 Hz band after only a few dialyses and are therefore consistent with an EEG frequency near to the normal range. There is a very low incidence of dialysis disequilibrium syndrome in patients undergoing CAPD. Compartmental shifts in fluid, electrolytes, and other solutes occur more slowly than with MHD. This process might induce a slow balancing of plasma and cerebral spinal fluid.

VEPs in CAPD patients had more stable wave shapes than in MHD patients. Similarly, from the study of AEPs, we can conclude that dialysis imbalance affects the electrocortical activity more in MHD than in CAPD, although in the long run morphological abnormalities of the tracing are evident in both dialysis styles.

The conduction velocities, peak latencies, and interpeak times recorded at cortical level by SEPs remained significantly delayed after both MHD and CAPD and sometimes deteriorated further in the long run.

In conclusion, with respect to the prevalence of central nervous system abnormalities, CAPD is certainly not inferior to MHD in controlling the clinical symptomatology. From the electrophysiological point of view, despite an adequate renal replacement therapy, uremic encephalopathy persists and, in the long run, may progress owing to a subclinical wasting syndrome that is frequently present in these patients.

Recently, it has become possible to investigate the role played by anemia in the altered brain function of CRF patients. The availability of recombinant human erythropoietin (rHuEPO) has offered a tool to test this hypothesis. Reports have already been published that show an improvement in P300 amplitudes and, in some cases, decreases in P300 latencies well correlated with rHuEPO increases in hematocrit levels (32,33). The P300 wave is a long-latency, event-related potential that remains somewhat prolonged in most dialysis patients. Its improvement by rHuEPO confirms the substantial role of anemia in uremic brain dysfunction, which may be particularly evident in the long run.

RENAL TRANSPLANTATION

It is generally agreed that successful renal transplantation is followed by a correction of previous neurological problems due to the elimination of retained toxic solutes and an improvement in metabolic status. The electrophysiological results are quite remarkable. A normalization of the P100 wave width of VEPs is observed, and the slowed central conduction recorded by SEPs shows a complete recovery 6 months after transplantation (11).

ENCEPHALOPATHY DUE TO ELECTROLYTE DISTURBANCES AND ACIDOSIS

Chronic renal diseases are frequently associated with electrolyte disturbances and metabolic acidosis, which can determine brain abnormalities not easily distinguishable from those related to uremic syndrome (4,34,35).

Hyponatremia

Hyponatremia, a decrease in serum sodium concentration below the normal range, is usually indicative of hypoosmolality of body fluids due to an excess of water compared to solutes.

Acute and chronic renal failure causes hyponatremia associated with normal or slightly expanded extracellular volume, as can be seen in uremic patients on dialysis treatment before the individual session. Congestive heart failure (frequently present during renal failure), nephrotic syndrome, or excess diuretics may be other causes of hyponatremia and hypoosmolality in patients with renal disease.

Neurological dysfunction is the principal manifestation of hyponatremia. It is due to intracellular movement of water leading to edema of brain cells and generally becomes manifest when the serum sodium concentration falls to 125 mmol/L or less. Its severity depends both on the degree of hyponatremia and on the rapidity with which it develops. The early symptoms, generally observed in chronic hyponatremia, include lethargy, weakness, and somnolence. As hyponatremia worsens or if it develops abruptly, these symptoms proceed rapidly to seizures, coma, and death if adequate treatment is not begun.

Appropriate therapy for the various types of hyponatremia has been outlined. When related to ARF or CRF and when present in dialyzed patients, therapy calls for a start to dialysis sessions. Hyponatremia associated with edema, as in congestive heart failure and the nephrotic syndrome, responds to effective treatment of the underlying disease. In patients with diuretic-induced hyponatremia, elimination of the drug and replacement of Na/K deficits may be sufficient.

Hypernatremia

Hypernatremia, an increase in the serum sodium concentration above the normal range, is indicative of a deficit in body water compared to sodium. Without exception, hypernatremia means that the body fluids are hypertonic.

It is rare in patients with renal failure, where it may occur accidentally during hemodialysis with high sodium dialysis bath. Abnormal renal wasting of water with inadequate intake of water leading to hypernatremia may occur secondarily to diabetes insipidus, osmotic diuresis, and the recovery phase of acute renal failure.

The major clinical feature of hypernatremia is central nervous system dysfunction resulting from brain cell shrinkage; confusion, neuromuscular excitability, seizures, or coma may result.

Hypernatremia itself is corrected by the patient drinking water if conscious and without gastrointestinal disturbance, or by intravenous infusion of 5% dextrose in water. In patients with associated sodium deficits, saline solutions should be infused. In addition, appropriate therapy for the underlying disease is essential.

Potassium disorders

Potassium disorders are not rare in renal disease. Renal tubular acidosis, Bartter's syndrome, Liddle's syndrome, and osmotic diuresis may be associated with hypokalemia, while ARF, oliguric CRF, and selective renal tubular potassium secretory defects may induce hyperkalemia.

Neverthless, neither hyponatremia nor hyperkalemia cause clearly recognizable clinical manifestations of brain dysfunction, although their major features consist in neuromuscular and cardiac changes.

Calcium disorders

Calcium disorders are the rule in CRF, patients being hypocalcemic owing to abnormalities of the vitamin D metabolism coupled with hyperphosphatemia. On the other hand, the ensuing secondary hyperparathyroidism produces an increased calcium content in various tissues such as the brain itself.

Decrease in the concentration of free calcium ions in plasma results in increased neuromuscular irritability and the tetany syndrome. Hypercalcemia and an increase in tissue calcium content may possibly disrupt cerebral function, causing anorexia, nausea, vomiting, hypotonia, depression, and occasionally lethargy and coma.

Central nervous system symptomatology due to calcium abnormalities needs to be controlled by treating the underlying metabolic abnormalities. In this context, hypercalcemia may represent a side effect of inadequate calcitriol treatment.

It is worth remembering that, in dialysis patients, acute hypercalcemia may occur accidentally in association with hypermagnesemia in the "hard water syndrome," which results from inadequate water treatment.

Metabolic acidosis

Renal failure, either acute or chronic, results in metabolic acidosis with an increased anion gap due to retention of sulphates and phosphates. In CRF, the principal defect is decreased ability to excrete ammonium as a result of progressive diminution of functioning renal mass.

In renal tubular acidosis with a relatively normal filtration rate, the defect is either proximal tubular bicarbonate wasting (proximal RTA) or an inability to generate an acid urine (distal RTA).

Chronic metabolic acidosis may produce only vague symptoms such as fatigue and anorexia not referrable to brain involvement.

Rapidly developing severe metabolic acidosis produces a variety of symptoms ranging from fatigue through confusion and stupor to coma. Secondary hyperventilation with the following loss of CO_2 from the blood and the cerebrospinal fluid may contribute to the clinical features.

Patients with ARF do not ordinarily require specific therapy for encephalopathic aspects of acidosis. Dialysis instituted to manage the renal failure should maintain an adequate plasma bicarbonate.

UREMIC POLYNEUROPATHY

Uremic peripheral neuropathy is a distal, usually symmetrical, mixed polyneuropathy that affects the lower limbs more frequently than the upper (2,36).

Clinical features

The earliest manifestation is *restless-legs syndrome*, characterized by sensations of crawling, prickling, and pruritus with an urge to move the legs and to walk around; these symptoms are worse at night.

The other main symptoms of polyneuropathy include burning-feet syndrome, cramps, paresthesias, and loss of the ankle jerks, followed by loss of the knee reflex.

In our experience, about 58% of severely uremic patients are symptom free, while dysesthesia is present in 15%, paresthesia in 12%, and signs of anesthesia in 6%. Full clinical examination does not show any alteration in 61% of cases, and in the remaining patients the main findings are hyporeflexia or areflexia and changes in vibratory sensitivity with normal perception.

Both subjective and objective symptoms appear with a frequency directly proportional to the degree and duration of renal insufficiency (37).

Electrophysiological findings

Results with SEPs indicate that a significant percentage of patients with CRF present a loss in velocity of peripheral nerve conduction. The intermediate tracts and the proximal fibers are not greatly affected (37,38). Generally, intracranial conduction along the short nervous fibers remains near normal, as mentioned in connection with uremic encephalopathy (20). Defective propagation of the impulse, responsible for a delayed cortical response despite perfectly conserved morphology, indicates axonal damage rather than a process of demyelinization. Conduction in the distal regions, recorded by motor (MNCV) and sensory (SNCV) nerve conduction velocities, is the most severely affected nervous system function. SNCV is more deranged than MNCV, and the peroneal nerve is more deranged than the median nerve (20,37–39). This neurophysiological picture is typical of central–peripheral axonopathy, also known as dying-back polyneuropathy (40).

Electromyographic examination (EMG) has proved of less interest and importance because the abnormalities cannot be quantified in the same way as conduction velocities can be measured. In uremia, different populations of motor unit potentials, compatible with a neurogenic cause, are present in patients on conservative treatment and in those on MHD (41). Another view is that measurement of vibratory perception thresholds is more suitable than nerve conduction velocity to evaluate uremic neuropathy (42).

Morphology

Biopsies of the sural nerve in CRF show axonal loss of both myelinated and unmyelinated fibers, with segmental demyelination and repair (43).

Surprisingly, in ARF no changes in nerve morphology have been observed (44).

Pathophysiology

Electrophysiological recordings confirm that uremia is responsible for distal degenerative axonopathy, with early onset in the more distal parts of the nerve cells with longer axonal continuations (dying-back polyneuropathy). The original damage probably arises in the gangliar cells and is related to metabolic disorders, thus affecting the flow of substances essential for cellular trophism in the more distal zones of the neuron. Abnormally retained catabolic products should not be considered the only factors responsible, nor should the other hypothetical uremic toxins, since they are presumably part of a wider metabolic derangement that alters impulse propagation at the most distal portions of long trajectory central and peripheral nerve fibers (5,11).

One striking difference between encephalopathy and polyneuropathy is revealed by the differing results of starting dialysis treatment. Uremic changes in the central nervous system are mainly functional and related to the inhibitory effect of uremic toxins on synaptic propagation, while in the peripheral nervous system they are structural and mainly related to the wasting syndrome of chronic uremia. This difference could explain why peripheral neuropathy does not react as favorably to dialysis treatment as encephalopathy.

Treatment

Clinical and electrophysiological findings have long shown that, in spite of conventional conservative treatment, uremic neuropathy persists and progresses (5,11).

DIETARY TREATMENT

The few studies specifically investigating the impact of dietary treatment on the natural history of uremic neuropathy have concluded that a very low nitrogen content needs to be supplemented with essential amino acids or a mixture of essential amino acids and ketoanalogues to exert a beneficial effect on polyneuropathy (28). In particular, a significantly faster MNCV and SNCV have been observed in uremic patients on a supplemented diet versus those treated with conventional low-nitrogen diet, MHD, or CAPD (Figure 1). Patients on such special diets have a very low BUN:serum creatinine ratio and conceivably a lesser amount of potentially neurotoxic retention products. In addition, the well-recognized anabolic effect, especially of branched-chain ketoacids, may enable the wasting effect of uremia on gangliar cells to be offset (45).

MHD AND CAPD

During adequate MHD, clinical polyneuropathy generally becomes stable or improves, despite differences in dialysis techniques and schedules. On long-term treatment, symptoms may appear de novo, despite good control of the

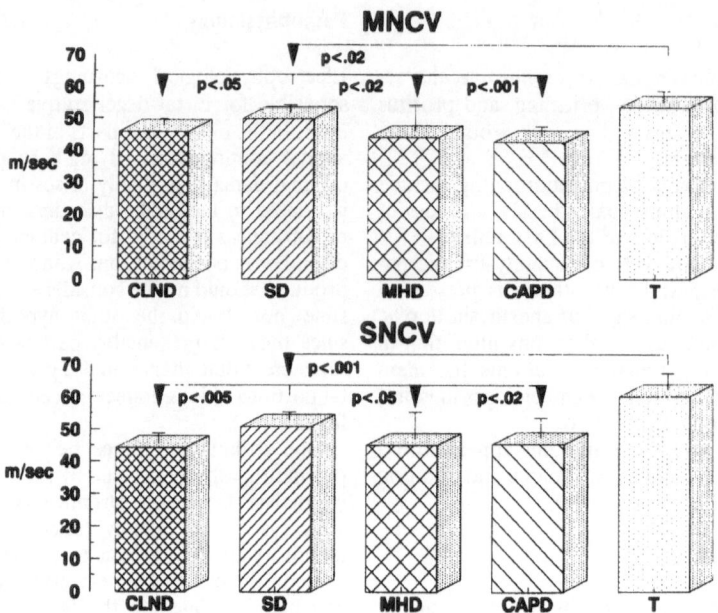

Figure 1. Effect of conservative and substitutive treatment on distal nervous conduction velocities (personal observations). Abbreviations: CLND, 16 patients on conventional low-nitrogen diet; SD, 12 patients on very-low-nitrogen diet supplemented with essential amino acids and ketoanalogues; MHD, 36 patients on regular dialysis treatment; CAPD, 11 patients on continuous ambulatory peritoneal dialysis; T, 16 transplanted patients. MNCV: motor nerve conduction velocity from peroneal nerve (normal values: 51.6 ± 3.6 m/sec); SNCV, sensory nerve conduction velocity from sural nerve (normal value: 52.3 ± 4.9 m/sec).

usual biochemical parameters of uremia; if the dialysis is not adequate, the neuropathy rapidly worsens (45,11,37). The net effect of MHD on nerve function is highly influenced by the condition of the patient before starting it. When MHD is given with a GFR around 10 mL/min, or slightly less provided the patient has been following a supplemented diet, clinical neuropathy is rare and no further progression usually takes place. In general, a mild case of polyneuropathy recovers completely; a moderate case recovers but may not return to normal, whereas a severe case often does not recover, probably because the retrograde chromatolytic changes have caused neuronal death, precluding nerve regeneration (23,36). Of great interest is the effect of a single dialysis, after which there occur a slight fall in the vibratory perception threshold, an increase in the amplitude of nerve action potentials, and a decrease in the relative refractory period (4). All these changes point to a reversal of functional membrane abnormalities due to the removal of potential neurotoxins. In this respect, greater effectiveness has been ascribed to the polyacrylonitrile dialyzer membrane compared to the more conventional regenerated cellulosic membrane (46). This difference appears to confirm the hypothesis of the middle molecules as major neurotoxins in uremic polyneuropathy. On this basis, a more favorable outcome should be ob-

tained by CAPD than by MHD. In actual fact, middle-sized molecules are removed more efficiently by CAPD than by other methods of dialysis on a weekly basis.

To pass from theory to clinical observation, it has been reported that MHD and CAPD do not yield any difference in the clinical score of the patients (47). Overall results for neurophysiological parameters tend to show a more beneficial course in CAPD patients, nerve conduction velocities remaining more stable over long periods in CAPD (48,49).

RENAL TRANSPLANTATION

After successful renal transplantation, clinical remission of peripheral neuropathy is the rule, with an early phase of rapid improvement followed by slow, gradual amelioration lasting many months. Full recovery is obtained in most patients as a result of nerve regeneration; only in cases with very severe neuropathy do sequelae of a nondisabling nature persist (50,51). The electrophysiological signs of peripheral nerve dysfunction likewise disappear in the majority of patients (52), in agreement with the remission of clinical neurological manifestations, thus demonstrating the superiority of a successful transplant over MHD or CAPD (Figure 1).

AUTONOMIC NERVOUS SYSTEM DYSFUNCTION IN UREMIA

Abnormalities of the autonomic nervous system (ANS) are often present in uremic patients, seem to correlate with peripheral neuropathy, and can involve both the parasympathetic and the sympathetic nervous systems. Plasma catecholamine concentration is high in chronic renal failure (53), and it may be indicative of an increased sympathetic nervous activity or, alternatively, it may be secondary to a reduced reuptake or reflect a diminished end-organ response (54). The manifestations of ANS dysfunction in uremia may include (55) changes in the function of sweat glands, an abnormal response to the Valsalva maneuver, a reduced baroreceptor sensitivity, orthostatic hypotension, non-volume-responsive intradialytic hypotension, an abnormal response to hand-grip exercise, a reduced nocturnal penile tumescence, and a reduced pressor response to vasoconstrictor agonists.

ANS dysfunction may already occur in chronic renal failure patients not on replacement therapy and may even be more pronounced in these patients than in those treated with maintenance hemodialysis (54). Particularly in nondiabetic uremic patients, the initiation of dialysis can induce an improvement in some ANS abnormalities. This improvement is at least partly related to the correction of the diminished end-organ responsiveness and may be less pronounced with continuous ambulatory peritoneal dialysis than with hemodialysis (56). After successful kidney transplantation, autonomic function generally improves, but it may also never return to normal (57). Since improvement of ANS abnormalities follows the initiation of chronic dialysis, it is important to provide all ESRD patients with opportune and adequate dialytic treatment.

NEUROLOGICAL COMPLICATIONS OF DIALYSIS

Dialysis disequilibrium syndrome

Dialysis disequilibrium syndrome (DDS) is an acute neurological syndrome occurring in patients with renal failure as a consequence of a rapid solute removal by dialysis therapy. The clinical manifestations of DDS usually occur during the later stages of a dialysis procedure or shortly thereafter, and the complete resolution may take hours to days. DDS has most often been associated with rapid hemodialysis, and very rarely with peritoneal dialysis (58). It is now more frequently observed in patients with acute renal failure being treated with rapid hemodialysis, but it may also occur in chronic renal failure patients initiating maintenance hemodialysis, especially when they are severely uremic and/or when short, high-efficiency hemodialysis is used. Considerable evidence suggests that DDS is a phenomenon only of patients initiating dialysis (59). When an alleged DDS occurs in a patient fully adjusted to a dialysis program, a complicating intracranial

disorder or errors in the composition of the dialysate should be considered (4).

In the pathogenesis of DDS, brain edema, intracellular brain acidosis, or a rise in cerebrospinal fluid (CSF) pressure may all play their part (60). DDS was initially attributed to a so-called *reverse urea effect* (58). It was thought that, during dialysis, urea was removed more rapidly from the blood than from the brain, thereby resulting in an osmotic gradient that caused cerebral edema and brain swelling, but it was subsequently shown that the rate of removal of urea from plasma parallels the rate of removal of urea from the brain. However, in experimental models, rapid hemodialysis induces a significant rise in brain osmolality and water content with cerebral edema (61); the increased brain osmolality has been attributed to osmotic particles of unknown nature, called *idiogenic osmoles*, and occurs in association with an intracellular acidosis of the brain (61). With rapid hemodialysis, this intracellular acidosis still persists despite the presence of controlled P_{CO_2} arterial levels (62), and there is also a fall in the pH of CSF, which, if associated with a concomitant decrease in the pH of the brain, could represent a major cause in the pathogenesis of DDS, since it may contribute to depression of the sensorium (60). Intracellular acidosis of the brain cells could lead to brain edema through alterations in the osmotic activity of intracellular cations (63).

Clinically, DDS in its mildest form may consist of headache, nausea, vomiting, restlessness, fatigue, and muscle cramping. In more severe cases, blurring of vision, disorientation, tremors, seizures (usually of the grand mal type, and more rarely focal), and cardiac arrhythmias have all been reported. Occasionally, seizures may lead to coma and death (64). The modern dialysis methods and the improved knowledge of DDS pathophysiology have both reduced the occurrence.

The EEG in DDS may be abnormal, showing bursts of symmetrical, bisynchronous rhythmic waves of medium-high voltage, particularly in the delta frequency range, with loss of normal alpha rhythm (65).

The diagnosis of DDS should always be a diagnosis by elimination, since many disorders can mimic the syndrome. These disorders include (60) subdural hematoma, uremia per se, dialysis dementia, cerebrovascular accident, copper intoxication, nonketotic hyperosmolar coma with hyperglycemia, hypoglycemia, hyponatremia, hyperparathyroidism with hypercalcemia, malignant hypertension, excessive ultrafiltration, malfunction of fluid-proportioning system, depletion syndrome, Wernicke's encephalopathy, and cardiac arrhythmia.

The mainstay of DDS management is minimizing rapid changes in plasma osmolality during dialysis, particularly when the latter is initiated in severely uremic patients, whether acute or chronic. DDS treatment has consisted of the addition to the dialysate, or in some cases the infusion into the patient, of osmotic agents such as glycerol, mannitol, glucose, fructose, sodium, and albumin (62,64,66,67). The substitution of bicarbonate for acetate in the dialysate

(68) and the use of a low rather than a high glucose concentration in the dialysate (67) may also lead to a reduction of DDS symptoms in some patients. In the management of DDS, it appears that prevention is essential. Preventive modalities at the start of hemodialysis, aimed at achieving a gradual correction of uremia, include use of short (2–3 hours) and frequent (every day) sessions of limited efficacy carried out with low blood flow rates (below 200 mL/min) and small surface area dialyzers. It is also advisable to keep the dialysate sodium concentration between 140 and 145 mmol/L, since it prevents a critical reduction in plasma osmolality during dialysis and results in a reduced occurrence of DDS (64).

In patients who have experienced seizures and in very severe uremic patients starting dialysis, the prophylactic administration of anticonvulsant drugs may be appropriate until the metabolic derangement is well controlled. Phenytoin should be given at an initial dosage of 10–15 mg/kg intravenously (the rate should not exceed 50 mg/min owing to the risk of cardiac arrhythmia, especially in elderly patients), followed by a maintenance therapy of 100 mg every 6–8 hours (7), with a careful monitoring of plasma drug concentration. Sodium valproate may be effective as well and should be given intravenously at an infusion of 400–800 mg over 3–5 minutes, followed by a maintenance dosage of 1–2 g daily (7). Despite a short half-life, a twice-daily dosage is generally sufficient, since sodium valproate has a prolonged pharmacological effect on the brain. Since the brain levels of phenytoin fall rapidly unless administered continuously, intravenous diazepam may be more effective in the suppression of acute seizures, since its effect lasts 30–60 minutes.

Dialytic encephalopathy

Dialytic encephalopathy (DE) is also called dialysis dementia. It is a progressive neurological disease that, unless recognized and treated early, is fatal, with a mean duration of 6 months from onset to death (69). DE has been almost exclusively observed in patients being treated with chronic hemodialysis, but it has also been reported in patients on peritoneal dialysis (70) and in nondialyzed uremic patients, both adult (71) and children (72). The syndrome has tended to occur in epidemic form in geographic clusters, at least partly due to contamination of the dialysate with aluminum (Al) (73).

The clinical features of DE typically have an insidious onset and manifest on average after 2–3 years on maintenance hemodialysis. Early in the course of the disease, the symptoms may fluctuate and characerically worsen towards the end and after (6–8 hours) the dialysis procedure, but subsequently they become constant and progressive. A disturbance of speech is very often the presenting clinical feature and usually consists of a combination of dysarthria and speech dyspraxia with stuttering and hesitancy. Other patients may show a true Broca's aphasia, although aphasia

and dysarthria may be found in the same patient (74). Dysgraphia and dyslexia are also common, whereas in the later stages of the disease muteness often occurs. Mental changes are very often associated with speech disturbances and may include depression, apathy, paranoia, memory failure, poor attention, daytime somnolence, and poor concentration. Other main features of DE are myoclonic jerks, asterixis, gait disturbances, and seizures. The disease is progressive and worsens with time, with development of global dementia and death as the usual outcome.

There are no confirmatory laboratory tests for the diagnosis of DE, and the principal investigative test is the EEG. EEG abnormalities are present in all cases of DE, may precede the clinical manifestations by 6 months, and are represented by generalized paroxysmal bursts of high-voltage delta activity with spikes and sharp waves, superimposed on a relatively normal background activity. The latter finding, during the progressive course of the disease, deteriorates to slow frequencies (75). Differential diagnosis includes metabolic encephalopathies, uremic encephalopathy, hypertensive encephalopathy, trace element intoxications, drug intoxications, structural neurological lesions, and dialysis disequilibrium syndrome.

There is much evidence to suggest a critical role for aluminum in the development of DE. In most outbreaks of the epidemic form of the disease, there have been reports of an elevated concentration of aluminum in the dialysate due to an inadequate treatment of the tap water used to prepare the dialysis fluid. Al content in the brain has been shown to be significantly higher in dialysis patients dying of DE than in patients dying of other causes (73), although overlapping may occur (3). During the course of dialysis, owing to the high plasma protein binding of Al, the high Al concentration in the dialysate results in the transfer of a large amount of the element to the patient across the dialysis membrane. The introduction of reverse osmosis for purification of the water used for dialysate has resulted in a dramatic drop in the incidence of DE, and epidemics of the disease are no longer seen, provided that dialysate Al levels are less than the recommended limits of 10 mcg/L (76).

The etiology of the sporadic cases of DE is more uncertain. The oral ingestion of aluminum-containing phosphate binders has been implicated in some cases (70–72). However, although large amounts of oral Al salts have been used in most uremic patients for treatment of hyperphosphatemia, DE is a relatively rare syndrome. This could mean that factors other than Al could be at work in those patients who develop DE (6).

The essence of DE management is prevention, since treatment of the syndrome is particularly difficult when clinically apparent. The use of deionizers and reverse osmosis filters for purification of the water used to reconstitute the dialysate is mandatory. Al dialysate levels no higher than 10 mcg/L are generally considered to be safe, but lower levels are preferable (77). Patients should be given no more than 3 g/day of oral aluminum gels at mealtimes, and the dosage should be adapted to the phosphate ingestion (78). The concomitant administration of Al compounds and citrate in any form must be avoided to prevent any greater absorption of Al (79).

Serum Al determination should be performed regularly, since it is the most cost-effective test to diagnose Al overload, although serum Al levels do not necessarily represent a reliable predictor of DE (7). If serum Al levels are greater than 100 mcg/L, it seems prudent to replace Al compounds with alternative phosphate binders such as calcium salts. This may require a reduction by 0.25 mmol/L in the calcium concentration in the dialysate.

Al is so strictly protein bound that it is inefficiently removed during routine hemodialysis; administration of the chelator deferoxamine (DFO), besides mobilizing tissue Al stores, increases the ultrafiltrable serum Al fraction by forming a low-molecular-weight (583 Da) aluminoxamine compound (80). DFO has been used with some success in the treatment of DE (81), and the therapy should be started early at the first signs of the disease, since in advanced, aggravated cases it may no longer be effective. Therapy with deferoxamine is not without some risk (82). Worsening of neurological manifestations soon after the beginning of DFO treatment has been documented, but most frequently this problem arises from the use of high doses of DFO in patients with severe Al toxicity, in whom a too rapid elimination of Al from the body tissue stores results in a transfer of the element to the central nervous system. Rapid infusion over less than 1 hour may induce headache, fatigue, hypotension, and abdominal pain. Other known complications of treatment with DFO include visual or auditory impairment as well as mucormycosis. To minimize the side effects of DFO treatment, it has recently been proposed (83) that a widely spaced, once-weekly administration of a low DFO dose (5 mg/kg) be given intravenously during the last 60 minutes of the dialysis session. Indeed, even at this low dosage, a sufficient chelation of Al has been demonstrated (84). Chelation therapy for 10–12 months may be required before there is any symptomatic improvement.

Diazepam or clonazepam are useful in controlling seizure and myoclonic activity, but they do not alter the course of the disease, nor is DE alleviated by an increased frequency of dialysis therapy. Renal transplantation may be beneficial in early encephalopathy, but it may also precipitate or accelerate the symptoms and the signs of the disease despite a good graft function (85). Parathyroidectomy was of benefit in one case report (86), but in 21 patients retrospectively evaluated, parathyroid status or parathyroidectomy had no influence on the outcome of the disease (87). Despite all the aforementioned styles of therapy, DE may continue to progress, and in the advanced stages of the disease psychological support by the dialysis unit staff to both affected and unaffected patients is very important (88).

Carpal tunnel syndrome

Carpal tunnel syndrome (CTS) is an entrapment neuropathy due to damage of the median nerve in the carpal tunnel in the wrist. CTS is rare during the first years of dialysis therapy, but it may affect 20% to 50% of uremic patients dialyzed for almost 10 years (89). Typically a long-term complication of hemodialysis treatment, CTS may also occasionally be seen in long-term CAPD patients (90). The clinical picture consists of paresthesia and aching of the first to the third fingers and of the radial side of the fourth finger. Symptoms are more pronounced at night, in the morning, and during hemodialysis procedure, and may be associated with pain in the joints of the upper limb. In more severe and advanced cases, atrophy of the proximal thenar muscles develops. Electrophysiological tests show a prolonged conduction time of the median nerve involving both the motor and the sensory fibers (91).

CTS is now considered to be a clinical manifestation of dialysis amyloidosis (92), a complication developing in the long-term dialysis patient that can include destructive arthropathy and pathological fractures. The deposition of amyloid in the tissues of the wrist causes the compression of the median nerve and results in CTS.

Relief from the symptoms may be obtained by wrist splints and by injection into the carpal tunnel of 0.75 mL of 1% lidocaine mixed with 0.75 mL of triamcinolone. Ultimately, especially if there is evidence of motor or sensory loss, surgery is necessary and usually curative, provided that CTS is diagnosed early, since in cases of prologed compression of the median nerve recovery may be not complete. Decompression with sectioning of the flexor retinaculum is an effective method of treatment (91). In recent years, an endoscopic technique has also been employed for the release of the carpal ligament (93). Even in cases of complete recovery, recurrence of CTS after several years often occurs.

Intracranial hemorrhage

Bleeding complications in the nervous system may occur in uremic patients, particularly in those on chronic hemodialysis. Besides head trauma, a long history of hypertension, the coagulation abnormalities of uremia, and the use of anticoagulants during hemodialysis are well-known risk factors.

SUBDURAL HEMATOMA

Subdural hematoma has an incidence of about 3% in hemodialysis patients (94). The collection of blood, usually venous, is bilateral in 15%–20% of cases and most often lies over the frontal and the parietal lobes. A severe, persisting headache is usually present and may be associated with nausea, vomiting, confusion, and drowsiness. In other cases, focal neurological abnormalities such as hemiparesis that may be prevailing. Signs of meningeal irritation, somnolence, and focal seizures may also be observed, as well as gait disturbances may become conspicuous (95). Patients can then lapse into coma.

Subdural hematoma can be visualized by CT scanning or MRI. The latter has some advantages over CT, since it is not affected by the hematoma becoming isodense with the brain or showing a volume-averaging effect with bone (6).

When subdural hematoma is suspected and surgical exploration indicated, it would be better to discontinue hemodialysis and use peritoneal dialysis (96). If this is not feasible, hemodialysis should be performed without any anticoagulation. In heparin-free hemodialysis, careful monitoring throughout the procedure, flushing of the dialyzer with saline solution (100–200 mL every 15–30 minutes), a high ultrafiltration rate (to remove the fluids given to the patient during flushing), and a blood flow as high as possible are all required. Alternatively, dialyzers with a low thrombogenicity such as those in ethylene-vinylalcohol copolymer may be successfully employed (97).

Treatment of subdural hematoma consists of surgical drainage or removal of the clot. Surgery may be curative, unless brain compression or herniation have occurred, but unfortunately the mortality rate still exceeds half the cases.

CEREBRAL HEMORRHAGE

In dialysis patients, cerebral hemorrhage is most often a massive extravasation into the brain tissue and has a poor prognosis. The clinical picture is characterized by a rapid onset, and may include nausea, vomiting, hemiparesis, signs of meningeal irritation, coma, and death. Therapeutic possibilities are very limited, and surgical drainage is often impractical due to the rapid worsening of the patient's condition.

SUBARACHNOID HEMORRHAGE

Subarachnoid hemorrhage is usually a fatal complication that could account for a substantial proportion of hemodialysis-related deaths (98). It is most often observed in patients affected by polycystic kidney disease with associated berry aneurism.

EPIDURAL HEMATOMA

Epidural hematoma causing spinal cord compression is characterized by the abrupt onset of bilateral weakness and loss of sensitivity of the legs. Since permanent paraplegia may result, surgical evacuation of the hematoma is urgently called for.

Werniche's encephalopathy

Wernicke's encephalopathy is an acute syndrome characterized by mental changes (apathy, inattention, inability to concentrate, confusion), ataxia, and abnormalities of ocular mobility (nystagmus, paresis of the lateral rectus, palsy of conjugate gaze). The syndrome may sometimes be associated with a Korsakoff psychosis, and in this case patients develop a loss of recent memory and tend to confabulate. Wernicke's encephalopathy has been reported in some dialysis patients (99) mostly before the routine supplementation of thiamine, a water-soluble vitamin that can be lost through the dialysis membrane.

The treatment of Wernicke's encephalopathy is represented by the intravenous administration of high doses of thiamine, which usually results in an improvement in symptoms (ocular disturbances) that may take hours to weeks. Since the response of mental changes to thiamine may be less favorable, adequate thiamine supplementation should always be given to dialysis patients, particularly those with restricted food intake.

SLEEP DISORDERS IN UREMIA

Sleep disorders are not rare in uremic patients and may influence the quality of life. A prevalent, specific sleep disorder in both chronic renal failure and hemodialysis patients is sleep apnea syndrome (SAS) (100), which is characterized by periodic episodes of cessation of airflow during sleep, accompanied by excessive daytime sleepiness, depression, fatigue, irritability, and headache. The incidence of SAS in hemodialysis patients may be as high as 30% (101), and the syndrome can be correctly diagnosed only by polysomnography, since uremia per se may induce an excessive daytime somnolence and nighttime wakefulness. Other sleep disorders that may affect dialysis patients include restless-legs syndrome (see Uremic Neuropathy above) and nocturnal myoclonus, characterized exclusively during sleeping by intermittent abrupt contractions of the leg muscles.

In uremic patients with symptoms suggestive of a sleep disorder, surgically correctable (tonsillar hypertrophy, nasal septum deviation, etc.), psychological, psychiatric, drug-induced, or metabolic (hypothyroidism) causes should be sought, since they may all result in poor sleep. Sedative and narcotic drugs and alcohol should be discontinued, since they may suppress ventilation (102). An effective therapy for SAS is represented by continuous positive airway pressure (CPAP) breathing (102). The CPAP system consists of a mask placed over the patient's nose with a large-bore tube attached to an air compressor fitted through an inspiratory port and with a tube emerging from an expiratory port that narrows to a fixed or a variable resistance, inducing regulated airway pressure. CPAP has also recently been used with benefit in hemodialysis patients (103), but further, broader studies are needed for evaluation of this therapy. In the treatment of nocturnal myoclonus and restless-legs syndrome, 0.5 mg of clonazepam at bedtime may be successful (4,104).

PSYCHOLOGICAL AND PSYCHIATRIC PROBLEMS IN ESRD

ESRD and its management are very frequently associated with psychological problems that may affect perception, intellectual functioning, state of consciousness, affective status, motor behavior, interpersonal relationships, and social functioning. The two main mechanisms that can produce psychological disturbances in uremic patients, and which can overlap, are represented by organic changes associated with ESRD altering CNS functioning and by the individual reaction to the chronic, progressive course of the disease and, ultimately, to replacement therapy. Throughout the course of ESRD, many patients complain of signs and symptoms consistent with an organic brain syndrome, such as tiredness, lethargy, slowed mentation, poor memory, and poor concentration. Psychotic features such as hallucinations, delusions, alterations in consciousness, and psychomotor agitation may be seen in more severe cases.

Regular dialytic treatment induces major changes in the lives of patients, and the way in which patients deal with these changes has a great influence on the psychological functioning. Adaptation to a new lifestyle and overcoming dependency on a machine may be particularly burdensome in some patients. Family relationships, predialysis functioning in term of coping style, and personality are factors found to be predictive of coping (105).

Depression is considered the most important clinical psychiatric problem in ESRD patients (106). It may manifest with a wide range and various combinations of symptoms, including hopelessness, depressed mood, lack of pleasure, loss of interest in daily life, sleep disturbance, loss of libido, appetite loss, and weight loss. In some cases, behavioral changes such as irritability, anger, and bad dreams may indicate an underlying depression. For a better accuracy of diagnosis, the focus of definition and measurement of depression in ESRD patients should emphasize the cognitive and affective aspects of depression rather than the somatic symptoms (107). Anxiety may also develop in some uremic patients, particularly prior to beginning dialysis. After maintenance hemodialysis is started, patients typically exhibit a euphoric sense of relief at the efficacy of the treatment and the discovery that they feel better. In some cases, after some months of dialysis, depression may occur again as the patients realize the long-term nature of their disease and that continued life is dependent on a machine. Over time, most will adjust to the new reality, although depression may be prolonged when patients are persistently uremic because of underdialysis (108).

Some patients may adapt poorly to maintenance dialysis regimen. Noncompliance with diet restrictions may be habitual in some and may result in excessive weight gain, fluid overload, salt overload, and hyperkalemia. Other patients may persistently demand to be removed from dialysis after only 1 or 2 hours, while others may attend irregularly for MHD. The most serious manifestation of patient inability to tolerate the stress of being ill is suicide, which has a higher incidence than in the general population. In addition, withdrawal from dialysis is not unusual, and may account for as much as 22% of all deaths of a dialysis population (109).

The beginning of MHD usually exerts a beneficial effect on overall neuropsychological and cognitive functioning. In particular, the symptoms associated with an organic brain syndrome are reported to improve as uremia improves. It is thus essential to avoid underdialysis, ensuring that all patients are dialyzed with an adequate and efficient dialytic therapy. Erythropoietin administration may be helpful, since it may result in an improvement of both the quality of life and the cognitive function of ESRD patients (110).

Patients with an organic brain syndrome associated with psychosis are indicated for pharmacotherapeutic management with phenothiazines. Haloperidol is the preferred drug generally, since it produces few anticholinergic side effects and little orthostatic hypotension. The dosage may range from 5 to 25 mg/day depending on the response, and no dosage reduction is usually needed, since the drug is metabolized by the liver. When anxiety is present, treatment with minor tranquilizers such as benzodiazapines may be beneficial.

Family support, optimal hemodialysis, and empathetic counseling may be sufficient to overcome transient severe depression (111). Social and psychological intervention is indicated for depressive symptoms in patients who do not meet psychiatric diagnostic criteria for a depressive disorder. Those patients who do not respond to the aforementioned therapy schedules, and those patients with a major depressive disorder, are candidates for pharmacological treatment with one of the tricyclic antidepressant medications such as imipramine, desipramine, and nortriptyline. Guidelines for their usage with dialysis patients have been recently reported (107). Imipramine and desipramine should initially be administered at a dosage of 25 mg/day, which may subsequently be increased up to 150–200 mg/day. For nortriptyline, whose initial dose is 10 mg/day, the full dosage is 75–100 mg/day. Since the therapeutic plasma level of these drugs is known, their concentration in plasma should be monitored for dosage adjustment to maintain the therapeutic range. Also, although the tricyclic antidepressant medications are primarily metabolized by the liver, therapeutic plasma levels may be achieved in ESRD patients by a lower dosage than in subjects with normal renal function (112). Side effects may include anticholinergic effects (constipation, dry mouth, blurred vision), postural hypotension, and quinidine-like effects on cardiac function and rhythm (113). Consultation with a psychiatrist can help the dialysis staff to deal with severely noncompliant patients.

Dialysis staff (both physicians and nurses), properly trained social workers, and psychologists or psychiatrists can play an important role in favoring adaptation to dialysis. Vocational, marital, and psychotherapeutic treatment may be helpful for the long-term support of dialysis patients, particularly those with disturbances in social functioning.

DISORDERS AFFECTING THE NERVOUS SYSTEM AND THE KIDNEY

We shall particularly consider conditions that have an impact on both renal and neurological function.

Primary neurological disease, apart from bladder dysfunction as a consequence of neurological deficit, rarely has any association with renal disease, yet the converse is certainly not true. Many conditions affecting the kidney have an associated effect on the nervous system.

The most common renal effect of damage to the nervous system is secondary to disordered bladder function, as a result of spinal cord disorders such as multiple sclerosis, trauma, or cord compression. Bladder symptoms develop in 80% of multiple sclerosis patients; the demyelination usually results in urgency, frequency, and incontinence with urinary tract infections. A few patients insidiously develop obstructive uropathy, and in those who notice retention of urine, regular control of renal function with ultrasound or intravenous urography is advised. Some patients with urinary retention may be able to manage intermittent self-catheterization, but in others, permanent catheterization, bladder neck resection, or urinary diversion may be required.

Dysproteinemias

MYELOMA

Myeloma is a widespread malignancy of plasma cells usually associated with the production of monoclonal protein in one of the immunoglobulin classes. Myeloma kidney is the result of tubulointerstitial damage caused by free light chains, and histological features include fractured casts in the tubular lumina, interstitial fibrosis, tubular atrophy, and foreign-body giant cells. Some improvement in renal function can be anticipated if a precipitant can be identified and suitable treatment instituted (114). Since renal failure may progress quite rapidly, aggressive treatment with rehydration, chemotherapy, and plasma exchange is recommended in patients who present with acute renal impairment (115). Myeloma patients are also at risk of developing AL amyloidosis which can be distinguished from deposition of the AA type of amyloid by immunofluorescence. Acute renal failure may be precipitated by infection and dehydration, hypercalcemia, or hyperuricaemia.

The neurological complications of multiple myeloma can be divided into three main groups: direct compression of nervous tissue, infiltration by myeloma, and associated or indirect complications. Complications from compression are the most common and may be due to protruding vertebral tumors, bone collapse, primary epidural tumor, expanding hematoma, or a large amyloid deposit. There is usually nerve root pain or dysfunction and signs and symptoms of cord or cauda compression, depending on the site. Myeloma masses may compress cranial nerves near their exit foramina, those most frequently affected being II, III, V, VI, and VII.

Polyneuropathy and amyloid involvement of the peripheral nervous system or carpal tunnel as remote effects of myeloma are common.

The treatment of multiple myeloma aims at reducing the number of neoplastic plasma cells. Adequate hydration is important to prevent or limit renal involvement. Local spinal compression may be treated by radiotherapy, if the compression is from bone collapse or surgical laminectomy or if extensive reconstructive surgery is indicated. Plasma cell reduction is achieved by chemotherapy with vincristine, cyclophosphamide, and prednisone. Persistently high paraproteins after this should be treated with intermittent melphalan and prednisone.

MONOCLONAL GAMMOPATHY

Peripheral neuropathy may occur in association with monoclonal gammopathy. The demyelinating segmental neuropathy, which causes coarse tremor, is usually of a motor and sensory, distal, symmetrical variety and is associated with marked slowing of conduction velocity.

WALDENSTROM'S MACROGLOBULINEMIA

Waldenstrom's macroglobulinemia is a rare lymphoproliferative disorder associated with the monoclonal immunoglobulin M peak on immunoelectrophoresis. In contrast to multiple myeloma, renal failure is rare in Waldenstrom's macroglobulinemia, but most patients show lymphoadenopathy and enlargement of the liver and/or spleen. Hyperviscosity syndrome is much more strongly associated with Waldenstrom's macroglobulinemia and may be accompanied by neurological complications, which occur in 25% of patients. The principal manifestations, in descending order of frequency, are retinopathy, generalized encephalopathy, multifocal strokes, meningitis, and cerebellar ataxia. Neuropathy and monoclonal gammopathy are also components of the POEMS syndrome (polyneuropathy, organomegaly, endocrinopathy, M-protein, and skin changes) (116). Cryoglobulinemia is also associated with neuropathy, which is often asymmetrical, with symptoms worse in cold weather.

Metabolic disorders

DIABETES MELLITUS

Diabetes mellitus is the most common serious metabolic disease in humans, affecting about 1% of the population.

The disease consists of hyperglycemia along with various hormonal abnormalities. Complications include blood vessel involvement, and end-organ involvement, especially the eyes, kidneys, and nerves. In the study by Fagerberg (117), 70% of patients suffered from central and peripheral neuropathy, of whom 89% also had a retinopathy, 93% a nephropathy, and 66% peripheral vascular disease. In all diabetics, with or without neuropathy, renal disease is a very frequent complication: diabetes is the second leading cause of ESRD in the United States (118).

Hypoglycemia must be considered first in the treated diabetic patient, and especially uremic diabetics may be more subject than others to insulin- or drug-induced hypoglycemia, which we deal with in more detail later.

Ketoacidosis occurs in the context of insulin deficiency; hyperglycemia is an essential component, but the production of ketoacids is dependent on high levels of glucagon, which promotes oxydation in the liver of the mobilized fatty acids from the fat stores of the body. Krane et al. (119) found subclinical brain swelling on CT scans of all the children studied immediately following treatment for diabetic ketoacidosis. This occurs due to an osmotic shift of water from the vascular to the brain compartment during treatment.

Hyperglycemic, hyperosmolar, nonketotic coma accounts for between 10% and 33% of episodes of diabetic coma (120,121). In the treatment of this condition, it is important to replace fluid volume and to restore urine flow. This is best done with normal saline solution; the serum osmolality should not be lowered abruptly, since this will cause a shift of fluid from the vascular into the tissue compartment and a further drop in circulating blood volume (122). Once the volume has been replaced, the serum osmolality can gradually be returned to normal over 48 hours. Small doses of insulin should be used.

Diabetes mellitus is a widely accepted risk factor for ischemic stroke. The mechanism of diabetic neuropathy is multifocal ischemia to the peripheral nerves. Conduction velocity in peripheral nerves seems to be reduced and accounts for the generalized symmetrical motor and sensory polyneuropathy, the commonest type of neuropathy in diabetic patients. However, many will also experience focal or multifocal neuropathies (123) that may affect the cranial nerves, particularly the third cranial nerve and the various nerve roots involving the trunk.

Diabetic amyotrophy sets in with fairly rapidly progressive pain and weakness involving the thigh muscles. There is a syndrome of small fiber neuropathy (123), in which very severe pain is accompanied by loss of pain and temperature sensation, with a certain preservation of the other modalities but particular involvement of the autonomic nervous system.

The results of treating diabetic patients with chronic hemodialysis or intermittent peritoneal dialysis are quite poor. Recently it has been shown that diabetic patients do quite well on continuous ambulatory peritoneal dialysis (124); in general, neuropathy remains unchanged.

While both diabetic and uremic polyneuropathy have in common a combination of axonal degeneration and segmental demyelination in the peripheral nerves, detailed electrophysiological studies have shown differences between the two neuropathies. Vibratory perception threshold increases with warming of the extremities in diabetic patients, but decreases in uremic patients (125).

The results of transplantation have been good if the kidney was from identical related donors, but in cadaveric transplantation the results have not been as good in diabetics as in nondiabetics (126). In a well-controlled study, Solders et al. (127) showed that polyneuropathy in diabetic patients with end-stage renal disease failed to improve, even in patients who had combined renal and pancreatic transplantation.

AMYLOIDOSIS

Peripheral neuropathy and renal failure commonly coexist in certain types of hereditary amyloidosis, and signs and symptoms usually begin in middle life. In the Type 1 variety, there is a motor and sensory polyneuropathy in which pain and temperature sensation are particularly affected. Autonomic signs are also prominent. There is associated renal, cardiac, and ocular (vitreous opacities) involvement. In the Type II variety, carpal tunnel syndrome is a prominent early feature, but a more diffuse polyneuropathy later develops, again with autonomic involvement, as well as heart disease and vitreous opacities. Type III has prominent renal involvement and peptic ulceration, and there is an associated motor and sensory polyneuropathy, particularly affecting pain and temperature. The Type IV variant starts as a cranial neuropathy, often accompanied by an ocular corneal lattice dystrophy.

FABRY'S DISEASE

Fabry's disease may appear as both peripheral neuropathy and renal failure. It is due to a deficiency of the enzyme alfa-galactosidase and is inherited through an X-linked, recessive pattern. The enzyme deficiency causes faulty breakdown of glycolipids, resulting in their deposition in tissues throughout the body. The skin becomes scaly and telangiectasic—so-called *angiokeratoma corporis diffusum*, chiefly present over the lower trunk and buttocks. Careful ophthalmological examination may reveal a corneal dystrophy and dilated conjunctival blood vessels. Ultimately, usually in later adult life, renal failure dominates the clinical picture, and chronic dialysis or renal transplantation may be necessary. The peripheral nerve involvement is quite distinctive, consisting of persistent aching in the limbs and outbreaks of burning pain, sometimes induced by emotional disturbances. There may be lack of sweating and resulting episodes of hyperthermia. Nerve biopsy shows a deposition of glycolipid in the perineurial and capillary endothelial cells and the dorsal root ganglion cells. Small myelinated and unmyelinated fibers are selectively lost. The pain may respond to phenytoin.

Vascular disorders

Vascular disease due to *hypertension* may cause renal impairment and accelerates atherosclerosis of the cerebral, cardiac, and major vessels. This may lead to occlusive stroke of the cerebral hemispheres and the brainstem.

There is an association between some vascular lesions of the brain and renal abnormalities: patients with *von Hippel–Lindau disease* may have cerebellar and spinal hemangioblastomas. Similarly, some forms of dominant polycystic kidney disease run risks of cerebral aneurysm on the order of 10%. With earlier and careful investigation, it is possible to identify the altered vessels and to weigh the need for surgical intervention.

Many vasculitic disorders affect the nervous system as well as the kidney. In polyarteritis nodosa and *Churg-Strauss vasculitis*, the central nervous system may be involved globally or focally in up to 50% of patients. Global effects include headache, aseptic meningitis, dementia, psychosis, and encephalopathy. The cerebrospinal fluid may show a pleocytosis. The characteristic peripheral nervous system lesion is mononeuritis multiplex, sometimes involving the cranial nerves, with typical lesions on nerve biopsy. However, a polyneuropathy may also occur, and muscle involvement is frequent (128).

In *Wegener's granulomatosis*, now classified as an antinuclear cytoplasmic antibody-positive vasculitis, neurological involvement occurs in 30%–50% of patients. This is a result of the vasculitic process causing thrombosis or hemorrhage or from the direct effects of granulomas breaking through into the central nervous system from the base of the skull.

The neurological effects of *collagen-vascular diseases* are relatively uniform, although the frequency of neurological dysfunction is much greater in systemic lupus erythematosus. The central effects may be generalized, such as dementia, or focal, such as chorea or hemiparesis. Cranial nerve lesions, especially trigeminal neuropathy and peripheral neuropathy, may also occur.

Clotting disorders

Thrombotic thrombocytopenic purpura, hemolytic–uremic syndrome, and *disseminated intravascular coagulation (DIC)* can all result in both occlusive stroke and intracerebral hemorrhage.

Thromboses may develop in DIC, and this could lead to ischemic damage in various organ systems, including the central nervous system and the kidney. Furthermore, there is a tendency to hemorrhage that could particularly affect the brain.

The treatment is primarily the correction of the underlying condition. Hematological therapy includes replacement of blood components. Giving more fibrinogen, however, may aggravate the DIC. Heparin deactivates thrombin, but there is a risk of hemorrhage.

Infectious diseases

SEPSIS

Sepsis can be defined as a systemic reaction to the presence of micro-organisms or their toxins in the blood or tissues (129). The brain, peripheral nerves, and kidneys are often involved, either together or separately, as part of the systemic reaction of multiple organ failure.

The general clinical features of sepsis commonly consist of a febrile response involving the cardiovascular and respiratory systems.

About two thirds of patients with sepsis may have evidence of encephalopathy. The clinical picture is that of a metabolic encephalopathy, and the level of consciousness varies from a confused state to coma. There is impairment of attention, concentration, memory, and writing in the encephalopathic patients who have been testable. Tremor, asterixis, and multifocal myoclonus occurs in 20% of noncomatose, encephalopathic patients. The EEG is sensitive to septic encephalopathy, and it often reveals features compatible with a metabolic encephalopathy. The clinical severity of the encephalopathy and the degree of EEG abnormality bears a significantly linear correlation with serum urea, creatinine, and bilirubin levels.

Polyneuropathy develops in patients suffering from sepsis and multiple organ failure. Due to the severe systemic disease, the polyneuropathy may be overlooked and can only be reliably demonstrated by electromyography and nerve-conduction studies. Occasionally, however, the neuropathy is so severe that there is a generalized, flaccid quadriplegia with sparing of cranial musculature that is obvious on clinical examination alone.

Since underlying pathology is a primary axonal degeneration of motor and sensory fibers, conduction velocity is little affected, and the chief manifestations are reduction in the amplitudes of muscle and sensory compound action potentials and signs of denervation on needle-electromyography-positive sharp waves and fibrillation potentials. The treatment of sepsis may aim at eradication of the infection responsible.

AIDS

There is increasing awareness of the association of renal failure with acquired immune deficiency syndrome (AIDS). Rao et al. (130) reported 78 cases of renal failure in 750 patients with AIDS (10.8%). The nervous system is involved in approximately 40% of patients with AIDS (131). It has been noted that the central nervous system is involved approximately 60% of the time and the peripheral nervous system 15% (132).

NEUROPSYCHIATRIC COMPLICATIONS OF DRUG TREATMENT IN RENAL PATIENTS

Diuretics

Hyponatremia, although seen relatively infrequently, may be particularly problematic in patients taking diuretics that work in the diluting segments of the nephron. A severe, chronic, diuretic-induced hyponatremia may lead to irreversible brain damage (133).

Loop diuretics can cause damage to the ear, and of these, ethacrynic acid appears to be the most harmful. The risk of ototoxicity is greatest when high doses of diuretics are used in patients with renal failure or when there is simultaneous administration with other ototoxic agents such as aminoglycosides.

Recombinant erythropoietin

The major adverse effect of erythropoietin administration in uremic patients is worsening hypertension, sometimes with hypertensive encephalopathy or seizures (134). These events are usually associated with initial high-dose erythropoietin therapy, often producing a rapid rise in hematocrit. To minimize the risks, the rise in hemoglobin should be kept to less than 0.5 g/dL/week.

Antimicrobials

Many antimicrobial agents are excreted by the kidney and may therefore accumulate in renal failure and produce neurological complications.

Penicillins, cephalosporins, and imipenen can cause encephalopathy (impaired consciousness, myoclonus, asterixis) or convulsions. Aminoglycosides, vancomicin, polymyxin B, and erythromicin can cause ototoxicity. Aminoglycoside toxicity has been more rarely associated with a peripheral neuropathy characterized by paresthesias in the extremities and around the mouth, which should be differentiated from neuromuscular blockade that may often represent an idiosyncratic drug effect (135). Nitrofurantoin, and possibly metronidazole, can cause peripheral neuropathy. To prevent the latter, when isoniazid is used, pyridoxine should be given (136). Decreased visual acuity and peripheral neuritis have been associated with ethambutol use. Nalidixic acid and tetracyclines can cause idiopathic intracranial hypertension (7). High doses of acyclovir can cause cerebral irritation, ataxia, and myoclonus.

Antihypertensive drugs

Peripheral vasodilators (nifedipine, prazosin, and hydralazine) can cause headache, while beta blockers (less frequently atenolol and nadolol, which do not cross the blood–brain barrier to any great extent) can cause lethargy and malaise that reverse as the drugs are discontinued.

Persistent use of nitroprusside in ESRD can cause seizures and myoclonus due to accumulation of its metabolite thiocyanate.

Drugs acting on the central nervous system

The effect of drugs acting on the central nervous system may be prolonged in uremic patients as a consequence of both changes in pharmacokinetics and an increased sensitivity due to uremia itself.

Immunosuppressive drugs

Acute side effects of corticosteroids occasionally include central nervous system changes such as psychosis and pseudotumor cerebri, which generally lessen or disappear as the dosage is tapered. Long-term steroid treatment may cause epidural lipomatosis, a condition characterized by deposits of fat that seem to cause spinal cord and root compression, resulting in signs of cord compression (137).

Since cyclosporin A (CsA) is lipophilic and penetrates the blood–brain barrier, it is to be expected that it can be neurotoxic. Involuntary fine hand tremors (the most common early neurological complication), and occasionally burning paresthesias in the soles and palms, tend to occur within the first 3 months of therapy and generally respond to dose reduction (138). Seizures can develop in a proportion of patients, usually in generalized tonic–clonic or grand mal forms (139). Seizures may sometimes be associated with a (usually reversible) encephalopathy characterized by confusion, hallucinations, and focal signs such as blindness or aphasia (140). Other reversible neurotoxic features of CsA therapy may include (141) cerebellar ataxia, often combined with tremor and confused state, and a spinal cord syndrome with either paraparesis, urinary retention, or sometimes extensor plantar responses. The development of central nervous system complications in CsA-treated patients should prompt checking the CsA and the magnesium concentration. Use of phenytoin, carbamazepine, or phenobarbital for seizure treatment may result in subtherapeutic CsA concentrations because these drugs induce a cytochrome P-450 that enhances CsA degradation (138).

OKT3 monoclonal antibodies

Use of OKT3 monoclonal antibodies for the treatment and/or prophylaxis of acute cellular rejection may be associated in the first few days of therapy with the occurrence of an aseptic meningitis consisting of headache, fever, stiff neck, and photophobia (142).

REFERENCES

1. Tyler HR: Neurological aspects of uremia. An overview. *Kidney Int* 7 (Suppl 2):S188–S193, 1975.

2. Raskin NH, Fishman RA: Neurologic disorders in renal failure. *N Engl J Med* 294:143–148, 1976.

3. Fraser CL, Arieff AL: Nervous system complications in uremia. *Ann Intern Med* 109:143–153, 1988.

4. Jennekens FGI, Jennekens-Schinkel A: Neurological aspects of dialysis patients. In: JF Maher, ed, *Replacement of Renal Function by Dialysis.* Kluwer Academic Publishers, Boston, pp 972–986, 1989.

5. Cappelli P, Di Paolo B, Albertazzi A: Neurological complications of the uremic syndrome. In: S Giovannetti, ed, *Nutritional Treatment of Chronic Renal Failure.* Kluwer Academic Publishers, Boston, pp 95–99, 1989.

6. Bolton CF, Young GB: *Neurological Complications of Renal Disease.* Butterworth Publishers, Boston, 1990.

7. Johnson M, Davison AM: The nervous system and the kidney. In: S Cameron, AM Davison, J-P Grunfeld, D Kerr, E Ritz, eds, *Oxford Textbook of Clinical Nephrology.* Oxford University Press, New York, pp 2323–2333, 1992.

8. Locke SJ, Merril JP, Tyler HR: Neurological complications of acute uremia. *Arch Intern Med* 108:75–86, 1961.

9. Ginn HE: Neurobehavioral dysfunction in uremia. *Kidney Int* 7 (Suppl 2):S217–S225, 1975.

10. Albertazzi A, Di Paolo B, Cappelli P, Spisni C, Del Rosso G: Evoked potentials in uremia. *Contrib Nephrol* 45:60–68, 1985.

11. Di Paolo B, Di Marco T, Cappelli P, Spisni C, Del Rosso G, Palmieri PF, Evangelista M, Albertazzi A: Electrophysiological aspects of nervous conduction in uremia. *Clin Nephrol* 29:253–260, 1988.

12. Teschan PE, Ginn HE, Bourne JR, Ward JW, Amel B, Nummally JC, Musso M, Vaughn WK: Quantitative indices of clinical uremia. *Kidney Int* 15:676–697, 1979.

13. Hagstam KE: EEG frequency content related to chemical blood parameters in chronic uremia. *Scand J Urol Nephrol* 7 (Suppl 1):1–9, 1971.

14. Albertazzi A, Di Paolo B, Del Rosso G, Gambi D, Rossini PM: Neurophysiological abnormalities in uraemic encephalopathy. *Proc Eur Dial Transplant Assoc Eur Ren Assoc* 18:652–657, 1981.

15. Rossini PM, Pirchio M, Treviso M, Gambi D, Di Paolo B, Albertazzi A: Checkerboard reversal pattern and flash VEPs in dialysed and nondialysed subjects. *Electroencephalogr Clin Neurophysiol* 52:435–444, 1981.

16. Weber B, Hacke W, Stiller S, Mann H: Evaluation of uremic neuropathy by visual (VEP) and brainstem auditory (BAEP) evoked potentials. *Trans Am Soc Artif Intern Organs* 31:586–589, 1985.

17. Brown JJ, Sufit RL, Sollinger HW: Visual evoked potential changes following renal transplantation. *Electroencephalogr Clin Neurophysiol* 66:101–107, 1987.

18. Rossini PM, Di Stefano E, Febbo A, Di Paolo B, Basciani M: Brainstem auditors evoked responses (BAERs) in patients with chronic renal failure. *Electroencephalogr Clin Neurophysiol* 57:507–514, 1984.

19. Komsuoglu SS, Mehta R, Jones LA, Harding GFA: Brainstem auditory evoked potentials in chronic renal failure and maintenance hemodialysis. *Neurology* 35:419–423, 1985.

20. Rossini PM, Treviso M, Di Stefano E, Di Paolo B: Nervous impulse propagation along peripheral and central fibres in patients with chronic renal failure. *Electroencephalogr Clin Neurophysiol* 56:293–303, 1983.

21. Albertazzi A, Di Paolo B, Amoroso L: Central and peripheral nervous system in dialysis patients: CAPD vs HD. In: G La Greca, S Chiaramonte, eds, *Peritoneal Dialysis.* Wichtig Editore, Milano, pp 281–286, 1988.

22. Olsen S: The brain in uremia. *Acta Psychiatr Neurol Scand* 36 (Suppl 156):3–129, 1961.

23. Arieff AI: Neurological manifestations of uremia. In: BM Brenner, FC Rector, eds, *The Kidney.* WB Saunders, Philadelphia, pp 1731–1756, 1986.

24. Akmal M, Goldstein DA, Multani S, Massry S, Massry SG: The role of uremia, brain Ca and PTH on change in EEG in chronic renal failure. *Am J Physiol* 246:F575, 1984.

25. Massry SG: Current status of the role of parathyroid hormone in uremic toxicity. *Contrib Nephrol* 49:1–11, 1985.

26. Mitch WE, Walser M: Nutritional therapy of the uremic patient. In: BM Brenner, FC Rector, eds, *The Kidney,* 4th ed. WB Saunders, Philadelphia, pp 2186–2222, 1991.

27. Bergstrom J, Lindblom U, Norèe L-O: Preservation of peripheral nerve function in severe uremia during treatment with low protein high calorie diet and surplus of essential amino acids. *Acta Neurol Scand* 51:99–109, 1975.

28. Cappelli P, Di Paolo B, Evangelista M, Di Marco T, Albertazzi A: Low-protein diet supplemented with essential amino acids and keto analogues. Effects on uremic polyneuropathy and encephalopathy. *Contrib Nephrol* 53:58–63, 1986.

29. Giovannetti S: Dietary treatment of chronic renal failure: Why is it not used more frequently? *Nephron* 40:1–12, 1985.

30. Cappelli P, Di Paolo B, Albertazzi A: Effects of nutritional treatment on the course of uremic neuropathy. In: S Giovannetti, ed, *Nutritional Treatment of Chronic Renal Failure.* Kluwer Academic Publishers, Boston, pp 255–257, 1989.

31. Rozeman CAM, Jonkman EJ, Poortvliet DCJ, Emmen HH, de Weerd AW, van der Maas APC, Tjandra YI, Beermann EM: Encephalopathy in patients on continuous ambulatory peritoneal dialysis and patients on chronic haemodialysis. *Nephrol Dial Transplant* 7:1213–1218, 1992.

32. Nissenson AR: Epoetin and cognitive function. *Am J Kidney Dis* 20 (Suppl 1):21–24, 1992.

33. Sagales T, Gimeno V, Planella MJ, Raguer N, Bartolome J: Effects of rHuEPO on Q-EEG and event-related potentials in chronic renal failure. *Kidney Int* 44:1109–1115, 1993.

34. Levinsky NG: Fluids and electrolytes—acidosis and alkalosis. In: JD Wilson, E Braunwald, KJ Isselbacher, RG Petersdorf, JB Martin, AS Fauci, RK Root, eds, *Harrison's Principles of Internal Medicine,* 12th ed. McGraw-Hill, New York, pp 278–295, 1991.

35. Andreoli TE: Disorders of fluid volume, electrolyte, and acid–base balance. In: JB Wyngaarden, LH Smith, JC Bennet, eds, *Cecil Textbook of Medicine,* 19th ed. WB Saunders, Philadelphia, pp 499–527, 1992.

36. Nielsen VK: The peripheral nerve function in chronic renal failure. I. Clinical signs and symptoms. *Acta Med Scand* 190:105–111, 1971.

37. Di Paolo B, Cappelli P, Spisni C, Albertazzi A, Rossini PM, Marchionno L, Gambi D: New electrophysiological assessments for the early diagnosis of encephalopathy and peripheral neuropathy in uremia. *Int J Tissue React* 4:301–307, 1982.

38. Nielsen VK: The peripheral nerve function in chronic renal failure. VI. Relationship between sensory and motor function and kidney function, azotemia, age, sex and clinical neuropathy. *Acta Med Scand* 194:455–462, 1973.

39. Ahonen RE: Peripheral neuropathy in uremic patients and in renal transplant recipients. *Acta Neuropathol* 54: 43–53, 1981.

40. Spencer PS, Schaumberg HH: Central–peripheral distal

axonopathy. The pathology of "dying-back" polyneuro-pathies. *Proc Neuropathol* 3:253–255, 1977.

41. Savazzi GM, Cambi V, Migone L, Marbini A, Govoni E, Bragaglia MM, Juvarra G, D'Aglio PP: The influence of uraemic neuropathy on muscle EMG, histoenzymatic and ultrastructural correlation. *Proc Eur Dial Transplant Assoc Eur Ren Assoc* 17:312–317, 1980.

42. Tegnèr R, Lindholm B: Vibratory perception threshold compared with nerve conduction velocity in the evaluation of uremic neuropathy. *Acta Neurol Scand* 71:290–297, 1985.

43. Dyck PJ, Johnson WJ, Lambert EH, O'Brien PC: Segmental demyelination secondary to axonal degeneration in uremic neuropathy. *Mayo Clin Proc* 46:400–531, 1971.

44. Rosales RL: Normal sural nerve morphometry in acute uremia. *J Neurol Neurosurg Psychiatry* 50:942–943, 1987.

45. Albertazzi A, Cappelli P, Bonomini M, Del Rosso G, Di Paolo B, Evangelista M, Palmieri PF: Role of essential amino acids and ketoanalogues in antagonizing uremic catabolism. *Contrib Nephrol* 98:167–173, 1992.

46. Violante F, Lorenzi S, Fusello M: Uremic neuropathy: clinical and neurophysiological investigation of dialysis patients using different chemical membranes. *Eur Neurol* 24:398–404, 1985.

47. Tegnér R, Lindholm B: Uremic polyneuropathy: different effects of hemodialysis and continuous ambulatory peritoneal dialysis. *Acta Med Scand* 218:409–416, 1985.

48. Yokota S, Takagi H, Kumano K, Sakai T: Peripheral nerve function in patients on CAPD as compared to hemodialysis. In: K Ota, ed, *Current Concepts in Peritoneal Dialysis*, Elsevier Science Publishers BV, Amsterdam, pp 587–592, 1992.

49. De Fijter CWH, Oe PL, Strijers RLM, Ven Der Meulen J, Ter Wu PM, Donker AJM: The course of uremia-associated peripheral neuropathy: chronic peritoneal dialysis (CPD) versus chronic hemodialysis (CHD). In: K Ota, ed, *Current Concepts in Peritoneal Dialysis*, Elsevier Science Publishers BV, Amsterdam, pp 593–597, 1992.

50. Nielsen VK: The peripheral nerve function in chronic renal failure. VII. Recovery after renal transplantation. *Acta Med Scand* 195:171–180, 1974.

51. Bolton CF: Electrophysiologic changes in uremic neuropathy after successful renal transplantation. *Neurology* 26:152–161, 1976.

52. Albertazzi A, Di Paolo B, Cappelli P, Evangelista M, Di Marco T, Varanese L: Uremic polyneuropathy: electrophysiologic findings after renal transplantation. *Transplant Proc* 17:121, 1985.

53. Brecht HM, Ernst W, Koch KM: Plasma noradrenaline levels in regular hemodialysis patients. *Proc EDTA* 12:281–289, 1975.

54. Campese VM, Romoff MS, Levitan D, Lane K, Massry SG: Mechanisms of autonomic nervous dysfunction in uremia. *Kidney Int* 20:246–253, 1981.

55. Campese VM, Massry SG: Autonomic nervous system. In: SG Massry, RJ Glassock, eds, *Textbook of Nephrology*. Williams & Wilkins, Baltimore, pp 1162–1165, 1989.

56. Zucchelli P, Sturani A, Zuccalà A, Santoro A, Degli Esposti E, Chiarini C: Dysfunction of the autonomic nervous system in patients with end-stage renal failure. *Contrib Nephrol* 45:69–81, 1985.

57. Wilson JA, Yalya TM, Giles GR, Davison AM: The effect of haemodialysis and transplantation on autonomic neuropathy. *Proc EDTA* 16:261–265, 1979.

58. Maher J, Schreiner G: Hazards and complications of dialysis. *N Engl J Med* 273:370–377, 1965.

59. Basil EC, Miller JDR, Koles Z, Grace M, Ulan RA: The effects of dialysis on brain water and EEG in stable chronic uremia. *Am J Kidney Dis* 9:462–469, 1987.

60. Arieff AI: Dialysis disequilibrium syndrome. In: SG Massry, RJ Glassock, eds, *Textbook of Nephrology*. Williams & Wilkins, Baltimore, pp 1168–1170, 1989.

61. Arieff AI, Massry SG, Barrientos A, Kleeman CR: Brain water and electrolyte metabolism in uremia: effects of slow and rapid hemodialysis. *Kidney Int* 4:177–187, 1973.

62. Arieff AI, Lazarowitz VC, Guisado R: Experimental dialysis disequilibrium syndrome: prevention with glycerol. *Kidney Int* 14:270–278, 1978.

63. Posner JB, Plum F: Spinal fluid pH and neurologic symptoms in systemic acidosis. *N Engl J Med* 277:605, 1977.

64. Port FK, Johnson WJ, Klass DW: Prevention of dialysis dysequilibrium syndrome by the use of high sodium concentration in the dialysate. *Kidney Int* 3:327–333, 1973.

65. Kennedy AC, Linton AL, Luke RG, Renfrew S: Electroencephalographic changes during hemodialysis. *Lancet* i:408–411, 1963.

66. Rosa AA, Shideman J, McHugh R, Duncan D, Kjellstrand CM: The importance of osmolality fall and ultrafiltration rate on hemodialysis side effects: influence of intravenous mannitol. *Nephron* 27:134–141, 1981.

67. Raju SF, White AR, Barness TT, Smith PP, Kirchner KA: Improvement in dysequilibrium symptoms during dialysis with low glucose dialysate. *Clin Nephrol* 18:126–129, 1982.

68. Pagel MD, Ahmad S, Vizzo JE, Scribner BH: Acetate and bicarbonate fluctuations and acetate intolerance during dialysis. *Kidney Int* 21:513–518, 1982.

69. Jack R, Rabin PL, McKinney TW: Dialysis encephalopathy: a review. *Int J Psychiatry Med* 13:309–326, 1983/1984.

70. Smith DB, Lewis JA, Burks JS, Alfrey AC: Dialysis encephalopathy in peritoneal dialysis. *JAMA* 244:365–366, 1980.

71. Dewberry FL, McKinney TD, Stone WJ: The dialysis dementia syndrome: report of fourteen cases and review of the literature. *Trans Am Soc Artif Intern Organs* 3:102–108, 1980.

72. Andreoli SP, Beegstein JM, Sherrard DJ: Aluminum intoxication from aluminum-containing phosphate binders in children with azotemia not undergoing dialysis. *N Engl J Med* 310:1079–1084, 1984.

73. Alfrey AC, LeGendre GR, Kaehney WD: The dialysis encephalopathy syndrome: possible aluminum intoxication. *N Engl J Med* 294:184–188, 1976.

74. Chokroverty S, Bruetman BE, Berger V, Reyes MG: Progressive dialytic encephalopathy. *J Neurol Neurosurg Psychiatry* 39:411–419, 1976.

75. Dunea G, Mahurkar SD, Mamdami B, Smith EC: Role of aluminum in dialysis dementia. *Ann Intern Med* 88:502–504, 1978.

76. Davison AM, Oli H, Walker GS, Lewins AM: Water supply, aluminum concentration, dialysis dementia and effect of reverse-osmosis water treatment. *Lancet* ii:785–786, 1982.

77. Mahoney CA, Arieff AI: Uremic encephalopathies: clinical, biochemical, and experimental features. *Am J Kidney Dis* 2:324–336, 1982.

78. Bommer J: Medical complications of the long-term dialysis patients. In: S Cameron, AM Davison, JP Grunfeld, D Kerr,

E Ritz, eds, *Oxford Textbook of Clinical Nephrology*. Oxford University Press, New York, pp 1436–1458, 1992.

79. Kirschbaum BB, Schoolwarth AC: Acute aluminum toxicity associated with oral citrate and aluminum-containing antacids. *Am J Med Sci* 297:9, 1989.

80. Vasilakakis DM, D'Haese PC, Lamberts LV, Lemoniatou E, Digenis PN, De Broe ME: Removal of aluminoxamine and ferrioxamine by charcoal hemoperfusion and hemodialysis. *Kidney Int* 41:1400–1407, 1992.

81. Ackrill P, Ralston AJ, Day JP, Hodge KC: Successful removal of aluminum from a patient with dialysis encephalopathy. *Lancet* ii:692–693, 1980.

82. Boelaert JR, de Locht M: Side-effects of desferrioxamine in dialysis patients. *Nephrol Dial Transplant Suppl* 1:43–46, 1993.

83. Consensus Conference: Diagnosis and treatment of aluminum overload in end-stage renal failure patients. *Nephrol Dial Transplant Suppl* 1:1–4, 1993.

84. Verpooten GA, D'Haese PC, Boelaert JR, Becaus I, Lamberts LV, De Broe ME: Pharmakokinetics of aluminoxamine and ferrioxamine and dose finding of desferrioxamine in haemodialysis patients. *Nephrol Dial Transplant* 7:931–938, 1992.

85. Davison AM, Giler GR: The effect of transplantation on dialysis dementia. *Proc EDTA* 16:407–412, 1979.

86. Ball JH, Butkus DE, Madison DS: Effect of subtotal parathyroidectomy on dialysis dementia. *Nephron* 18:151, 1977.

87. De Gencarelli NC, Cournot-Witmer G, Zingraff J, Drueke T: The role of parathyroid function and parathyroidectomy in the outcome of aluminum-related dialysis encephalopathy. *Nephrol Dial Transplant* 1:192–198, 1986.

88. Lewins AM: Aluminum intoxication. *Proc EDTNA* 10:219–220, 1982.

89. Pagani C, Zoerle C, Guaita MC, Bazzi C, Sorgato G, Torti G: Carpal tunnel syndrome in long-term dialyzed patients. *Contrib Nephrol* 45:82–96, 1985.

90. Maiorca R, Cancarini GC, Camerini C, Brunori G, Manili L, Movilli E, Feller P, Mombelloni S: Is CAPD competitive with hemodialysis for long term treatment of uraemic patients? *Nephrol Dial Transplant* 4:244–253, 1989.

91. Halter SK, De Lisa JA, Stolov W: Carpal tunnel syndrome in chronic renal dialysis patients. *Arch Phys Med Rehabil* 62:197–201, 1981.

92. Ritz E, Bommer J: Beta-2 microglobulin derived amyloid problems and perspectives. *Blood Purif* 6:61–68, 1988.

93. Chow JC: Endoscopic release of the carpal ligament: a new technique for carpal tunnel syndrome. *Arthroscopy* 5:19–24, 1989.

94. Bechar M, Lakke JP, Hem GK, van der Becks JW, Penning L: Subdural hematoma during long-term hemodialysis. *Arch Neurol* 26:513–518, 1972.

95. McLachlan RS, Bolton CF, Coates RK, Barnett HJM: Gait disturbance in chronic subdural hematoma. *Can Med Assoc J* 125:865–868, 1981.

96. Tietjen DP, Moore J Jr, Gouge JF: Hemodialysis-associated acute subdural hematoma: interim management with peritoneal dialysis. *Am J Nephrol* 7:478–485, 1987.

97. Tolkoff-Rubin NE, Nardini J, Fang LST, Rubin RH: Successful hemodialysis of patients at high risk of hemorrhage using the Eval dialyzer. *Dial Transplant* 15:125, 1986.

98. Rotter W, Roettger P: Comparative pathologic–anatomic study of cases of chronic global renal insufficiency with and without hemodialysis. *Clin Nephrol* 1:257, 1974.

99. Lopez RI, Collins GK: Wernicke's encephalopathy: a complication of chronic hemodialysis. *Arch Neurol* 18:248–259, 1968.

100. Kimmel PL, Miller G, Mendelson WB: Sleep apnoea syndrome in chronic renal disease. *Am J Med* 86:308–314, 1989.

101. Kimmel PL: Sleep disorders in hemodialysis patients. In: JP Bosch, JH Stein, eds, *Contemporary Issues in Nephrology. Vol. 27: Hemodialysis: high-efficiency treatments*. Churchill Livingstone, New York, pp 295–308, 1993.

102. Sullivan CE, Berthon-Jones M, Issa FG: Reversal of obstructive sleep apnea by continuous positive airway pressure applied through the nares. *Lancet* i:862, 1981.

103. Benz RL, Pressman MR, Schliefer CR, Peterson DD: Sleep disorder profiles in chronic renal failure patients: successful intervention with nasal continuous positive airway pressure (abstract). *Am J Kidney Dis* 20:A1, 1992.

104. Mitler MM, Browman CP, Menn SJ, et al.: Nocturnal myoclonus: treatment efficacy of clonazepam and ternazepam. *Sleep* 9:385, 1986.

105. Olsen CA: A statistical review of variables predictive of adjustment in hemodialysis patients. *Nephrol Nurse* 5:16–27, 1983.

106. Levenson JL, Glocheski S: Psychological factors affecting end-stage renal disease. *Psychosomatics* 32:382–389, 1991.

107. Kimmel PC, Weihs K, Peterson RA: Survival in hemodialysis patients: the role of depression. *J Am Soc Nephrol* 3:12–27, 1993.

108. Locsey L, Balogh L, Toth E: Psychological effects of chronic haemodialysis. *Int Urol Nephrol* 19:91–100, 1987.

109. Neu S, Kjellstrand CM: Stopping long-term dialysis: an empirical study of withdrawal of life-supporting treatment. *N Engl J Med* 314:14–20, 1986.

110. Wolcott DL, Marsh JT, La Rue A, Can C, Nissenson AR: Recombinant human erythropoietin therapy may improve quality of life and cognitive function in chronic hemodialysis patients. *Am J Kidney Dis* 14:478–485, 1989.

111. Friedman EA, Lundin AP III: Outcome and complication of chronic hemodialysis. In: RW Schrier, CW Gottschalk, eds, *Diseases of the Kidney*, 5th ed. Little, Brown, Boston, pp 3069–3095, 1993.

112. Kennedy SH, Craven JL, Rodin GM: Major depression in renal dialysis patients: an open trial of antidepressant therapy. *J Clin Psychiatry* 50:60–63, 1989.

113. Roose SP, Glassman AH, Dalack GW: Depression, heart disease, and tricyclic antidepressants. *J Clin Psychiatry* 50 (Suppl):12–16, 1989.

114. Pasquali S, Casanova S, Zucchelli A, Zucchelli P: Long-term survival patients with acute and severe renal failure due to multiple myeloma. *Clin Nephrol* 34:247–254, 1990.

115. Zucchelli P, Paquali S, Cagnoli L, Ferrari G: Controlled plasma exchange trial in acute renal failure due to multiple myeloma. *Kidney Int* 33:1175–1180, 1988.

116. Bardwick PA, Zvaifler NJ, Gill GN, Newman D, Greenway GD, Resnick DL: Plasma cell dyscrasia with polyneuropathy, organomegaly, endocrinopathy, M protein and skin changes: the POEMS syndrome, report on two cases and review of the literature. *Medicine (Baltimore)* 59:311–321, 1980.

117. Fagerburg SE: Diabetic neuropathy: a clinical and histologic study on the significance of vascular affections. *Acta Med Scand* 164 (Suppl 345):1–80, 1959.

118. Evans WE, Manninen DL, Garrison LP, et al.: The quality of life of patients with end-stage renal disease. *N Engl J Med* 312:553–558, 1985.

119. Krane EJ, Roackhoff MA, Wallman JD, Wolfsldorf JI: Subclinical brain swelling in children during treatment of diabetic ketoacidosis. *N Engl J Med* 312:1147–1151, 1985.

120. Keller V, Berger W, Troug P: Course and prognosis of 86 episodes of diabetic coma: a five year experience with a uniform schedule of treatment. *Diabetologia* 11:93–100, 1975.

121. Podolsky S: Hyperosmolar non-ketotic coma in the elderly diabetic. *Med Clin North Am* 62:815–828, 1978.

122. McCurdy DK: Hyperosmolar hyperglycaemic non-ketotic diabetic coma. *Med Clin North Am* 54:683–699, 1970.

123. Asbury AK: Focal and multifocal neuropathies of diabetes. In: PJ Dyck, PK Thomas, AK Asbury, et al., eds, *Diabetic Neuropathy*. WB Saunders, Philadelphia, pp 45–55, 1987.

124. Amair P, Khanna R, Leibel B, et al.: Continuous ambulatory peritoneal dialysis in diabetics with end-stage renal disease. *N Engl J Med* 306:625–630, 1982.

125. Tegnèr R: The effect of skin temperature on viibratory sensitivity in polyneuropathy. *J Neurol Neurosurg Psychiatry* 48:176–178, 1985.

126. Najarian JS, Sutherland DER, Simmons RL, et al.: Ten year experience with renal transplantation in juvenile onset diabetes. *Ann Surg* 190:487–500, 1979.

127. Solders G, Wilczek H, Gunnarsson R, et al.: Effects of combined pancreatic and renal transplantation on diabetic neuropathy; a two-year follow-up study. *Lancet* 2:1232–1235, 1987.

128. Moore PM, Fauci AS: Neurologic manifestations of systemic vasculitis: a retrospective and prospective study of the clinico-pathologic features and responses to therapy in 25 patients. *Am J Med* 71:517–524, 1981.

129. Sanford JP: Epidemiology and root of the problem. In: RK Root, MA Sande, eds, *Septic Shock*. Churchill Livingstone, New York, pp 1–11, 1985.

130. Rao TK, Friedman EA, Nicastri AD: The types of renal disease in acquired immune deficiency syndrome. *N Engl J Med* 316:1062–1068, 1987.

131. Bredesen DE, Levy RM, Rosenblum ML: Human immunodeficiency virus-related neurological dysfunction. In: MJ Aminoff, ed, *Neurology and General Medicine. The Neurological Aspects of Medical Disorders*, Chapter 37. Churchill Livingstone, New York, pp 673–679, 1989.

132. Miller RG, Parry GJ, Pfaeffl W, Lang W, Lippert R, Kiprov D: The spectrum of peripheral neuropathy associated with ARC and AIDS. *Muscle Nerve* 11:857–863, 1988.

133. Ayms JC, Krothapalli RK, Arieff AI: Treatment of symptomatic hyponatremia and its relation to brain damage. A prospective study. *N Engl J Med* 317:1190–1195, 1987.

134. Tomson CRV, Venning MC, Ward MK: Blood pressure and erythropoietin (letter). *Lancet* ii:351, 1988.

135. Sande MA, Mandell GL: Antimicrobial agents: the aminoglycosides. In: AG Gilman, LS Goodman, TW Rall, F Murad, eds, *Goodman and Gilman's The Pharmacological Basis of Therapeutics*, 7th ed, vol 51. Macmillian, New York, pp 1150–1169, 1985.

136. Cuss FMC, Carmichael DJS, Allington A, Hulme B: Tubercolosis in renal failure: a high incidence in patients born in the third world. *Clin Nephrol* 25:129–133, 1986.

137. Kaplan JG, Barasch E, Hirschfeld A, Ross L, Einberg K, Gordon M: Spinal epidural lipomatosis: a serious complication of iatrogenic Cushing's syndrome. *Neurology* 39:1031–1034, 1989.

138. Kahan BD, Flechner SM, Lorber MI, et al.: Complication of cyclosporine therapy. *World J Surg* 10:348–360, 1986.

139. Polson RJ, Powell-Jackson PR, Williams R: Convulsions associated with cyclosporin A in transplant recipients. *Br Med J* 290:1003, 1985.

140. Hughes RL: Cyclosporin-related central nervous system toxicity in cardiac transplantation. *N Engl J Med* 323:420–421, 1990.

141. Atkinson K, Biggs JC, Karveniza P, et al.: Spinal cord cerebellar-like syndromes associated with the use of cyclosporine in human recipients of allogenic marrow transplants. *Transplant Proc* 17:1673–1675, 1985.

142. Martin MA, Massanari M, Nighiem DD, Smith JL, Corry RJ: Nosocomial aseptic meningitis associated with administration of OKT3. *JAMA* 259:2002–2005, 1988.

CHAPTER 53

Hematologic Disorders in Renal Failure

J. RADERMACHER & KARL M. KOCH

INTRODUCTION

Even though renal failure also affects the function of white blood cells (1,2) and thrombocytes (3), renal anemia is the main hematologic disturbance of uremia for which well-founded possibilities of therapeutic intervention exist today. The basis for this exceptional and fortunate situation is our advanced understanding of the pathogenesis of renal anemia as well as recent progress in molecular biology. Since this book is devoted to therapy, this chapter will concentrate on renal anemia and its management.

CLINICAL FEATURES AND CONSEQUENCES

Anemia is one of the main clinical symptoms of renal failure, occurring in more than 80% of patients with end-stage renal failure. It becomes manifest when creatinine clearance has dropped to 30–40 mL/min/1.73 m^2, and its severity increases with further deterioration of excretory renal function. Renal anemia is normochromic and normocytic when no other aggravating factors such as iron deficiency or aluminium overload are coexisting with renal insufficiency. Renal anemia is hyporegenerative. The reticulocyte count, when corrected for normal hematocrit values, is inadequate.

The impact of renal anemia on physical and mental abilities is considerable and represents a major obstacle for the rehabilitation of patients in terminal renal failure. This observation applies even though the effect of anemia on tissue oxygenation may be partly balanced in uremic patients by a shift of the oxyhemoglobin dissociation curve to the right. This shift, which is attributed to acidosis and increased intraerythrocytotic levels of 2,3-diphosphoglycerate and other phosphates, reduces the peripheral affinity of hemoglobin for oxygen and thereby improves oxygen delivery to the tissues. A further compensating mechanism is an increase in cardiac output (4), which, when extremely severe, may result in heart failure due to a high output state even in the absence of underlying heart disease (5).

Accordingly, a typical echocardiographic finding in end-stage renal disease is an eccentric left ventricular hypertrophy (6), which is characteristic of volume overload (7). It is defined by a parallel increase in ventricular radius (end-diastolic diameter) and wall thickness, leaving the ratio between wall thickness and radius unchanged. Concentric hypertrophy (increase of wall thickness only), which is characteristic of pressure overload, can also be induced, since hypertension occurs in up to 80% of patients with end-stage renal disease and may combine with eccentric hypertrophy. Hypertension and the resulting hypertensive cardiomyopathy may compromise the ability to compensate for the reduced hemoglobin level by an increase in cardiac output. Also, many of the patients have advanced coronary artery disease, and even renal anemia of a moderate degree may be accompanied by myocardial hypoxia and angina.

PATHOGENESIS

The primary mechanism involved in the pathogenesis of the anemia of renal failure are hemolysis, inadequate production of erythropoietin, and possibly also an inhibition of the response of erythroid precursor cells to erythropoietin (8,9). In addition, secondary mechanisms such as blood loss, iron or folate deficiency, aluminum intoxication, drug effects, the anemia of chronic disease, marrow fibrosis resulting from hyperparathyroidism, hypersplenism, and toxic hemolysis may be operative.

Hemolysis

Hemolysis in terminal renal failure is of moderate degree, since red-cell survival in general is reduced by only 25%–30%. The accelerated destruction of red cells in uremia appears to be the result of the uremic environment, since cells from uremic subjects transfused in normal volunteers have a normal life span, whereas normal red cells transfused into uremic patients have a reduced life span. The cause for hemolysis appears to be extracellular and related to the effects of factors contained in the uremic plasma on membrane ATPase, on intracellular glutathione, and on the enzymes of the pentose phosphate shunt of erythrocytes. The malfunction of the pentose phosphate shunt and the resulting increase in oxidized glutathione renders erythrocytes vulnerable to hemoglobin oxidation with subsequent hemolysis. This defect may become especially critical when exogeneous oxidants are introduced via the dialysate or as medication. Thus, the use of chloramine-containing tap water for the production of dialysate can cause significant hemolysis in hemodialysis patients. Secondary hyperparathyroidism may also contribute to the reduction of red cell survival in uremia, since intact parathyroid hormone (PTH) or its 1–34 fragment increases the osmotic fragility of human red blood cells, probably by increasing cellular rigidity (10). Also, chronic uremic dogs have a shortened red cell survival that is normalized by parathyroidectomy (11). However, in the clinical setting, marrow fibrosis and not increased PTH serum level is the best predictor of the effect of subtotal parathyroidectomy on erythropoiesis, suggesting that hyperparathyroidism-associated marrow fibrosis and not PTH-induced hemolysis is the principal factor in the anemia associated with secondary hyperparathyroidism (12,13). Aggravation of hemolysis in renal failure may also be a consequence of additional pathologic processes like malignant hypertension or microangiopathy associated with various forms of systemic and renal vasculitis such as microscopic polyangiitis and Wegener's syndrome. Another mechanism causing an increase of erythrocyte rigidity with subsequent hemolysis in renal failure is intracellular phosphate depletion due to overtreatment with oral phosphate binders (14). There are a number of additional, less common mechanisms that occasionally may cause significant hemolysis, such as accidental exposure of blood to excess copper, zinc, formaldehyde, chloramine, and nitrates or to an overheated or very hypotonic dialysate in hemodialysis patients.

Erythropoietin deficiency

The mild hemolysis caused by renal failure alone, without the action of additional aggravating factors, should not result in anemia if the response of erythropoiesis is sufficient. However, erythropoiesis is impaired. The major reason for this phenomenon is insufficient production of erythropoietin in patients with advanced renal failure (15). Investigations applying specific radioimmunoassays showed that, in comparison to anemic patients without renal disease, patients with anemia of renal failure display an inadequate rise of the serum erythropoietin concentration (16–18).

The kidneys have been shown to produce about 80% of the erythropoietin in adult mammals (19); the rest is produced by the liver. The important role of erythropoietin deficiency in the pathogenesis of renal anemia is emphasized by the more severe degree of anemia observed in bilateral nephrectomized hemodialysis patients (20).

It is still unclear whether the inadequate production of erythropoietin is a consequence of progressive destruction of renal production sites of erythropoietin (most likely peritubular interstitial fibroblasts) (21) by the underlying renal disease or whether it is due to a dependence of erythropoietin formation on excretory renal function, or both. A simplified explanation for the second mechanism could be as follows (22): A decrease of glomerular filtration due to renal failure is associated with a decrease of tubular reabsorption and thereby also with a decrease of tubular oxygen consumption (23). This reduced oxygen consumption, would be perceived by an intrarenally located oxygen sensor (24), as an increase in blood or tissue PO_2, which in turn would reduce its stimulatory signal on erythropoietin-producing cells, with the consequence of a decrease in erythropoietin production.

Inhibition of erythropoiesis

In addition to the reduced availability of erythropoietin, inhibition of the response of erythroid precursor cells to erythropoietin has to be considered as a cause for the inadequate erythropoiesis in uremic patients.

The accumulation of inhibitors ("uremic toxins") within the uremic organism has been suggested by a number of clinical observations. First, elevated plasma levels of erythropoietin could be demonstrated in some anemic patients with end-stage renal disease (25–27), suggesting that the response of the bone marrow of these patients to erythropoietin is suppressed. Second, hematologic improvement can frequently be seen in patients with terminal renal failure after the induction of regular dialysis treatment. Hematocrit and red cell production as measured by erythrocyte iron turnover usually rise (28) in spite of a parallel decline of serum erythropoietin levels (29).

Attempts to identify endogenous "uremic" inhibitors of erythropoiesis have led to conflicting results (30). Amongst the many substances implicated (30), the most intensively investigated were the polyamines spermine, spermidine, and putrescine (31); parathyroid hormone; polar lipids; vitamin A; and prostaglandins. In spite of many observations supporting the involvement of these substances, the discussion is still controversial (9,32). One of the most relevant arguments against a significant role of uremic inhibitors in the pathogenesis of renal anemia is the observation that the response of erythropoiesis to recombinant human erythropoietin in normals and in uremic patients is not significantly different (33).

Secondary mechanisms

BLOOD LOSS

Hemodialysis patients have a small amount of blood loss during each dialysis, amounting to about 2 mL per dialyser (34) with additional loss from frequent blood sampling for hematological and biochemical measurements. When added to the normal loss from the gastrointestinal tract (5–7 mL) this blood loss amounts to a daily iron loss of 2–3 mg (0.7–1.1 g/year). However, in the older literature, average daily iron losses as high as 6 mg (2.1 g/year) have been reported in regular hemodialysis patients (35). In single cases, this iron loss may exceed possible iron uptake from food, since iron absorption in severe iron deficiency can only increase from a normal of 10% to a maximum of 50%–60% and since a normal diet contains only about 15 mg of iron. Therefore, monitoring of iron status is mandatory in hemodialysis patients.

IRON INSUFFICIENCY

Most guidelines for the monitoring of iron status have been established for patients treated with recombinant human erythropoietin (36) (see below), because iron insufficiency is the most common cause of a poor response of erythropoiesis to the recombinant hormone (37).

Iron deficiency may be either absolute (defined as a reduction in total body iron stores) or functional (implying adequate iron stores but a delay or failure to supply available iron the the marrow). Staining the bone marrow for hemosiderin gives the most accurate assessment of iron stores, but this procedure cannot be used for routine determination of iron status. Measurement of serum ferritin to quantify iron stores (38) and transferrin saturation as a measure of iron circulating in plasma (39) are the most widely used methods, but both have drawbacks (see below).

FOLATE DEFICIENCY

Folate deficiency results in megaloblastic anemia. The adequacy of folate stores is best estimated by red cell folate levels. The daily folate requirement is about 100 µg, an amount usually provided by a Western diet. However, folate is readily removed by hemodialysis, so hemodialysis patients were thought to require oral folate supplementation (40). In hemodialysis patients usually living on an almost normal mixed diet, however, no need for routine folic acid supplements could be observed (41), and therefore folate replacement should be restricted to malnourished patients. Folate is not removed in significant amounts by peritoneal dialysis.

ALUMINUM INTOXICATION

An additional antierythropoietic mechanism not directly linked to renal insufficiency can be aluminum intoxication, although this complication is becoming less common with modern methods of purifying the water used to prepare dialysate and with less frequent use of aluminium hydroxide as an oral phosphate binder. Aluminum induces a microcytic anemia, that, when observed in a patient with a normal iron status, should make one suspect that the patient's renal anemia may be aggravated by aluminum

intoxication. Other possible causes of microcytic anemia that must be kept in mind are malignancies or an inflammatory state. The exact pathogenesis of aluminum-associated anemia is not yet fully understood, but the available evidence strongly suggests that the toxic effects of aluminum on erythropoiesis involve inhibition of synthesis and ferrochelation of hemoglobin, perhaps as a result of Al binding to transferrin (42–44).

DRUGS

The interference of drugs with renal erythropoietin production is not well studied. Drugs acting on the proximal tubule (the presumed oxygen-sensing site) could affect erythropoietin production, and an attenuating effect of acetazolamide on erythropoietin formation has been shown in man (45). Angiotensin-converting enzyme inhibitors have been shown to inhibit erythropoietin production in rats (46), to lower serum erythropoietin concentration in healthy volunteers (47) and in patients with chronic nephropathy (48), and to worsen anemia in patients with chronic nephropathy (48,49). This effect may be brought about by ACE-inhibitor-induced renal hyperperfusion diminishing the hypoxic stimulus to erythropoietin formation (50) and can be therapeutically exploited (see below) in the treatment of transplantation-induced polycythemia (60). Inhibition of erythropoietin formation in response to hypoxia and anemia has also been shown with cyclooxygenase inhibitors in dogs and rats (51). Whether this effect also occurs in man is not known at present. Certain prostaglandins even seem to be involved in the pathogenesis of reduced bone marrow response to erythropoietin (52).

ANEMIA OF CHRONIC DISEASE

Chronic infection, inflammation, and neoplastic disorders have long been known to be associated with anemia (anemia of chronic disease (53)). Primary nonresponse to erythropoietin treatment has been observed with these disorders. This form of anemia is due to immune activation in reaction to foreign antigens, with the production of cytokines that directly inhibit erythropoiesis, liberation of iron from its stores, and erythropoietin production. Cytokines that have been predominantly involved as mediators of the anemia of chronic disease (ACD) are interleukin-1, gamma-interferon, and tumor necrosis factor-α. ACD is thus characterized by an underproduction of red blood cells and is found to be hypochromic and microcytic in up to 50% of patients. Most often, transferrin saturation is reduced in the presence of adequate iron stores (functional iron deficiency).

Recombinant human erythropoietin in high doses may overcome the resulting hyporesponsivness of the marrow; however, much larger doses than in the treatment of the anemia of CRF are needed for up to several weeks after resolution of the inflammatory response (54).

MANAGEMENT

The principles of treatment of renal anemia range from the more symptomatic measure of transfusion of red cells to complete cure by renal transplantation. Blood transfusions are only of temporary benefit and carry inherent risks such as exposure to the viruses of hepatitis and human immune deficiency, as well as the development of secondary hemochromatosis. Furthermore, blood transfusions have been shown to suppress endogenous erythropoietin secretion and may result in sensitization to HLA antigens. Renal transplantation in most cases is not available before a waiting period of variable length has passed, and not every regular dialysis patient, especially among the steadily growing population of older patients, is eligible for transplantation. As shown in Table 1, there exist a variety of therapeutic approaches between the two poles of blood transfusion and transplantation that either interfere with the pathogenesis of renal anemia itself or prevent or correct the effects of secondary aggravating mechanisms.

Transfusion

Frequent blood transfusion suppresses erythron activity (28) and hence increases subsequent transfusion requirements. The availability of recombinant erythropoietin obviates the need for regular transfusions in most chronic dialysis patients (55,56). Red cell transfusion should be reserved for acute symptomatic anemia with symptoms of tissue hypoxia such as angina and dyspnea that cannot wait for the more delayed effects of stimulation of erythropoiesis by erythropoietin substitution. All efforts should be made to avoid frequent blood transfusions, since they increase the risk of iron overload and blood-borne viral infections and expose the patient to the risk of antibody production to HLA antigens; therefore, they may reduce the chances of receiving a successful transplant.

Table 1. Principles of treatment of renal anemia

Blood transfusion
Erythropoietin supplementation
Iron supplementation
Removal of endogenous inhibitors of erythropoiesis and
   endogenous hemolytic toxins by extracorporeal renal
   replacement therapy or peritoneal dialysis
Removal of excess aluminum by desferrioxamine
Correction of hyperparathyroidism
Androgen therapy
Reduction of iatrogenic blood loss
Folate supplementation
Exclusion of physical and chemical hazards within the
   extracorporeal blood circuit
Renal transplantation

Erythropoietin supplementation

As a treatment focused on the primary pathogenesis, a very effective and promising therapy has become available in that recombinant human erythropoietin (r-HuEPO) has been produced for therapeutic application. When given intravenously or subcutaneously to regular hemodialysis patients, r-HuEPO caused a dramatic, dose-dependent improvement of erythropoiesis (57,58). It was even possible to keep hemoglobin levels normal after stopping blood transfusions in bilateral nephrectomized patients who had been in need of regular transfusions before. As shown in Figure 1, taken from one of the first trials performed in regular hemodialysis patients, hematocrit increases within a few weeks when r-HuEPO is given intravenously thrice a week. The speed of correction of renal anemia and the degree of normalization of hemoglobin levels are clearly dose dependent, and with high doses, complete correction of renal anemia is possible.

BENEFITS OF R-HUEPO THERAPY

The need for blood transfusion has decreased significantly—by about 75%—since the introduction of r-HuEPO treatment (55,56). Relief from blood transfusions with its associated risks (s.a.) is an obvious benefit. Reports of a significant fall of cytotoxic antibody levels after treatment with r-HuEPO in formerly polytransfused children and adults (59,60), highly immunized to HLA antigens, are just one example of the advantages of prevention of blood transfusion by r-HuEPO substitution.

The reversal of anemia with r-HuEPO treatment has also led to a significant improvement in the quality of life. Patients report an immediate feeling of well-being. This subjective finding has been supported by several objective findings. An improvement of exercise tolerance can be quantified by ergometry (Figure 2). Physical work capacity at a heart rate of 130 beats/min (PWC 130) was determined by bicycle ergometry in 15 regular hemodialysis patients with a mean age of 42.4 years (range 22–57) (61). When the mean hematocrit had risen from $23 \pm 4\%$ (SD) to $35 \pm 6\%$ approximately 12 weeks after starting r-HuEPO therapy, the mean PWC 130 rose significantly ($p < 0.05$) from 73 ± 28 watts to 98 ± 38 watts, a value just reaching the lower limit of the range obtained in healthy volunteers of comparable age. These results have been confirmed by other authors (62–64).

Other measures of the quality of life have also been reported to improve with the correction of anemia. Symptoms of anemia such as angina and tiredness may be relieved. Patients "feel less cold," and nutritional status improves (65), possibly due to increased physical activity resulting in increased appetite. Libido has been reported to return (66); associated changes of levels of relevant hormones are controversial (67). Cognitive function, as assessed by electrophysiological techniques, has been reported to improve (68). All these observations suggest

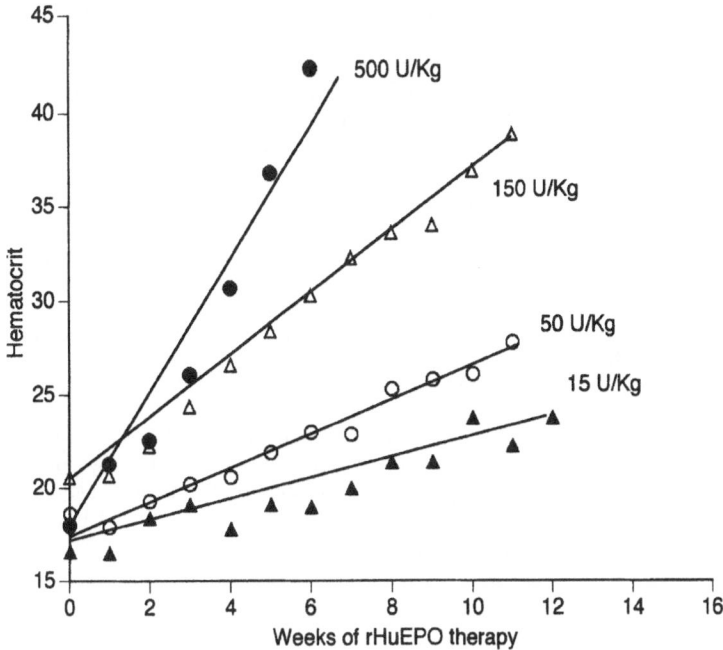

Figure 1. Increase of hematocrit at various doses of recombinant human erythropoietin (r-HuEPO). Four to five patients make up each treatment group, and the data points represent the mean weekly hematocrits for each group. From Eschbach et al. (57).

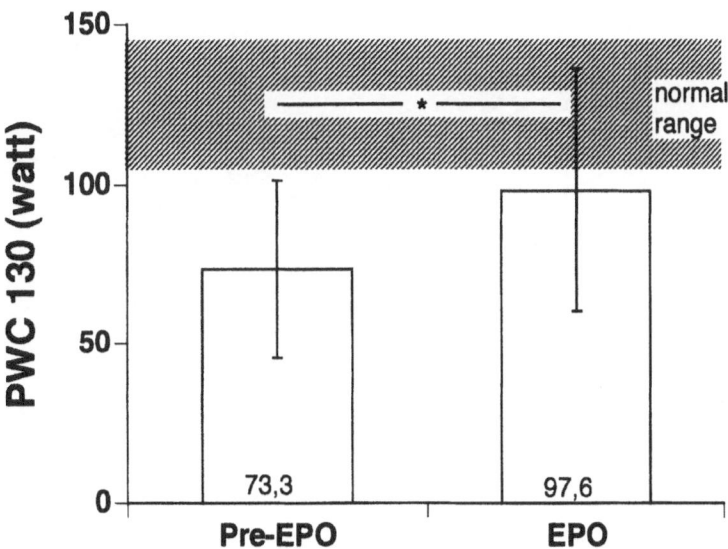

Figure 2. Physical work capacity at heart rate of 130 beats/min (PWC 130) in 15 regular hemodialysis patients before (pre-EPO) and during (EPO) treatment with recombinant human erythropoietin. Mean hematocrit pre-EPO, $23 \pm 4\%$; under EPO, $35 \pm 6\%$ (mean $\pm$ SD). * = $p < 0.05$, paired t-test.

that r-HuEPO substitution has a significant positive effect on rehabilitation in ESRD. This is also indicated by a reduction of hospitalization time (days spent in hospital) by as much as 50% in patients treated with r-HuEPO (65).

One of the main causes for the majority of the benefits of r-HuEPO therapy is an improvement in cardiovascular function. Cardiac output decreases toward the normal range (69), and this change is associated with normalization of left ventricular end-diastolic diameter (62,70–83). Left ventricular hypertrophy, as evidenced by an increase in left ventricular muscle mass, has been shown to decline with partial correction of renal anemia in many studies (Figure 3).

However, complete normalization of left ventricular muscle mass rarely occurred, which could have been due either to the only partial correction of anemia or to a counterproductive effect of hypertension (71), which sometimes develops under r-HuEPO treatment (see Adverse Effects of r-HuEPO Treatment below).

Left ventricular hypertrophy has been shown to be an important determinant of survival in patients on hemodialysis treatment (84,85). Furthermore, correction of anemia with r-HuEPO has been shown to reduce exercise-induced myocardial ischemia in hemodialysis patients with confirmed coronary artery disease, as evidenced by reduced exercise-induced ST-segment depression in the ECG (62,86). Both the reduction of left ventricular hypertrophy and the reduction of myocardial hypoxia with r-HuEPO treatment may have beneficial effects on cardiovascular death rate and overall survival in chronic renal failure patients. So far, the data on a reducing effect of r-HuEPO treatment on cardiovascular-related death are limited, and positive results after 3–5 years of r-HuEPO treatment were only reported for selected patients who may not have been representative of the general dialysis population (87). Therefore, further studies have to be awaited.

Finally, a normalization of uremia-associated abnormal hemostasis characterized by a prolonged bleeding time and abnormal in vitro platelet aggregation has been shown to occur (88) with r-HuEPO treatment in hemodialysis patients. The mechanisms underlying these derangements are

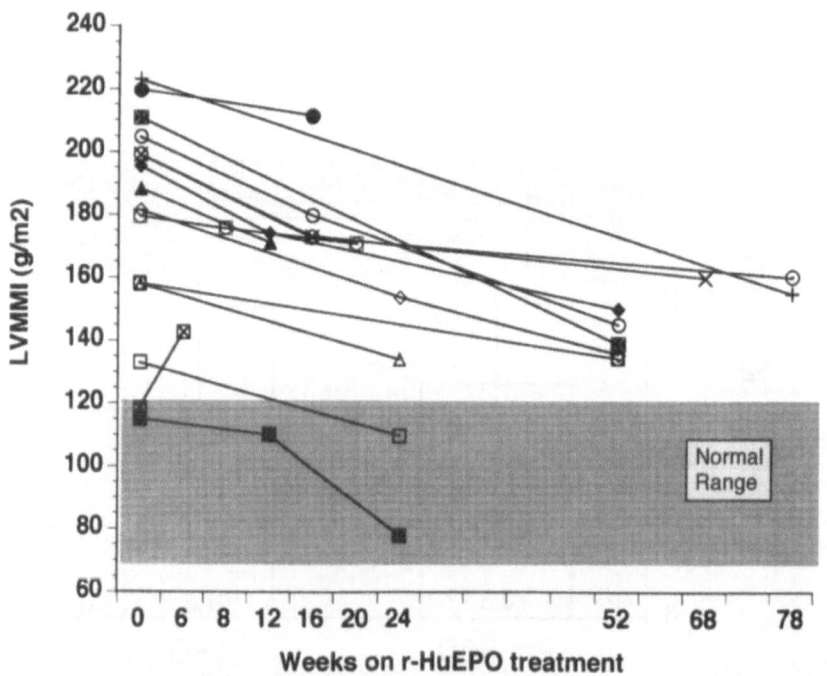

Figure 3. Reduction in left ventricular muscle mass index (LVMMI) with r-HuEPO treatment. Data taken from a total of 15 clinical studies (62,70–83). The symbols indicate the different studies.

not fully known; platelet dysfunction, altered platelet vessel interaction, and the anemia of uremia itself have all been implicated (89).

ADVERSE EFFECTS OF R-HUEPO THERAPY

The major side effects reported so far are listed in Table 2. An increase in blood pressure has been shown to occur in about 20% of r-HuEPO-treated patients (69) and may, in rare cases, be associated with hypertensive encephalopathy and seizures (90). In some patients, thrombosis of the vascular access site and other thrombotic events, together with a need for higher heparin doses to prevent clotting in the extracorporeal circulation, have been reported (57,58). There also were reports of an increase of predialysis serum concentrations of creatinine, urea, and phosphate, and in individual patients, severe hyperkalemia developed (57,58).

Antibody production against the recombinant hormone and resistance to its effect have only been reported for one patient (91).

A hypertensinogenic effect of r-HuEPO treatment has been reported almost exclusively in patients with renal disease and never in patients with anemic status of another etiology. In placebo-controlled trials of r-HuEPO in anemic dialysis patients, 24%–37% of placebo-treated patients as compared to 40%–58% of r-HuEPO-treated patients had to be started on antihypertensives, had to be placed on higher doses of antihypertensive medication, and/or experienced a rise in blood pressure of 10 mmHg or more ("blood pressure responders"), resulting in a net increase of the incidence of a "blood pressure response" due to r-HuEPO of 16%–21% (92,93). No common risk factor has been identified for the development of *hypertension* with r-HuEPO treatment. Whether a rise in hematocrit of more than 1.5% a week (i.e., speed of correction of anemia) results in an increased risk of induction or aggravation of hypertension is controversial (93,94). In the majority of studies, the rise of blood pressure following partial correction of anemia (target hematocrit 30%–35%) by r-HuEPO was accompanied by an inadequate increase in peripheral resistance, while cardiac index fell in blood pressure responders (s.a.) and nonresponders alike (69). The rise in peripheral resistance might be a consequence of three mechanisms. First, higher blood viscosity due to an increase of red cell mass causes a rise of total peripheral resistance. Second, improvement of tissue oxygenation due to higher oxygen transport capacity increases arteriolar vascular tone (95) and thereby vascular resistance. Third, r-HuEPO exerts vasoconstrictor effects either directly on smooth muscle cells or indirectly via a release of vasoactive substances from other cells. At least at target hematocrits below 35%, the role of whole-blood viscosity and/or reduction of hypoxic vasodilatation as the sole explanation for the development of hypertension is controversial. Neff et al. reported a progressive increase in blood pressure, with a stepwise increase of hematocrit from 20% to at least 40% with repetetive blood transfusions in hemodialysis patients. However, Pascual et al. and Williams et al. (96,97) were not able to observe hypertension when the anemia of uremia was corrected to a hematocrit of 30%–35% with blood transfusion (96,97) or anabolic steroids (96). A vasopressor effect of r-HuEPO, which could also be operative at target hematocrits below 35%, had formerly been thought to be unlikely, since erythropoietin receptors had only been shown on erythroid precursor cells. However, endothelial cells have been shown to possess a large number of low-affinity erythropoietin receptors (98), and a vasoconstrictor effect of r-HuEPO, even though with high doses, has been shown in isolated renal resistance vessels of nonuremic rats (99,100). Possible mediators of this vasopressor effect of r-HuEPO could be prostanoids (101,102) and/or endothelin (102–104). In this context, it is of interest that antiplatelet therapy has been reported to reduce the risk of development of hypertension associated with r-HuEPO treatment (105). It must be considered, though, that erythropoietin-treatment-induced hypertension is well established in uremic patients only. This finding suggests that the pressor effect of erythropoietin, if at all present, is a weak one that only can be observed in patients with terminal renal disease, who are especially prone to develop hypertension.

Thrombotic complications of r-HuEPO treatment, such as arteriovenous fistula or synthetic-graft thrombosis or dialyzer clotting, have been noted in the early clinical trials (106,107). Higher blood viscosity, an increase of thrombocyte size (108) or thrombocyte count (107,109)—although within the normal range—and the normalization of the uremic bleeding diathesis (3,110) have been discussed as pathogenetic explanation of these thrombotic complications. However, placebo-controlled studies of r-HuEPO have shown that these complications may be no more frequent in patients receiving r-HuEPO than in other uremic patients not receiving r-HuEPO (92,111–113), with the possible exception of an increase in synthetic-graft thrombosis in r-HuEPO-treated patients (113).

Higher predialysis serum concentrations of *urea, creatinine,* and *phosphate* as well as incidences of *hyperkalemia* have been reported under r-HuEPO treatment (114,115). These effects may be a consequence of reduced dialyzer clearance (up to 10%) due to higher hematocrits (114,115); however, improved appetite resulting in improved nutri-

Table 2. Treatment of anemia in regular hemodialysis patients by human recombinant erythropoietin: side effects

---

Hypertension
Hypertensive encephalopathy with seizures
Shunt thrombosis
Clotting within extracorporeal blood circuit
Increase of thrombocyte count
Increase of serum concentrations of phosphate, urea, creatinine, and potassium

---

tion with r-HuEPO treatment seems to be of greater importance (114,115).

Postinjection "flu-like" symptoms have been reported in a minority of hemodialysis patients treated with intravenous r-HuEPO (116). These symptoms are intermittent and mild and may be improved by slowing the injection rate (117).

THE OPTIMAL TIME TO START R-HUEPO TREATMENT

R-HuEPO treatment is nowadays started when symptomatic anemia develops and/or when hematocrit falls below 30%, which in most patients already occurs in the predialysis phase. Although animal studies have suggested that raising the hematocrit may accelerate progression of renal failure (118), human studies have not demonstrated any deterioration in renal function following partial correction of renal anemia with r-HuEPO (119–123). Hypertension, however, if induced or aggravated, has to be tightly controlled in predialysis patients in order to avoid unwanted progression of renal failure (119).

THE OPTIMAL ROUTE, FREQUENCY, AND DOSE OF
R-HUEPO ADMINISTRATION

In the initial studies, r-HuEPO was always given thrice weekly on the day of dialysis by the *intravenous route*. This route is convenient and comfortable for hemodialysis patients but less acceptable for predialysis patients or for patients on chronic ambulatory peritoneal dialysis. In these patients, thrice-weekly *subcutaneous* r-HuEPO effectively relieves anemia (124,125). The subcutaneous injections cause minimal discomfort, and sc r-HuEPO is usually administered by the patient himself. Even in hemodialysis patients with unproblematic intravenous access, subcutaneous application may be preferred to intravenous application due to a possible dose-saving effect of about 20% at the same target hematocrit (126–129). This economical advantage of the subcutaneous application form is controversial, however; equal dose requirements of intravenous versus subcutaneous r-HuEPO have also been described (130,131). The observed dose-saving effect of subcutaneous as opposed to intravenous application, in spite of a lesser bioavailability in the range of 23%–79%, may be explained by a more protracted resorption and elimination, resulting in a mean residence time of 33 hours as compared to 11 hours after intravenous application (132). Endogenous EPO levels are exceeded even 72 hours after sc r-HuEPO application. The bioavailability of r-HuEPO given intraperitoneally is even lower, with a range of 2.2–12% (129,132). Therefore, this mode of application cannot generally be recommended (133).

Regarding the *frequency of administration* of r-HuEPO, thrice-weekly application seems optimal for intravenous use (16). With the subcutaneous application, thrice-weekly application is the most common frequency used (126–128); however, r-HuEPO may still be effective when given in longer dose intervals but at higher doses, 1 or 2 times a week (123,128,134).

Starting *doses* in the range of 15–40 IU/kg three times a week seem to be sufficient to raise hematocrit. The effect on hematocrit may not become apparent until 2–4 weeks after initiation of therapy, so dose increases should not be considered during this time. To lower the risk of induction or aggravation of hypertension associated with r-HuEPO treatment, high initial doses of r-HuEPO are best avoided; this approach will help avoid both the risk of an increase in blood pressure associated with the rate of hemoglobin rise (s.a.) or the risk due to direct vasopressor actions of the hormone itself, since both effects should be dose dependent. When a target hematocrit of 30%–35% has been reached, r-HuEPO (maintenance) doses can frequently be reduced by 20%–30%.

THE OPTIMAL TARGET HEMATOCRIT WITH
R-HUEPO TREATMENT

A target hematocrit in the range of 30%–35% has presently found widespread acceptance. However, it still remains to be shown whether a further increase of hematocrit to the normal range is beneficial for the patient or whether it exposes him or her more to unwanted side effects of r-HuEPO treatment. Possible benefits are further improvement of physical capacity, increased rehabilitation, improved cardiovascular function, and ultimately improved survival. These possible benefits have to be weighed against the possible negative effects of r-HuEPO treatment, especially the development of severe hypertension, hypertension-associated encephalopathy (with seizures), and thrombotic complications. It must be considered that hematocrit determinations are usually performed before the start of hemodialysis treatment. Thus, a normal predialysis hematocrit, after correction of fluid overload by dialysis, could result in sudden and serious hemoconcentration, predisposing to rheological disturbances and thrombotic complications. Due to the physiological adaptation to anemia in uremia (shift of the oxyhemoglobin curve to the right), it may be unnecessary to bring hemoglobin levels to within the normal range to achieve maximal improvement in symptoms and performance. The results of further studies, some of which are already under way, have to be awaited before final recommendations on the optimal hematocrit level can be given. In this respect, a subgroup of uremic patients, those with polycystic kidney disease (PKD), may be of interest. These patients frequently have normal or near normal hematocrit levels in the presence of uremia. Although various cardiac and cerebral vascular abnormalities that should lead to an increase in cardiovascular and cerebrovascular mortality have been described in these patients, it has long been known that this patient group has the best chance of survival of all groups of uremic patients (135). This improved survival is not related to a better preservation of residudal renal function or a lower blood pressure (136). The chance of 5-year survival for 1459 patients with PKD was 49.2 ± 1.5% whereas for the group with the next best survival, namely, 5675 patients with glomerulonephritis, it was 36.4 ± 0.7%, a highly significant difference ($p < 0.0001$) (137). Reduced left ventricular hypertrophy, which may be associated with better survival rates, was not observed in patients with PKD (136); thus, a reduction in myocardial hypoxia due to the higher hemoglobin concentration could be the reason for the improved survival of patients with PKD.

On the basis of presently available data, target hematocrits of about 30%–35% can be recommended. It is possible that multicenter studies currently in progress will prove that complete normalization of uremic anemia in selected patients (e.g., no hypertension, no synthetic arteriovenous (AV) graft, no previous history of AV-shunt thrombosis) will be of further benefit without untoward side effects (138). The production of r-HuEPO and its clinical use represent a major breakthrough in the management of patients with uremia. The results of the clincial trials support the concept that erthropoietin deficiency is the primary mechanism in the pathogenesis of renal anemia.

Reduction of iatrogenic blood loss and iron supplementation

Of course, the management of anemia in terminal renal failure also includes the prevention and correction of iatrogenic aggravating factors. Excessive loss of blood for laboratory investigations, into the extracorporeal blood circuit, and from punctured access sites should be kept as low as possible. Monitoring of body iron stores by serum ferritin and transferrin saturation once or twice a year is indicated. When erythropoiesis is improving under treatment with human recombinant erythropoietin and iron demands are increasing, iron status should be controlled every 3–4 months.

As indicated above, serum ferritin levels and transferrin saturation are generally applied to monitor iron status. Both parameters, however, have limitations that should be taken into consideration.

Intracellular iron storage involves *ferritin*, a macromolecule with a large capacity for binding iron atoms. Circulating amounts of ferritin are directly correlated with the magnitude of iron stores and can be measured accurately by radioimmunoassay. A serum ferritin below 30µg/L reliably indicates absolute iron deficiency (38). However, several limitations must be appreciated. The threshold for iron deficiency in renal patients may be higher than in normal individuals; a serum ferritin below 80µg/L may already suggest iron deficiency (139). Furthermore, a normal or even high level of serum ferritin does not exclude *functional* iron deficiency (37). Finally, serum ferritin may be raised in inflammatory conditions and liver disease independent of iron stores (140). Levels as high as 1336µg/L have been found in hemodialysis patients with evidence of

depleted marrow iron stores (141). However, from the methods available to assess the adequacy of iron stores, ferritin is the best marker at present because it is easy to determine and because patients with low pretreatment ferritin levels (<100µg/L) will almost certainly require iron supplementation to support the requirements of the marrow during active erythropoiesis (36,37). Iron overload, either by overvigorous iron replacement or more commonly as the result of regular transfusion of red blood cells, is suggested by an elevated serum ferritin level (above 500µg/L).

It has been suggested by previous studies that the iron supply for erythropoiesis will be inadequate once the *transferrin saturation* decreases below 16% (142). However, like ferritin, transferrin saturation is not always an absolutely reliable marker of iron supply. At least in normal subjects, wide day-to-day fluctuations in transferrin saturation (15%–80%) have been shown to occur due to wide fluctuations in plasma iron concentration and unrelated to the assay used (143). Nevertheless, this parameter is widely used and, in combination with ferritin determinations, can be taken as a measure of the availability of iron to the marrow. If serum ferritin is high or normal and transferrin saturation is below 20% (36), functional iron deficiency may be suspected (i.e., iron is not released from its stores rapidly enough to support the demands of the bone marrow).

The amount of iron incorporated into heme in the proliferating erythroblasts cannot be directly measured. Hypochromatosis and microcytosis, however, are well-known markers of iron-deficient red cells. Reduced mean cell volume and mean cell hemoglobin concentration, parameters available with every whole-blood count, imply *advanced* iron deficiency, and an earlier marker is required to detect patients who might respond poorly to r-HuEPO treatment due to reduced iron stores. Modern autoanalyzers allow the measurement of the percentage of *hypochromic red cells* (defined as an individual cell hemoglobin concentration <28g/dL) in the circulation. A proportion of hypochromic red cells greater than 5%–10% appears to be a sensitive and early indicator of absolute or functional iron deficiency (144), allowing the assessment of iron uptake/utilization by the marrow and its incorporation into the proliferating erythroblasts. However, this method requires a modern coulter counter, which may not be available everywhere. Other tests as potential markers of iron insufficiency in hemodialysis patients, such as the red cell ferritin (145), serum transferrin receptor (146), free erythrocyte protoporphyrin levels (147), and red cell zinc protoporphyrin (148), lack widespread validation.

About 55%–66% of patients on r-HuEPO treatment will need iron supplementation at any given time (149,150). Iron supplementation can be given for three reasons: 1) prophylactically, to prevent the iron deficiency that may be expected to occur with r-HuEPO treatment; 2) as a treatment for absolute iron deficiency (ferritin below 100µg/L); and 3) as a treatment for functional iron insufficiency (adequate iron stores but insufficient or delayed liberation of iron from its stores, frequently indicated by a transferrin saturation below 20% or by more than 10% hypochromic red blood cells but normal ferritin (>100µg/L)). Iron supplementation can be performed either orally or intravenously. Regarding the optimal route of administration, there are conflicting data. Intestinal iron absorption is generally considered to be normal in uremic patients (151,152); therefore, oral iron supplementation (with 300–1000 mg of ferrous sulfate/day) is frequently preferred due to its convenience, rare serious side effects, and low cost. Only poor patient compliance, a slower correction of iron deficit compared to intravenous correction, and the possibility that phosphate binders and food interfere with the intestinal absorption of iron are thought to be disadvantages of this form of application. These disadvantages may explain an improved hemoglobin response in those hemodialysis patients receiving intravenous iron versus those receiving oral iron, leading to lower r-HuEPO dosage requirements (36,153). In certain constellations, intravenous iron supplementation should be preferred over oral supplementation: 1) if oral iron therapy fails to replete body iron stores (either due to a lack of compliance or due to interference of phosphate binders or food with intestinal absorption), 2) in the case of functional iron deficiency

(153,154), and 3) if the predicted iron deficit in a patient exceeds 200 mg. A nomogram has been devised by Van Wyck et al. (Figure 4) to estimate intravenous iron demand based on the initial hemoglobin and serum ferritin concentration (37).

A single dose of intravenous iron should not exceed 100 mg (155) and may be given I.V. over 2 minutes at the end of dialysis treatment (156).

Iron dextran is most widely used for parenteral iron supplementation in the United States, and most experience has been accumulated for this preparation. Anaphylactic shock may occur in 0.1%–1% of patients receiving parenteral iron (156–158); even death from anaphylaxia has been reported (159). These outcomes have led to the development of different preparations for parenteral iron supplementation in the hope of a reduced frequency of this serious side effect. Ferrous gluconate is frequently used in Germany; however, large-scale studies to evaluate whether there is a reduced frequency of anaphylactic reactions with this preparation have presently not been performed. To reduce the incidence of this dangerous complication, the patient should be tested with a small dose of I.V. iron (25 mg) and closely observed for 1 hour afterwards before the total dose is given. This test should be performed each time a new cycle of I.V. iron therapy is initiated (155).

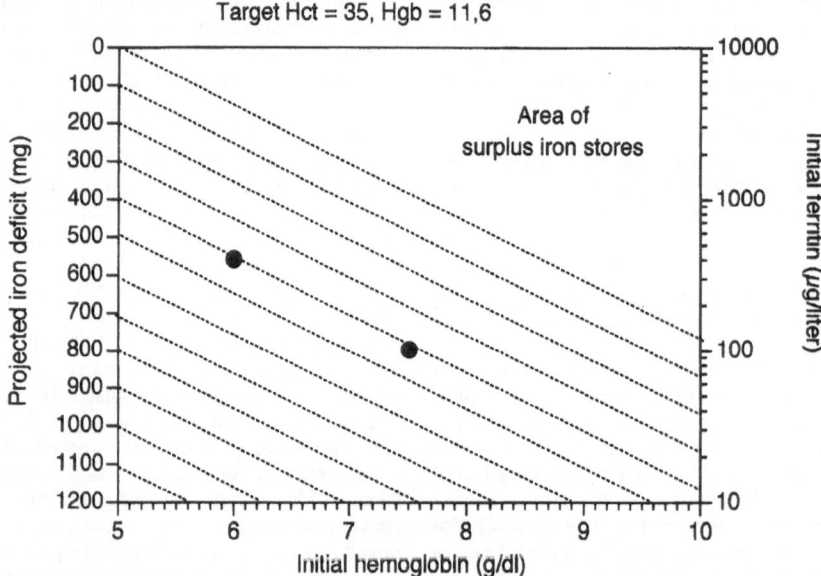

Figure 4. Nomogram for predicting net iron deficiency in anemic dialysis patients starting r-HuEPO treatment. A target hematocrit of 35% is assumed (hemoglobin approximately around 11.6g/dL) (taken from 37)).

To determine the projected iron deficiency, initial hemoglobin is plotted against initial ferritin concentration. The nearest isobar is located and followed to the left to find the corresponding deficit. For example, two patients, one with an initial hemoglobin of 7.5g/dL and a ferritin of 100mg/L and another with corresponding values for hemoglobin and ferritin of 6.0 and 300, respectively, will both be predicted to need 400mg more iron than available in their stores.

Some authors even advocate empirical substitution of 10 mg of iron intravenously with each dialysis session as maintenance therapy in order to prevent the development of iron deficiency under r-HuEPO treatment (160). This treatment will help to diminish dose-related anapylactoid reactions and exclude poor patient compliance with oral iron substitution. This form of iron supplementation would lead to a yearly dose of 1500 mg, whereas iron loss has been estimated to be around 2000 mg/year in hemodialysis patients in older studies (35) and 700–1100 mg in newer studies (34). Thus, in this form of iron substitution treatment as well, the adequacy of available iron has to be tested on a regular basis, in order to exclude both the development of iron deficiency and the development of iron overload.

Removal of inhibitors and toxins

All extracorporeal renal replacement therapies and peritoneal dialysis, in principle, could also interfere with the pathogenesis of anemia of renal failure, since they may remove toxins responsible for hemolysis and inhibition of erythropoiesis. Indeed, the clincial experience with all treatment modalities shows that a partial correction of the anemia is achieved. The improvement, however, falls significantly behind the results obtained with r-HuEPO treatment. This finding also applies to the speed of improvement, which is much faster with r-HuEPO therapy. The relative ineffectiveness of renal replacement therapies may be a consequence of our limited knowledge of the toxins involved and of the best way to remove them. The simple approach to improve detoxification therapy of uremia by raising the upper limit of the molecular size removed by diffusive and/or convective transport did not produce unequivocal results. For instance, no data exist to prove that hemofiltration or hemodiafiltration, which cover a larger molecular range of removal than hemodialysis with tight cellulosic membranes, are superior in correcting the anemia of renal failure. On the other hand, patients on continuous ambulatory peritoneal dialysis (CAPD), also a treatment with a larger molecular range of removal, display a faster rise in hematocrit and better absolute hematocrit levels than patients on standard hemodialysis with tight cellulosic membranes. This result could possibly be due to a better maintenance of residual kidney function in these patients. Furthermore, no blood loss due to venopuncture or into the dialyzer occurs in peritoneal dialysis patients. After 3–5 years on renal replacement therapy, however, there is no longer a significant difference between hemodialysis and peritoneal dialysis patients (161). When comparing hemoglobin levels between hemodialysis patients and patients on peritoneal dialysis, one has to take into account that, in hemodialysis samples for hemoglobin, measurements are usually taken immediately before dialysis when the patients are relatively hemodiluted, whereas no such difference exists in peritoneal dialysis patients. Comparison of red cell mass in hemodialysis and CAPD

patients suggests that there is little difference between the two modalities of treatment (162).

Removal of excess aluminium

When the inhibitor of erythropoiesis is known, as in the case of aluminum intoxication, treatment can be selective and effective. An aggravating effect of aluminum on the anemia of renal failure should always be suspected when, in regular hemodialysis, patient microcytotic anemia coincides with normal or elevated serum ferritin levels. The suspicion will be substantiated by a history of aluminum exposure orally or via dialysate and by further manifestations of aluminum intoxication, such as aluminum bone disease and encephalopathy, the latter being very rare since nephrologists became aware of the risks of aluminium intoxication in hemodialysis patients. The diagnosis of aluminium intoxication can be made by a bone biopsy (163) or by measuring elevated basal serum aluminum levels (>100 µg/L). However, the desferrioxamine (DFO) infusion test (10–20 mg/kg of DFO infused over 1 hour at the end of dialysis) may give more precise information on the aluminium load of a patient; aluminium intoxication may be assumed, if aluminium levels rise threefold above basal values or if the absolute increment is more than 200 µg/L (164). A successful therapeutic trial will retrospectively confirm the diagnosis of aluminium intoxication. The treatment of choice is the use of the chelator desferrioxamine (DFO) intravenously during the last 1–2 hours of hemodialysis or hemofiltration, or intraperitoneally overnight in CAPD patients. To limit the frequency of side effects, the dose should be limited to 1 g/week (10–20 mg/kg/week). DFO mobilizes aluminum as a soluble complex, which then is removed by the therapeutic dialytic or filtration procedure. The major side effects are hypotension, ocular toxicity and ototoxicity, and neurologic complications such as seizures (164). Very rarely, this treatment is associated with an increased susceptibility to yersiniosis and fungal infections such as mucormycosis. These side effects respond to temporary interruption of therapy, reduction of dose, or termination of therapy.

Correction of hyperparathyroidism

Despite a potential role for secondary hyperparathyroidism in the pathogenesis of the anemia of renal failure, parathyroidectomy is not indicated for the sole purpose of treating severe renal anemia. When other complications, however, necessitate subtotal removal of the parathyroids, an improvement of anemia may be a welcome side effect.

Androgen therapy

From the early 1970s until recently, a variety of androgens have been used in the treatment of the anemia of renal failure (165). Their positive effect is assumed to be mediated via increased erythropoietin production and increased proliferation of erythropoietin-sensitive stem cell populations (35). Not all patients, however, respond, and androgens have a high incidence of side effects such as virilization, prostatism, psychic disturbances, muscle and liver damage, and cholestasis in up to 25% of patients. The findings of Hendler et al. (166) suggest that the positive effect of androgens on erythropoiesis and red cell mass may not necessarily be associated with improved peripheral oxygenation, due to simultaneous effects on red cell metabolism. For these reasons, androgens are now rarely used in the treatment of uremic anemia.

Folate supplementation and other measures

Folate is lost into the dialysate from the blood. Therefore, folate deficiency and macrocytotic anemia may develop in patients with a low protein intake. Since the diet of regular dialysis patients is liberal and usually contains sufficient amounts of folate, folate deficiency and the need for oral folic acid supplementation are not common (41). Finally, the nephrologist should be aware that extracorporeal blood treatment carries many potential risks, predominantly in the form of contaminants of the blood and dialysate compartment, such as metals and chemicals that could cause red cell damage and hemolysis (s.a.).

Transplantation

The anemia of end-stage renal disease is usually reversed within 3 months of renal transplantation, provided that graft function is satisfactory. An increase in erythropoietin production is thought to play the major role in this correction (167). Serum erythropoietin levels rise within 3–4 days after transplantation, provided that graft function is satisfactory (168), and remain elevated until the anemia is corrected. Red cell aplasia has been reported with azathioprine use (169). This side effect is observed less frequently now because fewer patients are on azathioprine treatment and because, if azathioprine is given, it is usually given in in combination with cyclosporine in a reduced dose. However, severe anemia has been described with concomitant use of azathioprine and ACE inhibitors (170), probably due to a combination of the effect of azathioprine and reduced erythropoietin production with ACE inhibitors (s.a.). Persistent anemia is usually a consequence of insufficient graft function and may be treated with r-HuEPO. Hemolytic-uremic syndrome associated with cyclosporine use and autoimmune hemolysis caused by autoantibodies to ABO blood antigens are less frequent causes of anemia in renal transplantation.

POLYCYTHEMIA IN RENAL DISEASE

Secondary polycythemia can be due to renal disease. Lesions that can cause this include hypernephroma, obstruc-

tive uropathy, renal artery stenosis, Bartter's syndrome, and renal cystic disease. Polycythemia also occurs in 5%–10% of renal transplant patients. It is frequently due to overstimulation of the erythroid bone marrow by erythropoietin produced by the native kidneys (171), but occasionally transplanted kidney with renal artery stenosis may be the source of increased erythropoietin production. ACE inhibitors (50,172) and theophylline have been used to treat this special form of polycythemia. In a study (61) lasting 8 weeks, theophylline treatment reduced hematocrit in erythrocytotic renal transplant recipients from 58% to 46% in parallel with a decrease of serum erythropoietin concentration from 60 to 9 U/L. Sometimes even patients with end-stage renal disease will have normal hemoglobin concentration, spontaneous reversal of anemia, or even polycythemia. This situation is not unusual in dialysis patients with autosomal-dominant polycystic kidney disease, but it has also (though less frequently) been described in other dialysis patients with secondary cyst formation (*acquired* cystic disease) of the kidneys (173). In polycythemic patients of both groups, the presence of cysts often is associated with higher serum erythropoietin concentrations, and the cyst fluid of these patients has been found to contain high amounts of bioactive erythropoietin (173,174).

Renal artery stenosis reduces both renal oxgen supply and oxygen demand via reduction of renal blood flow. Both unchanged and increased erythropoietin and erythrocyte production have been observed (175).

WHITE BLOOD CELLS AND THROMBOCYTES IN RENAL FAILURE

Leukocyte function

Bacterial infection is one of the major causes of morbidity and mortality in patients with end-stage renal failure, amounting to about 20% (2). Infection is partly due to facilitated access of bacteria to tissues, either due to frequent puncture of the vascular access site in hemodialysis or due to bacterial peritonitis in chronic ambulatory peritoneal dialysis. Granulocyte and monocyte dysfunction in uremia (1,2)—especially in iron-overloaded patients—aggravates this problem. Reducing iron load with r-HuEPO treatment can partially reverse this defect in polymorphonuclear function (176). Granulocyte function, especially phagocytosis, adhesion, and the release of reactive oxygen species, may also be adversely affected by the use of bioincompatible dialysis membranes (2). This possibility has been suggested by studies comparing granulocyte function in patients on dialysis to uremic patients not on dialysis treatment (177) and by studies in which intradialytic changes in granulocyte function were tested with different dialysis membranes (2). It has also been shown that chronic hemodialysis with cellulosic membranes, as compared to other more biocompatible—mainly synthetic—membranes, may negatively affect monocyte macrophage and lymphocyte function (2). These advantages of more biocompatible membranes may be of clinical relevance, since a reduced mortality risk in chronic hemodialysis patients (178) and improved survival and faster recovery of renal function in acute renal failure (179) were reported to be associated with the use of biocompatible membranes.

Leukopenia not only may be a consequence of uremia itself but also may be caused by the use of cytotoxic drugs in the treatment of renal disease or after tranplantation; the disorder may also be due to viral infection. Short-term induction of leukopenia is regularly observed during dialysis with cellulosic dialysis membranes.

Thrombocyte function and hemostasis

Uremic patients suffer from a bleeding diathesis that is aggravated by the need for intermittent anticoagulation during dialysis treatment. The only defined defects to be found in the coagulation system are disturbances of platelet function, manifesting as prolonged bleeding time. The mechanism has not been explained; however, diminished platelet spreading, due to an inhibition of interaction between plasma von Willebrand factor and platelet glycoprotein IIb–IIIa, seems to be involved (180). The bleeding diathesis is improved by dialysis and by raising the hematocrit to more than 30%, either by transfusion or by r-HuEPO treatment (3). Infusion of conjugated estrogens at a dose of 0.6 mg/kg/day for 5 days has also been shown to have a beneficial effect on the bleeding diathesis of uremia, lasting for 3–14 days (181).

Not infrequently, nephrologists are faced with the problem of having to dialyze a bleeding patient. The simplest strategy in this case is to perform the dialysis without heparin at all. Before the start of dialysis, however, the dialyzer and the blood lines should be flushed with heparinized saline. Blood flow should be kept as high and dialysis time as short as possible. In the majority of cases, the dialysis can be completed without clotting of the extracorporeal circuit (182).

Thrombotic complications of renal disease

In patients with the nephrotic syndrome, thrombosis is an important clinical problem (see Chapter 31) and is caused by a combination of diminished plasma volume, physical inactivity, and hypercoagulopathy, resulting from increased concentrations of fibrinogen, Factors V and VIII, a deficiency of antithrombin III, and thrombocytosis. Clinical manifestations include renal vein thrombosis, deep venous thrombosis of limbs, pulmonary emboli, and arterial thromboses. As a general rule, nephrotic patients with thrombosis should receive anticoagulation (usually with warfarin) as long as they are nephrotic. Prophylactic anticoagulation in severly nephrotic patients with serum albumin less than 20 g/L is advised, as long as there are no contraindications.

REFERENCES

1. Lewis SL, Van Eps LWS: Neutrophil and monocyte alterations in chronic dialysis patients. *Am J Kidney Dis* 9:381–395, 1987.
2. Himmelfarb J, Hakim RM: Biocompatibility and risk of infection in haemodialysis patients. *Nephrol Dial Transplant* 9 (Suppl 2):138–144, 1994.
3. Vigano G, Benigni A, Mendogni D, Mingardi G, Mecca G, Remuzzi G: Recombinant human erythropoietin to correct uremic bleeding. *Am J Kidney Diseases* 18(1):44–49, 1991.
4. Neff MS, Kim KE, Persoff M: Hemodynamics of uremic anemia. *Circulation* 43:876–883, 1971.
5. Varat MA, Adolph RJ, Fowler NO: Cardiovascular effects of anemia. *Am Heart J* 83:415–426, 1972.
6. Silberberg JS, Rahal DP, Patton DR, Sniderman AD: Role of anemia in the pathogenesis of left ventricular hypertrophy in end-stage renal disease. *Am J Cardiol* 64(3):222–4, 1989.
7. Braunwald E: Pathophysiology of heart failure. In: E Braunwald, ed, *Heart Disease: A Textbook of Cardiovascular Medicine.* W.B. Saunders, Philadelphia, pp 393–403, 1992.
8. Eschbach J, Adamson J: Anemia of end-stage renal disease. *Kidney Int* 28:1–5, 1985.
9. Cambi V, David S: The hematopoietic system in renal failure. *Contrib Nephrol* 106:43–52, 1994.
10. Bogin E, Massry S, Levi J, Mdaldeti M, Bristol G, Smith J: Effect of parathyroid hormone on osmotic fragility of human erythrocytes. *J Clin Invest* 69:1017–1025, 1982.
11. Akmal M, Telfer N, Ansari A, Massry S: Red blood cell survival in chronic renal failure: role of secondary hyperparathyroidism. *J Clin Invest* 76:1695–1698, 1985.
12. Barbour GL: Effect of parathyroidectomy on anemia in chronic renal failure. *Arch Intern Med* 139:889–891, 1979.
13. Rao DS, Shih M-S, Mohini R: Effect of serum parathyroid hormone and bone marrow fibrosis on the response to erythropoietin in uremia. *N Engl J Med* 328:171–175, 1993.
14. Jacob H, Amsden T: Acute hemolytic anemia with rigid red cells in hypophosphatemia. *N Engl J Med* 285:1146–1150, 1971.
15. Eschbach JW: Erythropoietin: the promise and the facts. *Kidney Int* 45 (Suppl 44):S70–S76, 1994.
16. Cotes PM, Pippard MJ, Reid CD, Winearls CG, Oliver DO, Royston JP: Characterization of the anaemia of chronic renal failure and the mode of its correction by a preparation of human erythropoietin (r-HuEPO). An investigation of the pharmacokinetics of intravenous erythropoietin and its effects on erythrokinetics. *Q J Med* 70(262):113–37, 1989.
17. Garcia J, Ebbe S, Hollander L, Cutting H, Miller M, Cronkite E: Radioimmunoassay of erythropoietin: circulating levels in normal and polycythemic human beings. *J Lab Clin Med* 99:624–635, 1982.
18. McGonigle RJS, Wallin JD, Shadduck RK, Fisher JW: Erythropoietin deficiency and inhibition of erythropoiesis in renal insufficiency. *Kidney Int* 25:437–444, 1984.
19. Eckardt K-U, Tan CC, Ratcliffe PJ, Kurtz A: Accumulation of Erythropoietin mRNA in rat liver and kidneys. In: Bauer C, Koch KM, Scigalla P, Wieczorek L, eds, *Erythropoietin—Molecular Physiology and Clinical Applications.* Marcel Dekker, New York, pp 67–76, 1993.
20. Naets JP, Garcia JF, Tousaaint C, Buset M, Waks D: Radioimmunoassay of erythropoietin in chronic uraemia or anephric patients. *Scand J Haematol* 37:390–394, 1986.
21. Bachmann S, Le HM, Eckardt KU: Co-localization of eryth-

ropoietin mRNA and ecto-5'-nucleotidase immunoreactivity in peritubular cells of rat renal cortex indicates that fibroblasts produce erythropoietin. *J Histochem Cytochem* 41(3):335–341, 1993.

22. Eckardt KU, Kurtz A: The biological role, site, and regulation of erythropoietin production. *Adv Nephrol Necker Hosp* 21(203):203–233, 1992.

23. Eckardt K-U, Kurtz A, Bauer C: Regulation of erythropoietin formation is related to proximal tubular function. *Am J Physiol* 256:942–947, 1989.

24. Pagel H, Jelkmann W, Weiss C: A comparison of the effects of renal artery constriction and anemia on the production of erythropoietin. *Pflugers Arch* 413:62–66, 1988.

25. Caro J, Brown S, Miller O, Murray T, Erslev AJ: Erythropoietin levels in uremic nephric and anephric patients. *J Lab Clin Med* 93:449–458, 1979.

26. Radtke HW, Claussner A, Erbes PM, Scheuermann EH, Schoeppe W, Koch KM: Serum erythropoietin concentration in chronic renal failure: relationship to degree of anemia and excretory renal function. *Blood* 54:877–884, 1979.

27. Corazza F, Bergmann P, Dratawa M, Guns M, Fondu P: Responsiveness to recombinant erythropoietin therapy in end-stage renal disease—an analysis of the predictive value of several biological measurements, including circulating erythroid progenitors. *Nephrol Dial Transplant* 7:311–317, 1992.

28. Eschbach JW, Adamson JW, Cook JD: Disorders of red blood cell production in uremia. *Arch Intern Med* 126:812–815, 1970.

29. Radtke HW, Frei U, Erbes PM, Schoeppe W, Koch KM: Improving anemia by hemodialysis: effect on serum erythropoietin. *Kidney Int* 17:382–387, 1980.

30. Eschbach JW, Adamson JW: Hematologic consequences of renal failure. In: Brenner B, Rector FC, eds, *The Kidney*. WB Saunders, Philadelphia, pp 2019–2035, 1991.

31. Aoki I, Nishijima K, Homori M, Nakahara K, Higashi K, Ishikawa K: Responsiveness of bone marrow erythroid progenitors (CFU-E and BFU-E) to recombinant human erythropoietin (rh-Ep) in vitro in multiple myeloma. *Br J Haematol* 81:463–469, 1992.

32. Blumberg A: Pathogenese der renalen Anämie. *Nephron* 51 (Suppl 1):15–19, 1989.

33. Eschbach JW, Haley NR, Egrie JC, Adamson JW: A comparison of the responses to recombinant human erythropoietin in normal and uremic subjects. *Kidney Int* 43:407–416, 1992.

34. Frei U, Wilks MF, Boehmer S, Crisp LN, Schwarzrock R, Stiekema JC, Koch KM: Gastrointestinal blood loss in haemodialysis patients during use of a low-molecular-weight heparinoid anticoagulant. *Nephrol Dial Transplant* 3(4):435–439, 1988.

35. Koch KM, Pastyna WD, Shaldon S, Werner E: Anemia of the regular hemodialysis patient and its treatment. *Nephron* 14:405–419, 1974.

36. MacDougall IC: Monitoring of iron status and iron supplementation in patients treated with erythropoietin. *Curr Opin Nephrol Hypertens* 3(6):620–625, 1994.

37. Van Wyck DB, Stivelman JC, Ruiz J, Kirlin LF, Katz MA, Ogden DA: Iron status in patients receiving erythropoietin for dialysis associated anemia. *Kidney Int* 35:712–716, 1989.

38. Worwood M: Serum ferritin. *Clin Sci* 70:215–220, 1986.

39. Rosenberg ME: Role of transferrin measurement in monitoring iron status during recombinant human erythropoietin therapy. *Dial Transplant* 21:81–90, 1992.

40. Hampers CL, Streiff R, Nathan DG, Snyder D, Merrill JP: Megaloblastic hematopoiesis in uremia and in patients on long-term hemodialysis. *N Engl J Med* 276:551–554, 1967.

41. Ono K, Hisasue Y: Is folate supplementation necessary in hemodialysis patients on erythropoietin therapy. *Clin Nephrol* 38(5):290–292, 1992.

42. Kaiser L, Schwartz KA: Aluminium induced anemia. *Am J Kidney Dis* 6:348–352, 1985.

43. Swartz R, Dombrouski J, Burnatowska J, Hledin M, Mayor G: Microcytic anemia in dialysis patients: reversible marker of aluminium toxicity. *Am J Kidney Dis* 9:217–223, 1987.

44. Mladenovic J: Aluminium inhibits erythropoiesis in vitro. *J Clin Invest* 81:1661–1665, 1988.

45. Miller ME, Rort M, Parving HH, Howard D, Reddingt I, Valeri CR, Stohlman F: pH effect on erythropoietin response to hypoxia. *N Engl J Med* 288:706–710, 1973.

46. Onoyama K, Motomura K, Makita H, Kiyama S, Takata Y, Urabe A: Effects of long-term captopril on angiotensin II and erythropoietin levels and recovery from hemorrhagic anemia in rats. *Curr Ther Res* 41:472–477, 1987.

47. Pratt MC, Lewis BN, Walker RJ, Bailey RR, Shand BI, Livesey J: Effect of angiotensin converting enzyme inhibitors on erythropoietin concentrations in healthy volunteers. *Br J Clin Pharmacol* 34(4):363–365, 1992.

48. Kamper A-L, Nielsen OJ: Effect of enalapril on haemoglobin and serum erythropoietin in patients with chronic nephropathy. *Scand J Clin Lab Invest* 50:611–618, 1990.

49. Hirakata H, Onoyama K, Iseki K, Kumagai H, Fujimi S, Omae T: Worsening of anemia induced by long term use of captopril in hemodialysis patients. Am J Nephrol 4:355–360, 1984.

50. Graafland AD, Doorenbos CJ, Van Saase SJ: Enalapril-induced anemia in two kidney transplant recipients. *Transplant Int* 5(1):51–3, 1992.

51. Jelkmann W: Erythropoietin: structure, control of production, and function. *Physiol Rev* 72(2):449–89, 1992.

52. Taniguchi S, Shibuya T, Harada M, Niho Y: Prostaglandin-mediated suppression of in vitro growth of erythroid progenitor cells. *Kidney Int* 36(4):712–718, 1989.

53. Krantz SB: Pathogenesis and treatment of the anemia of chronic disease. *Am J Med Sci* 307(5):353–359, 1994.

54. Adamson JW, Eschbach JW: Management of the anaemia of chronic renal failure with recombinant human erythropoietin. *Q J Med* 73:1093–1101, 1989.

55. Powe NR, Griffiths RI, Greer JW, Watson AJ, Anderson GF, de LG, Herbert RJ, Eggers PW, Milam RA, Whelton PK: Early dosing practices and effectiveness of recombinant human erythropoietin. *Kidney Int* 43(5):1125–1133, 1993.

56. Goodnough LT, Strasburg D, Riddell J, Verbrugge D, Wish J: Has recombinant human erythropoietin therapy minimized red-cell transfusions in hemodialysis patients? *Clin Nephrol* 41(5):303–307, 1994.

57. Eschbach JW, Egrie JC, Downing MR, Browne JK, Adamson JW: Correction of the anemia of end stage renal disease with recombinant human erythropoietin. *N Engl J Med* 316:73–78, 1987.

58. Winearls CG, Oliver DO, Pippard MJ, Reid C, Downing MR, Cotes PM: Effect of human erythropoietin derived from recombinant DNA on the anaemia of patients maintained by chronic haemodialysis. *Lancet* 2:1175–1178, 1986.

59. Grimm PC, Sinai-Triemann L, Sekiya NM, Robertson LS,

Robinson BJ, Fine RN, Ettenger RB: Effects of recombinant human erythropoietin on HLA sensitization and cell mediated immunity. *Kidney Int* 38:12–18, 1990.

60. Ettenger RB, Marik J, Grimm P: The impact of recombinant human erythropoietin therapy on renal transplantation. *Am J Kidney Dis* 18 (4) (Suppl 1):57–61, 1991.

61. Frei U, Nonnast-Daniel B, Koch KM: Erythropoietin und Hypertonie. *Klin Wochenschr* 66(18):914–919, 1988.

62. MacDougall IC, Lewis NP, Saunders MJ, Cochlin DL, Davies ME, Hutton RD, Fox KAA, Coles GA, Williams JD: Long term cardiorespiratory effects of amelioration of renal anemia by erythropoietin. *Lancet* 335(8688):489–493, 1990.

63. Mayer G, Thum J, Cada EM, Stummvoll HK, Graf H: Working capacity is increased following recombinant human erythropoietin treatment. *Kidney Int* 34:525–528, 1988.

64. Barany P, Freyschuss U, Pettersson E, Bergstrom J: Treatment of anemia in haemodialysis patients with erythropoietin: long term effects on exercise capacity. *Clin Sci* 84:441–447, 1993.

65. Barany P, Pettersson E, Ahlberg M, Hultmann E, Bergstrom J: Nutritional assessment in anemic hemodialysis patients treated with recombinant human erythropoietin. *Clin Nephrol* 35:270–279, 1991.

66. Bommer J, Alexiou C, Müller-Bühl U, Eifert J, Ritz E: Recombinant human erythropoietin therapy in hemodialysis patients—dose determination and clinical experience. *Nephrol Dial Transplant* 2:238–242, 1987.

67. Bommer J, Kugel M, Schwbel B, Ritz E, Barth HP, Seelig R: Improved sexual function during recombinant human erythropoietin therapy. *Nephrol Dial Transplant* 5:204–207, 1990.

68. Marsh JT, Brown WS, Wolcott D, Carr CR, Harper R, Schweitzer SV, Nissenson AR: R-HuEPO treatment improves brain and cognitive function of anemic dialysis patients. *Kidney Int* 39:155–163, 1991.

69. Radermacher J, Koch KM: Erythropoietin and hypertension. In: Bauer C, Koch KM, Scigalla P, Wieczorek L, eds, *Erythropoietin—Molecular Physiology and Clinical Applications*. Marcel Dekker, New York, pp 129–152, 1993.

70. London GM, Zins B, Pannier B, Naret C, Berthelot J-M, Jacquot C, Safar M, Drueke T: Vascular changes in hemodialysis patients in response to recombinant human erythropoietin. *Kidney Int* 36:878–892, 1989.

71. Zehnder C, Zuber M, Sulzer M, Meyer B, Straumann E, Jenzer H-R, Blumberg A: Influence of long-term amelioration of anemia and blood pressure control on left ventricular hypertrophy in hemodialyzed patients. *Nephron* 61:21–25, 1992.

72. Pascual J, Teruel JL, Moya JL, Liano F, Jimenez MM, Ortuno J: Regression of left ventricular hypertrophy after partial correction of anemia with erythropoietin in patients on hemodialysis: a prospective study. *Clin Nephrol* 35(6):280–287, 1991.

73. Löw-Friedrich I, Grutzmacher P, Marz W, Bergmann M, Schoeppe W: Therapy with recombinant human erythropoietin reduces cardiac size and improves heart function in chronic hemodialysis patients. *Am J Nephrol* 11(1):54–60, 1991.

74. Satoh K, Masuda T, Ikeda Y, Kurokawa S, Kamata K, Kikawada R, Takamoto T, Marumo F: Hemodynamic changes by recombinant erythropoietin therapy in hemodialyzed patients. *Hypertension* 15(3):262–266, 1990.

75. McGregor E, McClaughlin K, Lowe GDO, Rodger RSC, Junor BJR, Briggs JD: abstract-Changes in blood viscosity,

and left ventricular mass with correction of anemia by renal transplantation and erythropoietin. *J Am Soc Nephrol* 2(3):382, 1991.

76. Klaus D, Schwarze D, Lederle RM, Saul F: Influence of erythropoietin in hemodynamics, left ventricular performance and neurohumoral factors in end-stage renal failure with left ventricular hypertrophy. *Nieren Hochdruckkr* 20(1):28–35, 1991.

77. Martinez VA, Bardaji A, Garcia C, Ridao C, Richart C, Oliver JA: Long-term myocardial effects of correction of anemia with recombinant human erythropoietin in aged patients on hemodialysis. *Am J Kidney Dis* 19(4):353–357, 1992.

78. Tagawa H, Nagano M, Saito H, Umezu M, Yamakado M: Echocardiographic findings in hemodialysis patients treated with recombinant human erythropoietin: proposal for a hematocrit most beneficial to hemodynamics. *Clin Nephrol* 35(1):35–38, 1991.

79. Silverberg JS, Racine N, Barre P, Sniderman AD: Regression of left ventricular hypertrophy in dialysis patients following correction of anemia with recombinant human erythropoietin. *Can J Cardiol* 6(1):S1–S4, 1989.

80. Löw I, Grutzmacher P, Bergmann M, Schoeppe W: Echocardiographic findings in patients on maintenance hemodialysis substituted with recombinant human erythropoietin. *Clin Nephrol* 31:26–30, 1989.

81. Canella G, LaCanna G, Sandrini M, Gaggiotti M, Nordio G, Movilli E, Mombelloni S, Visioli O, Maiorca R: Reversal of left ventricular hypertrophy following recombinant human erythropoietin treatment of anaemic dialysed uraemic patients. *Nephrol Dial Transplant* 6(1):31–37, 1991.

82. Schütterle G, Kramer W, Schfer R, Kaufmann J, Wizemann V: Cardiological findings in patients with end-stage renal failure under treatment with erythropoietin. In: Pagel H, Weiss C, Jelkmann W, eds, *Pathophysiology and Pharmacology of Erythropoietin*. Springer-Verlag, Berlin, Heidelberg, pp 177–180, 1992.

83. Wizemann V, Schäfer R, Kramer W: Follow-up of cardiac changes induced by anemia compensation in normotensive hemodialysis patients with left ventricular hypertrophy. *Nephron* 64:202–206, 1993.

84. Silberberg JS, Barre PE, Prichard SS, Sniderman AD: Impact of left ventricular hypertrophy on survival in end-stage renal disease. *Kidney Int* 36(2):286–290, 1989.

85. Sniderman AD, Silberberg J, Prichard S, Barré PE: Anemia and left ventricular function in end-stage renal disease. In: Parfrey PS, Harnett JD, eds, *Cardiac Dysfunction in Chronic Uremia*. Kluwer Academic Publishers, Boston, pp 161–170, 1992.

86. Wizemann V, Kaufmann J, Kramer W: Effect of erythropoietin on ischemia tolerance in anemic hemodialysis patients with confirmed coronary artery disease. *Nephron* 62:161–165, 1992.

87. Eschbach JW, Aquiling T, Haley NR, Fan MH, Blagg CR: The long-term effects of recombinant human erythropoietin on the cardiovascular system. *Clin Nephrol* 38 (Suppl 1):S98–S103, 1992.

88. El Shahawy M, Francis R, Akmal M, Massry SG: Recombinant human erythropoietin shortens the bleeding time and corrects the abnormal platelet aggregation in hemodialysis patients. *Clin Nephrol* 41(5):308–313, 1994.

89. Livio M, Boonigni A, Remuzzi G: Coagulation abnormalities in uremia. *Semin Nephrol* 5:82–90, 1985.

90. Edmunds ME, Walls J, Tucker B, Baker LR, Tomson CR, Ward M, Cunningham J, Moore R, Winearls CG: Seizures in haemodialysis patients treated with recombinant human erythropoietin. *Nephrol Dial Transplant* 4:1065–1069, 1989.

91. Bergrem H, Danielson BG, Eckardt K-U, Kutrtz A, Stridsberg M: A case of antierythropoietin antibodies following recombinant human erythropoietin treatment. In: Bauer C, Koch KM, Scigalla P, Wieczorek L, eds, *Erythropoietin—Molecular Physiology and Clinical Applications.* Marcel Dekker, New York, pp 265–273, 1993.

92. Bahlmann J, Schoter KH, Scigalla P, Gurland HJ, Hilfenhaus M, Koch KM, Muthny FA, Neumayer HH, Pommer W, Quelhorst E, Sieberth HG, Weber U: Morbidity and mortality in hemodialysis patients with and without erythropoietin treatment: a controlled study. *Contrib Nephrol* 88(90):90–106, 1991.

93. Abraham PA, Macres MG: Blood pressure in hemodialysis patients during amelioration of anemia with erythropoietin. *J Am Soc Nephrol* 2(4):927–936, 1991.

94. Canadian-Erythropoietin-Study-Group: Association between recombinant human erythropoietin and quality of life and exercise capacity of patients receiving haemodialysis. *Br Med J* 300(6724):573–578, 1990.

95. Duling BR, Pitman RN: Oxygen tension: dependent or independent variables in local control of blood flow? *Fed Proc* 34(11):2012–2019, 1975.

96. Pascual J, Teruel JL, Marcen R, Gamez C, Liano F, Ortuno J: Blood pressure after three different forms of correction of anemia in hemodialysis. *Int J Artif Organs* 15(7):393–396, 1992.

97. Williams B, Edmunds ME, Thompson JP, Burton PR, Feehally J, Walls J: Does increasing haemoglobin concentration and haematocrit have a pressor effect in dialysis patients. *Nephrol Dial Transplant* 4:878–891, 1989.

98. Anagnostou A, Lee ES, Kessimian N, Levinson R, Steiner M: Erythropoietin has a mitogenic and positive chemotactic effect on endothelial cells. *Proc Natl Acad Sci USA* 87:5978–5982, 1990.

99. Heidenreich S, Rahn KH, Zidek W: Direct vasopressor effect of recombinant human erythropoetin on renal vascular resistance. *Kidney Int* 39(2):259–265, 1991.

100. Tsukada H, Ishimitsu T, Ogawa Y, Sugimoto T, Yagi S: Direct vasopressor effects of erythropoietin in genetically hypertensive rats. *Life Sci* 52(17):1425–1434, 1993.

101. Radermacher J, Bode-Böger SM, Böger R, Frölich JC, Koch K-M: Erythropoietin enhances norepinephrine induced contractions via modulation in prostaglandin balance in rabbit and human arteries. *Blood Purif* 10(2):79–80, 1992.

102. Takayama K: Changes in endothelial vasoactive substances and blood coagulation and fibrinolysis functions under recombinant human erythropoietin therapy in hemodialysis patients. *Nippon Jinzo Gakkai Shi* 35(2):179–188, 1993.

103. Carlini R, Obialo CI, Rothstein M: Intravenous erythropoietin (rHuEPO) administration increases plasma endothelin and blood pressure in hemodialysis patients. *Am J Hypertens* 6(2):103–107, 1993.

104. Bode-Böger S, Böger RH, Kuhn M, Radermacher J, Frölich JC: Endothelin release and shift in prostaglandin balance are involved in the modulation of vascular tone by recombinant erythropoietin. *J Cardiovasc Pharmacol* 20 (Suppl 12):S25–S28, 1992.

105. Caravaca F, Pizarro JL, Arrobas M, Cubero JJ, Garcia MC,

Perez MM: Antiplatelet therapy and development of hypertension induced by recombinant human erythropoietin in uremic patients. *Kidney Int* 45(3):845–851, 1994.

106. Winearls CG: Treatment of anaemia in haemodialysis patients with recombinant erythropoietin. *Nephron* 51 (Supp l 1)):26–28, 1989.

107. Casati S, Passerini P, Campise MR, Graziani G, Cesana B, Perisic M, Ponticelli C: Benefits and risks of protracted treatment with human recombinant erythropoietin in patients having haemodialysis. *Br Med J Clin Res Ed* 295(6605):1017–1020, 1987.

108. Sharpe PC, Desai ZR, Morris TC: Increase in mean platelet volume in patients with chronic renal failure treated with erythropoietin. *J Clin Pathol* 47(2):159–161, 1994.

109. Bommer J, Müller-Bühl U, Ritz E, Eifert J: Recombinant human erythropoietin in anaemic patients on haemodialysis (letter). *Lancet* 1:392, 1987.

110. Wirtz JJJM, Van Esser JWJ, Hamulyak K, Leunissen KML, Van Hooff JP: The effects of recombinant human erythropoietin on hemostasis and fibrinolysis in hemodialysis patients. *Clin Nephrol* 38(5):277–282, 1992.

111. Bennett WM: A multicenter clinical trial of epoetin beta for anemia of end-stage renal disease. *J Am Soc Nephrol* 1(7):990–998, 1991.

112. Canadian-Erythropoietin-Study-Group: Effect of recombinant human erythropoietin therapy on blood pressure in hemodialysis patients. *Am J Nephrol* 11(1):23–26, 1991.

113. Churchill DN, Muirhead N, Goldstein M, Posen G, Fay W, Beecroft ML, Gorman J, Taylor DW: Probability of thrombosis of vascular access among hemodialysis patients treated with recombinant human erythropoietin. *J Am Soc Nephrol* 4(10):1809–1813, 1994.

114. Spinowitz BS, Arslanian J, Charytan C, Golden RA, Rascoff J, Galler M: Impact of epoetin beta on dialyzer clearance and heparin requirements. *Am J Kidney Dis* 18(6):668–673, 1991.

115. Veys N, Vanholder R, De Cuyper K, Ringoir S: Influence of erythropoietin on dialyzer reuse, heparin need, and urea kinetics in maintenance hemodialysis patients. *Am J Kidney Dis* 23(1):52–59, 1994.

116. Grützmacher P, Bergmann M, Weinreich T, Nattermann U, Reimers E, Pollok M: Beneficial and adverse effects of correction of anaemia by recombinant human erythropoietin in patients on maintenance haemodialysis. *Contrib Nephrol* 66:104–113, 1988.

117. Canaud B, Polito-Bouloux C, Garred LJ, Rivory J-P, Donnadieu P, Taib J, Florence P, Mion C: Recombinant human erythropoietin: 18 months experience in hemodialysis patients. *Am J Kidney Dis* 15(2):169–175, 1990.

118. Garcia DL, Anderson S, Rennke HG, Brenner BM: Anemia lessens and its prevention with recombinant human erythropoietin worsens glomerular injury and hypertension in rats with reduced renal mass. *Proc Natl Acad Sci USA* 85(16):6142–6146, 1988.

119. The US Recombinant Human Erythropoietin Predialysis Study Group: Double-blind, placebo-controlled study of the therapeutic use of recombinant human erythropoietin for anemia associated with chronic renal failure in predialysis patients. *Am J Kidney Dis* 18(1):50–59, 1991.

120. Abraham PA, Opsahl JA, Rachael KM, Asinger R, Halstenson CE: Renal function during erythropoietin therapy for anemia in predialysis chronic renal failure patients. *Am J Nephrol* 10:128–136, 1990.

121. Kleinmann KS, Schweitzer SU, Perdue ST, Bleifer KH, Abels RI: The use of recombinant human erythropoietin in the correction of anaemia in predialysis patients and its effect on renal function: a double-blind, placebo controlled trial. *Am J Kidney Dis* 14:486–495, 1989.

122. Lim VS: Recombinant human erythropoietin in predialysis patients. *Am J Kidney Dis* 18(4) (Suppl 1):34–37, 1991.

123. Austrian Multicenter Study Group of r-HuEPO in Predialysis Patients: Effectiveness and safety of recombinant human erythropoietin in predialysis patients. *Nephron* 61:399–403, 1992.

124. MacDougall IC, Davies ME, Hutton RD, Cavill I, Lewis NP, Coles GA, Williams JD: The treatment of renal anemia in CAPD patients with recombinant human erythropoietin. *Nephrol Dial Transplant* 5:950–955, 1990.

125. Frenken LAM, Verberckmoes R, Michielsen P, Koene RAP: Efficacy and tolerance of treatment with recombinant-human erythropoietin in chronic renal failure (pre-dialysis) patients. *Nephrol Dial Transplant* 4:782–786, 1989.

126. Ashai NI, Paganini EP, Wilson JM: Intravenous versus subcutaneous dosing of epoetin: a review of the literature. *Am J Kidney Dis* 22 (Suppl 1):23–31, 1993.

127. Wolfson M, Mundt DJ, Hawley GG: Recombinant human erythropoietin utilization in Department of Veterans Affairs dialysis units. *Am J Kidney Dis* 24(2):184–191, 1994.

128. Hörl WH: Optimal route of administration of erythropoietin in chronic renal failure patients: intravenous versus subcutaneous. *Acta Haematol* 1(16):16–19, 1992.

129. Macdougall IC, Roberts DE, Coles GA, Williams JD: Clinical pharmacokinetics of epoetin (recombinant human erythropoietin). *Clin Pharmacokinet* 20(2):99–113, 1991.

130. Taylor JE, Belch JJ, Fleming LW, Mactier RA, Henderson IS, Stewart WK: Erythropoietin response and route of administration. *Clin Nephrol* 41(5):297–302, 1994.

131. Hörl WH: Painless subcutaneous erythropoietin (rHuEPO) injection—is it the panacea. *Nephrol Dial Transplant* 9(9):1224–1225, 1994.

132. Kampf D, Kahl A, Passlick J, Pustelnik A, Eckardt K-U, Ehmer B, Jacobs C, Baumelou A, Grabensee B, Gahl GM: Single-dose kinetics of recombinant human erythropoietin after intravenous, subcutaneous and intraperitoneal administration. *Contrib Nephrol* 76:106–111, 1989.

133. Lai KN, Lui SF, Leung JC, Law E, Nicholls MG: Effect of subcutaneous and intraperitoneal administration of recombinant human erythropoietin on blood pressure and vasoactive hormones in patients on continuous ambulatory peritoneal dialysis. *Nephron* 57(4):394–400, 1991.

134. Schwartz AB, Kahn SB, Kelch KE, Pequignot E: RBC improved survival due to recombinant human erythropoietin explains effectiveness of less frequent, low dose subcutaneous therapy. *Clin Nephrol* 38(5):283–289, 1992.

135. Neff MS, Eiser AR, Slifkin RF, Baum M, Baez A, Gupta S, Amarga E: Patients surviving 10 years of hemodialysis. *Am J Med* 74(6):996–1004, 1983.

136. Ritz E, Zeier M, Schneider P, Jones E: Cardiovascular mortality of patients with polycystic kidney disease on dialysis: is there a lesson to learn? (editorial). *Nephron* 66(2):125–128, 1994.

137. Byrne C, Vernon P, Cohen JP: Effect of age and diagnosis on survival of older patients beginning chronic dialysis. *JAMA* 271(1):34–36, 1994.

138. Barany P, Svedenhag J, Freyschuss U, Bergström J: Physiological effects of correcting anemia in hemodialysis patients to a normal hemoglobin concentration (abstract). *Clin Invest* 72(5):B13, 1994.

139. Bell JD, Kincaid WR, Morgan RG, Bunce H, Alperin JB, Sarles HE, Remmers AR: Serum ferritin assay and bone-marrow iron stores in patients on maintenance hemodialysis. *Kidney Int* 17:237–241, 1980.

140. Birgegard G, Hallgren R, Killander A: Serum ferritin during infection: a longitudinal study. *Scand J Haematol* 21:333–340, 1978.

141. Ali M, Rigolosi R, Fayemi AO, Braun EV, Fascino J, Singer R: Failure of serum ferritin levels to predict bone-marrow iron content after intravenous iron-dextran therapy. *Lancet* i:652–655, 1982.

142. Bainton DF, Finch CA: The diagnosis of iron deficiency anemia. *Am J Med* 37:62–70, 1964.

143. Cavill I: Diagnostic methods. *Clin Haematol* 11:259–273, 1982.

144. Macdougall IC, Cavill I, Hulme B, Bain B, McGregor E, McKay P, Sanders E, Coles GA, Williams JD: Detection of functional iron deficiency during erythropoietin treatment: a new approach. *Br Med J* 304:225–226, 1992.

145. Cazzola M, Bergamaschi G, Barosi G, Bellotti V, Caldera D, Civiello MM, Quaglini S, Arosio P, Ascari E: Biological and clinical significance of red cell ferritin. *Blood* 62:1078–1087, 1983.

146. Beguin Y, Loo M, R Zik S, Sautois B, Lejune F, Rorive G, Fillet G: Early prediction of response to recombinant human erythropoietin in patients with the anemia of renal failure by serum transferrin receptor and fibrinogen. *Blood* 82:2010–2016, 1993.

147. Moreb J, Poportzer MM, Friedlander MM, Konijn AN, Hershko C: Evaluation of iron status in patients on chronic haemodialysis: relative usefulness of bone marrow haemosiderin, serum ferritin, transferrin saturation, mean corpuscular volume and red cell protoporphyrin. *Nephron* 35:196–200, 1983.

148. Garrett S, Worwood M: Zinc protoporphyrin and iron-deficient erythropoiesis. *Acta Haematol* 91(1):21–25, 1994.

149. Levin NW, Lazarus JM, Nissenson AR: National Cooperative rHu Erythropoietin Study in patients with chronic renal failure: an interim report. *Am J Kidney Dis* 22 (Suppl 1):3–12, 1993.

150. Anderson RJ, Melikian DM, Gambertoglio JG, Berns AS, Cadnapaphornchai J, Egan DJ, Goldberg JP, Henrich WL, Hicks DL, Kovaichik MT, Olin DB: Prescribing medication in long-term dialysis units. *Arch Int Med* 142:1305–1308, 1982.

151. Gokal R, Millard PR, Weatherall DJ, Callender STE, Ledingham JGG, Oliver DO: Iron metabolism in haemodialysis patients. *Q J Med* 48:369–391, 1979.

152. Cook JD, Dassenko S, Skikne BS: Serum transferrin receptor as an index of iron absorption. *J Lab Clin Med* 75:603–609, 1990.

153. Schaefer RM, Schaefer L: Management of iron substitution during r-HuEPO therapy in chronic renal failure patients. *Erythropoiesis* 3:71–75, 1992.

154. MacDougall IC, Hutton RD, Cavill I, Coles GA, Williams JD: Poor response to treatment of renal anemia with erythropoietin corrected by iron given intravenously. *Br Med J* 299:157–158, 1989.

155. Watson A: Iron management during treatment with recombinant human erythropoietin in chronic renal failure. *J Clin Pharmacol* 33:1134–1138, 1993.

156. Van Wyck DB: Iron management during recombinant human erythropoietin therapy. *Am J Kidney Dis* 14 (Suppl 1):9–13, 1989.

157. Auerbach M, Witt D, Toler W, Fierstein M, Lerner RG, Ballard H: Clinical use of the total dose intravenous infusion of iron dextran. *J Lab Clin Med* 111(5):566–570, 1988.

158. Porter J, Jick H: Drug-induced anaphylaxis, convulsions, deafness, and extrapyramidal symptoms. *Lancet* 1:587–588, 1977.

159. Zipf RJ: Fatal anaphylaxis after intravenous iron dextran. *J Forensic Sci* 20(2):326–333, 1975.

160. Granoleras C, Oulès R, Branger B, Fourcade J, Shaldon S: Iron supplementation of hemodialysis patients receiving recombinant human erythropoietin therapy. In: Bauer C, Koch KM, Scigalla P, Wieczorek L, eds, *Erythropoietin—Molecular Physiology and Clinical Applications*. Marcel Dekker, New York, pp 211–216, 1993.

161. Maiorca R, Cancarini G, Manili L, Brunorio G, Camerini C, Strada A, Feller P: CAPD is a first class treatment: results of an eight-year experience with a comparison of patient and method survival in CAPD and hemodialysis. *Clin Nephrol* 30 (Suppl 1):S3–S7, 1988.

162. Salahudeen AK, Keavey PM, Hawkins T, Wilkinson R: Is anemia during continous ambulatory peritoneal dialysis really better than during haemodialysis? *Lancet* ii:1046–1049, 1983.

163. Maluche HH, Faugere MC: Aluminium-related bone disease. *Blood Purif* 6:1–15, 1988.

164. McCarthy JT, Milliner DS, Johnson WJ: Clinical experience with desferrioxamine in dialysis patients with aluminium toxicity. *Q J Med* 74(275):257–276, 1990.

165. Neff MS, Goldberg J, Slifkin RF, Eiser AR, Calamia V: A comparison of androgens for anemia in patients on hemodialysis. *N Engl J Med* 304:871–875, 1981.

166. Hendler ED, Solomon L: Androgen therapy in hemodialysis patients: 1. Effects on red cell oxygen transport. *Kidney Int* 31:100–106, 1987.

167. Besarab A, Caro J, Jarrell BE, Francos G, Erslev AJ: Dynamics of erythropoiesis following renal transplantation. *Kidney Int* 32:526–536, 1987.

168. Eckardt K-U, Frei U, Kliem V, Bauer C, Koch KM, Kurtz A: Role of excretory graft function for erythropoietin formation after renal transplantation. *Eur J Clin Invest* 20:564–574, 1990.

169. McGrath BP, Ibels LS, Raik E, Hargrave M, Mahony JF, Stewart JH: Erythroid toxicity of azathioprine: macrocytosis and selective marrow hypoplasia. *Q J Med* 44:57–63, 1975.

170. Gossmann J, Kachel HG, Schoeppe W, Scheuermann EH: Anemia in renal transplant recipients caused by concomitant therapy with azathioprine and angiotensin-converting enzyme inhibitors. *Transplantation* 56(3):585–589, 1993.

171. Friman S, Nyberg G, Blohme I: Erythrocytosis after renal transplantation: treatment by removal of the native kidneys. *Nephrol Dial Transplant* 5(11):969–973, 1990.

172. Gaston RS, Julian BA, Curtis JJ: Posttransplant erythrocytosis: an enigma revisited. *Am J Kidney Dis* 24(1):1–11, 1994.

173. Fernandez A, Hortal L, Rodriguez JC, Vega N, Plaza C, Palop L: Anemia in dialysis: its relation to acquired cystic disease and serum levels of erythropoietin. *Am J Nephrol* 11:11–15, 1991.

174. Eckardt K-U, Möllmann M, Neumann R, Brunkhorst R, Burger H-U, Lonnemann G, Scholz H, Keusch G, Buchholz B, Frei U, Bauer C, Kurtz A: Erythropoietin in polycystic kidneys. *J Clin Invest* 84:1160–1166, 1989.

175. Luke RG, Kennedy AC, Stirling WB, MacDonald GA: Renal artery stenosis, hypertension and polycythemia. *Br Med J* 1:164–166, 1965.

176. Boelaert JR, Cantinieaux BF, Hariga CF, Fondu PG: Recombinant erythropoietin reverses polymorphonuclear granulocyte dysfunction in iron-overloaded dialysis patients. *Nephrol Dial Transplant* 5:504–507, 1990.

177. Greene HG, Ray C, Mauer MSM, Quie PG: The effect of hemodialysis on neutrophil chemotactic responsiveness. *Am J Nephrol* 88:971–974, 1976.

178. Hakim RM, Stannard D, Port F, Held P: The effect of the dialysis membrane on mortality of chronic hemodialysis patients (CHD) in the U.S. (abstract). *J Am Soc Nephrol* 5(3):451, 1994.

179. Hakim RM, Wingard RL, Parker RA: Effect of the dialysis membrane in the treatment of patients with acute renal failure. *N Engl J Med* 331:1338–1342, 1994.

180. Escolar G, Cases A, Bastida E, Garrido M, López J, Revert L, Castillo R, Ordinas A: Uremic platelets have a functional defect affecting the interaction of von Willebrand factor with glycoprotein IIb-IIIa. *Blood* 76:1336–1340, 1990.

181. Vigano G, Gaspari F, Locatelli M, Pusineri F, Bonati M, Remuzzi G: Dose-effect and pharmacokinetics of estrogens given to correct bleeding time in uremia. *Kidney Int* 34:853–858, 1988.

182. Sanders PW, Taylor H, Curtis JJ: Hemodialysis without anticoagulation. *Am J Kidney Dis* 5:32–35, 1985.

CHAPTER 53

Hematologic Disorders in Renal Failure

J. RADERMACHER & KARL M. KOCH

INTRODUCTION

Even though renal failure also affects the function of white blood cells (1,2) and thrombocytes (3), renal anemia is the main hematologic disturbance of uremia for which well-founded possibilities of therapeutic intervention exist today. The basis for this exceptional and fortunate situation is our advanced understanding of the pathogenesis of renal anemia as well as recent progress in molecular biology. Since this book is devoted to therapy, this chapter will concentrate on renal anemia and its management.

CLINICAL FEATURES AND CONSEQUENCES

Anemia is one of the main clinical symptoms of renal failure, occurring in more than 80% of patients with end-stage renal failure. It becomes manifest when creatinine clearance has dropped to $30-40\,mL/min/1.73\,m^2$, and its severity increases with further deterioration of excretory renal function. Renal anemia is normochromic and normocytic when no other aggravating factors such as iron deficiency or aluminium overload are coexisting with renal insufficiency. Renal anemia is hyporegenerative. The reticulocyte count, when corrected for normal hematocrit values, is inadequate.

The impact of renal anemia on physical and mental abilities is considerable and represents a major obstacle for the rehabilitation of patients in terminal renal failure. This observation applies even though the effect of anemia on tissue oxygenation may be partly balanced in uremic patients by a shift of the oxyhemoglobin dissociation curve to the right. This shift, which is attributed to acidosis and increased intraerythrocytotic levels of 2,3-diphosphoglycerate and other phosphates, reduces the peripheral affinity of hemoglobin for oxygen and thereby improves oxygen delivery to the tissues. A further compensating mechanism is an increase in cardiac output (4), which, when extremely severe, may result in heart failure due to a high output state even in the absence of underlying heart disease (5).

Accordingly, a typical echocardiographic finding in end-stage renal disease is an eccentric left ventricular hypertrophy (6), which is characteristic of volume overload (7). It is defined by a parallel increase in ventricular radius (end-diastolic diameter) and wall thickness, leaving the ratio between wall thickness and radius unchanged. Concentric hypertrophy (increase of wall thickness only), which is characteristic of pressure overload, can also be induced, since hypertension occurs in up to 80% of patients with end-stage renal disease and may combine with eccentric hypertrophy. Hypertension and the resulting hypertensive cardiomyopathy may compromise the ability to compensate for the reduced hemoglobin level by an increase in cardiac output. Also, many of the patients have advanced coronary artery disease, and even renal anemia of a moderate degree may be accompanied by myocardial hypoxia and angina.

PATHOGENESIS

The primary mechanism involved in the pathogenesis of the anemia of renal failure are hemolysis, inadequate production of erythropoietin, and possibly also an inhibition of the response of erythroid precursor cells to erythropoietin (8,9). In addition, secondary mechanisms such as blood loss, iron or folate deficiency, aluminum intoxication, drug effects, the anemia of chronic disease, marrow fibrosis resulting from hyperparathyroidism, hypersplenism, and toxic hemolysis may be operative.

Hemolysis

Hemolysis in terminal renal failure is of moderate degree, since red-cell survival in general is reduced by only 25%–30%. The accelerated destruction of red cells in uremia appears to be the result of the uremic environment, since cells from uremic subjects transfused in normal volunteers have a normal life span, whereas normal red cells transfused into uremic patients have a reduced life span. The cause for hemolysis appears to be extracellular and related

Suki, WN and Massry SG (eds), Suki and Massry's Therapy of Renal Diseases and Related Disorders, Third Edition. ISBN 978-1-4757-6634-9.

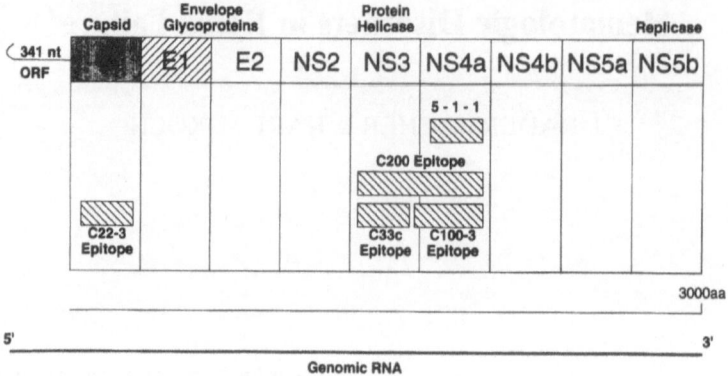

Figure 1. The organization of the hepatitis C viral genome. C, nucleocapsid gene; E1–E2, envelope genes; NS2–NS5, nonstructural genes involved in viral replication. The various epitopes correspond to antigenic regions of the genome that are determined serologically.

Table 1. Currently available assays for the diagnosis of HCV infection

Test system[a]	Detecting	Comments
Anti-HCV antibody assay		
EIA-I[b]	Anti-c100-3	Many false positive and negatives; 15–20-week interval postinoculation until seroconversion.
EIA-II[b]	Anti-c100-3, c200, c33c, c22-3	Greater sensitivity and earlier diagnosis (12–14 wks) than EIA-I.
RIBA[b]	Anti-5-1-1, c100-3, c33c, c22-3	Improved specificity vs. ELISA assays. Early diagnosis (similar to EIA-II).
Polymerase chain reaction		Only assay confirming active viral replication. Allows earliest
5'-NCR primers	HCV RNA	diagnosis of primary HCV infection (1–2 wks postinoculation).
NS3–4 primers	HCV RNA	Less sensitivity with NS3-4 primers.

[a] EIA, enzyme-linked immunoassay (ELISA); RIBA, recombinant immunoblot assay.
[b] Commercially licensed.

tion tests. This appears to be particularly true among immunosuppressed renal allograft recipients (6) and chronic hemodialysis patients (7,8) in whom active HCV infection has been demonstrated in the setting of persistently normal transaminases.

In addition to the inherent risk of progressive liver disease, patients with chronic HCV infection are at increased risk for HCV-associated complications. An increased incidence of hepatocellular carcinoma (HCC) has been noted in patients with cirrhosis secondary to HCV infection (9). The increased prevalence of both hepatitis B and hepatitis C infection in Japan enabled investigators to recognize an independent risk for HCC accompanying infection with either virus, as well as a synergistic increase in the risk of neoplasia in the setting of coinfection. Extrahepatic syndromes linked to HCV infection include essential cryoglobulinemia and several histologic types of glomerulonephritis (vide infra).

Diagnostic testing for HCV infection

IMMUNODIAGNOSIS

The molecular characterization and cloning of HCV led to the production of large quantities of viral protein from recombinant organisms. When purified, the recombinant polypeptide can be used to produce a capture assay for reactive antibody, indicating exposure of the individual to HCV (10). The first-generation anti-HCV immunoassay (ELISA I; Ortho Diagnostics) was licensed in May 1990 and incorporated the c100-3 polypeptide expressed in yeast (Table 1). The c100-3 epitope corresponds with almost all of the NS4 protein of the HCV genome (Figure 1). Antibody to this protein develops in nearly all cases of posttransfusion non-A, non-B hepatitis (1–3). A second-generation immunoassay (ELISA II; Ortho Diagnostics) is now commercially licensed and has replaced the ELISA I.

The ELISA II detects antibodies to proteins derived from three distinct regions of the HCV genome. The c200 recombinant antigen is an expression product of the NS3/NS4 region (Figure 1) and is derived from that region of the genome encoding both the c33c and c100-3 recombinant antigens. The c22-3 recombinant antigen is a product of the putative nucleocapsid region of the HCV genome. The recently licensed four-antigen recombinant immunoblot assay (RIBA) differs from the ELISA test system in that a nitrocellulose strip-based methodology is used that is capable of detecting antibodies to the recombinant HCV antigens 5-1-1, c100-3, c33c, and c22-3. During incubation of each strip with serum, anti-HCV antibodies will react to the corresponding antigen. Results are reported as reactive (reactivity with at least two antigen bands), indeterminate (reactivity with a single antigen band), or non-reactive (no reactive bands). A third generation assay, incorporating additional epitopes, has been recently licensed.

VIRAL RNA DETECTION

The application of polymerase chain reaction techniques to amplify reverse transcribed cDNA provided an opportunity to develop a very sensitive assay for viral RNA. The ability to detect small numbers of viral RNA molecules in the blood or tissue specimens by PCR represents an extremely sensitive assay for HCV infection (11). Several studies have conclusively demonstrated that primers specific for the 5'-untranslated region of the HCV genome are preferred, since this region is highly conserved among most worldwide HCV isolates studied to date (3). Polymerase chain reaction tests using primers from the NS3–4 region have been shown to be considerably less sensitive than assays incorporating primers from the 5'-untranslated section of the genome (12).

Clinical applications of anti-HCV diagnostic tests

By 1986, most blood banks incorporated ALT and anti-HBc screening to identify high-risk non-A, non-B hepatitis blood donors. The subsequent licensing of the first generation anti-HCV assay in 1990 and the earlier use of "surrogate marker" testing are both credited with reducing the incidence of HCV infection over the ensuing years (13). Currently, there are three assays licensed for commercial anti-HCV testing. The first-generation ELISA (EIA-I) was extremely successful in predicting whether coded sera contained the agent responsible for posttransfusion non-A, non-B hepatitis; however, there were many situations that gave rise to false-positive and false-negative results. Patients with hypergammaglobulinemia and autoimmune chronic active hepatitis often tested positive by EIA-I in the absence of HCV infection (14,15). False-negative tests have been seen in immunosuppressed individuals, patients with chronic renal failure, and patients with AIDS. The second-generation ELISA (EIA-II) has been demonstrated to provide increased sensitivity and an earlier detection of anti-HCV antibody when compared to the EIA-I (1,16,17). ELISA II testing shortens the "window" of seroconversion from approximately 18 to 14 weeks following exposure (16). The recombinant immunoblot assay (RIBA) increased the specificity of anti-HCV testing while maintaining the excellent sensitivity of the EIA-II (14,18). In a series reported by McHutchison et al. (17), all RIBA reactive samples were also positive by EIA-II testing. However, there does appear to be a slight reduction in specificity with the EIA-II, especially in patients at low risk for HCV infection. Validation of the value of the RIBA was provided by Esteban and coworkers (19). In their study, all RIBA-reactive patients had abnormal liver biopsies, although the severity of the histologic changes varied widely. Fully 69% of the RIBA positive patients had either chronic active hepatitis (CAH) or cirrhosis. Of note, 35% of the patients with CAH had persistently normal transaminases, emphasizing the importance of liver biopsy for proper diagnosis as well as the low sensitivity of liver enzymes for a diagnosis of ongoing infection. McGuinness and colleagues (12) screened 157 blood donors with anti-HCV assays and used PCR testing as a confirmatory test. Ninety percent of the patients who were RIBA reactive with abnormal liver function tests had detectable HCV RNA by PCR. This figure dropped to 54% in the RIBA-positive patients with normal liver enzymes. None of the ELISA-positive, RIBA-negative patients was PCR positive, confirming the superior specificity of the RIBA assay.

HCV infection in the ESRD patient

Hepatitis B virus (HBV) infection became the leading cause of liver disease in the ESRD population after the introduction of chronic hemodialysis and was responsible for several hepatitis epidemics. Even after the application of effective control measures for HBV infection, sporadic outbreaks of hepatitis in dialysis units continued to occur (20–24). The main agent responsible for these epidemics of non-A, non-B hepatitis, namely, the hepatitis C virus (HCV), was identified in 1989 (25). Subsequently, it has been possible to sequence most of the HCV genome (10,26).

SEROLOGIC AND MOLECULAR DETECTION OF HCV INFECTION

Anti-HCV testing in hemodialysis patients

The initial screening studies of ESRD patients (27–34) utilizing first-generation assays showed a prevalence of anti-HCV of between 5% and 29% (Table 2). In addition, two large series of over 1000 patients each were published in the form of letters to the editor (35,36). A study from Germany found that 112 of 1107 (10%) of the patients were anti-HCV positive. A much higher prevalence (22.2%) was observed in Japan using the same assay. In both studies, there were several patients that were never transfused.

Table 2. Initial studies of the prevalence of anti-HCV in hemo-dialysis units

Reference	Author	Year	Country	No. pts.	Anti-HCV positive (%)
27	Esteban	1989	Spain	42	20
28	Kuhnl	1990	Europe	387	5.4–12
29	Jeffers	1990	USA	90	12
30	Gilli	1990	Italy	144	18.4
31	Zeldis	1990	USA	102	16
32	Fairley	1990	Australia	205	5.9
33	Teruel	1990	Spain	64	17
34	Oguchi	1990	Japan	51	29

In our study (29), we evaluated 90 chronic hemodialysis patients and 37 staff members. The mean age of the patients was 54 ± 13 (range 25–87) years. There were 68 men and 22 women. Sixty-one patients were black. The mean duration of maintenance dialysis was 31 ± 36 months (range 1 month to 15 years). Transfusion records revealed that 87% of the patients had been transfused (mean 22 ± 38; range 0–269 units). Fifteen (17%) patients had a history of intravenous drug abuse (IVDA).

Of the 37 staff members screened, there were 28 women and 9 men. Their mean age was 42 ± 9 years, and they had worked an average of 12.5 years (range 1.2–35) in the medical environment and 7.9 years (range 0.2–18) in dialysis units. Anti-HCV was measured by the first-generation ELISA assay (10). Others markers were measured with commercially available kits.

Eleven patients (12%) were anti-HCV positive. Among the anti-HCV (+) patients, eight (73%) were positive for anti-HBc, one of whom was also HBsAg (+) and five of whom were anti-HBs (+). Among the 79 anti-HCV (−) patients, 33 (42%) were anti-HBs (+), one of whom was also HBsAg (+) and 27 of whom were anti-HBc (+). An analysis was made to determine whether the presence of anti-HCV and anti-HBc were related to each other. The odds ratio was 3.72, indicating the tendency for a higher prevalence of anti-HCV among anti-HBc-positive subjects. However, this figure did not reach statistical significance according to the criteria of the study ($p = 0.053$).

Risk factors in the 11 anti-HCV (+) patients included blood transfusions (all patients) and IVDA (eight patients). Nevertheless, 67 (85%) of anti-HCV (−) patients had a history of blood transfusions and 7 (10%) had a history of IVDA ($p = 0.348$ and $p = 0.00001$, odds ratio 27.4, respectively). The number of transfusions (anti-HCV (+) 59 ± 77; HCV (−) 16 ± 27) was significantly higher in the anti-HCV (+) patients, however ($p = 0.004$). Three of seven (43%) patients seropositive for anti-HCV tested positive for anti-HIV ($p = 0.003$, odds ratio 10.0).

Eight (10%) anti-HCV (−) and only two (18%) anti-HCV (+) patients had prior sporadic increases in serum in transaminase (ALT) levels. One of the anti-HCV (+) patients had chronic persistent hepatitis documented by liver biopsy, and the other had a history of chronic alcoholism, abnormal liver function tests, and stigmata of cirrhosis. At the time of the study, ALT was increased above normal levels in five patients (four anti-HCV (−), one anti-HCV (+); $p = 0.85$). The etiology of the increased ALT elevations was not established. The rest of the patients had no clinical or laboratory evidence of chronic liver disease; liver biopsies were not performed, however.

The main risk factors for HCV infection in our patients were intravenous drug abuse and, to a lesser degree, blood transfusions. Nevertheless, 84% of anti-HCV (−) patients also had received blood transfusions, and there were seven IVDA among them. The mean number of transfusions in the seven IVDA that were anti-HCV (−) was lower than that in the eight IVDA that were anti-HCV (+) (9 units vs. 65 units).

Anti-HBc, a marker of HBV infection, has been used as a surrogate marker for non-A, non-B hepatitis (37). Although of borderline statistical significance, this association was suggested by the results of the present study in that 8 of the 11 anti-HCV (+) patients were positive for anti-HBc. Sporadic prior increases or current elevations of ALT, however, did not correlate with anti-HCV positivity.

Anti-HCV in dialysis staff

Of the 37 staff members, none was anti-HCV (+) and seven (19%) were anti-HBc (+)/antiHBs (+). The prevalence of anti-HBc was significantly lower than that of the patients ($p = 0.001$). ALT levels were normal in all staff members. The personnel had a mean exposure period of 7.5 years in a dialysis setting, and 19% had evidence of previous exposure to HBV infection. However, none had serologic evidence of HCV infection, suggesting that HBV infection is greater than that of HCV infection in hemodialysis staff. Similar results have been reported by Oguchi et al. (34).

Second-generation assays in hemodialysis patients

To assess the improvement in detection of HCV infection afforded by second-generation assays, we tested serum samples from patients undergoing maintenance hemodialysis in a private dialysis unit using both a first- and a second-generation anti-HCV EIA (38). Specimens found to be repeatedly reactive by either EIA were assayed for antibodies to three HCV gene products, namely, c100-3, NS3, and core, by testing with experimental supplemental EIAs (Abbott Laboratories) and by MATRIX HCV.

There was 87.9% (87 of 99) agreement between the first- and second-generation HCV EIA. Of the 33 specimens that were repeatedly reactive by both assays, 21 were positive for antibodies to two gene products. Twelv specimens were repeatedly reactive by the HCV EIA-II. Of these 12 specimens, two were positive for antibodies to three gene products, five were positive for two gene products, three were positive for one gene product, and two specimens were indeterminate (i.e., not reactive for the same single gene product by both supplemental EIA and MATRIX HCV). None of the patients who had a reactive HCV EIA was found negative either by the supplemental EIA or by the MATRIX HCV test. The HCV EIA-II detected 10 more positive specimens than the first-generation HCV EIA, for an increase in detection from 33.3% to 43.4% (43 of 99); ($p = 0.14$). There were no differences in the clinical attributes of patients positive for both assays versus those who were positive only by the HCV EIA-II.

Table 3 shows the comparison between first- and second-generation EIAs initially reported from several dialysis centers (38–43). All studies show improved sensitivity with second-generation tests. The recombinant immunoblot assay (RIBA) has been used as a confirmatory test in some studies, giving indeterminate results in 2%–8% percent of the cases (43,44). In addition, Dentico et al. compared two second-generation EIAs (Ortho and Abbott) in 293 sera collected from dialysis patients (45). The agreement between the two tests was 98.3%. Ninety-two percent of reactive sera were confirmed using Ortho RIBA and 100% with Abbott supplemental tests. Third-generation assays incorporating additional epitopes have shown improves antibody detection.

Continuous ambulatory peritoneal dialysis

Studies in patients on chronic ambulatory peritoneal dialysis have shown a lower prevalence of HCV infection than those in patients on hemodialysis (40,46–49). In a study from Italy (40), the prevalence of HCV infection among CAPD patients was 17%, compared to 23% in hemodialysis patients. A more striking contrast (1.8% CAPD; 16.4% hemodialysis) was reported by Chan et al. (46). In another study (47), the prevalence of HCV infection in CAPD patients with a prior history of hemodialysis was higher (33%) than that in patients only receiving CAPD (5.9%). A lower prevalence of HCV infection on CAPD was also observed by Selgas et al. (48) and by Ng et al. (49), who evaluated their patients with a first-generation test (Ortho) followed by second-generation EIAs (Abbott and UBI).

HCV RNA detection in dialysis patients

In a recent study from our institution (50), blood samples from 63 patients undergoing hemodialysis were analyzed by HCV-cDNA/PCR, Abbott anti-HCV (EIA), and Abbott HCV Neutralization EIA Assays under code. Twenty-five percent (16 of 63) of the patients were anti-HCV (+). Of the 16 anti-HCV (+) patients, HCV RNA was detected in 5 (31%) with NS3 primers and in 12 (75%) with 5'-noncoding primers. Among the anti-HCV (–) patients, HCV RNA was detected in 2 of 47 (4.3%). For one of these patients, additional samples were obtained at 1 and 1.5 years after the initial testing, and both samples were HCV RNA (+) but remained anti-HCV (–). Eleven of the 19 patients with HCV infection (positive for anti-HCV and/or HCV RNA) had evidence of additional or other present or past viral infections. Ten were anti-HBc (+), three were HBV DNA (+) including one HBsAg (+) patient, and three were anti-HIV positive. In one patient, coinfection with HCV, HIV, and HBV was documented.

Table 4 summarizes several studies of HCV RNA in dialysis patients utilizing PCR (7,8,50–54). It is apparent that most anti-HCV (+) individuals are chronic viremic carriers as determined by PCR. HCV RNA (+) individuals may be potentially infectious and are at risk for the development of chronic active hepatitis (55–57).

In our study, HCV RNA was detected in two anti-HCV-negative patients, while no PCR positives were observed

Table 3. Comparison of selected studies of first- and second-generation EIAs in dialysis patients

Ref.	Author	Year	Country	EIA-I (% positive)	EIA-II (% positive)
36	de Medina	1992	USA	33.3	43.4
37	Mondelli	1992	Italy	31	55
38	Cantu	1992	Italy	11	21
39	Polywka	1992	Germany	15.7	16.9
40	Holzberger	1992	Germany	4.6	8.2
41	Chauveau	1993	France	31.3	55

Table 4. Detection of HCV RNA with PCR in dialysis patients

Ref.	Author	Year	Country	No. pts.	1st-generation EIA % (+)	2nd-generation EIA % (+)	HCV RNA % of HCV (+) pts.
48	Kuhns	1993	USA	63	—	25	
49	Li	1992	China	16	81.2	—	69.2
50	Sheu	1992	Taiwan	125	32	47.2	66
8	Chan	1993	Hong Kong	51	11.8	21.6	72.7
51	Sakamoto	1993	Japan	184	10.7	22	25[a]
52	Dussol	1993	France	145	—	29	52

[a] EIA first generation.

among the healthy control population. The data are consistent with a recent study from Japan in which HCV RNA was detected in 13 of 16 (81%) anti-HCV (+) patients, as well as in 7 of 14 anti-HCV (−) cases of chronic liver disease (56). In another study (53), HCV RNA was found in 6.1% of 164 c100-3 (−) dialysis patients. These results indicate that screening tests may underestimate the prevalence of HCV infection in dialysis patients. The presence of serum HCV RNA in seronegative patients may indicate early or chronic HCV infection not detected by current antibody assays. Alternatively, this phenomenon may be associated with the inability of immunodeficient uremic patients to mount or sustain a significant antibody response.

We recently evaluated the bDNA (58) test to quantitate HCV RNA in sera from 38 patients undergoing maintenance hemodialysis at the Miami Veterans Affairs Medical Center. Twelve of 38 (32%) patients were found to be anti-HCV reactive by ELISA. Nine of 12 (75%) were confirmed reactive, two (17%) were indeterminate, and one (8%) was nonreactive by RIBA. Eight of the nine (89%) reactive by RIBA were found to have detectable $(350 \, Eq/mL \times 10^3)$ HCV RNA levels (mean 3570 ± 3789 (SD); range 496–12,332). HCV RNA was not detected in one RIBA-reactive, the two indeterminate, and 26 nonreactive patients for anti-HCV. The two epitopes most commonly associated with HCV-RNA were c22 and c33c; c22 was detected in all patients and c33c in six of eight (75%), whereas 5-1-1 and/or c100-3 were detected in four of eight (50%) patients, respectively. HCV-RNA by RT-PCR confirmed results obtained by the bDNA assay.

Five of the nine confirmed anti-HCV-reactive patients had normal ALT (20–37 U/L). Liver biopsies were not performed. Two patients with detectable HCV RNA levels were infected with HIV. One of the patients had a CD4 of $77/mm^3$ (normal 685–1499) and exhibited the highest HCV RNA level $(12,322 \, Eq/mL \times 10^3)$.

Due to the technical difficulties inherent in the PCR, the bDNA assay could become a relatively simple and clinically acceptable test to evaluate HCV infection in dialysis patients. Although less sensitive than PCR at low levels of viremia, this quantitative assay may be useful to follow disease activity and to monitor the effect of antiviral therapy (59,60). In the latter study, patients with high levels of viremia acquired their infection by transfusion, were less likely to respond to interferon-α therapy, and were likely to manifest histological evidence of hepatic inflammation.

UNRESOLVED ISSUES

Incidence of HCV infection in dialysis patients

The National Surveillance of Hemodialysis Associated Diseases continues to show a low incidence of non-A, non-B hepatitis in the United States (61). In 1990, the incidence was 0.1%. In a recent study, the incidence of HCV infection in a dialysis unit was determined using a first-generation assay (62). Yearly incidence rates of 6.1%,

4.6%, 4.9%, 3.1%, 2.1%, and 2.2% were obtained using frozen sera collected between 1984 and 1990, respectively. A study of the incidence of anti-HCV positivity (confirmed by RIBA-II) was carried out between May 1991 and November 1992 in 15 Belgian hemodialysis units (63). The observed average yearly incidence was 1.7%. Three of eight seroconverters in this study did not receive transfusions, suggesting nosocomial transmission.

In a recent multicenter study of HCV infection in hemodialysis patients and staff, the cumulative incidence of infection as measured by first-generation assays was 4.6% over a period of 18 months (64). No staff members became positive, confirming previous studies (29,34) that demonstrated a low risk of HCV infection in dialysis staff. The validity of these estimates remains unclear due to the low sensitivity and specificity of transaminases and antibody tests and the variability of criteria for the diagnosis of liver disease. Definitive information about the incidence of HCV infection will not be available, however, until epidemiological studies are performed utilizing the recently introduced measurements of HCV RNA, HCV genotypes, and IgM antibodies to HCV antigens.

Risk factors

In most studies, duration of hemodialysis and transfusions have been the most important risks factors for the development of HCV infection in dialysis patients. Intravenous drug abusers have been found to have a high prevalence of HCV as well as HBV and HIV infection. Patients may have also acquired the infection at the time of a prior failed kidney transplant, either from blood transfusions or from an infected donor kidney. In some studies, however, a correlation with the history of blood transfusions has not been observed (64,65). For example, in the multicenter study (64), logistic regression analysis revealed that anti-HCV positivity correlated with length of time on dialysis, history of intravenous drugs, and history of non-A, non-B hepatitis. Anti-HCV positivity was not associated with history of blood transfusions, race, gender, or age.

In some, but not all studies, transminases and anti-HBc have been found to be surrogate markers for HCV infection. In the study of Willems et al. (66), 7 of 79 patients on hemodialysis were anti-HCV (+), and HCV RNA was detected in four. Transaminases were normal in all. Anti-HBc was detected in 27 of 72 (37%) patients without any marker and in four patients with markers for HCV infection. The authors concluded that surrogate markers (anti-HBc and transaminases) are not useful in the identification of HCV carriers in dialysis patients.

Outbreaks of HCV infection in dialysis units

There have been several outbreaks of HCV infection in dialysis units (67–70a,70b). It has been suggested that contamination of environmental surfaces, equipment, or poor universal precaution techniques of the dialysis staff might have been responsible for these outbreaks. In a well-investigated outbreak, it was determined that inadequate infection control measures might have been responsible for the spread of the infection (70). It appears that contamination of parts of the dialysis machines that are not accessible to routine cleansing is an uncommon event. Nevertheless, setting aside machines for anti-HCV (+) patients may decrease the incidence of infection in dialysis units with a high prevalence of HCV (71). Changing membranes on the venous pressure monitors from permeable PTFE to impermeable PVC, disinfection with 4% hypochlorite, and use of transducer protectors capable of withstanding high pressures are among the recommended measures (70,72). The evidence for transmission to household or sexual contacts is more limited and needs further study (73–78).

Infection control strategies

Current Centers for Disease Control (CDC) recommendations for the control of NANBH and hepatitis C in patients undergoing maintenance hemodialysis remain unchanged despite suggestive evidence of intradialytic spread (61). Routine screening of patients and staff for HCV infection is not advocated for infection control. The insensitivity of transaminase determinations and the recent discovery that most HCV (+) patients are viremic carriers should lead to reexamination of infection control policies in dialysis units. Although the infectivity of HCV appears to be less than that for HBV, presumably due to lower titer of virus in the blood, the potential for transmission in the dialysis setting has been documented. Furthermore, knowledge of the HCV status of dialysis patients may also be necessary to help diagnose the type of liver involvement and to determine the suitability of these patients for renal transplantation.

Progression to cirrhosis

In patients with posttransfusion hepatitis, persistent biochemical abnormalities occur in more than 50% of the patients, and as many as 20%–30% develop cirrhosis. It appears that progression to cirrhosis is not as high in anti-HCV (+) patients on chronic dialysis. In one study, however, 40% of anti-HCV (+) patients exhibited peripheral signs of chronic liver disease, 34% hepatomegaly and 9% splenomegaly (72). Unfortunately, there are few liver biopsy studies of patients with or without HCV infection on chronic dialysis. In the study of Alfurayh et al. (79), of 13 anti-HCV (+) patients who underwent a liver biopsy, six demonstrated chronic persistent hepatitis and the remaining seven showed changes of chronic active hepatitis. Gilli et al. (80) biopsied 12 hemodialysis patients with non-A, non-B hepatitis (six anti-HCV (+)) and found mild chronic active hepatitis in one and chronic persistent hepatitis or lesser findings in the other 11 patients. In a recent study from France (8), liver biopsy performed in 17 dialysis patients revealed chronic hepatitis in 16 cases (two had cir-

rhosis) and steatosis in one. In a study from Spain (81), several histopathologic patterns were observed in 33 liver biopsy specimens from anti-HCV (+) patients: cirrhosis ($n = 3$), chronic active hepatitis ($n = 14$), chronic persistent hepatitis ($n = 2$), hemosiderosis ($n = 5$), reactive hepatitis ($n = 6$), and others ($n = 3$).

It is recommended that all anti-HCV (+) hemodialysis patients being evaluated for renal transplantation undergo complete evaluation of liver function, including biopsy. This evaluation is felt to be necessary because the progression of liver disease in transplanted patients may accelerate due to unhampered viral replication during immunosuppressive therapy. For example, in the study of Rao et al. (82), 28% of transplanted patients exhibited early chronic active hepatitis and 21% advanced chronic active hepatitis. Progression to hepatocellular failure and death after a mean follow-up of 5.7 ± 3.9 years occurred in 35% of patients with early chronic active hepatitis and 60% of patients with advanced chronic active hepatitis. Unfortunately, testing for HCV infection was not performed, and recent studies have not confirmed an aggressive course in HCV-infected patients.

Therapy of HCV infection

Interferon-α2b has proved to be efficacious in the treatment of patients with chronic hepatitis C. Normalization of transaminases can be accomplished in approximately 45% of patients (83–85). However, once interferon therapy is stopped, relapse occurs in up to 80% of the patients, with sustained remission following interferon therapy in 15%–20% of patients over a period of 2–4 years. Biochemical remission is associated with virologic and histologic remission as well. The efficacy of IFN-α2b treatment for chronic hepatitis B is limited in immunocompromised patients (i.e., HIV positive) (86), but the response rate among immunocompromised patients with chronic hepatitis C has not been definitively characterized. Long-term, low-dose maintenance therapy is another approach that is being explored to improve viral clearance and amelioration of histologic progression.

There are few studies (87,87a,87b,87c) assessing the effectiveness of intravenous interferon-α2b in eliminating viremia and arresting the progression of liver disease in hemodialysis patients with chronic HCV infection. The authors concluded that the response rates where similar to those in nonuremic patients but the incidence of side effects was more pronounced. Eliminating viremia would be expected to slow the progression of liver disease and to reduce the chance of spread of infection in the dialysis setting.

TRANSPLANTATION

The success of renal transplantation as a therapy for end-stage renal disease has focused attention on factors affecting long-term patient and graft survival. Although the spectrum of liver disease following renal transplantation is varied (22,88–90), chronic liver disease contributes substantially to late posttransplant morbidity. The screening of large numbers of kidney recipients demonstrated that HCV was the causative agent for most cases of what had previously been referred to as posttransplant non-A, non-B hepatitis (91,92). Considering that 10%–30% of hemodialysis patients in the United States are anti-HCV positive (29,31), the pretransplant evaluation of these patients and the contribution of HCV infection to long-term patient outcome are important issues.

Transmission

Previous studies of asymptomatic blood donors have detected an anti-c100 seroprevalence of 0.5%–1.2%. Using the anti-c100 ELISA, Pereira and colleagues (93) reported that 1.8% of the cadaver organ donors in their series were anit-HCV positive. Using the same assay, we screened 484 donor serum samples and identified 89 positive specimens (18%), of which 33 (6.8%) were RIBA reactive (94). An obvious explanation for the discrepancy between these results is not readily available, although this may simply reflect significant differences in the geographic prevalence of HCV infection. In fact, data from a collaborative nationwide survey involving several organ procurement organizations has demonstrated a wide range of anti-HCV positivity (95). The observed higher prevalence of anti-HCV among cadaver organ donors when compared to the general community may reflect life-style and socioeconomic factors that are more prevalent among those individuals that become organ donors.

The transmission of HCV by solid-organ transplantation has been unequivocally demonstrated (94,96). However, there remain notable discrepancies in the reported incidence of transmission between centers. Pereira and coworkers (96) detected HCV RNA in 7 of 26 (27%) organ recipients preoperatively and 23 of 24 (96%) during follow-up after transplantation from an HCV carrier donor. They concluded that there was a high likelihood of transmission of HCV with solid organ transplantation. Although these data are compelling and undoubtedly represent true viral transmission in a certain number of cases, several questions remain unanswered from this study. It was unstated whether the patients received any blood products in the perioperative period. This point is especially relevant, since a number of these transplants were performed prior to the commercial licensing of the anti-c100 ELISA assay. Secondly, the inclusion of several liver recipients is not germaine to the question, since transmission will undoubtedly occur when studying a hepatotropic virus such as HCV. Finally, an analysis of historic, stored serum samples for HCV RNA generates many false-negative results; thus, any assessment of the extent of pretransplant viremia that relies on stored samples for purposes of comparison with freshly obtained posttransplant samples is likely to exaggerate the extent of seroconversion.

In our study (94), liver histology was available from 24 RIBA-positive organ donors. Chronic active or chronic persistent hepatitis was detected in 18 of 24 (75%) specimens, confirming that the majority of seropositive organ donors harbor active disease. Nevertheless, among the 27 kidney and heart recipients in whom the donor had either chronic active or chronic persistent hepatitis on biopsy (and HCV RNA in 13 of 15), only nine (33%) developed posttransplant liver dysfunction. Moreover, among 20 recipients of a kidney from an HCV-RNA-positive donor, only six (30%) developed biochemical evidence of liver disease. The remaining 14 patients maintained normal liver chemistries, with a mean follow-up of 27 ± 8 months. These findings contrast with the results of Pereira et al. (93), in which a high prevalence of liver disease in recipients of an organ from an HCV carrier donor was reported. Finally, we found no differences in 5-year patient and graft survival, regardless of the donor's serologic status.

A possible explanation for the discrepancy in reported HCV transmission may involve differences in organ preservation. The New England Organ Bank uses slush preservation, while we have always used pulsatile perfusion. Preliminary studies from our center have demonstrated a greater than 99% reduction in the viral load in the kidney and detectable HCV RNA in the perfusate after several hours of pulsatile perfusion (97). Conceivably, the reported differences in HCV transmission may be partly explainable on this basis, although other issues, including differing strain virulence patterns and recipient disease susceptibility associated with specific HLA specificities, require further study.

Seroprevalence of anti-HCV

Several investigators have reported the results of surveillance studies of anti-HCV among kidney recipients (Table 5). Using a second-generation anti-HCV assay, 17% of serum samples collected from the patients transplanted at our center were anti-HCV positive (98). This finding is consistent with reports from other centers in which 10%–49% of transplant patients were anti-HCV positive (6,91,92,94,99–104). These findings are not unexpected considering the high prevalence of anti-HCV among hemodialysis patients (8,34,39,43).

HCV RNA detection

In our series, HCV RNA was detected in the serum of 39 of 53 (74%) patients who were RIBA positive when transplanted. This is consistent with a recent report by Chan et al. (103) in which 95% of anti-HCV positive patients were viremic (Table 5). Also of note was the finding that 20 of 39 (52%) PCR-positive patients in our series maintained normal transaminases throughout their posttransplant follow-up. Ponz and colleagues detected liver disease in two thirds of the anti-HCV carriers transplanted at their center (99). Thus, between 33% and 51% of the anti-HCV-positive

Table 5. HCV infection in renal allograft recipients

Author (year, country)	Ref.	EIA-I no. pos/no. tested (%)	EIA-II no. pos/no. tested (%)	HCV RNA no. pos/no. EIA pos. (%)
Roth (1991, USA)	96	179/596 (30)	—	—
Ponz (1991, Spain)	97	32/67 (48)	—	—
Baur (1991, Germany)	98	27/272 (10)	—	—
Klauser (1992, Austria)	99	43/324 (13)	—	—
Huang (1992, China)	102	59/120 (49)	—	—
Morales (1992, Spain)	89	66/200 (33)	—	—
Pol (1992, France)	90	20/127 (24)	—	—
Stempel (1993, USA)	100	76/716 (11)	—	—
Chan (1993, Hong Kong)	101	—	19/185 (10)[a]	18/19 (95)
Roth (1994, USA)	6	—	109/641 (17)	39/53 (74)

[a] Recombinant immunoblot assay.
Reprinted from (193).

Table 6. Quantitative polymerase chain reaction and HCV strain identification[a]

	Posttransplant liver function[b]		
	Normal (n = 32)	Abnormal (n = 34)	p value
HCV RNA (copies/mL $\times 10^6$)	8.2 ± 13.8	6.9 ± 10.2	NS
Strain			
BK (n = 14)	7.8 ± 9.3 (5)	10.4 ± 16.4 (9)	NS
Hutch (n = 15)	6.4 ± 4.3 (8)	6.9 ± 4.8 (7)	NS
HCV-1 (n = 6)	16.7 ± 24.9 (5)	12 (1)	NS
HCV-M (n = 4)	2.1 ± 1.2 (2)	1.3 ± 0.3 (2)	NS
HCV-1/BK (n = 1)	8.8 (1)	—	
HCV-1/Hutch (n = 1)	—	8.8 (1)	

[a] Strain identification by restriction fragment length polymorphism of PCR product with confirmation by direct sequencing. Strain identification in patients with very low viral titers was not possible.
[b] Each value denotes the mean ± SD. Numbers in parentheses represent the number of patients in each group.
Reprinted from (193).

transplant recipients in these two reports maintained normal LFTs, emphasizing the low sensitivity of liver transaminases in the detection of active viral replication, a finding previously noted in hemodialysis patients (81). We recommend that every transplant patient with documented HCV infection and abnormal transaminases have a liver biopsy to morphologically characterize the extent of disease. This approach is supported by recent data from Rao et al. demonstrating histologic progression to cirrhosis in serial biopsies obtained from transplant patients with chronic active hepatitis (82). Until data are available describing the liver histology and clinical course in HCV-infected transplant patients with normal transaminases, recommendations on the timing and/or usefulness of a liver biopsy in this cohort of patients cannot be made.

Quantitative PCR analysis of fresh serum from the 39 HCV-RNA-positive patients in our series demonstrated that a wide range of viral copy number was present (0.13–88 $\times 10^6$/mL). Moreover, there was no correlation between HCV copy number and biochemical liver function abnormalities. This finding must be confirmed in a larger number of patients.

The rapid expansion of investigation in this field has led to the observation that HCV represents a variable group of agents, and multiple HCV strains have subsequently been identified worldwide (3). We detected HCV strains HCV-1, BK, Hutch, and HCV-M among our patients (Table 6), one of which (BK) was originally reported from Japan (105). Of interest, two patients were coinfected with two different strains of HCV. It will be important to study the clinical consequence of infection with multiple HCV strains. In our relatively small series, we were unable to detect any clinical patterns that would suggest differences in strain virulence. Nevertheless, the possibility that different HCV agents cause varying clinical outcomes requires investigation, especially in the immunosuppressed transplant recipient. An association between liver cirrhosis and hepatocellular carcinoma has been reported in HCV-infected Japanese patients (106), and a recent report of hepatocellular carcinoma developing in a Japanese renal allograft recipient (107) suggests that increased surveillance for cirrhosis and/or early carcinoma is warranted for the HCV-infected transplant recipient. This may be especially true for patients infected with Southeast Asian strains of HCV.

Coinfection with HBV and HCV

Huang and colleagues (104) screened 120 Chinese renal transplant recipients and found 49.2% to be anti-HCV positive, approximately half of whom were also HBsAg positive. Among the entire 120 patients, 34% developed chronic hepatitis, although this figure rose to 50% (14 of 28) in the coinfected patients. Furthermore, 21% of the dual-infected patients were found to have cirrhosis versus none in the HCV-positive and HBV-negative groups. The authors concluded that coinfection with HCV and HBV can lead to a particularly aggressive form of liver disease in renal allograft recipients.

The HCV-infected kidney recipient

We found RIBA positivity to be an independent predictor of posttransplant liver disease (6). Chan et al. (108) reported similar results, although 75% of their anti-HCV-positive patients developed liver dysfunction, in contrast to only 34% of our RIBA-positive cohort. We also observed a relationship between the dosage of ALG administered for induction therapy and the likelihood that the RIBA-positive patient would develop posttransplant liver disease. Antilymphocyte preparations are known to predispose to viral reactivation; thus, our findings are not surprising and emphasize the need to use these products with caution in the RIBA-positive transplant recipient.

Patients who were seropositive for anti-HCV were more heavily transfused and were more likely to experience serious infectious events and acute rejection episodes (Table 7). Prior studies have suggested that transplant recipients with active viral replication (i.e., cytomegalovirus) are further immunosuppressed as a consequence of an interaction between the viral infection and the host's immune responsiveness (109,110). Further study, however, is required to properly elucidate the mechanisms whereby HCV infection may interfere with the host's immune surveillance. Seemingly at odds with these findings was the nearly two-fold increase in acute rejection among the anti-HCV-positive patients. This finding contrasts with the results of Ponz et al. (99), who reported no difference in rejection rates between anti-HCV-positive and anti-HCV-negative patients. Although an explanation for our findings is not readily apparent, several possibilities exist. It is likely that the amount of immunosuppression the patients were receiving was markedly reduced following a serious infec-

Table 7. Univariate analysis according to perioperative anti-HCV serostatus

Variable	Anti-HCV[a]		
	Positive (n = 109)	Negative (n = 200)	p value
Age (years)	47 ± 11.3	42.9 ± 12.5	NS
Gender (male/female)	66/43	115/85	NS
Follow-up (months)	65.7 ± 28.9	81.3 ± 30.3	<0.001
Blood (no. units)[b]	9.5 ± 13.4	6.9 ± 5.7	<0.001
Preoperative LFT's[c]	3/109 (2.7)	1/200 (0.5)	NS
ALG (mg)[d]	6983 ± 6169	6451 ± 5750	NS
Infections[e]	24/109 (22)	26/200 (13)	0.03
Rejections	40/109 (37)	41/200 (20)	0.002
Abnormal LFT[f]	37/109 (34)	38/200 (19)	0.00

[a] Each value denotes mean ± SD. Number in parentheses are percentage. Anti-HCV detected by recombinant immunoblot assay.
[b] Preoperative blood transfusions.
[c] Abnormal pretransplant liver function tests.
[d] Total antilymphoblast globulin administered as induction therapy.
[e] Requiring hospitalization and antimicrobial therapy.
[f] Chronically abnormal liver function tests posttransplant.
Reprinted from (193).

tion, thus permitting an alloimmune response against the graft to occur. In fact, 10 of 24 (41%) RIBA-positive patients with infection experienced at least one rejection episode. Alternatively, HCV infection could initiate a process that results in the upregulation of MHC Class II antigen expression in the allograft. In this regard, kidney recipients with active cytomegalovirus infection have been described who either concomitantly or shortly thereafter developed acute rejection (111). In view of these risks, the anti-HCV-positive kidney recipient should be closely monitored for infection and allograft dysfunction. Furthermore, in light of the data linking ALG dosage with posttransplant liver dysfunction, the use of antilymphocyte preparations in the HCV-infected patient with allograft rejection becomes problematic. If possible, antilymphocyte products should not be used as first-line therapy to treat rejection in these individuals.

Transplant evaluation of the anti-HCV-seropositive ESRD patient

Although the anti-HCV-positive patient may be at increased risk for infection, rejection, and posttransplant liver disease, there has as yet not been a demonstrated difference in patient and graft survival. For this reason, HCV infection should not be considered a contraindication to renal transplantation. However, it is advisable that the evaluation of the anti-HCV-positive transplant candidate should include PCR testing, if available, and liver biopsy to histologically stage the patient's disease. The latter is recommended regardless of the transaminase levels. Furthermore, careful studies of the safety and efficacy of antiviral therapy (i.e., interferon) in the ESRD patient are needed to determine if a course of antiviral treatment should precede transplantation. Patients with minimal changes or chronic persistent hepatitis are clearly suitable for transplant; however, sufficient date are not yet available to determine whether the HCV-infected patient with chronic active hepatitis or early cirrhosis should be transplanted or should remain on dialysis.

HCV in clinical nephrology

GLOMERULONEPHRITIS

Several histologic forms of immune-complex-mediated glomerulonephritis have been linked to HBV infection. It is not surprising, therefore, that infection with HCV has been recently associated with the development of membranoproliferative (MPGN) and membranous glomerulonephritis (MGN).

Rollino and coworkers (112) were the first to associate HCV infection with an immune-complex type of glomerulonephritis. They screened 27 patients with MGN and found one who was anti-HCV seropositive. The patient entered remission following steroid plus chlorambucil therapy. MGN was also diagnosed in two bone-marrow recipients 9 and 18 months posttransplantation (113). Both recipients were PCR positive in both the serum and renal tissue.

Johnson et al. (114) described eight patients with immune-complex glomerulonephritis of the membranoproliferative pattern associated with active HCV infection. All eight patients had HCV RNA detected in the serum, elevated serum aminotransferase, and hypocomplementemia. Five of eight had circulating cryoglobulins, while three of four biopsies studied with electron microscopy showed organized, finely fibrillar, cylindric or immunotactoid-like structures compatible with cryoglobulins. Four patients were treated with interferon-α2b for 2–12 months duration. All converted to HCV RNA negative, and 3 of 4 had a decrease in urinary protein excretion to the normal range. The membranoproliferative pattern of glomerulonephritis has also been reported by two other investigators in association with HCV infection (115,116). Of interest is a recent case report in which heavy proteinuria developed 3 months after liver transplantation in a HCV-infected patient (116). Renal biopsy demonstrated changes compatible with MPGN. It is interesting to speculate why this patient's nephropathy manifested itself early after transplant, whereas the HCV infection had been present for a considerable period of time pre-transplant. Conceivably, the balance of antigen–antibody complexes was altered by the effect of immunosuppression on the circulating viral load.

These cases illustrate several important clinical points. Patients with chronic liver disease and evidence of HCV infection who have abnormal urinalysis findings may have an immune-complex glomerulonephritis. These patients should be tested for cryoglobulins, rheumatoid factor, and serum complement concentrations as part of their evaluation. Renal biopsy should be obtained to confirm the diagnosis and to assist in a decision to use interferon-α2b.

ESSENTIAL MIXED CRYOGLOBULINEMIA

The clinical syndrome of essential mixed cryoglobulinemia (EMC) is characterized by weakness, arthralgia, purpura, and, in some patients, an immune-complex glomerular lesion that has been referred to as *cryoglobulinemic glomerulonephritis* (117). Whereas 60%–75% of mixed cryoglobulinemias are associated with infectious or lymphophroliferative disorders, hepatobiliary disease, connective-tissue disease, or immunologically mediated glomerular disease, the remaining 30% have no underlying or associated disease.

Efforts to identify a single antigen in the serum of patients with EMC that is bound to polyclonal IgG and that then binds together with the polyclonal IgG to a polyclonal or monoclonal IgM have been unsuccessful. Some investigators have suggested an association between HBV infection and EMC, but these findings have not been consistently confirmed in subsequent studies.

Recently, several groups of investigators have detected a high prevalence of anti-HCV antibodies among patients with EMC (118–123) (Table 8). Moreover, several of these groups (118,119,124) have detected HCV RNA in anti-HCV-seronegative patients, confirming a significant incidence of false-negative serological testing for anti-HCV antibodies among patients with EMC. As summarized in Table 8, whereas 69% of patients with EMC were anti-HCV reactive using sensitive second-generation assays, 81% were HCV RNA positive by polymerase chain reaction.

In the study of Agnello and coworkers (118), quantitative assays of HCV RNA (Table 9) demonstrated that more than 99% of the HCV RNA in serum was cryoprecipitated. Furthermore, additional testing confirmed that the cryoprecipitation of HCV RNA from the serum was selective and specifically dependent on the Type II cryoglobulins in HCV-infected serum.

A definitive role for HCV immune complexes in the generation of the pathologic abnormalities of this disease awaits the demonstration of HCV antigens in the renal and vascular lesions that characterize EMC. Although the data available thus far suggest a strong association of HCV infection with EMC, conclusive studies must still be conducted.

If HCV is involved in the pathogenesis of EMC, then antiviral therapy may have a role in the treatment of patients with cryoglobulinemia. Several reports (118,125,126) have demonstrated a benefit of interferon with marked clinical improvement. Most of these reports are anecdotal and must be confirmed in larger series.

Table 8. Association of HCV with essential mixed cryoglobulinemia

Ref.	Type of mixed cryos	Serum HCV antibodies EIA[a] #pos/#tested (%)	RIBA[b] #pos/#tested (%)	HCV RNA #pos/#tested (%)	Cryoprecipitate HCV-Ab #pos/#tested (%)	HCV RNA #pos /#tested (%)
116	Type II	8/19 (42)	8/19 (42)	16/19 (84)	1/4 (25)[c]	4/4 (100)[c]
117	Type II	50/51 (98)	33/50 (66)[c]	13/16 (81)	21/51 (41)[d]	
118	Type II	21/30 (70)	21/30 (70)			
119	Type II and III	13/26 (50)	11/26 (42)			
120	Type II and III	129/161 (80)	88/100 (88)[c]			
120	Secondary	44/66 (70)				
121	Type II and III	28/52 (54)			7/28 (25)[c]	
122	Type II	13/15 (87)	13/15 (87)	5/7 (7)		
TOTAL		306/417 (73)	202/292 (69)	34/42 (81)	29/83 (35)	4/4 (100)

[a] Second-generation enzyme immunoassay.
[b] Recombinant immunoblot assay.
[c] All patients were anti-HCV positive.
[d] Prevalence of anti-HCV increased to 94% after removal of IgM RF from cryoprecipitate.
Reprinted from (193).

Table 9. Quantitative studies of HCV RNA in serum samples and cryoglobulins from patients with Type II cryoglobulinemia[a]

Cryocrit (%)	HCV RNA Serum	Supernatant after Cryoprecipitate	Cryoprecipitate	Relative HCV RNA concentration in cryoprecipitate[b]	Decrease in serum HCV RNA after cryoprecipitation (%)
4	22 ng/mL	0.015 ng/mL	15 ng/mL	1000	>99
8	50 pg/mL	0.030 pg/mL	30 pg/mL	1000	>99
4	7 pg/mL	0.006 ng/mL	NT[c]	NT	>99
1	700 pg/mL	0.080 pg/mL	NT	NT	>99

[a] Adapted from Agnello V, et al.: *N Engl J Med* 327:1490–1495, 1992.
[b] Values were calculated using the following equation:
    cryoprecipitate HCV RNA concentration/supernatant HCV RNA concentration.
[c] NT denotes not tested.

HEPATITIS B VIRUS

Hepatitis B virus (HBV) chronically infects over 5% of the world's population, with as many as 150–200 million people estimated to be persistent carriers of HBsAg. The majority of these carriers are in the Orient and sub-Saharan Africa, where HBV is endemic. Hepatitis B has been identified as a major cause of acute and chronic hepatitis, cirrhosis, and hepatocellular carcinoma (127). Furthermore, a variety of immunologically mediated disorders have been associated with HBV infection, including vasculitis and several morphologic patterns of glomerulonephritis.

Patients with chronic renal failure have consistently been shown to have a substantially higher prevalence of HBV infection than the general population. This is partly due to the aforementioned association of HBV with immune-mediated renal diseases, plus the historically high risk of acquiring HBV infection within the dialysis setting from either contaminated blood products or nosocomial transmission.

Dialysis

SEROLOGIC AND MOLECULAR EVIDENCE OF INFECTION

The impact of HBV infection in the hemodialysis population has been extensively evaluated. HBV infection evolves into a chronic HBsAg carrier state in 60% of uremic patients, with HBeAg detected in 70%–90%. Nationwide, the incidence of HBsAg positivity among dialysis patients has decreased from 3.0% in 1976 to 0.2% in 1990. Similarly, the prevalence of HBsAg has decreased from 7.8% to 1.2% during the same time period. Undoubtedly, the implementation of effective infection control strategies, including isolation of HBsAg-positive patients on dedicated machines, routine serologic screening, and routine disinfection procedures, have all had a major impact on the spread of HBV in the dialysis setting (128). Furthermore, the introduction of the plasma-derived hepatitis B vaccine in 1982 and the recombinant vaccine in 1986 further contributed to the declining incidence of HBV (vide infra).

In a study of 49 HBsAg positive hemodialysis patients, Harnett et al. (129) noted that only 19% converted to HBsAg negative during follow-up, a figure considerably less than the 90%–95% conversion rate reported for non-ESRD HBV-infected patients (130). In addition, 9 of 31 (29%) patients developed chronic hepatitis, although only 1 of 31 under age 50 died from complications of liver disease.

Evidence for active HBV replication was sought by Pao et al. (131) in a study of 239 hemodialysis patients. Whereas 42 of 239 (17%) were HBsAg positive, only 15 (35.7%) had detectable serum levels of HBV DNA. Of note, 22 of 197 (11.2%) HBsAg-negative patients were HBV DNA positive, a finding that brings into question the adequacy of HBsAg or anti-HBV antibodies to properly identify HBV infection in the uremic patient who may not be immunocompetent.

HBV VACCINATION

The introduction of a plasma-derived hepatitis B vaccine in 1982 and the genetically engineered recombinant hepatitis B vaccine in 1986 offered the exciting possibility of eradicating or severely reducing the spread of HBV infection within the dialysis population. Clearly, the success of such a program would be dependent on the implementation of effective vaccination programs in a group of patients who were immunocompetent and thus capable of generating anti-HBs antibodies. In healthy adults, more than 90% of hepatitis-B vaccinated patients respond with an anti-HBs titer greater than 10 mIU/mL, a level generally considered to offer protection. Unfortunately, neither the effective delivery of vaccination to most ESRD patients nor the hoped-for antibody response in those receiving the vaccine has been achieved.

Only 17% of hemodialysis patients were reported to have received the full, three-dose immunization schedule as of 1990 (132). In combination with this surprisingly low figure, numerous investigators have demonstrated that only 50%–60% of vaccinated ESRD patients actually develop protective titers of anti-HBs antibody (133–136). The combined impact of these two findings has resulted in a large number of hemodialysis patients remaining at risk to

acquire HBV infection more than a decade after the licensing of the first vaccine.

Most studies have noted an association between age and immunoresponsiveness to the hepatitis B vaccine. In one study (133), 64% of patients under age 40 developed adequate anti-HBs levels, in contrast to only 37% of the patients over age 60. A similar association was noted by Buti et al. (137), although the effect of age was not found in the study of Pasko (136). The antibody response to vaccine also appears to be lower in males then females. In a study by Stevens et al. (138), all female patients converted to anti-HBs positive, while only 76% of male patients became positive.

Patients on regular hemodialysis exhibit an impaired immune potential that mainly involves T-cell-mediated immune responses (139). These patients are particularly at risk to be nonresponders to the hepatitis B vaccine. In vaccine nonresponders, Meuer et al. (140) found impaired monocyte activity that failed to support the process of T-cell activation. In fact, the degree of monocyte dysfunction in vitro correlated with the patients' in vivo response to hepatitis B vaccine. Further evidence for an impaired immune response was reported in two other studies that detected higher IL-2 receptor expression in nonresponders than in those with higher anti-HBs levels (135,141).

Several groups have attempted to boost the immune response of nonresponders by administering an immunomodulator. Thymopentine was reported to significantly increase the percentage of vaccine responders in two different reports (142,143). Also of interest was a study by Sennesael et al. (139) in which a higher percentage of r-HuEPO-treated dialysis patients (80%) developed anti-HBs antibodies compared to controls (54%). Furthermore, patients receiving r-HuEPO consistently had higher anti-HBs titers than uremic controls. R-HuEPO-treated patients had a decrease in total number of lymphocytes and T cells; however, the decrease in the suppressor-cell subset was more pronounced, therefore tending to increase the helper: suppressor cell ratio. Thus, ample evidence is available to suggest that hepatitis B vaccine nonresponders are predominantly those patients with impaired immune responsiveness, and interventions aimed at enhancing their immune response may increase the percentage of patients successfully immunized.

Several groups have reported the follow-up of ESRD patients who initially responded to the hepatitis B vaccine (anti-HBs > 10 mIU/mL). Stevens et al. (133) found that 15% of the responding patients lost protective antibody on follow-up testing, a figure similar to the 21% seroconversion reported by Pasko et al. (136). The same authors also noted that one third of the responding patients had steadily declining anti-HBs titers, although still greater than 10 mIU/mL at 2 years postvaccination (136). In a study with 3-year follow-up, Buti and colleagues (137) reported that 18 of 44 (41%) responders had no detectable anti-HBs levels. Those who maintained immuno-reactivity were younger and had higher initial anti-HBs titers.

CURRENT RECOMMENDATIONS FOR VACCINATION AND
ROUTINE SEROLOGIC SCREENING

Patients and staff should continue to be screened for
HBsAg and anti-HBs when first being evaluated in the
unit. For hemodialysis patients, an increased number or
larger doses of the HB vaccine are required to induce a
protective antibody response in comparison to healthy
adults. Susceptible patients (HBsAg and anti-HBs negative) should receive 40 ug of the recombinant vaccine at 0,
1, and 6 months. Hemodialysis staff members appear to
respond in a manner similar to other health care workers
and need only receive 20 ug at each injection.

The falling incidence of hepatitis B infection in
hemodialysis centers in the United States and an increasing
use of the hepatitis B vaccine has resulted in a reduction in
the recommended frequency of routine serologic screening
(Table 10). Susceptible staff and patients (HBsAg and anti-
HBs negative) who have not yet received the vaccine, are
currently being vaccinated, or have not adequately responded to the vaccine should continue to have regular
HBsAg and anti-HBs testing. Susceptible patients should
continue to be tested for HBsAg monthly; however, anti-
HBs testing can be decreased to semiannually (144). Susceptible staff can be tested for HBsAg and anti-HBs
semiannually.

If unvaccinated patients are found to have protective
levels of anti-HBs, they need only be checked annually to
verify their immune statue. If their titers fall below 10 mIU/
mL, they should be vaccinated at that time. In contrast,
staff members with anti-HBs above 10 mIU/mL on two
separate occasions are considered immune and do not need
any further screening for anti-HBs.

Responding patients who developed a titer above
10 mIU/mL need only be tested annually thereafter to
confirm their status. Decreases in the titer of anti-HBs
below protective levels should be treated with a booster
injection.

Hepatitis-B-associated renal syndromes

Hepatitis B is a DNA virus that primarily infects the liver
and has been recognized as a leading cause of acute
and chronic hepatitis worldwide. The Australia antigen
(HBsAg) constitutes the envelope protein of HBV, while
other antigenic components include the hepatitis B core
antigen (HBsAg), hepatitis B e antigen (HBeAg), hepatitis
B x antigen (HBxAg), and DNA polymerase. During various phases of infection, antibodies to these antigens may be
detectable in serum. Immune complexes containing anti-
HBs, anti-HBe, anti-HBc, and anti-HBx can be found in
the sera and tissues of HBV-infected patients (145,146).
Not unexpectedly, immune-complex disease has been described in carriers of HBV and can present as glomerulonephritis, arthritis, and a vasculitis of the polyarteritis
nodosa pattern.

GLOMERULONEPHRITIS

In 1971, Combes et al. (147) first reported an association
between HBV infection and glomerulonephritis. A
variety of morphological lesions associated with HBV
infection have subsequently been described, including
membranous glomerulonephritis (MGN), membranoproliferative glomerulonephritis (MPGN), and mesangial proliferative glomerulonephritis.

The MGN seen in association with HBV usually occurs
in children, with a predominance in males. Acquisition of
HBV in children appears to be secondary to both vertical
transmission from infected mothers (148) and horizontal
transmission from infected siblings (149) in those geographic distributions where HBV remains endemic. Numerous reports from Japan and Southeast Asia have
documented that upwards of 80%–100% of children with
MGN have HBsAg antigenemia (149–154). In contrast,
only 30%–40% of adults with MGN are HBsAg positive
(153,155).

Table 10. Recommendations for serologic surveillance for hepatitis B in chronic hemodialysis centers

Vaccination and serologic status	Frequency of screening			
	HBsAg		Anti-HBs	
	Patients	Staff	Patients	Staff
Unvaccinated				
Susceptible	Monthly	Semiannually	Semiannually	Semiannually
HBsAg carrier	Annually	Annually	None	None
Anti-HBs positive	None	None	Annually	None
Vaccinees				
Anti-HBs positive	None	None	Annually	None
Low level or no anti-HBs	Monthly	Semiannually	Semiannually	Semiannually

Reprinted from (142).

Most patients with HBV-associated MGN have HBsAg and anti-HBc in the circulation (149,150,152,156,159). Furthermore, 60%–80% also have HBeAg, with the remainder being anti-HBe antibody positive (150,152,157,160–162). Most studies demonstrate hypocomplementemia in 20%–60% of patients and circulating immune complexes (CICs) in up to 80% of cases of childhood HBV MGN (157,161,162).

A recent review by Johnson and Couser (163) thoroughly discussed several different possibilities for the pathogenesis of HBV MGN. The major HBV antigens, including HBsAg, HBeAg, and HBcAg, have all been localized to the glomerular capillary wall in HBV MGN. This finding supports a mechanism in which HBV antigen containing immune complexes would localize to the subepithelial space either as a result of passive trapping of CICs or secondary to in situ formation of immune complexes. Size and charge properties of HBeAg and anti-HBe antibody favor a local process of immune-deposit formation involving HBeAg and antibody (163).

MPGN has been reported by multiple authors to be associated with HBV infection (152,162,163,165–169). Some studies have found an association of MPGN with the HBsAg carrier state (152,160,169), although a study from Hong Kong failed to find such an association (155).

Patients are often hypocomplementemic (152,164), and CICs may be present (168). Nephrotic syndrome and microhematuria are commonly part of the clinical presentation. Both hypertension and renal insufficiency may also be present (152). Histologically, the renal lesion resembles MPGN I, with subendothelial deposits and mild proliferation. In many cases, HBsAg has been localized to the glomerular capillary wall, whereas HBeAg has present in the capillary wall of one case of MPGN III (170).

Mesangial proliferative glomerulonephritis has been observed in HBV carriers in a greater frequency than expected, considering the prevalence of HBsAg. Both HBsAg and HBcAg have been localized to the mesangium (153,171). Unlike the probable scenario with HBV MGN in which in situ immune complex formation is likely, the pathogenesis of both HBV MPGN and HBV mesangial proliferative glomerulonephritis likely involves subendothelial and mesangial trapping of CICs (163).

VASCULITIS

In various series, the finding of HBsAg in the serum of patients with a polyarteritis nodosa- (PAN-) like syndrome has varied from 0% to 54% of cases (172–178). The HBV PAN syndrome generally presents several months following an episode of hepatitis with fever, arthralgias/arthritis, urticaria, and palpable purpura. Subsequently, a vasculitis may developed with involvement of one or many organs. Renal involvement can present with hypertension, hematuria, mild to severe proteinuria, and renal insufficiency.

The diagnosis of PAN can often be made by tissue bi-opsy, which demonstrates the local inflammation of small- and medium-sized arteries. Angiography to look for saccular or fusiform aneurysms especially of the renal vasculature, may be helpful.

The pathogenesis of HBV PAN has been extensively reviewed by Johnson (163) and appears to result from an accumulation of HBV antigen-containing CICs in the vasculature, with subsequent complement activation and infiltration by leukocytes.

TREATMENT OF HBV-RELATED SYNDROMES

The prognosis of PAN has been markedly improved by treatment with steroids and cytotoxic drugs (174,177,179,180). Most authors feel that patients with HBV PAN should be similarly treated, although careful studies of the role of immunosuppression in HBV PAN have not been done. Although immunosuppressive therapy is necessary to control the vasculitis, there is unquestionably a risk of maintaining the HBsAg carrier state and predisposing the patient to progressive liver disease.

The treatment of HBV MGN should be approached with the knowledge that spontaneous remission is not uncommon in children; up to 60% may remit without therapy (181). Furthermore, treatment with steroids has been associated with a longer persistence of cellular HBV DNA in peripheral blood mononuclear cells and increased viral replication (182,183). Thus, children with HBV MGN should be treated conservatively. Steroid therapy does not appear to be of benefit. In contrast, a recent study by Lai et al. (181) suggests that the course of HBV MGN in adults in regions where HBV is endemic may not be benign. Regardless of treatment, one third of patients had a relentless progression to chronic renal failure. Mixed results have been obtained with alpha interferon (183–186) in small numbers of patients. Others have treated patients with adenine arabinoside (187,188), but the use of this agent cannot be widely recommended at this time.

Transplantation

CLINICAL DISEASE

Liver disease has been recognized to be a major contributor to long-term patients morbidity and mortality following successful renal transplantation (22,88). The contribution of HBV infection to the overall effect of liver disease on long-term posttransplant outcome has been well defined (22,189–192). Parfrey et al. (22) reported that 14 of 26 (54%) HBsAg-positive patients died during a follow-up of 90.2 ± 8.9 months; 64% of these deaths were attributed to liver disease. Furthermore, 15 of 21 HBsAg-positive patients morphologically progressed to a more serious lesion on follow-up biopsies. A prospective study from Canada (190,191) followed 22 HBsAg-positive patients for a mean of 83 months posttransplant. None converted to anti-HBs positive, and 12 progressed to cirrhosis. Of note, 82% of those patients whose initial biopsy showed only reactive hepatitis or chronic persistent hepatitis progressed to chronic active hepatitis or cirrhosis on serially obtained biopsies. Also of interest is a study by Pol et al. (189) that examined the course of 122 HBsAg-positive patients. At the time of transplantation, liver biopsies demonstrated 80% (98 of 122) to already have chronic liver disease. Moreover, 12 of 16 patients whose initial biopsy was normal progressed to chronic hepatitis (11) or cirrhosis (1). Similarly aggressive patterns of progression were observed in patients whose initial biopsy showed chronic persistent or chronic active hepatitis.

Although progression and increased mortality have been observed in HBsAg-positive dialysis patients, the aggressiveness of HBV appears to be magnified under the influence of immunosuppression.

RECOMMENDATIONS

HBsAg-positive dialysis patients being considered for transplantation must be carefully evaluated. Initial testing should include studies for HBV DNA and HBeAg and a liver biopsy. Those with advanced morphological changes and active viral replication (HBV DNA positive) are at high risk to incur significant morbidity from liver disease in the years following transplantation and perhaps should be counseled to remain on dialysis. For patients with a more benign histology, the potential risks of long-term immunosuppression should be explained so that an individualized decision can be reached regarding the advisability of transplantation—a decision that takes into account the patient's age, comorbid illnesses, and course on dialysis up to that time.

REFERENCES

1. Aach RD, Stevens CE, Hollinger FB, Mosley JW, Peterson DA, Taylor PE, Johnson RG, Barbosa LH, Nemo GJ: Hepatitis C virus infection in post-transfusion hepatitis. An analysis with first and second-generation assays. *N Engl J Med* 325:1325–1329, 1991.
2. Alter HJ, Purcell RH, Shih SW, Melpolder JC, Houghton M, Choo Q-L, Kuo G: Detection of antibody to hepatitis C virus in prospectively followed transfusion recipients with acute and chronic non-A, non-B hepatitis. *N Engl J Med* 321:1494–1500, 1989.
3. Houghton M, Weiner A, Han J, Kuo G, Choo Q-L: Molecular biology of the hepatitis C viruses: implications for diagnosis, development and control of viral disease. *Hepatology* 14:381–388, 1991.
4. Esteban JI, Gonzalez A, Hernandez JM, Vildomiu L, Sánchez C, Lòpez-Talavera JC, Lucea D, Martin-Vega C, Vidal X, Esteban R, Guardia J: Evaluation of antibodies to hepatitis C virus in a study of transfusion associated hepatitis. *N Engl J Med* 323:1107–1112, 1990.
5. Alter MJ, Margolis HS, Krawczynski K, Judson FN, Mares A, Alexander WJ, Hu PY, Miller JK, Gerber MA, Sampliner RE, Meeks EL, Beach MJ: The natural history of community-acquired hepatitis C in the United States. *N Engl J Med* 327:1899–1905, 1992.
6. Roth D, Zucker K, Cirocco R, Demattos A, Burke GW, Nery J, Esquenazi V, Babischkin S, Miller J: The impact of hepatitis C virus infection on renal allograft recipients. *Kidney Int* 45:238–244, 1994.
7. Pol S, Romeo R, Zins B, Driss F, Lebkiri B, Carnot F, Berthelot P, Brichot C: Hepatitis C virus RNA in anti-HCV positive hemodialysis patients: significance and therapeutic implications. *Kideny Int* 44:1097–1100, 1993.
8. Chan TM, Lok ASF, Cheng IKP, Chan RT: Prevalence of hepatitis C virus infection in hemodialysis patients: a longitudinal study comparing the results of RNA and antibody assays. *Hepatology* 17:5–8, 1993.
9. Tsukarma H, Hiyama T, Tanaka S, Nakao M, Yabuuchi Y, Kitamura T, Nakanishi K, Fujimoto I, Inoue A, Yamazaki H, Kawashima T: Risk factors for hepatocellular carcinoma among patients with chronic liver disease. *N Engl J Med* 328:1797–1801, 1993.
10. Kuo G, Choo Q-L, Alter HJ, Gitnick GL, Redeker AG, Purcell RH, Miyamura T, Dienstag JL, Alter JM, Stevens CE, Tegtmeier GE, Bonino F, Colombo M, Lee W-S, Kuo C, Berger K, Shuster JR, Overby LR, Bradley DW, Houghton M: An assay for circulating antibodies to a major etiologic virus of human non-A, non-B hepatitis. *Science* 244:362–364, 1989.
11. Garson JA, Tedder RS, Briggs M, Tuke P, Glazebrook JA, Trute A, Parker D, Barbara JAJ, Contreras M, Aloysius S: Detection of hepatitis C viral sequences in blood donations by "nested" polymerase chain reaction and prediction of infectivity. *Lancet* 335:1419–1422, 1990.
12. McGuinness PH, Bishop GA, Lien A, Wiley B, Parsons C, McCaughan AW: Detection of serum hepatitis C virus RNA in HCV antibody-seropositive volunteer blood donors. *Hepatology* 18:485–490, 1993.
13. Donahue JG, Munoz A, Ness PM, Brown DE, Yawn DN, Mcallister HA, Reitz BA, Nelson KE: The declining risk of post-transfusion hepatitis C virus infection. *N Engl J Med* 327:369–373, 1992.
14. Alberti A, Chemello L, Cavaletto D, Tagger A, Canton A, Bizzaro N, Tagariello G, Ruol A: Antibody to hepatitis C virus and liver disease in volunteer blood donors. *Ann Intern Med* 114:1010–1012, 1991.
15. McFarlane IG, Smith HM, Johnson PJ, Bray GP, Vergani D, Williams R: Hepatitis C virus antibodies in chronic active hepatitis: pathogenetic factor or false-positive result? *Lancet* 335:754–757, 1990.
16. Farci P, London WT, Wong DC, Dawson GJ, Vallari DS, Engle R, Purcell RH: The natural history of infection with hepatitis C virus in chimpanzees: comparison of serologic responses measured with first and second generation assays and relationship to HCV viremia. *J Infect Dis* 165:1006–1011, 1992.
17. McHutchison JG, Person JL, Govindarajan S, Valinluck B, Gore T, Lee SR, Nelles M, Polito A, Chien D, DiNello R, Quan S, Kuo G, Redeker AG: Improved detection of hepatitis C virus antibodies in high-risk populations. *Hepatology* 15:19–25, 1992.
18. VanderPoel CL, Cuypers HTM, Reesink HW, Weiner AJ, Quan S, DiNello R, Boven JJP, Winkel I, Mulder-Folkerts D, Exel-Oehlers PJ, Schaasberg W, Leentvaar-Kuypers A, Polito A, Houghton M, Lelie P: Confirmation of hepatitis C virus infection by new four-antigen recombinant immunoblot assay. *Lancet* 337:317–319, 1991.

19. Esteban JI, Lòpez-Talavera JC, Genesca J, Madoz P, Viladomiu L, Muñiz E, Martin-Vega C, Rosell M, Allende H, Vidal X, Gonzalez A, Hernandez M, Esteban R, Guardia J: High rate of infectivity and liver disease in blood donors with antibodies to hepatitis C virus. *Ann Intern Med* 115:443–449, 1991.

20. Broyer M, Brunner FP, Brynger H, Fassbinder W, Guidlou PJ, Oules R, Rizzoni G, Selwood NH, Wing AJ: Combined report on regular dialysis and transplantation in Europe. *Proc Eur Dial Transplant Assoc* 16:50–52, 1985.

21. Shusterman N, Singer I: Infectious hepatitis in dialysis patients. *Am J Kidney Dis* 9:447–455, 1987.

22. Parfrey PS, Farge D, Forbes RD, Dandavino R, Kenick S, Guttman RD: Chronic hepatitis in end-stage renal disease: comparison of HBsAg-negative and HBsAg-positive patients. *Kidney Int* 28:959–967, 1985.

23. Koretz RL, Stone O, Mousa M, Gitnick G: The pursuit of hepatitis in dialysis units. *Am J Nephrol* 4:222–226, 1984.

24. Polakoff S: Hepatitis in dialysis units in the United Kingdom. A Public Health Laboratory Service Survey. *J Hyg (Lond)* 87:443–451, 1981.

25. Choo QL, Kuo G, Weiner AJ, Overby LR, Bradley DW, Houghton M: Isolation of a c-DNA clone derived from blood borne viral hepatitis genome. *Science* 244:262–264, 1989.

26. Choo QL, Weiner AJ, Overby LR, Kuo G, Houghton M, Bradley DW: Hepatitis C virus, the major causative agent for viral NANB hepatitis. *Br Med Bull* 46:423–441, 1990.

27. Esteban JI, Esteban R, Viladomiu L, Gonzalez A, Lopez-Talavera JC, Conzalez A, Hernandez JM, Roget M, Vargas V, Genesca J, Buti M, Guardia J: Hepatitis C virus antibodies among risk groups in Spain. *Lancet* 2:294–297, 1989.

28. Kuhnl P, Roggendorf M, Sibrowski W, Deinhardt F, Laufs R, Bornhovd K, Kalmar G, Seidl S, Bohm BO: Hepatitis C virus antibodies (HCV) in patients treated with chronic hemodialysis. *Beitr Infusionther* 26:27–29, 1990.

29. Jeffers LJ, Perez GO, de Medina MD, Ortiz-Interian CJ, Schiff ER, Reddy KR, Jimenez M, Bourgoignie JJ, Vaamonde CA, Duncan R, Houghton M, Choo QL, Kuo G: Hepatitis C infection in two urban hemodialysis units. *Kidney Int* 38:320–322, 1990.

30. Gilli P, Moretti M, Soffritti SM, Marchi N, Malacarne F, Bedani PL, DePaoli Vitali E, Fiocchi O, Menini C: Non-A, non-B hepatitis and anti-HCV antibodies in dialysis patients. *Int J Artif Organs* 13:737–741, 1990.

31. Zeldis J, Depner T, Kuramoto I, Gish, Holland P: The prevalence of hepatitis C virus antibodies among hemodialysis patients. *Ann Intern Med* 112:958–960, 1990.

32. Fairley CK, Leslie DE, Nicholson S, Gust: Epidemiology and hepatitis C virus in Victoria. *Med J Aust* 153:271–273, 1990.

33. Teruel JL, Fernandez Munoz R, Gamez C, Marcen A, Celma ML, Liano F, Ortuno J: Hepatitis C virus infection in patients treated by hemodialysis. *Med Clin (Barc)* 95:81–83, 1990.

34. Oguchi H, Miyasaka M, Tokunaga S, Hora K, Ichikawa S, Ochi T, Yamada K, Nagasawa M, Kanno Y, Aizawa T, Watanabe H, Yoshizawa S, Sato K, Terashima M, Yoshie T, Oguchi S, Tanaka E, Kiyosawa K, Furuta S: Hepatitis virus infection (HBV and HCV) in eleven Japanese hemodialysis units. *Clin Nephro* 38:36–43, 1992.

35. (letter to the editor). *Lancet* 335:1409, 1990.

36. (letter to the editor). *Lancet* 335:1409, 1990.

37. Lai KN, Tam JS, Llai FM, Lin HJ: Isolated presence of antibody to hepatitis B core antigen in dialysis patients: occurrence of subclinical hepatitis C. *Am J Kidney Dis* 13:370–376, 1989.

38. de Medina M, Ortiz C, Krenc C, Leete J, Vallari D, Hill M, LaRue S, Jimenez M, Anderson W, Schiff E, Perez G: Improved detection of antibodies to hepatitis C virus in dialysis patients using a second-generation enzyme immunoassay. *Am J Kidney Dis* 20:589–591, 1992.

39. Mondelli MU, Cristina G, Piazza V, Cerino A, Villa G, Salvadeo A: High prevelance of antibodies to hepatitis C virus in hemodialysis units using a second generation assay. *Nephron* 61:350–351, 1992.

40. Cantu P, Mangano S, Masini M, Limido A, Crovetti G, DeFilippo C: Prevalence of antibodies against hepatitis C virus in a dialysis unit. *Nephron* 61:337–338, 1992.

41. Polywka S, Kaars Wiele P, Schroeter E, Mandler J, Laufs R: Detection of antibodies to HCV: Comparison of a c100-3 EIA and the 2nd generation EIA. *Beitr Infusionther* 30:42–45, 1992.

42. Holzberger G, Seidl S, Peschke B, Scheuermann EH, Schoeppe W: Decreasing the risk of post-tranfusion non-A, non-B hepatitis by anti-HCV screening. *Beitr Infusionther* 30:46–48, 1992.

43. Chauveau P, Courouce AM, Lemarec N, Naret C, Poignet JL, Girault A, Ramdame M, Delons S: Antibodies to hepatitis C virus by second generation test in hemodialyzed patients. *Kidney Int Suppl* 41:149–152, 1993.

44. Knudsen F, Wantzin P, Rasmussen K, Ladefoged SD, Lokkegaard N, Rasmussen LS, Lassen A, Krogsgaard K: Hepatitis C in dialysis patients: relationship to blood transfusion, dialysis, and liver disease. *Kidney Int* 43:1353–1356, 1993.

45. Dentico P, Volpe A, Buongiorno R, Fiore G, Carbone M, Manno C, Pastore G, Schiraldi O: Detection of antibodies to HCV in hemodialysis patients using two second generation ELISA tests. *Ital J Gastroenterol* 25:19–22, 1993.

46. Chan TM, Lok AS, Cheng IK: Hepatitis C infection among dialysis patients: a comparison between patients on maintenance hemodialysis and continuous ambulatory peritoneal dialysis. *Nephrol Dial Transplant* 6:944–947, 1991.

47. Huang CC, Wu MS, Lin DY, Liaw YF: The prevalence of hepatitis C virus antibodies in patients treated with continuous ambulatory peritoneal dialysis. *Perit Dial Int* 12:31–33, 1992.

48. Selgas R, Martinez-Zapico R, Bajo MA, Romero JR, Munoz J, Rinon C, Miranda B, Miquel JL: Prevalence of hepatitis C antibodies (HCV) in a dialysis population at one center. *Perit Dial Int* 12:28–30, 1992.

49. Ng YY, Lee SD, Wu SC, Liu WT, Chia WL, Huang TP: The need for second generation anti-hepatitis C virus testing in uremic patients on continuous ambulatory peritoneal dialysis. *Perit Dial Int* 13:132–135, 1993.

50. Kuhns M, de Medina M, McNamara A, Jeffers LJ, Reddy ER, Silva M, Ortiz-Interian C, Jimenez M, Schiff E, Perez G: Detection of hepatitis C virus in hemodialysis patients. *J Am Soc Nephrol* 4:1491–1497, 1994.

51. Li JS: Hepatitis C virus infection in hemodialysis patients. *Chung Hua I Hsueh Tsa Chih* 72:655–701, 1992.

52. Sheu JC, Lee SH, Wang JT, Shih LN, Wang TH, Chen DS: Prevalence of anti-HCV and HCV viremia in hemodialysis patients in Taiwan. *J Med Virol* 37:108–112, 1992.

53. Sakamoto N, Enomoto N, Marumo F, Sato C: Prevalence of hepatitis C virus infection among long-term hemodialysis patients: detection of hepatitis C virus RNA in hemodialysis patients. *J Med Virol* 39:11–15, 1993.

54. Dussol B, Chicheportiche C, Cantaloube JF, Roubicek C, Biagini P, Berland Y: Detection of hepatitis C infection by

polymerase chain reaction among hemo-dialysis patients. *Am J Kidney Dis* 22:574–580, 1993.

55. Farci P, Alter H, Wong D, Miller R, Shih J, Jett B, Purcell R: A long-term study of hepatitis C virus replication in non-A, non-B hepatitis. *N Engl J Med* 325:98–104, 1991.

56. Kato N, Yokosuka O, Omata M, Hosoda K, Ohto M: Detection of hepatitis C virus ribonucleic acid in the serum by amplification with polymerase chain reaction. *J Clin Invest* 86:1764–1767, 1990.

57. Ulrich P, Romeo J, Lane P, Kelly I, Daniel L, Vyas G: Detection, semiquantitation, and genetic variation in hepatitis C virus sequences amplified from the plasma of blood donors with elevated alanine aminotransferase. *J Clin Invest* 86:1609–1614, 1990.

58. de Medina M, LaRue S, Hill M, Hunt W, Urdes M, Wilber JC, Johnson P, Xi XM, Jeffers LJ, Parker T, Reedy KR, Schiff ER, Perez G: Quantitative detection of hepatitis C virus in patients undergoing hemodialysis. ASAIO Journal 43:19–22, 1997.

59. Lau J YN, Davis GL, Kniffen J, Oian KP, Urdia M, Chan C, Mizokami M, Neuwald PD, Wiber JC: Significance of serum hepatitis C virus RNA levels in chronic hepatitis C. *Lancet* 341:1505–1508, 1993.

60. Hagiwara H, Hayashi N, Mita E, Takehara T, Kasahara A, Fusamoto H, Kamada T: Quantitative analysis of hepatitis C virus RNA in serum during interferon alfa therapy. *Gastroenterology* 104:877–883, 1993.

61. Favero M, Alter M, Bland L: In: JV Bennett, B Brachman, eds, *Hospital Infections*, 3rd ed. Little, Brown, Boston, 19:375–403.

62. Dentico P, Buongiorno R, Volpe A, Carlone A, Carbone M, Manno C, Proscia F, Pastore G, Schiraldi O: The prevalence and incidence of hepatitis C virus (HCV) in hemodialysis patients: study of risk factors. *Clin Nephrol* 38:49–52, 1992.

63. Jadoul M, Corner CH, Van Ypersele de Strihou CH, and the UCL collaborative group: Incidence and risk factors for hepatitis C seroconversion in hemodialysis: a prospective study. *Kidney Int* 44:1322–1326, 1993.

64. Niu MT, Coleman PJ, Alter MJ: Multicenter study of hepatitis C virus infection in chronic hemodialysis patients and hemodialysis center staff members. *J Am Soc Nephrol* 22:568–573, 1993.

65. Hardy NM, Sandroni S, Danielson S, Wilson WJ: Antibody to hepatitis C virus increases with time on hemodialysis. *Clin Nephrol* 38:44–48, 1992.

66. Willems M, de Jong G, Moshage H, Verresen L, Goubau P, Desmyter J, Yap SH: Surrogate markers are not useful for identification of HCV carriers in chronic hemodialysis patients. *J Med Virol* 35:303–306, 1991.

67. Gitnick G, Weiss S, Overby LR, Ling CM, Chairez R, Parsa K: Non-A, non-B hepatitis: a prospective study of a hemodialysis outbreak with evaluation of a serologic marker in patients and staff. *Hepatology* 3:625–630, 1983.

68. Chiaramonte S, Tagger A, Ribero ML, Grossi A, Milan M, La Greca G: Prevention of viral hepatitis in dialysis units: isolation and technical management of dialysis. *Nephron* 61:287–289, 1992.

69. Marchesi D, Arici C, Poletti E, Mingardi G, Minola E, Mecca G: Outbreak of non-A, non-B hepatitis in centre hemodialysis patients: a retrospective analysis. *Nephrol Dial Transplant* 3:795–799, 1988.

70. Niu MT Alter MJ, Kristensen C, Margolis HS: Outbreak of hemodialysis-associated non-A, non-B hepatitis and correlation with antibody to hepatitis C virus. *Am J Kidney Dis* 19:345–352, 1992.

70a. Stuyver L, Claeys H, Wysecer A, Arnherm WV, De Beenhouwer H, Uytendaele S, Beckers J, Matthys D, Leroux-Roels G, Maertens G, De Paepe M: Hepatitis Cuirus in hemodialysis unit: Molecular evidence for nosocomial transmission, *Kidney Intt* 49:889–895, 1996.

70b. Olmer M, Bouchouareb D, Zandotti C, de Mico P, de Lamballerie X: Transmission of the hepatitis B in a hemodialysis unit. *Clin Nephrol* 47:265–270, 1996.

71. Garcia-Valdecasas, J Bernal MC, Cerezo, Garcia F, Pereira BJG: Strategies to reduce the transmission of HCV infection in hemodialysis (HD) units. *J Am Soc Nephrol* 4:347, 1993.

72. Conway M, Catterall AP, Brown EA, Tibbs C, Gower PE, Curtis JR, Coleman JC, Murray-Lyon IM: Prevalence of antibodies to hepatitis C in dialysis patients and transplant recipients with possible routes of transmission. *Nephrol Dial Transplant* 7:1226–1229, 1992.

73. Everhart JE, Di Bisceglie AM, Murray LM, Alter HJ, Melpolder JJ, Kuo G, Hoofnagle JH: Risk for non-A, non-B (type C) hepatitis through sexual or household contact with chronic carriers. *Ann Intern Med* 112:544–545, 1990.

74. Riestra S, Carcaba V: Hepatitis C virus; evidence for sexual transmission. *Br Med J* 303:301–311, 1991.

75. Sanchez-Quijano A, Rey C, Aguado I, Pineda JA, Perez Romero M, Torres Y, Leal M, Lissen E: Hepatitis C infection in a sexually promiscuous group. *Eur J Clin Microbiol Infect Dis* 9:610–612, 1990.

76. Hess G, Massing A, Rossol S, Shutt H, Clemens R, Meyerzum-Buschenfelde KH: Hepatitis C virus and sexual transmission. *Lancet* 2:987, 1989.

77. Kamitsukasa H, Harada H, Yakura M, Fukuda A, Ohbayashi A, Saito I, Miyamura T, Choo OL, Houghton M, Kuo G: Intrafamilial transmission of hepatitis C virus. *Lancet* 2:98, 1989.

78. Ideo G, Bellati G, Pedraglio E, Bottelli R, Donzelli T, Putignano G: Intrafamilial transmission of hepatitis C virus. *Lancet* 1:353, 1990.

79. Alfurayh O, Sobh M, Buali A, Ali MA, Barri Y, Ounibi W, Taher S: Hepatitis C virus infection in chronic hemodialysis patients, a clinicopathologic study. *Nephrol Dial Transplant* 4:327–332, 1992.

80. Gilli P, Cavazzini L, Stabellini N, Malacarne F, Soffritti S, Storari A: Histological features of non-A, non-B hepatitis in hemodialysis patients. *Nephron* 61:296–297, 1992.

81. Caramelo C, Ortiz A, Aguilera B, Porres JC, Navas S, Marriott E, Alberola ML, Alamo C, Galera A, Garron MP, Gonzalez-Parra E, Fernandez de Gabriel MV, Oliva H, Carreno V: Liver disease in hemodialysis patients with antibodies to hepatitis C virus. *Am J Kidney Dis* 22:822–828, 1993.

82. Rao KV, Anderson WR, Kasiske BL, Dahl DC: Value of liver biopsy in the evaluation and management of chronic liver disease in renal transplant recipients. *Am J Med* 94:241 250, 1993.

83. Davis GL, Balart LA, Schiff ER, Lindsay K, Jacobson IM, Payne J, Dienstag JL, VanTheil DH, Tamburro C, Lefkowitch J, Albrecht J, Meschievitz C, Ortego TJ, Gibas A, and the Hepatitis Interventional Therapy Group: Treatment of chronic hepatitis C with recombinant interferon alpha: a multicenter randomized, controlled trial. *N Engl J Med* 321:1501–1506, 1989.

84. DiBisceglie AM, Martin P, Kassianides C, Llisker MM, Goodman Z, Banks SM, Hoofnagle JH: A randomized, double-blind, placebo-controlled trial of recombinant human alpha-interferon therapy for chronic non-A, non-B (type C) hepatitis. *Hepatology* 11:S36–S42, 1990.

85. Shindo M, DiBisceglie AM, Cheung L, Shih JW, Cristiano K, Feinstone SM, Hoofnagle JH: Decrease in serum hepatitis C viral RNA during alpha interferon therapy for chronic hepatitis C. *Ann Intern Med* 115:700–704, 1991.

86. McDonald J, Caruso L: Diminished responsiveness of male homosexual chronic hepatitis B virus carriers with HTLV-III antibodies to recombinant alpha interferon. *Hepatology* 7:719–723, 1987.

87. Koenig P, Umlauft F, Lhotta K, Weyrer K, Neyer U, Stummvoll HK, Vogel W, Brommeger R, Gruenewald K: Treatment of hemodialysis patients suffering from chronic HCV infection with interferon alpha. *J Am Soc Nephrol* 4:361, 1993.

87a. Ellis ME, Alfurayh O, Nalim MA, Sieck JO, Ali MA, Bermvil SS, Ali H, Barri Y, Ayub A, al Fadda M: Chronic non-A, non-B hepatitis complicated by end-stage renal failure treated with recombinant interferon alpha. *J Hepatol* 18:210–216, 1993.

87b. Pol S, Thiers V, Carnot F, Zins B, Romeo R, Berthelot P, Brechot C: Efficacy and tolerance of α-2b interferon therapy on HCV intection of hemodialyzed patients. *Kidney Int* 47:1412–1418, 1995.

87c. Raptopoulou-Gigi M, Spaia S, Garifallos A, Xerou P, Orphanou H, Zarafidou E, Petridou P, Vrettou H, Vagioras G, Galakitidou G, Mauroudi I, Efkarpidou A, Kortsaris A: Interferon α-2b treatment of chronic hepatitis C in hemodialysis patients. *Nephrol Dial Transplant* 10:1834–1837, 1995.

88. Weir MR, Kirkman RL, Strom TB, Tilney NL: Liver disease in recipients of long-functioning renal allografts. *Kidney Int* 28:839–844, 1985.

89. Boyce NW, Holdsworth SR, Hooke D, Thompson NM, Atkins RC: Non hepatitis B-associated liver disease in a renal transplant population. *Am J Kidney Dis* 11:307–312, 1988.

90. LaQuaglia MP, Tolkoff-Rubin NE, Dienstag JL, Dienstag JL, Cosimi B, Herrin JT, Kelly M, Rubin RH: Impact of hepatitis on renal transplantation. *Transplantation* 32:504–507, 1981.

91. Morales M, Campo C, Castellano G, Colina F, Andres A, Fuertes A, Praga M, Rodicio JL: Clinical implications of the presence of antibodies to hepatitis C after renal transplantation. *Transplant Proc* 24:78–80, 1992.

92. Pol S, Legendre C, Saltiel C, Carnot F, Bréchot C, Berthelot P, Mattlinger B, Kreis H: Hepatitis C virus in kidney recipients: epidemiology and impact on renal transplantation. *J Hepatol* 15:202–206, 1992.

93. Pereira BJG, Milford EL, Kirkman RL, Levey AS: Transmission of hepatitis C virus by organ transplantation. *N Engl J Med* 325:454–460, 1991.

94. Roth D, Fernandez JA, Babischkin S, Demattos A, Buck BE, Quan S, Olson L, Burke GW, Nery J, Esquenazi V, Schiff ER, Miller J: Detection of hepatitis C virus infection among cadaver organ donors: evidence for low transmission of disease. *Ann Intern Med* 117:470–475, 1992.

95. Pereira BJG, Kirkman RL, Wright TL, Wright TL, Bryan CF, Cooper ES, Griffith JL, Kelly MK, Light JA, Norman DJ, Schmid C, Van Thiel D, Werner BG, Wright CE, Levey AS: National collaborative study of anti-HCV in cadaver donors: reduced organ wastage using a second generation anti-HCV test. *J Am Soc Nephrol* 3:875A, 1992.

96. Pereira BJG, Milford EL, Kirkman RL, Quan S, Sayre KR, Johnson PJ, Wilber JC, Levey AS: Prevalence of hepatitis C virus RNA in organ donors positive for hepatitis C antibody and in the recipients of their organs. *N Engl J Med* 327:910–915, 1992.

97. Zucker K, Cirocco R, Roth D, Olson L, Burke GW, Nery J, Esquenazi V, Miller J: Depletion of hepatitis C virus from procured kidneys using pulsatile perfusion preservation. *Transplantation* 57:832–840, 1994.

98. Roth D, Fernandez JA, Burke GW, Esquenazi V, Miller J: Detection of antibody to hepatitis C virus in renal transplant recipients. *Transplantation* 51:396–400, 1991.

99. Ponz E, Campistol JM, Bruguera M, Barrera JM, Gil C, Pinto JB, Andreu J: Hepatitis C virus infection among kidney transplant recipients. *Kidney Int* 40:748–751, 1991.

100. Baur P, Daniel V, Pomer S, Scheurlen H, Opelz G, Roelcke D: Hepatitis C virus antibodies in patients after kidney transplantation. *Ann Hematol* 62:68–73, 1991.

101. Klauser R, Franz O, Traindl O, Pidlich J, Hay U, Watschinger B, Pohanka E, Kovank J: Hepatitis C antibody in renal transplant patients. *Transplant Proc* 24:286–288, 1992.

102. Stempel CA, Lake J, Kuo G, Vincenti F: Hepatitis C—its prevalence in end-stage renal failure patients and clinical course after kidney transplantation. *Transplantation* 55:273–276, 1993.

103. Chan T-M, Lok AS, Cheng KP, Chan RT: A prospective study of hepatitis C infection among renal transplant recipients. *Gastroenterology* 104:862–868, 1993.

104. Huang C-C, Liaw Y-F, Lai M-K, Chu S-H, Chuang C-K, Huang J-Y: The clinical outcome of hepatitis C virus antibody-positive renal allograft recipients. *Transplantation* 53:763–765, 1992.

105. Takamizawa A, Mori C, Fuke I, Manabe S, Murakami S, Fujita J, Onishi E, Andoh T, Yoshida I, Okayama H: Structure and organization of the hepatitis C virus genome isolated from human carries. *J Virology* 65:1105–1113, 1991.

106. Nishioka K, Watanabe J, Furuta S, Tanaka E, Iino S, Suzuki H, Tsuji T, Yano M, Kuo G, Choo Q, Houghton M, Oda T: A high prevalence of antibody to hepatitis C virus in patients with hepatocellular carcinoma in Japan. *Cancer* 67:429–433, 1991.

107. Arita S, Asano T, Suzuki T, Enomoto K, Kobayashi S, Kenmochi T, Ochiai T, Isono K, Sakamota K: Clinical study of hepatitis disorders in renal transplant recipients with special reference to hepatitis C. *Transplant Proc* 24:1538–1540, 1992.

108. Chan TM, Lok ASF, Cheng IKP: Hepatitis C in renal transplant recipients. *Transplantation* 52:810–813, 1991.

109. Linnemann CC, Kaufman CA, First MR, Schiff GM, Phair JP: Cellular immune response to cytomegalovirus infection after renal transplantation. *Infect Immunol* 22:176–180, 1978.

110. Rytel MW, Aguilar-Torres FG, Balay J, Heim LR: Assessment of the status of cell mediated immunity in cytomegalovirus infected renal allograft recipients. *Cell Immunol* 37:31–40, 1978.

111. Pouteil-Noble C, Ecochard R, Landrivon G, Hart J, Bacchi CE, Hartwell P, Couser WG, Corey L, Wener MH, Alpers CE, Weilson R: Cytomegalovirus infection—an etiological factor for rejection? *Transplantation* 55:851–857, 1993.

112. Rollino C, Roccatello D, Giachino O, Basolo B, Piccoli G: Hepatitis C virus infection and membranous glomerulonephritis. *Nephron* 59:319–320, 1991.

113. Davda R, Peterson J, Weiner R, Croker B, Lau JY: Membranous glomerulonephritis in association with hepatitis C virus infection. *Am J Kidney Dis* 22:452–455, 1993.

114. Johnson RJ, Gretch DR, Yamabe H, Hart J, Bacchi CE, Hartwell P, Couser WG, Corey L, Wener MH, Alpers CE, Wilson R: Membranoproliferative glomerulonephritis associated with hepatitis C virus infection. *N Engl J Med* 328:465–470, 1993.

115. Cottiero R, Westrick E, Weinberg M: Membranoproliferative glomerulonephritis type I associated with chronic hepatitis C virus infection. *J Am Soc Nephrol* 3:309A, 1992.

116. Burstein DM, Rodby RA: Membranoproliferative glomerulonephritis associated with hepatitis C virus infection. *J Am Soc Nephrol* 4:1288–1293, 1993.

117. D'Amico G, Colasanti G, Ferrario F, Sinico RA: Renal involvement in essential mixed cryoglobulinemia. *Kidney Int* 35:1004–1014, 1989.

118. Agnello V, Chung RT, Kaplan LM: A role for hepatitis C virus infection in type II cryoglobulinemia. *N Engl J Med* 327:1490–1495, 1992.

119. Misiani R, Bellavita P, Fenili D, Borelli G, Marchesi D, Massazza M, Vendramin G, Comotti B, Tanzi E, Ssudella G, Zanetti A: Hepatitis C virus infection in patients with essential mixed cryoglobulinemia. *Ann Intern Med* 117:573–577, 1992.

120. Disdier P, Harlé J-R, Weiller P-J: Cryoglobulinemia and hepatitis C infection. *Lancet* 338:1151–1152, 1991.

121. Dammacco F, Sansonno D: Antibodies to hepatitis C virus in essential mixed cryoglobulinemia. *Clin Exp Immunol* 87:352–356, 1992.

122. Galli M, Monti G, Monteverde A: Hepatitis C virus and mixed cryoglobulinemias. *Lancet* 1:989, 1992.

123. Ferri C, Greco F, Longobardo G: Antibodies to hepatitis C virus in patients with mixed cryoglobulinemia. *Arthritis Rheum* 34:1606–1610, 1991.

124. Pechére-Bertschi A, Perrin L, de Saussure P, Widmann JJ, Giostra E, Schifterli JA: Hepatitis C: a possible etiology for cryoglobulinemia type II. *Clin Exp Immunol* 89:419–422, 1992.

125. Bonomo L, Casato M, Afeltra A, Caccavo D: Treatment of idiopathic mixed cryoglobulinemia with alpha interferon. *Am J Med* 83:726–730, 1987.

126. Durand JM, Kaplanski G, Lefevre P, Richard MA, Andrac L, Trepo C, Soubeyrand J: Effect of interferon-α 2b on cryoglobulinemia related to hepatitis C virus infection. *J Infect Dis* 165:778–779, 1992.

127. Sherlock S: The natural history of hepatitis B. *Postgrad Med J* 63:7–11, 1987.

128. Alter MJ, Favero MS, Maynard JE: Impact of infection control strategies on the incidence of dialysis-associated hepatitis in the United States. *J Infect Dis* 153:1149–1151, 1986.

129. Harnett JD, Zeldis JB, Parfrey PS, Kennedy M, Sirca R, Steinman TI, Guttman RD: Hepatitis B disease in dialysis and transplant patients. *Transplantation* 44:369–376, 1987.

130. Neilson JO, Dietrichson O, Elling P, Christofferson P: Incidence and meaning of persistence of Australia antigen in patients with acute viral hepatitis: development of chronic hepatitis. *N Engl J Med* 285:1157–1160, 1971.

131. Pao CC, Yang W-L, Huang C-C, Hsu J-L, Lin S-S, Ken R, Chao Y, Sun C-F, Liaw Y-F, Lin J-Y: Hepatitis Type B

virus DNA in patients receiving hemodialysis: correlation with other HBV serological markers. *Nephron* 46:155–160, 1987.

132. Tokars JI, Alter MJ, Favero MS, Moyer LA, Bland LE: National surveillance of hemodialysis associated diseases in the United States 1990. *ASAIO J* 39:71–80, 1993.

133. Stevens CE, Alter HJ, Taylor PE, Zang EA, Harley EJ, Szmuness W, and the Dialysis Vaccine Trial Study Group: Hepatitis B vaccine in patients receiving hemodialysis. *N Engl J Med* 311:496–501, 1984.

134. Köhler H, Arnold W, Renschin G, Dormeyer H-H, Büschenfelde K-H: Active hepatitis B vaccination of dialysis patients and medical staff. *Kidney Int* 25:124–128, 1984.

135. Dumann H, Meuer S, Büschenfelde K-H, Köhler H: Hepatitis B vaccination and interleukin 2 receptor expression in chronic renal failure. *Kidney Int* 38:1164–1168, 1990.

136. Pasko MT, Bartholomew WR, Beam TR, Amsterdam D, Cunningham EE: Long-term evaluation of the hepatitis B vaccine (Heptavax-B) in hemodialysis patients. *Am J Kidney Dis* 11:326–331, 1988.

137. Buti M, Viladomiu L, Jardi R, Olmos A, Rodriguez JA, Bartolome J, Esteban R, Guardia J: Long-term immunogenecity and efficacy of hepatitis B vaccine in hemodialysis patients. *Am J Nephrol* 12:144–147, 1992.

138. Stevens CE, Szmuness W, Goodman AI, Weseley SA, Fotino, M: Hepatitis B vaccine: immune responses in hemodialysis patients. *Lancet* 2:1211–1213, 1980.

139. Sennesael JJ, Niepen P, Verbeeken DL: Treatment with recombinant human erythropoietin increases antibody titers after hepatitis B vaccination in dialysis patients. *Kidney Int* 40:121–128, 1991.

140. Meuer SC, Hauer M, Kurz P, Büschenfelde K-H, Köhler H: Selective blockade of the antigen-receptor-mediated pathway of T cell activation in patients with impaired primary immune responses. *J Clin Invest* 80:743–749, 1987.

141. Walz G, Kunzendorz U, Haller H, Keller F, Offermann G, Alasenic O: Factors influencing the response to hepatitis B vaccination of hemodialysis patients. *Nephron* 51:474–477, 1989.

142. Donati D, Gastaldi L: Controlled trial of thymopentin in hemodialysis patients who fail to respond to hepatits B vaccination. *Nephron* 50:133–136, 1988.

143. Melappioni M, Baldassani M, Saldini S, Radicioni R, Panichi N: Use of immunomodulators (thymopentine) in hepatitis B vaccine in elderly patients undergoing chronic hemodialysis. *Nephron* 61:358–359, 1992.

144. Moyer LA, Alter MJ, Favero MS: Hemodialysis-associated hepatitis B: revised recommendations for serologic screening. *Semin Dial* 3:201–204, 1990.

145. Almeida JD, Waterson AP: Immune complexes in hepatitis. *Lancet* 2:983–986, 1969.

146. Nowoslowski A, Krawzynski K, Nazarewicz T, Slusarczyk T: Immunopathological aspects of hepatitis type B. *Am J Med Sci* 270:229–239, 1975.

147. Combes B, Stastny P, Shorey J, Eigenbrodt EM, Barrera A, Hull AR, Carter NW: Glomerulonephritis with deposition of Australia antigen-antibody complexes in glomerular basement membrane. *Lancet* 2:234–237, 1971.

148. Takekoshi Y, Shida N, Saheki Y, Tanaka M, Satake Y, Matsumoto S: Strong association between membranous nephropathy and hepatitis B surface antigenemia in Japanese children. *Lancet* 2:1065–1068, 1978.

149. Hsu H-C, Lin G-H, Chong M-H, Chen C-H: Assocation of

hepatitis B surface (HBs) antigenemia and membranous nephropathy in children in Taiwan. *Clin Nephrol* 20:121–129, 1983.

150. Yoshikawa N, Ito H, Yamada Y, Hashimoto H, Katayama Y, Matsuyama S, Hasegawa O, Okada S, Hajikano H, Yoshizawa H, Mayumi M, Matsuo T: Membranous glomerulo-nephritis associated with hepatitis B antigen in children: a comparison with idiopathic membranous glomerulonephritis. *Clin Nephrol* 23:28–34, 1985.
151. Takekoshi Y, Tanaka M: Hepatitis B virus-associated glomerulonephritis in children. In: K Murakami, T Kitagawa, K Yabuta, T Sakai, eds, *Recent Advances in Pediatric Nephrology*. Excerpta Medica, New York, pp 293–298, 1987.
152. Lee HS, Choi Y, Yu SH, Koh HI, Kim MJ, Ko KW: A renal biopsy study of hepatitis B virus-associated nephropathy in Korea. *Kidney Int* 34:537–543, 1988.
153. Lai KN, Lai FM, Chan KW, Chow CB, Tong KL, Vallance-Owen J: The clinico-pathologic features of hepatitis B virus-associated glomerulonephritis. *Q J Med* 63:323–333, 1987.
154. Chow CB, Leung NK: Membranous glomerulonephritis in Hong Kong (letter). *Arch Dis Child* 59:693–694, 1984.
155. Sham MK, Rune KK, Yeung CK, Ng NL, Change WK, Chan MK: Hepatitis B induced glomerulonephritis, fact or fiction? *Aust N Z J Med* 15:356–358, 1985.
156. Southwest Pediatric Nephrology Study Group: Hepatitis B surface antigenemia in North American children with membranous glomerulonephropathy. *J Pediatr* 10:571–577, 1985.
157. Furuse A, Hattori S, Terashima T, Karashima S, Matsuda I: Circulating immune complex in glomerulo-nephropathy associated with hepatitis B virus infection. *Nephron* 31:212–228, 1982.
158. Collins AB, Bhan AK, Dienstag JL, Colvin RB, Haupert GT, Mushahwar IK, McCluskey RT: Hepatitis B immune complex glomerulonephritis: simultaneous glomerular deposition of hepatitis B surface and e antigens. *Clin Immunol Immunopathol* 26:137–153, 1983.
159. Takekoshi Y, Tanaka M, Miyakawa Y, Yoshizawa H, Takahashi K, Mayumi M: Free "small" and IgG-associated "large" hepatitis B e antigen in the serum and glomerular capillary walls of two patients with membranous glomerulonephritis. *N Engl J Med* 300:814–819, 1979.
160. Takekoshi Y, Shida N, Saheki Y, Tanaka M, Satake Y, Matsumoto S: Strong association between membranous nephropathy and hepatitis-B surface antigenaemia in Japanese children. *Lancet* 2:1065–1068, 1978.
161. Team of the Asian Study of Renal Disease in Children: Clinical suvey of hepatitis B antigenemia associated nephropathy in children. In: AB Gruskin, ME Norman, eds, *Pediatric Nephrology* (Proceedings of the Fifth International Pediatric Nephrology Symposium, held in Philadelphia, PA, October 6–10, 1980). Martinus Nijhoff Publishers, The Hague/Boston/London, pp 156–164, 1981.
162. Gregorek H, Jung H, Ulanowicz G, Madalinshi K: Immune complexes in sera of children with HCV-mediated glomerulonephritis. *Arch Immunol Ther Exp* 34:73–83, 1986.
163. Johnson RJ, Couser WG: Hepatitis B infection and renal disease: clinical immunopathogenetic and therapeutic considerations. *Kidney Int* 37:663–676, 1990.
164. Myers BD, Griffel B, Naveh D, Jankielowitz T, Klajman A: Membranoproliferative glomerulonephritis associated with persistent viral hepatitis. *Am J Clin Pathol* 59:222–228, 1973.

165. Knieser MR, Jenis EH, Lowenthal DT, Bancroft WH, Burns W, Shalhoub R: Pathogenesis of renal disease associated with viral hepatitis. *Arch Pathol* 97:193–200, 1974.
166. Wysznska T, Jung H, Madalinski K, Morzycka M: Hepatits B mediated glomerulonephritis in children. *Int J Pediatr Nephrol* 5:147–150, 1984.
167. Nagy J, Bajtai G, Brasch H, Süle T, Ambrus M, Deák G, Hámori A: The role of hepatitis B surface antigen in the pathogenesis of glomerulopathies. *Clin Nephrol* 12:109–116, 1979.
168. Lev M, Kleinkecht C, Droz D, Drueke T: Glomerular nephropathies and hepatitis B virus infection. In: J-F Bach, J Crosnier, J-L Funck-Brentano, J-P Grunfeld, MH Maxwell, eds, *Advances in Nephrology*, vol 11. Year Book Medical Publishers, Chicago, pp 341–370, 1982.
169. Brzosko W, Nazarewicz T, Krawczynski K, Morzycka M, Nowoslawski A: Glomerulonephritis associated with hepatitis-B surface antigen immune complexes in children. *Lancet* 2:477–482, 1974.
170. Amemiya S, Ito H, Kato K, Sakaguchi H, Hasegawa O, Hajikano H: A case of membranous proliferative glomerulonephritis type III (Burkholder) with the deposition of both HBeAg and HBsAg. *Int J Pediatr Nephrol* 4:267–273, 1983.
171. Lai KN, Lai FM, Lo S, Ho CP, Chan KW: IgA nephropathy associated with hepatitis B virus antigenemia. *Nephron* 47:141–143, 1987.
172. Trepo C, Thivolet J: Hepatitis associated antigen and periarteritis nodosa (PAN). *Vox Sang* 19:410–411, 1970.
173. Gocke DJ, Hsu K, Morgan C, Bombardieri S, Lockshin M, Christian CL: Vasculitis in association with Australia antigen. *J Exp Med* 134:330–335, 1971.
174. Sack M, Cassidy JT, Bole GG: Prognostic factors in polyarteritis. *J Rheumatol* 2:411–420, 1975.
175. Ewald EA, Griffin D, McCune WJ: Correlation of angiographic abnormalities with disease manifestations and disease severity in polyarteritis nodosa. *J Rheumatol* 14:952–956, 1987.
176. Cohen RD, Conn DT, Ilstrup DM: Clinical features, prognosis, and response to treatment in polyarteritis. *Mayo Clin Proc* 55:146–155, 1980.
177. Fauci AS, Katz P, Haynes BF, Wolff SM: Cyclophosphamide therapy of severe systemic necrotizing vasculitis. *N Engl J Med* 301:235–238, 1979.
178. Trepo CG, Zuckerman AJ, Bird RC, Prince AM: The role of circulating hepatitis B antigen/antibody immune complexes in the pathogenesis of vascular and hepatic manifestations in polyarteritis nodosa. *J Clin Pathol* 27:863–868, 1974.
179. Frohnert PP, Sheps SG: Long-term follow-up study of periarteritis nodosa. *Am J Med* 43:8–14, 1967.
180. Leib ES, Restivo C, Paulus HE: Immunosuppressive and corticosteroid therapy of polyarteritis nodosa. *Am J Med* 7:941–947, 1979.
181. Lai KN, Li PKT, Lui SF, Ch B, Au TG, Tam JSL, Tong KL, Lai F: Membranous nephropathy related to hepatitis B virus in adults. *N Engl J Med* 324:1457–1463, 1991.
182. Lin C-Y: Clinical features and natural course of HBV-related glomerulopathy in children. *Kidney Int* 40:S46–S53, 1991.
183. Garcia G, Scullard G, Smith C, Weissberg, J, Alexander S, Robinson WS, Gregory P, Merigan TC: Preliminary observation of hepatitis B-associated membranous glomerulonephritis treated with leukocyte interferon. *Hepatology* 5:317–320, 1985.

184. Mizushima N, Kanai K, Matsuda H, Matsumoto M, Tamakoshi K, Hidemasa I, Nakajima T, Yoshimi T, Kimura M, Nagase M: Improvement of proteinuria in a case of hepatitis B-associated glomeruloepphritis after treatment with interferon. *Gastroenterology* 92:524–526, 1987.

185. De Man RA, Schalm SW, Van Der Heijden AJ, Ten Kate FWJ, Wolff ED, Heijtink RA: Improvement of hepatitis B-associated glomerulonephritis after antiviral combination therapy. *J Hepatol* 8:367–372, 1989.

186. Lisker-Melman M, Webb D, Di Bisceglie AM, Kassianides C, Martin P, Rustgi V, Waggoner JG, Park Y, Hoofnagle JH: Glomerulonephritis caused by chronic hepatitis B virus infection: treatment with recombinant human alpha-interferon. *Ann Intern Med* 111:479–483, 1989.

187. Esteban R, Buti M, Valles M, Allende H, Guardia J: Hepatitis B-associated membranous glomerulonephritis treated with adenine arabinoside monophosphate (letter). *Hepatology* 6:762–763, 1986.

188. Lin C-Y, Lo S: Treatment of hepatitis B virus-associated membranous nephropathy with adenine arabinoside and thymic extract. *Kidney Int* 39:301–306, 1991.

189. Pol S, Debure A, Degott C, Carnot F, Legendre C, Brechot C, Kreis H: Chronic hepatitis in kidney allograft recipients. *Lancet* 335:878–880, 1990.

190. Parfrey PS, Forbes RDC, Hutchinson TA, Kenick S, Farge D, Dauphinee WD, Seely JF, Guttman RD: The impact of renal transplantation on the course of hepatitis B liver disease. *Transplantation* 39:610–615, 1985.

191. Parfrey PS, Forbes RDC, Hutchinson TA, Beaudoin JG, Dauphinee WD, Hollomby DJ, Guttman RD: The clinical and pathological course of hepatitis B liver disease in renal transplant recipients. *Transplantation* 37:461–466, 1984.

192. Degos F, Degott C, Bedrossian J, Camilieri JP, Barbanel C, Dubour A, Rueff B, Benhamou JP, Kreis H: Is renal transplantation involved in post-transplantation liver disease? *Transplantation* 29:100–102, 1980.

193. Roth D: Hepatitis C virus: The Nephrologist's view. *Am J Kid Dis* 25:3–16, 1995.

CHAPTER 55

Acute, Intermittent, and Cycled Peritoneal Dialysis

JOSE A. DIAZ-BUXO

INTRODUCTION

Peritoneal dialysis (PD) is the oldest modality of renal replacement therapy and the first successful effort in replacing the function of a vital internal organ. Since its first clinical application in 1923 for the treatment of a patient with acute renal insufficiency (1), much progress has been made, which can be divided into three categories: 1) improved access to the peritoneal cavity; 2) development of modern equipment, including cyclers, connectors, and disposable tubing; and 3) better understanding of peritoneal physiology and kinetics, leading to the formulation of improved prescriptions for PD.

PD has played an important role in the treatment of acute renal failure (ARF). Prior to the advent of hemodialysis (HD), PD was reserved for patients with a reasonable chance of recovery of renal function. However, despite the advances and availability of HD, PD continues to be used in the treatment of the patient with ARF due to its maintenance of a steady physiologic state, its continued ultrafiltration (UF), and the fact that it can be provided without the use of systemic heparinization.

The automated forms of PD have also found a place in the extensive renal therapeutic armamentarium for chronic use. Continuous cyclic peritoneal dialysis (CCPD) has become the most commonly used type of dialysis among infants and young children in many countries. The use of CCPD increased during the second half of the 1980s and now accounts for approximately 10% of the combined CAPD/CCPD group of patients in the U.S. (2). The growth of automated PD is surpassing that of CAPD during the past few years. This is likely due to recent adjustments indialysis adequacy standards and the ability of automated PD regimes to provide higher clearances of small solutes.

This chapter will focus on the therapeutics of PD, with a limited background on the rationale for dialysis prescription and tools for the calculation of the magnitude of fluid and solute removal for specific schedules of dialysis.

ACUTE PERITONEAL DIALYSIS

PD is an attractive option for the treatment of ARF (3,4). It can be performed in practically any hospital and does not require specialized equipment or surgical skills. It is the preferred modality of dialysis for small children (5,6) due to the difficulties in obtaining adequate circulatory access for HD and the technical difficulties in matching the size of the hemodialyzer to the child's surface area. Although acute PD is a relatively simple procedure, the clinician should be knowledgeable about its limitations and potential complications and must always pay strict attention to sterile technique.

Indications and contraindications

The most frequent indications for acute PD are ARF and its common manifestations—uremic syndrome, hyperkalemia, extracellular fluid overload, and metabolic acidosis; isolated electrolytic disorders, where conservative therapy is ineffective; and intractable congestive heart failure (CHF). PD is the preferred method of renal replacement in patients with bleeding disorders and in those in whom heparinization is contraindicated, in those with unstable cardiovascular systems, and in patients with poor or abused peripheral and central veins that are not suitable as vascular access for HD.

The indications for dialysis in ARF are usually relative, and the decision to start therapy is often made in the setting of progressive azotemia, long before life-threatening complications present. Since ARF frequently occurs as a consequence, or concomitantly, with sepsis, surgery, and malnutrition, the patient is often hypercatabolic (7). Due to the limitations of PD in achieving solute removal (vide infra), it is recommended that PD be started early in order to facilitate adequate nutrition and prevent further catabolism. Although a specific BUN level is seldom the indication for PD, levels in excess of 100 mg/dL should be

Suki, WN and Massry SG (eds), Suki and Massry's Therapy of Renal Diseases and Related Disorders, Third Edition. ISBN 978-1-4757-6634-9.
©1998, Kluwer Academic Publishers, Boston/Dordrecht/London. All rights reserved.

monitored closely and be considered in the decision to commence therapy.

Severe hyperkalemia (potassium $\geq 6\,mEq/L$) that cannot be treated or has not responded to conservative management (sodium polysterene sulfonate, bicarbonate, glucose/insulin infusions) is an indication for acute dialysis. Evidence of myocardial toxicity should immediately trigger initiation of therapy; however, an occasional patient may have severe hyperkalemia in the absence of clinical cardiovascular manifestations or electrocardiographic abnormalities such as tall T waves, prolonged PR intervals, QRS widening, or cardiac arrhythmias.

Acute PD may also correct electrolytic aberrations, which are less frequent and are usually controlled with pharmacologic therapy. Severe hyponatremia typically responds to administration of hypertonic saline or to water intake restriction. Conversely, hypernatremia is treated by administration of free water. However, in the presence of overhydration and advanced renal insufficiency, dialysis may be indicated. Acute PD with low calcium concentrations or a calcium-free solution can correct hypercalcemia (8–10). If hypercalcemia is life-threatening, the use of HD with a low-calcium bath is recommended.

Overhydration manifested by peripheral edema (or sacral edema in bedridden patients), elevations in central venous pressure, pulmonary rales, cardiac gallops, pleural effusions, and ascites is a common indication for PD. Acute PD has proven of benefit in the temporary treatment of patients with cardiomyopathy and life-threatening congestive failure in the absence of renal failure (11–15). It may also benefit nephrotic patients with cardiopulmonary compromise who are awaiting the benefits of specific therapy for parenchymal renal disease.

PD has been successfully used in the treatment of acute drug intoxication (16,17). Certain substances can enhance drug removal when added to the dialysate. Examples of accepted practices to augment drug removal by PD are 1) alteration of dialysate pH to enhance anion diffusion (18); 2) addition of albumin to the dialysate to increase protein binding and prevent reabsorption of the toxin (19,20); and 3) intraperitoneal administration of vasoactive agents to augment peritoneal clearances (17). Despite the proven benefit of PD in the treatment of acute intoxication, it is known that its effectiveness is only a fraction of that of HD or hemoperfusion. PD should be reserved for the treatment of drug overdoses when hemoperfusion or HD are unavailable or contraindicated.

Miscellaneous indications for acute PD include profound hypothermia, which can be reversed by slowly increasing core temperature (21–23); acute pancreatitis (24,25), often associated with oliguric renal failure; prolonged hypoglycemia associated with the use of oral hypoglycemic agents (26); hepatic coma (27); and psoriasis (28).

Although there are no absolute contraindications for acute PD, several conditions may interfere with adequate dialysate flow or peritoneal access. In the immediate postoperative period, PD may prove impossible due to the presence of drains or profuse leakage around the surgical wound. The presence of adhesions from previous inflammatory processes or surgery could make peritoneal access impossible and may limit peritoneal surface area. Similarly, intra-abdominal masses, large polycystic kidneys, or extreme obesity may impair fluid dynamics. Finally, conditions such as severe pulmonary disease and diaphragmatic, abdominal, or inguinal hernias may be aggravated by the increased abdominal pressure generated by dialysate infusion.

Acute peritoneal access

INSERTION OF ACUTE PERITONEAL CATHETERS

Peritoneal access for acute dialysis can be readily obtained by insertion of a semirigid catheter under local anesthesia. Strict sterile precautions should be observed, and the operator and assistants must wear masks and sterile gloves. The abdomen is prepared in the usual manner by shaving the area between the umbilicus and symphysis pubis and cleansing the area with povidone-iodine. A local anesthetic is injected in the midline 2–3 cm under the umbilicus. A small stab wound is made and extended to the fascial plane. If the patient is conscious, he or she is requested to cooperate by performing a Valsalva maneuver in order to stiffen the anterior abdominal wall. The catheter, with stylet in place, is inserted into the stab wound and directed slightly caudad into the peritoneum. In order to avoid bowel perforation, it is recommended that the operator uses one hand to thrust the catheter into the abdominal cavity, while the other hand holds the catheter 2–3 cm from its distal end. As the catheter and stylet are pushed through the fibrous tissues of the anterior abdominal wall and peritoneum, resistance increases. Once the peritoneum is pierced, a sudden "pop" is felt, signaling entrance into the peritoneal cavity. At this point, the stylet can be withdrawn and the catheter advanced towards the left lower quadrant or other dependent area in the pelvis. The advance of the catheter should be smooth. Whenever resistance is encountered, rotary or back-and-forth motion should be used to facilitate placement and prevent visceral perforation. The system can then be tested by infusing dialysate and obtaining adequate return.

Some clinicians prefer to fill up the abdominal cavity with 2–3 L of dialysate, prior to insertion of the catheter, in order to obtain abdominal distention, which both approximates the peritoneum against the abdominal wall and allows the bowel to float in the solution, making the procedure safer. This maneuver has been criticized by others who contend that the risk of visceral perforation is greater with the use of a sharp needle for the infusion of dialysate than with a blunt stylet.

Once the semirigid catheter is in place, a small metal ring is fitted around the external shaft of the catheter to limit the path of the catheter into the abdominal wall. This same disk can be used to properly anchor the catheter to the abdominal wall with adhesive tape.

Semirigid catheters can be used for several days; however, it is recommended that the catheter be removed between sessions of acute PD. Due to the inconvenience of multiple punctures and the potential risks involved in catheter insertion, some centers have elected to insert single- or double-cuff Tenckhoff catheters if repeated procedures are anticipated. The techniques for insertion of permanent catheters are described in Chapter 57. Therefore, only the Seldinger technique will be described here.

IMPLANTATION OF THE TENCKHOFF CATHETER USING THE SELDINGER TECHNIQUE

The abdomen is shaved and cleansed with povidone-iodine. One percent xylocaine is used for local anesthesia. A 3–4-cm midline incision is created approximately 3 cm below the umbilicus for midline insertion or paramedial over the left belly of the rectus muscle. A 16-gauge plastic needle with stylet is used to enter the peritoneal cavity. The stylet is removed, and the Seldinger wire is inserted through the needle. If no obstruction is encountered, the Seldinger wire is advanced into the peritoneal cavity and the needle is removed. A disposable dilator with catheter sheath is slid over the wire and forced into the peritoneal cavity, with the patient exerting a Valsalva maneuver while the wire is held with the other hand. Once inside the peritoneal cavity the wire and the dilator are removed while the base of the sheath is firmly held against the anterior abdominal wall. The sheath is now directed towards the left lower quadrant while a straight or curled catheter is introduced intraluminally. The sheath is then split and removed from the peritoneal cavity while the catheter is held in place. The catheter is tested for patency by irrigating it with dialysate solution and observing the rate and clarity of the outflow. The inner cuff of the catheter is placed over the rectus fascia and a purse-string suture is tied around the cuff, assuring proper anchoring but avoiding collapse of the catheter lumen by excessive tension.

A straight or semicircular subcutaneous tunnel is created with a straight or semiflexible probe, and the outer end of the catheter is pulled through a small skin puncture. The catheter is pulled through the incision, leaving the outer cuff 2–3 cm from the skin exit site. The midline incision is now closed, and the abdominal cavity is drained.

Peritoneal dialysis solutions

Commercial dialysate is available from several manufacturers in containers varying in size from 0.25 L for pediatric use to 6 L. Table 1 provides the formulation for different dialysate solutions. Standard commercial dialysate is usually utilized during acute PD.

Reverse osmosis (RO) systems use a dialysate concentrate that is diluted 19 times to produce the final dialysate. A 2-L bottle of concentrate is diluted to make 40 L of dialysate. The concentration of solutes in the final solution is similar to commercially available dialysate. When rapid cycling with extremely short dwell times (less than 30 minutes) is performed in combination with hypertonic glucose solutions, greater removal of extracellular water is accomplished, leading to hypernatremia (29,30). This can be prevented with the use of a low sodium dialysate.

Technique and schedules for acute peritoneal dialysis

INTERMITTENT PERITONEAL DIALYSIS (IPD)

The oldest and simplest technique for the provision of IPD consists of the periodic manual infusion of commercial dialysate from crystal or plastic containers into the peritoneal cavity and its drainage into a calibrated collecting device with the use of a closed tubing set. The initial exchange volume for adults can be set at 1 L and gradually increased to 2 L if comfortably tolerated by the patient and if no pericatheter leaks are observed. Variable dwell times and dialysate flow rates can be utilized. For practical purposes, dialysate flow of 2–3 L/h of dialysate can be obtained using infusion and dwell times of 20–30 minutes and drain times of 15–20 minutes. Manual IPD is usually carried on for approximately 24–48 hours and repeated whenever necessary.

IPD can be more conveniently performed with the use of an automated RO delivery system or a dialysate cycler (see chronic IPD). These devices allow provision of automated peritoneal dialysis (APD) with excellent control of flow, dwell time, and drainage time. Modern equipment is also available which can determine UF.

CLINICAL EXPERIENCE WITH IPD IN THE TREATMENT OF ARF

IPD is considered an acceptable alternative to HD for the treatment of patients with ARF (4,31). The mortality rate in various series has been comparable to that of HD (3,31). Control of biochemical parameters has been acceptable except in cases of extreme hypercatabolism. Fluid removal can be easily manipulated by altering the dialysate flow and the osmolality of the solution. Although heparin is usually recommended in order to avoid catheter obstruction from fibrin strands, the use of intraperitoneal heparin does not result in systemic heparinization (32,33).

Table 1. Peritoneal dialysis solutions

	Units	IPD concentrate[a]	Standard dialysate[b]
Volume	(L)	2	0.25, 0.5, 1, 1.5, 2, 2.5, 3, 5, 6
Glucose	(%)	1.5, 2.5	1.5, 2.5, 4.25
Sodium	(mEq/L)	118–132	132
Potassium	(mEq/L)	0	0
Calcium	(mEq/L)	3.5	2.5–3.5
Magnesium	(mEq/L)	1	0.5–1.5
Acetate	(mEq/L)	35	—
Lactate	(mEq/L)	—	35–40

[a] Concentration resulting after 1:19 dilution.
[b] Dialysate used for acute and chronic IPD, CAPD, CCPD, and NPD.

IPD, being a high-flow peritoneal system, provides relatively high small-molecule removal. The following sample prescription for IPD using an automated delivery system demonstrates its efficiency for creatinine clearance:

Length of session—24 hours
Dialysate flow—24, 2 L exchanges/session (48 L/session)
Exchange duration—1 hour (inflow time 5 minutes, dwell time 40 minutes, drainage time 15 minutes)
Dialysate—1.5% dextrose, sodium 132 mEq/L, chloride 101 mEq/L, calcium 3.5 mEq/L, magnesium 1.5 mEq/L, lactate 37 mEq/L
Dialysate: plasma creatinine ratio—0.3
Drainage volume—48 L + 4.2 L ultrafiltrate = 52.2 L
Creatinine clearance = 52.2 L × 0.3 = 15.7 L/day

The net UF accomplished with IPD can be easily altered by either increasing the dextrose concentration of the solution or reducing the dwell time. Figure 1 can be used to estimate the net UF, urea, and creatinine clearances with variable dwell times.

CONTINUOUS EQUILIBRATION PERITONEAL DIALYSIS (CEPD)

CEPD is a low-flow, continuous system that maintains stable levels of nitrogenous waste products and a steady hydration status, thus making parenteral alimentation and the regular infusion of intravenous medications feasible (34–39). The kinetics of CEPD are similar to continuous ambulatory peritoneal dialysis (CAPD). The use of a cycler to administer dialysate exchanges assures precise scheduling and reduces nursing labor.

A typical dialysis schedule for adults consists of a 2-L dialysate/exchange using standard solutions for a total length of exchange of 2–4 hours. Variable UF is achieved by adjusting the dialysate dextrose concentration and length of dwell. The following sample prescription illustrates the efficiency of the system:

Dialysate flow—6 2-L exchanges/day (12 L/day)
Exchange duration—4 hours (inflow 10 minutes, dwell 210 minutes, drain 20 minutes)
Dialysate—2.5% dextrose standard solution
Dialysate: plasma urea ratio—0.88
Drainage volume—12 L dialysate + 3 L ultrafiltrate = 15 L
Urea clearance = 15 L × 0.88 = 13 L/day

The reduced urea removal of CEPD compared to IPD is readily compensated by the fact that it is carried continuously. The steady state attained with this technique makes it particularly valuable for critical care patients in need of parenteral alimentation and those with unstable cardiovascular systems.

Complications of acute peritoneal dialysis (Table 2)

INFECTIOUS COMPLICATIONS

Peritonitis

Although peritonitis is a relatively common complication of acute PD, it is much less frequent than in chronic PD.

The rate of peritonitis is dependent on the length of the procedure, its frequency, maintenance of sterile control, and the presence of concomitant infection of the skin in proximity to the catheter exit site. Immunocompromised patients, those with abdominal stomas, and those with poorly healed wounds are more susceptible to this complication.

The incidence of peritonitis in recent series ranges between 1.2% and 2.5% of all procedures (3). The first signs of peritonitis are a cloudy outflow, abdominal pain or tenderness, and fever. Prompt diagnosis and treatment usually result in complete eradication of the infection without significant sequela. The therapy of peritonitis is discussed in Chapter 58.

Exit-site infections

Catheter exit site infections are infrequent when acute semirigid catheters are used due to the short length of implantation of these catheters. The presence of a catheter exit-site infection is an indication for immediate removal of the semirigid catheter and replacement in a different location. When exit-site infections are diagnosed with permanent catheters, immediate antibiotic therapy should be initiated and the area cleansed on a regular basis with peroxide and povidone-iodine. If there is tenderness,

Table 2. Complications of acute peritoneal dialysis

Infectious complications
  Peritonitis
  Catheter exit-site infections

Catheter-related complications
  Laceration of internal organs
  Dialysate leaks
  Catheter obstruction
    One-way
    Complete

Mechanical complications
  Abdominal pain
  Shoulder pain
  Hernia

Medical complications
  Cardiovascular
    Dehydration
    Overhydration
    Arrhythmias
  Pulmonary
    Effusion
    Atelectasis
    Aspiration
    Pneumonia
  Neurologic
    Disequilibrium syndrome
  Metabolic
    Hyperglycemia
    Hypernatremia

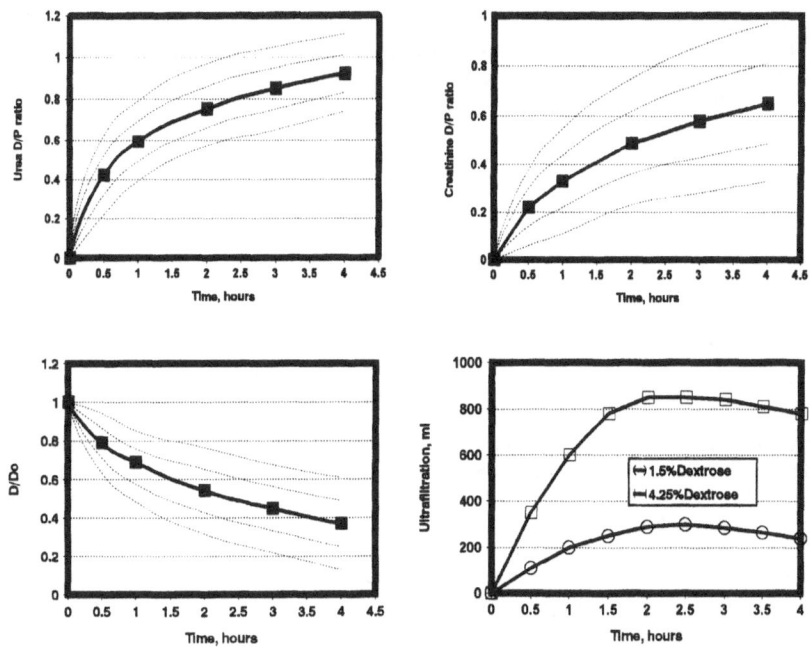

Figure 1. Dialysate to plasma (D/P) ratios for urea and creatinine; timed dextrose concentration/ initial dextrose concentration (D/Do); and net ultrafiltration obtained with 1.5% and 4.25% dextrose solutions. A 2.5% dextrose solution was used to calculate D/P ratios and D/Do. Dotted lines denote ±1 and 2 SD from the mean.

erythema, or extrusion of purulent material from the subcutaneous tunnel, the catheter should be removed and antibiotics continued for at least 1 week following clinical healing of the infection.

CATHETER-RELATED COMPLICATIONS

Laceration of internal organs

Perforation of a viscus or laceration of a blood vessel may occur during catheter implantation. Laceration of a blood vessel is immediately manifested by a bloody peritoneal outflow. If the initial peritoneal outflow is clear but turns progressively darker, it suggests minor bleeding from the anterior abdominal wall. The addition of heparin, 500–1000 units/L of dialysate, is recommended to prevent occlusion of the catheter from blood clots or fibrin. Rapid dialysate exchanges are used to clear intraperitoneal blood and to assess the severity and activity of the bleeder. In most cases, bleeding is self-limited and does not interfere with the procedure. However, it is imperative to monitor the patient's vital signs, dialysate outflow, and hemoglobin concentration at frequent intervals while bleeding persists.

The perforation of an internal viscus may be more difficult to diagnose. A whistling sound through the peritoneal catheter during the initial entrance into the peritoneal cavity suggests perforation of the large bowel and extrusion of colonic gas. The catheter should be removed and a new catheter inserted at a different site. If puncture of the large bowel is suspected, the patient should be treated with prophylactic antibiotics to cover enteric organisms including anaerobic bacteria. If intestinal content is suspected in the outflow, the sample should be immediately inspected under the microscope to verify the diagnosis. Intestinal or bladder perforation not recognized at the time of catheter insertion is usually manifested by either diarrhea or profuse urination after infusion of dialysate. In those circumstances, dialysate cultures should be obtained, the catheter should be removed and replaced in an adequate location, and the patient should be treated with antibiotics. Cloudy fluid shortly after insertion of the catheter and confirmation of polymicrobial peritonitis are suggestive of bowel perforation.

Dialysate leaks

Extravasation of dialysate around the catheter is a common complication of acute dialysis and is encountered in approximately 20% of patients (40–42). This complication can be partially prevented by controlling the size of the initial incision and avoiding frequent manipulation of the catheter. When leaks occur, the exchange volume should be reduced in order to lower intra-abdominal pressure.

The presence of a dialysate leak may be a source of discomfort to the patient and to the paramedical personnel caring for them but is seldom of any significant consequence. A large leak may interfere with proper determination of fluid balance.

Preperitoneal leaks may cause dissection of the peritoneum into the scrotum or vulva, resulting in significant edema. Action should be taken depending on the severity and rate of fluid accumulation. The first step in managing this complication is to reduce the volume of the exchange. Progressive edema may dictate removal of the catheter and temporary discontinuation of peritoneal dialysis.

Catheter obstruction

One-way or ball-valve obstruction is more commonly seen with intermittent than with continuous peritoneal dialysis (CPD) (43). This complication is characterized by easy dialysate inflow but poor or no outflow. The most common causes of one-way obstruction are wrapping of the omentum around the catheter, introduction of the catheter into a small compartment created by adhesions, or a catheter resting against the pelvic or abdominal wall. The use of enemas to stimulate the bowel and omentum, changing the position of the patient in bed, or manipulation of the catheter often corrects the problem.

Complete catheter obstruction to inflow and outflow suggests an intraluminal blood or fibrin clot or kinking of the catheter. If a clot is suspected, brisk infusion of 20–30 mL of dialysate or saline usually corrects the problem. A sharp kink in the catheter is best corrected by manipulation or replacement of the catheter.

OTHER MECHANICAL COMPLICATIONS

Abdominal pain

Many patients complain of diffuse abdominal pain or shoulder pain shortly after initiation of acute PD. The pain is most severe during inflow and subsides during dwell. Inflow pain is more frequently seen with high-flow acute PD using the automated equipment. This type of pain is often relieved by adjustment of the dialysate pH to 6.5–7 with sodium hydroxide (44). In some instances, abdominal pain is not due to the acidity of dialysate but to the hypertonicity of the dialysate. A 1% or 2% xylocaine solution added to the dialysate (5 mL/L) may relieve the pain. Severe pain on inflow that increases in proportion to dialysate infusion suggests that the catheter tip may be located inside a peritoneal compartment. An air contrast study or Tenckhoff cannulography should help diagnose this condition (45).

Shoulder pain can result from introduction of air into the peritoneal cavity during insertion of the catheter. This type of pain usually subsides spontaneously. However, if the pain persists, the air bubble can be displaced by filling the peritoneal cavity with dialysate and manipulating the patient's position into Trendelenburg while letting the air escape through the catheter.

Hernias

A hernia may manifest shortly after initiation of acute PD in patients who already have a weak anterior abdominal wall or weak inguinal rings. Nevertheless, it is relatively rare when compared to chronic PD.

MEDICAL COMPLICATIONS

Cardiovascular complications

Acute PD can result in dehydration or overhydration of the patient if careful monitoring of the hydration status is not maintained. Dehydration can always be corrected by infusion of intravenous fluids, reduction of the dialysate osmolality, or both. Overhydration can be corrected by reducing the dialysate dwell time and/or increasing the dialysate glucose concentration. Cardiac arrhythmias may be the consequence of fluctuations in hydration status, hyperkalemia, or hypokalemia.

Pulmonary complications

Pleural effusions manifesting immediately after initiation of PD suggest a pleuroperitoneal communication. The diagnosis can be readily made by draining the peritoneal cavity and obtaining a chest x-ray. If the level of a pleural effusion fluctuates with the volume of intraperitoneal dialysate, the complication is confirmed. If this relationship is not so clear, infusion of a small amount of radioactive material into the peritoneal cavity with appearance of the radioisotope in the pleural cavity is diagnostic (46). In such circumstances, the peritoneal cavity should be drained and dialysis discontinued.

Basal atelectasis, pneumonia, and aspiration are occasional complications of acute PD (47).

Metabolic complications

Severe hyperglycemia and a hyperosmolar state can occur in diabetic patients during acute peritoneal dialysis, particularly when hypertonic solutions are used. Careful monitoring of blood sugar, intraperitoneal or intravenous infusion of insulin, and reduction of the dialysate glucose concentration usually correct this complication.

Neurologic complications

The disequilibrium syndrome is seldom seen with acute PD. It is usually manifested by headaches, nausea, vomiting, hypertension, seizures, and coma. This syndrome is the consequence of cerebral edema that may occur when a rapid osmotic gradient is created between the brain and the extracellular compartment due to the lag in removal of urea across the blood–brain barrier (48).

Confusion, irritability, generalized weakness, and cloudy sensorium can be a complication of hypernatremia when very short dwell times and standard solutions are used. This complication can be prevented by adjusting the dialysate sodium concentration (29).

CHRONIC PERITONEAL DIALYSIS

Since the introduction of CAPD, the proportion of end-stage renal disease (ESRD) patients undergoing PD has increased steeply. The development of safe and permanent PD catheters, improved connectology, dialysate in plastic containers of variable volume, more physiologic PD solutions, and introduction of new dialysis techniques have been responsible for this accelerated growth. The larger population of patients requiring assistance with procedures and the recognition of certain conditions that require high-flow PD have fostered the use of APD. Compared to the entire ESRD populations' annual increase of 11% for 1988 to 1990, the number of patients treated with CCPD increased more rapidly (33%/year) than the overall rate of change (49). Interest in other forms of APD such as nocturnal PD (NPD) hybrid modalities (PD Plus) and tidal PD (TPD) is reflected in the recent literature, but the number of patients on these modalities is limited.

Peritoneal access

The peritoneal catheter designed by Tenckhoff and Schechter (50) has become the most popular means of providing adequate peritoneal access. The catheter consists of a silastic tube with one or two Dacron cuffs for anchoring and a straight or curled configuration.

The Tenckhoff peritoneal catheter can be inserted in the original manner using a special trocar (51), surgically (52), under peritoneoscopy (53), or using the Seldinger technique (54).

Several modifications to the Tenckhoff catheter have been introduced, including the curled catheter and those with disks, balloons, and other devices in the distal end, designed to avoid omental wrapping or to improve dialysate drainage. Other catheters have been designed to improve flow dynamics. An important modification of the original design has been the incorporation of a Swan-neck or pan-handle subcutaneous segment to eliminate the stress generated by the catheter against the tissues when a semiarcuate subcutaneous tunnel is utilized (55,56). More recently, a new catheter implantation technique has been described by Moncrief et al. (57). The new technique consists of surgical implantation of the catheter, with the segment that would ordinarily be brought out through the skin in the standard implantation technique being completely buried under the skin in a subcutaneous tunnel. The wound

is closed, leaving no exit site for several weeks. Four to six weeks postoperatively, a small incision is made 2 cm distal to the subcutaneous cuff and perpendicular to the long axis of the catheter. The distal segment of the catheter is then brought out through the skin. The rationale behind this technique is to allow complete healing at the level of the external subcutaneous cuff in an attempt to prevent migration of bacteria through the tunnel and to prevent exit-site infections and peritonitis. The details of catheter placement and management are covered in Chapter 57.

BREAK-IN TECHNIQUE

Many protocols have been suggested for the care and use of a new peritoneal catheter (58,59). Some centers recommend a period of rest of 24 hours to 1 week before using the catheter or as long as 6 weeks following implantation. Although these protocols allow time for healing and avoidance of pericatheter or incisional dialysate leaks, they have the disadvantage of preventing the immediate use of the catheter and the early diagnosis of catheter dysfunction. Whether the catheter is used immediately or a healing period is allowed, the use of 500–1000 units of heparin per L of dialysate is recommended to avoid clotting of the catheter lumen with fibrin strands.

Many centers use the catheter immediately after implantation. In our experience with more than 800 catheters using the traditional Tenckhoff methodology, Seldinger technique, peritoneoscopy, or surgical technique, the majority of catheters can be used immediately after implantation, with an incidence of leakage of less than 4%. The volume of dialysate during the first few days of use should be limited to 1 L in normal-size adults in order to minimize intra-abdominal pressure and consequent discomfort and pericatheter leaks. The dialysate volume can be gradually increased to 2 or 3 L/exchange as tolerated by the patient. The sutures should be removed within 10 days or whenever proper healing is noted.

Peritoneal dialysis delivery systems

REVERSE OSMOSIS PROPORTIONING SYSTEMS

The RO proportioning system combines an RO water treatment device with a product water–dialysate concentrate proportioning unit (60). Tap water is filtered to remove sediment or particulate matter prior to entering the RO pump. The water is then forced through an RO membrane where pyrogens and trace elements are removed to form the product water. The product water is then mixed with dialysate concentrate at a 19:1 ratio to produce dialysate. These systems allow automated delivery of dialysate to the patient and can be programmed to provide specific rates of inflow, dwell times, and variable drain periods. Although the RO proportioning systems provide the convenience of automated dialysis delivery in a reliable and safe manner, the complexity of the system, their large size, the high initial purchase price, high cost of maintenance, relatively long training period, and complex sterilization procedure required have hindered their popularity. These systems are seldom used today and usually reserved for use in the hospital or for acute IPD.

PERITONEAL DIALYSIS CYCLERS

Most cyclers are designed after Lasker's original concept using the principles of gravity infusion and drainage (61). Peritoneal cyclers automatically deliver a prescribed volume of commercial dialysate and allow variable dwell and drain times. Their simplicity and short procedural requirements have made them readily acceptable for home use for IPD, CCPD, NPD, and TPD. A cycler consists of three main parts: the stand/base, heater cabinet, and control unit. Dialysate flow from the bags or bottles takes place by gravity or by using a partially pump-driven system to deliver dialysate to an overhead bag. The partially pump-dependent systems propel the dialysate from a large dialysate bag to a smaller dialysate container usually lying on a heating cradle that often also serves as a scale to determine the volume to be infused into the patient. This modification has the advantage of allowing the use of larger dialysate containers and reducing cost. It also eliminates the effort of lifting a heavy bag from the floor to a level above the patient's bed.

Totally pump-driven systems use pumps both to instill dialysate into the patient and to drain the spent dialysate. Such systems have been avoided in the past for fear of abdominal overdistention or suction of intraperitoneal structures through the catheter. A new cycler has been recently introduced using strategically placed positive and negative pressure monitors that have rendered the system safe. The possible advantages of these systems are the faster instillation and removal of fluid from the peritoneal cavity and their potential to provide sufficient stirring of the fluid in the peritoneal cavity to overcome the effect of unstirred layers of dialysate and thus improve dialysis efficiency.

While the primary functions of a cycler are to deliver a measured volume of dialysate into the peritoneal cavity, to allow the delivered dialysate to dwell in the peritoneal cavity for a prescribed period of time, and to drain the used or spent dialysate from the peritoneal cavity, most modern cyclers provide important secondary functions. The selection of a cycler and the vast array of accessories depends on the patient's specific needs. Some of the available features of modern cyclers include warming of solutions to body temperature; calculation of fluid balance and net UF; safety monitors and alarms for temperature, fluid balance, power failure, dialysate flow obstruction, and insufficient dialysate; built-in programs to determine modality of dialysis; real-time graphic displays of dialysate delivered and drained; automatic elimination of superfluous drain time and proportional increase in dwell time allotted for that cycle; selection of dialysate glucose concentration and volume for a particular cycle; data storage and telephone

transmission of dialytic events to the center; use of large dialysate containers; direct drainage into a tray, drain, or drainage bag; built-in kinetic programs; and oversized visual displays and computerized voice recognition systems for the sight impaired. The increase in cost and potential complexity of these options demand the medical team's input into the selection of a cycler.

Intermittent peritoneal dialysis

Chronic IPD was mostly used in the 1970s before the introduction of CAPD and CCPD. IPD represented the first automated modality of PD capable of providing long-term renal replacement. Some of the factors that influenced the selection of IPD included its relative simplicity, no need for venipunctures or blood access, avoidance of systemic heparinization, and gradual removal of nitrogenous products and water. The rate of peritonitis was generally low at approximately 0.3% of all dialyses (62,63). Although the initial clinical experience claimed control of biochemical parameters and mortality rates similar to chronic HD for the first years of therapy (63), the long-term experience was very disappointing. The mortality rate after 2 years exceeded 50%, and the mortality among diabetic patients was significantly higher (64).

The typical IPD prescription is a 10-hour session every other night or three times per week, using dialysate flow rates of 2–4 L/hour delivered via an RO proportioning unit or a PD cycler. Although adequate UF can usually be accomplished, total solute removal is less than desirable, as noted in Table 3. Patients with residual renal function (RRF) (GFR 3–5 mL/min) can benefit from supplementary IPD and often remain healthy; however, anuric patients and those with minimal renal function eventually develop uremic complications and malnutrition (64–66).

Table 3. Comparative clearances of selected solutes obtained with various modalities of peritoneal dialysis (in L/day)

	C_{urea}	$C_{creatinine}$	Dialysate flow
Acute PD	25	16	24, 2-L exchanges/24 hr
CAPD	8.2	6.2	4, 2-L exchanges/24 hr
CCPD	8.1	6.1	Nocturnal: 4, 2-L exchanges (10 hr) Diurnal: 1, 2-L exchange (14 hr)
PD Plus	14.2	10.7	Nocturnal: 4, 2.75-L exchanges (10 hr) Diurnal: 2, 2-L exchanges (14 h)
NPD	8.2	5.2	12, 2-L exchanges or 24 L/8 hr
TPD	8.2	5.2	TV[a] 1.0 RV[b] 1.0 or 24 L/8 hr
	9.4	6.2	TV 1.5 RV 1.5 or 24 L/8 hr

[a] TV, tidal volume.
[b] RV, reserve volume.

The use of chronic IPD has plummeted due to the inadequate dialysis it provides, the high cost of dialysate, other disposables and equipment, and the introduction of simpler and more effective forms of PD. IPD is now reserved for patients with RRF, those who refuse CPD, and the few that require hospital dialysis due to their unstable medical condition and unfavorable socioeconomic environment.

Continuous cyclic peritoneal dialysis (CCPD)

The introduction of CEPD by Popovich et al. in l976 offered a potential solution to the problem of inadequate dialysis (67). Although the clearances offered by CAPD are rather limited, the continuous nature of the treatment overcomes this problem, achieving total weekly clearances definitely superior to those of IPD for small molecules and greater than those of IPD or HD for middle-size molecules (Table 3). Notwithstanding CAPD's simplicity, ability to maintain a steady physiologic state, and adequate UF, multiple drawbacks, such as the long and interrupted procedural time and high rate of peritonitis, stimulated the development of CCPD (68,69).

TECHNIQUE

CCPD provides CPD and is a virtual reversal of CAPD. The schedule consists of a long diurnal dwell exchange and multiple shorter nocturnal exchanges delivered by a peritoneal cycler. Before retiring at night, the patient prepares the peritoneal cycler with the necessary dialysate and sets the cycler controls that determine the volume of each exchange, the duration of dwell, and drainage. The connection between the cycler's patient line and the peritoneal catheter takes place under aseptic control. During the night, the patient receives three to five exchanges of variable volumes (2–3 L/exchange). Standard dialysis solution containing 1.5%–4.25% dextrose is used for the nocturnal exchanges (Table 2). The last exchange consists of hypertonic (4.25%) solution. The nocturnal cycles last approximately 10 hours. In the morning, the patient disconnects the cycler line from the catheter after infusing 1500–2000 mL of hypertonic solution. The disconnection can be achieved by traditional methodology or with the external occlusion technique, which is much simpler and faster to perform (70). The diurnal exchange lasts approximately 14 hours.

CLINICAL EXPERIENCE

The clinical experience with CCPD has been similar to that reported with CAPD in terms of hematologic and biochemical profiles (68,69,71–73). The incidence of the majority of complications related to PD has also been similar among CAPD and CCPD patients. Therefore, only those complications or outcomes that differ between the two therapies will be discussed in this chapter.

A low percentage of patients have developed frank hypertriglyceridemia and/or obesity while undergoing CCPD. A possible explanation for this phenomenon lies in the increased UF per gram of absorbed glucose observed with shorter peritoneal cycles (74). The shorter nocturnal cycles of CCPD accomplish UF earlier in the cycler, while dialysate glucose concentrations are higher. Therefore, the same or higher UF is attained with lower glucose absorption.

No prospective studies have been conducted comparing nutritional status among CAPD and CCPD patients. However, preliminary data from our center suggest that there are no significant differences and that patient-specific differences are mostly related to dialysis dose, RRF, and comorbid factors rather than to the type of dialysis modality. Peritoneal protein losses in uninfected patients average 6–9 g/day, a figure is similar to that reported for noninfected CAPD patients (74,75).

The peritonitis rates have been reported to be significantly lower than with CAPD in most adult series (70). In our series, the rate of peritonitis has been one episode every 2 years. This experience is not exclusive to our institution and has been corroborated or surpassed by other centers primarily caring for adult patients (76). Holley et al. have also reported a lower rate of catheter exit-site infections with CCPD (76).

Several factors that may explain the lower rate of peritonitis among CCPD patients should be mentioned. The fact that all connections for CCPD take place only once daily in the home environment may allow better aseptic control, greater concentration, the possible use of a partner, and less stress on the patient and his or her relatives. The number of actual connections can be reduced by utilizing large-volume dialysate containers. In vitro and clinical experiences strongly suggest that part of the reason for the lower rate of peritonitis and particularly for reduction in peritonitis with *Staphylococcus epidermidis* is the direction of flow (77,78). Since the first event to occur during a connection in CCPD is an outflow of spent dialysate, it is likely that the potential contamination is flushed by the spent dialysate. The experience with CAPD Y-sets has confirmed this hypothesis by significantly lowering the peritonitis rates for CAPD patients as well (79–82). It is possible that the long diurnal dwell of CCPD allows repopulation of the peritoneal resident macrophages and provides a better host immune defense. We have reported elevated peritoneal fluid cell counts in noninfected patients following the diurnal cycle of CCPD (72). Vlaanderen et al. have also reported an increase in the number of phagocytes with longer dwell times and an increase in opsonic activity and IgG levels (83). Finally, the prolonged dwell time of CCPD is also associated with a fall in glucose concentration at the end of the cycle. Since the lower glucose concentration may enhance macrophage phagocytic function, it is conceivable that the prolonged dwell time of CCPD and the periods of rest between PD sessions in NPD and TPD may be associated with improved peritoneal host defenses (84).

CCPD is capable of providing adequate dialysis for patients with normal peritoneal permeability. CCPD pro-

Table 4. Indications for CCPD

Patient preference
  Employed, active patients
  Unwilling or unable to perform exchanges
  Poor eye–hand coordination
  Need for partner
  Psychological (self-image)
Children
Poor compliance with number of exchanges
Frequent peritonitis
Hernias
Chronic low-back pain
Severe cardiopulmonary compromise
Recurrent catheter exit-site leakage

---

vides solute clearances similar to CAPD (Table 3). The minor differences observed may not be of clinical importance and could be corrected by increasing dialysate flow during the nocturnal cycles. The cumulative patient and technique survival for nondiabetic patients on CCPD exceeds 80% at 3 years for patient survival and 60% for technique survival (64). In our program, these figures are comparable to those of CAPD and hemodialysis.

INDICATIONS AND CONTRAINDICATIONS

The major indications for CCPD are summarized in Table 4. Most patients select CCPD due to the daytime freedom that it allows, the improved self-image provided by the freedom from bags and procedural exchanges during the day, and the reduced fatigue from the procedure.

CCPD has become the most common form of therapy for pediatric use in many large centers. The main reasons for this preference are that this procedure allows the participation of a parent in performing connections and disconnections, as well as daytime freedom for school and recreational activities, while retaining all the other advantages inherent in CPD.

Additional advantages of CCPD relate to the physical effects of a reduced intra-abdominal volume. Aside from the direct correlation between intra-abdominal volume and pressure, it has been shown that position further influences intra-abdominal pressure (85,86). The same volume of dialysate increases the intra-abdominal pressure when the patient changes from the supine to the standing or sitting position. An increase in intraabdominal pressure can lead to a higher incidence of abdominal discomfort, lumbosacral strain, pericatheter leaks, and hernias. Many patients with these complications benefit from a reduced diurnal intra-abdominal volume.

PD Plus, Quantum and other hybrid modalities

In order to enhance the efficiency of PD, new regimes have been developed incorporating features of CAPD and CCPD (87). These modalities of therapy combine diurnal

manual exchanges and automated nocturnal exchanges using very simple and inexpensive cyclers and large volume dialysis containers to reduce cost. These modalities optimize dwell time by eliminating the long diurnal cycles of CCPD or long nocturnal cycles of CAPD and the very short cycles of CCPD, thereby improving utilization of the dialysis solution. They commonly use large volume nocturnal exchanges. Larger exchange volumes and dialysis in the supine position are known to increase the mass transfer area coefficient (MTAC), thus improving small solute clearance (88, 89). Larger dialysate volumes are also better tolerated in the supine position than sitting or standing.

TECHNIQUE

PD Plus consists of three or four nocturnal exchanges and two diurnal exchanges. The nocturnal exchanges and the first morning exchange are delivered by the cycler. The second diurnal exchange can be done manually or obtained from the cycler if it is equipped with a pause feature. The diurnal exchange volume is typically 2 L in adults and the dwell time between 6 and 8 hours. The nocturnal exchange volumes should be as high as comfortably tolerated by the patient, usually 2.5 to 3.5 L. The total dialysis solution volume ranges between 12 and 15 L/day.

Other modalities use typical CAPD exchanges during the day and provide an additional nocturnal exchange using a very simple cycling device (Quantum). The nocturnal exchange volumes should be increased as tolerated by the patient.

CLINICAL EXPERIENCE

The limited experience with these modalities has demonstrated a significant increase in small solute clearance as compared to CAPD or CCPD (87). The enhancement of clearances is proportionally greater than the increase in volume of dialysis solution due to the larger exchange volumes utilized. Preliminary reports suggest good patient acceptance. The main disadvantage of these systems is that they require a cycler as well as diurnal exchanges. The great advantage is their ability to deliver higher dialysis dose for large and anuric patients. These regimes can provide adequate PD (weekly $Kt/V_{urea} \geq 2.0$) for anuric patients weighing 90 to 100 Kg, depending on their peritoneal transport rates.

Nocturnal peritoneal dialysis (NPD)

Nightly PD is similar to IPD but is performed nightly (74). The total exchange time is 8–10 hours, using cycle times of 20–60 minutes. Although NPD has the disadvantages of not being able to provide a steady physiologic state, is expensive due to the high dialysate flow, and requires a delivery system capable of infusing large amounts of dialysate during every session, it has some specific indications. The indications fall into two main categories:

Table 5. Complications of chronic peritoneal dialysis

Infectious complications
  Peritonitis
  Exit-site and tunnel infections
Catheter-related complications
  Abdominal pain
  Bloody outflow
  Pericatheter leaks
  Perforations or lacerations of blood vessels and internal
    organs
  Catheter obstruction
    One-way
    Complete
Peritoneal membrane dysfunction
  Ultrafiltration failure
  Peritoneal sclerosis
Complications due to increased intra-abdominal pressure
  Dialysate leaks
  Hernias
  Low back pain
  Gastroesophageal reflux
  Hemorrhoids
  Pulmonary compromise
  Cardiac compromise
Inadequate dialysis
Medical complications
  Metabolic
    Protein malnutrition
    Obesity
    Hyperlipoproteinemia
    Renal osteodystrophy
  Neurologic
    Disequilibrium syndrome
    Peripheral neuropathy
    Dialysis dementia
  Hematologic
    Anemia

---

a high peritoneal membrane permeability and mechanical indications.

Patients with high peritoneal permeability accomplish osmotic equilibration within a relative short dwell period. Consequently, UF becomes inadequate and absorption of dialysate takes place. The use of short dwell times leads to drainage of the fluid while the peritoneal osmotic gradient is still effective. Solute equilibration also takes place faster than in normal permeability states, thus allowing adequate solute removal with shorter dwell times. Therefore, a patient with high peritoneal permeability can achieve adequate UF and solute removal with a high-flow, short-dwell schedule, while the long dwell periods of CAPD and CCPD may prove detrimental.

Patients suffering from abdominal leaks and hernias, bladder prolapse, low back pain, and restrictive lung disease may be intolerant of the increased intra-abdominal pressure associated with the infusion of 1 or 2 L of dialysate during the day while the patient is sitting or standing.

These patients may tolerate equal volumes of dialysate in the supine position, as provided by NPD.

Table 3 provides the average clearances obtained with NPD in patients with normal permeability using 24 L of dialysate over an 8-hour period. The daily clearances for urea are similar as those obtained with CAPD or CCPD. However, the clearance for creatinine and larger molecules is significantly lower despite the high dialysate flow.

The clinical experience with NPD is limited, preventing any firm conclusions regarding the long-term safety and efficiency of this technique. However, there are preliminary data to suggest that patients with increased peritoneal permeability who remain on PD may develop further deterioration of peritoneal membrane function (90). It has also been speculated that this group of patients may eventually develop peritoneal sclerosis.

Tidal peritoneal dialysis (TPD)

TPD is a variation of APD that consists of maintaining a constant reserve volume of dialysis solution in the peritoneal cavity at all times and an additional tidal volume of dialysate that is intermittently cycled in and out of the peritoneal cavity (91,92). The rationale behind this technique is that a sufficient reserve volume in contact with the peritoneal membrane at all times, as well as the additional tidal volume, which assures adequate mixing of the dialysate and frequent restoration of the dialysate/plasma gradient, will enhance peritoneal clearance.

The early experience suggested higher small-solute clearances than with CAPD or CCPD (93,94). However, more recent experience suggests that the higher exchange volumes (3 L instead of 2 L used for CAPD) account for the enhanced clearances (95–96). Other studies have demonstrated that, indeed, an increase in exchange volume may significantly enhance the transperitoneal mass transfer of small solutes (88,89). The main disadvantages of this procedure are the need for a specially modified cycler, which is regulated by volume rather than time, and the extremely high dialysate flows, both of which result in additional cost.

Complications of chronic peritoneal dialysis (Table 5)

PERITONITIS

Peritonitis remains the most common complication of chronic PD. However, significant differences in the incidence of this complication have been reported for IPD, CCPD, and CAPD. The peritonitis rate for IPD is approximately 0.3% of all procedures, or one episode of peritonitis every 2–3 years (62,63). The peritonitis rate for CCPD in most large adult series has been in the range of one episode every 1.5–2 years (70). Peritonitis rates for CAPD remain higher and approximate one episode every year with the standard spike technique but have drastically improved with the use of the CAPD Y-sets. Port et al. have recently reported an incidence of 1.05 episodes per year for CAPD with standard spike connectors and 0.58 episodes per year for CAPD Y-set (97). Peritonitis and PD infectious complications are discussed in detail in Chapter 58.

CATHETER-RELATED COMPLICATIONS

Abdominal pain can present immediately after insertion of the peritoneal catheter or late during treatment of the chronic PD patient. The pain can be related to pressure of the catheter against the abdominal or pelvic wall and usually subsides after a few days or weeks on PD. Introduction of the catheter into a small peritoneal compartment formed by previous adhesions can also cause pain on inflow. These complications should always be suspected when the pain increases as a function of the volume of peritoneal dialysate infused. The problem should be corrected by removal and replacement of the catheter. Abdominal pain associated with the use of acetate-containing dialysate concentrate or commercial dialysate is very uncommon at present, since these solutions are seldom used. The problem can be remedied by the addition of sodium hydroxide to increase the pH to between 6 and 7 (44). Abdominal pain and peritoneal eosinophilia have been noted to occur shortly after insertion of a new PD catheter. Daugirdas et al. have demonstrated a direct relationship between the infusion of intraperitoneal air and this syndrome (98). The symptoms usually subside spontaneously and do not require specific therapy.

Bloody peritoneal outflow occurring immediately after insertion of a peritoneal catheter suggests laceration of a major blood vessel or continuous oozing from the anterior abdominal wall at the site of the peritoneal catheter entrance. Therapy will depend on the severity and persistence of the bleeding. Close monitoring of the dialysate outflow and the hemoglobin concentration should be maintained and exploratory laparotomy considered if the bleeding persists or results in a significant hemoglobin drop. The late presentation of peritoneal bleeding should be viewed in a different manner. The possibility of erosion of the peritoneal catheter into a blood vessel or spleen is rare but possible. Displacement of the Tenckhoff catheter to the left upper quadrant associated with severe intraperitoneal

bleeding due to rupture of the spleen has been reported (99). Hemoperitoneum during CPD has also been ascribed to postradiation peritoneal injury (100). Recurrent bloody peritoneal outflow, with or without associated vaginal bleeding, is not uncommon among women of menstruating age undergoing CPD. This phenomenon is often referred to as retrograde menstruation and does not require specific therapy.

Dialysate leaks around the catheter exit site are common complications of PD. Patients who suffer from malnutrition or debilitating diseases or who are under the effects of corticosteroid therapy are at high risk. Internal dialysate leaks manifested by infiltration of dialysate into the anterior abdominal wall, scrotum, and vulva usually occur shortly after catheter implantation and suggest leakage around the catheter entrance into the peritoneum. Reduction in the volume of dialysate or temporary discontinuation of PD usually corrects the problem. Persistence of leakage after these maneuvers suggests a larger tear in the peritoneal entrance or a pinhole in the catheter itself, resulting in continuous leakage. In such instances, the catheter must be removed and replaced with a new device, preferably after allowing a 10- to 14-day rest to assure proper healing of the original incision. The use of technetium-99m scintigraphy or CT scanning of the abdomen has been proposed for the diagnosis of dialysate leakage (101,102). Although this procedure has a high diagnostic yield in cases of pleuroperitoneal communications and open processus vaginalis, it is seldom diagnostic in cases of small cracks or pinholes in the Tenckhoff catheter itself (103).

Late dialysate leaks are less common and probably are due to increased intra-abdominal pressure (vide infra). The complication can be adequately treated in most cases by either decreasing the dialysate volume, interrupting PD with temporary transfer to HD, or using IPD or NPD. Removal and reimplantation of the catheter is seldom necessary. Vaginal leakage of dialysate by way of the fallopian tubes and uterus has been observed both in asymptomatic women and in association with peritonitis (104). Although women have the potential anatomic vaginoperitoneal communication, this complication has been rare.

Table 6. Therapeutic recommendations based on PET results

Solute transport	$D/P_{creat, 4hr}$[a]	$D/P_{urea, 4hr}$	D_4/D_0[b]	Ultrafiltration	Recommended therapy
Normal	0.50–0.80	1.0–0.84	0.25–0.49	Adequate	CAPD, CCPD
High	0.81–0.95	≥1.0	0.24–0.12	Low	NPD
Low	0.49–0.34	0.83–0.73	0.50–0.62	High	Increase Vip[c] (CAPD, CCPD, TPD)
Very high	≥0.96	≥1.0	≤0.11	Very low	Transfer to HD
Very low	≤0.33	≤0.72	≥0.63	Variable	Transfer to HD

[a] D/P, dialysate/plasma ratio of solute.
[b] D_4/D_0, glucose concentration in dialysate at 4 hours/glucose concentration in dialysate at the end of infusion.
[c] Vip, exchange volume or intraperitoneal volume.

Early perforation or laceration of an internal organ is relatively rare. The criteria for diagnosis are similar to those introduced above under Complications of Acute Peritoneal Access. The organs most frequently injured are the bowel, bladder, liver, kidney (renal cysts), and blood vessels. Perforation of the bowel and mesenteric vessels is most likely to occur in patients who have undergone previous abdominal surgery and have developed adhesions and fixation of the organ to the anterior abdominal wall. Also at higher risks are patients with bowel distention due to paralytic ileus, toxic magacolon, or bowel obstruction. Recognition of visceral perforation requires prompt removal of the catheter, with or without reinsertion, appropriate peritoneal cultures, prophylactic antibiotic therapy, and close observation. If symptoms of peritoneal inflammation manifest within the first 48 hours, suggesting continuous leakage of visceral content and peritoneal contamination, consideration should be given to exploratory laparotomy.

Perforation or laceration of internal organs as a late complication of the peritoneal catheter is uncommon. However, erosion of the catheter into the colon has been reported as late as 9 months after insertion of the catheter (105). Erosion of the catheter into the pelvic wall with eventual vaginal penetration has also been reported after 17 months of successful chronic PD (106). The causative factors offered to explain these complications include pressure necrosis due to the continuous pressure of the catheter against tissue and chemical irritation caused by the jet current during dialysate infusion. Malnutrition and peritonitis may serve as predisposing factors.

Catheter obstruction can be partial or complete. The most common type of catheter dysfunction is the one-way or ball-valve type. The diagnosis and correct therapy for these complications are similar to those described for acute peritoneal access. One-way obstruction has been reported to be the cause of catheter failure in 14%–23% of the cases (43,107,108). However, this complication is more frequent in patients undergoing IPD than in those on CPD (43). The likely explanation for this difference is that the fluid is always present during CPD and reduces the concentration of fibrin strands and prevents omental wrapping around the peritoneal catheter.

PERITONEAL MEMBRANE DYSFUNCTION

Although many patients can remain on PD for as long as 8 or 10 years, others have developed evidence of peritoneal membrane dysfunction (109,110). With the increased use of PD as a chronic means of renal replacement, the incidence of this type of complication has increased, particularly among those with a high rate of infectious complications. A recent prospective long-term study of patients undergoing chronic PD for at least 3 years has shown remarkably stable mass transfer coefficients for urea without significant differences between the first and the fifth year of therapy. On the other hand, peritoneal UF capacity signifi-

cantly decreased over that period of time and correlated well with the accumulated days of peritoneal inflammation (111). This study suggests that after 5–11 years, the human peritoneum shows functional stability in patients with low rates of peritoneal inflammation. The earliest and most frequently recognized form of peritoneal dysfunction is the syndrome of UF failure. This condition has been characterized as an increase in peritoneal permeability, which results in rapid absorption of dialysate glucose with prompt blunting of the osmotic gradient between dialysate and plasma. The transport of solutes remains intact, but failure to achieve UF of water precludes adequate PD. Many investigators have suggested that the use of acetate in dialysate solutions is a causative factor for this condition (110,112,113). Although the data are not conclusive, there is enough circumstantial evidence to implicate acetate as a possible etiology. This syndrome has been much more frequently seen in France than in North America but has been diagnosed in isolated patients throughout the world. Whether this condition progresses to the more serious complication of peritoneal membrane thickening and sclerosis is uncertain.

The wealth of data today suggest that the etiology of peritoneal UF failure may be multifactorial, that it may be present at the initiation of PD in some patients or may gradually develop in others, that a temporary transfer to HD or the use of IPD or NPD may restore normal permeability in some patients (114), and that a few patients may progress to peritoneal sclerosis if PD is continued (90,115,116). Proper evaluation of peritoneal permeability is indicated in any patient who fails to achieve adequate water UF with CAPD or CCPD and in those who progressively require a higher proportion of hypertonic exchanges in order to accomplish the same UF. If peritoneal hyperpermeability is diagnosed, a transfer to higher-flow dialysis using shorter dwell times and elimination of the long diurnal dwells of CCPD or long nocturnal dwells of CAPD is indicated.

The application of the standard peritoneal equilibration test (PET) at the initiation of PD and periodically thereafter has proven of great benefit in the evaluation of peritoneal transport and in the modification of the dialysis prescription (117). Table 6 summarizes the therapeutic recommendations for patients undergoing PD based on PET results. Patients with a normal solute transport can be maintained on CPD (CAPD or CCPD) and should achieve adequate UF and toxin removal. High transporters benefit from a transfer to NPD due to its frequent and short exchanges enhancing UF. Patients with moderately low solute transport may be managed with an increase in exchange volume while remaining on CAPD, CCPD, or TPD. Those with extremely high or low solute transfer rates should be transferred to HD in order to achieve adequate UF and solute removal.

A more dreadful complication of PD is peritoneal sclerosis. In this condition, the peritoneal membrane becomes thickened, eventually leading to strangulation of the bowel by the formation of a leathery cocoon that envelopes all intra-abdominal organs. The condition has been reported in patients on IPD, CAPD, and CCPD (118). Peritoneal sclerosis eventually leads to decreased solute and water movement across the peritoneal membrane due to loss of peritoneal permeability or surface area. Repeated episodes of peritonitis, the use of acetate solutions, regular use of hyperosmolar dialysate, chlorhexidine, plasticizers, and particulate matter in the dialysate have all been implicated as etiologic factors. Peritoneal sclerosis has also been associated with the use of other pharmacologic agents such as propranolol and oxprenolol. There is no specific therapy for this condition, which may prove fatal in its most advanced forms.

COMPLICATIONS DUE TO INCREASED INTRA-ABDOMINAL PRESSURE (IAP)

IAP is directly proportional to the volume of dialysate infused intraperitoneally (119). Changes in position further affect IAP (85,86). The highest IAP is observed with the patient in the sitting position, followed by the standing and supine positions. This phenomenon probably explains the higher incidence of certain complications in patients undergoing CAPD and those on CCPD using high diurnal volumes, as compared to those undergoing IPD or NPD. Additional factors that influence the rate of development of these complications include intra-abdominal masses such as large polycystic kidneys, previous abdominal surgery, weak abdominal walls from malnutrition, and multiparity.

Late dialysate leaks are often a product of these circumstances. Similarly, hernias, whether incisional, umbilical, inguinal, abdominal, or diaphragmatic, can be observed with relatively high frequency. Although the incidence of abdominal hernias with CAPD and CCPD using exchanges of 2 or more liters has been reported to be 9%–12% (120,121), the incidence is 2%–3% among patients on IPD and those on CCPD with reduced diurnal volumes (43).

Low back pain can present de novo or may be aggravated by the infusion of large volumes of intra-abdominal fluid. High IAP increases the lordotic curvature, which is associated with lumbosacral strain and pain (122). The use of exercise to strengthen the paravertebral and the anterior abdominal wall muscles may help prevent or ameliorate these symptoms. However, if symptomatology persists, a reduction in the exchange volume is indicated.

Increased IAP can affect changes in cardiac and pulmonary function. Gotloib et al. have demonstrated a significant decrease in cardiac output and stroke volume in response to increase in IAP. Mean arterial blood pressure increased as a consequence of a significant increase in peripheral resistance (119). Alpert et al. have shown that in CAPD patients with left ventricular hypertrophy, intraperitoneal volumes exceeding 2 L produce a significant decrease in left ventricular systolic function due to preload reduction, probably from increasing IAP (123). Neverthe-

less, for practical purposes, the infusion of 2 L of dialysate intraperitoneally does not adversely affect hemodynamics in most patients (124).

Increases in intra-abdominal volume and IAP may also result in pulmonary compromise. Marked deterioration of vital capacity, forced vital capacity, and forced expiratory volume at 1 second have been reported in some patients with intraperitoneal volumes in excess of 2 L (86,125). In our experience, very few patients with chronic obstructive pulmonary disease tolerate dialysate volumes in excess of 2 L in the sitting position.

Other symptoms that are occasionally associated with increased IAP include gastroesophageal reflux and hemorrhoidal discomfort.

Intolerance to high IAP can be corrected by reducing the exchange volume of the diurnal cycles of CCPD. However, the total elimination of the diurnal cycles and transfer to NPD is not recommended in patients with normal peritoneal solute transport, since this will result in a significant decrease in solute clearance and particularly of larger molecules (126).

INADEQUATE DIALYSIS

Insufficient dialysis is perhaps the most common and least recognized complication of long-term PD. Most patients initiate renal replacement therapy with significant RRF. After a period of several years, RRF diminishes, and by the end of the third year it is usually insignificant. While some patients of small size and with adequate peritoneal transport can maintain nitrogen balance with standard regimens of CAPD and CCPD, many patients require modifications in their peritoneal prescription to maintain nitrogen balance.

During the past few years, great interest in defining the adequacy of PD has been expressed in the literature. A strong correlation between the dialysis dose and protein intake or normalized protein catabolic rate (NPCR) has been demonstrated by various investigators (127–131). A recent analysis of 132 patients from 15 dialysis centers using urea kinetic modeling (UKM) showed that RRF comprised 25% of the total KT for these patients and that the mean total KT/V was 0.28 or the equivalent of thrice-weekly HD KT/V of 1.07; however, 67% of the values were less than 1 (132). The mean NPCR was 0.8 and showed a significant correlation with total KT/V. These data suggest that a significant number of patients are receiving less than adequate dialysis using HD criteria. It also corroborates the strong correlation between dialysis dose and protein intake. A large number of patients were ingesting less protein than is generally considered adequate. In view of the fact that RRF contributed 25% of the total urea clearance, it is likely that the number of inadequately dialyzed patients would increase with time on dialysis. The current recommendations for PD adequacy, based on theoretical constructs and clinical outcome studies are to provide a weekly $k+/V_{urea} \geq 2.0$ and/or $C_{creatinine} \geq 60 L/1.73M^2$ (133).

APD offers great flexibility of prescription and allows significant increases in solute clearance by increasing either total dialysate flow or the volume of dialysate exchange, or both. Larger volumes of dialysate are better tolerated with the patient in the supine position than while sitting or standing, offering an additional advantage of APD over CAPD.

Medical complications

METABOLIC COMPLICATIONS

Protein malnutrition is a frequent complication of chronic PD. An international study of nutrition among CAPD patients showed an incidence of moderate or severe malnutrition of 41% (134). Causes of malnutrition unique to PD include abdominal distention, excessive glucose absorption from dialysate, and protein losses into the dialysate. Most important, however, is the possibility of inadequate dialysis and consequent anorexia from residual uremia. While dialysate protein loss varies widely among patients, it averages 6–10 g/day (75). During episodes of peritonitis, the protein losses may increase drastically and may significantly contribute to protein depletion. The strong relationship between normalized total urea clearance (KT/V_{urea}), and NPCR and the aforementioned observation that RRF makes a significant contribution to KT/V_{urea} in a large proportion of patients dictate alterations in the dialysis prescription as RRF diminishes in order to prevent malnutrition.

Close monitoring of plasma protein concentration is recommended. Evidence of progressive protein malnutrition should alert the physician to intervene with either dietary supplementation, alteration in dialysis prescription, or temporary discontinuation of PD. Although the use of intraperitoneal administration of amino acids has been explored, no long-term studies have been published. Amino acid solutions have been shown to provide adequate UF, comparable to glucose, and transient improvement in plasma amino acid concentrations (135). However, they also result in an increased metabolic acid load and azotemia.

The caloric load of patients undergoing chronic PD can be markedly increased in patients using high dextrose concentrations in their dialysate. Patients undergoing chronic PD receive 20%–35% of their daily caloric intake from intraperitoneal glucose absorption (136). This can result in obesity or uncontrolled hyperglycemia in diabetics. The constant infusion of glucose can also lead to lipid abnormalities such as hypertriglyceridemia. This problem is best approached by controlling dietary salt intake and thus reducing the need for high UF; the use of shorter dwell times, which increases the UF/glucose absorption ratio; and dietary restriction of carbohydrates.

There has been concern about the possibility of a depletion syndrome in patients undergoing chronic PD due to peritoneal losses of important nutrients such as vitamin B_{12}.

Although the equilibration and losses of certain vitamins through dialysate outflow have been studied, the lack of exhaustive studies in this area precludes firm recommendations for vitamin supplementation. The same general guidelines recommended for vitamin supplementation among HD patients have been temporarily used in the treatment of the chronic PD patient.

Renal osteodystrophy is one of the most frequent and crippling complications of uremia. This complication usually develops long before the patient reaches end-stage renal disease and starts dialysis. The particular influences of chronic PD on renal osteodystrophy have not been well characterized. Multiple studies have provided conflicting results (137–140). However, it is apparent that both osteitis fibrosa and osteomalacia are prevalent among patients undergoing chronic PD. The availability and common use of active forms of vitamin D by the oral route or parenterally has significantly reduced the incidence and severity of osteitis fibrosa. The management of this complication is similar for both HD and PD patients (see Chapter 51).

Specific neurologic, psychiatric, and hematologic complications are discussed in Chapters 52 and 53.

REFERENCES

1. Ganter G: Ueber die Beseitigung giftiger Stoffe aus dem Blute durch Dialyse. *Munch Med Wochschr* 70-II:1478–1480, 1923.
2. *USRDS Annual Data Report of the National Institute of Health, March 1993.* National Institute of Diabetes and Digestive and Kidney Diseases, Bethesda, MD, 1993.
3. Firmat J, Zucchini A: Peritoneal dialysis in acute renal failure. *Contrib Nephrol* 17:33–38, 1979.
4. Mathew TH: Comparison of peritoneal dialysis and haemodialysis in acute renal failure. In: RC Atkins, NM Thomson, PC Farrell, eds, *Peritoneal Dialysis.* Churchill Livingstone, Edinburgh, pp 80–86, 1981.
5. Segar WE, Gibson RK, Rhamy R: Peritoneal dialysis in infants and small children. *Pediatrics* 27:603–613, 1961.
6. Chan JCM, Campbell RA: Peritoneal dialysis in children, a survey of its indications and applications. *Clin Pediatr* 12:131–139, 1973.
7. Cameron JS, Ogg C, Trounce JR: Peritoneal dialysis in hypercatabolic acute renal failure. *Lancet* 1:1188–1191, 1967.
8. Stolz ML, Nolph KD, Maher JF: Factors affecting calcium removal with calcium-free peritoneal dialysate. *J Lab Clin Med* 78:389–398, 1971.
9. Counts SJ, Baylink DJ, Shen FH, Sherrard DJ, Hickman RO: Vitamin D intoxication in an anephric child. *Ann Intern Med* 82:196–200, 1975.
10. Cruz C, Schmidt R, Dumler F, VanDellen S, Duncan H, Kleerekoper M: Successful treatment of hypercalcemia and tumoral calcifications with calcium-free peritoneal dialysis. *Perit Dial Int* 12:109, 1992.
11. Mailloux LU, Swartz CD, Onesti GO, Heider C, Ramirez O, Brest A: Peritoneal dialysis for refractory congestive heart failure. *JAMA* 199:873–878, 1967.

12. Cairns KB, Porter GA, Kloster FE, Bristow JD, Griswold HE: Clinical and hemodynamic results of peritoneal dialysis for severe cardiac failure. *Am Heart J* 76:227–234, 1968.

13. Raja RM, Krasnoff SO, Moros JG, Kramer MS, Robenbaum JL: Repeated peritoneal dialysis in treatment of heart failure. *JAMA* 213:2268–2269, 1970.

14. Shapira J, Lang R, Jutrin I, Robson M, Ravid M: Peritoneal dialysis in refractory congestive heart failure, Part I: Intermittent peritoneal dialysis. *Perit Dial Bull* 3:130–132, 1983.

15. Robson M, Biro A, Knobel B, Schai G, Ravid M: Peritoneal dialysis in refractory congestive heart failure, Part II: Continuous ambulatory peritoneal dialysis. *Perit Dial Bull* 3:133–134, 1983.

16. Winchester JF, Gelfand MC, Knepshield JH, Schreiner GE: Dialysis and hemoperfusion of poisons and drugs—update. *Trans Am Soc Artif Intern Organs* 23:762–842, 1977.

17. Maher JF: Principles of dialysis and dialysis of drugs. *Am J Med* 62:475–481, 1977.

18. Knochel JP, Mason AD: Effect of alkalinization on peritoneal diffusion of uric acid. *Am J Physiol* 210:1160–1162, 1966.

19. Campion DS, North JDK: Effect of protein binding of barbituates on their rate of removal during peritoneal dialysis. *J Lab Clin Med* 66:549–563, 1965.

20. Etteldorf JN, Dobbins WT, Summitt RL, Rainwater WT, Fischer RL: Intermittent peritoneal dialysis using 5% albumin in the treatment of salicylate intoxication in children. *J Pediatr* 58:226–236, 1961.

21. Reuler JB, Parker RA: Peritoneal dialysis in the management of hypothermia. *JAMA* 240:2289–2290, 1978.

22. Zawada ET: Treatment of profound hypothermia with peritoneal dialysis. *Dial Transplant* 9:255–256, 1980.

23. O'Connor J: The treatment of profound hypothermia with peritoneal dialysis. *Perit Dial Bull* 2:171–173, 1982.

24. Wall AJ: Peritoneal dialysis in the treatment of severe acute pancreatitis. *Med J Aust* 52:281–283, 1965.

25. Glenn LD, Nolph KD: Treatment of pancreatitis with peritoneal dialysis. *Perit Dial Bull* 2:63–68, 1982.

26. Skoutakis VA, Black WD, Acchiardo SR, Wood GC: Peritoneal dialysis in the treatment of acetohexamide induced hypoglycemia. *Am J Hosp Pharm* 34:68–70, 1977.

27. Sidek M, Sieberth HG, Schmitz G, Redlich A: Extrarenal indications for peritoneal dialysis. *Proc Eur Dial Transplant Assoc* 3:355, 1966.

28. Twardowski ZJ, Nolph KD, Rubin J, Anderson PC: Peritoneal dialysis for psorasis, an uncontrolled study. *Ann Intern Med* 88:349–351, 1978.

29. Shen FH, Sherrard DJ, Scollard D, Merritt A, Curtis FK: Thirst, relative hypernatremia, and excessive weight gain in maintenance peritoneal dialysis. *Trans Am Soc Artif Intern Organs* 24:142–149, 1978.

30. Nolph KD, Sorkin ML, Moore H: Autoregulation of sodium and potassium removed during continuous ambulatory peritoneal dialysis. *Trans Am Soc Artif Intern Organ* 26:334–338, 1980.

31. Stewart JH, Tuckwell LA, Sinnett PF, Edwards KDG, Whyte HM: Peritoneal and haemodialysis: A comparison of their morbidity and of their mortality suffered by dialysed patients. *Q J Med* 35:406–420, 1966.

32. Furman KL, Gomperts ED, Hockley J: Activity of intraperitoneal heparin during peritoneal dialysis. *Clin Nephrol* 9:15–18, 1978.

33. Thayssen P, Pindborg T: Peritoneal dialysis and heparin. *Scand J Urol Nephrol* 12:73–74, 1978.

34. Posen GA, Luisello J: Continuous equilibration peritoneal dialysis in the treatment of acute renal failure. *Perit Dial Bull* 1:6–7, 1980.

35. Katirtzoglou A, Digenis G, Mayopoulou-Symvoulidis D, Zervaris D, Symvoulidis A, Komninos Z: Continuous equilibration peritoneal dialysis versus acute peritoneal dialysis. In: GM Gahl, M Kessel, KD Nolph, eds, *Advances in Peritoneal Dialysis*. Excerpta Medica, Amsterdam, pp 122–125, 1981.

36. Katirtzoglou A, Kontesis P, Maopoulou-Symvoulidis D, Digenis GE, Symvoulidis A, Komninos Z: Continuous equilibration peritoneal dialysis in hypercatabolic renal failure. *Perit Dial Bull* 3:178–180, 1983.

37. Trevino-Becerra A, Munoz P, Avilez C: Equilibrium peritoneal dialysis (EPD) in acute renal failure (ARF) secondary to rhabdiomyolysis (sic). *Perit Dial Bull* 7:244–246, 1987.

38. Steiner RW: Continuous equilibration peritoneal dialysis in acute renal failure. *Perit Dial Int* 9:5–7, 1989.

39. Nolph KD: Continuous *versus* intermittent therapy for acute renal failure. *Trans Am Soc Artif Intern Organs* 34:54–55, 1988.

40. Maher JF, Schreiner GE: Hazards and complications of dialysis. *N Engl J Med* 273:370–377, 1965.

41. Vaamonde CA, Michael VF, Metzger RA, Carrd KE: Complications of acute peritoneal dialysis. *J Chron Dis* 28:637–659, 1975.

42. Valk TW, Swartz RD, Hsu CH: Peritoneal dialysis in acute renal failure: analysis of outcome and complications. *Dial Transplant* 9:64–68, 1980.

43. Diaz-Buxo JA, Geissinger WT: Single cuff versus double cuff Tenckhoff catheter. *Perit Dial Bull* 4:S100–S102, 1984.

44. Gutman RA: Automated peritoneal dialysis for home use. *Q J Med* 47:261–280, 1978.

45. Tucker CT, Cunningham JT, Nichols AM, Greer CF, Bailey CT: Cannulography with peritoneal air contrast study. *Contemp Dial* 3:9–16, 1982.

46. O'Connor J, Rutland M: Demonstration of pleuroperitoneal communication with radionuclide magnification in a CAPD patient. *Perit Dial Bull* 1:153, 1981.

47. Berlyne GM, Lee HA, Ralston AJ, Woodlock JA: Pulmonary complications of peritoneal dialysis. *Lancet* 2:75–78, 1966.

48. Port F, Johnson WJ, Klass DW: Prevention of dialysis disequilibrium syndrome by use of high sodium concentration in the dialysate. *Kidney Int* 3:327–333, 1973.

49. Excerpts from the 1993 USRDS Annual Data Report. *Am J Kidney Dis* 22:38–45, 1993.

50. Tenckhoff H, Schechter H: A bacteriologically safe peritoneal access device. *Trans Am Soc Artif Intern Organs* 14:181–186, 1968.

51. Diaz-Buxo JA: Acute intermittent and cycled peritoneal dialysis. In: WN Suki, SG Massry, eds, *Therapy of Renal Diseases and Related Disorders*, 2nd ed. Kluwer Academic Publishers, Boston, pp 739–753, 1991.

52. Scott DF, Marshall VC: Insertion and complications of Tenckhoff catheters—surgical aspects. In: RC Atkins, NM Thomson, PC Farrell, eds, *Peritoneal Dialysis*. Churchill Livingstone, Edinburg, pp 61–72, 1981.

53. Ash SR, Handt AE, Bloch R: Peritoneoscopic placement of the Tenckhoff catheter: further clinical experience. *Perit Dial Bull* 3:8–12, 1983.

54. Zappacosta AR, Perras ST: Seldinger technique for Tenckhoff catheter placement. *Perit Dial Bull* 6:S24, 1986.

55. Twardowski ZJ, Prowant BF, Khanna R, Nichols WK, Nolph KD: Long-term experience with Swan-neck Missouri catheters. *Trans Am Soc Artif Intern Organs* 36:M491–M494, 1990.

56. Cruz C: Clinical experience with a new peritoneal access device. In: K Ota, JF Maher, JF Winchester, P Hirszel, eds, *Current Concepts in Peritoneal Dialysis*. Elsevier Science Publishers, Amsterdam, pp 164–169, 1992.

57. Moncrief JW, Popovich RP, Dasgupta M, Costeerton JW, Simmons E, Moncrief V: Reduction in peritonitis incidence in continuous ambulatory peritoneal dialysis with a new catheter and implantation technique. *Perit Dial Int* 13:S329–S331, 1993.

58. Khanna R: Is a break-in period necessary following peritoneal catheter insertion? A break-in period is recommended. *Semin Dial* 5:197–199, 1992.

59. Ash SR: Is a break-in period necessary following peritoneal catheter insertion? A break-in period is unnecessary. *Semin Dial* 5:199–201, 1992.

60. Diaz-Buxo JA: Peritoneal dialysis reverse osmosis machines and cyclers. In: AR Nissenson, RN Fine, eds, *Dialysis Therapy*. Hanley & Belfus, Philadelphia, pp 41–46, 1986.

61. Lasker N, McCauley EP, Passarotti CT: Chronic peritoneal dialysis. *Trans Am Soc Artif Intern Organs* 12:94–97, 1966.

62. Boen ST: Overview and history of peritoneal dialysis. *Dial Transplant* 6:12–18, 1977.

63. Diaz-Buxo JA, Chandler JT, Farmer CD, Smith DL: Chronic peritoneal dialysis at home—a comparison with hemodialysis. *Trans Am Soc Artif Intern Organs* 23:191–193, 1977.

64. Diaz-Buxo JA, Walker PJ, Chandler JT, Burgess WP, Farmer CD: Experience with intermittent peritoneal dialysis and continuous cyclic peritoneal dialysis. *Am J Kidney Dis* 4:242–248, 1984.

65. Schmidt RW, Blumenkrantz MJ: IPD, CAPD, CCPD, CRPD—peritoneal dialysis: Past, present and future. *Int J Artif Organs* 4:124–129, 1981.

66. Ghantous WN, Salkin MS, Adelson BN, Ghantous S, McGinnis K, Valenziano A, Cronin M: Limitations of peritoneal dialysis in the treatment of ESRD patients. *Trans Am Soc Artif Intern Organs* 25:100–103, 1979.

67. Popovich RP, Moncrief JW, Decherd JF, Bomar JB, Pyle WK: The definition of a novel portable/wearable equilibrium peritoneal dialysis technique (abstract). *Am Soc Artif Intern Organs* 5:64, 1976.

68. Diaz-Buxo JA, Farmer CD, Walker PJ, Chandler JT, Holt KL: Continuous cyclic peritoneal dialysis—a preliminary report. *Artif Organs* 5:157–161, 1981.

69. Price C, Suki W: New modifications of peritoneal dialysis: options in the treatment of patients with renal failure. *Am J Nephrol* 1:97–104, 1981.

70. Diaz-Buxo JA, Walker PJ, Burgess WP, Chandler JT, Farmer CD, Holt KL: Current status of CCPD in the prevention of peritonitis. In: R Khanna, KD Nolph, B Prowant, ZJ Twardowski, DG Oreopoulos, eds, *Advances in Continuous Ambulatory Peritoneal Dialysis*. University Of Toronto Press, Toronto, pp 145–148, 1986.

71. Price CG, Suki WN: New modifications of peritoneal dialysis: options in the treatment of patients with renal failure. *Am J Nephrol* 1:97–104, 1981.

72. Diaz-Buxo JA: Continuous ambulatory and continuous cycling peritoneal dialysis. In: G LaGreca, S Chiaramonte, A Fabris, M Feriani, C Ronco, eds, *Peritoneal Dialysis*. Wichtig Editore, Milano, pp 257–264, 1985.

73. Diaz-Buxo JA: Current status of CCPD (editorial). *Perit Dial Int* 9:9–14, 1989.

74. Twardowski ZJ, Nolph KD, Khanna R, Gluck Z, Prowant BF, Ryan LP: Daily clearances with continuous ambulatory peritoneal dialysis and nightly peritoneal dialysis. *Trans Am Soc Artif Intern Organs* 32:575–580, 1986.

75. Blumenkrantz MJ, Gahl GM, Kopple JD, Kamdar AV, Jones MR, Kessel M, Coburn JW: Protein losses during peritoneal dialysis. *Kidney Int* 19:593–602, 1981.

76. Holley JL, Bernardini J, Piraino B: Continuous cycling peritoneal dialysis is associated with lower rates of catheter infections than continuous ambulatory peritoneal dialysis. *Am J Kidney Dis* 16:133–136, 1990.

77. Verger C, Luzar MA: In vitro study of CAPD Y-line system. In: R Khanna, KD Nolph, BF Prowant, ZJ Twardowski, DG Oreopoulos, eds, *Advances in Continuous Ambulatory Peritoneal Dialysis*. University of Toronto Press, Toronto, pp 160–164, 1986.

78. Verger C, Faller B, Ryckelynck JPH, Cam G, Pierre D: Comparison between the efficacy of CAPD Y-lines without "in-line" disinfectant and standard systems: a multicenter prospective controlled trial. *Perit Dial Bull* 7:S82, 1987.

79. Bazzato G, Landini S, Coli U, Lucatello S, Francasso A, Moracchiello M: A new technique of continuous ambulatory peritoneal dialysis (CAPD): double-bag system for freedom to the patient and significant reduction of peritonitis. *Clin Nephrol* 13:251–254, 1988.

80. Diaz-Buxo JA, Walshe JJ, Flanigan M: Multicenter experience with Y-set CAPD system (Freedom Set) (abstract). *Perit Dial Bull* 7:S23, 1987.

81. Maiorca R, Cancarini GC, Broccoli R, et al.: Prospective controlled trial of a Y-connector and disinfectant to prevent peritonitis in continuous ambulatory peritoneal dialysis. *Lancet* 2:642–644, 1983.

82. Suki WN, Walshe JJ, Ashebrook DW, Gentile DE, Tucker CT, Ash S, Ahmad S: Multicenter evaluation of a bagless CAPD system. Trans Am Soc Artif Intern Organs 32:572–574, 1986.

83. Vlaanderen K, de Fijter CW, Bos HJ, van der Meulen J, Beelen RH, Oe PL, Verbrugh HA: The effect of dwell time on peritoneal phagocytic defense of chronic peritoneal dialysis patients. In: R Khanna, K Nolph, B Prowant, Z Twardowski, D Oreopoulos, eds, *Advances in Peritoneal Dialysis*. University of Toronto Press, Toronto, pp 151–153, 1989.

84. de Fijter CW, Verbrugh HA, Peters ED, Oe PL, van der Meulen J, Donker AJ, Verhoef J: Another reason to restrict the use of a hypertonic glucose-bases peritoneal dialysis fluid: Its impact on peritoneal macrophage function in vivo. In: R Khanna, K Nolph, B Prowant, Z Twardowski, D Oreopoulos, eds, *Advances in Peritoneal Dialysis*. University of Toronto Press, Toronto, pp 150–153, 1991.

85. Diaz-Buxo JA: CCPD is even better than CAPD. *Kidney Int* 28:S26–S28, 1985.

86. Twardowski ZJ, Prowant BF, Nolph KD, Martinez AJ, Lampton RN: High volume, low freqency continuous ambulatory peritoneal dialysis. *Kidney Int* 23:64–70, 1983.

87. Diaz-Buxo JA: Enhancement of peritoneal dialysis: The PD Plus concept. *Am J Kidney Dis* 27:92–98, 1996.

88. Brandes J, Emerson P, Campbell D, Keshaviah P: The relationship between body size, fill volume and mass transfer

area coefficient (MTAC) in PD (abstract). *J Am Soc Nephrol* 3:407, 1992.

89. Schoenfeld P, Diaz-Buxo JA, Keen M, Gotch FA: The effect of body position (P), surface area (BSA), and intraperitoneal exchange volume (Vip) on the peritoneal transport constant (KoA) (abstract). *J Am Soc Nephrol* 4:416, 1993.

90. Diaz-Buxo JA: Peritoneal sclerosis in a woman on continuous cyclic peritoneal dialysis. *Semin Dial* 5:317–320, 1992.

91. Di Paolo N: Semicontinuous peritoneal dialysis with a subcutaneous peritoneal catheter. *Dial Transplant* 7:834–838, 1978.

92. Frock J, Twardowski Z, Nolph K, Khanna R, Prowant B, Dobbie J, Serkes K, Kennley R, Witsoe D, Garber J: Tidal peritoneal dialysis (abstract). *Kidney Int* 31:250, 1987.

93. Twardowski ZJ, Nolph K, Khanna R, Prowant B, Frock J, Dobbie J, Serkes K, Kenley R, Witsoe D, Garber J: Eight hr tidal peritoneal dialysis (TPD) matches 24 hr CAPD and surpasses 8 hr nightly intermittent peritoneal dialysis (NIPD) clearances (C) (abstract). Perit Dial Bull 7:S79, 1987.

94. Twardowski ZJ, Nolph KD, Khanna R, Prowant BF, Frock JT, Dobbie JW, Kenley RS, Serkes KD, Witsoe DA, Garber JW: Tidal peritoneal dialysis. In: MM Avram, C Giordano, eds, *Ambulatory Peritoneal Dialysis.* Plenum, New York, pp 145–149, 1990.

95. Shah J, Lane D, Shrivastava D, Berlyne GM, Barth RH: Isovolemic tidal technique does not increase clearances in intermittent peritoneal dialysis (IPD) (abstract). *J Am Soc Nephrol* 3:419, 1992.

96. Balaskas EV, Izatt S, Chu M, Oreopoulos DG: Tidal volume peritoneal dialysis versus intermittent peritoneal dialysis. In: R Khanna, KD Nolph, BF Prowant, ZJ Twardowski, DG Oreopoulos, eds, *Advances in Peritoneal Dialysis.* Multimed, Toronto, pp 105–109, 1993.

97. Port FK, Held PJ, Nolph KD, Turenne MN, Wolfe RA: Risk of peritonitis and technique failure by CAPD connection technique: a national study. *Kidney Int* 42:967–974, 1992.

98. Daugirdas JT, Leehey DJ, Popli S, Gandhi VC, Zayas I, Hoffman W, Ing TS: Induction of peritoneal fluid eosinophilia by intraperitoneal air in patients on continuous ambulatory peritoneal dialysis. *N Engl J Med* 313:1481, 1985.

99. Abaete de los Santos C, Von Eye O, d'Avila D, Mottin CC: Rupture of the spleen: a complication of continuous ambulatory peritoneal dialysis. *Perit Dial Bull* 6:203–204, 1986.

100. Hassell LH, Moore J, Conklin JJ: Hemoperitoneum during continuous ambulatory peritoneal dialysis: A possible complication of radiation induced peritoneal injury. *Clin Nephrol* 21:241–243, 1984.

101. Orfei R, Seybold K, Blumberg A: Genital edema in patients undergoing continuous ambulatory peritoneal dialysis. *Perit Dial Bull* 4:251–252, 1984.

102. Twardowski ZJ, Tully RJ, Nichols WK, Sunderrajan S: Computerized tomography CT in the diagnosis of subcutaneous leaks during continuous ambulatory peritoneal dialysis. *Perit Dial Bull* 4:163–166, 1984.

103. Schleifer CR, Smink RD, Baum SF: Dialysate leakage with a negative Technetium scan—a diagnostic dilemma. *Perit Dial Bull* 5:255–256, 1985.

104. Coward RA, Gokal R, Wise M, Mallick NP, Warrell D: Peritonitis associated with vaginal leakage of dialysis fluid in continuous ambulatory peritoneal dialysis. *Br Med J* 284:1529, 1982.

105. Watson LC, Thompson JC: Erosion of the colon by a long-dwelling peritoneal dialysis catheter. *JAMA* 243:2156–2157, 1980.

106. Diaz-Buxo JA, Burgess WP, Walker PJ: Peritoneovaginal fistula—unusual complication of peritoneal dialysis. *Perit Dial Bull* 3:142–143, 1983.

107. Bierman MH, Kasperbauer J, Kusek A, Hammeke MD, Fitzgibbons RJ, Egan: Peritoneal catheter survival and complications in end-stage renal disease. *Perit Dial Bull* 5:229–233, 1985.

108. Odor A, Alessio-Robles LP, Leuchter J, Mendoza A, Bordes J, Wadgymar A, Gonzalez RF, Peon FC: Experience with 150 consecutive permanent peritoneal catheters in patients on CAPD. *Perit Dial Bull* 5:226–229, 1985.

109. Diaz-Buxo JA, Chandler JT, Farmer CD, Walker PJ, Holt KL, Burgess WP, Orr SL: Long-term observation of peritoneal clearances in patients undergoing peritoneal dialysis. *ASAIO J* 6:21–25, 1983.

110. International Cooperative Study Group: A survey of ultrafiltation in continuous ambulatory peritoneal dialysis. *Perit Dial Bull* 4:137–142, 1984.

111. Selgas R, Fernandez-Reyes MJ, Bosque E, Bajo MA, Borrego F, Jimenez C, Del Peso G, de Alvaro F: Functional longevity of the human peritoneum: how long is continuous peritoneal dialysis possible? Results of a prospective medium long-term study. *Am J Kidney Dis* 23:64–73, 1994.

112. Faller B, Marichal JF: Loss of ultrafiltration in continuous ambulatory peritoneal dialysis: a role for acetate. *Perit Dial Bull* 4:10–13, 1984.

113. Nielsen LH, Nolph KD, Khanna R, Moore H: Sclerosing peritonitis on CAPD; the acetate-lactate controversy (abstract). *Am J Nephrol* 17:82A, 1984.

114. de Alvaro F, Castro MJ, Dapena F, Bajo MA, Fernandez-Reyes MJ, Romero JR, Jimenez C, Miranda B, Selgas R: Peritoneal resting is beneficial in peritoneal hyperpermeability and ultrafiltration failure. In: R Khanna, KD Nolph, BF Prowant, ZJ Twardowski, DG Oreopoulos, eds, *Advances in Peritoneal Dialysis.* Multimed, Toronto, pp 56–61, 1993.

115. Manuel MA: Failure of ultrafiltration in patients on CAPD. *Perit Dial Bull* 3:S38–S40, 1983.

116. Hasbargen JA, Smith BJ, Rodgers DJ: Ultrafiltration failure at the initation of CAPD. *Perit Dial Bull* 6:46–47, 1986.

117. Twardowski ZJ, Nolph KD, Khanna R, et al.: Peritoneal equilibration test. *Perit Dial Bull* 7:138, 1987.

118. Junor BJR, Briggs JD, Forwell MA, Dobbie JW, Henderson I: Sclerosing peritonitis—The contribution of chlorhexidine in alcohol. *Perit Dial Bull* 5:101–104, 1985.

119. Gotloib LA, Mines M, Garmizo L, Varka I: Hemodynamic effects of increasing intra-abdominal pressure in peritoneal dialysis. *Perit Dial Bull* 1:41–43, 1981.

120. Wetherington GM, Leapman SB, Robison RJ, Filo RS: Abdominal wall and inguinal hernias in continuous ambulatory peritoneal dialysis patients. *Am J Surg* 150:357–360, 1985.

121. Rocco MV, Stone WJ: Abdominal hernias in chronic peritoneal dialysis patients: a review. *Perit Dial Bull* 5:171–174, 1985.

122. Goodman CD, Husserl FE: Etiology, prevention and treatment of back pain in patients undergoing continuous ambulatory peritoneal dialysis. *Perit Dial Bull* 1:119–122, 1981.

123. Alpert MA, Franklin JO, Twardowski ZJ, Khanna R: Effect of increasing intra-abdominal pressure and posture on left ventricular function in patients on CAPD. *Kidney Int* 31:248, 1987.

124. Diaz-Buxo JA: Is peritoneal dialysis the best choice for patients with severe heart disease? *Int J Artif Organs* 15:573–578, 1992.

125. Gotloib LA, Garmizo L, Varak T, Mines M: Reduction of vital capacity due to increased intra-abdominal pressure during peritoneal dialysis. *Perit Dial Bull* 1:63–64, 1981.

126. Diaz-Buxo JA, Farmer CD, Chandler JT, Walker PJ, Burgess WP: CCPD: wet is better than dry. In: MM Avram, C Giordano, eds, *Ambulatory Peritoneal Dialysis.* Plenum Medical, New York, pp 259–263, 1990.

127. Teehan BP, Schleifer CR, Brown JM, Sigler MH, Raimondo J: Urea kinetic analysis and clinical outcome in CAPD: a five year longitudinal study. In: R Khanna, KD Nolph, BF Prowant, et al., eds, *Advances in Peritoneal Dialysis.* University of Toronto Press, Toronto, pp 181–185, 1990.

128. Tattersall JE, Doyle S, Greenwood RN, Farrington K: Urea kinetic modeling (UKM) and underdialysis in CAPD patients. *J Am Soc Nephrol* 3:420, 1992.

129. Grefberg N, Danielson BG, Nilsson P, Wahlberg J: Comparison of two catheters for peritoneal access in patients undergoing continuous ambulatory peritoneal dialysis (CAPD). *Scand J Urol Nephrol* 17:343–346, 1983.

130. Lameire NH, Vanholder R, Veyt D, Lambert MC, Ringoir S: A longitudinal, five year survey of urea kinetic parameters in CAPD patients. *Kidney Int* 42:426–432, 1992.

131. Bergström J, Alvestrand A, Lindholm B, Tranaeus A: Relationship between KT/V and protein catabolic rate is different in continuous peritoneal dialysis and haemodialysis patients (abstract). *J Am Soc Nephrol* 2:358, 1991.

132. Gotch F, Gentile DE, Schoenfeld PY: CAPD prescription in current clinical practice. In: R Khanna, KD Nolph, BF Prowant, ZJ Twardowski, DG Oreopoulos, eds, *Advances in Peritoneal Dialysis.* University of Toronto Press, Toronto, pp 69–72, 1993.

133. Canada-USA (CANUSA) Peritoneal Dialysis Study Group: Adequacy of dialysis and nutrition in continuous peritoneal dialysis: Association with clinical outcomes. *J Am Soc Nephrol* 7:198–207, 1996.

134. Young GA, Kopple JD, Lindholm B, et al.: Nutritional assessment of continuous ambulatory peritoneal dialysis patients: an international study. *Am J Kidney Dis* 17:462–471, 1991.

135. Williams PF, Marliss EB, Anderson GH, et al.: Amino acid absorption following intraperitoneal administration in CAPD patients. *Perit Dial Bull* 2:124–130, 1982.

136. Grodstein GP, Blumenkrantz MJ, Kopple JD, Moran JK, Coburn JW: Glucose absorption during continuous ambulatory peritoneal dialysis. *Kidney Int* 19:564–567, 1981.

137. Delmez JA, Fallon MD, Bergfeld MA, Gearing BK, Dougan CS, Teitelbaum SL: Continuous ambulatory peritoneal dialysis and bone. *Kidney Int* 30:379–384, 1986.

138. Buccianti G, Bianchi ML, Valenti G: Progress of renal osteodystrophy during continuous ambulatory peritoneal dialysis. *Clin Nephrol* 22:279–283, 1984.

139. Campese V, Easterling RE, Finkelstein F, Mattern W, Ogden DA, Steiner RW, Oreopoulos DG: Renal osteodystrophy and the status of albumin and other trace metals in CAPD: a panel review. *Perit Dial Bull* 4:129–136, 1984.

140. Taber T, Hageman T, York S, Miller R: Removal of aluminum with intraperitoneal deferoxamine. *Perit Dial Bull* 6:213–216, 1986.

CHAPTER 56

Continuous Ambulatory Peritoneal Dialysis

RAMESH KHANNA, ROBERT MACTIER & KARL D. NOLPH

INTRODUCTION

The potential use of the peritoneum as a dialyzing membrane was recognized as early as 1923 (1,2). Nevertheless, not until a permanent indwelling peritoneal catheter was developed in 1964 by Palmer et al. (3) and later modified by Tenckhoff (4) did long-term intermittent peritoneal dialysis (IPD) become a practical alternative to hemodialysis. However, probably mainly due to inadequate dialysis, the cumulative technique survival on IPD was low (5), and hemodialysis remained the predominant form of dialysis therapy.

The concept of portable/wearable equilibrium peritoneal dialysis was introduced by Popovich and Moncrief in 1976 (6). Initial clinical studies with four or five 2–1 exchanges per day showed that adequate steady-state control of uremia, sodium and water balance, hyperkalemia, and acidosis could be achieved in patients with end-stage renal failure, and this technique was retermed *continuous ambulatory peritoneal dialysis* (CAPD) (7). Oreopoulos replaced the use of glass bottles containing dialysis solution with a polyvinylchloride (PVC) bag, which could be rolled up when empty and carried under the clothing without being disconnected from the transfer set (8). After equilibrating for the selected dwell time (4–10 hours), the dialysate was drained into the PVC bag, and the connection–disconnection procedure was repeated using an aseptic, nontouch technique. This development markedly reduced the peritonitis rate, and apart from further minor modifications, this basic CAPD system (peritoneal catheter, transfer set, and PVC bag containing dialysis solution) remains unchanged today.

CAPD now has an established role in renal replacement therapy (9); as of the end of 1993, there were industrial estimates of nearly 80,000 patients maintained on chronic peritoneal dialysis (PD) worldwide (10). The annual growth rate for the chronic PD patient population from 1990 through 1993 was estimated at 17% per year. Of the nearly 80,000 patients maintained on chronic PD at the end of 1993, nearly 28,000 were in the United States. The percentage of the total dialysis population on chronic PD range from 91% in Mexico to 6% in Japan; this percentage was 17% in the U.S.A. In the U.S.A. at the time of the 1993 survey, nearly 22,000 patients were on continuous ambulatory peritoneal dialysis (CAPD) and about 6000 on automated peritoneal dialysis (APD) including nightly intermittent peritoneal dialysis (NIPD) and cyclic peritoneal dialysis (CCPD). Factors identified as being of paramount importance in a successful CAPD program include

1. Patient selection
2. Peritoneal access
3. Patient training and education
4. Individualized dialysis
5. Avoidance of complications

PATIENT SELECTION

Advantages of CAPD

CAPD offers the patient with end-stage renal disease a relatively simple home dialysis therapy that does not require routine vascular access, a machine, a supervising partner, limitation of activity during dialysis, or rigid dietary restriction. CAPD provides steady-state control of serum biochemistry and fluid balance, thus avoiding the problems of transcellular disequilibrium, interdialysis weight gain, and hemodynamic instability that are observed with intermittent dialysis therapies. A comparison of solute clearances with CAPD (four exchanges and 10–1 dialysate drain volume per day) and of hemodialysis with cellulose membranes (12 hr/week) is shown in Table 1. The low solute clearance rates in CAPD are due to the very low dialysate flow rate (7 mL/min) and are compensated for by dialysis being performed continuously (11). Weekly removal of solutes of molecular weight greater than 100 daltons (creatinine = 113) is higher with CAPD, since the peritoneum has a greater permeability to larger solutes than standard hemodialysis membranes and since serum solute concentrations decrease markedly during hemodialysis, reducing solute mass transfer at a given clearance rate. Consequently, it has been proposed that great

Suki, WN and Massry SG (eds), Suki and Massry's Therapy of Renal Diseases and Related Disorders, Third Edition. ISBN 978-1-4757-6634-9.
©*1998, Kluwer Academic Publishers, Boston/Dordrecht/London. All rights reserved.*

Table 1. Comparison of solute clearances in CAPD and hemodialysis

Solute (molecular weight)	CAPD		Hemodialysis	
	mL/min	L/wk	mL/min	L/wk
Urea (60)	7	70	150	108
Creatinine (113)	6	60	120	86
Vitamin B_{12} (1355)	4	42	17	12
Inulin (5200)	2.6	26	5.5	4

removal of uremic toxins, such as middle molecules, with CAPD (12) may improve well-being and reduce the severity of anemia, the incidence of pericarditis, and the progression of peripheral neuropathy (13–17). An additional benefit to patients on CAPD is the longer preservation of residual renal function compared to those on hemodialysis; it is suggested that during hemodialysis, blood membrane interaction releases IL-2, tumor necrosis factor, and cytokines, which are injurious to residual nephrons and cause rapid loss of residual renal function (18). A further benefit for the community in this modern age of financial restraint in health care is that CAPD has a lower initial capital expenditure and annual maintenance costs than hemodialysis (19) and has enabled the number of patients receiving dialysis to be expanded in some countries (20,21).

Indications and contraindications

The aforementioned medical advantages make CAPD a more appropriate initial therapy than hemodialysis for children (22) and probably for some patients with cardiac failure (23) or diabetes (24,25). Moreover, intraperitoneal administration of insulin in diabetic CAPD patients can improve control of blood glucose, and CAPD avoids the need for systemic heparinization, which may increase the risk of retinal or vitreous hemorrhage (24,26,27). Social factors and complications encountered with hemodialysis may also influence the decision in favor of beginning or transferring to CAPD (Table 2). It was feared that CAPD immediately prior to renal transplantation would predispose the patient to peritonitis, but this has not been verified (28,29), and indeed CAPD has been advocated by some as the preferred dialysis therapy for patients who are likely to receive an allograft in the near future (9). However, as with home hemodialysis, patient motivation for self-treatment is essential in CAPD, and the patient has to be able to perform the dialysis schedule correctly and safely. The latter need not apply if a partner is willing to be trained to perform the exchanges for the patient every day. The major and minor contraindications to CAPD are summarized in Table 3. The only absolute contraindication to CAPD is extensive peritoneal fibrosis. An assessment of the advantages and disadvantages of each mode of dialysis will help determine the dialysis therapy best suited for the individual patient. Since CAPD is self-dialysis, it is emphasized that

Table 2. Indications for CAPD

1. Age of patient	Children
	Elderly
2. Medical complications	Diabetes
	Cardiac failure
	Anephric/severe anemia (refusing blood transfusion)
	Recurrent hemorrhage
3. Psychosocial factors	Patient choice
	Self-motivated
	Long distance from in-center dialysis
	Freedom to travel
4. Transfer from hemodialysis	No vascular access
	Uncontrolled hypertension
	Hemodynamic instability
	High interdialysis weight gain
	Postdialysis dysequilibrium syndrome
	Dialysis-associated ascites
5. Awaiting transplantation	

Table 3. Contraindications for CAPD

Major	Minor
1. Extensive peritoneal fibrosis	Chronic obstructive pulmonary disease
2. Recent major abdominal surgery	Peripheral vascular disease
3. Inflammatory bowel disease	Diverticulosis
4. Colostomy, ileal conduit	Hernias
5. Immunosuppressed	Polycystic kidney disease
6. Poor motivation	Systemic vasculitis
7. Psychosis[a]	Hyperlipidemia
8. Impaired intellect[a]	Obesity
9. Crippling arthritis of hand[a]	Lumbar backache
10. Neurological deficit[a]	Protein malnutrition
11. Blindness[a]	

[a] For self-therapy only.

"patient selection" should refer to the dialysis choice of the patient as well as the physician.

PERITONEAL ACCESS

Catheters are described in detail in another chapter in this book.

PATIENT TRAINING AND EDUCATION

The success of a CAPD program depends on proper patient training and education (30), and a well-trained and dedicated nursing team with a special interest in peritoneal dialysis facilitates achieving these objectives (31). Training is best conducted on an outpatient and one-to-one basis by the nurse who will later follow up the patient at home. In addition to systematic training in aseptic technique, patients require a basic knowledge of the CAPD system and education in early recognition of complications and in simple problem solving. These teaching goals are aided by providing patients with a training manual containing protocols for unit procedures dealing with CAPD techniques and complications. The time taken to train a CAPD patient varies but averages 10 days and is dependent on many factors, including age, mental alertness (state of uremia), presence of physical handicaps, and level of family support. After completion of training, the patient's progress is assessed at regular clinic visits. Home visits and telephone calls by the patient's nurse and social worker provide further patient support during intervals between clinic attendances (32).

INDIVIDUALIZED DIALYSIS

Adequacy

In peritoneal dialysis, the rate of equilibration of dialysate solutes with plasma depends on the solute molecular weight (7). Accordingly, in CAPD, small-molecular-weight solutes such as urea almost completely equilibrate with the plasma within 4 hours (dialysate/plasma urea = 1), whereas larger solutes continue to equilibrate until the end of the dwell time (Figure 1) (33). The mass transfer of solutes not present in the infused dialysis solution is equal to the drained dialysate solute concentration multiplied by the daily drain volume. Thus the daily net removal of small solutes in CAPD is primarily determined by the daily drain volume (dialysate flow rate), while the mass transfer rates of larger solutes are predominantly influenced by the patient's peritoneal permeability–area product (34). If the exchange dwell time is reduced below 3 hours (Figure 1), the mass transfer of small solutes is also influenced by peritoneal permeability multiplied by area.

The peritoneum is a composite biologic "membrane" (capillary endothelium and endothelial basement membrane, interstitium, and mesothelium) that is subjected to chronic reuse during CAPD. Consequently, not only is there interindividual variation in the peritoneal permeability–area product but also the peritoneal membrane transport kinetics of each patient may change with time. Moreover, the dialysis requirements of CAPD patients also vary and depend on several factors, including body weight, dietary protein intake, catabolic rate, and residual renal clearance. Thus individualized dialysis schedules are recommended to ensure that CAPD patients with differing peritoneal transport and dialysis requirements all receive adequate dialysis (35).

After the peritoneal catheter break-in period, most adult patients on CAPD are initially prescribed four 2–1 ex-

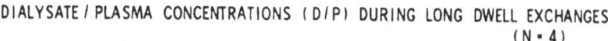

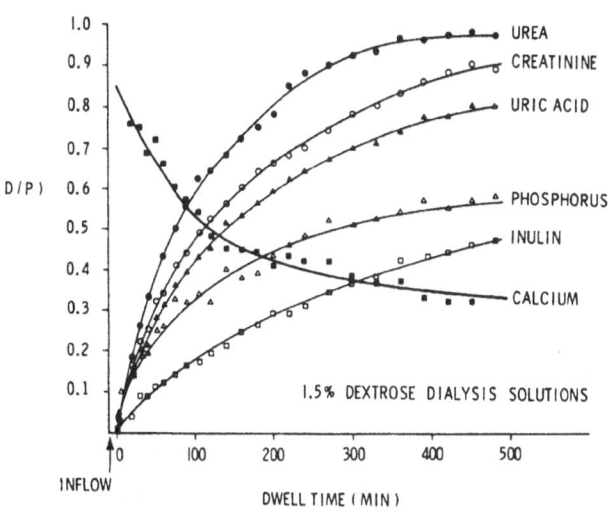

Figure 1. Equilibration of dialysate and plasma solute concentrations during long-dwell exchanges using 2L of 1.5% dextrose dialysis solution. Reproduced with permission from Nolph et al. (33).

changes per day, a regimen that commonly results in dialysate drain volumes and urea clearances of around 10 L/day. Dialysis solution tonicity and/or volume can be increased until there are no symptoms attributable to uremia and the desired biochemical values are achieved. Hypertonic exchanges increase solute clearances by increasing both the drain volume and the peritoneal permeability–area product (36). Furthermore, the peritoneal permeability–area product remains increased for several exchanges after the dialysate osmolality is reduced (37). Large adult patients can usually tolerate 2.5-L or 3.0-L exchanges, provided that there are no contraindications to a further increase in intra-abdominal pressure (38). Alternatively, solute clearances on CAPD can be augmented by increasing the number of exchanges per day. However, the inconvenience of the extra exchange procedures each day negates their therapeutic application for most CAPD patients.

CAPD creatinine clearance rates by dialysis average 6 mL/min, and so a renal creatinine clearance at the beginning of dialysis of only 1–2 mL/min makes a significant contribution to the total clearance. Moreover, for each decrease in residual renal urea clearance of 1 mL/min, the CAPD urea clearance (essentially drain volume) must be increased by 1.44 L/day to maintain the same total urea clearance. Consequently, residual renal function should be conserved for as long as possible, and nephrotoxic drugs, such as aminoglycosides and nonsteroidal anti-inflammatory drugs, should be prescribed with caution. If the dialysis schedule remains unchanged during progressive loss of residual renal function, underdialysis may occur. Furthermore, inadequate dialysis may not be recognized early unless the nutritional intake and status are routinely assessed, since the concomitant anorexia results in failure to adhere to recommended protein and calorie intakes, resulting in reduced urea nitrogen appearance rate as well as muscle wasting and thus in relatively stable or low serum urea nitrogen and creatinine levels. Nevertheless, underdialysis usually manifests as a rise in serum urea nitrogen and creatinine, especially if there is an acute decline in total daily clearances.

KT/V UREA

A quantitative approach to CAPD focuses on small-solute clearances like urea rather than on hypothetical middle molecules (39). Figure 2A shows the weekly clearances of solutes over a range of molecular weights in CAPD patients using different numbers of 2-L exchanges. Increasing the number of exchanges can alleviate uremic symptoms in patients who eventually lose residual renal function. Figure 2A shows that such maneuvers mainly have an impact on the weekly clearances of small-molecular-weight solutes, which are dependent on dialysate volume. The larger-molecular-weight solute clearances are more dependent on membrane area and permeability. Based on patient survivals and numerous clinical outcomes, including dietary protein intakes, a composite KT/V urea (urea clearance normalized for the total body water) scale for hemodialysis (HD) and peritoneal dialysis has been developed (Figure 2B). An HD KT/V per treatment of 1.4 (4.2 per week with thrice-weekly therapy) corresponds to a weekly KT/V urea for peritoneal dialysis of 2.1. One explanation for the greater weekly clearance requirement with HD therapy is that the control of peak body fluid concentrations of small-molecular-weight solutes is important and that an intermittent therapy such as HD requires greater clearances to maintain the serum concentrations of small solutes at or below the steady-state concentrations of CAPD, assuming that solute generation rates are equal.

Similarly, the importance of protein intake in the adequacy of dialysis is reflected by the observation that a protein catabolic rate (PCR) below 0.8 gm/kg lean body

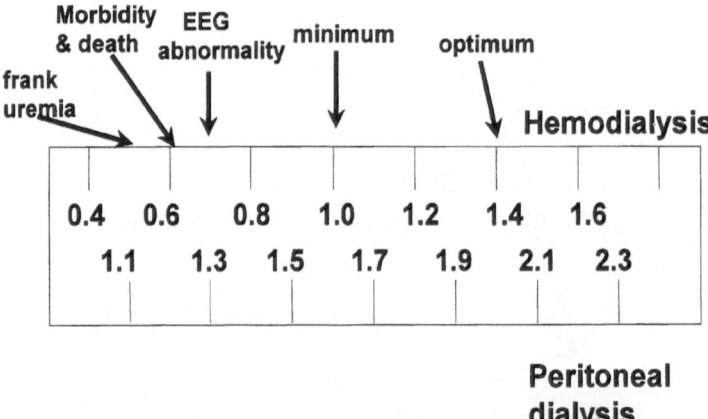

Figure 2. (**A**) Weekly clearances of solutes over a range of molecular weights in CAPD patients. (**B**) A composite KT/V urea scale for hemodialysis (HD) and peritoneal dialysis. Reproduced with permission from P. Keshaviah (39).

weight/day is associated with a high morbidity in hemodialysis patients. Several studies have shown a close correlation between the PCR and dietary protein intake (DPI) by history. Well-dialyzed hemodialysis patients that eat well and have a good nutritional status usually have a PCR of 1 or above. Their serum albumin is in the normal range. The serum albumin is a good predictor of long-term survival in dialysis patients. Increasing the urea clearance in CAPD or in HD increases the net PCR (40). It is recommended that regular urea kinetic modeling be performed on all patients regardless of the treatment modality, and if the PCR is low, a cause for this finding should be sought. If no obvious cause is found, consideration should be given to raising the KT/V urea, regardless of the current level. We have recommended that a minimum target of 2.1 of KT/V urea for CAPD is reasonable if protein intakes in excess of 0.8 g/kg normalized body weight are to be achieved in most CAPD patients (41).

TOTAL CREATININE CLEARANCE

Net mean peritoneal clearance is determined for a continuous treatment (CAPD or CCPD) by dividing the amount of creatinine removed through dialysis per unit time (mass transfer rate) by the concentration of creatinine in the serum:

$$C_{cr} = \frac{(D_t \times V_t) - (D_0 \times V_0)}{P}$$

where D_t and D_0 = final and infused dialysis solution creatinine concentrations, respectively; V_t and V_0 = final and initial dialysis solution volumes, respectively; and P = serum creatinine concentration.

Since the infused solution is devoid of creatinine, the equation can be simplified as follows:

$$C_{cr} = \frac{(D_t \times V_t)}{P}$$

This clearance expresses the volume of serum cleared of creatinine per unit time (usually expressed as mL/min) by the peritoneal membrane. Clearance is influenced by dialysis flow rate, ultrafiltration, and membrane area and permeability, and is independent of blood concentration. Mean net clearance rate may be calculated per exchange, per day, or per week. The true instantaneous clearance rate is highest at the beginning of dialysis and approaches zero at equilibrium.

Residual renal function contributes to the overall clearance of small- and middle-molecular-weight solutes and fluid removal. Since the renal creatinine clearance overestimates the glomerular filtration rate (GFR) in chronic renal failure patients, the mean of renal creatinine and urea clearance may be added to the peritoneal creatinine clearance to estimate the combined or total creatinine clearance provided to a patient by peritoneal dialysis and GFR. It is our clinical impression that tubular creatinine secretion is not a marker of the excretion of small-molecular-weight uremic toxins.

We recommend a minimum target of 65 L/week/1.73 m² body surface area of combined peritoneal and GFR creatinine clearance (41).

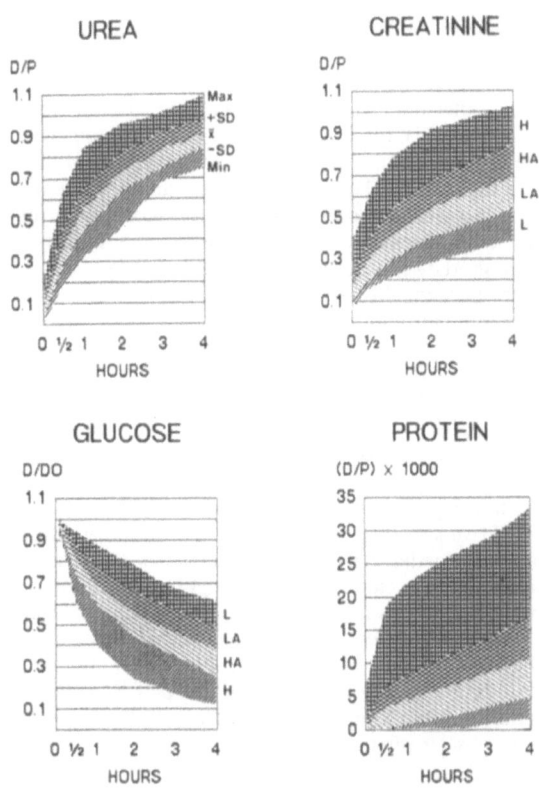

Figure 3. Equilibration curves during standardized 4-hour exchanges using 2 L of 2.5% dextrose dialysis solution (*n* = 103). The mean and mean ± 1 SD solute ratios categorize patients with high (H), high average (HA), low average (LA), and low (L) peritoneal transport. Reproduced with permission from Twardowski et al. (43).

Table 4. Clinical applications of standardized peritoneal equilibration test

1. Peritoneal membrane classification
2. Monitor peritoneal membrane transport function
3. Selection of peritoneal dialysis regimen
4. Diagnose peritoneal membrane acute injury
5. Diagnose cause of inadequate ultrafiltration
6. Diagnose cause of inadequate solute clearance
7. Estimate D/P ratio at time t from the PET curve
8. Assess patient compliance

PERITONEAL EQUILIBRATION TEST

Studies of transperitoneal solute and fluid transport during standardized exchanges (2-L, 2.5% dextrose dialysis solution with a 4-hour dwell time) provide a clinically useful index of the peritoneal permeability–area product and are helpful in selecting the patient's individualized dialysis schedule (42,43). Equilibration curves relating the dialysate/plasma urea nitrogen, creatinine, and protein, as well as sequential/initial dialysate glucose, concentration ratios to dwell time show wide interindividual variation, but reference values are available (Figure 3).

Baseline equilibration studies, performed soon after beginning CAPD, can have a number of clinical applications (Table 4), including prediction of the adequacy of dialysis on standard CAPD after the loss of residual renal function. Patients with high peritoneal solute transport (more than 1 SD above the mean in Figure 3) usually require four or more short dwell exchanges during the day (daytime ambulatory peritoneal dialysis, or DAPD) in order to capture maximum ultrafiltration and solute clearances. Patients with low peritoneal solute transport (more than 1 SD below the mean) are at risk of underdialysis on standard CAPD after the loss of residual function, especially if they are of high body weight. These patients often require dialysate outflow volumes of at least 11–12 L/day. Patients with average peritoneal transport rates (within 1 SD of the mean in Figure 3) can usually be maintained on standard CAPD unless they have a very high body weight, are catabolic, or have a significant change in the peritoneal permeability–area product. The latter can be confirmed by repeating the standardized equilibration test, and the dialysis schedule should be modified appropriately. These alterations in peritoneal transport have been observed infrequently but may reflect underlying pathologic changes in the peritoneum and may forewarn of the future development of sclerosing peritonitis (44).

Ultrafiltration

In peritoneal dialysis, ultrafiltration is induced by the transperitoneal osmotic gradient of the hypertonic (glucose) dialysis solution (45). The ultrafiltration rate decreases exponentially from the beginning of the exchange due to dissipation of the osmotic gradient by absorption of dialysate glucose and dilution of dialysate glucose by the ultrafiltrate (45). The peritoneal cavity lymphatics, in contrast, absorb intraperitoneal fluid at a near constant rate during the long dwell exchanges of CAPD (46). Consequently, the maximum net ultrafiltration volume is observed before osmotic equilibrium is reached, when the transperitoneal ultrafiltration and lymphatic absorption rates are equal (47). Thereafter, the reabsorption (predominantly by lymphatic flow rate) exceeds the transperitoneal ultrafiltration rate, and intraperitoneal fluid volume decreases (47). For any given patient, increasing the tonicity and volume of the dialysis solution increases

Ultrafiltration (UF) Related to Dwell Time With 2 and 3L Volumes, 1.5, 2.5, and 4.25% Glucose Concentrations

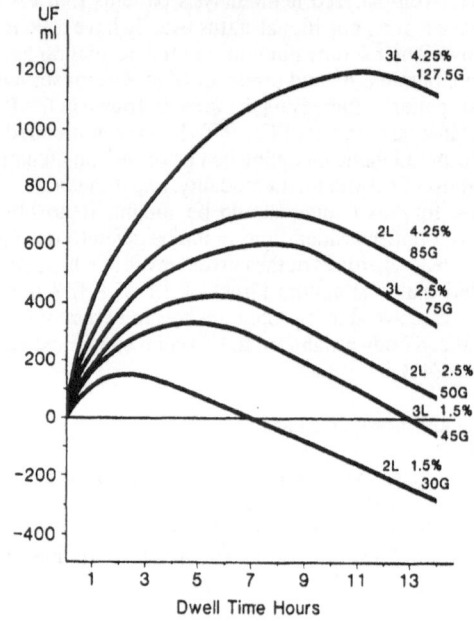

Figure 4. Effect of volume and tonicity of dextrose dialysis solution on net ultrafiltration during the dwell time. Reproduced with permission from Twardowski et al. (48).

the maximum intraperitoneal volume, increases the absorbed glucose load, and prolongs the exchange dwell time until net fluid absorption occurs (Figure 4) (48).

Fluid balance is achieved when the daily net ultrafiltration and residual urine volumes balance fluid intake. Excessive fluid intake, necessitating extra hypertonic exchanges and an increased obligatory glucose load from the dialysis solution, should be discouraged. High-dose furosemide may be prescribed to try to preserve residual urine volumes for as long as possible after the onset of dialysis (49) and so minimize the need for hypertonic exchanges. However, as residual renal function decreases, the increased number of hypertonic exchanges needed to ensure fluid balance augment peritoneal small-solute clearances as well as drain volumes and thus help prevent underdialysis. Nevertheless, with the loss of residual urine volume, some patients continue to have insufficient ultrafiltration despite extra hypertonic exchanges (50,51). Standardized peritoneal equilibrium studies (Figure 3) can often delineate the cause of loss of ultrafiltration, especially if a baseline study is available for comparison (42,43). The diagnosis and recommended therapy for each causes of failure of ultrafiltration is summarized in Figure 5. Apparent loss of ultrafiltration is observed in patients with a

Repeat PET in Fluid Retention

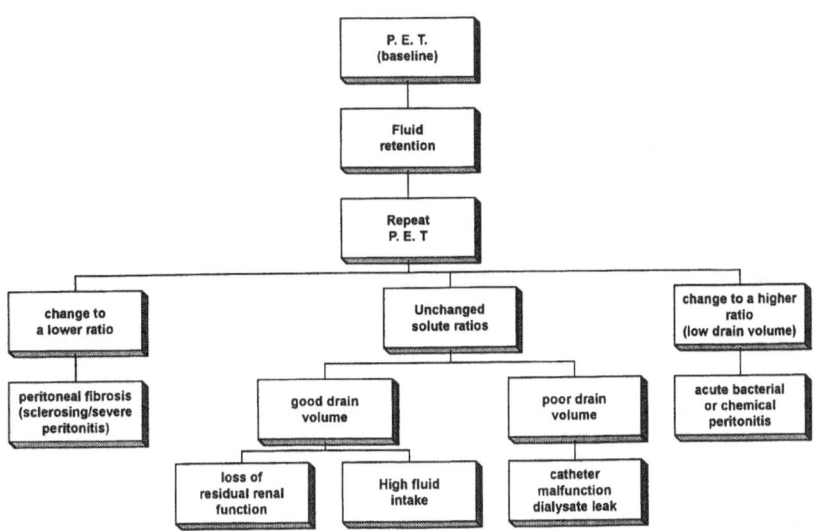

Figure 5. Diagnostic value of repeat standardized equilibration studies in CAPD patients with apparent and actual loss of ultrafiltration.

high peritoneal permeability–area product when they lose residual urine volume or in patients with an injudiciously high fluid intake. Actual loss of ultrafiltration occurs when the daily cumulative peritoneal cavity lymphatic absorption (47) and/or dialysate leakage (52) equals or exceeds the daily net transperitoneal ultrafiltration. Extraperitoneal dialysate leaks may occur with a pericatheter leak. Consequently, in the absence of a dialysate leak, true failure of ultrafiltration is observed when transperitoneal water transport is relatively low (53) and/or peritoneal cavity lymphatic drainage is relatively high (54). Leaving the peritoneal cavity empty overnight and resting the peritoneum may reverse, at least in part, peritoneal hyperpermeability changes and so increase transperitoneal ultrafiltration (42), but at present there is no therapy to consistently reduce lymphatic absorption during CAPD.

Alternatively excessive ultrafiltration may lead to a sudden weight loss and orthostatic tachycardia and hypotension. This outcome is most likely to occur when the patient with a reduced fluid intake or increased gastrointestinal fluid losses continues to use several hypertonic exchanges each day. Since extraperitoneal fluid is absorbed at around 50 mL/hr after osmotic equilibrium is approached (55,56), minor dehydration can be corrected by using 1.5% glucose exchanges with a prolonged dwell time (8–12 hours). Chronic orthostatic hypotension unrelated to a recent negative fluid balance may indicate sodium depletion (57).

Control of blood pressure and sodium balance

The improvement in blood pressure control on CAPD is attributed to daily controlled ultrafiltration, which can maintain patients at near dry body weight (13,58). A reduction in blood pressure is most marked in the first weeks of CAPD (58) and emphasizes the importance of volume status in the pathogenesis of hypertension in end-stage renal disease. Indeed, hypertension can often be controlled without antihypertensive therapy, despite an increase in plasma renin and aldosterone levels (59). CAPD results in daily net removal of sodium as well as water. Peritoneal mass transfer of sodium can be readily calculated for each exchange using the following formula:

(drain volume × drained dialysate sodium concentration) — (infusion volume × infused dialysate sodium concentration).

The dialysate sodium concentration decreases during the first 2–3 hours of each exchange due to solute sieving with ultrafiltration (60) and thereafter approaches Gibbs–Donnan equilibrium with serum sodium by diffusion (61). Thus, net ultrafiltration of 1.0–1.5 L/day of dialysate at the standard infused dialysate sodium concentration (132 mEq/L) will result in sodium losses of 132–198 mEq/day. Consequently, CAPD patients with high daily ultrafiltration volumes require a liberal dietary sodium intake to avoid sodium depletion. If serum sodium decreases, sodium removal decreases, tending to autoregulate net sodium removal (61). Nevertheless, symptomatic hypotension in nondiabetic CAPD patients has been attributed to sodium depletion (62) and, in a small series of such patients, symptoms improved and exchangeable sodium increased with sodium supplementation (57).

Acid–base balance

Commercial peritoneal dialysis solutions for CAPD contain lactate as a buffer base. A dialysis solution lactate concentration of 40 mEq/L can maintain the serum concentration of total CO_2 at 28 mEq/L in most patients using four 2-L exchanges per day (63), whereas with solutions containing 35 mEq/L of lactate, serum total CO_2 averages 22 mEq/L (13). There is interindividual variation, however, and the dialysate lactate concentration for CAPD patients needs to be individualized. It has been reported that acidosis is better controlled by CAPD than by other forms of dialysis (64).

Dialysis solutions containing acetate are no longer commercially available. Acetate solutions have been withdrawn, since their long-term use has been associated with increased absorption of dialysate glucose and loss of ultrafiltration (51,65). The development of sclerosing peritonitis in some patients has been linked with exposure to acetate-containing dialysis solutions, but a causative role remains unproven (66,67).

Bicarbonate has not been used routinely in CAPD, since insoluble calcium and magnesium salts form in the dialysis solution during storage. This problem can be avoided if sodium bicarbonate and buffer-free dialysis solution are stored in separate compartments in the dialysis bag and are not mixed until immediately prior to infusion (68). However, the clinical application of this formulation remains to be evaluated.

Prevention of hyperkalemia

In CAPD patients, serum potassium is maintained at the level where dietary intake is balanced by dialysate, fecal, and urinary losses. Hyperkalemia is observed infrequently, even though potassium intake is usually 70–80 mEq/day and dialysate losses average only 35 mEq/day (61). This discrepancy has been explained by an increase in fecal potassium losses during CAPD and by a concurrent increase in dialysate potassium losses as serum potassium rises (61). Indeed, metabolic balance studies in CAPD patients have shown that a positive potassium balance was not observed until the potassium intake exceeded 67 mEq/day (69).

Mineral metabolism

Transperitoneal transport of calcium depends on the direction of the concentration gradient between the dialysate and serum ionized calcium. In normocalcemic patients, peritoneal dialysis solutions containing 3.5 mEq/L of calcium result in a positive calcium balance during 1.5% dextrose exchanges (70,71) but a net removal of calcium during more hypertonic exchanges due to convection with ultrafiltration. Thus daily peritoneal mass transfer of calcium depends on the osmolality of the exchanges used each day as well as on the serum ionized calcium concentration. Most normocalcemic CAPD patients using three 1.5% dextrose and one 4.25% dextrose exchanges per day have a daily net uptake of calcium from the dialysate (69,70).

The rate of diffusion of phosphate into the dialysate is slower than predicted from its molecular weight (MW = 98) and is attributed to its hydration shell and anionic charge (Figure 1). Nevertheless, with the long dwell exchanges of CAPD, 250–350 mg of phosphorus are removed in the dialysate each day (70). Most patients on an adequate protein diet will ingest 800–1200 mg of phosphorous per day, and, assuming 50% phosphorus absorption and no residual renal function, will need to use phosphate binders to remove 150–250 mg phosphorus each day. After serum phosphorus has been lowered below 6.0 mg/dL with dialysis and aluminum-containing phosphate binders, calcium carbonate can be prescribed with food in increasing dosages until serum ionized or total calcium is in the upper-normal rate (72). Hypercalcemia is a frequent occurrence when calcium is used as the phosphate-binding agent (73). Dialysis solution containing calcium at 1.25 mmol/L has considerably reduced hypercalcemic complications seen when calcium is used as the phosphate-binding agent (74). Phosphate control and parathyroid suppression were reported to be better with the use of both calcium carbonate and low-calcium dialysis solution.

We use only calcium phosphate binders such as calcium carbonate or calcium acetate whenever possible to control serum phosphate. Sometimes hypercalcemia requires some aluminum phosphate binders as well. We avoid calcium binders when serum phosphate exceeds 6 mg/dL (fearing metastatic calcification) and use aluminum binder only until aluminum, diet, and dialysis manipulation reduce serum phosphate and allow conversion from aluminum to calcium binder. This therapeutic approach helps ensure adequate calcium supplementation, while the use of calcium carbonate as a phosphate binder (75) lessens the requirement for aluminum-containing antacids. The latter is important, since cumulative aluminum intake from aluminum-containing phosphate binders is the major determinant of serum aluminum levels in CAPD patients maintained on dialysis solutions containing less than 15 ug/L aluminum (76,77). Net removal of aluminum has been observed with the currently available dialysis solutions (78,79) and may explain the infrequent reports of overt aluminum toxicity in adult CAPD patients (80) unless they have been exposed to dialysate contaminated with aluminum (81). Reducing the dialysate magnesium concentration from 1.5 to 0.5 mEq/L prevents magnesium uptake from the dialysate during 1.5% dextrose exchanges (71) and corrects hypermagnesemia. Low dialysate magnesium concentration may enable magnesium hydroxide to be used as a phosphate binder for patients on CAPD (82).

1,25-dihydroxycholecalciferol levels are often reduced at the beginning of CAPD (83) and 25-hydroxycholecalciferol levels may fall during CAPD due to losses in the dialysate (84,85). However, therapy with vitamin D analogues has the potential hazards of worsening hyperphosphatemia, hypercalcemia, and metastatic calcification, and has usually been reserved for CAPD patients with worsening secondary hyperparathyroidism despite optimum existing therapy or osteomalacia unrelated to aluminum toxicity. With this overall management strategy, most patients on CAPD show an improvement in radiologic and histologic features of renal bone disease (72,84). Recently there has been a trend for oral pulse calcitriol treatment for patients on CAPD to decrease parathyroid hormone concentrations (86). However, indiscriminate use of calcitriol in CAPD patients may predispose to low-turnover bone disease (86). It is recommended that serum levels of intact parathyroid hormone be maintained between 1.5 and 2.5 times the upper limits of normal; lower levels seem to be associated with increased risk of adynamic (low-turnover) bone disease.

Bone histology assessment has revealed an increasing incidence of aplastic bone disease in patients treated with CAPD as compared to those treated with hemodialysis (87). Some of the factors contributing to the higher incidence of low-turnover bone disease in PD may be lower mean parathyroid hormone concentrations compared to HD patients, older age, higher prevalence of diabetes, and a shorter duration of dialysis. Although osteomalacia, one of the low-turnover bone diseases, is commonly associated with aluminum toxicity, the other low-turnover disorder, it is just as likely to be seen in the absence of aluminum. It is suggested that in the absence of aluminum, low-turnover bone disease may not be particularly dysfunctional but merely the bone response to aggressive parathyroid hormone control. Usually, such patients are asymptomatic. Until more is known about this disorder, caution should be exercised in efforts to treat the lesion. Since aplastic bone lesion patients are often prone to hypercalcemia, some caution should be taken with oral calcium intake and use of higher dialysis solution calcium concentrations.

Daily dietary requirements of CAPD patients

The nutritional requirements of patients on CAPD are significantly influenced by losses of proteins, amino acids, and water-soluble vitamins into the dialysate and by absorption of glucose from the dialysate (88). Protein losses in the dialysis solution range from 6 to 12 g/day and are unrelated to dietary protein intake or ultrafiltration volume (89–91). Dialysate protein losses remain relatively constant in the same patients but markedly increase during episodes of peritonitis (92,93). Amino acid losses in the dialysate reflect the plasma amino-acid profile and range from 2.0 to 3.5 g/day (94–96). Nevertheless, CAPD patients

are noted to be in neutral or positive nitrogen balance, with protein intakes as low as 0.7 g/kg body weight/day (97). The anabolic effects of glucose absorption from the peritoneal cavity, stable metabolite levels, improved control of acidosis, avoidance of cytokine release due to blood-membrane incompatibility, and good middle-molecule removal in CAPD may explain in part why CAPD patients seem to tolerate lower weekly urea clearances and lower protein intakes than do hemodialysis patients. Nevertheless, low serum albumin is an independent predictor of morbidity, as evidenced by increased frequency of hospitalization (98). The strongest predictors of a low albumin state are diabetes, high peritoneal transport rate, older age, lower body weight, and shorter time on CAPD (99). It is important to emphasize here the role of a skilled dietician for ongoing assessment of patient caloric and protein intakes and for ensuring an adequate dialysis prescription (100).

Serum levels of vitamin C, vitamin B_1, vitamin B_6, and folic acid decrease in CAPD patients not receiving vitamin supplementation to the diet (101,102). Absorption of intraperitoneal glucose varies from 100 to 200 g/day depending on the number, volume, and tonicity of dextrose dialysis solutions used each day (103,104). This obligatory glucose load promotes insulin secretion and anabolism in CAPD patients (104) but has the disadvantages of also predisposing the patients to obesity, impaired glucose tolerance, and hypertriglyceridemia (105–107).

CAPD patients without peritonitis are in a neutral to positive nitrogen balance while on a diet providing at least

Table 5. Daily dietary allowances for CAPD patients

Energy (diet and dialysate)	35–42 kcal/kg normalized body weight
Protein	1.2–1.3 g/kg normalized body weight
Carbohydrate (diet)	35% of ingested calories
Fat	Remainder of nonprotein ingested calories
Polyunsaturated: saturated fatty acid	1.5 : 1
Minerals	
Calcium	At least 1000–1400 mg
Phosphorus	800–1200 mg
Magnesium	200–300 mg
Sodium and water	As tolerated to achieve fluid balance
Potassium	70–80 mEq
Ferrous sulphate	200 mg
Supplemental vitamins	
Ascorbic acid	100 mg
Pyridoxine HCl	10 mg
Thiamine HCl	2 mg
Folic acid	1 mg
Other water-soluble vitamins	Recommended daily allowances
Fat-soluble vitamins (A, D, E, K)	None routinely

1.2 g protein/kg/day (69,108). Fifty percent of the daily protein intake should be of high biologic value to replace the dialysate losses of essential amino acids (94,100). Several other dietary manipulations have been proposed to lessen the risk of metabolic complications (105–107) and at the same time to maintain adequate nutrition: only 35% of ingested calories should be in the form of carbohydrate, fat intake should be mainly polyunsaturated fatty acids, and daily total calorie (diet and dialysate) and protein intakes should reflect the patient's normalized rather than actual weight. Trace element supplements are not recommended unless there is both biochemical and clinical evidence of a deficiency state (109). These considerations provide a rationale for the daily dietary allowances currently advocated for CAPD patients (Table 5).

COMPLICATIONS

Peritonitis

Peritonitis is the most common acute complication of CAPD (Table 6) and is the major cause of technique failure (10). More than half of all patients using standard manual exchange procedures experience at least one episode of peritonitis during the first year of CAPD. The host defenses of the peritoneal cavity are compromised by CAPD and thus predispose patients to develop peritonitis (110):

Table 6. Complications of CAPD

1. Peritonitis
    Bacterial
    Fungal
    Eosinophilic
    Culture negative
2. Catheter-related
    Exit-site and/or tunnel infection
    External cuff extrusion
    Inflow and/or outflow obstruction
    Dialysis solution inflow pain
3. Related to increased intra-abdominal pressure
    Abdominal hernia
    Abdominal wall or genital edema
    Massive hydrothorax
    Cardiorespiratory compromise
    Hiatus hernia
    Hemorrhoids
4. Membrane failure
    Inadequate ultrafiltration and/or inadequate dialysis
    Sclerosing peritonitis
5. Metabolic
    Protein depletion
    Hyperlipidemia and obesity
6. Medical
    Cardiovascular disease
    Progression of renal osteodystrophy

1. The peritoneal catheter provides a ready route for recurrent intraperitoneal contamination with skin commensals and opportunistic organisms
2. The dialysate concentrations of opsonins (IgG and C3) and resident peritoneal macrophages are diluted by the daily exchange of large volumes of dialysis solution (111,112)
3. The intraperitoneal volume of dialysis solution impairs the localization of infection within the peritoneal cavity by the omentum
4. The phagocytic and bactericidal activity of intraperitoneal polymorphonuclear leukocytes is suppressed by the acidic pH and hypertonicity of freshly infused dialysate (113)

Passive immunization with intraperitoneal IgG may reduce the incidence of peritonitis (114), especially in patients with very low opsonic activity in the dialysate, but this possibility needs further evaluation. Existing improvements in connector technology and aseptic technique may have contributed to the gradual decrease in peritonitis rates of patients in the U.S.A. to one episode every 12–24 patient months (115). Detailed discussion of peritonitis is provided elsewhere in this book.

Catheter-related complications

The prevention and treatment of catheter-related complications (Table 6) is described in detail in Chapter 57.

Complications related to increased intra-abdominal pressure

ABDOMINAL HERNIA

Increased intra-abdominal pressure with CAPD may predispose the patient to develop an abdominal hernia. Alternatively, the initiation of peritoneal dialysis may facilitate the clinical presentation of a previously unrecognized hernia. More than 10% of CAPD patients develop a hernia, and all forms of abdominal hernia have been reported (116,117). The elderly, multiparous women, and patients on steroids appear to be more prone to develop hernias on CAPD (118). Incisional hernias are more common with midline insertion of the peritoneal catheter (119), and paramedian placement is now preferred (119,120).

Abdominal hernias should be carefully looked for and repaired before peritoneal dialysis is begun. If patients develop hernias after starting CAPD, temporary transfer to hemodialysis or low-volume supine IPD is required until the surgical repair is healed. Thereafter, most patients are able to resume CAPD.

DIALYSATE LEAKAGE

Pericatheter external dialysate leaks most commonly occur during the first weeks after catheter insertion. The incidence of these dialysate leaks is reduced if peritoneal dialysis can be delayed for 7–10 days, if low dialysate volumes are used in the break-in period, and if a paramedian rather than a midline approach is used for catheter insertion (119,120). Patients with internal dialysate leaks usually present with a combination of abdominal wall or genital edema, a sudden decrease in dialysate drain volume, and a rapid weight gain. The most common sites of leakage are around the peritoneal entrance of the catheter, through previous scars, or through an open processus vaginalis and, if not evident clinically, can be localized using computerized tomography with contrast added to the dialysis solution (52). External dialysate leaks usually resolve after the patient has been changed temporarily to hemodialysis or supine IPD. Internal dialysate leaks are much more likely to persist when CAPD is resumed and then to require surgical intervention. Genital edema usually indicates a patent processus vaginalis and merits surgical correction. Occasionally, genital edema without a cough impulse may be the initial presentation of an inguinal hernia (121).

MASSIVE HYDROTHORAX

Transdiaphragmatic leakage of dialysate is an uncommon but serious complication that usually requires that CAPD be discontinued. Acute hydrothorax almost always occurs on the right side and usually presents within hours to a few weeks of beginning peritoneal dialysis (122,123). The pleural fluid glucose concentration is high, and the protein concentration is low (123). The presence of a pleuroperitoneal communication can often be confirmed by radionuclide scanning using technetium-99 m-labeled macroaggregated albumin added to the dialysis solution (122,124). However, anatomic evidence of either an acquired or congenital pleuroperitoneal connection can be found at autopsy in only some of the patients (123,124). Thoracocentesis may be required for acute respiratory distress or, if less acute, the effusion may be allowed to resolve spontaneously once peritoneal dialysis is discontinued. The patient should be transferred from CAPD permanently, since hydrothorax is likely to reoccur if peritoneal dialysis is reinstituted at a later date (124). Alternatively, sclerosing agents can be instilled into the pleural cavity in an attempt to close the leak (125), but the long-term success of this approach needs confirmation.

CARDIORESPIRATORY COMPROMISE

Increased intra-abdominal pressure and intraperitoneal fluid volume during CAPD may compromise pulmonary and cardiac function. Nevertheless, in adult CAPD patients at stable dry weight, vital capacity (126), maximum expiratory flow rate (127), and left ventricular function (128) are not significantly changed with standard volumes of dialysis solution (2.0–2.51). These parameters are not adversely influenced in most patients until infusion volumes of dialysis solution are at least 31 (126,128). However, in the supine position, some patients may experience dyspnea and a reduction in vital capacity at lower infusion volumes (126,38). Patients with a low body surface area or a poor cardiopulmonary reserve (chronic obstructive pulmonary disease, pulmonary edema) are unlikely to tolerate infusion volumes greater than 2 L and, indeed, may require lower dialysate volumes.

Membrane failure

INADEQUATE ULTRAFILTRATION AND/OR
INADEQUATE DIALYSIS

The ability of the peritoneum to function as a long-term dialysis membrane is not well established. The durability of the peritoneum in CAPD may be adversely influenced by continuous exposure to unphysiologic dialysis solutions, intercurrent episodes of peritonitis, and/or coincident drug therapy. In vitro, glucose was found to inhibit proliferation of human mesothelial cells in a dose–dependent manner (129). Reversibility of this effect was inversely proportional to exposure time. Heat sterilization of peritoneal dialysis fluid causes glucose to degrade and may cause membrane toxicity (130). There is now evidence to suggest that a glucose polymer solution has improved biocompatibility compared with glucose-monomer-based solutions (131). Nevertheless, at least in North America and Australasia, peritoneal solute transport has rarely been reported to decline significantly with time on CAPD (43,132–134). Loss of ultrafiltration (true and apparent) is more common (65); true loss of ultrafiltration is often related to increased membrane transport and rapid glucose absorption, perhaps reflecting increased area and/or permeability. However, a change in peritoneal membrane transport is only one of the potential mechanisms of ultrafiltration failure in CAPD patients. A persistent increase in the peritoneal permeability–area product, resulting in rapid glucose absorption from the dialysate, early dissipation for the osmotic gradient, and decreased ultrafiltration volume, has been observed most frequently in Europe (44) and is termed *Type I membrane failure* (135). Almost complete equilibration of solutes during the dwell time compensates in part for the reduction in the dialysate drain volume and helps maintain adequate solute removal. This pattern of peritoneal transport is simulated transiently during peritonitis (92,93). Hypertonic dialysis solutions containing acetate or lactate induce vasodilatation, and their long-term use may predispose to increased peritoneal permeability (136). Several clinical studies from Europe have implicated acetate-containing dialysis solution as a risk factor for gradual loss of ultrafiltration (50,51), and this finding has been supported by an international survey of ultrafiltration in CAPD patients (65). However, the ultrafiltration volume did not correlate with the number of prior episodes of peritonitis (65).

The formation of fibrous adhesions or peritoneal sclerosis following most episodes of peritonitis is probably limited, since peritoneal transport is usually unchanged and there is no interference with dialysate inflow and outflow. However, massive adhesion formation may occasionally complicate refractory peritonitis, especially if due to Staphylococcus aureus or fungi, and prevent reinstitution of peritoneal dialysis (132). In addition to mechanical complications (loculation of intraperitoneal fluid, abdominal pain during dialysate infusion, bowel obstruction), extensive adhesions can lead to an acute reduction the peritoneal permeability–area product and initially to a greater reduction in solute transport than ultrafiltration (Type II membrane failure). It is emphasized that, in the absence of laparotomy, intraperitoneal adhesions are only diagnosed early after peritonitis if complications develop, but remain unassessed in patients who are initially asymptomatic on peritoneal dialysis.

SCLEROSING PERITONITIS

Sclerosing peritonitis is characterized by the development of progressive peritoneal sclerosis and may be unrelated to an episode of acute infectious peritonitis (137,138). Clinical features include Type II membrane failure, relapsing culture-negative peritonitis, and/or acute bowel obstruction. At laparotomy, dense laminated fibrous tissue may be found around the viscera (encapsulating peritonitis), in the peritoneum, or even within the bowel wall (137,139). Peritoneal fibrosis may progress despite cessation of CAPD, and patients may first develop symptoms while on chronic hemodialysis. The etiology remains unknown but is most likely to be multifactorial. The clustering of cases within some centers suggests that local exogenous factors may be important, but an international survey has failed to identify a common etiology (140). Factors associated with the occurrence of sclerosing peritonitis include severe or recurrent episodes of peritonitis leading to the cessation of CAPD, increased past incidence of Staphylococcus aureus peritonitis, potential dialysate contamination with antiseptics, beta-blocker therapy, and exposure to acetate-containing dialysis solutions (137,140,141). An increase in peritoneal permeability (Type I membrane failure) has been claimed to precede symptomatic sclerosing peritonitis (44,142). If peritoneal dialysis is discontinued and the catheter is removed at this stage or before acute complications develop, progression of peritoneal sclerosis may be halted. For patients presenting with acute or subacute bowel obstruction, mortality exceeds 50% despite surgical intervention and cessation of peritoneal dialysis (137,138).

Metabolic complication

PROTEIN DEPLETION

Persistent anorexia, nausea, and early satiety are not uncommon symptoms in CAPD patients and may lead to chronic protein and/or calorie malnutrition. Dietary assessment, serial anthropometric measurements, and biochemical monitoring (serum albumin and transferrin) are invaluable for the early detection of undernutrition in patients on CAPD. With progressive loss of residual renal function, underdialysis on CAPD and undernutrition are often interrelated (64). Dietary protein intake in stable CAPD patients can be estimated from the measurement of urea nitrogen appearance (UNA) (143,144), where

UNA (g/day) = Serum urea nitrogen (gm/dL) × total serum urea clearance (L/day) and

Total urea clearance (L/day) = drain volume (L/day) + residual renal urea clearance (L/day).

Urea N appearance (essentially equal to urea generation in CAPD) is used to calculate net protein catabolic rate (PCR), which is also a good estimation of dietary protein intake:

PCR (g/day) = 10.76 (G_U + 1.46),
    where G_U = urea generation rate (mg/min),
GU = the mg of urea in the 24 hour (urine + dialystate) / 1440, and
Urea nitrogen × (60/28) = urea

These results help verify the dietary history and establish whether an increase in dietary protein intake and/or dialysis clearance is required. If, despite adequate dialysis, the daily nutritional intake remains poor (Table 5), temporary enteral or parenteral nutritional supplementation may be required. Alternatively, in the future, amino acids may be administered in the dialysis solution (145,146).

HYPERLIPIDEMIA AND OBESITY

Hyperlipidemia is common in uremic patients and is due, at least in part, to reduced activity of serum lipoprotein lipase and hepatic lipase (147). Compared to HD cohorts, CAPD patients have significantly higher total cholesterol, apo A1, and apo B levels, as well as a lower ratios of apo A-1 to apo B levels, suggesting CAPD patients have more atherogenic lipoprotein profiles than HD patients (148,149). Dyslipoproteinemia would be expected to worsen during CAPD due to the additional glucose load from the dialysate (103) and hyperinsulinemia (150). Indeed, the prevalence of hypertriglyceridemia and de novo hypercholesterolemia in patients during their first year of CAPD is reported to be 60%–80% and 20%–30%, respectively (83,107). However, except in a small subgroup of patients (107), hyperlipidemia reaches a peak after 3–12 months of CAPD and thereafter falls to pretreatment levels (83,107).

Patients also frequently gain more than 5 kg in weight during the first year on CAPD (13,105). Despite evidence of net anabolism and an increase in lean body mass after beginning CAPD (151,152), the major proportion of this weight gain appears to be increased body fat (105,153). Nevertheless, most patients do not become obese during CAPD, but rather tend to return to their premorbid nonuremic weight (153).

For CAPD patients who require treatment for hyperlipidemia and/or obesity, the oral carbohydrate intake can be restricted and exercise can be increased (106,154). Decreasing oral fluid intake will reduce the number of hypertonic exchanges required and will limit the dialysate glucose load, but the reduced dialysate drain volume will also decrease the small-solute clearances (34). An alternative osmotic agent would be invaluable for such patients (48,155). Lipid-lowering drugs such as clofibrate should be prescribed with caution to uremic patients, since side effects are common. CAPD patients with hypercholesterolemia and hyper-triglyceridemia may be treated with simvastatin, a competitive inhibitor of 2-hydroxy-3-methyl glutaryl coenzyme A reductase, with significant reduction in total cholesterol, LDL cholesterol, and apolipoprotein B and increase in HDL cholesterol (156). Gemfibrozil in doses of 300 mg once or twice a day also significantly reduces total and LDL cholesterol (157). What is unclear is the benefit of such reduction in the incidence of atherosclerosis and atherosclerotic complications in dialysis patients.

Medical complications

CARDIOVASCULAR DISEASE

Cardiovascular disease is by far the major cause of death in CAPD patients (158). This outcome may be related to the high proportion of at-risk patients selected for CAPD (diabetic, known cardiac disease, elderly) and/or the acceleration of atherogenesis by metabolic sequelae of CAPD (hyperlipidemia, hyperinsulinemia). Indeed, more than 25% of patients now beginning CAPD in the U.S.A. are diabetic (10). However, when standardized dialysis populations (15–55 years, nondiabetic, normotensive, no malignancy) are compared, no difference in actuarial patient survival is observed between CAPD and hemodialysis (159,160). Therefore, it is unlikely that the choice of the dialysis modality per se significantly alters the risk of cardiovascular disease in patients with end-stage renal failure. Primary and secondary prevention of cardiovascular risk factors before and after beginning dialysis is much more likely to lessen cardiovascular morbidity and mortality.

PATIENT SURVIVAL

The Michigan registry compared survivals in CAPD and HD patients in Michigan during the 1980s (*n* = 4288) (161). By 1989, one third of incident end-stage renal disease patients 20–59 years of age were using CAPD at the fourth month of ESRD. CAPD patients with glomerulonephritis as the cause of their ESRD had lower mortality rates than their HD counterparts; there were no differences in survival between HD and CAPD in patients with hypertension and other reported causes of ESRD. Among young diabetics, long-term mortality was shown to be lower for patients using CAPD. An Italian study reported that patient survivals adjusted for pretreatment differences in populations are similar for CAPD and HD (162). Their findings suggest that older patients have a lower risk of death on CAPD than on HD. Although the CAPD patient may be marginally more immunocompetent than the HD

patient, kidney graft survival in CAPD patients is equal to that in HD patients in most reports covered in a recent extensive review (163).

CONCLUSION

During the past 15 years of CAPD, improvements in patient selection, modifications in catheter design and implantation, an increased range of dialysis solutions and schedules, and a significant reduction in complications have all contributed to increased patient and technique survival. Significant reduction in the incidence of peritonitis has allowed researchers to focus on setting adequacy standards and improving the efficiency of peritoneal dialysis. CAPD now has a well-established role in the short- to medium-term management of patients with end-stage renal failure and in the provision of an integrated renal replacement program. Currently, about 17% of ESRD patients worldwide receive chronic PD, with a wide range from country to country.

REFERENCES

1. Putnam J: The living peritoneum as a dialyzing membrane. *Am J Physiol* 63:548–565, 1923.
2. Ganter G: Uber die beseitigung gigtiger stoffe dein blute durch dialyse. *Munch Med Wochenschr* 70:1478–1480, 1923.
3. Palmer RA, Quinton WE, Gray JF: Prolonged peritoneal dialysis for renalfailure. *Lancet* 1:700–702, 1964.
4. Tenckhoff H, Schechter H: A bacteriologically safe peritoneal access device. *Trans Am Soc Artif Intern Organs* 14:181–186, 1968.
5. Ahmad S, Gallagher N, Shen F: Intermittent peritoneal dialysis: status reassessed. *Trans Am Soc Artif Intern Organs* 25:86–88, 1979.
6. Popovich RP, Moncrief JW, Decherd JF, et al.: The definition of a novel portable/wearable equilibrium dialysis technique. *Trans Am Soc Artif Intern Organs* 5:64A, 1976.
7. Popovich RP, Moncrief JW, Nolph KD, et al.: Continuous ambulatory peritoneal dialysis. *Ann Intern Med* 88:449–456, 1978.
8. Oreopoulos DG, Robson M, Izatt S, et al.: A simple and safe technique for continuous ambulatory peritoneal dialysis. *Trans Am Soc Artif Intern Organs* 24:484–489, 1978.
9. Gokal R: World-wide experience, cost effectiveness and future of CAPD—its role in renal replacement therapy. In: R Gokal, ed, *Continuous Ambulatory Peritoneal Dialysis*. Churchill Livingstone, Edinburgh, pp 349–369, 1986.
10. *1993 World-wide Registry Update*. Baxter Healthcare, Deerfield, IL, 1993.
11. Nolph KD, Popovich RP, Moncrief JW: Theoretical and practical implications of continuous ambulatory peritoneal dialysis. *Nephron* 21:117–122, 1978.
12. Bergstrom J, Asaba H, Furst P, et al.: Middle molecules in chronic uremic patients treated with continuous ambulatory peritoneal dialyis. *Perit Dial Bull* 3:S7–S9, 1983.
13. Nolph KD, Sorkin M, Rubin J, et al.: Continuous ambulatory peritoneal dialysis: three-year experience at one center. *Ann Intern Med* 92:609–613, 1980.

14. Zappacosta AR, Caro J, Erslev A: Normalization of hematocrit in patients with end-stage renal disease on continuous ambulatory peritoneal dialysis. The role of erythropoietin. *Am J Med* 72:53–57, 1982.

15. De Paepe MBJ, Schelstraete KGH, Ringoir SMG, et al.: Influence of continuous ambulatory peritoneal dialysis on the anemia of end-stage renal disease. *Kidney Int* 27:744–748,1983.

16. Sunderrajan S, Nolph KD: Longitudinal study of nerve conduction velocities during continuous ambulatory peritoneal dialysis. *Perit Dial Bull* 5:48–50, 1985.

17. Kim D, Blair G, Wu G, et al.: Electrophysiological studies of nerve function in patients on CAPD over long periods. *Perit Dial Bull* 5:45–48, 1985.

18. Rottembourg J: Residual renal function and recovery of renal function in patients treated by CAPD. *Kidney Int* 43 (Suppl 40):S106–A110, 1993.

19. Levery AS, Harrington JT: Continuous peritoneal dialysis for chronic renal failure. *Medicine (Baltimore)* 61:330–339, 1982.

20. Gokal R, Marsh F: Survey of CAPD in UK-1982. *Perit Dial Bull* 4:240–243, 1984.

21. Nichols AJ, Waldek S, Plats MM, et al.: Impact of CAPD on treatment of renal failure in patients over 60. *Br Med J* 288:18–19, 1984.

22. Fine RN: Peritoneal dialsis update. *J Pediatr* 100:1–7, 1982.

23. Rubin J, Bell R: Continuous ambulatory peritoneal dialysis as treatment of severe congestive heart failure in the face of chronic renal failure. *Arch Intern Med* 146:1533–2538, 1986.

24. Amair P, Khanna R, Leibel B, et al: Continuous ambulatory peritoneal dialysis in diabetics with end-stage renal disease. *N Engl J Med* 306:625–630, 1982.

25. Khanna R: Dialysis considerations for diabetic patients. *Kidney Int* 43 (Suppl 40):S58–S64, 1993.

26. Flynn CT, Nanson JA: Intraperitoneal insulin with CAPD—an artifical pancreas. *Trans Am Soc Artif Intern Organs* 25:114–117, 1979.

27. Madden MA, Zimmerman SW, Simpson DP: CAPD in diabetes mellitus—the risks and benefits of intraperitoneal insulin. *Am J Nephrol* 2:133–139, 1982.

28. Gokal R, Ramos JM, Veitch P, et al.: Renal transplantation in patients on continuous ambulatory peritoneal dialysis. *Proc Eur Dial Tranplant Assoc* 18:222–227, 1981.

29. Stephanidis CJ, Balfe JW, Arbus GS, et al.: Renal translantation in children treated with continuous ambulatory peritoneal dialysis. *Perit Dial Bull* 3:5–8, 1983.

30. Moncrief JW, Sorrels PAJ, Druger VG, et al.: Development of training programs for continuous ambulatory peritoneal dialysis—historical review. In: M Legrain, ed, *Continuous Ambulatory Peritoneal Dialysis.* Excerpta Medica, Amsterdam, pp 149–151, 1980.

31. Oreopoulos DG: Requirements for the organisation of a CAPD Program. *Nephron* 24:261–263, 1979.

32. Moon J, Uttley L, Mano J, et al.: Home CAPD nurse, an asset to a CAPD programme? In: JF Maher, JF Winchester, eds, *Frontiers in Peritoneal Dialysis.* Field Rich and Associates, New York, pp 360–363, 1986.

33. Nolph KD, Twardowski ZJ, Popovich RP, et al.: Equilibration of peritoneal dialysis solutions during long dwell exchanges. *J Lab Clin Med* 93:246–256, 1979.

34. Nolph KD, Popovich RP, Ghods AJ, et al.: Determinants of low clearances of small solutes during peritoneal dialysis. *Kidney Int* 13:117–123, 1978.

35. Twardowski ZJ: Individualized dialysis for CAPD patients. *Uremia Invest* 8:35–43, 1984.

36. Henderson LW: Peritoneal ultrafiltration dialysis: enhanced urea transfer using hypertonic peritoneal dialysis fluid. *J Clin Invest* 45:950–955, 1966.

37. Henderson LW, Nolph KD: Altered permeability of the peritoneal membrane after using hypertonic peritoneal dialysis fluid. *J Clin Invest* 48:992–1001, 1983.

38. Twardowski ZJ, Prowant B, Nolph KD, et al.: High volume, low frequency continuous ambulatory peritoneal dialysis. *Kidney Int* 23:64–70, 1983.

39. Keshaviah P: Adequacy of PD: a quantitative approach. *Kidney Int* 42 (Suppl 32):S160–S164, 1992.

40. Lindsay RM, Spanner E, Heidenheim RP, LeFebvre JM, Hodsman A, Baird J, Allison MEM: Which comes first, KT/V or PCR—chicken or egg? *Kidney Int* 42 (Suppl 38):S32–S36, 1992.

41. Nolph KD: Small solute clearances and clinical outcomes in CAPD. *Perit Dial Int* 12:343–345, 1992.

42. Khanna R, Nolph KD: Ultrafiltration failure and sclerosing peritonitis in peritoneal dialysis patients. In: AR Nissenson, RN Fine, eds, *Dialysis Therapy.* Hanley and Belfus, Philadelphia, pp 122–125, 1986.

43. Twardowski ZJ, Nolph KD, Khanna R, et al.: Peritoneal equilibration test. *Perit Dial Bull* 7:138–147, 1987.

44. Werger C, Larpent L, Dumontet M: Prognostic value of peritoneal equilibration curves in CAPD patients. In: JF Maher, JF Winchester, eds, *Frontiers in Peritoneal Dialysis.* Field, Rich and Associates, New York, pp 88–93, 1986.

45. Nolph KD, Miller FN, Pyle WK, et al.: An hypothesis to explain the ultrafiltration characterisitics of peritoneal dialysis. *Kidney Int* 20:543–548, 1981.

46. Mactier RA, Khanna R, Twardowski Z, et al.: Role of peritoneal cavity lymphatic absorption in peritoneal dialysis. *Kidney Int*, in press.

47. Mactier RA, Khanna R, Twardowski Z, et al.: Lymphatic absorption in CAPD. *Kidney Int* 31:252A, 1987.

48. Twardowski ZJ, Khanna R, Nolph KD: Osmotic agents and ultrafiltration in peritoneal dialysis. *Nephron* 42:93–101, 1986.

49. Rottembourg J, El shahat Y, Agrafiotis A, et al.: Continuous ambulatory perioneal dialysis in insulin-dependent diabetic patients. A 40-month experience. *Kidney Int* 23:40–45, 1983.

50. Slingeneyer A, Canaud B, Mion C: Permanent loss of ultrafiltration capacity of the peritoneum in long-term peritoneal dialysis: an epidemiological study. *Nephron* 33:133–138, 1983.

51. Faller B, Marichal JF: Loss of ultrafiltration in continuous ambulatory peritoneal dialysis: a role for acetate. *Perit Dial Bull* 4:10–13, 1984.

52. Twardowski ZJ, Tully RJ, Nichols WK, et al.: Computerized tomography in the diagnosis of subcutaneous leak sites during CAPD. *Perit Dial Bull* 4:163–166, 1984.

53. Wideroe TE, Smeby LC, Mjaaland S, et al.: Long-term changes in transperitoneal water transport during continuous ambulatory peritoneal dialysis. *Nephron* 38:238–247, 1984.

54. Mactier RA, Khannna R, Twardowski Z, et al.: Ultrafiltration failure in CAPD due to excessive peritoneal cavity lymphatic absorption. *Am J Kidney Dis*, in press.

55. Pyle WK, Popovich RP, Moncrief JW: Mass transfer evaluation in peritoneal dialysis. In: JW Moncrief, RP

Popovich, eds, *CAPD Update*. Masson, New York, pp 35–52, 1981.

56. Twardowski Z, Ksiazek A, Majdan M, et al.: Kinetics of continuous ambulatory peritoneal dialysis (CAPD) with four exchanges per day. *Clin Nephrol* 15:119–130, 1981.

57. Leenen FHH, Shah P, Boer WH, et al.: Hypotension in CAPD: an approach to treatment. *Perit Dial Bull* 3:S33–S35, 1983.

58. Young MA, Nolph KD, Dutton S, et al.: Anti-hypertensive drug requirements in continuous ambulatory peritoneal dialysis. *Perit Dial Bull* 4:85–88, 1984.

59. Glasson PH, Favre H, Valloton MB: Response of blood pressure and the renin–angiotensin–aldosterone system to chronic ambulatory peritoneal dialysis in hypertensive end-stage renal failure. *Clin Sci* 63:S207–209, 1982.

60. Nolph KD, Hano JE, Teschan PE: Peritoneal sodium transport during hypertonic peritoneal dialysis: physiologic mechanisms and clinical implications. *Ann Intern Med* 70:931–941, 1969.

61. Nolph KD, Sorkin MI, Moore H: Autoregulation of sodium and potassium removal during continuous ambulatory peritoneal dialysis. *Trans Am Soc Artif Intern Organs* 6:334–337, 1980.

62. Marquez-Julio A, Dombros N, Osmond D, et al.: Hypotension in patients on continuous ambulatory peritoneal dialysis. In: M Legrain, ed, *Proceedings of the First International Symposium on CAPD*. Excerpta Medica, Amsterdam, pp 263–267, 1979.

63. Nolph KD, Prowant B, Serkes KD, et al.: Multicenter evaluation of a new peritoneal dialysis solution with a high lactate and a low magnesium concentration. *Perit Dial Bull* 3:63–65, 1983.

64. Nissenson AR: Acid–base homeostasis in peritoneal dialysis patients. *Int J Artif Organs* 7:175–176, 1984.

65. An International Cooperative Study (Third Report): A survey of ultrafiltration in CAPD. In: R Khanna, KD Nolph, B Prowant, ZJ Twardowski, DG Oreopoulos, eds, *Advances in Continuous Ambulatory Peritoneal Dialysis*. University of Toronto Press, Toronto, pp 79–86, 1985.

66. Gandhi VC, Humayun HM, Ing TS, et al.: Sclerotic thickening of the peritoneal membrane in maintenance peritoneal dialysis patients. *Arch Intern Med* 140:1201–1203, 1980.

67. Novello AC, Port FK: Sclerosing encapsulating peritonitis. *Int J Artif Organs* 9:393–396, 1986.

68. Feriani M, Biasioli S, Boring D, et al.: Bicarbonate buffer for CAPD solutions. *Trans Am Soc Artif Organs* 31:668–672, 1985.

69. Blumenkrantz MJ, Kopple JD, Mora JK, et al.: Metabolic balance studies and dietary protein requirements in patients undergoing continuous ambulatory peritoneal dialysis. *Kidney Int* 21:849–861, 1982.

70. Delmez JA, Slatopolsky E, Martin KJ, et al.: Minerals, vitamin D, and parathyroid hormone in CAPD. *Kidney Int* 21:862–867, 1982.

71. Parker A, Nolph KD: Magnesium and calcium transfer during CAPD. *Trans Am Soc Artif Intern Organs* 26:194–196, 1980.

72. Cassidy MJD, Owen JP, Ellis HA, et al.: Renal osteodystrophy and metastatic calcification in long-term CAPD. *Q J Med* 213:29–48, 1985.

73. Davenport A, Goel S, Mackenzie JC: Audit of the use of calcium carbonate as a phosphate binder in 100 patients treated with continuous ambulatory peritoneal dialysis.

Nephrol Dial Transplant 7:632–635, 1992.

74. Hutchison AJ, Freemont AJ, Boulton HF, Gokal R: Low-calcium dialysis fluid and oral calcium carbonate in CAPD: a method of controlling hyperphosphatemia whilst minimizing aluminum exposure and hypercalcemia. *Nephrol Dial Transplant* 7:1219–1225, 1992.

75. Slatopolsky E, Weerts C, Lopez-Hilder S, et al.: Calcium carbonate as a phosphate binder in patients with chronic renal failure undergoing dialysis. *N Engl J Med* 315:157–161, 1986.

76. Mactier RA, Nolph KD, Khanna R, et al.: Risk factors for hyperaluminemia in continuous ambulatory peritoneal dialysis. *Perit Dial Bull* 6:188–193, 1986.

77. Salusky IB, Coburn JB, Paunier L, et al.: Role of aluminum hydroxide in raising serum aluminum levels in children undergoing CAPD. *J Pediatr* 105:717–720, 1984.

78. Rottembourg J, Gallego JL, Jaudon M, et al.: Serum concentration and peritoneal mass transfer of aluminum during treatment by continuous ambulatory peritoneal dialysis. *Kidney Int* 24:99–924, 1984.

79. Sorkin MI, Nolph KD, Anderson HO, et al.: Aluminum mass transfer during continuous ambulatory peritoneal dialysis. *Perit Dial Bull* 1:91–94, 1981.

80. Bertholf RL, Roman, JM, Brown S, et al.: Aluminum hydroxide induced osteomalacia, encephalopathy and hyperaluminemia in CAPD, treatment with desferrioxamine. *Perit Dial Bull* 4:30–32, 1984.

81. Cumming AD, Simpson G, Bell D, et al.: Acute aluminum intoxication in patients on continuous ambulatory peritoneal dialysis. *Lancet* 1:103–104, 1982.

82. Guillot AP, Hood BL, Runge CF, et al.: Use of magnesium containing phosphate binders in patients with end-stage renal disease on maintenance hemodialysis. *Nephron* 30:114–117, 1982.

83. Nolph KD, Ryan L, Prowant B, et al.: A cross-sectional assessment of serum vitamin D and triglyceride concentration in a CAPD population. *Perit Dial Bull* 4:232–237, 1984.

84. Gokal R, Ramos JM, Ellis HA, et al.: Histological renal osteodystrophy, and 25 hydroxycholecalciferol and aluminum levels in patients on continuous ambulatory peritoneal dialysis. *Kidney Int* 23:15–21, 1983.

85. Aloni Y, Shany S, Chaimovitz C: Losses of 25-hydroxy vitamin D in peritoneal fluid: possible mechanisms for bone disease in uremic patients treated with CAPD. *Miner Electrolyte Metab* 9:82–86, 1983.

86. Delmez JA: Calcitriol and secondary hyperparathyroidism in continuous ambulatory peritoneal dialysis patients. *Perit Dial Int* 13:95–97, 1993.

87. Sherrard DJ, Hercz G, Pei Y, Maloney NA, Greenwood C, Manuel A, Saiphoo C, Fenton SS, Segre GV: The spectrum of bone disease in end-stage renal failure: an evolving disorder. *Kidney Int* 43:436–442, 1993.

88. Kopple JD, Blumenkrnatz MJ: Nutritional requirements for patients undergoing continuous ambulatory peritoneal dialysis. *Kidney Int* 24:S295–S302, 1983.

89. Dulaney JT, Hatch FE: Peritoneal dialysis and loss of proteins: a review. *Kidney Int* 26:253–262, 1984.

90. Rubin J, Nolph KD, Arfania D, et al.: Protein losses in continuous ambulatory peritoneal dialysis. *Nephron* 28:218–221, 1981.

91. Blumenkrantz MJ, Gahl GM, Kopple JD, et al.: Protein losses during peritoneal dialysis. *Kidney Int* 19:593–602, 1981.

92. Rubin J, Ray R, Barnes T, et al.: Peritoneal abnormalities during infectious episodes of continuous ambulatory peritoneal dialysis. *Nephron* 29:124–127, 1981.

93. Kredict RT, Zuyderhoudt FMJ, Bocschoten EW, et al.: Alterations in peritoneal transport of water and solutes during peritonitis in continuous ambulatory peritoneal dialysis patients. *Eur J Clin Invest*, in press.

94. Dombros N, Oren A, Marliss EB, et al.: Plasma amino acid profiles and amino acid losses in patients undergoing CAPD. *Perit Dial Bull* 2:27–32, 1982.

95. Giordano C, De Santo NG, Capodicasa G, et al.: Amino acid losses during CAPD. *Clin Nephrol* 14:230–232, 1980.

96. Kopple JD, Blumenkrantz MJ, Jones MR, et al.: Plasma amino acid levels and amino acid losses during continuous ambulatory peritoneal dialysis. *Am J Clin Nutr* 36:395–402, 1982.

97. Lindhom B, Bergstrom J: Nutritional aspects on peritoneal dialysis. *Kidney Int* 42 (Suppl 38):S165–S171, ••.

98. Bergstrom J, Lindhom B: Nutrition and adequacy of dialysis: how do hemodialysis and CAPD compare? *Kidney Int* 43 (Suppl 40):S39–S50, 1993.

99. Blake PG, Flowerdew G, Blake RM, Oreopoulos DG: Serum albumin in patients on continuous ambulatory peritoneal dialysis: predictors and correlations with outcomes. *J Am Soc Nephrol* 3:1501–1507, 1993.

100. Zaltzman JS, Fenton SSA: Continuous ambulatory peritoneal dialysis and nutritional adequacy. *Semin Dial* 5:257–260, 1992.

101. Blumberg A, Hanck A, Sander G: Vitamin nutrition in patients on continuous ambulatory peritoneal dialysis. *Clin Nephrol* 20:244–250, 1983.

102. Henderson IS, Leung ACT, Shenkin A: Vitamin status in continuous ambulatory peritoneal dialysis. *Perit Dial Bull* 4:143–145, 1984.

103. Grodstein GP, Blumenkrantz MJ, Kopple JD, et al.: Glucose absorption during continuous ambulatory peritoneal dialysis. *Kidney Int* 19:564–567, 1981.

104. Von Baeyer H, Gahl GM, Riedinger H, et al.: Adaptation of CAPD patients to the continuous peritoneal energy uptake. *Kidney Int* 23:29–34, 1983.

105. Young GA, Hobson SM, Young SM, et al.: Adverse effects of hypertonic dialysis fluid during CAPD. *Lancet* 2:1421, 1983.

106. Cattran DC, Steiner GS, Fenton SSA, et al.: Dialysis hyperlipemia: response to dietary manipulations. *Clin Nephrol* 13:177–182, 1980.

107. Ramos JM, Heaton A, Mc Gurk JC, et al.: Sequential changes in serum lipids and their subfractions in patients receiving continuous ambulatory peritoneal dialysis. *Nephron* 35:20–23, 1983.

108. Giordano C, De Santo NG, Pluvio M, et al.: Protein requirement of patients on CAPD: a study of nitrogen balance. *Int J Artif Organs* 3:11–14, 1980.

109. Thomson NM, Stenens BJ, Humphery TJ, et al.: Comparison of trace elements in peritoneal dialysis, hemodialysis and uremia. *Kidney Int* 23:9–14, 1983.

110. Keane WF, Peterson PK: Host defense mechanisms of the peritoneal cavity and continuous ambulatory peritoneal dialysis. *Perit Dial Bull* 4:122–127, 1984.

111. Deane WF, Comty CM, Verbrugh HA, et al.: Opsonic deficiency of peritoneal dialysis effluent in contiuous ambulatory peritoneal dialysis. *Kidney Int* 25:539–543, 1984.

112. Verbrugh HA, Keane WF, Hoikal JR, et al.: Peritoneal macrophage and opsonins: antibacterial defense in patients on chronic peritoneal dialysis. *J Infect Dis* 147:1018–1029, 1983.

113. Duwe AK, Vas SI, Weatherhead JW: Effect of the composition of peritoneal dialysis fluid on chemiluminescence, phagocytosis and bactericidal activity in vitro. *Infect Immun* 33:130–135, 1981.

114. Lamperi S, Carozzi S: Defective opsonic activity of peritoneal effluent during continuous ambulatory peritoneal dialysis. *Perit Dial Bull* 6:87–92, 1986.

115. Khanna, R, Nolph KD, Prowant BF, Twardowski ZJ: Computer interactive session: peritonitis. In: R Khanna, ed, *Advances in Peritoneal Dialysis*. Peritoneal Publications, Toronto, in press.

116. Chan MK, Biallod RA, Tanner A, et al.: Abdominal hernias in patients receiving continuous ambulatory peritoneal dialysis. *Br Med J* 283:826. 1981.

117. Rubin J, Raju S, Teal N, et al.: Abdominal hernia in patients undergoing continuous ambulatory peritoneal dialysis. *Arch Intern Med* 142:1453–1455, 1982.

118. Digenis GE, Khanna R, Mathews R, et al.: Abdominal hernia in patients undergoing CAPD. *Perit Dial Bull* 2:115–118, 1982.

119. Helfrich GB, Pechan BW, Alifani MR, et al.: Reduced catheter complications with lateral placement. *Perit Dial Bull* 3:S2–S4, 1983.

120. Khanna R, Oreopoulos DG: Peritoneal access using the Toronto Western Hospital permanent catheter. *Perspect Perit Dial* 1:4–6, 1983.

121. Cooper JC, Nicholls AJ, Simms AG, et al.: Genital edema in patients treated by continuous ambulatory peritoneal dialysis: an unusual presentation of inguinal hernia. *Br Med J* 286:1923–1924, 1983.

122. Singh S, Vaidya P, Dale A, et al.: Massive hydrothorax complicating continuous ambulatory peritoneal dialysis. *Nephron* 34:168–172, 1983.

123. Grefberg N, Danielson BG, Benson L, et al.: Right-sided hydrothorax complicating peritoneal dialysis. *Nephron* 34:130–134, 1983.

124. Spadaro JJ, Thakur V, Nolh KD: Technetium-99m-labelled macroaggragated albumin in demonstration of transdiaphragmatic leakage of dialysate in peritoneal dialysis. *Am J Nephrol* 2:36–38, 1982.

125. Rudnick MR, Coyle JF, Beck LH, et al.: Acute massive hydrothorax complicating peritoneal dialysis, report of 2 cases and review of the literature. *Clin Nephrol* 12:38–44, 1979.

126. Twardowski ZJ, Khanna R, Nolph KD, et al.: Intraabdominal pressures during natural activities in patients treated with continuous ambulatory peritoneal dialysis. *Nephron* 44:129–135, 1986.

127. Epstein SW, Inouye T, Robson M, et al.: Effect of peritoneal dialysis fluid on ventilatory function. *Perit Dial Bull* 2:120–122, 1982.

128. Franklin JO, Alpert MA, Twardowski ZJ, et al.: Effect of intraperitoneal infusion volume and posture on left ventricular systolic junction in patients on continuous ambulatory peritoneal dialysis. *J Am Soc Artif Intern Organs* 15:49A, 1986.

129. Breborowicz A, Rodela H, Oreopoulos DG: Toxicity of osmotic studies on human mesothelial cells in vitro. *Kidney Int* 41:1280–1285, 1992.

130. Martison E, Weislander A, Kjellstrand P, Boberg U: Toxicity

of heat sterilized peritoneal dialysis fluids is derived from degradation of glucose. *ASAIO J* 38:M370–M372, 1993.

131. De Fijter CWH, Verbrugh HA, Oe LP, Heezius E, Donker AJM, Verhoef J, Gokal R: Biocompatibility of a glucose-polymer-containing peritoneal dialysis fluid. *Am J Kidney Dis* 21:411–418, 1993.

132. Gokal R, Ramos JM, Francis DMA, et al.: Peritonitis in continuous ambulatory peritoneal dialysis. *Lancet* 2:1388–1391, 1982.

133. Spencer PC, Farrell PC: Solute and water kinetics in CAPD. In: R Gokal, ed, *Continuous Ambulatory Peritoneal Dialysis*. Churchill Livingstone, Edinburgh, pp 38–55, 1986.

134. Gilmour J, Wu G, Khanna R, et al.: Long-term continuous ambulatory peritoneal dialysis. *Perit Dial Bull* 5:112–118, 1985.

135. Khanna R, Mcneely DJ, Oreopoulos DG, et al.: Treating fungal infections: fungal peritonitis in CAPD. *Br Med J* 280:1147–1148, 1980.

136. Miller FN, Nolph Kd, Joshua IG, Weigman DL, Harris PD, Anderson DB: Hyperosmolality, acetate and lactate: dilatory factors during peritoneal dialysis. *Kidney Int* 20:397–402, 1981.

137. Slingeneyer A, Faller B, Beraud JT: Progressive sclerosing peritonitis: late and severe complication of maintenance peritoneal dialysis. *Tran Am Soc Artif Intern Organs* 29:633–638, 1983.

138. Rottembourg J, Gahl GM, Piognet JL, et al.: Severe abdominal complications in patients undergoing continuous ambulatory peritoneal dialysis. *Proc Eur Dial Transplant Assoc* 20:236–241, 1983.

139. Bradley JA, Mcwhinnie DL, Hamiton DNH, et al.: Sclerosing obstructive peritonitis after continuous ambulatory peritoneal dialysis. *Lancet* 2:113–114, 1983.

140. Slingeneyer A, Ellie M: Co-operative international study on sclerosing encapsulating peritonitis: preliminary report. In: R Khanna, KD Nolph, B Prowant, et al., eds, *Advances in Continuous Ambulatory Peritoneal Dialysis*. University of Toronto Press, Toronto, pp 118–123, 1985.

141. Junor BJR, Briggs JD, Forwell MA, et al.: Sclerosing peritonitis: Role of chlorhexedine in alcohol. *Perit Dial Bull* 5:101–104, 1985.

142. Verger C, Brunschvicg O, Le Carpentier Y, et al.: Structural and ultrastructural peritoneal membrane changes and permeability alterations during CAPD. *Proc Eur Dial Transplant Assoc* 18:199–203, 1981.

143. Gahl GM, Von Baeyer H, Averdunk R, et al.: Outpatient evaluation of dietary intake and nitrogen removal in continuous ambulatory peritoneal dialysis. *Ann Intern Med* 94:643–646, 1981.

144. Blumenkrantz MJ, Kopple JD, Moran JK, et al.: Nitrogen and urea metabolism during continuous ambulatory peritoneal dialysis. *Kidney Int* 20:78–82, 1981.

145. Williams P, Marliss E, Anderson GH, et al.: Amino acid absorption following intraperitoneal administration in CAPD patients. *Perit Dial Bull* 3:66–73, 1982.

146. Oren A, Wu G, Anderson GH, et al.: Effective use of amino acid dialysate over 4 weeks in CAPD patients. *Perit Dial Bull* 3:66–73, 1983.

147. Chan MK, Varghese Z, Moorhead JF: Lipid abnormalities in ureamia, dialysis and transplantation. *Kidney Int* 19:625–637, 1981.

148. Avram MM, Golwasser P, Burrel DE, Antignani A, Fein PA, Mittman N: The uremic dyslipidemia: a cross-sectional and longitudinal study. *Am J Kidney Dis* 20:324–335, 1992.

149. Kandoussi A, Cachera C, Pagniez D, Fruchart JC, Tacquet A: Apo AIV in plasma and dialysate fluid of CAPD patients: comparison with other apolipoproteins. *Nephrol Dial Transplant* 7:1026–1029, 1992.

150. Heaton A, Johnston DG, Burrin JM, et al.: Carbohydrate and lipid metabolism during continuous ambulatory peritoneal dialysis (CAPD): the effect of a single cycle. *Clin Sci* 65:539–545, 1983.

151. Williams P, Kay R, Harrison J, et al.: Nutritional and anthropometric assessment of patient on CAPD over 1 year: contrasting changes in total body nitrogen and potassium. *Perit Dial Bull* 1:82–87, 1981.

152. Rubin J, Flynn MA, Nolph KD: Total body potassium—a guide to nutritional health in patients undergoing continuous ambulatory peritoneal dialysis. *Am J Clin Nutr* 34:94–98, 1981.

153. Rubin J, Kirchner K, Barnes T, et al.: Evaluation of continuous ambulatory peritoneal dialysis. *Am J Kidney Dis* 3:199–204, 1983.

154. Turgan C, Feehally J, Bennett S, et al.: Accelerated hypertriglyceridemia in patients on continuous ambulatory peritoneal dialysis—a preventable abnormality. *Int J Artif Organs* 4:158–160, 1981.

155. Wu G: Osmotic agents for peritoneal dialysis solution. *Perit Dial Bull* 2:151–154, 1982.

156. Wanner C, Lubrich-Birkner I, Summ O, Wieland H, Schollmeyer P: Effect of simvastatin on qualitative changes of lipoprotein metabolism in CAPD patients. *Nephron* 62:40–46, 1992.

157. Elisaf MS, Dardamanis MA, Papagalanis ND, Siamopoulos KC: Lipid abnormalities in chronic uremic patients. Response to treatment with gemfibrozil. *Perit Dial Int* 13:101–108, 1993.

158. Canadian Renal Failure Register: *Kidney Foundation of Canada-1986 Report.* 1987.

159. Wing AJ, Broyer M , Brunner FP, et al.: Combined report on regular dialysis and transplantation in Europe. *Proc Eur Dial Transplant Assoc* 20:2–75, 1983.

160. Hutchison TA, Thomas DC, MacGibbon B: Predicting survival in adults with end-stage renal disease: an age equivalent index. *Ann Intern Med* 96:417–423, 1982.

161. Nelson CB, Port FK, Wolfe RA, Guire KE: Comparison of continuous ambulatory peritoneal dialysis and hemodialysis patient survival with evaluation of trends during the 1980s. *J Am Soc Nephrol* 3:1147–1155, 1992.

162. Maiorca R, Cancarini GC, Brunori G, Camarini C, Manili L: Morbidity and mortality of CAPD and hemodialysis. *Kidney Int* 43 (Suppl 40):S4–S15, 1993.

163. Winchester JF, Rotellar C, Goggins M, Robino D, Alijani MR, Rokowski TA, Argy WP: Transplantation in peritoneal dialysis and hemodialysis. *Kidney Int* 43 (Suppl 40):S101–S105, 1993.

CHAPTER 57

Peritoneal Catheter Placement and Management

ZBYLUT J. TWARDOWSKI

INTRODUCTION

The peritoneal catheter is a lifeline for the peritoneal dialysis patient. The double-cuff Tenckhoff catheter, developed in 1968 for treatment of patients with intermittent peritoneal dialysis (1), is also widely used for continuous ambulatory peritoneal dialysis (CAPD); however, catheter-related complications are increased in CAPD due to higher intra-abdominal pressure and numerous daily manipulations. Such complications as catheter-tip migration, dialysate leaks, and exit-site infections are not uncommon. An in-depth review of the peritoneal catheter history, theoretical background of catheter design, implantation, complications, and care was recently published (2). This chapter will present practical aspects of design, implantation, and care of the rigid and most commonly used soft catheters.

RIGID CATHETERS

The two most widely used rigid catheters in North America are the Stylocath (Abbott Laboratories, North Chicago, IL 60064, U.S.A.) and the Trocath (Baxter Healthcare Corporation, Deerfield, IL 60015, U.S.A.).

Preinsertion patient assessment and preparation

When the need to start peritoneal dialysis is urgent, one may elect to access the peritoneal cavity through a rigid catheter. This catheter could be inserted at the bedside, with very minimal preparation. Equipment required for paracentesis is all that is needed.

Bedside insertion should not be offered to patients who are extremely obese or have had previous abdominal surgery, since abdominal adhesions increase the risk of inadvertent viscus perforation. In addition, this approach should not be taken in children except by an experienced pediatric nephrologist or nephrologist with a pediatrician in attendance. If a nephrologist implants the catheter, a surgeon should be on standby in case of complications. The

patient should receive preoperative sedation and have nothing to eat or drink for at least 12 hours prior to the procedure.

All observers and persons in the immediate area, including the patient, should wear surgical masks. Those patients who experience discomfort while completely supine should raise their heads slightly. If the patient is conscious, it may be useful to familiarize him or her with the Valsalva maneuver. The operator and assistant(s) should "scrub, gown, and glove." A "circulating" nurse should be present to assist.

Insertion

With all sterile precautions taken, a small stab wound (2–3 mm) is made in the midline under local anesthesia, 2–3 cm below the umbilicus. The stab wound should be small so that the abdominal wall holds the catheter firmly and minimizes dialysis solution leak. With the stylet in place, the catheter is forced through the abdominal wall by a short thrust or preferably with a rotary motion. The operator will recognize the loss of resistance as a "pop" as soon as the peritoneal cavity is entered. While the catheter is being thrust through the abdominal wall, its tip is directed towards the coccyx. Because successful perforation of the abdominal wall for introduction of the catheter requires a sensitive "feel" for the pressure applied, infusion of 2–3 L of dialysate will distend the abdomen, which in turn will facilitate this maneuver. Some infuse 2 L of dialysis fluid via a small gauge needle prior to stylet puncture. A cooperative patient can also assist in successful perforation by voluntarily contracting the abdominal musculature.

Once the peritoneal cavity has been entered, the stylet is withdrawn a few centimeters and the catheter is advanced deep into the pelvis. If the operator encounters resistance while the catheter is being advanced, or if the patient complains of pain, the advance in this direction should be stopped and another direction tried. If this is still not possible, 2 or 3 L of dialysis solution may be infused into the peritoneal cavity, if this has not been done. Infusion can be via the catheter if the holes in the distal end are in the

Suki, WN and Massry SG (eds), Suki and Massry's Therapy of Renal Diseases and Related Disorders, Third Edition. ISBN 978-1-4757-6634-9.
©*1998, Kluwer Academic Publishers, Boston/Dordrecht/London. All rights reserved.*

cavity. This infusion accomplishes two important objectives: first, it facilitates recognition of the "true" intraperitoneal space; and second, dialysis solution in the peritoneal cavity reduces the likelihood of viscus perforation by moving the intra-abdominal contents away from the advancing catheter. After one or two good in-and-out exchanges, the catheter is firmly secured to the skin with the aid of a metal disc.

Complications

Table 1 shows complications of rigid catheter insertion. Following catheter implantation, bloody effluent appears after the first exchange in approximately 30% of cases (3,4). This bleeding (usually minor) comes from the small vessels in the abdominal wall. After three to four exchanges, bleeding usually stops unless the procedure has damaged a major vessel or the patient has a bleeding disorder. Pressure applied over the catheter insertion site usually controls minor bleeding. Occasionally, a transfusion of fresh blood will stop the bleeding. If the bleeding is copious, it may obstruct the catheter; in this event, it is a common practice to add 1000 units of heparin to each liter of dialysate to minimize the risk of obstruction. Heparin (MW 15,000 daltons) is poorly absorbed from the peritoneal cavity and does not influence systemic coagulation, but prevents clot formation in the peritoneal cavity.

Dialysis solution leak is encountered in 14%–36% of patients after rigid catheter insertion (3–5). Frequent manipulation of the catheter to improve drainage increases the risk of dialysis solution leak from the catheter exit site. Such leaks may also occur when the catheter is not properly secured to the skin. The risk of external leak is higher in elderly or debilitated patients who have lax abdominal walls. The presence of a large intra-abdominal mass, such as polycystic kidneys, may raise the intra-abdominal pressure to high levels and promote an external dialysis solution leak after the standard 2-L volume has been instilled.

Fluid may extravasate into the abdominal wall, particularly in patients who have had a previous abdominal operation or multiple catheter insertions. This complication usually results from tears in the peritoneum or represents an infusion of dialysate into the potential space between

Table 1. Complications of rigid catheter insertion

Bleeding
Dialysis solution leak
Poor drainage
Extraperitoneal space penetration
Viscus perforation
Peritonitis
Abdominal pain
Loss of rigid catheter in the peritoneum

---

the layers of abdominal wall. Uncommonly, dialysis fluid may enter the pleural cavity (6–8). In such cases, peritoneal dialysis is usually discontinued, and the patients are switched to hemodialysis. Acute hydrothorax results from either a traumatic or a congenital defect in the diaphragm.

Inadequate drainage is frequent during initial dialysis and may be due to one or more of the following factors: loss of siphon effect, one-way obstruction, and incorrect placement of the catheter. One-way (outflow) catheter obstruction may have multiple causes. Fibrin or blood clots may be trapped in the catheter and block the terminal holes, especially when dialysis is complicated by major hemorrhage or peritonitis. Poor outflow may also reflect extrinsic pressure on the catheter from adjacent organs such as a sigmoid colon full of feces or a distended bladder. Omental wrapping is likely if the catheter is misplaced into the upper abdomen.

Occasionally, accidental penetration of the extraperitoneal space by the catheter may cause poor drainage. In such a situation, continued infusion produces further dissection, and the fluid may become trapped and no longer be available for drainage. Loculation of fluid, another cause of poor drainage, is encountered in patients who have had previous intra-abdominal operations or peritonitis. Such loculation not only diminishes the surface area available for dialysis but also may seriously reduce ultrafiltration capacity. The incidence of this complication is low, varying between 0.5% and 1.3% (5,9,10).

Perforation or laceration of internal organs during bedside insertion of the catheter has been frequently reported. Lacerated or perforated organs include the bowel, bladder, liver, a polycystic kidney, aorta, mesenteric artery, and hernia sac (9–15). Abdominal distention due to paralytic ileus or bowel obstruction may predispose the patient to bowel perforation. Those who are unconscious, cachectic or heavily sedated are also at high risk. Clinical evidence of bowel perforation includes sudden, sharp, or severe abdominal pain followed by watery diarrhea and poor drainage of the dialysis solution, which may be cloudy, foul-smelling, or mixed with fecal material. Such a situation requires prompt removal of the catheter and then allowing the perforation to seal off completely in about 12–24 hours.

The incidence of peritonitis when the stylet catheter was used was 2.5% of all the dialyses (16). The incidence of peritonitis almost doubled when the duration of dialysis was longer than 60 hours.

Abdominal pain may be encountered in as many as 56%–75% of patients with the first use of the catheter (3). There are many causes of abdominal pain, but catheter-related pain occurs when the catheter impinges on any of the viscera. Pain may occur during inflow and outflow of dialysis solution and also when the solution is dwelling. Outflow pain is due to entrapment of omentum in the catheter during the siphoning action of fluid drainage. Constant pain during dialysis indicates pressure effects on intra-abdominal organs and often produces continuous rectal or low back pain. This complaint calls for an adjustment in catheter position.

Loss of a part or all of the rigid catheter has been reported following its manipulation with the trocar in place (3,12,16). Its distal end may be amputated after intra-abdominal kinking of the catheter, followed by manipulation. However, the presence of broken catheters within the abdominal cavity does not cause symptoms or ill effects. During laparoscopy, broken catheters have been found lying freely in the peritoneal cavity without causing a peritoneal reaction or have been found walled off by mesentery without an inflammatory reaction. On a routine postmortem examination, Stein (17) discovered such a catheter in a patient who had had previous peritoneal dialysis. Exploration to retrieve the catheter is unnecessary because laparotomy is more hazardous than leaving the catheter in a severely ill patient. The incidence of catheter loss into the peritoneal cavity has been greatly reduced since the introduction of a design that incorporates a metal disc with a central hole.

SOFT CATHETERS

A Computer Interactive Session carried on during the XIVth Annual Peritoneal Dialysis Conference in Orlando, Florida, on January 24, 1994, revealed preferences and practices of 650–690 respondents voting on questions related to peritoneal catheters (18).

Table 2 presents the numbers and percentages of persons who answered positively to a question about whether they used a particular catheter at least once in 1993. Since the total number of respondents was 660–670 and the number of positive answers was 1552, the program of each respondent used 2–3 types of catheters on average. Compared to the surveys conducted in 1987 (19) and 1989 (20), the most striking change was an increase in the use of catheters with the bent intramural segment, particularly the swan-neck catheters. Whereas no catheters with bent intraperitoneal segment were included in the 1997 report and only 12% of these catheters were used in 1989, over 30% of these catheters were used in 1993. An increase in

Table 2. Number and percentages of catheters used in 1993 according to the computer interactive survey, Orlando, 1994[a]

Catheter type	North America		Europe		Rest of the world		Total	
	Number	Percent	Number	Percent	Number	Percent	Number	Percent
Tenckhoff, double-cuff, coiled	234	23.1	60	24.5	39	13.4	333	21.5
Tenckhoff, double-cuff, straight	144	14.2	61	24.9	80	27.4	285	18.4
Tenckhoff, single-cuff, straight	75	7.4	15	6.1	30	10.3	120	7.7
Tenckhoff, single-cuff, coiled	93	9.2	5	2.0	16	5.5	114	7.3
Total Tenckhoff	546	53.8	141	57.6	165	56.5	852	54.9
Swan-neck Tenckhoff coiled	98	9.7	13	5.3	21	7.2	132	8.5
Swan-neck Tenckhoff straight	29	2.9	34	13.9	34	11.6	97	6.3
Swan-neck Missouri coiled	44	4.3	8	3.3	7	2.4	59	3.8
Swan-neck Missouri straight	25	2.5	13	5.3	13	4.5	51	3.3
Swan-neck presternal	11	1.1	0	0.0	3	1.0	14	0.9
Swan-neck Moncrief–Popovich	51	5.0	9	3.7	9	3.1	69	4.4
Swan-neck other	34	3.3	6	2.4	8	2.7	48	3.1
Total swan neck	292	28.8	83	33.9	95	32.5	470	30.3
Cruz	73	7.2	2	0.8	6	2.1	81	5.2
Toronto Western Hospital	32	3.2	9	3.7	9	3.1	50	3.2
Gore-Tex	16	1.6	0	0.0	2	0.7	18	1.2
Ash	13	1.3	2	0.8	1	0.3	16	1.0
Valli	2	0.2	1	0.4	2	0.7	5	0.3
Other	41	4.0	7	2.9	12	4.1	60	3.9
Other than Tenckhoff/swan neck	177	17.4	21	8.6	32	11.0	230	14.8
Grand total	1015	100.0	245	100.0	292	100.0	1552	100.0

[a] Modified from (18), with permission. See text for explanations.

the use of catheters with the coiled intraperitoneal segment was also significant in North America (21.9% in 1987, 40.1% in 1989, and 52.3% in 1993). The Tenckhoff catheter continued to be the most popular, although its use was decreasing. The remaining catheters were used in small numbers. A vast majority of nephrologists remained convinced of the superiority of double-cuff catheters over single-cuff ones, and the use of the former continued to exceed 70% (18).

Straight and coiled Tenckhoff catheters

The Tenckhoff catheter, developed in 1968 (1), consists of silicon rubber tubing with a 2.6 mm internal diameter and a 5-mm external diameter (Figure 1). The catheter is provided with one or two polyester (Dacron®), 1-cm-long cuffs. The overall length of the adult straight double-cuff catheter is about 40 cm. The lengths of segments are as follows: intraperitoneal, about 15 cm; intercuff, 5–7 cm; external, 16 cm. The intraperitoneal segment has an open end and multiple 0.5-mm perforations at a distance of 11 cm from the tip. The coiled Tenckhoff catheter differs from the straight in having a coiled, 18.5-cm-long perforated distal end. The coiled catheter reduces the inflow infusion "jet effect" and pressure discomfort. All Tenckhoff catheters are provided with a barium-impregnated radiopaque stripe to assist in radiological visualization of the catheter. The catheters are manufactured by numerous companies, including the Quinton Instrument Co. (2121 Terry Ave., Seattle, WA 98121, U.S.A.) and the Accurate Surgical Instruments Co. (588–590 Richmond St. W., Toronto, Ontario, Canada M5V 1Y9).

Swan-neck catheters

Swan-neck catheters feature a permanent bend between cuffs (Table 3, Figure 1) (21,22). The catheter was dubbed *swan-neck* due to its shape. As a result of this design, catheters can be placed in an arcuate tunnel in an unstressed condition with both external and internal segments of the tunnel directed downward. A downward-directed exit, two cuffs, and a short sinus reduce exit/tunnel infection rates. A permanent bend between cuffs eliminates the Silastic® resilience force or the "shape memory" that tends to extrude the external cuff. A downward peritoneal entrance tends to keep the tip in the true pelvis, reducing its migration. Insertion through the rectus muscle decreases pericatheter leaks. Lower exit/tunnel infection rates curtail peritonitis episodes. Finally, swan-neck catheters with a coiled intraperitoneal segment minimize infusion and pressure pain. Swan-neck catheters are manufactured by the Accurate Surgical Instruments Co.

SWAN-NECK TENCKHOFF STRAIGHT AND COILED

The Tenckhoff type of swan-neck peritoneal dialysis catheter is provided with two Dacron® cuffs (Figure 1). It differs from the double-cuff Tenckhoff catheter only by being permanently bent between cuffs (22). This type of catheter may be inserted at the bedside and does not require surgical insertion; however, a subcutaneous tunnel has to be created in the same way as for other swan-neck catheters. The intraperitoneal segment of the swan-neck coiled catheter is identical to that of the Tenckhoff coiled catheter.

SWAN-NECK MISSOURI STRAIGHT

The swan-neck Missouri catheter (Figure 1) has a flange and bead circumferentially surrounding the catheter just below the internal cuff; the flange and bead are slanted approximately 45° relative to the axis of the catheter. The catheters for left and right tunnels are mirror images of

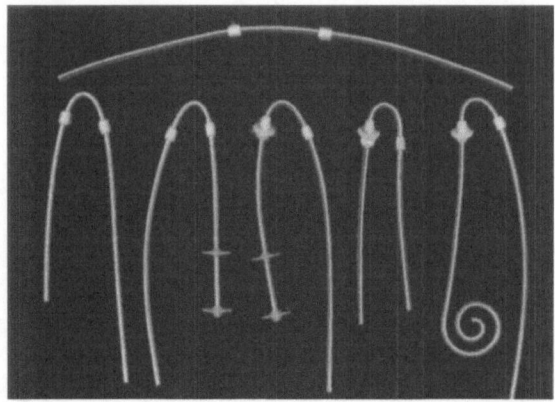

Figure 1. **Top:** Double-cuff Tenckhoff catheter with straight intraperitoneal segment. **Bottom:** Five catheters, each with a bent intramural segment. (From left: 1) swan-neck straight Tenckhoff, 2) swan-neck Tenckhoff with intraperitoneal discs, 3) swan-neck with bead, flange, and intraperitoneal discs for left tunnel, 4) swan-neck Missouri 2 straight for left tunnel, 5) swan-neck Missouri 2 coiled for left tunnel.

Table 3. Swan-neck catheter features preventing complications

Complication	Features preventing complication
Exit/tunnel infection	Downward exit, double cuff, short sinus
External cuff extrusion	Permanent bend between cuffs
Intraperitoneal tip migration	Downward intraperitoneal entrance
Pericatheter leak	Insertion through the rectus muscle
Peritonitis	Decreased tunnel infections
Infusion/pressure pain	Coiled intraperitoneal tip

each other. A swan-neck Missouri 2 catheter with a 5-cm intercuff distance is used in average-to-obese people. The intraperitoneal segment is 21.5 cm long in the swan-neck Missouri 2 long catheters. A swan-neck Missouri 3 catheter with a 3-cm intercuff distance is used in lean-to-average persons.

SWAN-NECK MISSOURI COILED

Because some patients experienced pain with straight catheters, we have modified the intraperitoneal segment of the catheters, replacing the straight segment with a coiled one. The intraperitoneal segment in all swan-neck coiled catheters is 34 cm from the bead to the tip of the coil. Swan-neck Missouri 2 coiled catheters with the 5-cm intercuff distance (Figure 2) are used in average-to-obese people. Swan-neck Missouri 3 coiled catheters with the 3-cm intercuff distance (Figure 2) are used in lean-to-average persons. The catheters for left and right tunnels are mirror images of each other (Figure 2). The overall survival of straight and coiled swan-neck Missouri catheters is not significantly different, but none of the patients experienced infusion or pressure pain with coiled catheters, whereas this complication occurred in several patients who had catheters with straight intraperitoneal segments (23). Swan-neck catheters are also available in smaller sizes for children and infants.

SWAN-NECK PRESTERNAL

The swan-neck presternal catheter is a modified swan-neck Missouri coil catheter. It differs in a major way from the swan-neck Missouri catheter in the length of the subcuta-

neous tunnel. The catheter (Figure 3) is composed of two silicon rubber tubes that are to be connected end to end at the time of implantation (24,25). The implanted lower (abdominal) tube constitutes the intraperitoneal catheter segment and a part of the intramural segment. The upper or chest tube constitutes the remaining part of the intramural segment and the external catheter segment. The lower tube is identical to the swan-neck Missouri catheter, with the exception that it is not bent and does not have a second cuff. The proximal end of the lower tube is straight, with a redundant length to be trimmed to the patient's size at the time of implantation. A titanium connector, provided in a package, is to be coupled with the distal part of the upper or chest part at the time of implantation.

The upper tube carries two porous cuffs, a superficial and a middle or central, spaced 5 cm apart. The tube between the cuffs has a permanently bent section defining an arc angle of 180°. The distal lumen of the upper tube communicates with the proximal lumen of the lower tube through the titanium connector. The tubing grip of the titanium connector is so strong that the two parts of the catheter, especially after connection reinforcement with a Prolene suture, practically cannot separate spontaneously in the tunnel (26). The swan-neck presternal catheter is

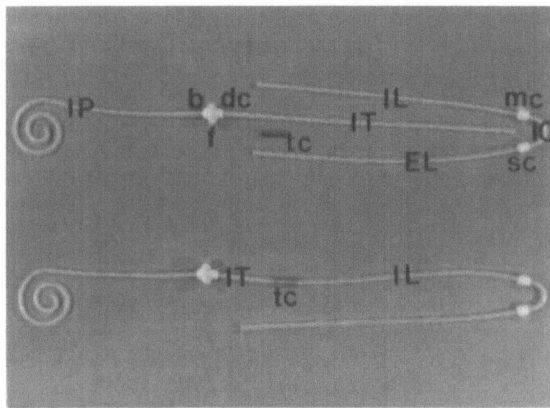

Figure 3. Two tubes of the swan-neck presternal peritoneal catheter before (top) and after (bottom) connection. Both tubes and bead are made of silicon rubber molded in the shapes as shown. A flange and all cuffs are made of woven polyester fibers. The proximal (upper, chest) tube (**PT**) consists of an intratunnel limb (**IL**), medial (center) cuff (**mc**), intercuff segment (**IC**), superficial cuff (**sc**), and external limb (**EL**); 1–2 cm of the external limb adjacent to the superficial cuff is intended to be in the sinus tract of the tunnel (from the cuff to the exit). The distal (abdominal, lower) tube (**DT**) consists of an intratunnel segment (**IT**), deep (distal, preperitoneal) cuff (**dc**), flange (**f**), bead (**b**), and intraperitoneal segment (**IP**). After implantation (bottom), the intratunnel limb (**IL**) of the chest tube and the intratunnel segment (**IT**) of the abdominal tube are trimmed to the size of the tunnel and coupled with the titanium connector (**tc**).

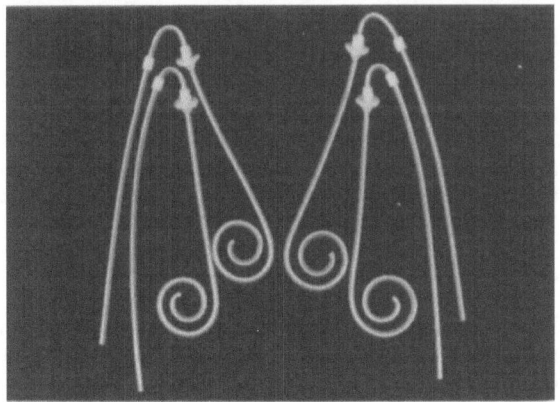

Figure 2. Swan-neck Missouri 2 (upper) and 3 (lower) catheters with coiled intraperitoneal segments. Left-tunnel catheters to the right; right-tunnel catheters to the left. The intercuff distance is 5 cm in Missouri 2 and 3 cm in Missouri 3 catheters. Stripes are to the front. The catheters for left and right tunnels are mirror images of each other. Reproduced from (88), with permission.

available for children and infants. Tubing diameter is smaller for pediatric patients.

This catheter was designed primarily to decrease infectious complications. The chest is a sturdy structure with minimal wall motion; the catheter exit located on the chest wall is subjected to minimal movements, decreasing chances of trauma and contamination. Also, in patients with abdominal ostomies and in children with diapers, a chest exit location decreases chances of contamination. Moreover, a loose garment is usually worn on the chest, so there is less pressure on the exit. Clinical surgical experience indicates that wounds heal better after thoracic surgery than after abdominal surgery; this outcome may be related to less chest mobility or some other reasons. Obese patients have higher exit-site infection rates and a tendency toward poor wound healing, particularly after abdominal surgery. The subcutaneous fat layer is several times thinner on the chest than on the abdomen. If fat thickness *per se* is responsible for quality of healing and susceptibility to infection, then chest location may be preferred for obese patients. All these favorable factors, together with easy exit-site care using a magnifying mirror, significantly reduce exit-site infections. The catheter chest location of the exit is particularly advantageous in small children due to the greater distance from diapers and is subjected to less trauma during crawling/creeping. The catheter is also advantageous for psychosocial reasons. A chest exit location allows a deep tub bath without the risk of exit contamination. Although the exit site can be located in the presternal or parasternal area, we will usually refer to this catheter as presternal for the sake of simplicity. A long catheter tunnel combined with three cuffs may hinder pericatheter bacterial penetration into the peritoneal cavity, thus reducing the incidence of peritonitis (24–27).

MONCRIEF–POPOVICH CATHETER

This catheter is a modified swan-neck Tenckhoff coiled catheter with a longer subcutaneous cuff (2.5 cm instead of 1 cm). This catheter is most commonly used in conjunction with the Moncrief–Popovich implantation technique (see below).

OTHER SWAN-NECK CATHETERS

Other swan-neck catheters include those with intraperitoneal discs (Figure 1), a deep cuff at the top of the bend and catheters, and single instead of double cuffs. Only small numbers of these catheters were used in 1993 (Table 2).

RADIOPAQUE STRIPE

The slanted flange and bead and the bent tunnel segment require that the swan-neck Missouri catheters for right and left tunnels be mirror images of each other (Figure 2). In order to facilitate recognition of the right and left Missouri catheters, each tubing has a radiopaque stripe in front of the catheter. In the swan-neck presternal catheter, the stripe also facilitates proper alignment of the lower and upper tubes. The stripe is also useful during insertion and postimplantation care, facilitating recognition of catheter twisting. Due to this last feature, Tenckhoff and Moncrief-Popovich catheters are also provided with the stripe. Right and left swan-neck Tenckhoff catheters differ only with respect to the position of the stripe. Unlike swan-neck Missouri catheters, the swan-neck Tenckhoff catheter intended for the right or left tunnel may be implanted with an opposite tunnel. In this case, the stripe should be kept in back of the catheter. Nevertheless, to retain uniformity of the stripe position, it is recommended that swan-neck Tenckhoff catheters be inserted with the corresponding tunnel direction (right tunnel with right catheter, left tunnel with left catheter).

Other catheters

As seen in Table 2, Cruz (28), Toronto Western Hospital (29), Ash (Lifecath, Column disc) (30) Valli (31), and Gore-Tex (32) catheters were used in small numbers in 1993.

IMPLANTATION OF SOFT CATHETERS

Since rigid catheters are associated with a high frequency of dialysis solution leaks and poor drainage (necessitating frequent catheter manipulation and resultant peritonitis), some centers prefer to insert single- or double-cuff Tenckhoff or swan-neck Tenckhoff catheters for the treatment of acute renal failure. Tenckhoff recommended using a single-cuff catheter for acute cases (1). For treatment of chronic renal failure, only soft catheters are used.

Patient preparation

ACUTE DIALYSIS

Patient assessment and preparation before soft catheter implantation for treatment of acute renal failure are the same as those before rigid catheter insertion.

CHRONIC DIALYSIS

Patient preparation before catheter implantation for treatment of chronic renal failure is more elaborate (22,24,33,34). In most cases, chest and/or abdominal hair should be removed with an electric shaver one day prior to surgery.

Skin-marking stencils have been developed to facilitate the creation of proper tunnels for swan-neck catheters (22). These stencils are available for swan-neck Missouri 2, swan-neck Missouri 3, and swan-neck Tenckhoff catheters. In order to maximize the advantages of the swan-neck design, the catheter tunnels must follow the precise shape of the catheters; the stencils follow exactly the shape of the intramural segments of the catheters. The stencils can be flipped to be used for right or left catheters. The holes for exit-site markings are located 2 cm and 1 cm from the cuff. A 2-cm mark is used for average or obese persons, and a 1-cm mark is suitable for lean and small persons. Stencils for swan-neck Tenckhoff catheters also reflect precisely the shape of their intramural segments.

Abdominal exit

The patient's belt line is identified, preferably in the sitting or standing position, with slacks or pants as usually worn (22). Taking into consideration the size and shape of the abdomen, the presence of previous scars, right or left hand-edness, and the patient's preference, a tunnel is marked (using a swan-neck catheter stencil) with an exit hole at least 2 cm from the belt line. Skin markings may be made with any good surgical marker.

Since women usually wear a belt above the umbilicus, their stencils are usually marked below their belt lines. The catheter should not be subjected to excessive motion with patient activities, and there should not be pressure on the tunnel when the patient bends forward. In obese people with pendulous abdomens, it is mandatory to insert the catheter above the skin fold so that they can see the exit for its care. Men usually prefer a belt line below the umbilicus, and there may not be enough space below the belt line; therefore, a stencil is frequently marked above the belt line in male patients. The label of the chosen catheter type is written on the belly of the patient. A band with the catheter label is also attached to the patient's left wrist.

One gram of vancomycin is given by slow intravenous infusion within 24 hours prior to surgery. On the evening preceding the surgery, a tap-water enema is administered and the patient takes a shower. Skin markings may require correction if they become faint after the shower. Cephalosporins (1.0 g I.V. 1 hr preoperatively repeated 12 hours postoperatively) also constitute appropriate prophylactic therapy (33,34).

Presternal exit

Depending on the size of the patient, the abdominal cuff and flange location is marked over the rectus muscle (24). To secure the catheter tip position in the true pelvis but without excessive pressure on the pelvic peritoneum, the position of the cuff should be above the umbilicus in small persons and at the level of or slightly below the umbilicus in tall persons. To determine a preferable position of the deep cuff, a coiled catheter tip is placed on the pubic bone and the cuff position is marked. On the chest, a superficial cuff is marked at the second or third intercostal space and the exit 3 cm from the cuff in the presternal or parasternal area. It is preferable not to cross the midline in patients likely to have heart surgery. Care is taken to avoid an exit

site too close to the bra area in females. Prophylactic antibiotics, shower, and enema are used in the same way as for abdominal exit (24).

Catheter preparation

Immediately before implantation, the catheter is removed from the sterile peel pack and immersed in sterile saline. Dacron® cuffs and the flange are gently squeezed to remove air (22,24). Thoroughly wetted cuffs provide markedly better tissue ingrowth compared to dry, air-containing cuffs (35).

Implantation method

BLIND (TENCKHOFF TROCAR)

When the catheter is inserted at the bedside, a sterile procedure must be strictly followed. A 2–3-cm incision is made in the skin at the insertion site (e.g., the midline 2 cm inferior to the umbilicus). This places the site of entry at the linea alba, a point of minimal vascularity and tissue resistance (36). The lateral margins of either rectus muscle are alternative sites because they are also relatively avascular. It should be remembered that the placement through the belly of the rectus muscle using blind insertion may cause injury to the inferior or superior epigastric artery.

Through the skin incision, the wound is extended to the linea alba with blunt dissection using a curved hemostat. At this time, an anchoring suture is inserted in the fascia. The peritoneal cavity is entered with a priming needle (a "catheter over a needle," venicath-type needle or a stylet peritoneal catheter) into the superior aspect of the wound and through the linea alba. One must take care to ensure intraperitoneal placement of the priming of all hole outlets of the priming device. Separation of the parietal peritoneal membrane from the preperitoneal tissue will result in preperitoneal infusion of dialysis fluid, making any further intraperitoneal infusion of dialysis impossible. Furthermore, the resulting expansion of the preperitoneal pocket is extremely painful. When dialysis-solution infusion produces pain, the operator should suspect preperitoneal instillation; however, the heavily sedated patient may not be able to voice objections. At this time, poor dialysis solution inflow may also indicate that hole outlets are lodged in a preperitoneal position, although one should also expect a moderate restriction of flow, given the relatively small lumen of the access catheter.

Following sterile connection of the administration tubing, 2–3 L of dialysis solution are infused into the peritoneal cavity until the patient feels distended. While dialysate is being instilled to the desired volume, the Tenckhoff catheter should be prepared by wetting it with a small volume of normal saline. Air from the cuffs is removed by squeezing. A wetted stiffening stilette is inserted into the catheter, thus straightening and "stiffening" it to permit introduction of the catheter into the Tenckhoff trocar, and beyond it into its correct intra-abdominal position.

It is useful to start perforation of the linea alba with a smaller trocar or dilator rather than a needle, thereby facilitating introduction of the larger Tenckhoff trocar. The trocar (available from Quinton Instruments, Co) consists of a sharp, stainless steel stylet; a solid, wide, open-ended barrel; and two side pieces with handles (36). With firm but gentle pressure and a twisting action, the trocar with its pointed stylet in place is pushed into the peritoneal cavity via the small perforation. Immediately after the resistance ceases (indicating entrance into the peritoneal cavity), the obturator is removed. Then the true intraperitoneal placement should be recognized by the welling up of dialysis solution into the barrel of the trocar. If the operator has instilled enough dialysis solution during the priming procedure, he or she should insert the trocar until its wider portion comes to rest on the linea alba. This portion should not enter the peritoneal cavity, thus keeping the perforation at the desired diameter. This larger barrel not only is designed to accept the Tenckhoff catheter but also allows for the passage of the Dacron® cuffs.

The catheter is threaded on a stiffening stilette. About 1 cm of catheter is left beyond the tip of the stilette to protect the bowels. Proper placement of the catheter in the pelvis will greatly facilitate siphon drainage. In order to produce favorable results, it is critical that the following details, though seemingly trivial, are followed. As the catheter is introduced into the trocar on its way to the abdominal cavity, the tip should be passed smoothly beyond the trocar. Careful, gentle, and angular movement of the trocar and stiffened catheter (adjusting its intra-abdominal position and relationship to abdominal contents) may be needed to achieve easy passage of the catheter deep into pelvis.

After the catheter has completed its internal course, the detachable trocar barrel should be removed, leaving the split side-pieces in situ for easier manipulation until the final positioning is satisfactory. At this point, the stiffening stilette should be removed while the operator holds the catheter firmly in place. Once the desired depth of placement is achieved, the remaining catheter is fed into the peritoneal cavity while slowly withdrawing the stiffening stilette until the preperitoneal (inner or deep) Dacron® cuff comes to rest on the linea alba. Then the trocar is separated into its two longitudinal sections and withdrawn, leaving the catheter cuff in proper position. The ideal location for the internal cuff is at the preperitoneal level. However, if the catheter is intended for short-term use (while the patient recovers from an acute renal failure event), the location of the deep cuff at the preperitoneal level is not as critical as in the case of chronic long-term use.

Catheter patency is tested in the same manner described in the surgical procedure. When the function is deemed satisfactory, the catheter is secured in place to the linea alba with an anchoring suture before preparing for the creation of the subcutaneous tunnel toward the proposed exit site.

After choosing the catheter exit site, a stab wound (not an incision) is made using a blade, taking care to penetrate only the skin. The opening should be just the size of the catheter. A site should be chosen that will permit the creation of a tunnel of an appropriate length and shape for the catheter. A subcutaneous tunnel is created using a malleable uterine sound or the Faller guide, care being taken to manipulate the catheter gently. For the swan-neck Tenckhoff catheter, the tunnel must follow the skin marking made prior to the insertion. The outer cuff should be positioned approximately 1–2 cm from the skin exit. The recommended method for tunnel creation for the swan-neck Tenckhoff catheter is to make a superior subcutaneous pocket as described for surgical insertion (see below) and to penetrate the exit with the piercing trocar. The titanium connector is then inserted into the end of the catheter. The skin of the insertion wound is sutured and appropriate surgical dressings applied. Dressings are applied for at least 1 week while leaving an accessible length of catheter in order to permit the catheter to be handled without disturbing the dressings.

PERITONEOSCOPIC

The use of peritoneoscopy for peritoneal catheter placement was developed by Ash at Lafayette, Indiana (37,38). The basic equipment required for this type of insertion (manufactured and distributed by Medigroup Inc.) includes a 2.2-mm-diameter, 15-cm-long Y-TEC peritoneoscope with a 2.5-mm steel cannula with internal trocar and a spiral-wound Quill catheter guide surrounding the cannula (37). The Tenckhoff and swan-neck Tenckhoff (straight and coiled) catheters may be implanted with this technique. Like blind insertion, the procedure is performed through a single abdominal puncture. No fluid is instilled before insertion of the cannula and the trocar into the abdomen (through the medial or lateral border of the rectus). The trocar is removed, and the scope is inserted through the cannula. After the intraperitoneal location is assured through observation of the motion of glistening surfaces, the scope is removed and 600 cm³ of air placed in the peritoneal cavity, with the patient in the Trendelenburg position. The scope is reinserted and, during continuous observation, the scope, Quill, and cannula are advanced into the clearest space and the most open direction between the parietal and visceral peritoneum. Following this, the scope and cannula are removed, and the Quill catheter guide is left in place. The next step in the procedure involves the dilation of the Quill and musculature to approximately half a centimeter, which is large enough to allow the catheter to be easily inserted through the rectus muscle and the cuff to be advanced into the muscle. The catheter follows the path previously viewed by the peritoneoscope as directed by the Quill guide. As long as the Quill guide stays in position, the catheter will advance into the desired place.

The catheter is advanced on a stylet and is actually "dilating" its way until the cuff arrives and stops at the muscular layer. Placing the cuff in the musculature can be accomplished using a pair of hemostats advancing the cuff within the Quill guide. Thereafter, the Quill guide is removed, hydraulic function of the catheter checked, the tunnel made subcutaneously using a trocar, and the catheter brought out through the exit site—similar to the surgical insertion technique.

SELDINGER (GUIDE WIRE) AND PEEL-AWAY SHEATH

The essential instruments for this technique include a guide needle attached to a syringe, a Seldinger guide wire, and a tapered dilator with surrounding scored peel-away sheath (39–43). The necessary equipment and videos can be obtained through Cook Critical Care, Division of Cook Inc., P.O. Box 489, Bloomington, IN 47402, U.S.A. This technique may be used for insertion of straight and coiled Tenckhoff catheters as well as for swan-neck Tenckhoff straight and coiled catheters. The preinsertion patient preparation is similar to the one described for rigid catheter insertion. The procedure may be done with (39) or without (40–43) prefilling the abdomen with dialysis solution. Prefilling of the abdomen is accomplished through a temporary peritoneal catheter.

In the dry method, a 2-cm incision is made and the "dry" abdomen is entered with an 18-gauge needle (e.g., the Verres needle as used for laparoscopy). A guide wire is passed through the needle and the needle is withdrawn. The introducer (dilator) with sheath is passed over the guide wire. After the dilator–sheath is inserted, the dilator is removed, leaving the sheath in place. The Tenckhoff or swan-neck Tenckhoff catheter, stiffened by a partially inserted blunt stiffening stilette, is then directed down into the sheath (42,43). The catheter may be introduced without stiffening (40,41). As the cuff advances, the sheath is split by pulling tabs on its opposing sides. Splitting the sheath allows the cuff to advance to a position next to the abdominal wall. By further splitting and retraction, the sheath is removed from its position around the catheter. The subcutaneous tunnel is then created as in surgical placement. With this technique, the incidence of early leak is very low. However, high risks of viscus perforation and improper placement of catheter are the drawbacks of this technique.

SURGICAL (BY DISSECTION)

Surgeons perform 87% of catheter implantations, and the majority of the procedures (73%) are done by surgical dissection (18). Dissective placement is mandatory for catheters with stabilizing devices at the parietal surfaces (swan-neck Missouri and swan-neck presternal). The paramedian approach through the rectus muscle, currently used in our center, will be described (22,24,44).

General anesthesia is avoided, if possible, because it predisposes patients to vomiting and constipation and re-quires voluntary coughing during the postoperative period as a part of pulmonary atelectasis prevention; coughing, vomiting, and straining markedly increase intra-abdominal pressures and predispose patients to abdominal leaks (45). The patient frequently receives propofol 100 µg/kg/min intravenously for 6 minutes to initiate monitored anesthesia care sedation prior to catheter placement and a maintenance dose of 25–50 µg/kg/min thereafter.

The surgical preparation of the abdominal wall consists of a threefold scrub with Betadine suds, pat drying, and threefold painting with Betadine alcohol solutions and again pat drying. Skin markings are usually very faint after surgical preparation and require remarking with a sterile surgical pen. Finally, the abdomen is covered with a sterile, transparent surgical drape. The skin and surrounding tissues of the tunnel are anesthetized with 1% lidocaine.

A 3–4-cm transverse incision is made through the skin and the subcutaneous tissue. A perfect hemostasis, preferably using cauterization, is mandatory. The anterior rectus sheath is exposed and infiltrated with 1% lidocaine. A transverse incision is made in the anterior rectus sheath (Figure 4). The rectus muscle fibers are separated bluntly in the direction of the fibers down to the posterior rectus sheath. Self-retaining retractors are helpful to hold muscle fibers away from the operative field. The sheath is infiltrated with 1% lidocaine. A purse-string nonabsorbable suture of 2–0 monofilament is placed through the posterior rectus sheath, transversalis fascia, and the peritoneum. A 5-mm incision, reaching the peritoneal cavity, is made with a scalpel and stretched slightly (Figure 5).

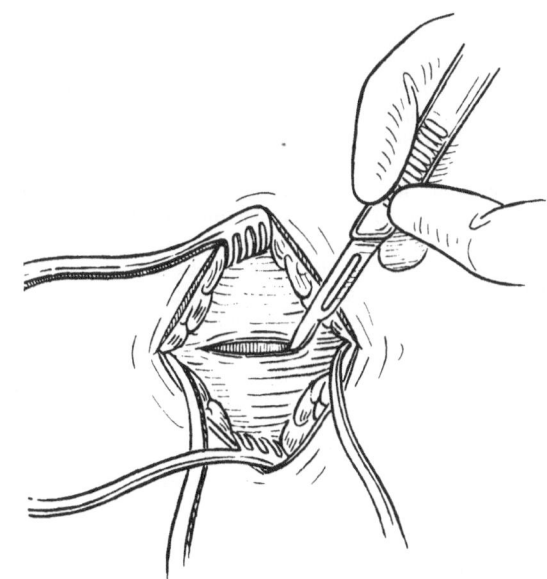

Figure 4. An incision through the anterior rectus sheath. (Figures 4–7 are reproduced from (97), with permission.)

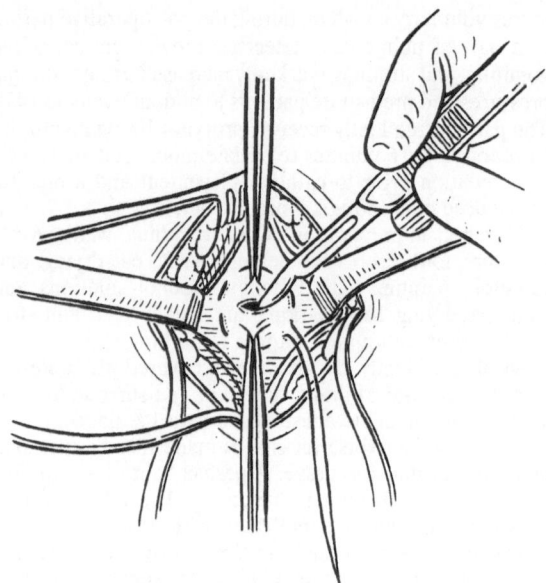

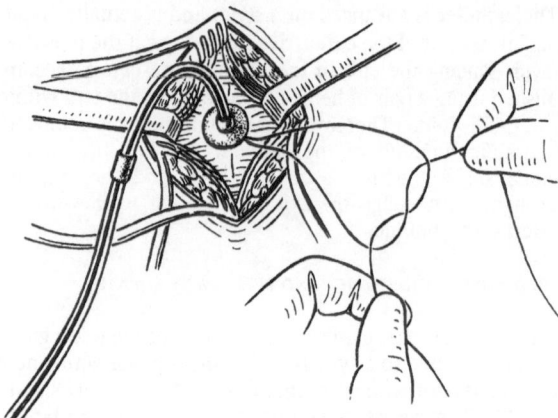

Figure 6. Purse-string suture is tightened between the bead and the flange.

Figure 5. The posterior rectus sheath has been exposed, a purse-string suture has been made, and an incision reaching the peritoneal cavity is being created.

The catheter is threaded on a long, blunt stiffening stilette. About 1 cm of catheter is left beyond the tip of the stilette to protect the bowels. The edges of the opening are lifted. The catheter is inserted through the opening and introduced into the opposite deep pelvis if there is no resistance. The patient may feel some pressure on the bladder or rectum. When the catheter with stilette is about one half to three quarters inserted, the stilette is removed, and the catheter continues to be pushed into the pelvis.

Using a combination of retraction on the peritoneal edge and pushing, the bead is introduced into the peritoneal cavity. The flange is placed flat on the posterior rectus sheath, and a purse-string suture of peritoneum and rectus fascia is tied securely between the bead and the flange (Figure 6). The stripe must be positioned anteriorly, and the flange is anchored with four 2–0 monofilament, nonabsorbable sutures into the posterior rectus sheath at the 6, 9, 12, and 3 o'clock positions (Figure 7). The relationship of the catheter to the tissue structures of the abdominal wall is shown in Figure 8.

The self-retaining retractors are removed, and the deep or internal cuff is buried among the muscle fibers. A small stab wound is made in the anterior rectus sheath above the transverse incision. The catheter is grasped with a hemostat and pulled through the stab incision (Figure 9). The stripe is positioned anteriorly. The remaining procedure differs for the swan-neck Missouri and swan-neck presternal catheter.

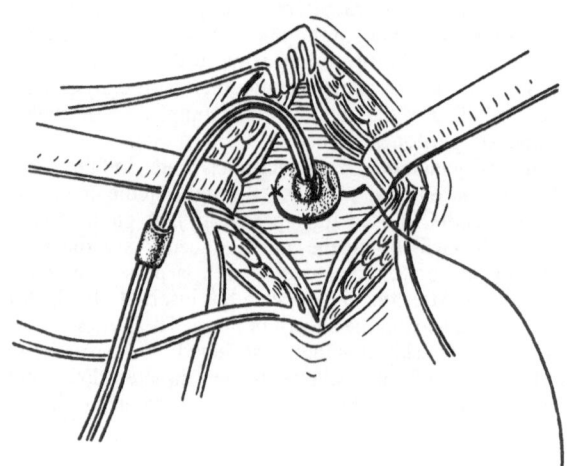

Figure 7. The flange is anchored with four 2–0 monofilament nonabsorbable sutures.

Swan-neck Missouri

A titanium adapter is attached to the catheter, and an extension tube is connected to the adapter (22,44). A 1-L bag of sterile saline or dialysis solution containing 1000 units of heparin is spiked via the extension tubing, and the solution is infused. The wound is checked for leaks and inspected for hemostasis. The transverse incision in the anterior rectus sheath is sewn with 2–0 monofilament nonabsorbable suture.

A superior subcutaneous pocket is made to the level of skin marking to accommodate the bent portion of the catheter and the external cuff (Figure 10). The catheter tunnel extending from the cuff to the skin exit should have a

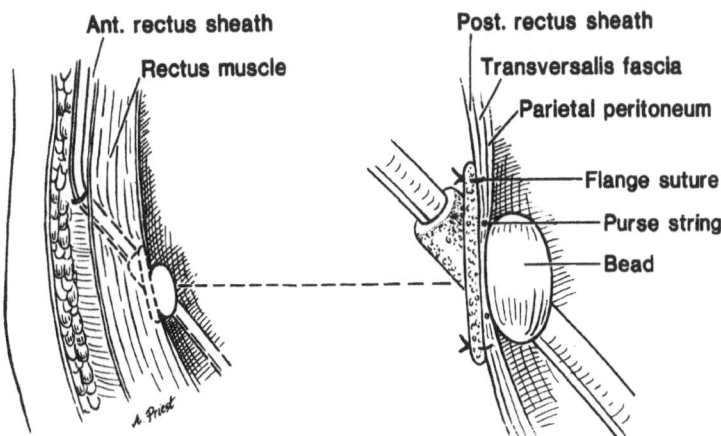

Figure 8. Schematic drawing to indicate relative position of catheter in abdominal wall and relationship of bead and flange to peritoneum/posterior rectus sheath. Reproduced from (25), with permission.

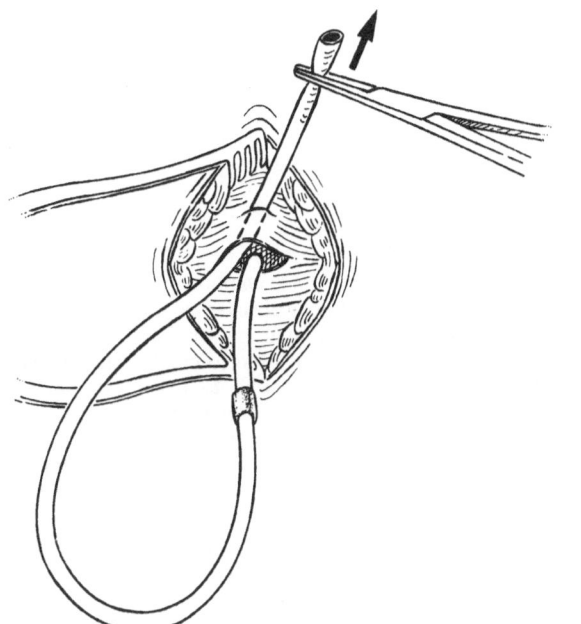

Figure 9. The catheter is passed through the incision centered above the transverse incision. (Figures 9–11 are reproduced from (97), with permission.)

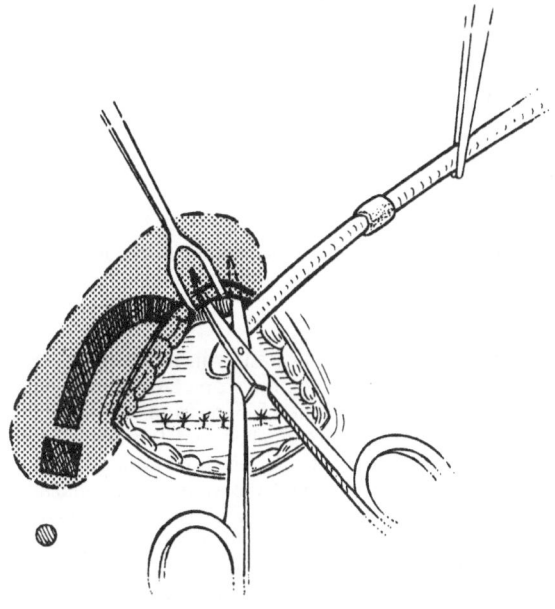

Figure 10. A subcutaneous pocket is made to accommodate the bent portion of the catheter and the external cuff.

diameter close to that of catheter tubing. Thus, the last portion of the tunnel (from external cuff to the exit) should be made with a piercing trocar, e.g., the Faller trocar (Accurate Surgical Instruments Co.), or a 3/16′ (4.76 mm, F 15) trocar for Hemovac system (Zimmer Mfg. Co., 11235

Manchester Road, St. Louis, MO 63122) of external diameter similar to that of the catheter tubing (22,24). The titanium adaptor is detached, a trocar is attached and carefully passed through the pocket, and the external exit is indicated by the stencil mark (Figure 11). The bent portion

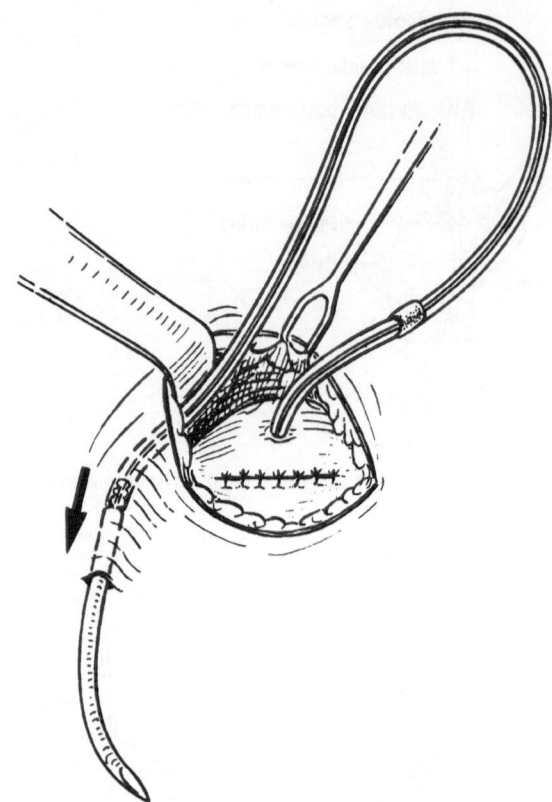

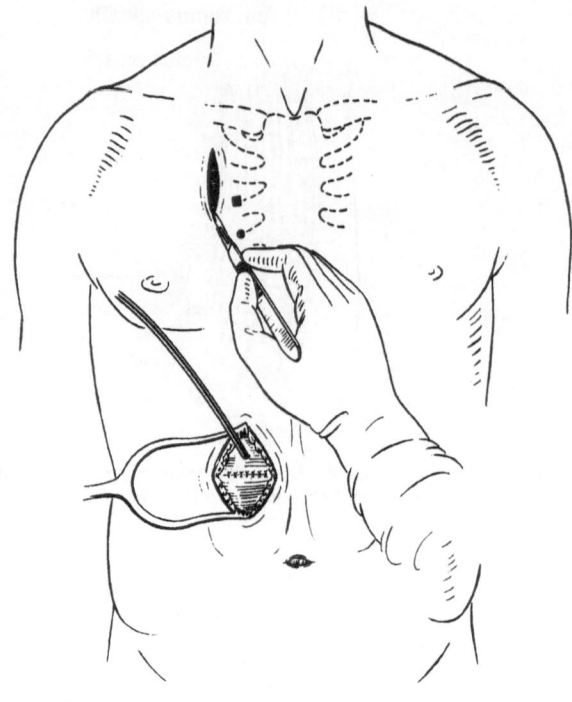

Figure 12. Vertical incision over the sternum. (Figures 12–15 are reproduced from (25), with permission.)

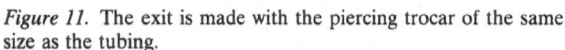

Figure 11. The exit is made with the piercing trocar of the same size as the tubing.

of the catheter is positioned carefully in the subcutaneous pocket. Care is taken to keep the stripe facing frontward. The external cuff is positioned 2–3 cm from the skin exit. The titanium adaptor is reattached and the dialysate is drained. At least 200 mL of solution should drain within 1 minute. If good flow is obtained, the wound is irrigated and the skin incision is closed with absorbable subcuticular sutures. The incision is covered with Steri-strips and several layers of high-absorbency gauze dressings and is secured with Tegaderm®, which also immobilizes the catheter. The dressing is to be left in place for a week. In cases with bleeding or large drainage from the incision or exit, the dressing should be changed earlier.

Swan-neck presternal

A vertical 3–4-cm incision is made in the parasternal area (Figure 12) or over the sternum at the level of the second and third rib (24,25). Using a combination of sharp and blunt dissection, two small subcutaneous pockets are made on both sides of the incision to accommodate the bent section of the upper (chest) tube of the catheter. The pock-

ets are dissected enough to accommodate the middle and superficial cuffs. Careful hemostasis is essential.

A Scanlan tunneler (Scanlan International, 1 Scanlan Plaza, St. Paul, MN 56107) is used to create a tunnel extending from the abdominal wall to the presternal or parasternal area to join the upper and lower tube. A tunneler to accommodate grafts up to 8 mm is suitable for presternal catheter implantation. The tunneler, developed for tunneling vascular grafts, consists of an outside sheath, a blunt tip, and a spring clamp. Depending on the size of the patient, either a green (51 cm long) or an orange (30 cm long) tunneler may be used. A spring clamp serves to stiffen the tunneler as it is pushed through the subcutaneous tissue and to grasp and pull an upper tube through the sheath (24). The tunneler is pushed from the abdominal incision to the chest one (Figure 13). The tunnel path is carefully guided. The blunt tip of the outside sheath is removed. Keeping the stripe in front as a guide, the abdominal end of the upper tube is grasped with the spring clamp and pulled caudally through the sheath, and the sheath is removed by pulling in the caudal direction.

The middle cuff of the upper tube is carefully placed under the stencil mark. When the catheter is appropriately positioned, the desired lengths of the tubes are measured and the tubes are trimmed. Enough length on each tube

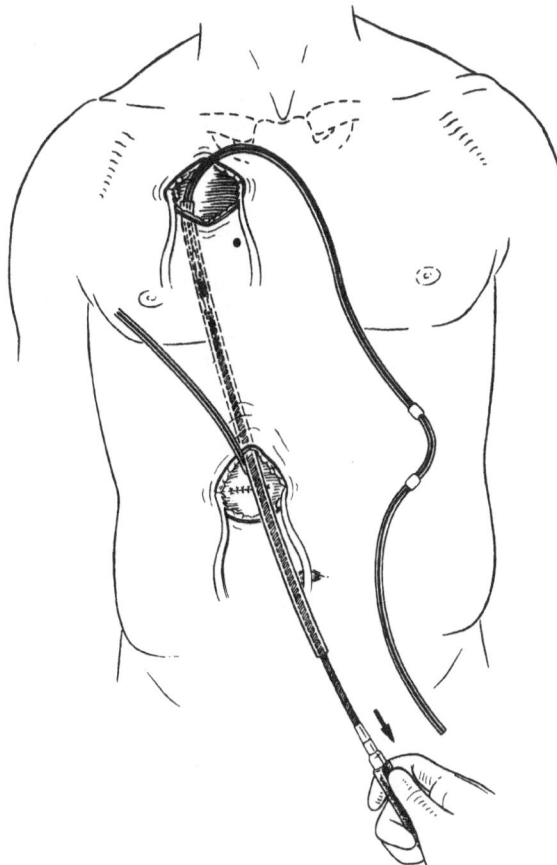

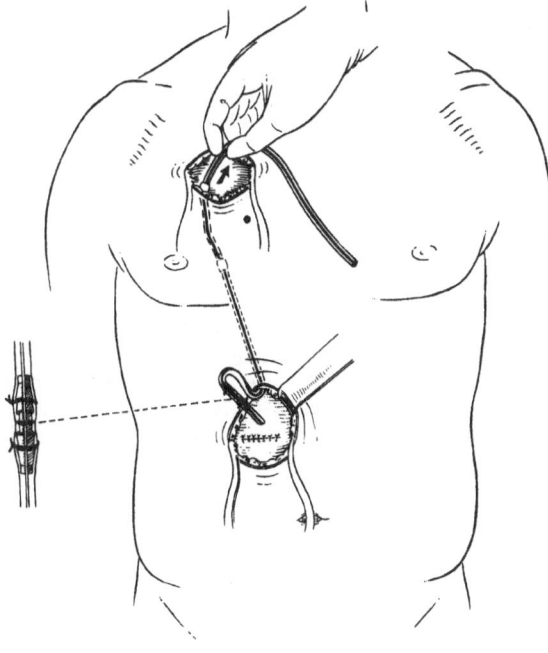

Figure 14. Both portions of the catheter are tied together over the titanium connector, and the catheter is pulled cephalad.

Figure 13. A tunnel between the abdominal and chest incisions is made with a Scanlan tunneling device, and the upper tube is pulled caudally through the sheath.

should be left to facilitate connection. The titanium connector is inserted into the upper tube and secured with a Zero-Prolene suture placed over the groove. Then the connector is inserted into the lower tube. The stripes on both tubes are facing up. The tie is now placed on the lower tube over the groove of the titanium connector. Both sutures are tied together (Figure 14), and the titanium connector is positioned in the subcutaneous tissue approximately 5–8 cm above the rectus sheath incision.

A trocar of the same size as the catheter tubing is attached and carefully passed through the pocket and the external exit indicated by the stencil mark (Figure 15). The stripe is facing front. The trocar is disconnected. The bent portion of the catheter is carefully positioned in the subcutaneous pocket. The titanium Luer lock connector is attached. One liter of normal saline is infused through the infusion set and drained immediately. Outflow should be approximately 200 mL in 1 minute. The wounds are checked for leaks, irrigated, and inspected for

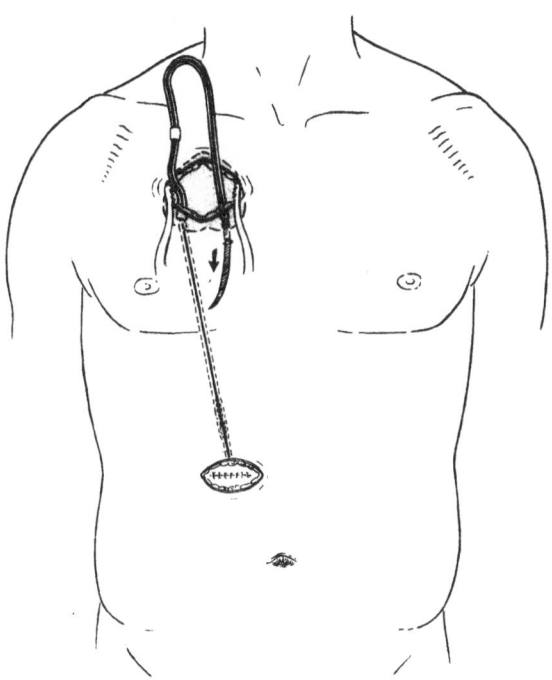

Figure 15. Schematic view of the presternal catheter after implantation.

hemostasis. The transverse incision in the anterior rectus sheath is sewn with 2–0 monofilament nonabsorbable suture. Skin incisions are again inspected for hemostasis. Any bleeding vessels are cauterized, and the incisions are closed with absorbable subcuticular sutures. The operative site is covered with several layers of high-absorbency gauze dressings and secured with Tegaderm®, which also immobilizes the catheter. The dressing is to be left in place for a week.

Swan-neck Tenckhoff

A procedure described for the swan-neck Missouri catheter is generally followed. Since the catheter does not have a flange and bead, the catheter is introduced into the peritoneal cavity to the level of the deep cuff. The cuff is positioned longitudinally on the posterior rectus sheath, with the stripe facing front. If the left catheter is used for the right tunnel and vice versa, the stripe must be positioned posteriorly. The subcutaneous pocket is made in the same way as for the swan-neck Missouri catheter.

Tenckhoff

The technique is similar to that for the swan-neck Tenckhoff catheter; however, because there is no intercuff bend, the anterior stripe position is not essential and the subcutaneous pocket is not needed. Instead, a straight or laterally curved tunnel is made with the help of a piercing trocar. The subcutaneous cuff is positioned 2–3 cm from the exit.

Moncrief–Popovich technique

This is a new technique that allows tissue ingrowth into the cuff material without exposure to the skin surface area. Unlike any other technique, the distal (external segment) of the catheter is completely buried and remains in the subcutaneous tunnel until exteriorized after 3–8 weeks after catheter insertion (46). A video demonstrating the technique is available from the Austin Biomedical Research Institute (47). Using swan-neck catheters with this technique, Moncrief and coworkers reported a significant reduction in peritonitis incidence (46).

CATHETER BREAK-IN AND CATHETER CARE

Tyton ties and a tension tool (Tyton Corporation, P.O. Box 23055, 7930 Faulkner Road, Milwaukee, WI 53223, U.S.A.), routinely used to secure bundles of electrical wirings and available in department stores, are used to prevent disconnection of the titanium adaptor from the tubing. A 4-inch tie is placed around the distal end of the catheter over the adapter. Care is taken to place the tie in the groove between adapter ridges and not over a ridge. Then the tie is tightened with the tension tool, which also trims the excess length. The locking segment is located at the stripe, which will be positioned at the front of the patient. This keeps the added bulk away from the patient (22,24,48).

Tyton ties are not needed if a two-part titanium connector (Accurate Surgical Instruments Co.) is used. Such a connector has an outer screw that prevents accidental disconnection of the connector from the tubing.

Immediate intraperitoneal segment care

In the recovery room, the position of the catheter is checked by a plain x-ray of the abdomen. No catheter kink in the tunnel and the catheter tip in the true pelvis usually predict an excellent catheter function.

Peritoneal dialysis

In the ward, the patient is attached to the cycler to perform additional exchanges. Each liter of dialysis solution contains 1000 units of heparin. One-half-liter or one-liter volumes of dialysis solutions are used for the first supine peritoneal dialysis. Usual cycler settings are 10 minutes fill time, 0 minutes dwell, and 12 minutes outflow. The dialysate is usually blood tinged during the first cycler exchange. No dwell exchanges are continued until the dialysate is clear. If immediate peritoneal dialysis is needed, the patient continues on a cycler in the strict supine position, with dwell time prolonged to 30–40 min. The present author does not commence peritoneal dialysis in the vertical position sooner than 10 days postimplantation; thus, CAPD or a last-bag CCPD are not used for 10 days. The patient may be maintained on hemodialysis through the temporary access for logistical reasons before peritoneal dialysis training can be started or may require hemodialysis due to the catheter malfunction (see below).

Exit

HEALING

Since 1988, we have been studying the healing process of the exit after catheter implantation. Forty-three exits in 41 patients were examined weekly for 6 weeks with a magnifying loupe and macrophotographed. Cultures were taken from sterile saline sinus washouts, periexit smears, and nares. A detailed report of the study with over 100 color pictures of the various exit appearances has been recently published (49,50). A brief summary of the findings will be provided here.

In optimally healing exits, at 1 week postimplantation, slight tenderness is present in about one third of exits, a scab is visible in almost all exits, and epidermis surrounding the exit orifice is pale pink or pink. A small amount of serosanguineous, bloody or serous drainage is visible around the exit in about half of patients. There is no swelling. Drainage inside the sinus is visible in almost all sinuses and is similar in character to that seen outside. There is no epithelium visible in the sinus; the sinus is lined with a white tissue, which resembles aponeurosis.

External drainage abates by week 2 and is absent by week 3. Scabs diminish by week 3 and are not seen after week 4. Exit color remains pale pink or pink throughout the 6-week period. Drainage in the sinus diminishes, and most sinuses are dry at week 6. Sinus lining remains flat but is gradually transformed into plain granulation tissue. Epithelium starts entering the sinus at week 2 or week 3, progresses steadily, and covers at least half of the visible sinus tract by 5 weeks after implantation. Epithelium is fragile and pale pink, or occasionally white.

Early infected exits do not show signs of healing (progression of epithelium, decrease in drainage amount). Instead, drainage changes to purulent, sinus lining becomes composed of granulation tissue at week 1 or week 2, and the tissue becomes slightly or frankly exuberant. The presence of purulent drainage and/or slightly exuberant granulation tissue in the sinus alone, without external drainage, is sufficient for diagnosis of early infection.

Early colonization of the exit was the most significant factor in determining the healing pattern: the later the colonization, the better the healing. Positive culture from either washout or periexit smear 1 week after implantation was associated with early exit infection, a higher peritonitis rate, and a high probability of catheter loss due to an exit/tunnel infection. Based on these results, we postulated that prophylactic antibiotics should be used for at least 2 weeks after catheter implantation and sterile exit-dressing procedure for the entire healing time of approximately 6 weeks (49).

CARE

Early care

To delay bacterial colonization of the exit site and to minimize trauma, the dressing should not be changed frequently. The surgical dressing is gently removed after 1 week. Sterile nonionic surfactant or saline is used to help gauze removal if the gauze is attached to the scab. If the scab is forcibly removed, then the epidermal layer is broken, a new scab has to be made, and the epidermization is prolonged. Care must be taken to avoid catheter pulling or twisting.

Cleansing agents should not only decrease the number of bacteria but also be harmless to the body defenses. Strong oxidants like povidone-iodine and hydrogen peroxide are cytotoxic to mammalian cells and should not be used (51,52). Nonionic, amphophilic, nontoxic surfactants, widely used in burn wound care, facilitate necrotic tissue removal without jeopardizing body defense mechanisms (53). In agreement with the experience of others (54), we found 20% Poloxamer 188 (Shur-Clens ; Calgon Vestal Laboratories, St. Louis, MO, U.S.A.) to be innocuous, yet excellent in cleansing the exit from contaminants.

The exit and the skin surrounding the catheter are cleansed, patted dry with sterile gauze, covered with several layers of gauze dressings, and secured with air-permeable tape. The dressing is changed after another week. The quality of healing should be evaluated until the exit is healed. Weekly dressing changes may be continued throughout the 6-week healing period if drainage is minimal or absent and epithelium progresses steadily. There are two reasons for infrequent dressing changes: firstly, each dressing change may introduce bacteria into the exit even though a sterile procedure is used, and secondly, the less manipulation of the catheter, the lower chance of exit trauma. In cases with excessive bleeding or a large quantity of drainage from the incision or exit, the dressing should be changed earlier and more frequently.

If healing is not progressing as desired, it is likely that the exit is already colonized, and a clinical culture should be taken. The frequency of dressing changes should be increased to every other day because the major rationale for infrequent dressing changes (avoidance of exit colonization) no longer exists, and more frequent cleansing of the exit will decrease the number of bacteria. If the amount of drainage is minimal, local antibiotics according to sensitivity may be sufficient. With large drainage and overt infection, systemic antibiotics are necessary. Antibiotics should be adjusted according to the sensitivity results. The patient may shower only before the dressing change; otherwise, he or she must take sponge baths and avoid exit wetting.

Protecting the catheter from mechanical stress seems to be extremely important, especially during break-in. Catheters should be anchored in such a way that the patient's movements are only minimally transmitted to the exit. The method of catheter immobilization is individualized, depending on exit location and shape of the abdomen. Immobilization of the catheter in the chest is easier but also has to be individualized.

Late care

Late care, after the healing process is completed, is simpler. The results of a prospective study indicate that cleaning with soap and water is the least expensive and tends to prevent infections better than povidone-iodine painting and hydrogen peroxide cleaning (55). After cleansing, the exit has to be patted dry with sterile gauze and well immobilized. Most of our patients use a dressing cover for 6–12 months after implantation. Patients are then allowed to omit use of a cover dressing, if desired. We could not find any reason why in some patients an uncovered exit seems to do better and in others worse.

We recommend that our patients use only a shower and avoid submersion in water, particularly in a Jacuzzi, hot tub, or public pool, unless watertight exit protection can be implemented. Prolonged submersion in water containing high concentrations of bacteria frequently leads to severe infection with consequent loss of catheter. Swimming in the ocean or in well-sterilized private pools is less dangerous than swimming in public pools. Exit care must be performed immediately after a shower or water submersion, with particular attention to obtaining a well-dried exit. The surrounding skin is coated with a skin protector and secured with Tegaderm®. Patients with the swan-neck presternal catheter may take a hot-tub bath without exit-site submersion. Due to this feature, this catheter was dubbed the "bathtub" catheter (25).

SOFT-CATHETER COMPLICATIONS

Early complications

Early complications after soft-catheter insertion are similar to those after implantation of the rigid catheter, but their frequency is lower, particularly with surgical and peritoneoscopic insertion.

BLEEDING

Blood tinged dialysate is common postimplantation, but severe bleeding occurs very rarely with surgical insertion.

DIALYSATE LEAK

Dialysate leaks are unlikely if ambulatory peritoneal dialysis is postponed for at least 10 days after implantation (56). This complication is particularly rare with the swan-neck Missouri and swan-neck presternal catheters. Early leak is usually external and may be confused with serous drainage from the exit. A diagnosis of a leak is supported by a drainage glucose concentration higher than the simultaneously measured blood glucose concentration.

OBSTRUCTION

Table 4 presents the most common causes of obstruction and their treatment. Two-way peritoneal catheter obstruction is usually due to a closed tubing clamp or kinking of the catheter or extension tubing. The catheter lumen may also be completely blocked by fibrin or blood clots, especially when dialysis is complicated by major hemorrhage or peritonitis. One-way obstruction of the peritoneal catheter is usually equated with the failure to drain; fluid can be infused, but cannot be drained. Poor outflow may be due to extrinsic pressure on the catheter tip from adjacent organs, such as a sigmoid colon full of feces or a distended bladder. Omental wrapping is likely if the catheter is misplaced into the upper abdomen. A fibrin or blood clot also may be responsible for a one-way obstruction when only a few proximal side holes remain open and can be easily blocked by adjacent organs. Emptying the bladder and using laxatives may restore catheter function if there is occlusion by bladder or bowel. A clot may be prevented by rinsing out blood from the peritoneal cavity and using heparin, and/or the clot may be dislodged by pushing into the peritoneal cavity or pulling by suction using a syringe filled with hep-

Table 4. Early catheter obstruction

Cause	Prevention/treatment
Occlusion by bowel	Laxatives
Occlusion by bladder	Empty bladder
Clot	Rinse out blood
	Heparin, urokinase
	Dislodge
Omental wrap	Partial omentectomy
Multiple adhesions	Adhesiolysis
Kink in the tunnel	Surgical correction

arinized saline. If these maneuvers are unsuccessful, the catheter may be filled with urokinase (Abbokinase) 5000 IU diluted in normal saline. Urokinase may open the obstruction in 10%–15% of cases (57). Catheter kinking in the tunnel usually is associated with two-way obstruction, is recognizable on abdominal x-ray in two views, and requires surgical correction as soon as the diagnosis is made.

A reversed one-way peritoneal catheter obstruction, where the fluid can be drained but the next infusion cannot be performed, is almost unheard of. Recently we have observed such a case (58). The catheter tip was obstructed with a clot, which caused inflow obstruction. This clot was removed by suction with a syringe. We speculated that the clot was firmly anchored in the catheter tip and that only a few proximal side holes were opened. The outflow was not obstructed because the catheter tip must have been located in a large pocket of free space. The clot behaved like an accordion. During drainage, the clot became stretched and narrowed (like an accordion bellow in extension), and fluid was able to flow through some of the side holes. During infusion, the clot buckled up and widened (like a compressed accordion bellow), completely occluding the central lumen and side holes.

Another reason for obstruction may be catheter adherence to the peritoneum. This complication was found in children who have undergone partial omentectomy at the time of insertion of a single-cuff, straight Tenckhoff catheter. Relocation of such catheters may be attempted with a so-called *whiplash* technique (59). After localization of the catheter adherence site, using a strict sterile technique, a blunted steel trocar is inserted into the catheter and gently advanced until the trocar tip is 5–7 cm proximal to the tip of the catheter. Using a deep cuff as a fulcrum and using short and rapid whiplash motions, the catheter is then freed from the adherence point. The catheter tip is then, under fluoroscopy, relocated to a new site. A modification of this method using a pliable copper thread was successfully used in adults (60). A catheter that has migrated to the upper abdomen may be relocated using a guide wire (61, 62). Although these methods may obviate the need for surgery, they are not without risks. The guide wire may break during manipulations, perforate the catheter, and lead to recurrent peritonitis. We do not use these procedures in our institution, considering them too risky.

Catheter migration out of the true pelvis is seen frequently on abdominal x-rays done for various reasons in patients with functioning catheters (63). While about 20% of x-rays showed the catheter tip translocated to the upper abdomen, only 20% of these translocated catheters (4% of the total) were obstructed. The remaining functioning malpositioned catheters were either permanently translocated or repositioned spontaneously to the true pelvis. About 3% of catheters in our series were obstructed with the tip in the true pelvis (64).

While the great majority of malpositioned catheters are not obstructed, a catheter with its tip in the upper abdomen is still about six times more likely to be obstructed than a normally positioned catheter. The migration of the catheter tip may, however, be the result of the obstruction rather than its cause; omentum entangling the catheter tip may be responsible for its translocation.

If the catheter is not kinked but does not function for 2 weeks even after the above-described maneuvers have been tried, omental wrapping or multiple adhesions are most likely, and omentectomy or adhesiolysis through laparoscopy may be required. In our experience, if this method fails to restore catheter function, the peritoneum is not fit for peritoneal dialysis due to massive adhesions. Replacement of the catheter in such a situation is worthless. The patient has to be transferred to hemodialysis.

VISCUS PERFORATION AND PERITONITIS

Viscus perforation is unheard of with surgical catheter insertion. Early peritonitis with a soft catheter is half of that reported with a rigid catheter, even in treatment of acute renal failure (65).

ABDOMINAL PAIN

Minimal pain after catheter insertion usually can be controlled with mild analgesics such as acetaminophen. Opiates must be avoided because they cause constipation and, frequently, vomiting. Vomiting and straining increase intra-abdominal pressure and predispose the patient to pericatheter leaks (45). Abdominal pain at the catheter tip is more likely with straight catheters due to the "jet effect" and tip pressure. This pain usually subsides within a few days; however, it may become chronic and require treatment (see below).

Late complications

Complications are not randomly distributed throughout the life of the catheter. Whereas leaks and malfunctions occur shortly after catheter implantation, infectious complications lead to catheter failure later (23).

EXIT-SITE INFECTION

There has been no single definition of exit-site infection that has achieved universal approval. The most widely accepted is that published by Pierratos in 1984 (66), which was agreed upon by the vast majority of Peritoneal Dialysis Bulletin Editorial Board members. Pierratos defined exit-site infection as follows: "Redness or skin induration or purulent discharge from the exit-site. Formation of the crust around the exit may not indicate infection. Positive cultures from the exit site in the absence of inflammation do not indicate infection." The definition implies the presence of infection in the instances where laboratory cultures are negative and rejects the existence of infection based on a positive culture without inflammation.

The definition also suggests that there are only two possible exit conditions, namely, infected and uninfected; however, contrary to the situation encountered with diagnosis of peritonitis, the distinction between infected and noninfected exit may not be obvious. There is no difficulty in the diagnosis of peritonitis; dialysate contains either a small number of cells when uninfected or a large number of cells, mostly granulocytes, when infected. Normal dialysate does not contain microorganisms; a correctly performed culture is usually positive in peritonitis. Bacterial peritonitis cannot be cured without antibiotics. Attempts to classify exit appearance into two categories (infected and not infected) is difficult, if not impossible, because infected and uninfected exit appearances overlap. This overlap is due to the peculiarity of tissue reaction to the foreign body penetrating the skin and stems from the delicate balance between bacteria in the sinus and host defenses. Low-grade exit infection may abate without systemic antibiotics.

From 1988 to 1994, we performed 565 evaluations of 61 healed exit sites in 56 patients. The exit and the sinus were inspected using a Zeiss prism loupe with 4.5 × magnification for the presence, absence, intensity, and/or characteristics of specific attributes such as swelling, color, crust, drainage, granulation tissue, and epithelium in the sinus. Pictures of the external exit and the visible sinus tract were then drawn, and photographs of the exit site and visible sinus tract were taken. As a result of this study, we introduced a new classification of exit-site appearance. A detailed description of this classification was reported elsewhere (67,68); only a brief synopsis will be given here.

The classification is based on the cardinal signs of inflammation: *calor* (heat), *rubor* (redness), *turgor* (swelling), and *dolor* (pain). Additional features, specific for an exit of any skin-penetrating foreign body, are drainage, regression of epidermis, and exuberance (profuse overgrowth) of granulation tissue ("proud flesh"). Granulation tissue is defined as exuberant if it is bulging, soft, and vascularized and if it bleeds easily. Culture results do not influence exit classification. Positive cultures in exits not inflamed indicate colonization, not infection. Cultures are commonly negative from infected exits on antibiotic therapy. However, inflammation in almost all cases is caused by infection, regardless of culture results. Inflammatory response to tubing itself or to local irritants is rare.

Improvement or deterioration of inflammation is associated with respective decreases or increases of pain, induration, drainage, exuberant granulation tissue, and/or regression or progression of epithelium in the sinus. Increased lightness (pink, pale pink) or darkness (deep black, brown) and a decrease in color diameter indicate improvement; an increase in red color saturation and diameter indicates deterioration. Ultimately, five categories of exit appearances have been established: perfect, good, equivocal, acutely inflamed, and chronically inflamed. Two special categories also were established: traumatized exit and external-cuff infection with or without exit infection. The most salient feature of infected exits is drainage. In equivocal exits, the drainage may be discerned only in the sinus but cannot be expressed outside. Features of traumatized exit depend on the intensity of trauma and time of examination. Common features of trauma are pain, bleeding, scab, and deterioration of exit appearance. Prophylactic antibiotics are recommended in exit trauma.

Good and perfect exits require daily or every other day cleansing and protection from trauma. Although equivocal exits may recover spontaneously, it is prudent to treat them with systemic antibiotics. Acute and chronic exit infections need systemic antibiotics according to culture and sensitivity results. The length of treatment depends on exit appearance. It is unwise to stop antibiotics before a good exit appearance is achieved.

Excellent results were reported with the use of local hypertonic saline compresses in cases that failed prolonged antibiotic therapy (69). These consist of exit-site applications of gauze pads soaked with warm 3% sodium chloride for 5–10 minutes three times daily. The authors recommend courses of 2–4 weeks followed by at least one daily application indefinitely in chronic infections.

External cuff infection without exit infection is characterized by the presence of various combinations of intermittent or chronic purulent, bloody, or gluey drainage, usually seen outside; intermittently or chronically macerated epithelium in the visible sinus; and proud flesh deep inside the visible sinus. Unlike chronic exit infection, the visible sinus may be completely or partly covered with epithelium, and the exit on external examination can look normal. Drainage in the sinus may be seen only after pressure on the cuff. The tissue around the cuff may be indurated on palpation.

Tenckhoff observed that tunnel infection with Dacron cuff involvement cannot be cured (36); however, the life of the catheter may be prolonged by treatment with systemic antibiotics and/or cuff shaving (67,70). Cuff shaving should be attempted if prolonged treatment with antibiotics fails. The perfect timing of catheter removal is difficult to ascertain. It would be desirable to avoid peritonitis associated with tunnel infection, so early removal would be advisable. On the other hand, apparently complete remissions tempt one to postpone the removal, and patients are also reluctant to have catheters removed. In patients with limited life expectancies and in those who may remain on peritoneal dialysis only a short time (transplant candidates), it may be reasonable to postpone catheter removal. In patients who

are expected to remain a long time on peritoneal dialysis, once the diagnosis of cuff infection is established and cure is not achieved, removal of the catheter should be strongly recommended.

In cases of chronic exit infection, it is difficult to determine by exit evaluation whether there is cuff involvement. Ultrasound has been recommended as a valuable tool in diagnosing tunnel infections (71,72). These authors found a statistically significant correlation between positive ultrasound for pericatheter fluid collection and loss of catheter due to tunnel infection; however, the specificity of the method was not high: only 44%–80% of cases with positive findings for tunnel infection required catheter removal. In three cases, we used ultrasound with Doppler, but only in one case was the study positive for fluid collection and increased vascularity. In the other two cases, ultrasound results did not confirm the presence of fluid collection despite cuff infection diagnosed clinically and confirmed by pathological examination after catheter removal. A technique with higher specificity and sensitivity is needed.

Local antibiotics in acute or chronic infection are of little value because they cannot achieve proper local concentrations before being washed away with large drainage; antibiotics administered systemically can provide therapeutic concentrations locally by being excreted into the drainage. Local antibiotics can achieve high concentrations in the sinus in equivocal, good, or perfect exits but may be useful only in equivocal exits and/or in patients with recurrent acute infections after an acute episode subsides. We have had good experience with mupirocin ointment for gram-positive organisms and Neosporin (neomycin, bacitracin, polymyxin) or gentamicin ophthalmic solution or ointment for gram-positive and gram-negative organisms.

EXTERNAL-CUFF EXTRUSION

The main cause of cuff extrusion is placement of the external segment of the catheter in any shape other than its natural design with the cuff too close to the exit. Due to the resilience force of the silicon rubber, the catheter tends to slowly assume its original shape and may push the cuff out of the sinus. If the cuff is not infected, it is left alone; however, the cuff usually becomes infected during this process and requires systemic antibiotics or even surgical intervention. Topical mupirocin may markedly delay cuff infection. If there is no peritonitis or deep-cuff infection, then the catheter may be saved, at least for some time, by shaving off the infected cuff (70). Infection is another cause of cuff extrusion. In this instance, the cuff becomes infected while still in the sinus and extruded by tissue retraction around the cuff. Two such extrusions were observed with swan-neck Missouri catheters (23).

CATHETER OBSTRUCTION

"Capture" of the catheter by active omentum may cause outflow obstruction. Obstruction from this cause, in the absence of peritonitis, when it occurs is usually a postoperative event (related to a new catheter). The present author has never seen an obstruction (in the absence of peritonitis) due to omental capture as a late event and believes that a foreign body (e.g., Silastic) is more prone to attract omentum very early. In the due course of time, with or without use, a proteinaceous (not bacterial) biofilm catheter coating may make the Silastic less foreign to omental tissue. Slow drainage due to catheter translocation, occlusion by bowel, or fibrin clot formation occurs from time to time in some patients. Laxatives and/or addition of heparin 500 U/L to the dialysis solution are usually successful in restoring good catheter function. Some patients have permanently translocated the catheter out of the true pelvis. If the catheter functions (even with slower drainage), the present author does not attempt to reposition the catheter. In patients on nocturnal peritoneal dialysis, where fast drainage is particularly important, it is prudent to use a tidal mode of cycler dialysis in such a situation. The fluid flow mechanics are better compared to a complete-drain, intermittent-flow technique. Since there is always some sump volume in the peritoneal cavity, dialysate flow is fast throughout the tidal exchange (73).

PERICATHETER LEAK

Dialysis solution leaks may occur months or even years after starting CAPD. The management of a late leak is similar to that described for early leaks. However, most cases of late leak are refractory to conservative therapy and require surgical repair. Pericatheter leaks are more likely with midline catheter insertion than with rectus muscle insertion (21,74). Similar to the acute leak, this complication is rarely seen with the catheters provided with a bead and polyester flange at the deep cuff (swan-neck Missouri, swan-neck presternal, Toronto Western Hospital catheter). We have not observed a single late pericatheter leak with 181 swan-neck Missouri catheters (23).

Contrary to the early leaks, which are usually external, the late leaks infiltrate the abdominal wall. The acute leak causes a sudden drop of ultrafiltration and usually occurs after sudden increase in intra-abdominal pressure (heavy lifting, coughing, or straining). The leak may be mild and intermittent. Such a leak may be difficult to localize. Immediately after leak occurrence, the patient may be in good fluid balance without edema in the lower extremities. Abdominal wall edema reveals itself with skin dimpling resembling that of an orange (*peau d'orange*) and a spongy feeling on palpation. A chronic leak is usually a sequela of an acute leak but may occur gradually. The patient is usually fluid overloaded due to poor ultrafiltration.

The best method of leak localization is CT scan with intraperitoneal contrast (75,76). Prior to the study, the peritoneal cavity is drained completely. A fresh bag of 2 L dialysis solution is prepared, 100 mL of 60% diatrizoate meglumine is injected into the dialysis solution bag through the injection port, and the solution is mixed and infused into the peritoneal cavity. No oral or intravenous contrast material is needed. To increase intra-abdominal pressure (45), the patients should stand up, walk, strain, cough, and bend over for at least 30 minutes, then assume the supine position on the CT table. The images are taken every 6 mm, each with a 6-mm slice thickness in the region of the suspected leak; in other regions, the images are taken every 12 or 24 mm, each with a 12-mm slice thickness. An example of a leak through an incisional hernia is shown in Figures 16 and 17.

PERITONITIS

Bacteria that cause peritonitis or bacteria that have migrated around the catheter may colonize the intraperitoneal segment of the catheter. These bacteria synthesize biofilm, which protects them from host mechanisms and antibiotics. It is believed that such colonization may lead to recurrent peritonitis with the same organism (77).

Recurrent peritonitis may be also the result of deep cuff infection with formation of microabscesses (78). Finally, bowel trauma by the catheter may lead to peritonitis (79).

INFUSION OR PRESSURE PAIN

Coiled catheters are less likely than the straight ones to induce infusion pain. The pain is usually most intense at the beginning of infusion and at the end of drainage. In the majority of cases, the pain is transient and disappears within a few weeks. Table 5 shows the maneuvers used by the present author to alleviate the pain. Decreased infusion rate is frequently helpful. If pain occurs only at the beginning of inflow and the end of outflow, incomplete drainage and/or tidal mode for nightly peritoneal dialysis may be successful (73). Alkalization of fluid with sodium bicarbonate or use of lidocaine is sometimes effective. If all these maneuvers are ineffective, the catheter has to be replaced. The replacement catheter should be a coiled one, and the catheter should be implanted in such a way that no undue pressure is exerted at the tip. Outflow pain is usually secondary to a negative pressure exerted on the peritoneum.

UNUSUAL COMPLICATIONS

Organ erosion

Damage of the internal organ leading to intra-abdominal bleeding and/or peritonitis, as well as genital edema due to

Table 5. Maneuvers to alleviate infusion pain

Slower infusion rate
Incomplete drainage
Tidal mode for nightly peritoneal dialysis
Solution alkalization (Na bicarbonate: 2–5 mEq/L)
1% Lidocaine–2.5 mL/L (50 mg/exchange)
Catheter replacement

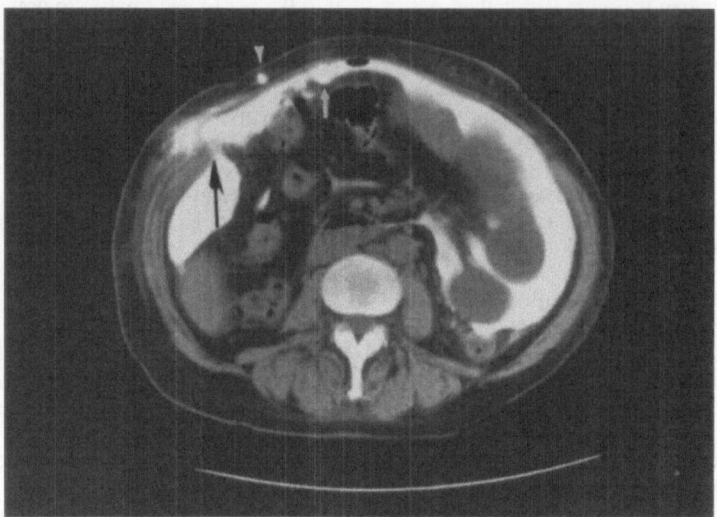

Figure 16. CT scan of the abdomen after infusion of 2 L of contrasted dialysate showing peritoneal dialysate leak in the right abdominal wall between rectus and oblique muscles (black arrow). The protrusion of contrast points into the small incisional hernia through which the leak occurred. The bead of the swan-neck Missouri catheter (white arrow) is at a distance from the fluid extravasation. White arrowhead points into the intramural segment of the catheter.

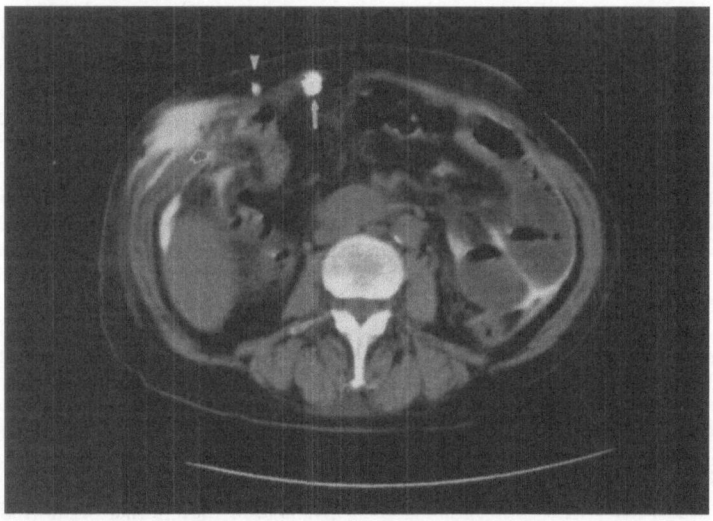

Figure 17. Contrast retained in the subcutaneous tissue after the dialysate has been drained. The distinction between extravasation (open arrow), the intramural catheter segment (white arrowhead), and the bead (white arrow) is clearly seen and indicates that the leak is not around the catheter. (Leak site through incisional hernia confirmed and repaired surgically.)

peritoneal laceration, have been reported as late catheter complications of straight Tenckhoff and Toronto Western Hospital catheters (79–83). These complications most likely are due to the pressure exerted by the "soft" but resilient tubing with a pointed tubing end of the straight Tenckhoff catheter or the relatively sharp Silastic discs of the Toronto Western Hospital catheter. In most instances, the catheters had not been used for 1–12 weeks before this complication was diagnosed (81,82). No such complications have been reported with coiled (curled) catheters.

Mechanical accidents

Golper and Carpenter (83) reported two instances of catheters being accidentally cut with scissors. The present author has observed several such instances, despite our teaching that scissors should not be used during dressing changes. Silicon rubber will not self-seal if punctured, and such instances occur during the implantation procedure and shaving of the cuff.

To avoid system contamination the catheter should be clamped immediately. If the damage is at least 15 mm from the exit, the catheter may be saved using a peritoneal catheter repair kit available from the Quinton Instrument Co. While the catheter is repaired, a sterile procedure must be strictly followed. The operator should "scrub, mask, and glove." A "circulating" nurse should be present to assist. The operating field has to be well protected with sterile towels, and the catheter should be wrapped with Betadine®-soaked gauze for 5 minutes. The catheter is transversely cut with a sterile blade proximal to the damaged site. The catheter clamp is released and the catheter is squeezed with fingers. The patient is asked to strain to allow dialysate flow from the peritoneal cavity. The flowing dialysate will flush eventual contaminants. While the fluid is still flowing, the Teflon® tubing of the repair kit is inserted into the catheter as far as possible. Then the silicon rubber tubing of the repair kit is clamped to stop dialysate flow. The connection is dried with gauze. A mold is positioned over the connection and filled with sterile silicon glue. The extension tubing is connected to the catheter in the usual way. The glue cures for 72 hours. Using this method, the present author has been able to save eight catheters over an 11-year period.

Material breakdown

There are reports of problems arising from the physical properties of the catheter material. The inclusion of barium sulphate throughout the entire catheter to render it radiopaque has been reported to make the catheter brittle (84). Currently the catheters contain only a stripe of barium sulfate and seem to be less prone to this mode of failure. Silicon rubber catheters have been observed to stretch, crack, or become brittle with age or after repeated exposure to Betadine® (84). The present author has observed four such instances. One nine-year-old catheter broke at the skin level and had to be replaced. This catheter, subjected to five years of Betadine® exposure, became discolored and brittle. Another catheter, six years old, became stretched approximately 6 cm from the exit. This catheter, never subjected to Betadine®, did not break and could be repaired. The third catheter broke twice at the age of 7 and 9 years. This catheter was repaired successfully twice and survived 11 years until removed after suc-

cessful kidney transplantation. The fourth catheter broke twice in the proximity of the stripe at the age of 3 and 5 years and was also successfully repaired.

Polyurethane is even more likely to be damaged with aging due to so-called *environmental stress cracking (ESC)*. As its name suggests, ESC leads to microcracks in the surface materials of a device, the result of corrosive forces of the living organism. Once the process begins, ultimate failure is inevitable (85).

Allergic reaction

Eosinophilic peritonitis occurs most frequently during the postimplantation period. Although there are many possible causes for this condition (such as blood, air, and antibiotics), one cannot exclude a reaction to Silastic® tubing. After implantation, the Silastic® tubing is gradually covered with proteinaceous biofilm. The coated catheter is less likely to cause an allergic reaction. Allergic eosinophilic dermatitis due to silicon rubber has been reported (86,87).

INDICATIONS FOR CATHETER REMOVAL

The need for catheter removal occurs under various conditions. These may be broadly categorized under two headings: catheter malfunction and complicating medical conditions with a functioning catheter. Finally, the catheter may be removed electively because it is not needed.

Malfunction

The decision to remove the catheter is usually made only when conservative measures to restore function have failed. Catheter malfunction requiring catheter removal may be seen in the following conditions: 1) intraluminal obstruction with blood or fibrin clot or omental tissue incarceration, 2) catheter-tip migration out of the pelvis with poor drainage, 3) a catheter kink along its course, and 4) catheter tip caught in adhesions following severe peritonitis. In these situations, there usually are both inflow and outflow draining problems. An accidental break in the continuity of the catheter that cannot be repaired will also require catheter removal.

Functioning catheter with a complication

Under the following conditions, catheters may have to be removed: 1) recurrent peritonitis with no identifiable cause, 2) peritonitis due to exit-site and/or tunnel infection, 3) catheter with persistent exit-site infection, 4) tunnel infection and abscess, 5) late recurrent dialysate leak through the exit site or into the layers of the abdominal wall, 6) unusual peritonitis, i.e., tuberculosis, fungal, etc., 7) bowel perforation with multiple organism peritonitis, 8) refractory peritonitis of other causes, 9) severe abdominal pain either due to the catheter impinging on internal organs or during solution inflow, and 10) catheter-cuff extrusion with infection.

Functioning catheter that is no longer needed

This situation is encountered after a successful renal transplantation or after peritoneal dialysis is discontinued because dialysis is no longer needed or when the patient transfers to another form of dialysis.

Removal method

UNCUFFED CATHETER

Removal of the uncuffed catheter is a simple procedure. After cutting an anchoring suture, the catheter is simply pulled out and the opening is covered with a sterile dressing.

CUFFED CATHETERS

A Tenckhoff catheter inserted through the midline may be removed at the bedside. After preparation of the operating field, local anesthesia is applied around the cuffs, the incisions are reopened, the cuffs are excised, and the catheter is pulled. The incisions of catheters removed for cuff/tunnel infection should be packed open and allowed to heal by second intention. In this author's experience, calcium–sodium alginate fibers (Kaltostat Wound Dressing) are excellent for wound packing. The fibers absorb exudate very efficiently, control minor bleeding, and protect the wound from contamination. Once-daily dressing change is usually sufficient for wound packing with the fibers.

The catheters inserted through the belly of the rectus muscle require surgical dissection in the operating room. Although the catheter can be removed using a local anesthetic, patient comfort usually dictates a general anesthetic, particularly for the Toronto Western Hospital and swan-neck Missouri catheters. After an appropriate surgical scrub and routine draping, the incision is reopened. The anterior rectus fascia is reopened along the site of the previous incision, and the catheter/cuff/flange is sharply dissected free of the ingrown rectus muscle. The previously placed four quadrant sutures in the flange and the pursestring sutures are cut and, with traction and continued sharp dissection, the abdominal portion of the catheter is removed. The remaining small opening into the abdomen is closed with 0 or 00 Prolene™ sutures. The anterior fascia is re-approximated in a similar fashion. Depending on the clinical indication for removal, the incision may either be closed or packed open and allowed to heal by second intention.

SWAN-NECK PRESTERNAL CATHETER

Removal of a swan-neck presternal peritoneal dialysis catheter is a surgical procedure performed in the operating room, preferably with general anesthesia. After an appropriate surgical scrub and routine draping of both the chest and abdomen, both the chest and abdominal incisions are reopened. Bleeding is controlled with electrocautery. Using blunt and sharp dissection, the two cuffs at the bent portion of the catheter are freed from the adjacent subcutaneous tissue. Working from the abdominal incision, the catheter is divided between sutures *above* the titanium connector. The chest portion of the catheter is pulled out in a cephalad direction through the chest (parasternal) incision. The abdominal part of the catheter is then removed in an identical way as described for the swan-neck Missouri and Toronto Western Hospital catheters . Depending on the clinical indication for removal, the two incisions may either be closed or packed open and allowed to heal by second intention.

LONG-TERM RESULTS

National CAPD Registry survey

In 1987, the National CAPD Registry of the National Institutes of Health reported the results of a survey that attempted to determine the natural history of implanted peritoneal catheters and to estimate the survival distribution of different types of catheters (19). The survey also estimated the frequency of catheter complications as well as reasons for catheter removal. Standard straight ($n = 957$; 64%) and curled ($n = 330$; 22%) Tenckhoff catheters, as well as Toronto Western Hospital catheters ($n = 94$; 6%), Column-disc or Ash ($n = 49$; 3%), Gore-Tex ($n = 28$; 2%), and others ($n = 2$; 0.1%), composed the catheters reported for the survey. The survey did not clearly show major differences in catheter survival among various types of catheters. The probability of catheter survival at 6, 12, 18, 24, and 36 months for the double-cuff standard straight Tenckhoff catheter was 80%, 70%, 60%, 51%, and 33%, respectively; for standard curled Tenckhoff catheters, the survival rate was 85%, 69%, 51%, 43%, and 34%, respectively; and for the double-cuff Toronto Western catheter, the survival rate was 80%, 69%, 52%, 35%, and 22%, respectively. The probability of survival at 6, 12, 18, and 24 months for the column-disc catheter was 81%, 71%, 59%, 47%, respectively. None of the Toronto Western Hospital catheters was removed due to a drainage problem; however, they were most likely to be removed due to peritonitis. The reason for the high failure rate due to peritonitis is unclear but is probably related to the presence of intraperitoneal discs. Column-disc catheters had a high rate of failure due to peritonitis and obstruction but the lowest rate of failure due to exit/tunnel infections. This survey also found that exit-site infection and peritonitis were disproportionately distributed among the cuff types. Exit-site infections were reported in proportionately more patients using a single subcutaneously placed cuff (13%) than in patients using a double cuff (7%). Gore-tex catheters, which were designed to lower exit-site infections, had an extremely high failure rate due to infections.

Swan-neck catheters

At the University of Missouri, Columbia, between August 1985 and September 1991, 181 swan-neck catheters were implanted in three Columbia hospitals and cared for by the technique described above. Survival and complications were monitored prospectively. The prospectively collected data with the swan-neck catheters and retrospectively collected data with Tenckhoff and Toronto Western Hospital catheters were compared (23,88).

There were 148 Tenckhoff and Toronto Western Hospital catheters, 27 swan-neck prototypes, 105 swan-neck Missouri 2 and straight, and 49 swan-neck Missouri 2 and 3 coiled (curled). The overall respective observation periods of Tenckhoff and Toronto Western Hospital catheters, swan-neck prototypes, swan-neck Missouri 2 and 3 straight, and swan-neck Missouri 2 and 3 coiled were 1859, 427, 1487, and 305 catheter-months. The probability of catheter survival at 6, 12, 18, 24, and 36 months for Tenckhoff and Toronto Western Hospital catheters was 75%, 61%, 52%, 48%, 29%, respectively, similar to that reported by the CAPD Registry Special Survey (19); for swan-neck Missouri 2 and 3 straight, the probability was 93%, 85%, 79%, 68%, and 61%; and for swan-neck Missouri 2 and 3 curled, the probability was 88% and 88% at 6 and 12 months respectively.

The survival probability of swan-neck Missouri straight and coiled catheters was significantly higher than that of Tenckhoff and Toronto Western Hospital catheters. Compared to the CAPD Registry Special Survey (19), in our series more Tenckhoff and Toronto Western catheters were removed due to obstruction, but fewer due to peritonitis. The overall removal percentage was similar.

Swan-neck Missouri 2 and 3 with straight intraperitoneal segments yielded markedly better results. The estimated survival probability at 3 years doubled compared to previously used Tenckhoff and Toronto Western Hospital catheters. Improvement was noted in malfunctions, leaks, cuff extrusions, and exit/tunnel infections. Cuff extrusion occurred only in two swan-neck straight catheters, in both instances after exit-site infection, not due to catheter resilience. This finding was a notable reversal of the event sequence compared to previously used catheters, where cuff extrusion usually preceded exit/tunnel infection.

The results regarding survival and removal rates with swan-neck coiled catheters were not significantly different from that of the swan-neck Missouri 2 and 3 straight catheters. Nevertheless, there are two major advantages with these catheters, the same as with other coiled catheters: a decrease in the incidence of infusion pain due to a "jet effect" and pain related to straight-catheter tip pressure on the peritoneum experienced by some patients.

Low complication rates and higher probability of survival with swan-neck catheters compared to other cath-

eters have been reported also by others (89–92). A prospective comparison by life-table analysis of 25 double-cuff Tenckhoff and 25 swan-neck catheters showed patient survival of 75% and 79%, respectively, at 12 months and dialysis technique survival of 80% and 82%, respectively (93). The groups were too small to reveal the statistical significance of differences. Lye et al. (94) reported significantly lower exit-site infection rates with swan-neck catheters, and insignificantly worse catheter survival and tip migrations with Tenckhoff catheters.

Preliminary experiences with swan-neck presternal catheters in adults and in children were very encouraging (25,26,95). The results of the 4-year prospective, nonrandomized comparison between swan-neck presternal catheters and swan-neck abdominal catheters in one center have been recently published (96).

Presternal catheters tended to perform better regarding exit and tunnel infections, even though they were implanted in several patients in whom regular catheters with the exit on the abdomen would be difficult or impossible to implant. Two-year survival probability of presternal catheters was 0.88 ± 0.14 (SE). Recurrent/refractory peritonitis was the only reason for catheter failure. The differences in results between presternal and abdominal catheters were statistically insignificant; only the use of antibiotics for exit infection was significantly higher with abdominal catheters. Patient acceptance of the exit position was excellent.

United States Renal Data System report 1992

In a national study of all patients starting CAPD therapy in the United States during January through June 1989, the prevailing catheter practices were appraised and the peritonitis risk was assessed by catheter-related factors in 2807 patients followed for up to 21 months (20). Of these patients, 44% used a straight intraperitoneal segment with no bend, 40% used a curled (coiled) catheter with no bend, 12% used a catheter with "a preformed bend" (swan neck) with either straight or curled intraperitoneal segment. Four percent of patients used "other" (Lifecath and unspecified) catheters. Double-cuff catheters were used in 78%, single deep-cuff in 13%, and single superficial in 5%, and data were not available in 10% of patients. Surgeons and nephrologists implanted 88% and 10% of these catheters, respectively (data for 2% unavailable). Surgical dissection was used in 74% of cases, peritoneoscopy in 6%, and blind (trocar or guide wire) in 8%. Midline insertion was used in 20%, paramedian in 33%, and lateral in 14% of these cases. Prophylactic antibiotics were used in 43% of insertions; data were not available in 28%, and the antibiotics were not used in 29% of cases. This study did not assess catheter survival and all complications; only the relative risk of a first peritonitis episode was analyzed using Cox proportional hazards model. The relative risk of peritonitis was essentially identical for straight, curled, and bent catheters; the risk was significantly higher for "other" catheters. When the analysis was repeated with adjustment for possible center effect, the peritonitis risk was significantly, lower (40%) among patients having catheters with "a permanent bend" (swan neck) (Port F, oral communication during the XVth Annual PD Conference, Orlando, FL, January 25, 1994). In comparison to the double-cuff catheter, the risk of peritonitis was 16% and 31% higher for single deep-cuff and single superficial-cuff catheters, respectively. Insertion by a nephrologist was associated with a 15% higher peritonitis risk as compared to insertion by a surgeon.

CONCLUDING REMARKS

Peritoneal catheters are lifelines for peritoneal dialysis patients. Soft catheters are gradually replacing rigid catheters in the treatment of acute renal failure. Soft catheters are used exclusively for the treatment of chronic renal failure. The Tenckhoff catheter continues to be the most widely used catheter, although its use is decreasing in favor of swan-neck catheters. Surgical implantation virtually eliminated such early complications as bowel perforation or massive bleeding. Other complications, such as obstruction, pericatheter leaks, and superficial cuff extrusions have been markedly reduced in recent years, particularly with the use of swan-neck catheters and insertion through the rectus muscle instead of the midline.

The exit should be located in a place only minimally subjected to pressure and movement. Prophylactic antibiotic prior to implantation and a meticulous sterile surgical technique with perfect hemostasis prevent early infection. Healing of the exit lasts 4–8 weeks. During this time, a nonocclusive (air-permeable) dressing changed weekly is recommended. After the exit is healed, the simplest and best method of care is protection from trauma, cleansing with water and liquid soap containing mild disinfectant, and avoidance of gross exit contamination. Early antibiotics with mild infection prevent severe infection leading to catheter loss. Whereas supine peritoneal dialysis may be started immediately postimplantation, ambulatory peritoneal dialysis should be postponed for at least 10 days after implantation to avoid early leaks. The success of the catheter depends on meticulous adherence to the details of catheter insertion and postimplantation care.

REFERENCES

1. Tenckhoff J, Schechter H: A bacteriologically safe peritoneal access device. *Trans Am Soc Artif Intern Organs* 14:181–187, 1968.
2. Twardowski ZJ, Khanna R: Peritoneal dialysis access and exit site care. In: R Gokal, KD Nolph, eds, *The Textbook of Peritoneal Dialysis*. Kluwer Academic Publishers, Dordrecht, The Netherlands, pp 271–314, 1994.
3. Vaamonde CA, Michael VF, Metzger RA, Carrol KE: Complications of acute peritoneal dialysis. *J Chron Dis* 28:637–659, 1975.
4. Valk TW, Swartz RD, Hsu CH: Peritoneal dialysis in acute renal failure: analysis of outcome and complications. *Dial Transplant* 9:48–54, 1980.
5. Maher JF, Schreiner GE: Hazards and complications of dialysis. *N Engl J Med* 273:370–377, 1965.
6. Edward SR, Unger AM: Acute hydrothorax a new complication of peritoneal dialysis. *JAMA* 199:853–855, 1967.
7. Finn R, Jowett EW: Acute hydrothorax: complication of peritoneal dialysis. *Br Med J* 2:94, 1970.
8. Holm J, Lieden B, Lindgrist B: Unilateral effusion—a rare complication of peritoneal dialysis. *Scand J Urol Nephrol* 5:84–85, 1971.
9. Ribot S, Jacobs MG, Frankel HJ, Bernstein A: Complications of peritoneal dialysis. *Am J Med Sci* 252:505–517, 1966.
10. Mion CM, Boen ST: Analysis of factors responsible for the formation of adhesions during chronic peritoneal dialysis. *Am J Med Sci* 250:675–679, 1965.
11. Matalon R, Levine S, Eisinger RP: Hazards in routine use of peritoneal dialysis. *NY State J Med* 71:219–224, 1971.
12. Henderson LW: Peritoneal dialysis. In: SG Massry, AL Sellers, eds, *Clinical Aspects of Uraemia and Dialysis*. Charles C. Thomas, Springfield, IL, p 574, 1976.
13. Simkin EP, Wright FK: Perforating injuries of the bowel complicating peritoneal catheter insertion. *Lancet* 1:61–67, 1968.
14. Krebs RA, Burtiss BB: Bowel perforation. *JAMA* 198:486–487, 1966.
15. Rigalosi RS, Maher JF, Schreiner GE: Intestinal perforation during peritoneal dialysis. *Ann Intern Med* 70:1013–1015, 1964.
16. Smith E, Chamberlain MJ: Complications of peritoneal dialysis. *Br Med J* 1:126–127, 1965.
17. Stein MF Jr: Intraperitoneal loss of dialysis catheter. *Ann Intern Med* 71:869–870, 1969.
18. Twardowski ZJ, Nolph KD, Khanna R, Prowant BF: Computer interaction: catheters. In: R Khanna, *Advances in Peritoneal Dialysis. Selected Papers from the Fourteenth Annual Conference on Peritoneal Dialysis, Orlando, Florida, January, 1994*, vol 10. Peritoneal Dialysis Publications, Toronto, pp 11–18, 1994.
19. Lindblad AS, Hamilton RW, Novak JW: Complications of peritoneal catheters. In: AS Lindblad, JW Novak, KD Nolph, eds, *Continuous Ambulatory Peritoneal Dialysis in the USA—Final Report of the National CAPD Registry*. Kluwer Academic Publishers, Dordrecht, pp 157–166, 1989.
20. U. S. Renal Data System, USRDS 1992 Annual Data Report, VI. Catheter-related factors and peritonitis risk in CAPD patients. *Am J Kidney Dis* 5 (Suppl 2):48–54, 1992.
21. Twardowski ZJ, Nolph KD, Khanna R, Prowant BF, Ryan LP: The need for a "Swan Neck" permanently bent, arcuate peritoneal dialysis catheter. *Perit Dial Bull* 5:219–223, 1985.
22. Twardowski ZJ, Nichols WK, Khanna R, Nolph KD: *Swan Neck Missouri Peritoneal Dialysis Catheters: Design, Insertion, and Break-in.* Video produced by the Academic Support Center, University of Missouri, Columbia, MO, U.S.A., 1993. (Available through Accurate Surgical Instruments Co., 588–590 Richmond St. W., Toronto, Ontario, Canada M5V 1Y9.)
23. Twardowski ZJ, Prowant BF, Nichols WK, Nolph KD, Khanna R: Six year experience with swan neck catheter. *Perit Dial Int* 12:384–389, 1992.
24. Twardowski ZJ, Nichols WK, Khanna R, Nolph KD: *Swan Neck Presternal Peritoneal Dialysis Catheter: Design, Insertion, and Break-in.* Video produced by the Academic Support Center, University of Missouri, Columbia, MO, U.S.A., 1993.

(Available through Accurate Surgical Instruments Co., 588–590 Richmond St. W., Toronto, Ontario, Canada M5V 1Y9.)

25. Twardowski ZJ, Nichols WK, Nolph KD, Khanna R: Swan neck presternal ("bath tub") catheter for peritoneal dialysis. In: R Khanna, KD Nolph, BF Prowant, ZJ Twardowski, DG Oreopoulos, eds, *Advances in Peritoneal Dialysis. Selected Papers from the Twelfth Annual Conference on Peritoneal Dialysis, Seattle, Washington, February 1992*, vol 8. Peritoneal Dialysis Bulletin, Toronto, pp 316–324, 1992.

26. Twardowski ZJ, Nichols WK, Nolph KD, Khanna R: Swan neck presternal peritoneal dialysis catheter. Selected topics from the VIth ISPD Congress, Thessaloniki, Greece, October 1–4, 1992. *Perit Dial Int* 13 (Suppl 2):S130–S132, 1993.

27. Twardowski ZJ, Khanna R, Nolph KD, Nichols WK: *Peritoneal Dialysis Catheter: Principles of Design, Implantation, and Early Care.* Video produced by the Academic Support Center, University of Missouri, Columbia, MO, U.S.A., 1993. (Available through Accurate Surgical Instruments Co., 588–590 Richmond St. W., Toronto, Ontario, Canada M5V 1Y9.)

28. Cruz C: Clinical experience with a new peritoneal access device (the Cruz™ catheter). In: K Ota, J Maher, J Winchester, P Hirszel, K Ito, T Suzuki, eds, *Current Concepts in Peritoneal Dialysis: Proceedings of the Fifth Congress of the International Society for Peritoneal Dialysis, Kyoto, July 21–24, 1990.* Excerpta Medica, Amsterdam, London, New York, Tokyo, pp 164–169, 1992.

29. Oreopoulos DG, Izatt S, Zellerman G, Karanicolas S, Mathews RE: A prospective study of the effectiveness of three permanent peritoneal catheters. *Proc Clin Dial Transplant Forum* 6:96–100, 1976.

30. Ash SR, Johnson H, Hartman J, Granger J, Koszuta J, Sell L, Dhein C, Blevins W, Thornhill JA: The column disc peritoneal catheter. A peritoneal access device with improved drainage. *ASAIO J* 3:109–115, 1980.

31. Valli A, Andreotti C, Degetto P, Midiri R, Mazzon M, Rovati C, Valentini A, Crescimanno U, Depaoli Vitali E, Manili L, Camerini C: 48-months' experience with Valli-2 catheter. In: R Khanna, KD Nolph, BF Prowant, ZJ Twardowski, DG Oreopoulos, eds, *Advances in Continuous Ambulatory Peritoneal Dialysis. Selected papers from the Eight Annual CAPD Conference, Kansas City, Missouri, February 1988.* Peritoneal Dialysis Bulletin, Toronto, pp 292–297, 1988.

32. Ogden DA, Benavente G, Wheeler D, Zukoski CF: Experience with the right angle Gore-Tex® peritoneal dialysis catheter. In: R Khanna, KD Nolph, BF Prowant, ZJ Twardowski, GD Oreopoulos, eds, *Advances in Continuous Ambulatory Peritoneal Dialysis.* Selected papers from the Sixth Annual CAPD Conference, Kansas City, Missouri, February 1986. Peritoneal Dialysis Bulletin, Toronto, pp 155–159, 1986.

33. Oreopoulos DG, Helfrich GB, Khanna R, Lum GM, Matthews R, Paulsen K, Twardowski ZJ, Vas SI: Peritoneal catheters and exit-site practices: current recommendations. *Perit Dial Bull* 7:130–138, 1987.

34. Gokal R, Ash SR, Helfrich GB, Holmes CJ, Joffe P, Nichols WK, Oreopoulos DG, Riella MC, Slingeneyer A, Twardowski ZJ, Vas SI: Peritoneal catheters and exit-site practices: toward optimum peritoneal access. *Perit Dial Int* 13:29–39, 1992.

35. Poirier VL, Daly BDT, Dasse KA, Haudenschild CC, Fine RE: Elimination of tunnel infection. In: JF Maher, JF Winchester, eds, *Frontiers in Peritoneal Dialysis. Proceedings of the III International Symposium on Peritoneal Dialysis. Washington, D.C., 1984*, Field, Rich & Assoc., New York, pp 210–217, 1986.

36. Tenckhoff H: Home peritoneal dialysis. In: SG Massry, AL Sellers, eds, *Clinical Aspects of Uremia and Dialysis.* Charles C Thomas, Springfield, IL, pp 583–615, 1976.

37. Ash SR, Daugirdas JT: Peritoneal access devices. In: JT Daugirdas, TS Ing, eds, *Handbook of Dialysis.* Little, Brown, Boston, pp 194–218, 1988.

38. Ash S: *Y-TEC Peritoneoscopic Implantation of the Peritoneal Dialysis Catheter.* Video produced by Medigroup Inc., North Aurora, IL 60542-1720, U.S.A., 1993.

39. Gonzales AR, Goltz GM, Eaton CL, Ratajeski G, Olin JW: The peel away method for insertion of Tenckhoff catheter (abstract). *Am Soc Nephrol* 16:119A, 1983.

40. Updike S, O'Brien M, Peterson W, Zimmerman S: Placement of catheter using pacemaker-like introducer with peel-away sleeve (abstract). *Am Soc Nephrol* 17:87A, 1984.

41. Updike S, Zimmerman S, O'Brien M, Peterson W: *Peel-Away@ Sheath Technique for Placing Peritoneal Dialysis Catheters.* Video produced by Television Studio, School of Nursing, University of Wisconsin, Madison, WI, U.S.A., 1984.

42. Zappacosta AR, Perras ST, Closkey GM: Seldinger technique for Tenckhoff catheter placement. *ASAIO Trans* 37:13–15, 1991.

43. Zappacosta AR: *Seldinger Technique for Placement of the Tenckhoff Catheter.* Video produced by the Bryn Mawr Hospital, Bryn Mawr, PA, 1984.

44. Twardowski ZJ, Khanna R: Swan neck peritoneal dialysis catheter. In: VE Andreucci, ed, *Vascular and Peritoneal Access for Dialysis.* Kluwer Academic Publishers, Boston/Dordrecht/London, pp 271–289, 1989.

45. Twardowski ZJ, Khanna R, Nolph KD, Scalamogna A, Metzler MH, Schneider TW, Prowant BF, Ryan LP: Intraabdominal pressure during natural activities in patients treated with continuous ambulatory peritoneal dialysis. *Nephron* 44:129–135, 1986.

46. Moncrief JW, Popovich RP, Broadrick LJ, He ZZ, Simmons EE, Tate RA: Moncrief–Popovich catheter: a new peritoneal access technique for patients on peritoneal dialysis. *ASAIO J* 39:62–65, 1993.

47. *Moncrief-Popovich Catheter.* Video produced by Austin Biomedical Research Institute, 4211 Medical Parkway, Austin, TX, 78756, U.S.A.

48. Schmidt LM, Craig PC, Prowant BF, Twardowski ZJ: A simple method of preventing accidental disconnection at the peritoneal catheter adapter junction. *Perit Dial Int* 10:309–310, 1990.

49. Twardowski ZJ, Prowant BF: Exit-site healing post catheter implantation. *Perit Dial Int* 16 (Suppl 3):S51–S70, 1996.

50. Twardowski ZJ, Prowant BF: Appearance and classification of healing peritoneal catheter exit sites. *Perit Dial Int* 16 (Suppl 3):S71–S93, 1996.

51. Van den Broek PJ, Buys LF, Van Furth R: Interaction of povidone-iodine compounds, phagocytic cells, and macroorganisms. *Antimicrob Agents Chemother* 22:593–597, 1982.

52. Iwasaki N, Kamoi K, Bae RD, Tsutsui T: Cytotoxicity of povidone-iodine on cultured mammalian cells. *J Jpn Assoc Periodont* 31:836–842, 1989.

53. Laufman H: Current use of skin and wound cleansers and antiseptics. *Am J Surg* 157:359–365, 1989.

54. Bryant CA, Rodeheaver GT, Reem EM, Nitcher LS, Kennedy JC, Edlich RF: Search for a nontoxic surgical scrub solution for periorbital lacerations. *Ann Emerg Med* 13:317–319, 1984.

55. Prowant BF, Schmidt LM, Twardowski ZJ, Griebel CK, Bur-

rows L, Ryan LP, Satalowich RJ: Peritoneal dialysis catheter exit site care. *Am Nephrol; Nurs Assoc J* 15:219–222, 1988.

56. Twardowski ZJ, Ryan LP, Kennedy JM: Catheter break-in for continuous ambulatory peritoneal dialysis—University of Missouri experience. *Perit Dial Bull* 4 (Suppl 3):S 110–S 111, 1984.

57. Ash SR, Carr DJ, Diaz-Buxo JA: Peritoneal access devices: hydraulic function and compatibility. In: AR Nissenson, RN Fine, DE Gentile, eds, *Clinical Dialysis 2nd ed.* Appleton & Lange, Norwalk, CT, pp 212–239, 1990.

58. Twardowski ZJ, Pasley K: Reversed one-way obstruction of the peritoneal catheter (the accordion clot). *Perit Dial Int* 14:296–297, 1994.

59. O'Regan S, Garel L, Patriquin H, Yazbeck S: Outflow obstruction: whiplash technique for catheter mobilization. *Perit Dial Int* 8:265–268, 1988.

60. Honkanen E, Eklund B, Laasonen L, Ylinen K, Grönhagen-Riska C: Reposition of a displaced peritoneal catheter: The Helsinki whiplash method. In: R Khanna, KD Nolph, BF Prowant, ZJ Twardowski, DG Oreopoulos, eds, *Advances in Peritoneal Dialysis. Selected Papers from the Tenth Annual Conference on Peritoneal Dialysis, Dallas, Texas, February 1990*, vol 6. Peritoneal Dialysis Bulletin, Toronto, pp 159–164, 1990.

61. Schleifer CR, Ziemek H, Teehan BP, Benz RL, Sigler MH, Gilgore GS: Migration of peritoneal catheters: personal experience and a survey of 72 other units. *Perit Dial Bull* 7:189–193, 1987.

62. Yoshihara K, Yoshi S, Miyagi S: Alpha replacement method for the displacement of the swan neck catheter. In: R Khanna, KD Nolph, BF Prowant, ZJ Twardowski, DG Oreopoulos, eds, *Advances in Peritoneal Dialysis. Selected Papers from the Thirteenth Annual Conference on Peritoneal Dialysis, San Diego, California, March 1993*, vol 9. Peritoneal Dialysis Bulletin, Toronto, pp 227–230, 1993.

63. Ersoy FF, Twardowski ZJ, Satalovich RJ, Ketchersid T: A retrospective analysis of catheter position and function in 91 CAPD patients. *Perit Dial Int* 14:409–410, 1994.

64. Twardowski ZJ: Malposition and poor drainage of peritoneal catheters. *Semin Dial* 3:57, 1990.

65. Goldsmith HJ, Edwards EC, Moorhead PJ, Wright FK: Difficulties encountered in intermittent dialysis for chronic renal failure. *Br J Urol* 38:625–634, 1966.

66. Pierratos A: Peritoneal dialysis glossary. *Perit Dial Bull* 4:2–3, 1984.

67. Twardowski ZJ, Prowant BF: Exit-site study methods and results. *Perit Dial Int* 16 (Suppl 3):S6–S31, 1996.

68. Twardowski ZJ, Prowant BF: Classification of normal and diseased exit sites. *Perit Dial Int* 16 (Suppl 3):S32–S50, 1996.

69. Strauss FG, Holmes D, Nortman DF, Friedman S: Hypertonic saline compresses: therapy for complicated exit site infections. In: R Khanna, KD Nolph, BF Prowant, ZJ Twardowski, DG Oreopoulos, eds, *Advances in Peritoneal Dialysis. Selected Papers from the Thirteenth Annual Conference on Peritoneal Dialysis, San Diego, California, March 1993*, vol 9. Peritoneal Dialysis Bulletin, Toronto, pp 248–250, 1993.

70. Nichols WK, Nolph KD: A technique for managing exit site and cuff infection in Tenckhoff catheters. *Perit Dial Bull* 3 (Suppl 4):S4–S5, 1983.

71. Domico J, Warman M, Jaykamur S, Sorkin MI: Is ultrasonography useful in predicting catheter loss? In: R Khanna, KD Nolph, BF Prowant, ZJ Twardowski, DG Oreopoulos, eds, *Advances in Peritoneal Dialysis. Selected*

Papers from the Thirteenth Annual Conference on Peritoneal Dialysis, San Diego, California. March 1993. Peritoneal Dialysis Bulletin, Toronto, pp 231–232, 1993.

72. Plum J, Sudkamp S, Grabensee G: Results of ultrasound-assisted diagnosis of tunnel infections in continuous ambulatory peritoneal dialysis. *Am J Kidney Dis* 23:99–104, 1994.

73. Twardowski ZJ: Tidal peritoneal dialysis. In: RN Fine, AR Nissenson, eds, *Dialysis Therapy.* Hanley & Belfus, Philadelphia, pp 153–156, 1993.

74. Helfrich GB, Pechan BW, Alijani MR, Bernard WF, Rakowski TA, Winchester JF: Reduced catheter complications with lateral placement. *Perit Dial Bull* 3 (Suppl 4):S2–S4, 1983.

75. Twardowski ZJ, Tully RJ, Nichols WK, Sunderrajan S: Computerized tomography in the diagnosis of subcutaneous leak sites during continuous ambulatory peritoneal dialysis (CAPD). *Perit Dial Bull* 4:163–166, 1984.

76. Twardowski ZJ, Tully RJ, Ersoy FF, Dedhia NM: Computerized tomography with and without intraperitoneal contrast for determination of intraabdominal fluid distribution and diagnosis of complications in peritoneal dialysis patients. *ASAIO Trans* 36:95–103, 1990.

77. Dasgupta MK, Bettcher KB, Ulan RA, Burns V, Lam K, Dossetor JB, Costerton JW: Relationship of adherent bacterial biofilms to peritonitis in chronic ambulatory peritoneal dialysis. *Perit Dial Bull* 7:168–173, 1987.

78. Dimitriadis A, Antoniou S, Toliou T, Papadopoulos C: Tissue reaction to deep cuff of Tenckhoff catheter and peritonitis. In: R Khanna, KD Nolph, BF Prowant, ZJ Twardowski, DG Oreopoulos, eds, *Advances in Peritoneal Dialysis. Selected Papers from the Tenth Annual Conference on Peritoneal Dialysis, Dallas, Texas, February 1990*, vol 6. Peritoneal Dialysis Bulletin, Toronto, pp 155–158, 1990.

79. Grefberg N, Danielson BG, Nilsson P, Wahlberg J: An unusual complication of the Toronto Western Hospital catheter (letter). *Perit Dial Bull* 3:219, 1983.

80. della Volpe M, Iberti M, Ortensia A, Veronesi GV: Erosion of the sigmoid by a permanent peritoneal catheter (letter). *Perit Dial Bull* 4:108, 1984.

81. Jamison MH, Fleming SJ, Ackrill P, Schofield PF: Erosion of rectum by Tenckhoff catheter. *Br J Surg* 75:360, 1988.

82. Brady HR, Abraham G, Oreopoulos DG, Cardella CJ: Bowel erosion due to a dormant peritoneal catheter in immunosuppressed renal transplant recipients. *Perit Dial Int* 8:163–165, 1988.

83. Golper TA, Carpenter J: Accidents with Tenckhoff catheters. *Ann Intern Med* 95:121–122, 1981.

84. Ward RA, Klein E, Wathen RL, eds, Peritoneal catheters. In: Investigation of the risks and hazards with devices associated with peritoneal dialysis and sorbent regenerated dialysate delivery systems. *Perit Dial Bull* 3 (Suppl 3):S9–S17, 1983.

85. Szycher M, Siciliano AA, Reed AM: Polyurethane in medical devices. *Med Design Material* 18–25, 1991.

86. Kurihara S, Tani Y, Tatcishi K, Yuri T, Kitada II, Sugishita N, Fukuda Y, Ishikawa I, Shinoda A, Hayakawa Y: Allergic eosinophilic dermatitis due to silicone rubber: a rare but troublesome complication of the Tenckhoff catheter. *Perit Dial Bull* 5:65–67, 1985.

87. Prowant BF, Schmidt LM, Twardowski ZJ, Taylor HM, Ryan LP, Satalowich RJ, Burrows L, Griebel CK, Burrows LM: Use of exudate smears for diagnosis of peritoneal catheter exit site infection. In: MM Avram, C Giordano, eds, *Ambulatory Peri-*

toneal Dialysis—Proceedings of the IVth Congress of the International Society for Peritoneal Dialysis, Venice, Italy, June 29–July 2, 1987. Plenum Publishing, New York, pp 220–222, 1990.

88. Twardowski ZJ, Prowant BF, Khanna R, Nichols WK, Nolph KD: Long-term experience with Swan Neck Missouri catheters. *ASAIO Trans* 36:M491–M494, 1990.

89. Bozkurt F, Keller E, Schollmeyer P: Swan Neck peritoneal dialysis catheter can reduce complications in CAPD patients. Abstracts of the IVth Congress of the International Society for Peritoneal Dialysis, Venice, Italy, June 29–July 2, 1987. *Perit Dial Bull* 7 (Suppl 2):S9, 1987.

90. Gucek A, Bren FA, Lindic J, Premru V, Kveder R: CAPD catheter survival: our 9-year experience (abstract). *Perit Dial Int* 12 (Suppl 2):S49, 1992.

91. Hwang TL, Huang CC: Comparison of swan neck catheter with Tenckhoff catheter for CAPD. *Adv Perit Dial* 10:203–205, 1994.

92. Nube MJ, De Vet JA, Van Geelen JA: Bacterial and clinical sequelae of the Twin bag system in continuous ambulatory peritoneal dialysis. A single centre study. *Neth J Med* 44:191–197, 1994.

93. Ahlmén J, Brunes L, Schönborg C: A randomized comparison of two peritoneal dialysis catheters. *ASAIO 1993 Abstracts. 39th Annual Meeting, New Orleans Hilton Hotel, New Orleans, Louisiana, April 29–30 & May 1, 1993,* p 110, 1993.

94. Lye WC, Kour NW, van den Straaten J, Leong SO, Lee EJC: A prospective randomized comparison of the swan neck coiled and straight Tenckhoff catheters in patients on CAPD. *Perit Dial Int* 15 (Suppl):S57, 1995.

95. Sieniawska M, Blaim M, Warchol S: Swan-neck presternal catheter for continuous ambulatory peritoneal dialysis in children. *Pediatr Nephrol* 7:557–558, 1993.

96. Twardowski ZJ, Prowant BF, Pickett B, Nichols WK, Nolph KD, Khanna R: Four-year experience with swan neck presternal peritoneal dialysis catheter. *Am J Kidney Dis* 27(1):99–105, 1996.

97. Ash SR, Nichols WK: Placement, repair, and removal of chronic peritoneal catheters. In: R Gokal, KD Nolph, ed, *The Textbook of Peritoneal Dialysis.* Kluwer Academic Publishers, Dordrecht, The Netherlands, pp 315–333, 1994.

CHAPTER 58

Peritonitis and Other Complications

CHARLES E. HALSTENSON & WILLIAM F. KEANE

INCIDENCE

Infection is the most frequent clinical complication in patients with end-stage renal disease maintained on peritoneal dialysis (1). These infections include bacterial and fungal peritonitis as well as exit-site and catheter tunnel infections. The incidence of peritonitis is 3 to 5 times higher in patients maintained on continuous ambulatory peritoneal dialysis (CAPD) than in those on intermittent peritoneal dialysis and contributes to the morbidity and mortality of patients receiving CAPD therapy (2). During the 1980s the incidence of peritonitis was about 1.3 episodes per patient per year (3). This rate has declined over time with the introduction of various types of disconnect systems (4). These disconnect systems have predominantly decreased the risk of peritonitis due to skin organisms, e.g., coagulase-negative staphylococcus. The Y set, an example of disconnect technology, has also been associated with a decrease in the peritonitis rate to 1 episode per 24–36 months (5,6).

PATHOGENESIS

The main pathways for infection of the peritoneal cavity are exogenous contamination through the lumen of the catheter or across the abdominal wall (Table 1). Contamination during an exchange procedure of the connection between the dialysis bag and transfer set is an important cause of peritonitis. Recognition of this led to developments of improved connect–disconnect technology and an apparent reduction in peritonitis rates. However, peritonitis (usually gram-negative organisms) has been associated with intra-abdominal pathology, e.g., cholecystitis, diverticulitis, and pancreatitis.

The distribution of organisms isolated from CAPD peritonitis is of predominantly gram-positive organisms (Table 2) (7,8). The most commonly isolated organisms are coagulase-negative staphylococci. The introduction of the newer "flush before fill' technology has changed the distribution of organisms causing peritonitis, reducing the contribution of gram-positive skin organisms with a slight, proportionate increase in gram-negative organisms. A minority of peritoneal infections occur as a result of an intra-abdominal event such as diverticular disease, acute cholecystitis, ischemic bowel, or perforated viscus. Fungal peritonitis is a relatively rare, yet well-defined cause of CAPD-associated peritonitis (9).

Catheter exit-site and tunnel infections are events frequently associated with recurrent peritonitis and catheter failure (10). The major portal of entry into the peritoneal cavity is migration around the catheter insertion site. From 2% to 8.6% of peritonitis episodes are estimated to arise from exit-site and tunnel infections (11).

In addition to exogenous touch contamination, another source of bacteria that might contribute to the development of peritonitis is the presence of catheter biofilm (12). Biofilm is an adherent substance composed of bacteria encased in microbial-produced extracellular polysaccharides. It appears that the presence of biofilm per se on the catheters does not necessarily lead to peritonitis (13), but its presence, probably on all catheters, may contribute biological products that may alter host defense mechanisms.

HOST DEFENSE MECHANISMS

An understanding of cellular and humoral defenses against microbial invasion has provided potential methods to prevent peritonitis (14). The peritoneal membrane lines the interior of the abdominal wall and consists of a surface layer of mesothelial cells that lie on a basement membrane with deeper layers of capillaries and lymphatics (Figure 1). Transport through the peritoneal membrane moves from the capillaries through the basement membrane via intracellular junctions. Transport of particles may be either through cellular junctions or through pinocytosis by mesothelial cells (15). The primary route for movement of small particles from the peritoneum is via the lymphatics. During peritonitis, the primary flow is towards the peritoneal cavity (16), which may explain the low rate of bacteremia in peritoneal patients during peritonitis.

Suki, WN and Massry SG (eds), Suki and Massry's Therapy of Renal Diseases and Related Disorders, Third Edition. ISBN 978-1-4757-6634-9.
©1998, *Kluwer Academic Publishers, Boston/Dordrecht/London.* All rights reserved.

Table 1. Routes of infections in CAPD patients

Route	Organism	%
Transluminal	S. epidermidis	30–40
	Acinetobacter	
Periluminal	S. epidermidis	20–30
	S. aureus	
	Pseudomonas	
	Yeast	
Transmural	Enteric gram-negative	25–30
	Anaerobes	
Hematogenous	Streptococcus	5–10
	M. tuberculosis	
Ascending	Yeast	2–5
	Lactobacillus	

Table 2. Distribution of organisms isolated from peritonitis episodes

Organism	%
Coagulase negative staphylococci	30–40
Staphylococcus aureus	20
Streptococcus sp	10–15
Neisseria sp	1–2
Diphtheroid sp	1–2
E. coli	5–10
Pseudomonas sp	5–10
Enterococcus	3–6
Klebsiella sp	1–3
Proteus sp	3–6
Acinetobacter sp	2–5
Anaerobic organisms	2–5
Fungi	2–10
Other (mycobacteria, etc.)	2–5
Culture negative	0–30

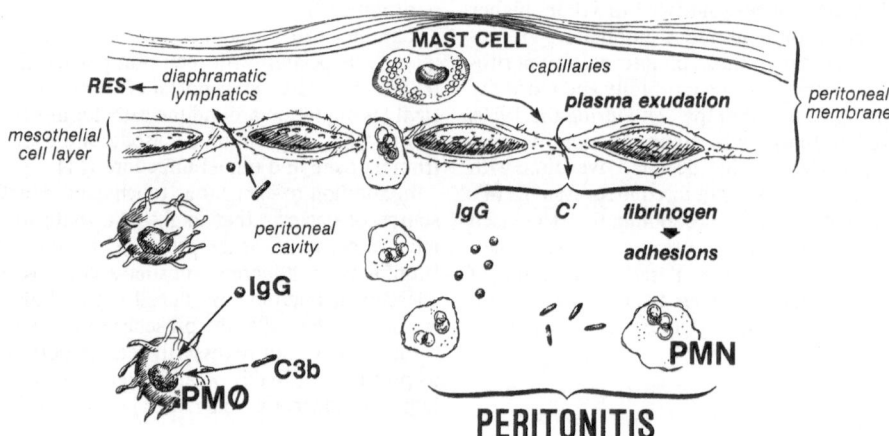

Figure 1. Schematic representation of the major host defense mechanism of the peritoneal cavity. Bacteria may be removed from the peritoneal cavity via lymphatics in the diaphragmatic serosa, and these organisms are eventually phagocytized and killed by macrophages of the reticuloendothelial system (RES). Peritoneal macrophages (PMØ) are able to phagocytize and kill opsonized bacteria. When these defenses are overwhelmed, however, peritonitis develops—a process characterized by exudation of polymorphonuclear leukocytes (PMN) and plasma into the peritoneal cavity. (From: PK Peterson, WF Keane: Infections in chronic peritoneal dialysis patients. In: JS Remington, MN Swartz, eds, *Corrent Clinical Topics in Infectious Diseases*, vol. 6. McGraw-Hill, New York, 1985. Reproduced with permission.)

HUMORAL FACTORS

Immunoglobulins and complement are present in normal peritoneal fluid. Most studies of CAPD have demonstrated near normal serum levels of immunoglobulins (17). However, the peritoneal concentrations appear diluted due to the volume of the dialysis fluid (17–19). There are decreased levels of opsonins and other factors needed for immunological reactions in the peritoneal cavity (17–19). This relative lack of opsonins has been postulated to be a factor in repeated episodes of peritonitis in the high-risk patient (19–21). The inability to produce adequate amounts of interleukin-1 and the release of large amounts of prostaglandin E_2 by the macrophages of certain patients has also been postulated as contributing to the development of recurrent peritonitis by downregulating macrophage phagocytic activity (22).

CELLULAR FACTORS

Mesothelial and mononuclear cells are important in the normal self-clearing mechanism of the peritoneal cavity. During inflammation, a large number of active phagocytic polymorphonuclear cells enter the peritoneal cavity, aiding in the removal of bacteria (23–25). Low pH and high osmo-

Table 3. Pharmacokinetics of antibiotics in CAPD patients and proposed regimens for the treatment of CAPD peritonitis

	Half-life (H)			Dose (per 70 kg adult)[a]		
					Maintenance	
	Normal	ESRD	CAPD	Initial (mg/2-L bag)	Intermittent (mg/2-L bag per dosing interval)	Continuous (mg/2-L bag)
Aminoglycosides						
Amikacin	1.6	39	40	500	120/day	12–24
Gentamicin	2.2	53	32	70–140	40/day	8–16
Netilmicin	2.1	42	18	70–140	40/day	8–16
Tobramycin	2.5	58	36	70–140	40/day	8–16
Cephalosporins						
First generation						
Cefazolin	2.2	28	30	500–1000	1000/day	250–500
Cefonicid	4.0	68	50	250	ND	50
Cephalothin	0.2	3.7	ND	1000	ND	200
Cephradine	0.9	12	ND	500	ND	250
Cephalexin	0.8	19	9	1000 p.o.	500/QID p.o.	NA
Second generation						
Cefamandole	1.0	10	8.0	1000	1000/day	500
Cefmenoxime	1.3	11.3	6.0	2000	1000/day	100
Cefoxitin	0.8	20	15	1000	ND	200
Cefuroxime	1.3	18	15	1000	400/day I.V./p.o.	150–400
Third generation						
Cefixime	3.2	11.5	15	400 p.o.	400/day p.o.	NA
Cefoperazone	1.8	2.3	2.2	2000	ND	400–1000
Cefotaxime	0.9	2.5	2.4	2000	2000/day	500
Cefsulodin	1.8	11	11	1000	500/day	50
Ceftazidime	1.8	26	13	1000	1000/day	250
Ceftizoxime	1.6	28	11	1000	1000/day	250
Ceftriaxone	8.0	15	12	1000	1000/day	250–500
Moxalactam	2.2	20	16	1000	1000/day	350
Penicillins						
Azlocillin	0.9	5.1	ND	500	ND	500
Mezlocillin	1.0	4.3	ND	3000 I.V.	3000/BID I.V.	500
Piperacillin	1.2	3.9	2.4	4000 I.V.	4000/BID I.V.	500
Ticarcillin	1.2	15	ND	1000–2000	2000/BID	250
Quinolones						
Ciprofloxacin	4.0	8.0	11	500 p.o.	500/TID p.o.	50
Fleroxacin	13	27	27	800 p.o.	400/d p.o.	NA
Ofloxacin	7.0	30	25	400 p.o.	200/d p.o.	NA
Vancomycin and others						
Vancomycin	6.9	161	92	1000–2000	1–2000/7 day	30–50
Teicoplanin	50	260	260	400	400/BID	40[b]
Aztreonam	2.0	7.0	9.3	1000	1000/day	500
Clindamycin	2.8	2.8	ND	300	ND	300
Erythromycin	2.1	4.0	ND	ND	500/QID p.o.	150
Metronidazole	7.9	7.7	11	500 p.o./I.V.	500/TID p.o./I.V.	ND
Minocycline	15.5	20	ND	NA	100/BID p.o.	NA
Rifampin	4.0	8.0	ND	600 p.o.	600/d. p.o.	NA
Antifungal agents						
Amphotericin B	360	360	ND	NA	20–30/day I.V.	2–8
Flucytosine	4.2	115	ND	2000–3000 p.o.	1000/day p.o.	NA
Fluconazole	22	125	72	NA	150 mg q 2 day	ND
Ketoconazole	2.0	1.8	2.4	400 p.o.	200–800/day p.o.	NA
Miconazole	24	25	ND	200	ND	100–200

Table 3 (Continued).

| | Half-life (H) | | | Dose (per 70 kg adult)[a] | | |
| | | | | | Maintenance | |
	Normal	ESRD	CAPD	Initial (mg/2-L bag)	Intermittent (mg/2-L bag per dosing interval)	Continuous (mg/2-L bag)
Amphicillin	1.3	15	9.5	1000–2000	1000/BID	100
Sulbactam	1.0	19	9.7	1000–2000	1000/BID	100
Imipenem	0.9	3.0	6.4	1000	500/BID	200
Cilistatin	0.8	15	19	500–1000	500/BID	100–200
Sulfamethoxazole	10	13	14	1600 p.o.	1600/1–2 day p.o.	400
Trimethoprim	14	33	34	320 p.o.	320/1–2 day p.o.	80

[a] The route of administration is intraperitoneal unless otherwise specified. The pharmacokinetic data and proposed dosage regimens presented here are based on published literature reviewed through April 1992.
There is no evidence that mixing different antibiotics in dialysis fluid (except for aminoglycosides and penicillins) is deleterious for the drugs or patients. However, the same syringe should not be used to mix antibiotics.
[b] This is in each bay × 7 days, then in 2 bags/day × 7 days, and then in 1 bag/day × 7 days.
ESRD, creatinine clearance < 10 mL/min, patient not on dialysis; NA, not applicable; ND, no data; I.V., intravenous; p.o., oral; day, once a day; BID, twice a day; TID, three times a day; QID, four times a day. Reproduced from (31), permission.

lality of the dialysis fluid decrease, temporarily, the efficacy of phagocytic cells (26–29). The ratio of bacteria to cell is diluted in the peritoneal cavity during peritoneal dialysis; thus, the chance of phagocytosis is diminished. The role of eosinophils and lymphocyte mediators in peritoneal defenses is not clear. Whether the altered production of mediators or inhibitors of cell immunity contributes to the susceptibility of end-stage renal disease patients to infection has been continually debated (22).

CLINICAL PRESENTATION—INITIAL ASSESSMENT

The suggestive signs of peritonitis are cloudy fluid, abdominal pain, or increased temperature. If there is no increase in peritoneal white blood cells (WBCs) or more than 100 polymorphonuclear neutrophils/mm^3 and the differential is normal and no bacteria are seen on Gram stain, immediate initiation of therapy is not necessary. In contrast, patients with cloudy fluid accompanied by abdominal pain or fever require prompt initiation of therapy, and diagnostic laboratory studies should be obtained expeditiously. However, neither the differential nor the magnitude of the WBC elevation has been shown to be helpful in predicting the putative causative microorganism. A Gram stain is positive in approximately 9%–40% of episodes of peritonitis and, when positive, is predictive of the type of organism in approximately 85% of cases. A Gram stain is particularly useful in early recognition of fungal peritonitis. Culture of dialysate effluent should be obtained as soon as possible, but availability of culture results should not delay initiation of therapy.

CLINICAL COURSE OF PERITONITIS— TREATMENT OF PERITONITIS

Many different antimicrobial agents have been used to treat CAPD peritonitis (30,31) (Table 3). Antibiotics usually have been administered intraperitoneally or intravenously, and a variety of different dosing regimens have been suggested. No single regimen has been shown to be the most efficacious in appropriate clinical trials.

It is recognized that many patients treated with CAPD reside in locations that are remote from medical facilities, and, thus, may not be seen expeditiously after onset of symptoms nor have immediately available microbiologic and laboratory diagnostic services. Since most clinicians agree that prompt initiation of therapy for peritonitis is critical, these facts will necessitate reliance on immediate patient reporting of symptomatology to the dialysis center. Prompt initiation of therapy by these patients remote from the center is of obvious importance and requires the availability of antimicrobials in the patient's home. Instructions for reporting of symptomatology and utilization of home antimicrobial therapy should be considered part of CAPD patient training.

INITIAL ANTIBIOTIC SELECTION

Gram-positive organisms on Gram stain

For the treatment of a presumed gram-positive peritonitis, vancomycin in a dose of 2 g in one 6-hr exchange every 7 days would provide adequate bacteriocidal activity in both serum and dialysate for almost all gram-positive organisms

(30). A broad clinical experience has now been obtained with an intermittent dosing regimen that has demonstrated the efficacy of this approach (30). Alternatively, vancomycin may be administered continuously utilizing a regimen of 30–50 mg/L in each exchange. Recent concern has been focused on vancomycin resistant microorganisms thus, precenting new treatment dilemmas.

The cost of vancomycin treatment may be prohibitive in certain parts of the world. Alternatively, the use of a first-generation cephalosporin is probably acceptable for clinical care when used with an initial loading dose of 500 mg/L I.P. and a maintenance dose of 125 mg/L I.P. in each subsequent exchange (31). However, it is important to recognize that the worldwide prevalence of methicillin-(thus, cephalosporin-) resistant coagulase negative staphylococci is increasing.

Gram stain negative or not done; grem-negative organisms

Therapeutic regimens most commonly used as initial therapies for peritonitis, when the causal organism is unknown, have utilized two agents. Vancomycin administered intraperitoneally may be utilized in combination with intraperitoneal ceftazidime or an aminoglycoside (30) (Table 3). These combinations appear equally efficacious.

The aminoglycosides, gentamicin, tobramycin, and netilmicin appear to have equal efficacy. A single daily dose of these agents has been shown to be efficacious and less toxic in other patients with severe systemic infections (32). Increased bacterial killing rates associated with a prolonged postantibiotic effect are obtained using once-daily dosing, while toxic drug accumulation in renal and cochlear tissues is minimized. In contrast, continuous administration results in sustained, but low, serum levels that are less bactericidal and favor toxic accumulation of these agents in renal and cochlear tissues. Prolonged or closely spaced, repetitive courses with aminoglycosides should be avoided in these patients. While these principles of dosing using intravenously administered aminoglycosides have been demonstrated to be efficacious in nonuremic patients, clinical trials in CAPD-related peritonitis demonstrating comparable efficacy of intermittent intraperitoneal dosing compared to the more traditional intraperitoneal dosing, i.e., in each exchange, are limited and have only recently been reported. Haqqie et al. reported effective treatment of a small number of CAPD patients with peritonitis in outpatient treatment with once-daily gentamicin (0.6 mg/kg I.P.) dosing in combination with once-weekly vancomycin (30 mg/kg I.P.) dosing (33).

Gram stain reveals yeast

Although the mainstay of therapy for fungal peritonitis in the past has been amphotericin, its toxicity has frequently precluded its effective use. Experience with the newer imidizoles/triazoles and flucytosine has suggested that these agents are well tolerated and are efficacious. When used in combination, these agents appear to have a synergistic effect and have demonstrated cure rates similar to those reported with amphotericin B (30). Treatment for 4–6 weeks is recommended (31). However, if clinical improvement does not occur within 4–7 days of therapy, the catheter should be removed. Therapy should then be continued for an additional 10 days after catheter removal.

MODIFICATION OF TREATMENT REGIMEN ONCE CULTURE AND SENSITIVITY RESULTS ARE KNOWN

Gram-positive microorganisms cultured

The choice of alternative antibiotic therapy should be guided by sensitivity patterns (31). If *S. aureus* is identified and clinical improvement is not seen within 4–5 days, rifampin, 600 mg p.o. daily, should be added to the regimen and therapy continued for 3 weeks. In those patients in whom an enterococcus is identified, an aminoglycoside should be used in addition to vancomycin.

Cultures are negative

Occasionally (10%–15%), cultures may be negative, related to a variety of technical or clinical reasons. Experience would indicate that if the patient is clinically improving after 4–5 days, and there is no suggestion of gram-negative organisms on Gram stain, only vancomycin need be continued and that the second antibiotic (ceftazidime/aminoglycoside) can be discontinued. Duration of therapy should be for 2 weeks. If, on the other hand, no clinical improvement occurs, repeat evaluation is mandatory, and consideration should be given to catheter removal.

Gram-negative microorganisms cultured

If the culture report reveals gram-negative organisms, it is imperative to consider the possibility of intra-abdominal pathology necessitating surgical exploration. If a single gram-negative organism, such as *E. coli, Klebsiella, Proteus*, or *Pseudomonas* is obtained, it is not necessary to continue the vancomycin. An aminoglycoside alone or ceftazidime alone should be used. Utilization of these antimicrobial agents must be guided by in vitro sensitivity testing.

Finally, if *Pseudomonas aeruginosa* or *Xanthomonas* are identified, therapy with at least two agents that have activity against *Pseudomonas* or *Xanthomonas* should be used. Intravenous piperacillin, 4 g every 12 hr, can be added to ceftazidime or an aminoglycoside, although other effective agents are available for *Pseudomonas* infection. Clinical experience has demonstrated that *Pseudomonas* peritonitis in CAPD patients is extremely difficult to cure, particularly when it develops as a consequence of a catheter-related infection (30). In this setting, antibiotic treatment without catheter removal has a low likelihood of therapeutic success. *Xanthomonas* organisms require special attention since they display sensitivity to only a few antimicrobial agents. Therapy for *Pseudomonas/Xanthomonas* peritonitis is recommended for 3–4 weeks if the patient is clinically improving.

PROPHYLACTIC THERAPIES

There is some evidence now that nasal carriage of *S. aureus* is associated with an increased risk of exit-site infection and peritonitis due to this organism. However, the natural history of nasal carriage in uremic peritoneal dialysis patients is not known, and hence, eradication of nasal carriage using naseptin or mupirocin creams is empirical. The use of these topical agents may be associated with changes in the structural integrity of the dialysis catheter (34). The use of mupirocin at the exit site may be as effective with fewer side effects in reducing *S. aureus* catheter infections as oral rifampin every 3 months (35).

Whether prophylactic immunization against staphylococci would change the incidence of peritonitis has been frequently discussed. However, recent data in 124 CAPD patients demonstrated no beneficial protective response following vaccination for the prevention of staphylococcal peritonitis (36).

TREATMENT OF EXIT-SITE AND TUNNEL INFECTIONS

An exit-site infection is defined by the presence of purulent drainage and erythema of the skin at the catheter–epidermal interface. The presence of erythema alone may be an early indication of infection, and topical therapy with chlorhexidin, mupirocin, or hydrogen peroxide should be initiated. However, Gram stain and culture should be performed only when purulent drainage is present. There is a paucity of information regarding therapeutic efficacy of any agent in patients with these infections. Nonetheless, if gram-positive organisms are present, either oral cephalexin or cephradine or parenteral vancomycin are indicated. Vancomycin may be used either intravenously in a single dose of 1 g for adults or 2 g intraperitoneally (Table 3). The length of time that exit-site infections should be treated has not been established. However, it should be noted that fungal peritonitis has been associated with prolonged use of antibiotics or multiple drug regimens. If Gram stain reveals gram-negative organisms, a *Pseudomonas* exit-site infection should be suspected. In adults, oral ciprofloxacin, 500 mg three times a day orally, has been recommended. Patients should be advised that ciprofloxacin should not be administered at the same time that phosphate binders are taken, since this may dramatically reduce absorption. In the pediatric population, ceftazidime in the recommended doses should be used.

Once results of the culture are obtained, antibiotic therapy should be modified accordingly. For gram-positive infections, if clinical signs of improvement are not evident in 1 week, rifampin, 600 mg p.o. daily, should be added. If *S. aureus* site infection persists (purulent drainage and erythema) for 2–3 weeks despite adequate antibiotic therapy, exploration of the tunnel and removal of the external cuff should be considered. If this maneuver fails to cure the exit-site infection, the catheter should be removed. Similarly, if a gram-negative exit-site infection persists for 2–3 weeks, removal of the catheter is appropriate. If *Pseudomonas/Xanthomonas* exit-site infection is demonstrated, it is unlikely that it will respond to antimicrobial therapy, and early catheter removal should be considered.

SUMMARY

Recent experience has shown a decline in the rate of CAPD-related peritonitis. Advances in catheter technology, connect systems, patient training, and diagnostic and therapeutic methods may lead to a further reduction in peritonitis rates. Recent changes in the treatment recommendations should be consulted for current therapeutic recommendations (37).

REFERENCES

1. Nolph KD, Cutler SJ, Steinberg SM, Novak JW, Hirschman GH: Factors associated with morbidity and mortality among patients on CAPD. *ASAIO Trans* 33:57–65, 1987.
2. Excerpts from United States Renal Data System 1993 Annual Data Report. *Am J Kidney Dis* 22:53–57, 1993.
3. Nolph KD, Lindblad AS, Novak JW: Current concepts. Continuous ambulatory peritoneal dialysis. Clinical Coordinating Center, National Institutes of Health Continuous Ambulatory Peritoneal Dialysis Registry. *N Engl J Med* 318:1595–1600, 1988.
4. Bernardini J, Holley JL, Johnston JR, Perlmutter JA, Piraino B: An analysis of ten-year trends in infections in adults on continuous ambulatory peritoneal dialysis (CAPD). *Clin Nephrol* 36:29–34, 1991.
5. Fellin G, Gentile MG, Manna GM: Peritonitis prevention: Y connector and sodium hypochlorite. Three years' experience. Report of the Italian Study Group. In: R Khanna, KD Nolph, B Prowant, ZJ Twardowski, DG Oreopoulis, eds, Advances in Peritoneal Dialysis. Peritoneal Dialysis International, Toronto, pp 114–118, 1987.
6. Churchill DN, Taylor DW, Vas SI, Oreopoulos DG, Bettcher KB, Fenton SSA, Fine A, Lavoie S, Page D, Wu G, Beecroft ML, Pemberton R, Wilczynski NL, deVeber GA, Williams W: Peritonitis in continuous ambulatory peritoneal dialysis (CAPD): a multicenter randomized clinical trial comparing the Y-connector disinfectant system to standard systems. *Perit Dial Int* 9:159–163, 1989.
7. Michael J, Adu D, Frier LD, McIntyre M: Bacteriological

spectrum of CAPD peritonitis. *Contrib Nephrol* 57:41–44, 1987.

8. Golper TA, Hartstein AI: Analysis of the causative pathogens in uncomplicated CAPD-associated peritonitis: duration of therapy, relapses, and prognosis. *Am J Kidney Dis* 7:141–145, 1986.

9. Rubin J, Kirschner K, Walsh D, et al.: Fungal peritonitis during continuous ambulatory peritoneal dialysis: a report of 17 cases. *Am J Kidney Dis* 10:361–368, 1987.

10. Scalamogna A, Castelnovo C, De Vecchi A, Ponticelli C: Exit-site and tunnel infections in continuous ambulatory peritoneal dialysis patients. *Am J Kidney Dis* 18:674–677, 1991.

11. Mion C, Slingeneyer A, Canaud B: Peritonitis. In: R Gokal, ed, *Continuous Ambulatory Peritoneal Dialysis,*. Churchill Livingstone, New York, pp 163–217, 1986.

12. Marrie TJ, Noble MA, Costerton JW: Examination of the morphology of bacteria adhering to peritoneal dialysis catheters by scanning and transmission electron microscopy. *J Clin Microbiol* 18:1388–1398, 1983.

13. Dasgupta MK, Bettcher KB, Ulan RA, Burns V, Lam K, Dossetor JB, Costerton JW: Relationship of adherent bacterial biofilms to peritonitis in chronic ambulatory peritoneal dialysis. *Perit Dial Bull* 7:168–173, 1987.

14. Harrison M, Keane WF: Host defense mechanisms in CAPD-associated peritonitis. *Semin Dial* 2:117–121, 1989.

15. Cotran RS, Karnovsky MJ: Ultrastructural studies on the permeability of the mesothelium to horseradish peroxidase. *J Cell Biol* 37:123–137, 1968.

16. Casley-Smith JR: An electron microscopical study of the passage of ions through the endothelium of lymphatic and blood capillaries, and through the mesothelium. *Q J Exp Physiol Cogn Med Sci* 52:105–113, 1967.

17. Gilmour J, Tymiansky R, Pierratos A, Vas S, Klein M, Khanna R, Digenis D, Cuff S, Oreopoulos DG: Changes in some inflammatory proteins during peritonitis in CAPD patients. *Perit Dial Bull* 3:201–204, 1983.

18. Rubin J, Lin LM, Lewis R, Cruse J, Bower JD: Host defense mechanisms in continuous ambulatory peritoneal dialysis. *Clin Nephrol* 20:140–144, 1983.

19. Verbrugh HA, Keane WA, Hoidal JR, Freiberg MR, Elliot GR, Peterson PK: Peritoneal macrophages and opsonins: antibacterial defense in patients on chronic peritoneal dialysis. *J Infect Dis* 147:1018–1029, 1983.

20. Clark LA, Easmon CS: Opsonic activity of intravenous immunoglobulin preparations against Staphylococcus epidermidis. *J Clin Pathol* 39:856–860, 1986.

21. Lamperi S, Carozzi S: Defective opsonic activity of peritoneal effluent during continuous ambulatory peritoneal dialysis (CAPD): importance and prevention. *Perit Dial Bull* 6:87–92, 1986.

22. Lamperi S, Carozzi S: Suppressor resident peritoneal macrophages and peritonitis incidence in continuous ambulatory peritoneal dialysis. *Nephron* 44:219–225, 1986.

23. Peterson PK, Gaziano E, Devalon M, Peterson LA, Keane WF: Antimicrobial activities of dialysate elicited and resident human peritoneal macrophages. *Infect Immunol* 49:212–218, 1985.

24. Wierusz-Wysocka B, Wysocki H, Michta G, Wykretowicz A, Czarnecki R, Baczyk K: Phagocytosis and neutrophil bactericidal capacity in patients with uremia. *Folia Haematol* 111:589–594, 1984.

25. Huttunen K, Lampainen E, Silvennoinen-Kassinen S, Tiilikainen A: The neutrophil function of uremic patients treated by hemodialysis or CAPD. *Scand J Urol Nephrol* 18:167–172, 1984.

26. Duwea K, Vas SI, Weatherhead JW: The effect of the composition of peritoneal dialysis fluid on chemiluminescence phagocytosis and bactericidal activity *in vitro. Infect Immunol* 33:130–135, 1981.

27. Harvey DM, Sheppard KJ, Morgan AG, Fletcher J: Effect of dialysate fluids on phagocytosis and killing by normal neutrophils. *J Clin Microbiol* 25:1424–1427, 1987.

28. McGregor SJ, Brock JH, Briggs JD, Junor BJ: Bactericidal activity of peritoneal macrophages from continuous ambulatory dialysis patients. *Nephrol Dial Transplant* 2:104–108, 1987.

29. Alobaidi HM, Coles GA, Davies M, Lloyd D: Host defense in continuous ambulatory peritoneal dialysis: the effect of dialysate on phagocyte function. *Nephrol Dial Transplant* 1:16–21, 1986.

30. Millikin SP, Matzke GR, Keane WF: Antimicrobial treatment of peritonitis associated with continuous ambulatory peritoneal dialysis. *Perit Dial Int* 11:252–260, 1991.

31. Keane WF, Everett ED, Golper TA, Gokal R, Halstenson C, Kawaguchi Y, Riella M, Vas S, Verbrugh HA: Peritoneal dialysis-related peritonitis treatment recommendations. 1993 update. The Ad Hoc Advisory Committee on Peritonitis Management. International Society for Peritoneal Dialysis. *Perit Dial Int* 13:14–28, 1993.

32. Gilbert DN: Once-daily aminoglycoside therapy. *Antimicrob Agents Chemother* 35:399–405, 1991.

33. Haqqie SS, Bailie GR, Eisele G: Once-daily gentamicin and once-weekly vancomycin intraperitoneally to treat CAPD peritonitis (abstract). *Perit Dial Int* 14:S79, 1994.

34. Weaver ME, Dunbeck DC: Mupirocin (Bactroban) causes permanent structural changes in peritoneal dialysis catheters (abstract). *Perit Dial Int* 14:S20, 1994.

35. Piraino B, Barnardini J, Lutes R, Johnston J, Holley J: Randomized trial of mupirocin at exit site vs oral rifampin to prevent S. Aureus catheter infections (abstract). *Perit Dial Int* 14:S27

36. Poole-Warren LA, Hallett MD, Hone PW, Burden SH, Farrell PC: Vaccination for the prevention of CAPD-associated staphylococcal infection: results of a prospective multicentre clinical trial. *Clin Nephrol* 35:198–206, 1991.

37. Keane WP: *Peritoneal Dialysis International* 16:557–573, 1996.

CHAPTER 59

Dialysis Access: Temporary and Permanent

H. DAVID SHORT, WADE R. ROSENBERG, & GEORGE P. NOON

INTRODUCTION

The evolution of dialysis techniques continues to parallel the development of access devices that may be used on a short-term or a long-term basis. In the brief time since the first edition of this chapter, certain technologies have been relegated to the history of surgery, while new access devices are currently available that bridge the gap between short-term temporary dialysis and chronic dialysis. In this chapter, we will summarize the surgical techniques for inserting and maintaining access devices that we currently utilize for hemodialysis and peritoneal dialysis.

We continue to emphasize that in renal failure patients, dialysis access is a vital technology. Although surgery for establishing access may seem technically minor, when access is no longer available, patients come to the end of their clinical course. Efforts should begin with insertion of the first dialysis access device to conserve dialysis access sites. With proper care and foresight, in most patients, dialysis can be provided for many years.

HEMODIALYSIS

Considerable progress has been made in providing devices for angioaccess since the demonstration by Kolff of the clinical feasibility of hemodialysis (1). Early efforts were restricted to cannulation of peripheral vessels with metal or glass cannulas under direct vision. Because the cannulas thrombosed after use and the vessels had to be ligated when the cannulas were removed, dialysis was limited by the number of peripheral vessels available. This, in effect, meant that only temporary renal failure could be treated.

The introduction in 1960 of the indwelling arteriovenous cannula by Scribner and associates represented the first dialysis access device that could used repeatedly for chronic dialysis (2). This conceptual change was made possible by technological advances of improved biomaterials and the widespread availability of heparin. At present, angioaccess devices can be roughly divided into those for temporary use and those for permanent use. Angioaccess devices for temporary (both short- and intermediate-term) use are utilized temporarily for patients with acute renal failure in whom return of renal function may reasonably be expected. These devices are also useful for patients with chronic renal failure as a temporary measure until a permanent device is available for chronic dialysis. Intermediate-term devices, although useful in some patients for the long term, may require particularly high maintenance when used chronically. Permanent devices make up the majority of devices used for chronic hemodialysis.

Temporary

SHORT-TERM USE

Effective dialysis can be accomplished utilizing cannulas inserted percutaneously into peripheral or central vessels. Early clinical use involved outflow catheters introduced into brachial or femoral arteries, with inflow provided by other catheters introduced into the central or peripheral veins. It later became evident that inflow and outflow could both be provided by percutaneous cannulation of large central veins, avoiding the problems inherent in arterial cannulation.

Shunts

Until the introduction of effective percutaneous catheters, the silastic arteriovenous shunts were the angioaccess of choice for immediate use. Although historically these shunts were a major advance, they are rarely used now in this country. The most popular of the shunts, the Scribner shunt (2), is composed of standardized silastic tubing with teflon connectors and teflon vessel tips of varying sizes and lengths. The outflow of the shunt is provided by direct cannulation of a peripheral artery just proximal to the wrist or ankle and inflow through another cannula in a suitable peripheral vein. These cannulas are connected externally by a teflon connector that can be disconnected for dialysis. Shunts are easily inserted using local anesthesia and can provide immediate dialysis. Ultimately they fail within

Suki, WN and Massry SG (eds), Suki and Massry's Therapy of Renal Diseases and Related Disorders, Third Edition. ISBN 978-1-4757-6634-9.
©*1998, Kluwer Academic Publishers, Boston/Dordrecht/London. All rights reserved.*

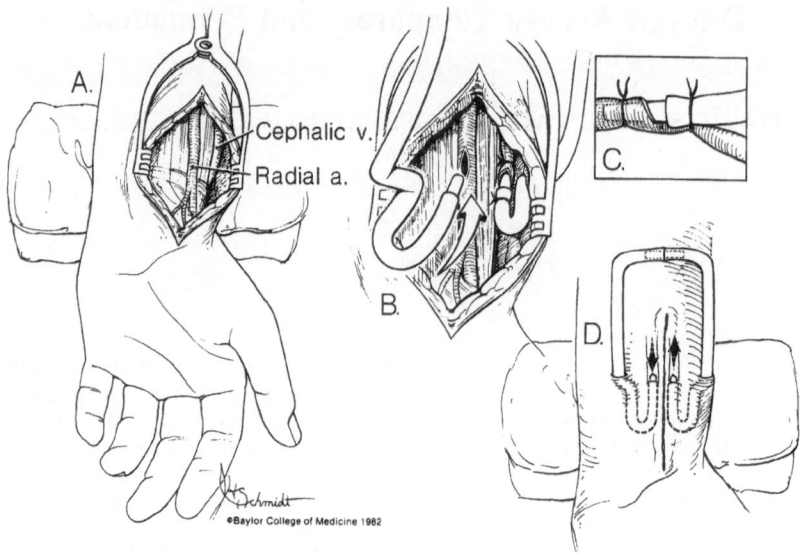

Figure 1. Technique of insertion of hemodialysis cannulas in the radial artery and cephalic vein. **A.** Artery and vein exposed. **B.** Cannulas inserted in the artery and vein. **C.** Cannulas fixed in place with suture ligature. **D.** Cannulas connected while not dialyzing.

weeks or months and so must be considered short-term devices (see Operative Techniques below and Figure 1).

Percutaneous catheters

Separate cannulas may be used in two different veins for outflow and inflow, or a single, large-bore catheter may be used for both. The large catheters can be inserted directly into the subclavian, internal jugular, or femoral vein over a guidewire using the Seldinger technique (3). Single-lumen catheters provide outflow and inflow alternately with recycle. Double-lumen catheters have one lumen for outflow, with another separate lumen that supplies inflow simultaneously. In our experience, double-lumen catheters achieve superior performance and are currently our access of choice for temporary or immediate hemodialysis (Figure 2).

Separate catheters can also be used percutaneously in the arterial and venous systems for continuous arteriovenous hemofiltration (CAVH). Large-bore percutaneous catheters inserted in the common femoral artery and vein are connected in series with a hemoconcentrator for patients with renal insufficiency and fluid overload. Driven by the pressure of the arterial system, this provides a continuous removal of extracellular water, the rate of which may be controlled using a programmable pump on the filtrate line .

Even with meticulous care, the insertion site or tract of catheters inserted for dialysis or CAVH will invariably become contaminated with bacteria. This outcome always limits catheters inserted percutaneously to temporary usage.

INTERMEDIATE-TERM USE

The addition of a velour cuff to subcutaneously tunneled catheters has revolutionized the use of intravascular devices for all sorts of applications. The cuff, which is positioned in the subcutaneous tract, allows fibroblastic ingrowth, preventing ascending infection of the catheter tract. For hemodialysis, these catheters are available for intermediate- or long-term use but can be used immediately after insertion. As such, these catheters conceptually represent a bridge between temporary and permanent devices for hemodialysis. These catheters are inserted using local anesthesia in the operating room under sterile conditions and may be inserted into the central venous circulation through the subclavian, internal jugular, or femoral veins (Figure 3). The velour cuff is placed in the subcutaneous tunnel immediately subjacent to the exit site, close enough to facilitate later removal but deep enough to avoid cuff extrusion. The advent of peel-apart introducer sheaths has greatly facilitated the insertion of these catheters. With the increased use of large-bore central venous catheters for hemodialysis, the incidence of subclavian vein stenosis or thrombosis has become more common. For this reason, the internal jugular vein or femoral vein is preferable to the subclavian vein for temporary catheter insertion. Although tunneled silastic catheters have been used in some patients for longer than a year, they generally require much higher maintenance than chronic fistulas. For this reason, these catheters have found their greatest utility as an intermediate-term device.

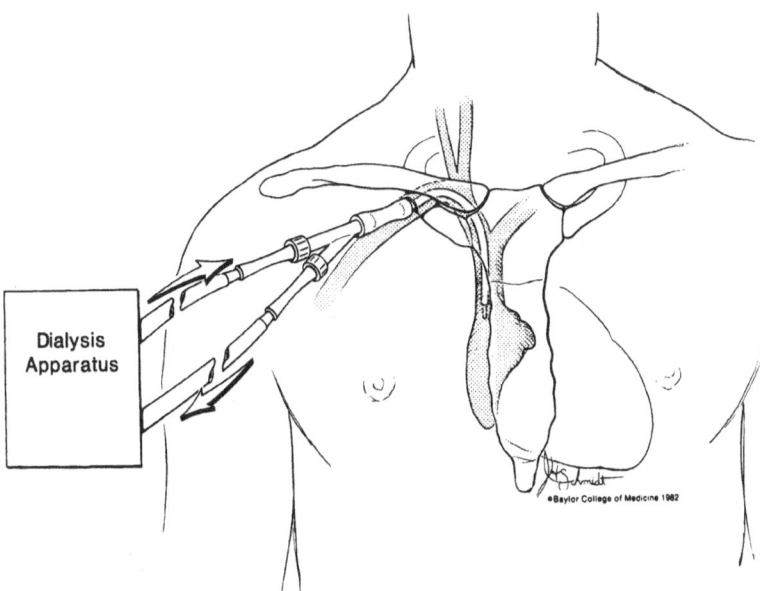

Figure 2. Double-lumen hemodialysis catheter introduced via the right subclavian evin.

COMPLICATIONS OF SHORT-TERM AND
INTERMEDIATE-TERM DEVICES

Infection

Infection is a common complication of intravascular catheters inserted percutaneously for any purpose. Subcutaneous tunneling and the addition of a subcutaneous cuff, with or without antimicrobial activity has dramatically reduced the incidence of infections but has not eliminated infections entirely. Infections may present with redness or exudate at the exit site, or as systemic sepsis. These infections generally resolve with removal of the catheter and a short course of
antibiotics.

Stenosis/thrombosis

The incidence of subclavian vein stenosis and thrombosis increased after the introduction of large-bore, percutaneous dialysis catheters. Stenosis and thrombosis are manifested by poor dialysis through the catheter or edema in the upper extremity and are easily demonstrated by injecting radiocontrast through the catheter. Edema in the upper extremity may resolve with minimally invasive techniques such as thrombolytic therapy, percutaneous balloon angioplasty, or stenting. If the stenosis is above a functioning fistula or if thrombosis propagates to involve the jugular if innominate veins, the disorders likely will not respond to minimal efforts (see Surgical Correction of Venous Obstruction below).

Permanent

At the present time, most long-term dialysis is achieved by means of arteriovenous fistula. In the parlance of angioaccess, fistulas differ from shunts in that fistulas are totally internal, whereas shunts are at least partially external. Fistulas may involve either a direct arteriovenous anastomosis or a conduit of tissue of prosthetic origin. Most fistulas require some delay before use, so if immediate hemodialysis is required, short-term devices are used simultaneously.

PRIMARY FISTULAS

Direct arteriovenous anastomosis between the radial artery and cephalic vein for dialysis access was first described by Brescia (4). Blood flowing from the radial artery distends the superficial venous system of the arm. After the veins dilate sufficiently, they may be used for hemodialysis outflow and inflow by means of needles inserted percutaneously. Since several weeks to months are required for the veins to dilate, the veins are generally not available for immediate use. An exception to this is when a previously constructed radial–cephalic shunt has been in place long enough for venous dilatation to occur. After direct arteriovenous anastomosis, the veins remain dilated, and immediate dialysis is possible.

Primary arteriovenous fistulas have several advantages over graft fistulas. First, no foreign material except suture is implanted, so infection is rare. Second, patency rates are higher with primary arteriovenous fistulas. Finally, primary

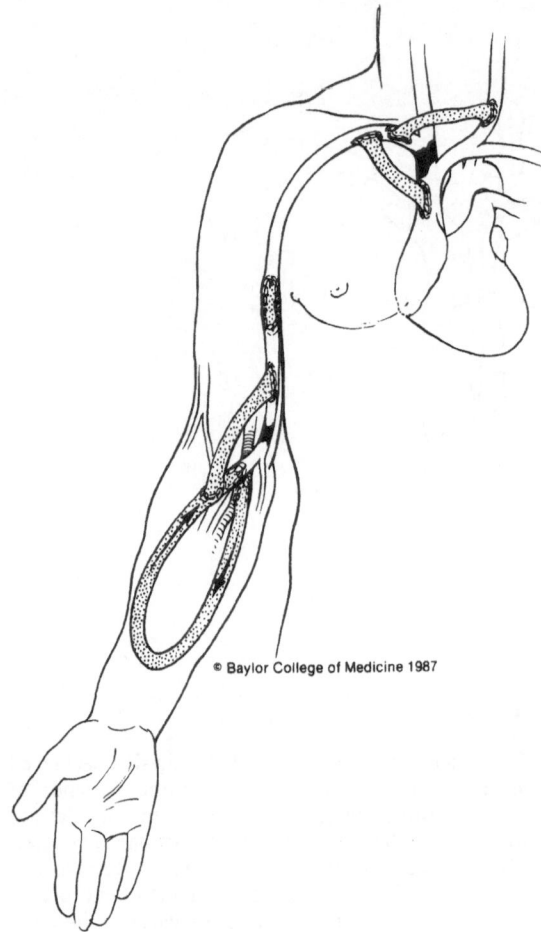

© Baylor College of Medicine 1987

Figure 3. Subcutancously tunneled catheter with velour cuff.

arteriovenous fistulas require very little maintenance. These are such attractive features that we use primary fistulas whenever possible, but proper selection of suitable candidates requires considerable judgment.

If arterial flow into the fistula is inadequate, thrombosis usually occurs. If the flow is only marginal or limited by fixed obstruction, the veins may never dilate enough to be usable. Older patients with arteriosclerosis may not be good candidates for a radial–cephalic fistula for this reason. Patients who have small arm veins, or whose veins have been obliterated by frequent vein punctures or phlebitis, are not suitable candidates for primary arteriovenous fistulas. Finally, patients with very fat arms and deep veins may not be good candidates for primary fistulas because the veins are not easy to access.

Some patients may have inadequate veins in the distal portion of the arm, but adequate veins more proximally.

Primary fistulas constructed using the brachial artery and cephalic or basilic veins have been recommended by some authors, although we would initially prefer to use a graft in this situation. The key to initial success with primary arteriovenous fistulas is selection of patients with adequate arteries and veins with which to construct satisfactory fistulas.

Operative techniques (Figure 4)

Construction of a primary radial–cephalic fistula can be accomplished using local anesthesia supplemented with mild intravenous sedation. A single longitudinal incision placed between the course of the cephalic vein and radial artery is adequate to expose both vessels. Each vessel is mobilized for several centimeters so that it may be anastomosed without tension. The anastomosis may be constructed as a side-to-side, end-vein to side-artery, end-artery to side-vein, or end-to-end configuration. Whenever contemplating interruption of the radial artery, the existence of an intact palmar arch with normal ulnar flow must be ascertained to avoid ischemia of the hand.

Systemic anticoagulation with intravenous heparin is used to prevent clot formation during the creation of the fistula. Topical papaverine is also sometimes employed to reduce vessel spasm, which may make the anastomosis more difficult and also may result in low flow and thrombosis of the fistula. The cephalic vein is clamped distally and opened with a longitudinal incision. It may not be necessary to clamp the vein proximally if valves prevent backflow. Dilators of up to 4 mm in diameter are gently passed proximally to ensure adequate lumen size and patency. Flushing the vein proximally with heparinized saline will allow estimation of venous resistance. The artery is then clamped proximally and distally. The artery is opened longitudinally and then anastomosed to the vein using a running 7–0 or 8–0 polypropylene suture and loop magnification. As the suture line is completed, before tying, the dilator is again passed proximally in each vessel to ensure patency. The artery and vein are then flushed to remove any clot or debris, the clamps are removed, and the suture line is tied. At this point, there should be an easily palpable pulse and thrill in the vein proximal to the anastomosis. Each of the limbs is checked to be sure that it lies without kinking or undue tension. Protamine sulfate is given to reverse the heparin, and when hemostasis is adequate, the wound is closed in two layers.

Complications

Complications with primary arteriovenous fistulas are uncommon. Because they are constructed with autogenous tissue, infections almost never occur. When they do, they are usually superficial wound infections and the fistulas continue to function.

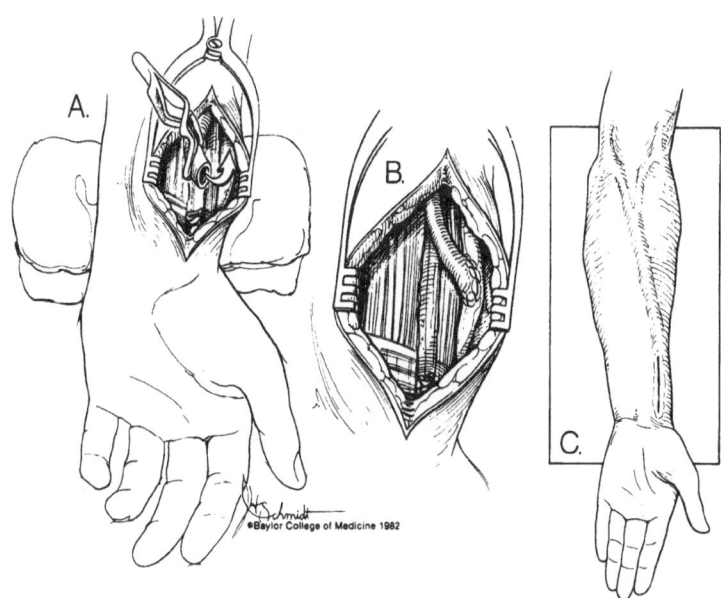

Figure 4. Construction of an arteriovenous fistula for hemodialysis utillizing the radial artery and cephalic vein. **A.** readial artery isolated and transected. **B.** An end-artery to side-vein anastomosis. **C.** Cephalic vein distends and is used for dialysis.

Thrombosis. Thrombosis is the most common complication of primary arteriovenous fistulas. If it occurs early, either the vessels were inadequate to support flow or a technical error has been committed. If thrombosis occurs late, obstruction of flow by localized stenosis in the venous system or hyperplasia at the anastomosis should be suspected. Sometimes, in critically ill patients, an episode of hypotension may be enough to cause thrombosis in an adequately functioning fistula. Thrombosis in native vessels should be corrected as soon as possible because undue delay may make correction impossible. We generally employ systemic heparinization for thrombectomy. These cases may be prolonged and tedious, and systemic heparinization prevents rethrombosis in the limbs after the clot is removed and obviates the need for excessive flushing.

The anastomosis should be exposed and inspected. A twist or kink severe enough to cause thrombosis should be obvious on initial inspection. In a new fistula, the anastomosis is taken down to thrombectomize the afferent and efferent limbs. In an older fistula, a longitudinal incision in the vein at the level of the anastomosis may be adequate. The thrombus is easily removed with a #2, #3 or #4 Fogarty catheter. A #4 Fogarty catheter has a balloon diameter of 9 mm, generally larger than any radial artery. Care must be taken when using this catheter not to overdistend and damage the radial artery. Inflow from the radial artery adequate enough to sustain a fistula is easily estimated by merely flushing this vessel.

Thrombosis of an older fistula is often due to poor outflow with increasing venous resistance. After the venous limb has been disobliterated, it may be checked for stenosis by passing dilators or a Fogarty catheter or by flushing heparinized saline into the venous limb. Resistance to the flow of saline is a clue to obstruction somewhere in the venous limb. If the exact location of stenosis is not easily determined, intraoperative venography after thrombectomy may localize the area responsible for thrombosis. Localized areas of venous obstruction may be amenable to patch-graft angioplasty or segmental resection and repair by primary anastomosis or graft interposition (Figure 5). Fistulas that have functioned well initially but thrombose later are worth strenuous attempts at repair, even if this requires graft interposition in the arterial or venous limbs. If flow can be reestablished in these cases, function can often be restored for prolonged periods (Figure 6). However, primary fistulas that fail very early and require elaborate reconstruction are probably best abandoned in favor of a graft fistula. If it can be determined whether the failure is due to inadequate inflow or outflow, that limb can be replaced with a conduit to a more proximal vessel.

Aneurysms. Aneurysms may occur along the course of the venous limb of primary fistulas. These may be true aneurysms due to dilatation of the vein by arterial pressure, or false aneurysms formed by frequent punctures for dialysis. In contrast to graft fistulas, aneurysms of primary fistulas rarely cause problems that require surgical correction.

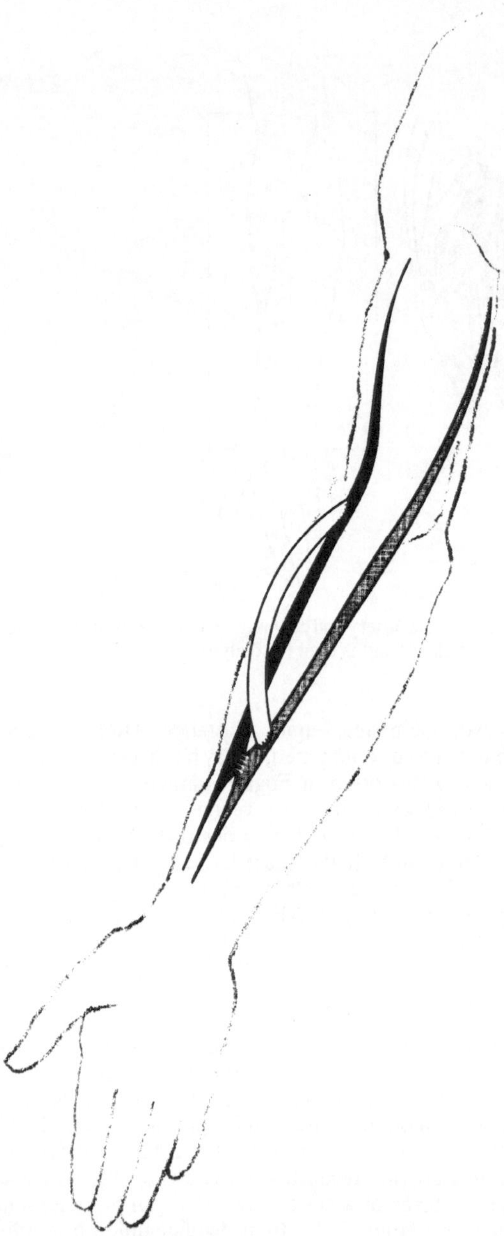

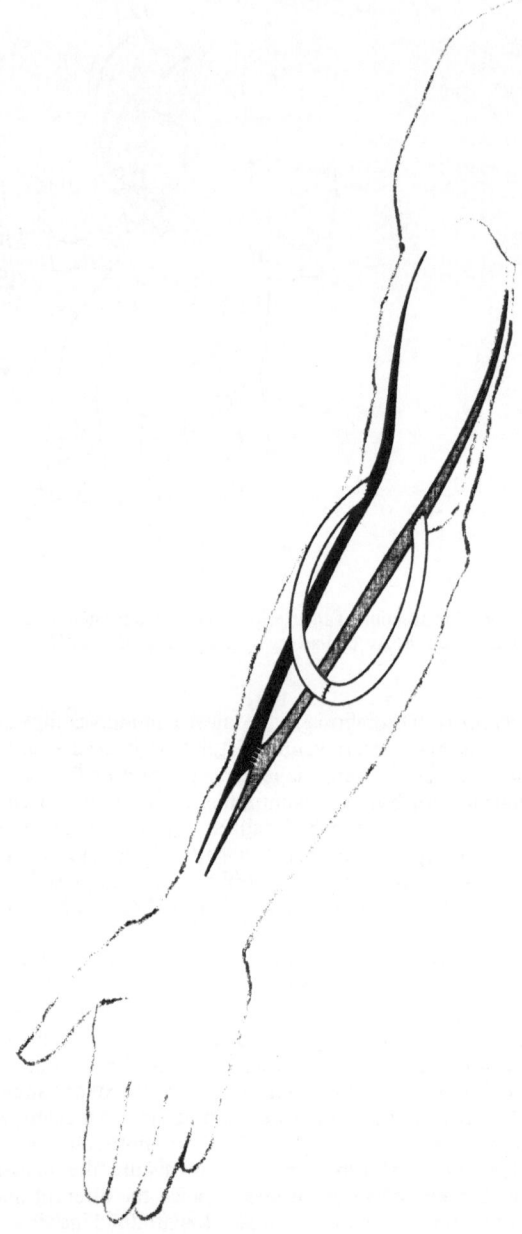

Figure 5. Graft interposition repair of primary fistula.

Figure 6. Conversim of primary Fistula to loop graftfistula.

Venous hypertension

The success of primary arteriovenous fistulas depends upon flow to dilate prominently proximal veins enough to be used for dialysis. Sometimes, however, the venous dilatation occurs in the distal veins across the dorsum of the hand. It may occur less commonly in end-vein to side artery, and it can occur without apparent proximal obstruction in the cephalic vein. In these cases, presumably there is less resistance exists in the distal cephalic vein than the proximal cephalic vein, and blood flows preferentially, or at least equally across the hand. Edema of the hand may be quite severe and may produce nonhealing ulcers on the digits. Ligation of the cephalic vein distal to the anastomosis may be required to relieve the venous hypertension causing the hand edema. Venous hypertension of later onset in a previously well-functioning fistula should alert one to the development of proximal venous stenosis. Palpation of the vein for a pressure differential may localize the area of obstruction. A "fistulogram" performed at this time should reveal the area of obstruction, and timely surgical intervention will not only relieve the obstruction but also help avoid future thrombosis.

GRAFT FISTULA

Although primary fistulas may function satisfactorily for many years, ultimately they, like shunts, fail as distal vessels fail. The solution to the problem of inadequate distal peripheral vessels has been aided by the introduction of graft fistulas. These large-caliber conduits, anastomosed to more proximal vessels, provide adequate flow for hemodialysis. They are placed subcutaneously, so puncture is easy, and repeated puncture causes no direct damage to the native circulation. Because there is a tunnel through which the graft is placed, early puncture of the graft for dialysis can result in perigraft hematoma until healing around the graft has occurred. For this reason, a period of several weeks is required for graft "maturation." If immediate dialysis is required, it is best supplied by some other access.

Graft fistulas are inserted in the operating room, using local anesthesia with intravenous sedation. Prophylactic antibiotics with activity against gram-positive organisms are begun before the procedure. In patients with some renal function, we generally use a cephalosporin antibiotic; cephalosporins have cidal activity and a low incidence of toxicity or allergy. In patients with no renal function, vancomycin is a good alternative. This drug is nondialyzable, so only one dose is needed; in addition, its major toxicity (nephrotoxicity) is no factor in functionally anephric patients.

Historically, various conduits have been used for graft fistulas: autogenous or homograft veins, and Dacron and bovine grafts (5). Our present choice of graft material is a PTFE straight tube graft (6). This graft is easy to use, readily available, and has low porosity. This last feature is important whenever systemic heparinization is used for graft insertion. PTFE grafts have demonstrated good patency rates over long periods of time. Grafts allowed to mature show a low incidence of false aneurysm formation, and true aneurysms are now rare. In addition, graft infections, should they occur, are easier to control with less risk of hemorrhage compared with the other graft materials available. We generally prefer 8-mm grafts because they are easy to puncture and it is easy maintain a large lumen after neotintima has formed. six-mm grafts are preferable in patients with small native vessels or in diabetics in whome the risk of steal is increased.

Operative technique (Figure 7)

Grafts are generally placed as loops on the volar aspect of the nondominant forearm. The vessels are exposed through a single transverse incision in the antecubital fossa distal to the flexion crease. Since finding an adequate vein is more often problematic than finding an adequate artery, the vein sought first. The cephalic, basilic, or median cubital veins are used most commonly. If none of these is adequate, the deep brachial veins around the artery are used.

The brachial artery is exposed by incising the aponeurosis of the biceps muscle and is mobilized proximally and distally for several centimeters. The arterial anastomosis is usually performed first. The brachial artery is clamped proximally and distally and is opened through a longitudinal arteriotomy. The graft is anastomosed with a running 7–0 Prolene suture. After the suture line is completed, the brachial artery is flushed through the graft to remove any clot of debris. Heparinized saline is then flushed back through the graft, which is then clamped just distal to the anastomosis with a rubber-shod hemostat. At this point, blood flow is reestablished though the brachial artery.

Some authors have recommended primary construction of a straight graft, sewing the arterial anastomosis on the radial or ulnar artery and the venous anastomosis at the antecubital fossa. If the graft becomes infected, the entire graft can be removed and the vessel sacrificed, if necessary, to control the infection. There may also be a decrease incidence of steal. In our experience, these circumstances do not compensate for the lesser flow provided by the radial or ulnar artery.

After infiltrating the path in the arm with xylocaine, the graft is then passed through a subcutaneous loop in the forearm. This process is facilitated by making a second incision at the apex of the loop. The graft is first delivered from the incision in the antecubital fossa into the distal incision, then back into the incision in the antecubital fossa near the selected vein. This may be done using a special tunneler or a long, narrow clamp. Care should be taken to avoid kinking or twisting the graft. If systemic heparinization is employed, it is helpful to develop this tract before anticoagulation is undertaken.

With the arterial anastomosis completed first, it is possible at this point to remove the proximal clamp and, compressing the graft distally, to fill the graft with blood. The arterial pressure will distend the graft filled with heparinized blood, showing how it lies in the subcutaneous tunnel.

The vein is then clamped proximally and distally. It is opened through a longitudinal incision, and dilators of up to 4 mm are passed proximally to check for any areas of unsuspected stenosis. Heparinized saline is flushed proximally in the vein. Any resistance to flow should alert one to significant proximal venous obstruction, which could lead to early graft thrombosis. If the vein is satisfactory, the graft is cut to length and sutured to the venotomy with a running 7–0 Prolene suture. When this suture line is com-

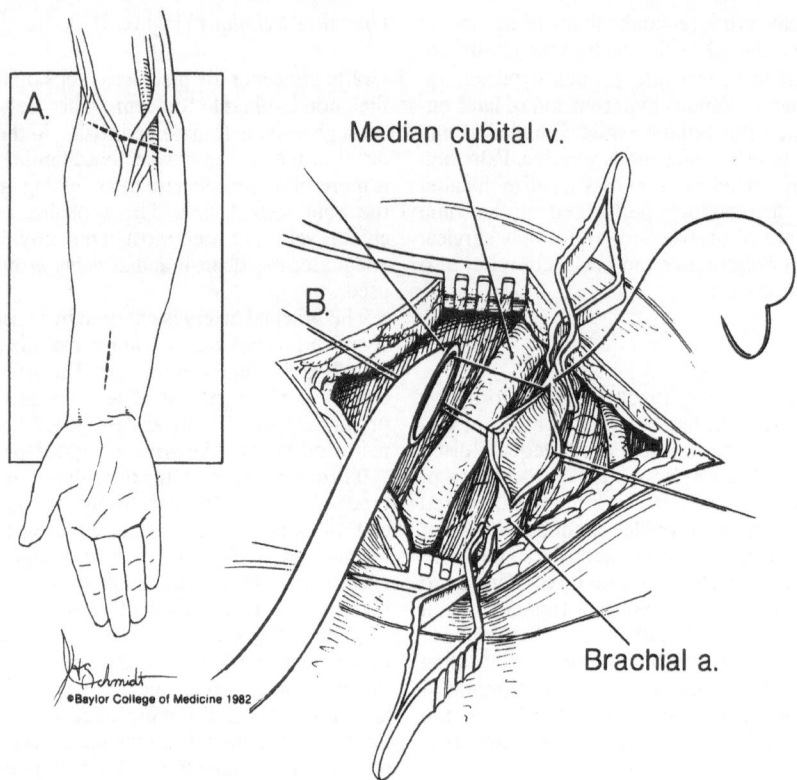

Figure 7. **A.** Incisions used for implantation of hemodialysis access graft. **B.** Anastomosis of the graft to the brachial artery. **C,D.** Graft is tunneled subcutaneously in the forearm. **E.** Graft is anastomosed to the median cubital vein. **F.** Functioning graft at completion of the procedure.

pleted, the clamps are removed, establishing flow from the brachial artery through the graft into the vein. There should be a palpable pulse and thrill in the vein at this time. The outflow from the vein may be so good that the graft pulse is very weak. Momentary compression of the vein or graft will then produce an increased graft pulse, demonstrating adequate inflow with low outflow resistance. Other causes of low graft pressure are poor arterial inflow, graft thrombosis, twisting or kinking, and hypotension.

There is generally very little bleeding from the suture line using 7–0 suture. When hemostasis is adequate, the wounds are then closed over the graft in two layers, completing the procedure.

Complications

Some of the operative techniques for complications differ from those used with the original procedures and need special emphasis. The operative correction of complications of graft fistulas can usually be accomplished using local anesthesia with intravenous sedation. This procedure is performed in the operating room using strict sterile technique. We routinely employ antibiotics directed against gram-positive organisms in the perioperative period. In cases of known infection, we use antibiotics with documented activity against the offending organism. Because the operation may be prolonged or complicated, systemic anticoagulation with heparin is often used, which allows the graft to be clamped at any level without fear of thrombosis and minimizes the blood loss due to flushing. Once reconstruction is accomplished, the heparin is reversed with protamine sulfate to decrease the risk of bleeding or hematoma formation.

Extensive dissection during graft revision may create dead spaces adjacent to the graft. To avoid hematoma formation or perigraft fluid collection, small closed-suction drains are sometimes inserted. These are fashioned from butterfly I.V. catheters by cutting off the hub and cutting several side holes in the tubing. These catheters are brought out through the wound, and the needles are inserted into sterile vacutainer tubes. The drains are removed from the wound whenever drainage ceases, usually about 2 or 3 days later.

Angiograms are employed frequently in the evaluation of graft complications. The cause of edema or high graft resistance by venous obstruction may be diagnosed by and arm, where grafts are implanted. Doppler studies at the wrist or digital pulse volume recordings may demonstrate markedly reduced flow, which augments to normal with temporary graft compression. In the absence of abnormal peripheral nerve studies, this finding is evidence for a steal syndrome contributing to the symptom of hand pain distal to a dialysis fistula. Duplex scanning may be used to directly image areas of aneurysm formation, pseudointimal buildup, or other sites of obstruction.

Occlusion. Graft occlusion is the most common complication of graft fistulas. Thrombosis can be dealt with on an elective basis because, in contrast to thrombosis in a native vessel, the thrombus does not become adherent to the graft. In fact, PTFE grafts can often be disobliterated months after occlusion. When occlusion occurs early after insertion, technical problems, poor inflow or runoff, or hypotension should be suspected. The graft must be examined, and if an obvious technical problem exists, it must be corrected. After thrombectomy, the adequacy of arterial inflow and venous outflow should be reassessed. Poor inflow from the brachial artery should be a rare cause of early graft occlusion; it is easily evaluated by flushing the brachial artery, and it should have been obvious at the time of initial graft insertion. Inflow that was initially brisk but diminished after graft insertion should alert one to the possibility of iatrogenic stenosis or dissection of the brachial artery. Efforts should then be directed toward the detection and correction of these technical errors.

Poor venous outflow may be due to venous narrowing near the anastomosis or more proximally in the vein. Passing dilators proximally in the vein will give an estimation of the lumen of the vein, and flushing heparinized saline proximally can give an appreciation of the impedence to flow. Stenosis of the vein may be correctable with patch angioplasty or may require graft interposition proximally to the same vein or a different vein to establish adequate outflow.

If no obvious cause of early graft occlusion is found, intraoperative angiography of the graft may be performed after thrombectomy renders the graft functional. This procedure may demonstrate areas of stenosis that were not demonstrable by any other means.

Late graft occlusion may be precipitated by obvious causes. Occlusion may result from a period of hypotension in a critically ill patient. Once the cause of hypotension is corrected and the patient is stable, reestablishment of graft patency is easily accomplished by simple thrombectomy. Thrombosis of a graft can also result from placement of a compression dressing or blood pressure cuff above the graft. Should thrombosis occur, simple thrombectomy will again reestablish graft patency. Early puncture of a PTFE graft can result in perigraft hematoma formation before "maturation" of the graft has occurred. We generally allow 2–4 weeks of healing around a graft before use. If hematoma formation with occlusion does occur, the hematoma must be evacuated when thrombectomy of the graft is performed.

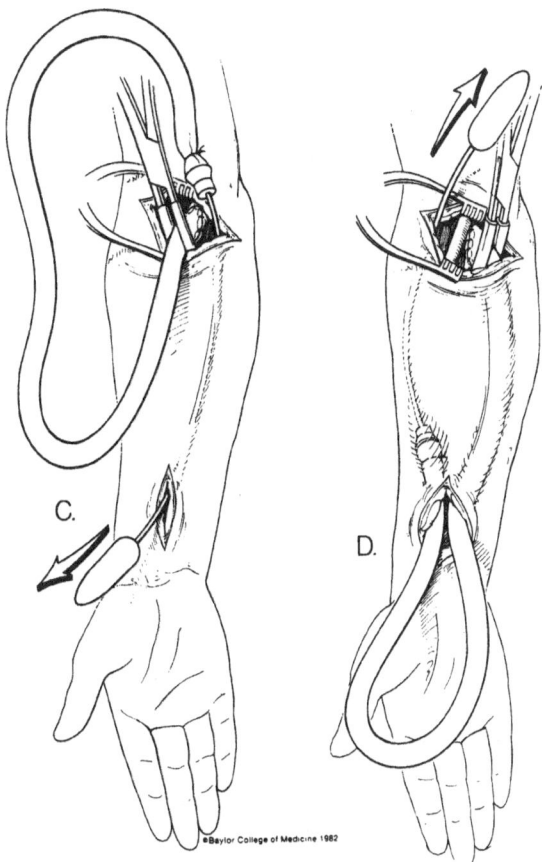

Figure 7. (continued).

angiography, which helps to plan elective revision to relieve edema, and high resistance and may help to prevent subsequent graft thrombosis. Intraoperatively, after thrombectomy of a graft, angiography may demonstrate mechanical causes for graft thrombosis that cannot be discerned by other methods. Unusual graft configurations or diffuse venous dilitation can be distinguished from an aneurysm of the graft or native vessels, thereby avoiding unnecessary exploration of what externally appears to be an aneurysm.

Thrombolytic therapy. Streptokinase or urokinase may have a role in the treatment of thrombosis of grafts due to iatrogenic factors or hypotension. However, if the graft has occluded spontaneously, thrombolysis will not suffice, because invariably a problem exists that requires surgical correction.

Noninvasive studies. Noninvasive vascular studies play a part in the differentiation of pain syndromes in the hand

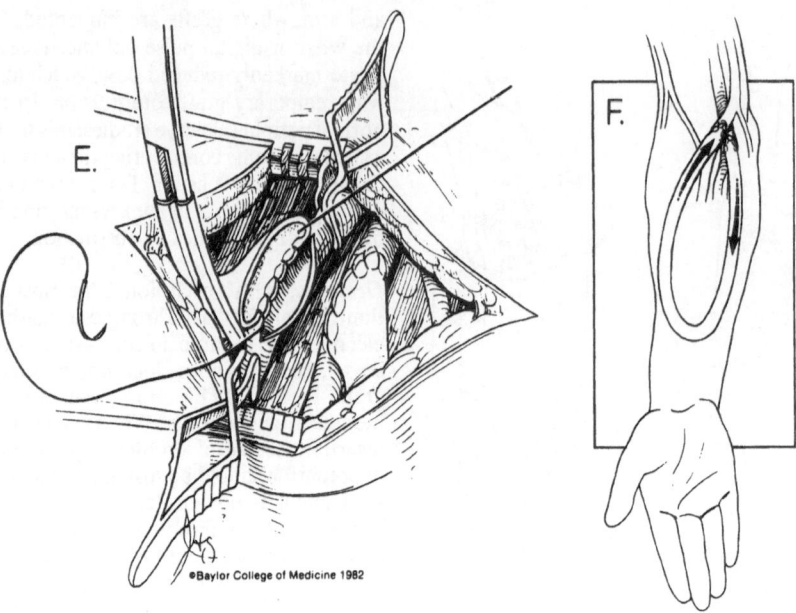

Figure 7. (continued).

Prevention of compression occlusion of the graft by bandages or hematoma should be possible through proper education of the medical staff who deal with chronic renal failure patients.

Most late graft occlusions occur without an obvious precipitating event. Reexploration of the graft is necessary, which generally exposes the venous anastomosis first (Figure 8). The most common etiology in the circumstance is pseudointimal buildup, especially at the venous anastomosis. After the patient is systemically anticoagulated with heparin, the graft is opened just proximal to the venous anastomosis using a longitudinal incision. The thrombectomy is accomplished with a 5F or 7F Fogarty catheter. Use of a large catheter with only partial balloon inflation is helpful, because the balloon will not be as easily disrupted by the rough inner surface of the graft. Care must be taken to avoid overdistention and injury to native vessels. Dilators may then be passed through the anastomosis and up into the vein to identify any areas of narrowing. Narrowing of the anastomosis due to pseudointimal buildup is corrected by patch-graft angioplasty. The incision is extended through the anastomosis and onto the vein past the pseudointimal buildup. The Fogarty catheter is passed proximally into the graft to remove the thrombus back to the arterial anastomosis. The graft is flushed to remove any clot or debris and can be clamped, since the patient is systemically heparinized. Finally, the incision is closed using a Gore-Tex patch and running 5-0, 6-0, or 7-0 Prolene suture. Occasionally it will be difficult to pass the Fogarty catheter back to the arterial anastomosis and to adequately

thrombectomize the graft. In this case, a second incision is made in the graft, near the arterial anastomosis, and the catheter is then passed in both directions to remove the thrombus. Control of bleeding from the brachial artery during thrombectomy is easy with simple manual compression. The incision on the arterial limb of the graft, however, should be placed far enough from the arterial anastomosis so that after thrombectomy the graft can be clamped for proximal control. This obviates any need for direct exposure or clamping of the native artery. In some patients, pseudointimal buildup within the graft becomes calcified or rough in areas frequently punctured. We have employed intraluminal scrapers to dislodge this pseudointima and smooth the intraluminal surface.

If the venous anastomosis and outflow appear adequate, the arterial anastomosis and inflow should be evaluated. Although uncommon, pseudointimal buildup at the arterial anastomosis can produce sufficient narrowing to precipitate thrombosis. This is corrected by extending the graft incision through the arterial anastomosis and performing a patch-graft angioplasty. Proximal control of the brachial artery in these cases must be established either by exposing the vessel and clamping it directly or by inserting balloon catheters to occluded the lumen while sewing on the patch.

Whenever a patch-graft angioplasty is performed on the arterial or venous anastomosis, the running suture of the previous anastomosis is obviously divided. This is not a problem in a healed graft, because separation of the graft from the native vessel with false aneurysm formation does

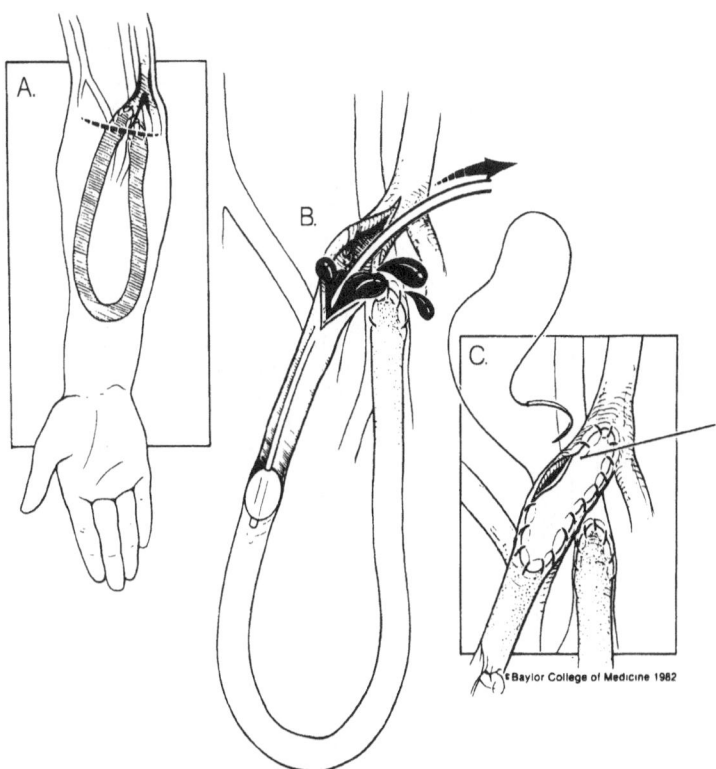

Figure 8. **A.** Thrombosis of a hemodialysis access graft secondary to intimal hyperplasia at the venous anastomosis. **B.** Thrombectomy performed. **C.** Patch-graft angioplasty of the venous anastomosis.

not occur. However, if possible, the new suture can be tied to the old or interrupted sutures can be placed on either side of the incision to secure it.

Venous obstruction more proximal in the arm may lead to graft occlusion. Localized areas can sometimes be dilated, or, once identified, can be exposed directly and treated with local patch angioplasty. Serial obstructions of long narrow segments in the upper arm vein are best treated by bypass. A Gore-Tex interposition from the venous limb of the dialysis graft to the vein above the obstruction or to another vein in the upper arm will reestablish the outflow. We have experienced no difficulty with graft occlusions due to the interposition grafts extended across the flexion crease of the antecubital fossa.

Infection. Dialysis graft infections may be localized or may involve the entire graft. Before graft maturation occurs, infections often involve the entire length of the graft. These infections may require total graft removal for control, but because fibroblastic ingrowth has not occurred, it may be accomplished relatively easily. After healing around the graft has occurred, infections are often localized by the firm adherence of surrounding tissue to the graft. These infections are often at a puncture site or an area of skin break-

down over a false aneurysm. If the infection can be controlled by the administration of appropriate antibiotics, the wound may heal over the exposed graft. If healing does not occur, a cure may be accomplished in a three-step proceedure. Initially, the infection is incised and drained, and the graft is defunctionalized. Later, the contaminated segment is excised and the wound allowed to heal. Finally, the graft is reconstructed through uninfected tissue. This conservative approach to graft infection is really only applicable to PTFE grafts because biologic grafts have a much greater risk of rupture or hemorrhage. Ultimately, even some PTFE grafts have to be ligated and removed due to bleeding or uncontrollable sepsis.

Aneurysms (Figure 9). True aneurysms are much more common with bovine grafts and vein conduits. False aneurysms from punctures occur with equal frequency in biologic and prosthetic grafts. Aneurysms can cause problems of bleeding, skin ulceration with infection, or graft thrombosis and are best repaired before complications arise. Segmental resection and graft interposition are usually employed. Proximal and distal control may be gained by direct exposure of the graft on both sides of the aneurysm. An alternative is temporary compression of the graft

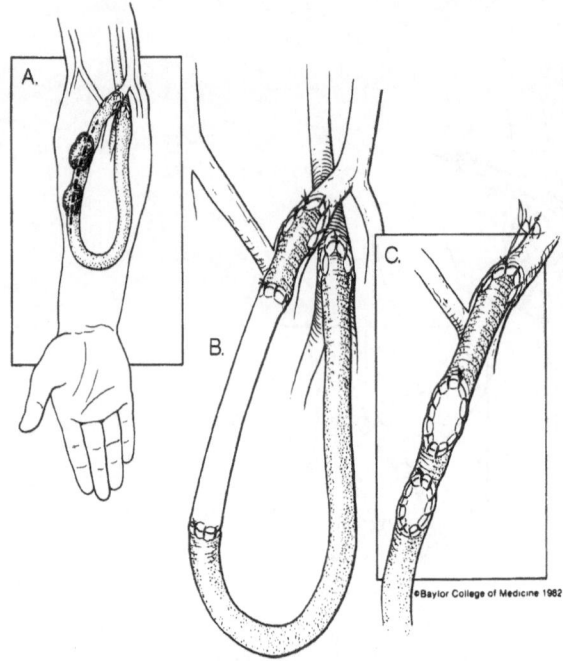

Figure 9. **A.** Aneurysms of a hemodialysis access graft. **B.** Resection of aneurysms and graft replacement. **C.** Resection of aneurysm and patch-graft angioplasty.

while the aneurysm is opened directly. Balloon catheters may then be inserted into the graft for proximal and distal control. After gaining control, the aneurysm is resected and a segment of Gore-Tex is interposed using 4–0 Prolene for the anastomosis. Drains may be employed around the graft to avoid fluid collection in the space created by the aneurysm resection.

Steal. When resistance is very low in an arteriovenous graft fistula, diminished flow in the hand may occur. This will be manifested by a painful, cool, pale hand, with diminished or absent radial pulse. Momentary compression of the graft will restore a normal radial pulse, demonstrating the existence of a steal syndrome. Patients may complain of numbness or parathesias in the hand, which must be distinguished from neuropathy or carpal tunnel syndrome. When symptoms occur immediately after graft insertion, they usually improve with time, and expectant treatment is warranted. In a few cases, the graft has to be ligated to relieve the symptoms or, rarely, reverse ischemic changes in the hand.

Congestive failure. On very rare occasions, flow through a graft fistula will compose so much of the cardiac output that congestive failure occurs. This outcome usually takes place in patients with limited cardiac reserve from intrinsic cardiac disease. It may be possible to limit flow though the graft by narrowing the graft or interposing a smaller segment of graft. If this does not suffice, the graft will require ligation and dialysis must be supplied by other means.

Edema. Edema, along with erythema and tenderness, around a newly inserted Gore-Tex graft fistula is common. The swelling may extend into the upper arm and down to the hand, and may be accompanied by low-grade fever. This inflammatory reaction usually resolves spontaneously in several weeks, but is aided by elevation of the extremity. Edema that is persistent or appears late is abnormal. Persistent inflammation, high fevers, or purulent drainage may signify infection. A Gram stain and cultures should be taken and appropriate antibiotic coverage instituted. Edema without inflammation is rarely due to lymphatic obstruction and may be the first clue to venous outflow obstruction. If allowed to go untreated, severe skin changes, including brawny edema and ulceration, can occur. Graft angiography should be employed to localize areas of venous obstruction.

SURGICAL CORRECTION OF VENOUS OBSTRUCTION (Figure 10)

Obstruction to the venous outflow at any level above a functioning arteriovenous fistula can result in severe edema of the extremity below the level of obstruction. The higher the level of venous obstruction, the more of the arm will be involved in the edema process. A localized area of stenosis in the arm vein may be treated with patch angioplasty or localized bypasses, balloon angioplasty, or stents. Stenosis in the central circulation at the level of the subclavian or innominate vein may require bypasses to other veins in the central venous circulation to correct upper-extremity edema. Occasionally a functioning graft will have to be ligated in order to allow the resolution of upper-extremity edema. In spite of the persistent obstruction of the central venous circulation, ligation of the functioning graft normally will provide adequate resolution of edema in the extremity. Edema that has been allowed to progress to severe degrees may be slow to resolve, even after the obstruction has been relieved (Figure 8).

Increased resistance

Increased resistance and high venous pressures on dialysis may also be an early clue to venous outflow obstruction. If relieved early, graft thrombosis may be averted. Graft angiography is very useful to demonstrate areas of obstruction that may be amenable to correction, either by surgery, balloon dilitation, or stenting.

Pain

Persistent pain or late development of pain in the hand below a graft fistula is an occasional complaint. Since some of the causes are remediable, it is important to estab-

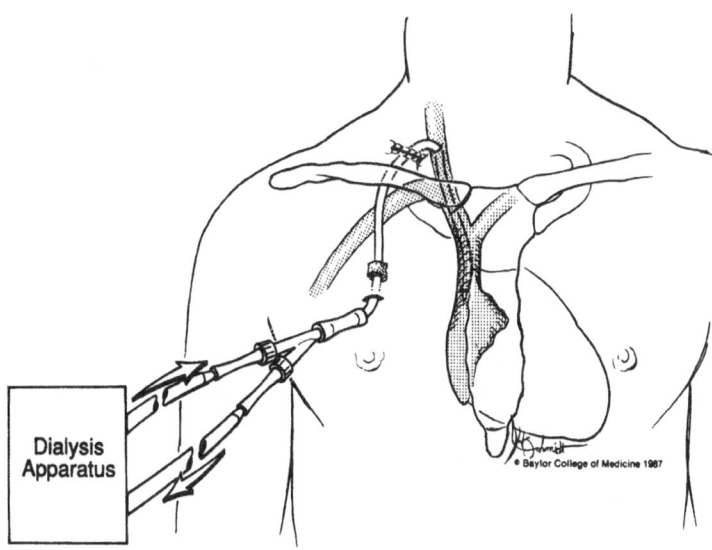

Figure 10. Surgical correction of venous obstruction.

lish the etiology in each specific case. Angiography, noninvasive vascular studies, and nerve conduction studies are helpful to distinguish the various syndrome that may cause pain.

Generalized neuropathy in renal failure patients may cause hand pain. Neuropathic pain is especially common in diabetic patients, but so is steal syndrome. Nerve conduction studies should show decreased nerve conduction in all the nerves in the arm and in the other extremities as well. This type of pain is difficult to treat, and surgery has no role in the therapy.

Accumulating case reports in the literature indicate that carpal tunnel syndrome associated with functioning dialysis fistulas may be more common than is generally appreciated. Hand pain is in the median nerve distribution, and nerve conduction studies show decreased conduction across the wrist. Frequently, the transverse carpel ligament is very thick and densely calcified. Open carpal tunnel release will relieve the pain. It is important to distinguish this syndrome from other neuropathy, because proper surgical treatment can provide a lasting cure.

Occasionally, pain may be due to direct entrapment of nerves at the site of insertion of a graft. Conduction studies will show dysfunction of the nerve below the site of insertion, and exploration of the nerve with neurolysis can provide lasting relief.

The steal syndrome may produce hand pain that is difficult to distinguish from neuropathic pain. Normal nerve conduction testing along with noninvasive vascular studies that show diminished perfusion identify steal as the probable cause of pain. The pathophysiology and approach to relief of the steal syndrome is described elsewhere in this chapter.

PERITONEAL DIALYSIS

As with hemodialysis, the possibility of dialysis by means of the peritoneal cavity has been known for many years (7), but the popularization of this technique has awaited the development of reliable hardware. Peritoneal dialysis has an advantage in that it may be used immediately, and also can be used as a chronic dialysis access. Because the dialysate is left in the peritoneal cavity while equilibrium is taking place, the patient is not inseparably linked to the dialysis machine. Finally, because no direct access to the bloodstream is involved, peritoneal dialysis does not represent as much of a hazard or require quite as rigid supervision.

The device we currently use for peritoneal dialysis is a Tenckhoff catheter with two Dacron cuffs (8). The peritoneal end of the catheter has numerous small holes to facilitate inflow and drainage. The two cuffs are designed to receive fibrobastic ingrowth: one at the fascial level to establish a watertight seal and the other subjacent to the skin to prevent infection along the catheter.

Operative technique (Figure 11)

The catheters are placed with local anesthesia using mild intravenous sedation, but in the operating room, using strict sterile technique. Antibiotic prophylaxis for gram-positive organisms is used routinely. In patients with no prior abdominal surgery, the catheter is placed subumbilically, through a midline incision. If previous surgery has been performed through a lower abdominal midline incision, a paramedian muscle splitting incision or a supraumbilical midline incision may be used. The perito-

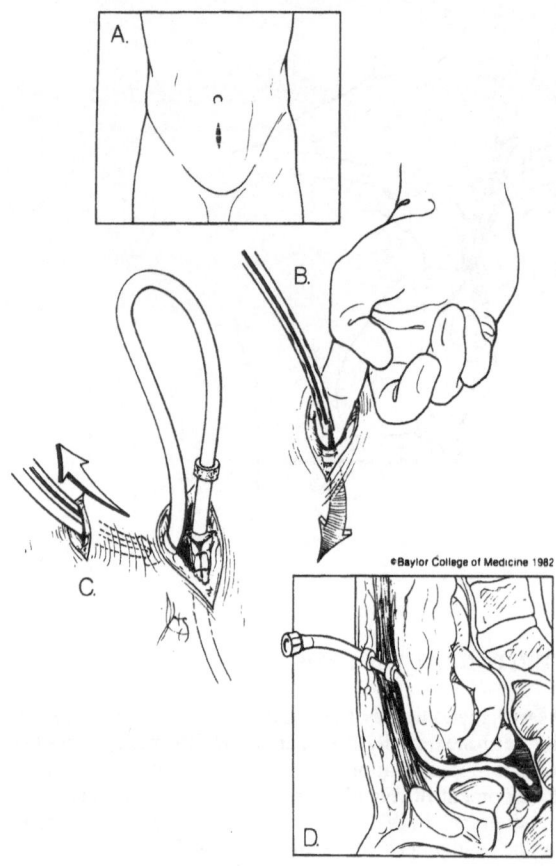

© Baylor College of Medicine 1982

Figure 11. Technique of insertion of a double-cuff peritoneal dialysis catheter. **A.** Lower abdominal incision. **B.** Peritoneum entered and digitally explored and catheter inserted into pelvis using a stilette. **C.** The deep cuff is incorporated in the abdominal closure. The catheter is pulled through a separate stab-wound exit site. **D.** Position of catheter after completion of the procedure.

neal cavity should be opened under direct vision, and digital exploration ensures that an adequate free peritoneal cavity exists for catheter insertion. The peritoneal end of the catheter is gently introduced and positioned in the pelvis. This process is facilitated by a stilette that is temporarily inserted into the catheter. Once the catheter is positioned, it is irrigated and aspirated to ascertain free flow. Meticulous watertight fascial closure is accomplished using interrupted sutures, catching a stitch or two in the deep cuff to fix the catheter at the fascial level. The external end is then brought out through a separate stab wound lateral to the incision. This exit site should be placed such that the catheter is not kinked in the subcutaneous tissue and such that the superficial cuff is far enough beneath the skin that it will not later erode through the skin. At this point, the catheter is again irrigated to ensure adequate flow, and if it

is satisfactory the catheter is capped. The wound is then closed in layers, completing the procedure.

Local care of the exit site, including daily dressing changes and the use of povidone-iodine ointment, is important to prevent the development of infection of the exit site. This treatment is usually continued at least until healing around the site has occurred (about 7–10 days). Meticulous sterile technique is also important at the connector to prevent the development of peritonitis.

Complications

INFECTION

Infection is one of the most common complications of peritoneal dialysis, and may be a localized infection of the exit site or generalized peritonitis. Because the catheter is a foreign body, infections are frequently difficult to eradicate and are the most common indication for catheter removal. Infections may be caused by gram-positive cocci, gram-negative rods, or fungi. Knowledge of specific pathogens and their antibiotic sensitivities is important in treating the infections if any hope of cure without catheter removal is to be expected.

Patients with peritonitis frequently have high fevers and marked abdominal tenderness. Dialysis may be continued during the episode of peritonitis, and indeed antibiotics may be delivered along with the dialysate. Patients who do not respond to appropriate antibiotics in several days or who have recurrent infections may need to have their catheter removed to control the infection. In our experience, infections due to *Pseudomonas* or *Candida* species usually will not resolve without removing the catheter.

Patients with exit-site infections usually do not manifest systemic symptoms, but if the infection spreads, generalized peritonitis may ensue. Attempts to suppress exit-site infections are worthwhile, but frequently catheter removal is required. Incision and drainage of the exit site and removal of the subcutaneous cuff will resolve the infection in 50% of the cases. If there is persistent or recurrent infection, the catheter must be removed.

The previous implant incision is reopened under local anesthesia and the fascia is exposed. The fascial cuff has to be dissected free from the fascia to get the catheter out. The wound is irrigated with povidine-iodine, then closed. We generally prefer to wait several weeks before reinsertion of another peritoneal dialysis catheter after infection has precipitated removal, and we avoid using the previous incision, regardless of how well healed it appears. If dialysis is required during the waiting period, a central vein hemodialysis catheter for dialysis is inserted unless a permanent hemoaccess is present.

LEAKING

Secure fascial closure around the catheter is important to prevent leaking during dialysis. Waiting several days before using the catheter is helpful to allow some healing to occur, although this delay is not always necessary. The use of small exchange volumes initially may also minimize leaking around a newly implanted PD catheter. New catheters that leak may be revised by exploring the incision and placing more fascial sutures to establish a watertight closure. Recurrent leaking or leaking in a chronic catheter is often the first clue to the presence of infection.

POOR OUTFLOW

Poor outflow is a common problem with chronic peritoneal dialysis. Usually the dialysis will flow easily into the peritoneal cavity, but returns slowly or not at all. This can be due to a poor position of the catheter. The catheter position can be checked with a plain x-ray of the abdomen. Sometimes a previously well-placed catheter will be seen to have moved or kinked, presumably as a result of intestinal motility. Contrast injected through the catheter using x-ray or image intensification may demonstrate the cause of poor outflow in catheters that appear well positioned on plain film. In cases where the position of the catheter appears to be acceptable, the holes in the catheter may be occluded by omental fat or by fibrin or protein. Streptokinase infusion may improve the outflow in the later cases, but in the former case repositioning is usually necessary. When repositioning a catheter, it is helpful to go through a separate incision that is lateral to the previous incision used for insertion. In this way, the fascial closure around the catheter and the previously healed wound are not disrupted. The laparoscope may be used in this situation to demonstrate the cause of catheter dysfunction. Both repositioning of the catheter and removing omentum wrapped around the catheter may be accomplished with the scope.

POOR DIALYSIS

Finally, there are some patients who either initially, or later as a result of recurrent peritonitis, have obliteration of their free peritoneal cavity. They do not have enough absorptive surface to dialyze adequately. These patients should be recognized as poor candidates for peritoneal dialysis so that provisions for hemodialysis may be made.

INTESTINAL PERFORATION

Intestinal perforation is fortunately a rare complication of peritoneal dialysis. The use of temporary dialysis catheters with sharp stilettes designed for blind insertion through the fascia make the complication more frequent. However, insertion under direct vision into the peritoneal cavity should not result in this complication. Overzealous attempts to free up the peritoneal cavity by blunt dissection could cause intestinal perforation at the time of insertion, but the soft Teflon catheter used for chronic peritoneal dialysis will not erode into the bowel lumen.

BLEEDING

Bleeding from various sources may be encountered after Tenckhoff catheter insertion. Bleeding at the exit site is usually from small subcutaneous blood vessels and, if clotting studies are normal, is of little significance. Significant bleeding, however, may occur in the peritoneal cavity. Early after surgery, it is usually from the incision or from adhesions disrupted during catheter insertion. Later, spontaneous intraperitoneal bleeding can occur, presumably due to the disruption of omental vessels by the catheter. Peritoneal bleeding from any of these cause almost always resolves spontaneously, and reexploration to control hemorrhage is rare.

PAIN

Some patients experience pain during the inflow or outflow of the peritoneal dialysate. For the most part, pain on inflow is the discomfort of distention of the peritoneal cavity. Patients gradually become accustomed to this sensation, and it becomes subjectively tolerable. Pain on outflow is due to catheter impingement upon an intra-abdominal viscus or entrapment of omentum in the holes of the catheter. Blind maneuvers to reposition the catheter, such as changing the patient's position, rapid flushing of the catheter, or enemas, may resolve the problem. Contrast material injected through the catheter may show the position of the catheter and the organ involved. Conservative measures are usually successful in resolving this complication, but ultimately, in some patients, surgical repositioning of the catheter may be necessary.

REFERENCES

1. Kolff WJ, Berk HTJ, ter-Welle M, van der Leg JW, van Dijk EC, van Nordwijk J: The artificial kidney: a dialyser with a great area. *Acta Med Scand* 117:121, 1944.
2. Scribner BH, Caner JEZ, Buri R, Quinton W: The technique of continuous hemodialysis. *Trans Am Soc Artif Intern Organs* 12:220, 1966.
3. Uldall PR, Dyck RF, Woods F: A subclavian cannula for temporary vascular access for hemodialysis or plasmapheresis. *Dial Transplant* 8(10):963, 1979.
4. Brescia MJ, Cimino JE, Appel K, Hurwich BJ: Chronic hemodialysis using vein puncture and a surgically created arteriovenous fistual. *N Engl J Med* 275:1089, 1966.
5. Lefrak EA, Noon GP: Surgical technique for creation of an arteriovenous fistula using a looped bovine graft. *Ann Surg* 182:782, 1975.
6. Rapaport A, Noon GP, McCollum CH: Polytetrafluoroethylene (PTEE) grafts for haemodialysis in chronic renal failure. *Aust NZ J Surg* 51:562, 1981.
7. Frank HA, Seligman AM, Fine J: Treatment of uremia after acute renal failure by peritoneal irrigation. *JAMA* 130:703, 1946.
8. Striker GE, Tenckhoff H: A transcutaneous prosthesis for prolonged access to the peritoneal cavity. *Surgery* 69:71, 1971.

CHAPTER 60

Dialyzers, Dialysates, and Water Treatment

NUHAD ISMAIL, BRYAN BECKER, & RAYMOND M. HAKIM

GENERAL PRINCIPLES

Hemodialysis is a complex process performed with apparent simplicity. The major extracorporeal components of this therapy are dialyzers, dialysate, and water treatment systems. In this chapter, we will present a brief synopsis of dialyzers and their operative features and will discuss dialysate composition and water treatment systems.

Dialyzers are devices that obey the laws of mass transfer across semipermeable membranes. Contemporary dialysis membranes have evolved from their primitive ancestors into highly efficient structures capable of tremendous solute transport and water removal. Such membranes are the cornerstone of the hemodialysis procedure.

A hemodialyzer is schematically a semipermeable membrane separating blood and dialysate compartments. The process of hemodialysis is simply the interface of blood with a balanced solution (the dialysate) across this membrane.

Two important membrane properties are diffusion and ultrafiltration. Diffusion is the movement of solutes from one compartment to another, relying on a concentration gradient between the two compartments. During hemodialysis, effective blood flow (Q_B) also determines mass solute removal from blood in concert with the differences between the afferent and efferent concentrations of solute, traditionally labelled as *arterial* and *venous* (C_A and C_V). The definition of dialyzer clearance (K) is similar to the principles of creatinine clearance in the normal kidney, calculated as the amount of creatinine removed ($U_{cr}V/P_{cr}$), where U_{cr} is the concentration of creatinine and V is the volume of urine, divided by the driving force, plasma creatinine concentration, P_{cr}. Thus, dialyzer clearance is

$$K = (Q_B)(C_A - C_V)/C_A$$

where Q_B = blood flow rate to dialyzer,
           C_A = inlet (to dialyzer) blood concentration,
           C_V = outlet (to dialyzer) blood concentration.

This equation, however, neglects the contribution of fluid removal during the dialytic process. This phenomenon, ul-trafiltration, involves the bulk movement of solute and solvent across the dialysis membrane. The driving force for ultrafiltration is the hydrostatic pressure gradient across the membrane, the transmembrane pressure (TMP). With ultrafiltration, blood flow leaving the dialyzer (Q_{Bo}) is less than blood flow entering the dialyzer (Q_{Bi}). The difference between these values represents ultrafiltration (Q_{UF}). This fact can be incorporated into the above equation to yield a more precise definition of clearance:

$$Q_{UF} = Q_{Bi} - Q_{Bo}$$

where Q_{Bo} = blood flow leaving the dialyzer
           Q_{Bi} = blood flow entering the dialyzer

$$K = \frac{\left[Q_{Bi}(C_A) - (Q_{Bo})(C_V)\right]}{C_A} = \frac{\left[Q_{Bo}(C_A - C_V) + (Q_{UF})\right]}{C_A}$$

True clearance should be calculated by using the concentration in the aqueous compartment of blood and the concentration of solute in that compartment. Since solutes diffusing out of blood will appear in the dialysate, it is possible to calculate clearance for solutes not present in the incoming dialysate (e.g., urea) as $K = Q_{Do}(C_{Do})/C_A$ where C_{Do} and Q_{Do} are the concentration of solute in the dialysate outlet and the effluent dialysate flow, respectively. Although this equation provides a simple concept for determining clearance, the necessity of measuring low concentrations of any substance in the dialysate increases the error of measurement.

DIALYZERS

Dialyzer characteristics

The classical view of membranes as an inert diffusive–convective structure has evolved into a greater understanding of dialysis membranes that encompasses the physical characteristics, the biocompatible properties, and adsorptive properties associated with such membranes. The ideal dialyzer membrane should be defined through each of these properties (see Table 1). Optimal diffusive–convective properties include rapid diffusion of small solutes, se-

Suki, WN and Massry SG (eds), Suki and Massry's Therapy of Renal Diseases and Related Disorders, Third Edition. ISBN 978-1-4757-6634-9.
©*1998, Kluwer Academic Publishers, Boston/Dordrecht/London. All rights reserved.*

Table 1. Characteristics of an ideal dialyzer membrane

High diffusion coefficients of small solutes
Selective permeability to middle- and large-molecular-weight
    molecules
Facile water permeability for easy control of ultrafiltration
Selective adsorption of proteins
Completely inert, without bioreactivity
Easy to use with reproducible efficacy

lective permeability to middle- and large-molecular-weight molecules, and adequate water permeability for easy control of ultrafiltration. The adsorptive properties of such a membrane should manifest a dual nature. Indiscriminant protein binding is detrimental to membrane function, interfering with plasma proteins, decreasing membrane efficacy by altering diffusion capacity, and modifying systemic drug stores. Some adsorptive properties however, may be beneficial, e.g., the removal of β_2-microglobulin, the protein associated with dialysis-related amyloidosis (1,2). Therefore, an ideal membrane would exhibit such selective adsorption. An ideal membrane also would be completely inert, without bioreactivity. Finally, such a dialyzer should be easy to use and should have reproducible efficacy. This entails physical stability and operating characteristics allowing for its insertion into the dialytic system with a predictable and beneficial result.

Available dialyzer membranes can divided into cellulosic and synthetic membranes. Each manifests a different physical and biochemical profile. Hydrophilicity and charge are two major characteristics that influence transport across the membrane (3). Hydrophilicity, or membrane wettability, is due to hydrogen bonding between terminal carboxyl (COOH), amino (NH_2), or hydroxyl (OH^-) groups on the membrane and water. Hydrophilicity is generally associated with decreased protein adsorption. Polyacrylonitrile (PAN), polyamide (PA), and polymethylmethacrylate (PMMA) all have low hydrophilicity and appreciable protein adsorption, while cellulose-based membranes have greater hydrophilicity and low adsorptive properties (4).

Membrane surface charge results from the dissociation of acidic groups or the quaternation of amino compounds in water (4). The balance of these electrical forces determines the net surface charge on the membrane. Surface charge significantly influences membrane function by altering the sieving of charged solutes (5).

Other traits that affect dialyzer function are membrane thickness and symmetry. Membrane permeability is inversely proportional to membrane thickness and directly proportional to the membrane's intrinsic diffusion coefficient. A thinner membrane provides the logical means for increasing diffusive flux.

Most synthetic membranes are thicker than their less permeable cellulosic counterparts. However, synthetic membranes also display greater intrinsic diffusion coefficients, and they maintain their thickness when wet, while cuprophane and cellulose acetate membranes swell when wet (6,7).

Membranes also can be asymmetric with the smooth "skin" on the side that interacts with blood, in contradistinction to symmetric membranes in which both sides of the membrane are similar. Symmetry or asymmetry is obtained by altering membrane precipitation during manufacturing (4). Commonly used asymmetric membranes include polyamide (PA) and polysulfone (PS). This property allows for greater diffusive permeability—hence, the utility of asymmetric membranes for hemofiltration.

The chemical composition of membranes influences many of the aforementioned properties. Cellulose and its derivatives, cuprophan and cellulose acetate, remain the most commonly used used membranes for dialysis, although their use appears to be declining. Cellulose, extracted from cotton linters with cellobiose, is a natural linear condensation of D-glucose polymer. After cellulose is obtained, it is shunted into membrane production. First, the polymer is formed; then it undergoes controlled precipitation; and finally, it is manufactured. Each step affords an opportunity to alter membrane characteristics with attendant functional effects. After cellulose is dissolved initially in sodium hydroxide, it is regenerated and the membrane formed in an acid bath. Cuprophan is generated differently, with the initial solvent being an ammonium solution of copper hydroxide. Copper–ammonia–cellulose complexes are then extruded into an acid bath, producing a membrane with cuprammonium radicals in the midst of its structure. This modification yields greater diffusion and ultrafiltration capabilities for cuprophan membranes as compared to straight cellulose. Glycerine content added during the extrusion process also affects these characteristics. The glycerine content of cuprophan is usually about 5%. Increasing this value adds greater solute and flux capacities to the membrane.

Cellulose acetate membranes are manufactured with acetylation preceding the acid-bath production step. Acetylation also increases ultrafiltration and solute transport. All cellulose membranes have hydroxyl radicals at the surface, which increase the hydrophilicity of the membrane as well. Using hydroxyl masking techniques to alter this characteristic enhances the hydrophobicity of the membrane and increases protein adsorption, though it remains very low (8).

Synthetic membranes have several differences from cellulose-based dialyzers. PAN membranes have marked asymmetry, with consequent high filtration rates. They do, however, bind blood proteins and alter their filtration efficiency. PAN and polycarbonate–polyether membranes maintain structural integrity and flexibility well during use, allowing for their utility in hemofiltration. The latter membranes (not commercially available in the United States) also are characterized by minimal thrombogenicity (9). The polycarbonate–polyether copolymer is formed asymmetrically and has wettability. PAN membranes demonstrate greater wettability, with higher filtration rates and greater diffusive permeability (10). Membranes constructed from PMMA and polysulfone (PS) also have many of these characteristics.

Dialyzer types

Three forms of dialyzers have been used for hemodialysis. Plate dialyzers provided the means for dialysis early in its history. These dialyzers consist of a number of sheets of membranes separated by a spacer in rectangular compartments placed in parallel alignment. This arrangement allows for low blood-flow resistance and controlled ultrafiltration. Coil dialyzers are constructed from one or several pieces of membrane tubing wound around a central core. A support screen maintains the tubing positioning and allows for dialysate flow on the outside of these tubings. Blood flows through the tubing while dialysate flows through this supporting screen. Coil dialyzers have a high blood-flow resistance and, due to their compliance, variable ultrafiltration rates. They are rarely used in the United States.

Hollow-fiber dialyzers are the most common dialyzers in use today. These consist of several thousand (10,000–15,000) hollow fibers wrapped in a bundle inside a plastic jacket. Each fiber has a diameter of 200–300 μm. Blood flows through the fibers while dialysate flows outside the fibers, typically in a countercurrent fashion. Hollow-fiber dialyzers are easy to use and provide low blood-flow resistance, excellent mass transfer, low compliance, and controllable ultrafiltration. They have low priming volumes as well, generally 100–150 mL. Finally, hollow-fiber dialyzers are easier to reuse compared to the other types of dialyzers.

While the hollow-fiber construction offers convenience and efficiency, there have been some disadvantages to these membranes. Blood left in these dialyzers previously was difficult to clear, resulting in increased clotting and blood loss. However, this has diminished greatly with the introduction of newer hollow-fiber dialyzers. Hollow-fiber dialyzers also require potting compound to anchor fibers to the dialyzer. This compound acts as a "sink" and can make it more difficult to remove ethylene oxide or formaldehyde used in the reprocessing of these dialyzers. This difficulty can be overcome by allowing longer degassing of membranes sterilized by this method or the use of alternative sterilization modes, e.g., steam or gamma irradiation (11).

Large-surface-area dialyzers, generally using synthetic membranes with high permeability, comprose a subset of hollow-fiber dialyzers. These so-called *high-flux* dialyzers have greater surface area than their hollow-fiber counterparts, with similar low priming volumes. Their utility obviously lies in their provision of increased clearance for certain solutes; however, their marked permeability requires special devices and monitoring to control the rate of ultrafiltration.

A multitude of dialyzers are currently available (see Table 2). As mentioned, most are hollow-fiber dialyzers. Each dialyzer includes a specification sheet that describes the pertinent operating information for the dialyzer: the ultrafiltration coefficient (K_{UF}); the clearance of certain molecules, such as creatinine, phosphate, vitamin B_{12}, and urea; the membrane surface area; priming volume; and fiber thickness and length.

The K_{UF} is the number of milliliters per hour ultrafiltration achieved for every mmHg of TMP. For example, if the K_{UF} is 4.0, the TMP required to remove 1000 mL/hr is 250 mmHg. This pressure is assessed at the midpoint of the fibers. Since most hollow-fiber dialyzers have pressure drops across the fibers, since blood is pushed by the blood pump at high pressures (generally 300–350 mmHg) and exits the dialyzers at pressures approximating 100 mmHg, a "natural" TMP of 100–150 mmHg is possible. Thus, with ultrafiltration coefficients exceeding 5 mL/mmHg/hr, there is an obligate loss of 500 mL/hr. Patients on such dialyzers with ultrafiltration requirements that are less than 500 mL/hr will therefore require replacement of the excess fluid loss. Consequently, when the K_{UF} is high (>6.0), as with most synthetic membranes, ultrafiltration monitoring is necessary to prevent errors in the amount of ultrafiltrate

Table 2. Representative listing of commonly used hollow-fiber dialyzers[a]

Model	Membrane	K_{UF}	In vitro KoA (urea)	Surface area (M^2)	Urea clearance ($Q_B = 200$)
Cobe 400	Cellulose	5.3	520	0.9	173
Terumo C-101	Cellulose	3.5	520	1.0	171
Fresenius F-80	Polysulfone	60	945	1.8	192
Toray B1-1.6-H	PMMA	12	720	1.6	186
Gambro polyflux 130	Polyamide	45	590	1.3	181
Gambro/Hospal Biospan-1800-S	AN69	18	270	0.6	137

[a] For a more extensive list of commonly used dialyzer membranes, refer to (47).

removed. The values for K_{UF} supplied by manufacturers are derived from in vitro data and usually underestimate the actual clinical K_{UF} by 5%–30% (12).

Solute clearance values accompany the dialyzer specifications and are determined by in vitro testing as well that utilizes aqueous solutions. Clearance values usually are supplied for urea, creatinine, and vitamin B_{12}. Dialyzer urea clearance is frequently reported at various blood flow rates, e.g., 200, 300, and 400 mL/min (although most commonly at 200 mL/min, but at a particular dialysate flow rate, usually 500 mL/min). Creatinine clearance often will approximate 80% of urea clearance. The clearance of vitamin B_{12} denotes the ability for the membrane to allow the passage of larger-moleculas-weight solutes. High-flux and high-efficiency dialyzers increase vitamin B_{12} clearance significantly (>100 mL/min at a blood flow of 200 mL/min) compared to standard dialyzers (30–60 mL/min at a blood flow of 200 mL/min). For most dialyzers, the equivalent in vivo clearance is 20%–25% less than the in vitro clearance.

Each dialyzer also has a mass transfer coefficient (KoA) which provides a gauge of dialyzer efficiency. KoA determines the interrelationship between clearance and the flow rates for blood and dialysate and therefore allows the estimation of the in-vitro clearance at any given blood and dialysate flow. KoA values range from 200–300, which are only sufficient for small patients, to more than 700, which are standard for high-efficiency dialyzers. In vivo urea clearance can be determined by measuring the arterial and venous concentrations of a solute simultaneously at a given blood flow rate; however, these values often are significantly lower (approximately 25%) than the in vitro clearance data supplied by the dialyzer specification sheets.

Obviously, dialyzer specification sheets provide useful information about the function and efficiency of membranes, but their data cannot be completely extrapolated to the in vivo dialysis setting (12). Such information is best utilized as a guide for choosing a specific dialyzer and determining the general effectiveness of the dialysis delivered with this membrane.

Biocompatibility

Biocompatibility is best defined as the sum of the interactions between blood and the hemodialysis circuit. The artificial components of hemodialysis are "foreign"; therefore, when blood encounters these materials, it initiates an inflammatory response. Often, these reactions are minimal, and the membrane can be termed *biocompatible*. On other occasions, however, severe reactions can lead to patient morbidity and even the risk of death. The importance of this concept for hemodialysis patients lies in their repetitive exposure to the "nonself" structures of the dialysis circuit. Thus, the chronicity of contact may transform even mild interactions to deleterious and detrimental clinical sequelae in the long term (Table 3).

When blood encounters the hemodialysis membrane,

Table 3. Sequelae of hemodialysis membrane bioincompatibility

1. Complement activation
   a. Release of C3a and C5a leading to smooth muscle contraction, increased vascular permeability, and histamine release from mast cells
   b. Formation of membrane attack complex (C5b-9)
   c. Neutrophil activation with degranulation, production of reactive oxygen species, increased expression of adhesion molecules, increased arachidonic acid metabolism
   d. Monocyte activation
   Clinical sequelae—"First-Use syndrome," dialysis-related B_2-m amyloid production, dialysis-associated neutropenia
2. Contact pathway activation
   a. Development of circulating complexes of high-molecular-weight kininogen (HMWK) complexing with pre-kallikrein
   b. Bradykinin production
   Clinical sequelae—anaphylactoid reactions in patients using angiotensin-converting enzyme inhibitors
3. Other
   Increased incidence of infection
   Increased morbidity and mortality
4. Possible
   Increased rate of decline in residual renal function
   Pulmonary fibrosis
   Decreased erythrocyte survival

several reactions are triggered, including the complement cascade, the coagulation cascade, and the contact-phase reaction (13). In addition, evidence suggests that neutrophils, monocytes, and platelets that directly contact membranes become activated, leading to the upregulation of adhesion receptors (14), cytokine release (15), and the generation of cyclooxygenase metabolites (16).

The acute effects of these events can be profound. Dialysis-related neutropenia, hypoxemia, and anaphylaxis have all been described (17,18). The finding that complement activation occurs during hemodialysis via the alternative pathway provides the pathophysiology for these phenomena. It is noteworthy that cellulose-based membranes generally result in a far greater activation of complement than noncellulose-derived membranes.

The products of complement activation, C3a and C5a, have been termed *anaphylatoxin*. These proteins produce intense vasoconstriction and anaphylaxis in some animal models—hence, their designation. Blood exposed to cellulose membranes has been experimentally infused into animals, with resulting ischemic electrocardiographic changes, elevations in pulmonary artery pressure, histamine release, and increased vascular permeability (19). When C5a was introduced in similar fashion, many similar findings were present, suggesting that C5a was the primary mediator of these complement-induced effects.

The clinical relevance of this has been well examined in

the context of patient exposure to new cellulosic dialyzers. Many studies have documented a significant difference in the incidence of symptoms, e.g., chest pain or dyspnea, in patients dialyzed with new cellulosic membranes compared to reprocessed membranes that do not activate complement as extensively (19). Another study also has demonstrated elevated levels of C3a and C5a in patients experiencing adverse symptomatology compared to other patients dialyzing with the same membrane surface (20). It has been postulated that this difference may be responsible for the *First Use syndrome*. This syndrome affects patients early in their dialysis session and has been subdivided based upon the extent of their symptoms (21). Type A manifests itself usually very early in the dialysis treatment as dyspnea, cramping, angioedema, and pruritus. Its incidence approximates 5/100,000. Type B often occurs after about 1 hour of hemodialysis with the onset of back pain or chest pain. Both forms of the First Use syndrome can be prevented by instituting an appropriate reuse program for dialyzers or switching to more biocompatible membranes (21). Interestingly, a similar syndrome has been associated with the use of PAN membranes in hemodialysis patients receiving angiotensin-converting enzyme inhibitors (22). This reaction is believed to be secondary to the bradykinin-generating effects of the membrane in combination with converting enzyme inhibitors, which also inhibit the kininase enzymes, resulting in high concentrations of bradykinin in the circulation, profound hypotension, and cardiopulmonary arrest.

Complement proteins generated upon exposure to hemodialysis membranes also induce neutrophil and monocyte activation (23). Neutrophils thus stimulated produce reactive oxygen species that may be involved in a variety of pathogenetic pathways in dialysis patients, including progressive pulmonary fibrosis, atherogenesis, and potentially carcinogenesis (24). Neutrophil activation also results in upregulation of adhesion receptors and, consequently, granulocyte adherence to the vasculature, primarily the pulmonary vasculature. Cell aggregates can lead to thromboembolic events (25) or decreases in peak expiratory flow rates and P_{O_2}, two events observed in patients dialyzing with new cellulosic membranes (26).

In contrast to the aforementioned acute syndromes, the chronic sequelae associated with bioincompatibility are less dramatic but no less potent in their deleterious effects. The accumulation of amyloid fibrils, consisting of β_2-microglobulin fibrils, has been recognized in chronic hemodialysis since the mid-1980s (27). This form of amyloidosis manifests itself as patients develop carpal tunnel syndrome, arthropathy, lytic bony lesions, and pathologic fractures. Available evidence suggests that membrane bioincompatibility may be directly involved in the evolution of this process. Several studies have shown an increased incidence of β_2-microglobulin-related amyloidosis in patients dialyzed with cellulosic membranes (28–30). The pathogenesis of β_2-microglobulin-related amyloidosis appears to be multifactorial and is associated

with an increase in mononuclear cell synthesis and release of β_2-microglobulin after contact with celluslosic membranes (31). In addition, cellulosic membranes may enhance the polymerization of β_2-microglobulin fibrils by stimulating the release of proteases from leukocytes (32). Furthermore, these membranes do not adsorb or clear β_2-microglobulin readily from the circulation (33).

Membrane bioincompatibility also appears to affect recovery from acute renal failure. Conger et al., as well as Solez et al., initially advanced the notion that dialysis may alter the pace of recovery in acute renal failure (34,35). Both studies examined renal histopathology in individuals with acute renal failure who required lengthy courses of hemodialysis. Fresh areas of acute tubular necrosis were evident despite the fact that the initial injury was remote. Certain investigators have implicated infiltrating leukocytes in this ongoing injury, accompanying acute renal failure (36,37). It appears, therefore, that cellulosic membranes, because they activate complement and leukocytes, may contribute significantly to this injury, thereby delaying recovery in acute renal failure. Studies in animals with reversible acute renal failure have shown that renal recovery is slower when animals have been exposed to cellulosic membranes than when they have been exposed to biocompatible membranes (38).

Biocompatible membranes also appear to reduce the incidence of infections in hemodialysis patients (39). This may be due, in part, to alterations in cellular immunity. Chronic dialysis with cellulosic membranes further depresses T-cell function and decreases the expression of high-affinity interleukin-2 (IL-2) receptors on mononuclear cells. Changing to a more biocompatible membrane, PMMA, allows these receptors to increase in number to near normal levels (40). Other investigators have also found decreased natural killer (NK) function in patients dialyzed with bioincompatible membranes as well as decreased IL-2 generation and a decreased proliferative response (41,42).

Several studies have also suggested the possibility that bioincompatibility may be a catabolic stimulus in chronic hemodialysis patients. Exposure to cellulosic membranes appears to increase net protein catabolism, whereas PS or PAN membranes do not affect protein catabolism (43,44). Moreover, patients dialyzed with biocompatible membranes appear to have greater protein intake than patients dialyzed with cellulosic membranes (45). Though further studies are necessary to establish the extent to which bioincompatibility alone accounts for these findings, these observations support the contention that biocompatibility directly affects the catabolic nature of hemodialysis.

Clearly, then, biocompatibility is very important for understanding and optimizing membrane use. In addition to the above list, biocompatibility may affect residual renal function, long-term pulmonary changes, and erythrocyte survival (13). Maybe most important, biocompatibility appears to alter patient morbidity and mortality. Retrospective analyses suggest that patients dialyzing with cuprophane membranes experience more in-hospital days and increased annual mortality than patients who dialyze with PAN membranes (40,46). Biocompatibility therefore should be a consideration, along with membrane clearance, K_{UF}, and KoA, when choosing a dialyzer for a patient.

DIALYSATE COMPOSITION

The composition of the dialysis solution has undergone substantial changes since the inception of hemodialysis. Table 4 shows the dialysate composition generally used in the U.S. today. One of the major aims of hemodialysis is the restoration of normal ion concentrations (via diffusional transfer between dialysis fluid and blood). To accomplish this goal, the level of individual ions in the dialysate can be set to approximate the desired levels in plasma water. For calcium and magnesium, dialysate levels are set for the *diffusible* fraction found in plasma water.

A discussion of the principles governing the concentrations of each major dialysate component follows.

Dialysate glucose

In the early 1960s, high glucose concentrations in the dialysis fluid (>100 mmol/L, or >1.8 g/dL) were used to provide osmotic pressure for water removal. More recently, efficacious and accurate hydraulic ultrafiltration (UF) has made glucose-mediated osmotic water extraction unnecessary. Since the studies by Mendelssohn et al. (48) in 1967 that demonstrated inefficient UF with high dialysate glucose concentrations (>3.2 g/dL) and increased risks for hyperosmolar syndrome, postdialysis hypoglycemia, and hyponatremia with such glucose concentrations, the use of high dialysate glucose has been abandoned.

Contemporary dialysis fluids range from glucose-free to isoglycemic (5–5.5 mmol/L, or 90–100 mg/dL) or slightly hyperglycemic (5.5–11.0 mmol/L, or 100–200 mg/dL) (49). Most noninsulin-dependent patients tolerate dialysis with glucose-free dialysate without ill effects, despite losing 25–30 g of glucose across the dialyzer. A few studies, however, have shown that this glucose loss may adversely affect intermediary metabolism of carbohydrates and proteins (50,51).

The adverse effects of glucose-free dialysate include a reduction in plasma glucose, a corresponding decrease in plasma insulin levels, and a marked decrease in lactate and pyruvate levels. Acetoacetate and beta-hydroxybutyrate levels also increase dramatically, with consequent ketogenesis and, ultimately, gluconeogenesis. These biochemical measures often are sufficient to maintain serum glucose in the physiologic range. Nevertheless, hypoglycemia may develop during the use of glucose-free dialysate, especially in the presence of cachexia, sepsis,

Table 4. Composition of standard acetate and bicarbonate dialysate solutions

Solute	Acetate dialysate (mEq/L)	Bicarbonate dialysate (mEq/L)	Comments
Sodium	135–145	135–145	Bicarbonate dialysate offers hemodynamic advantage over acetate if dialysate sodium <135 Sodium-gradient dialysis confers no advantage to high-sodium dialysate (140–145 mEq/L); may confer advantage in patients with low urea transfercoefficient[b]
Potassium	0–4.0	0–4.0	Avoid dialysate K < 2 mEq/L in arrhythmia-prone patients[c]
Chloride	100–119	100–124	
Calcium[a]	2.5–3.5	2.5–3.5	Individualize: 3.5 mEq/L for hemodynamic stability 2.5 mEq/L for hypercalcemia prone on calcium salts and vitamin D
Magnesium	0.5–1.0	0.5–10	
Acetate	35–38	2.0–4.0	Avoid in patients unable to metabolize acetate[d]
Bicarbonate	0	30–38	Dialysate of choice for all critically ill patients
Dextrose (mmol/L)	5.5–11.0	5.5–11.0	Avoid dialysate-free dextrose in gluconeogenesis-impaired patients, diabetics, malnourished patients, and acetate dialysate patients
(mg/dL)	100–200	100–200	
P_{CO_2} (mmHg)	0.5	40–100	High P_{CO2} prevents hypocapnea-induced hypoventilation and dialysis-associated hypoxemia.
pH	Variable	7.0–7.4	Prevents calcium and magnesium microprecipitation

[a] 2.5–3.5 meq/L = 1.25–1.75 mmol/L = 5.0–7.0 mg/dL.
[b] Average urea mass transfer coefficient = 800 mL/min.
[c] Patients with left ventricular hypertrophy, impaired LV function, acute MI, and patients on digoxin.
[d] Elderly, reduced muscle mass, malnourished, especially with high-flux.

diabetes mellitus, or drugs such as aspirin or propranolol (52,53). Ganda et al. (54) found a 30% reduction in whole-blood amino acid levels in patients dialyzed against a glucose-free dialysate. The most significant decline (60%) occurred in alanine, the major amino acid precursor in gluconeogenesis. Other investigators have also linked glucose-free dialysate to hemodialysis catabolism. Kopple measured twice as much free amino acid with a glucose-free dialysate as compared to a glucose concentration 450 mg/dL in dialysate (55). Using kinetic modeling, Ward et al. found a 27% increase in intradialytic protein catabolism, compared to nondialysis days, in patients dialyzed with glucose-free dialysate (56).

Available data at present also indicate that dialysate glucose does not play a significant role in determining total cholesterol levels in noninsulin-dependent hemodialysis patients. On the other hand, while it is possible that high glucose concentrations may aggravate the hypertriglyceridemia of ESRD, there is little evidence to suggest that physiologic dialysate glucose (≤ 200 mg/dL) has a notable adverse effect (57,58).

Dialysate glucose may affect other aspects of the dialysis procedure:

1. Increased dialytic potassium removal with glucose-free dialysate (53). The proposed mechanism is that decreased insulin levels result from glucose-free dialysate, leading to potassium egress from intracellular stores and, consequently, increased dialytic [K^+] removal.
2. Addition of glucose to dialysate fluid may lessen the risk of dialysis disequilibrium syndrome. In a study by Ramirez et al. (59), abnormal EEG tracings were observed in two of seven patients with normal baseline EEG when dialyzed without glucose, but not when dialysate contained 200 mg/dL glucose.
3. Dialysate glucose promotes microbial growth within the dialysate, particularly with the use of highly permeable dialyzer membranes or when central proportioning systems are used.
4. Though the presence of glucose minimizes some of the disturbances of acetate-based hemodialysis (50), there may be less need for dextrose in bicarbonate-based dialysis. In a study by Ward et al. (56), less postdialysis fatigue occurred when glucose-containing (200 mg/dL) dialysate was used, as compared to glucose-free dialysis.

In summary, a dialysate glucose concentration of 100–200 mg/dL is optimal and is recommended in most patients with gluconeogenic defects. Such a dialysate glucose also may be beneficial in malnourished patients who often experience increased dialysis catabolism with no glucose in dialysis. Finally, dialysate glucose concentrations of 100–200 mg/dL are essential for insulin-dependent diabetic patients, who comprose approximately 30% of all hemodialysis patients in the U.S. While such levels of glucose do not prevent hypoglycemia, particularly if insulin doses are high, they may attenuate the frequency of hypoglycemia.

Dialysate sodium

The pivotal role that plasma osmolality plays in maintaining hemodynamic stability during hemodialysis (HD) is now well established (60–63) (Figure 1). Such a role became apparent when investigators began comparing the hemodynamic changes induced by conventional dialysis, ultrafiltration (UF) and sequential UF dialysis. Isoosmolar fluid removal clearly improved hemodynamic stability. During hemodialysis, the fall in extracellular osmolality is more rapid than corresponding changes in intracellular osmolality, resulting in fluid shifts from ECF to ICF, exacerbating volume depletion. This decline in P_{osm} is more apparent when solute removal is rapid and is not counteracted by diffusion of sodium from the dialysate to the blood. Use of low sodium dialysate (<135 mEq/L) further favors this ICF shift as plasma becomes more hypoosmolar consequent to sodium movement from plasma to dialysate.

The reduction in P_V with both UF and HD also leads to an increase in plasma oncotic pressure and a decrease in capillary hydrostatic pressure. Both forces mobilize fluid from extravascular spaces. The degree to which P_V decreases thus depends not only on the rate of UF and ICF shifts, but also on the plasma refilling rate (PRR) from intracellular and interstitial fluid compartments. In turn, the PRR depends on several factors, most importantly, dialysate sodium concentration. By maintaining a relatively constant plasma osmolality, a high dialysate sodium minimizes water movement intracellular during dialysis, therefore better preserving plasma volume (59,63).

It has now been clearly established that maintaining constant plasma osmolality (P_{osm}) enhances blood pressure stability during dialysis (66–68). Numerous investigators also have demonstrated that hemodynamic stability during dialysis is improved when dialysate sodium concentration is increased to at least 135 mEq/L (56,69). The use of a lower dialysate-sodium in routine maintenance hemodialysis therefore has now been abandoned.

MECHANISMS BY WHICH HIGH DIALYSATE SODIUM IMPROVES HEMODYNAMIC STABILITY

Hyposmolality impairs peripheral vasoconstriction during volume removal and exacerbates autonomic insufficiency. Hence, by maintaining a stable P_{osm}, high dialysate sodium favorably influences compensatory mechanisms during volume removal (60).

Improving hemodynamic stability with high dialysate sodium is clinically paralleled by an increased tolerance to hemodialysis, namely, a reduction in cramping, nausea, vomiting, and headaches (68–70). Despite greater interdialytic weight gains and increased P_{Na} and P_{osm} in patients dialyzed with dialysate sodium of 144 mEq/L, Henrich et al. (70) found no increase in blood pressure or signs of volume overload. In addition, despite greater weight removal, higher dialysate sodium was associated

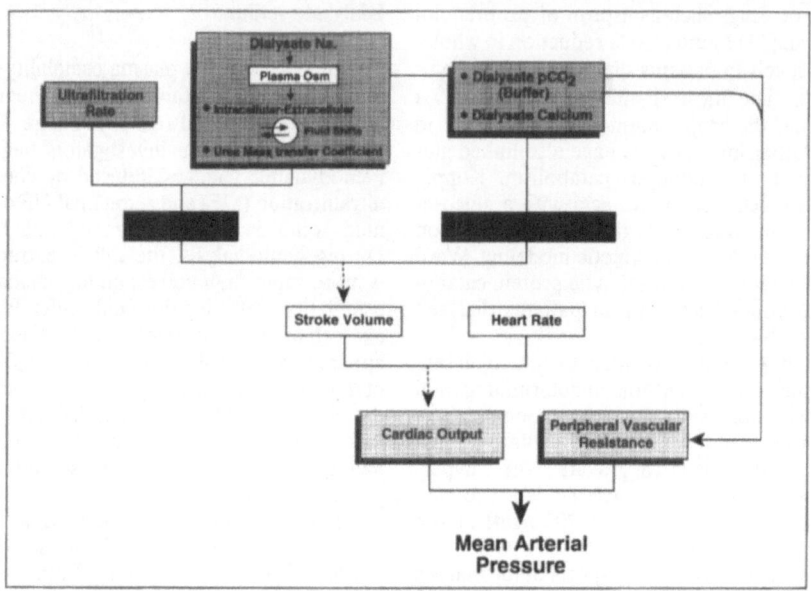

Figure 1. Determinants of systemic blood pressure and effects of dialysate composition on systemic hemodynamics. During ultrafiltration and/or dialysis, reduction of plasma volume will result in hypotension if compensatory changes in myocardial contractility, heart rate, or peripheral vascular resistance do not occur. During conventional dialysis, the reduction in plasma osmolality favors fluid shift from ECF to ICF, exacerbating the volume depleting effects of dialysis. This is further augmented by using low dialysate sodium (<130–135 mEq/L) and in patients with reduced urea mass transfer coefficients. Low dialysate calcium and/or hypoventilation/hypoxemia due to low P_{CO_2} reduce myocardial contractility. Low dialysate sodium and IL-2 impair compensatory peripheral vasoconstriction. The role of acetate on myocardial contractility is controversial.

with less hypotensive episodes compared to low dialysate sodium (132 mEq/L). Based upon these data, it is reasonable to use a dialysate Na concentration of 140–145 mEq/L, gauging the optimal dialysate Na concentration to each patient's overall clinical picture, i.e., blood pressure, weight gains, and symptoms on dialysis.

SODIUM-GRADIENT HEMODIALYSIS

In this model, a high dialysate sodium is used during the first hour or so of dialysis and then is progressively reduced toward isotonic levels through the remainder of the HD session. Sodium modeling thus allows the greatest influx of sodium to the patient at a time when the flux of urea and other solutes from the body are greatest. Using this technique, Dumler et al. (71) noted fewer symptomatic hypotensive episodes. Others, however, have not found any hemodynamic advantage for sodium-gradient dialysis compared to a fixed high-sodium dialysate (72–74). In the study by Daugirdas et al., there was a significant difference in the interdialytic weight gains for the three treatments (72). These data suggested that a sodium-gradient dialysis offers little advantage over a constant dialysate sodium of 140–145 mEq/L. Sodium-gradient dialysis may offer its greatest benefits in two clinical situations: 1) the initial

dialysis session for a patient with advanced renal insufficiency and an extremely elevated urea concentration (>200 mg/dL), in which case sodium modeling might decrease the risk of dialysis disequilibrium syndrome (60,75); and 2) patients with a low urea mass transfer coefficient, who exhibit a delay in urea equilibration between ICF and ECF compartments (76). Sodium-gradient dialysis may allow for more balanced urea and volume transfer.

Dialysate buffer

The 1980s witnessed an increase in the use of bicarbonate dialysis. According to the 1994 report by the Centers for Disease Control on hemodialysis-associated diseases in the U.S. (77), the reported use of bicarbonate as the primary method of dialysis among centers increased from 22% in 1986 to 94% in 1992.

Bicarbonate dialysis is considered the dialytic treatment of choice in critically ill patients, conferring many benefits over acetate dialysis in these patients, including a lower incidence of arterial hypotension, less hypoxemia, and improved left ventricular stroke work (78–81). Hakim et al. have also investigated the effects of acetate and bicarbonate dialysate on intradialytic and interdialytic morbidity in chronic dialysis patients (82). Using equivalent sodium concentrations and osmolality with each dialysate buffer in a single-pass delivery system, they found less hypoxemia and less hypotensive episodes with bicarbonate dialysis. They also found that older patients with recurrent hypotension and low muscle mass are a subset of patients who particularly benefit from bicarbonate dialysate. These patients appear to metabolize acetate more slowly (possibly because of decreased muscle mass) and have significantly lower postdialysis bicarbonate concentrations than asymptomatic patients undergoing acetate dialysis.

Acetate metabolism predominantly occurs in the liver and in skeletal muscle. While healthy individuals can metabolize acetate at a rate up to 300 mM/hr, chronic hemodialysis patients can only metabolize acetate at a markedly reduced rate, 3–3.5 mM/hr (83,84). Using larger-surface-area dialyzers and increased blood flow rates further enhances the transfer of acetate to the patient and may result in increased acetate exposure for the patient (79).

Other mechanisms by which acetate buffer results in hemodynamic instability include the following:
1. direct vasodilation, possibly by the conversion of acetate to adenosine, results in decreased PVR and thereby can decrease preload and cardiac filling (60).
2. Stimulating the release of interleukin-1, a vasodilatory compound (85), may cause hemodynamic instability.
3. An association with arterial hypoxemia and increases in oxygen consumption (86,87) may lead to myocardial hypoperfusion (88). A role for dialysate delivery systems has also been suggested in this. Vaziri et al. have shown that a change from a single-pass system to recirculation with cellulose membranes can reduce hypoxemia during acetate dialysis (89) because the rate of acetate entry (and bicarbonate loss) is less with recirculating systems.

   In acetate dialysis, hypoxemia results from the transfer of CO_2 across the dialysis membrane, from blood to dialysate, with consequent reflex hypoventilation. There is a decrease in the respiratory quotient

   $$\frac{(CO_2 \text{ produced})}{(O_2 \text{ consumed})},$$

   again resulting in hypocapnia and hypoventilation. Bicarbonate dialysate solutions, however, have elevated P_{CO_2} levels, and this prevents reflex hypoventilation and hypoxemia. Nonetheless, when the bicarbonate concentration exceeds 35 mEq/L in the dialysate, hypoventilation may also result from metabolic alkalosis.
4. Finally, acetate dialysate may have a myocardial depressant effect. Although controversy exists concerning the overall effects of acetate and bicarbonate buffers on myocardial performance, these conflicting results can be reconciled if one carefully reviews the independent effects of dialysate sodium, volume removal, and the type of patients (average weight, male vs. female, age, etc.) studied. Several studies have found that the vascular instability with acetate dialysis is generally improved with use of higher sodium dialysate concentration. Wehle et al. (66) documented no added benefit of bicarbonate over acetate with the use of dialysate sodium of 145 mEq/L. In males (veterans), Henrich et al. found strikingly similar hemodynamic parameters in both acetate and bicarbonate dialyzed patients when dialysate sodium was 140 mEq/L (90). Using a dialysate sodium of 130 mEq/L, Velez found better tolerance to bicarbonate, but no difference with a dialysate sodium of 140 mEq/L (91). With isovolemic dialysis, Mehta et al. (92) also found no difference in ventricular function with either buffer.

In conclusion, bicarbonate dialysis is the dialysate buffer of choice and confers advantages in critically ill patients. In chronic stable hemodialysis patients, bicarbonate buffer may not offer added hemodynamic benefit when the dialysate sodium is 140 mEq/L, or more. Patients who are unable to metabolize acetate well—elderly patients, patients with reduced muscle mass, malnourished patients, and possibly females—tolerate bicarbonate dialysate better (82,93). These patients may be particularly intolerant to acetate with the use of high-flux dialysis due to the high influx of acetate with these dialyzers. Finally, it should be noted that no studies have demonstrated an advantage for acetate over bicarbonate dialysis.

Dialysate calcium

Because dialysate calcium equilibrates with the diffusible (ionized) fraction of calcium in the plasma, a dialysate calcium of 2.5 mEq/L is equivalent to serum calcium of 10 mg/dL.

The use of a high dialysate calcium (3.5 mEq/L) or low dialysate calcium (≤2.5 mEq/L) entails separate advantages and risks (Table 4). The choice of a dialysate calcium concentration requires an understanding of these benefits and risks. In advanced chronic renal failure, the serum calcium concentrations are often reduced. The pathophysiology of this hypocalcemia is multifactorial and is discussed extensively elsewhere (94,95). Numerous studies have shown a beneficial effect of high dialysate calcium on the indices of metabolic bone disease as well as a reduction in parathyroid hormone (PTH) levels (96,97).

High-dialysate calcium has also been shown to improve hemodynamic stability during dialysis (98,99). Increased dialysate calcium augments SV and CO without changing PVR (100). Henrich et al. studied the mechanism of dialysate calcium-related increased left vertricular function using echocardiography. They found significant improvement in left ventricular end-diastolic volume, left ventricular end-systolic volume, and the velocity of circumferential fiber shortening when dialysate calcium was increased from 4.4 to 7.4 mg/dL (101). This led to an increase in plasma ionized calcium from 4.4 to 5.4 mg/dL. A similar increase in plasma ionized calcium and myocardial contractility was also reported by Lang et al. (102).

The current management of hyperphosphatemia and

secondary hyperparathyroidism entails calcium-based phosphate binders and oral or intravenous 1,25 dihydroxy vitamin D_3 (103–105). One of its main limitations is the development of hypercalcemia (106). A high calcium dialysate can accentuate this complication, limiting the usefulness of this therapy. Recently, there has been renewed interest in lowering dialysate calcium during combined therapy with vitamin D sterols and calcium-based phosphate binders. With a dialysate calcium concentration of 2.5 mEq/L, Slatopolsky and colleagues (107) have been able to successfully use high-dose calcium carbonate to control hyperphosphatemia without the development of hypercalcemia. Other investigators have reduced the extent of secondary hyperparathyroidism with low dialysate calcium in combination with either high doses of calcium-containing phosphate binders (108) or oral 1,25-dihydroxy vitamin D_3 (109). Mild hypotension has been reported with the use of such dialysate calcium concentrations in these instances (98,107).

In summary, in a hemodynamically stable patient, and, particularly, in those prone to hypercalcemia during treatment with vitamin D and calcium salts, a dialysate calcium concentration of 2.5–2.7 mEq/L is recommended.

Dialysate potassium

Although the gastrointestinal tract contributes to potassium excretion, dialysis is the primary route for potassium elimination for patients on hemodialysis (110,111). While the amount of potassium removed during hemodialysis is highly variable, the rate of potassium removal is largely a function of the concentration gradient between blood and dialysate. Blood and dialysate flow rates, dialyzer efficiency, and factors affecting the transcellular distribution of $[K^+]$, pH, insulin, and catecholamines are also important.

Typically, 50–80 mEq of potassium are removed with each dialysis treatment (112). The majority of dialyzed $[K^+]$ originates within cells and must traverse cell membranes before crossing the dialyzer membrane. Several investigators have found that plasma $[K^+]$ concentrations "rebound" following dialysis within 5 hours, with values averaging 30% greater than immediate postdialysis $[K^+]$ values (113–115). This postdialysis rebound has several clinical implications. Most importantly, the immediate postdialysis $[K^+]$ value should not be considered "safe" at levels of 5.5 mEq/L or more, since plasma $[K^+]$ concentrations can climb into the hyperkalemic range in the hours following dialysis. This possibility mandates repeat serum $[K^+]$ measurements several hours after hemodialysis. In addition, $[K^+]$ supplementation to treat postdialysis hypokalemia should be discouraged in light of this anticipated rebound.

The rebound in plasma $[K^+]$ following hemodialysis reflects a two-compartment model. Most authors believe that the transit of $[K^+]$ across cell membranes is the limiting factor in $[K^+]$ removal during dialysis, since it is slower than external transfer. As a result, dysequilibrium is established,

with the $[K^+]$ transfer from intracellular to extracellular [ICF/ECF] compartments during dialysis failing to replenish the external $[K^+]$ transfer to the dialysate. Net internal transfer continues following the termination of dialysis until a new steady-state ICF/ECF $[K^+]$ gradient is established.

Because internal $[K^+]$ transfer is affected by many factors, the acid–base status of the hemodialysis patient must be considered when choosing a dialysate $[K^+]$ concentration. EC acidosis promotes $[K^+]$ egress from cells, while alkalosis causes cellular $[K^+]$ uptake. This point is particularly important in hypokalemic patients with metabolic acidosis. In contrast to acidemia, dialysate base composition (acetate or bicarbonate) has no effect on $[K^+]$ removal during hemodialysis.

Plasma tonicity also can affect $[K^+]$ distribution. Hypertonic saline or mannitol, used in the treatment of hypotension or muscle cramps during dialysis, favors $[K^+]$ removal during dialysis, since tonicity favors $[K^+]$ movement into EC spaces and, consequently, its dialysance.

Glucose-free dialysate lowers plasma insulin concentrations and promotes $[K^+]$ movement from cells to EC space, making $[K^+]$ available for dialytic removal. Ward et al. found that $[K^+]$ removal during glucose-free dialysis was 28%–32% greater than that removed with 200 mg/dL glucose dialysate (50).

Low dialysate $[K^+]$ can precipitate ventricular ectopy. This outcome is most pronounced in patients with left ventricular hypertrophy, impaired left ventricular function, or in patients taking digoxin (117). The frequency of arrhythmias is greatest during the first 2 hours of dialysis, when $[K^+]$ flux is greatest. This observation suggests that a "sequential" reduction in dialysate $[K^+]$ during hemodialysis may be safer for removing $[K^+]$ in the arrhythmia-prone patient.

Finally, the dialysis membrane is not always the great "equalizer" for potassium. Dialyzing patients with total body $[K^+]$ depletion can worsen preexisting hypokalemia when concurrent metabolic acidosis is corrected with parenteral bicarbonate during dialysis. Hypokalemia, in this situation, can also be exacerbated by the concurrent use of high glucose dialysate (118).

In summary, the amount of potassium removed during dialysis is difficult to predict but typically ranges between 50 and 80 mEq per treatment when dialysate potassium is 2 mEq/L. Physicians caring for hemodialysis patients should be aware of the postdialysis $[K^+]$ rebound, and plasma $[K^+]$ values should be monitored in the hours following dialysis when an anticipated $[K^+]$ rebound may pose a problem. For patients at risk for arrhythmias, the use of dialysate $[K^+]$ less than 2 mEq/L should be avoided. Finally, prior to instituting digoxin therapy for a hemodialysis patient, the potential risk: benefit ratio of such therapy should be carefully assessed, since hemodialysis patients experience considerable variability in $[K^+]$ concentrations.

WATER TREATMENT

Hemodialysis patients have compromised urinary excretion, yet, on average, they are exposed to nearly 400 L of dialysis water weekly. The nonselective diffusion of solute across dialysis membranes potentially exposes these patients to the hazards of chemical contaminants in the water used for dialysis. Although further treatment of municipal water used by dialysis centers would produce higher-quality water for safer dialysis, such water treatment systems (WTSs) may invoke additional hazards if malfunction or user error occurs.

Recent technological advances in dialysis practices, including high-flux and high-efficiency dialysis, ever-increasing dialyzer reuse, and bicarbonate dialysate (119,120), have heightened awareness about the safety of dialysis water. Fortunately, the aforementioned dialysis practices have been paralleled by continuous advancement in reverse osmosis (RO) membrane technology. RO membranes in WTSs represent an effective barrier to endotoxin and bacteria with clear benefits over simple deionization.

In the final part of this chapter, we discuss the essential components of WTSs and their associated hazards as well as the AAMI Standards for product water that is safe for HD (Table 5). We also discuss the pathogenesis of dialysis-related pyrogenic reactions.

Hazards associated with dialysis water

The medical literature, the FDA's Medical Device Reporting and Device Experience Network files, and investiga-

Table 5. Risks associated with improperly treated water used for dialysis

Contaminant	Toxic effects
Aluminum	Dialysis dementia
	Osteomalacia
	Aplastic bone disease
	Pseudohyperparathyroidism
	Cardiomyopathy
	Anemia
Chloramines	Hemolysis
	Anemia
	Methemoglobinemia
Sodium azide	Severe hypotension
Fluoride	Osteomalacia
	Osteoporosis
	Cardiac arrest, arrhythmias
Calcium/magnesium	Hard-water syndrome
Nitrates	Methemoglobinemia
Copper	Hemolysis
	Liver damage
Zinc	Anemia
Formaldehyde	Hemolytic anemia
Microbial/endotoxin	Pyrogenic reactions

Modified from (120–139,153–163).

tions by the Centers for Disease Control (CDC) contain numerous reports of patient injury or death associated with improperly treated or inadequately monitored water used for hemodialysis.

Chemical contaminants in water

Aluminum sulfate is used as a flocculent in municipal water treatment. Maximal suggested aluminum levels in dialysate water are 10 µg/L. Reports of severe bone disease (osteomalacia and aplastic bone disease) and fatal dialysis encephalopathy (dialysis dementia) have been associated with high levels of aluminum in the water supply (121–123). Fortunately, there has been a continued decline in the incidence and case-fatality rate of dialysis dementia (119,120). Since RO is theoretically the most efficient way to remove aluminum from water, the declining incidence of dialysis dementia may be due to increasing use of RO water treatment prior to dialysate preparation.

Chloramines are used as bactericidal agents in municipal water treatment. Chloramines denature hemoglobin by direct oxidation as well as by inhibiting the hexose monophosphate shunt. In 1988, the FDA reported 44 cases of hemolysis due to inadequate chloramine removal in Philadelphia (125). Hemolysis, Heinz-body hemolytic anemias, and methemoglobinemia also have been reported in association with chloramine exposure (126,127).

Sodium azide exposure resulted in an epidemic of hypotension in a New York state dialysis facility (128). Sodiumazide was used as an admixture with glycerine as a preservative solution for WTS ultrafilters.

An RO system was installed in one center when inadequately deionization-treated fluoridated city water exposure led to fluoride intoxication in eight patients and one death (129). Even at the recommended level of 1 mg/L, continued fluoride exposure can cause osteomalacia and bone disease in dialysis patients (130). In a recent FDA safety alert, mechanical failure of deionizing tanks led to inadequate fluoride removal in a dialysis facility in Chicago, resulting in acute cardiac death in three patients (131).

Finally, excess calcium and magnesium in dialysate water have been associated with the *hard water syndrome*—a constellation of symptoms including nausea, vomiting, weakness, flushing, and fluctuations in blood pressure (132,133).

Several other adverse effects related to chemical contaminants have resulted from nitrates (methemoglobinemia with cyanosis and hypertension) (134), copper (hemolytic anemia) (135,136), and zinc (137). A syndrome of anemia, nausea, vomiting, fever, and high zinc levels has been correlated with the use of galvanized iron in the WTS and distribution system. Formaldehyde toxicity has occurred secondary to improper disinfectant use and leaching from sediment filters. This has resulted in hemolytic anemia and even death in one report (138,139).

Table 6. Components, advantages, risks, and AAMI recommendations for users of hemodialysis water treatment systems

Component	Advantages	Bacterial proliferation (other risk)	AAMI recommendations
Sediment filters	Removes particulate matter	+	Opaque housings Pressure gauges, pre and post filters Monitor pressure drop (ΔP) Charge filters when $\Delta P > 10$ lbs/sq. Inch Monitor for bacteria
Water softener	(1) Removes calcium & magnesium (2) Protects against scalling of RO system	+	Automatic regeneration with "bypass" Use pellet salt designed for softeners Check timer before dialysis Check hardness before dialysis
Carbon filters	Absorbs chlorine & chloramine	+	Use disposable carbon (GAC) Use two GAC tanks in series Each GAC tank with EBCT of 3–5 min 5-μ filters downstream Monitor for exhaustion; replace exhausted tanks (backup system replaces spent tank when chloramine level >0.1 mg/L) Monitor for bacteria
Reverse osmosis	(1) Rejects univalent & divalent Ions (2) Filters bacteria	+	Must produce AAMI-quality water Audible/visual alarms Monitor salt passage (2 × initial) (Salt passage = 100 − rejection rate) Monitor pretreatment
Deionization	Removes all types of cations & anions	+	Continuously monitor resistivity (<1 megohm/cm) Temperature compensated monitor Visual & audible alarm GAC upstream Don't use industrial or process resin
Disinfection	Prevention of endotoxemia & pyrogenic reactions	Anti-N-like antibody formation (formaldehyde)	See Table (11)
		Anaphylactoid reactions (ACE/Renalin/reprocessing)	4% formaldehyde, 24 hours contact time 1–2% formaldehyde, 40°C, 24 hours Renalin/diacide (FDA approved sterilants)

GAC, granular activated carbon; EBCT, empty bed contact time; GAC maximum mesh size 12 × 40 and minimum iodine number of 900; ACE, angiotensin-converting enzyme inhibitor.

Essential components of water purification

The efficiency of a water purification system depends on the capacity of the system, the nature of the incoming water supply, seasonal variations in municipal water quality, and the desired quality of product water. Figure 2 is representative of a typical water treatment system. In the section below, we will discuss the various components of the water treatment system in the order they are used in most dialysis units.

TEMPERATURE BLENDING VALVES

Temperature blending valves are used to mix incoming hot and cold water to provide an optimum water temperature for downstream components. Most RO membranes work most effectively at 77°F; water colder than 77°F will reduce the flow rate of the RO system, while water that is too hot (>100°F) may damage RO membranes and cause hemolysis.

FILTERS

Filters remove particle matter from water and consist of three types: sand filters, which remove particles ranging from 25 to 100μm; cartridge filters capable of extracting particles from 1 to 100μm in size; and submicron membrane filters, which can remove particles as small as 0.25μm. Five-μm filters are generally accepted as the size necessary to provide adequate protection for equipment and water treatment. Sediment filters may be placed downstream of carbon filters and are usually placed just before RO membranes.

WATER SOFTENERS

Water softening is used to remove calcium, magnesium, and other polyvalent cations from the feedwater. Water softeners are usually sodium-containing cation exchange resins. Calcium and magnesium are removed from the water in exchange for sodium. In extremely hard water, the

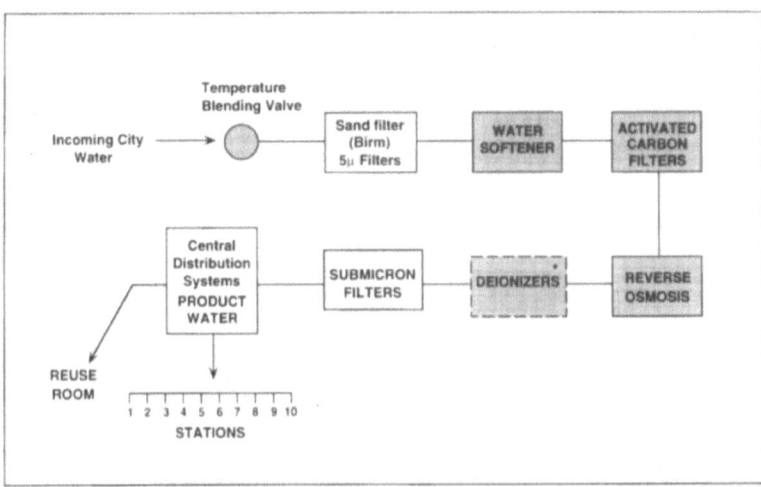

Figure 2. Components of water treatment system for hemodialysis. Deionizers are optional if reverse osmosis (RO) produces water of adequate quality. Granular activated carbon filters are always placed pre-RO system to reduce water hardness and prevent scaling of RO membranes. Deionization does not remove bacteria and endotoxin and should always be followed by ultrafiltration or submicron filters.

amount of sodium released can become problematic. The concentration of sodium released can be calculated:

$$Na(mEq/l) = \text{total hardness as } CaCO_3\,(mg/L)/50.$$

In addition to preventing the hard-water syndrome, the practical rationale for removing calcium and magnesium is to prevent these ions from depositing on the RO system, resulting in its malfunction. When the resin is exhausted, regeneration is accomplished by exposure to a brine solution. If the water softener is regenerated on site, water treatment equipment must contain bypass valves to ensure that regeneration does not occur during dialysis with consequent hypernatremia (140).

CARBON FILTRATION

Granular activated carbon (GAC) will absorb chlorine, chloramines, and other organic substances from water. Since carbon filters are highly porous with a high affinity for organic material, they can be contaminated with bacteria if they are not serviced properly or exchanged frequently. The size of an activated carbon bed requires an understanding of empty bed contact time (EBCT). The EBCT is calculated as

$$EBCT = \left[V \right]\!\left[7.48(\text{gallons})/\text{ft}^3 \right]/Q,$$

where V = volume of carbon required in cubic feet and Q = water flow rate (gallons/minute). The recommended EBCT for chlorine removal is 6 minutes and for chloramine removal 10 minutes.

The FDA recommends that two tanks filled with GAC

be used in series. Each tank should have an EBCT of 3–5 minutes. When the first GAC filter has a chloramine concentration in the effluent filter greater than 0.1 mg/L, it should be replaced within 72 hours. Similarly, if the chloramine level in the effluent of the second tank exceeds 0.1 mg/L, the water must not be used for dialysis (141,142).

REVERSE OSMOSIS

RO applies the principles of high hydrostatic pressure across a semipermeable membrane to a solution to prepare a purified solvent. This process rejects 90%–95% of univalent ions (e.g. Na^+) and 95%–99% of divalent ions, as well as microbiologic contaminants. Accordingly, 2%–10% of the dissolved ions will pass through the membrane into the product dialysate water. RO generally produces water that is safe for dialysis, but, in some instances, the quantity of dissolved salts in the dialysate water may exceed maximum safety concentrations. RO membrane technology advanced greatly in the late 1970s with the development of thin film composite (TFC) membranes, which offered several advantages over celluloid acetate and polyamide membranes. The TFC membranes were more resilient to frequent cleaning and/or sanitization with stronger chemical agents. The finished water quality is thus higher in terms of total dissolved solid rejections.

When an RO device is used as a pretreatment to deionization, it serves primarily as an economic device to provide longer service life for the deionization system. Subsequent deionization of permeate (product) RO water is usually unnecessary.

DEIONIZATION

Like water softeners, ionizers also work by ion exchange principles; however, deionizers remove all types of cations and anions. The cation exchange resin is in the form of $[H^+]$ ion (exchanging Na^+, K^+, Mg^{++}); the anion exchange resin is $[OH^-]$ (exchanging HCO_3^-, Cl^-, F^-, and SO_4^{2-}). The dual-bed system contains two tanks, one with an anion resin, the other with a cation resin. The mix-bed system results in a better water quality than the dual-bed system, though it is more expensive.

Deionizer efficacy is monitored by measuring the resistivity of the effluent. As resistivity varies with temperature, resistivity monitors also must be temperature-compensated to gauge deionization efficacy. AAMI standards specify that product water should have a specific resistivity of 1 megaohm/cm or more at 25°C. When the deionization system is exhausted, previously adsorbed ions can elute into the effluent, causing ion-related toxicities. Reports of fluoride, aluminum, and copper intoxications have all appeared as a consequence of unrecognized deionizer exhaustion (135,143). For a complete listing, the reader is referred to the AAMI/American National Standards (144).

Microbiology of hemodialysis systems

Water used by HD centers is usually obtained from the community water supply, which may be derived from ground and/or surface water. Both sources can contain high concentrations of bacteria and endotoxin. Community water treatment plans may reduce the number of bacteria in water but often do not reduce the endotoxin concentration. In addition to the water supply, all components of the WTS itself (except ultraviolet light) can harbor bacteria and endotoxin contamination (145,146).

The primary microbial contaminants of dialysis fluids are naturally occurring water bacteria. These include gram-negative bacteria and nontuberculous mycobacteria (Table 7). These bacteria can survive and multiply in water containing little organic matter, such as deionized or RO-treated water (145). In 1984, the CDC conducted a study of chronic HD units in the U.S. to determine the prevalence of nontuberculous mycobacteria in the water systems. The results showed that nontuberculous mycobacteria were present in the water of 83% of the centers surveyed (147).

Disinfection strategies for HD systems are targeted at gram-negative bacteria. Although bacteria may be inactivated by exposure to chemical germicides, bacterial endotoxins may remain in the HD system. Endotoxins are produced by bacteria and can persist despite the absence of bacteria. Although nontuberculous mycobacteria do not produce endotoxins, they are, compared to gram-negative bacteria, more resistant to chemical germicides and have been responsible for patient infections as a result of inadequately disinfected dialyzers (145–150).

Sterilization is a procedure that leads to the total de-

Table 7. Naturally occurring water bacteria commonly found in hemodialysis systems

Gram-negative bacteria	Nontuberculous mycobacteria
Pseudomonas	Mycobacterium chelonae
Flavobacterium	M. fortuitum
Acinetobacter	M. gordonae
Alcaligenes	M. scrofulaceum
Xanthomonas	M. avium
Serratia	M. abscessus
Achromobacter	M. intracellularis
Aeromonas	

struction of microorganisms, including highly resistant bacterial spores. Disinfection is defined as a process that eliminates most recognizable bacterial pathogens but not necessarily highly resistant microorganisms (151,152). Disinfection processes can be either high-level, intermediate, or low-level, depending on germicidal activity. High-level disinfection inactivates all microorganisms except bacterial spores. Low-level disinfection inactivates many, but not all, microorganisms and reduces the bacterial population to a level considered to be safe. Disinfection of WTS components and water dialysate distribution systems generally requires only low-level procedures. On the other hand, in dialyzer reprocessing, high-level disinfection is practiced and entails a sufficient concentration of germicidal agents for adequate contact time to eradicate nearly all microorganisms.

Pyrogenic reactions during hemodialysis

Pyrogenic reactions (PRs) developing during or after dialysis treatment are frequently recognized. In two recent studies, the frequency of dialysis-related PRs associated with bacterial contamination of the dialysate ranged from 1% to 5% (120,151). Incidence rates have been reported as high as 12% (152). Recently, Gordon et al. (153) identified a low incidence of PRs in a prospective study evaluating patients receiving all modes of HD treatments with bicarbonate dialysate. The dialysate contained high concentrations of bacteria and endotoxin. The authors reported 19 PRs among 18 patients in 268 HD treatments. They also found no statistically significant difference in PR rates by treatment modality (conventional 0.5/1000 versus high-efficiency 0.9/1000 versus high-flux (1.2/1000 treatments). It is noteworthy that in this study, the integrity of dialysis membranes was evaluated prospectively, preventing the subsequent use of damaged dialyzers. Also, only one type of hollow-fiber dialyzer (PS) was used for high-flux dialysis. The findings of this study therefore, cannot be generalized to all types of high-flux membranes. In addition, because high-flux treatments accounted for only 10% of the study treatments, it is possible that a longer observation period might have resulted in greater differences in adverse event rates between conventional and high-flux treatments. Finally, it is important to note that the incidence of PRs in high-flux dialysis was twice that of conventional dialysis.

The variable incidence of PRs may be due to different definitions of this disorder (152). Most authors, however, would agree that a case of PR can be defined as the onset of objective chills (or rigors) and/or fever (oral temperature >37.8°C (100°F)) in a previously afebrile patient with no recorded signs or symptoms of infection before dialysis (120,152–153). Hypotension (decrease in systolic blood pressure >30 mmHg) is included by some authors (153). Other less frequent signs are headache, myalgias, nausea, and vomiting. The symptoms usually begin 30–60 minutes into the dialysis treatment and, unless they are extreme, stop shortly after the treatment.

In the early 1970s, it was reported that severe PRs in HD patients correlated with the degree of bacterial contamination in the dialysate (154). A recent multicenter study in the U.S. by Klein et al. (155) demonstrated that 35.5% of water samples and 19% of dialysate samples did not comply with AAMI standards (≤200 colony forming units (CFU)/mL in water, 2000 CFU/mL in dialysate). In the same study, the endotoxin concentrations in dialysate measured by the Limulus Amoebocyte lysate assay (LAL) exceeded 5 endotoxin units/mL (1 ng/mL) in 6% of samples. Furthermore, there was no correlation between bacterial growth and endotoxin concentrations in water or dialysate samples. Likewise, in the study by Favero et al. (154), PRs correlated with the amount of bacterial growth in the dialysate but not necessarily with endotoxin levels. From these studies, one can speculate that low levels of bacterial growth can be associated with high endotoxin concentration. Presumably, bacteria adhere to and grow in the dialysis tubing and release endotoxin and endotoxin fragments into the dialysate. It is noteworthy that PRs may not necessarily correlate with the positive tests for endotoxin. There are many laboratory tests for endotoxin, the most common being the LAL assay. However, the sensitivity of this test, particularly for endotoxin fragments, has been questioned. More sensitive tests, such as the release of cytokines by mononuclear cells in response to endotoxin, have been advocated.

PRs also have been reported with higher frequency in association with other factors aside from bacterial and endotoxin dialysate contamination (see Table 8). Dialyzer reuse has been correlated with PRs in some studies. Theoretically, RO use and membrane integrity monitoring should lead to a decrease in the incidence of PRs.

Changing dialysis practices have had an impact on the number of PRs. In the 1991 CDC report on dialysis-associated diseases in the U.S., the use of bicarbonate dialysis and high-flux dialysis was associated with a higher risk of PRs (120). Notably, in dialysis units that used bicarbonate dialysis, a higher frequency of PRs occurred only in centers that also performed high-flux dialysis. Centers that prepared their own bicarbonate dialysate also were more likely to report PRs than centers that used commercially prepared bicarbonate dialysate.

Table 8. Risk factors for pyrogenic reactions

Bacterial and endotoxin contamination of dialysate
Bicarbonate dialysate (center prepared > commercial)
Dialyzer reuse (especially > 40), large centers (>40 patients)
Manual reprocessing of dialyzers
Failure to check dialyzer membrane integrity frequently (air-pressure leak test)
Inadequate admixture of germicide
Inadequate concentration and contact time for germicide
High-flux/high-efficiency dialysis

The method for preparing bicarbonate dialysate entails potential contamination hazards (156). Acetate dialysate is prepared from a single concentrate at a concentration that prohibits bacterial growth (4.8 M). Bicarbonate dialysate, however, must be prepared from two concentrates: an acid concentrate with a pH of 2.8 that is not conducive to bacterial growth and a 1.2-M bicarbonate concentrate with a neutral pH. Bicarbonate concentrates can support the growth of halo-tolerant endotoxin-producing gram-negative organisms. As many as 10^5–10^6 CFU/mL can develop in liquid bicarbonate in as few as 10 days after preparation. Halophile gram-negative rods are facultative anaerobes and can be difficult to culture using standard media. Increased microbial recovery from liquid bicarbonate concentrate can be achieved by supplementing Standard Method Agar with 0.2 M NaCl and 0.4 M NaHCO₃.

Due to the innate capability of liquid bicarbonate concentrate (LBC) to support bacterial proliferation, active quality assurance should be exercised in its manufacture and use. LBC should be used as soon as possible after manufacture or receipt by the dialysis center. If LBC is placed in storage tanks, the tanks and distribution lines should be disinfected at least twice weekly.

Finally, some reuse practices have been associated with PRs independent of high-flux dialyzer use, especially with large number of reuses of the dialyzer (120). Manual dialyzer reprocessing has been associated with a higher incidence of PRs compared to automated reprocessing (151). Manual reprocessing can allow dialyzer membrane defects to go undetected because testing for dialyzer membrane integrity is generally not performed with this technique.

In conclusion, a number of risk factors interact to cause PRs (Table 8). However, the overall quality of dialysis at individual centers may be more important than any single factor in determining PR occurrence. One recent study has demonstrated that units that simply filter hemodialysis fluid can remove bacteria and endotoxin reducing by two-fold the incidence of PRs among patients receiving high-flux, high-efficiency, or conventional HD (157).

Outbreaks of pyrogenic reactions

Several outbreaks of patient infection and PRs have been reported in patients during HD treatment (158–161). Many of these were the result of substandard reprocessing or poor water quality (152). Inadequate mixing of germicide or the use of a new germicide also has been implicated in several of these outbreaks (153,162).

In the report by Gordon et al. (153), the water used for rinsing dialyzers and diluting the disinfectant germicide contained high levels of endotoxin (>10^4 CFU/mL). After dialyzer reuse was discontinued at the center, the PR incidence fell to its preepidemic level.

In 1986, six dialysis centers reported outbreaks of PRs and septicemia associated with the use of a new germicide, chlorine dioxide. This chemical, though effective for disinfecting dialyzers, degraded cellulosic dialyzer membranes, with consequent membrane leakage (163). Centers that reported using chlorine dioxide also employed manual reprocessing, and most of these centers reused dialyzers more than 20 times. Manual dialyzer reprocessing has consistently been associated a with higher frequency of PRs (161). Alter and colleagues also reported that centers using Renalin to manually reprocess dialyzers more than 20 times had more clusters of PRs than centers that reused less than 20 times and used automated systems or 4% formaldehyde for reprocessing (161). Outbreaks of gram-negative bacteremia and PRs have also occurred due to failure to admix Renalin adequately during dilution (153).

Errors in the design and maintenance of a WTS were responsible for 29 PRs and 5 episodes of *Pseudomonas* bacteremia in another center (163). Damage to RO membranes contributed to this outbreak, leading to the recommendation of a thorough inspection for RO damage whenever the RO system removes less than 90%–95% of total dissolved solids.

Finally, though HD has been safely conducted outside the hospital or dialysis center setting, fatal endotoxemia occurred in dialysis patients at summer camp (164), illustrating the importance of dialysis WTSs in different environmental conditions.

In a recent CDC investigation of a dialysis-associated epidemic of nontuberculous mycobacterial infection, it was apparent that nominal 2% formaldehyde did not effectively eradicate these organisms within 36 hours (159). Another outbreak of systemic mycobacterial infection occurred when high-flux dialyzers were contaminated with mycobacteria during manual reprocessing and were then disinfected with a weak concentration of a commercial disinfectant (165). Additional studies have shown that if the concentration of formaldehyde is increased to 4%, none of the strains of mycobacteria survives at room temperature beyond 24 hours (166). It is possible that these infections may have been related to an improper mixing of the formaldehyde solution such that the final concentration was less than the intended concentration.

Finally, there is increasing evidence that lower concentrations of formaldehyde, e.g., 1%, can provide effective strength if the dialyzers are kept at temperatures of 37–40°C. (167).

In summary, ensuring the use of product water that meets AAMI standards, proper dialyzer reuse, appropriate germicide concentrations, and adequate exposure time and temperature are all necessary to reduce endotoxemia and PRs during dialysis. Use of commercial bicarbonate dialysate soon after receipt by dialysis centers is also vital to prevent bacterial proliferation. With these principles in mind, dialyzer reuse and high-flux, high-efficiency dialysis are likely to continue to be efficient and cost-effective in the future with even fewer microbial hazards.

Pathogenesis of pyrogenic reactions

Three lines of evidence implicate endotoxins in the pathogenesis of PRs: 1) antibodies in HD patients to endotoxins elaborated by bacteria in dialysate (168,169); 2) limulus lysate reactivity in plasma from HD patients experiencing pyrexia (170,171); and 3) the association of PRs with HD fluids contaminated with gram-negative bacteria (154,171).

Given the pore diameters of a dialysis membrane, it is unlikely that microorganisms cross intact dialyzer membranes. Instead, it is more probable that endotoxins or other pyrogenic substances in dialysis fluid gain access to the patients' bloodstream across the dialysis membrane (171,172).

Some of these substances are bacterial pyrogens released by gram-negative bacteria (Table 9) (173). They include lipopolysaccharide (LPS), its subunit, layer A, other LPS fragments, peptidoglycans, muramylpeptides, exotoxins, and exotoxin fragments.

Assays for determining pyrogen permeability include the LAL assay, the mononuclear cell (MNC) assay, radiolabeled LPS fragments, and neutrophil activation. Despite the sensitivity of the LAL assay many bacterial substances, so-called *endotoxin fragments* (Table 9), are small enough to penetrate even tight cellulosic membranes but cannot be detected in the LAL assay. Measuring in vitro cytokine production by MNCs is a most sensitive and specific assay and allows detection of these small-molecular-weight substances (174–176).

Table 9. Pyrogenic bacterial substances and assays to test pyrogen permeability of dialysis membranes

Bacterial substance	MW (kDa)	LAL assay[a]	MNC assay[b]	Inhibition by polymyxin B[c]
LPS	>100	+	+	+
Lipid-A related LPS fragments	2–4	+	+	+
Peptidoglycans	1–20	–	+	–
Muramylpeptides	0.4–1	–	+	–
Exotoxins	20–50	–	+	–
Exotoxin fragments	<5	–	+	–

[a] Specific but poorly sensitive. False positives with charged plasma proteins.
[b] Highly sensitive.
[c] Distinguishes lipid-A related & non-lipid A related pyrogens in MNC cytokine induction.
Modified, from Lonnemann (ref. 176).

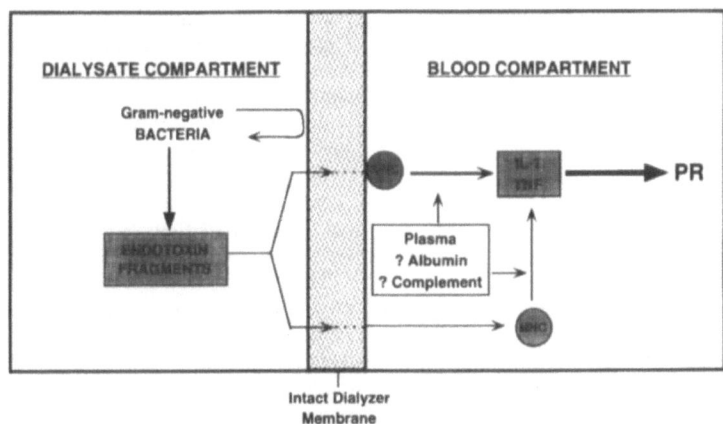

Figure 3. Pathogenesis of pyrogenic reactions (PRs) during hemodialysis. Living microorganisms cannot cross intact dialyzer membranes. Gram-negative organisms produce endotoxins and endotoxin fragments. Non-tuberculous mycobacteria may contaminate dialyzers. They do not produce endotoxin. At high concentrations, endotoxin can cross cellulosic and high-flux dialyzer membranes. In the presence of plasma, albumin, or complement, these fragments induce monocytes to produce IL-1 and TNF-α. Large fragments also may interact with monocytes at the dialyzer membrane interface. Cytokines may then induce a febrile reaction.

Table 10. Factors influencing dialyzer membrane pyrogen permeability

---

Dialyzer membrane type
Dialysate microorganism species
Bacterial and endotoxin dose
Plasma proteins in blood compartment
Pyrogen adsorption to dialyzer membrane
Pryogen test employed
    LAL versus MNC cytokine production versus radiolabeled
    LPS

LAL, limulus Ameobocyte lysate test; MNC, mononuclear cells; LPS, lipopolysaccharide.

Various studies have been unable to detect the passage of endotoxin in dialysate across intact dialyzer membranes during conventional or high-flux dialysis (177–179). Gordon et al. found a low incidence of PRs with each modality, despite elevated concentrations of bacteria (19,000 CFU/mL) and endotoxin (390 pg/mL) (153). They also observed a low positive predictive value for the LAL assay. They suggested that detectable levels of endotoxin were not the cause of PRs. Others have also concluded that HD-associated pyrexia is not simply due to the transfer of endotoxin across intact dialyzers (179).

Bacterial products including endotoxins induce human MNCs to produce interleukin-1 (IL-1) and tumor necrosis factor-alpha (TNF-α), two cytokines integral in the immune response (173). Investigations using in vitro hemodialysis have demonstrate that cultured MNCs produce significant amounts of IL-1 when LPS is in the dialysate (179).

Lonneman et al. also studied whether LPS fragments or plasma proteins were involved in MNC cytokine induction (176,181). They found that LPS-like fragments from E. coli can cross the dialyzer membrane. However, plasma needed to be present in the blood side for cytokine induction. The role of plasma in this interaction, however, is still not completely understood. Plasma proteins, e.g., LPS-binding proteins and complement, can be activated by regenerated cellulosic membranes (181). They can also amplify MNC cytokine production in response to small concentrations of LPS fragments (181–184). These proteins, however, do not have cytokine-inducing activity per se (175,181). These data suggest that many factors influence the permeability of dialysis membranes to pyrogens (Table 10).

In summary, evidence suggests that endotoxin fragments can transit intact hemodialysis membranes and induce MNC cytokine production, particularly in the presence of plasma. The latter substances may be the cause of febrile reactions on hemodialysis (Figure 3). However, because many studies of dialyzer membrane pyrogen permeability have used exceedingly high challenge doses, firm conclusions about the pathogenesis of PRs in vivo cannot yet be deduced from these data.

AAMI STANDARDS FOR HEMODIALYSIS WATER QUALITY

A summary of the AAMI's recommendations for safe and proper water treatment and the use of WTS components is listed in Table 11. With referance to water for dialysis, current federal regulations state, "Water used for dialysis

Table 11. AAMI hemodialysis water quality standards[a]

A. Microbiologic and endotoxin standards for dialysis fluids

Type of fluid	Microbial count (CFU/mL)[b]	Endotoxin (EU/mL)[c]
Water to prepare dialysate	≤200	No standard
Dialysate	≤2000	No standard
Water to rinse & reprocess dialyzers	≤200	≤5[d]
Water to prepare dialyzer disinfectant	≤200	≤5[d]

B. Chemical contaminants monitoring

Contaminant	Suggested maximum level (mg/L)
Calcium	2 (0.1 mEq/L)
Magnesium	4 (0.3 mEq/L)
Sodium	70 (3 mEq/L)[e]
Potassium	8 (0.2 mEq/L)
Fluoride	0.2
Chlorine	0.5
Chloramines	0.1
Nitrates	2
Sulfate	100
Copper, barium, zinc	0.1 each
Aluminum	0.01
Arsenic, lead, silver	0.005 each
Cadmium	0.001
Chromium	0.014
Selenium	0.09
Mercury	0.002

[a] Association for the Advancement of Medical Instrumentation, American National Standards: *AAMI Standard and Recommended Practices. Vol. 3: Dialysis.* Arlington, VA, 1993.
[b] CFU, colony-forming units.
[c] EU, endotoxin units.
[d] 5 EU = 1 ng.
[e] 230 mq/L (10 mEq/L) where Na concentration of the concentrate has been reduced to compensate for excess Na in the water as long as conductivity of water is being continuously monitored.

purposes is analyzed periodically and treated as necessary to maintain a continuous water supply that is biologically and chemically compatible with acceptable dialysis techniques. Records of test results and equipment maintenance are maintained in the facility" (42 CFR 405.2140 (a) 5). The standard notes that assay frequency should be based upon the type of water-refining system utilized by the facility. In practice, state or HCFA surveyors interpret the federal regulation to mean "the facility performs an AAMI chemical contaminants analysis at least yearly and does bacterial monitoring at least monthly." A more aggressive assay schedule should be performed when influent city-water quality varies or when changes occur in functioning system components (e.g., new systems, modification of previous system, or when clinical indications suggest PRs or septicemias due to bacterial contamination).

Microbiologic samples should be assayed by the spread-plate or membrane filtration technique. If a spread-plate technique is used, the sample must be quantitatively measured with a pipette, not a calibrated loop. Because the calibrated loop places such a small amount on the culture plate (0.001 mL or 0.01 mL), it cannot provide the necessary test sensitivity. Culture results, therefore, may grossly underestimate the actual levels of bacterial contamination. A pipette delivers much larger volume, 0.01–0.5 mL, to the culture medium, thereby enhancing the culture's sensitivity for documenting bacterial growth.

The current AAMI Standards recommend that culture medium should be trypticase soy agar (incubated at 35–37°C, with colony counts after 48 hours). In a recent study, bacterial growth of dialysate samples in standard culture media, trypticase soy agar, or plate-count agar was compared to results obtained in a nutrient-poor R2A medium, cultured at 25° for 96 hours (191). Several typical water bacteria grew better or more selectively on R2A agar. The growth of common water microorganisms can be 100–1000-fold higher on nutrient-poor media compared to standard agar. Thus, bacterial contamination of dialysate fluid may be underinterpreted using standard clinical bacteriological methods. Endotoxin concentrations should be determined by the LAL assay (192).

Internal fluid pathways should be disinfected weekly, the RO unit monthly. One to two percent aqueous formaldehyde, glutaraldehyde, or chlorine-based disinfectants produce consistent disinfection for internal fluid pathways. Hot water (>80°C or 176°F) is an alternative and avoids the hazards associated with chemical germicides.

Disinfection strategies for dialyzer reprocessing are quite different from those targeted to the water supply. While low-level disinfection is adequate for WTS components, high-level disinfection is mandatory for dialyzer reprocessing. Water monitoring for reprocessing hemodialyzers therefore requires more stringent criteria. While there are no AAMI standards for endotoxin levels in water used to prepare dialysate, water for rinsing, reprocessing, and disinfecting dialyzers should contain less than 5 endotoxin units/mL (1 ng/mL).

The recognition that nontuberculous mycobacteria can be resistant to certain germicides and still cause infection spurred the establishment of current safety microbiologic standards for dialyzer reprocessing. After reverse ultrafiltration and cleaning with sodium hypochlorite bleach <1%, or with H_2O_2 ≤ 3% and peracetic acid ≤2%, manual or automated pressure tests for leaks should be performed. Dialyzers should then undergo disinfection/sterilization. Germicides are generally instilled into the blood and dialysate compartments and remain in contact for at least 24 hours. The three most commonly used agents are 4% formaldehyde, peracetic-acid–hydrogen-peroxide–acetic-acid mixture (Renalin®) and glutaraldehyde (Diacide®). A 2% formaldehyde solution should not be used because some mycobacteria can survive in 2% formaldehyde at room temperature. However, even 1% solutions of formaldehyde may have excellent germicidal efficacy when dialyzers are incubated at 40°C for 24 hours (193). Heat sterilization (105° for 20 hours) for reprocessing certain polysulfone membranes also has been successful (194). Some clinical concerns have appeared in association with dialyzer reprocessing. Anti-N-like antibody formation can be produced when residual dialyzer formaldehyde levels are high (195). These have been associated with hemolysis and early transplant failure. However, no such reports have appeared since the use of more sensitive detecting of residual formaldehyde. Potential anaphylactoid reactions have also been noted in patients taking ACE inhibitors who underwent hemodialysis with dialyzers reprocessed with Renalin (196) or bleach (197). These reactions likely reflect the characteristic of the membrane, rather than the sterilant.

Increased mortality associated with manual dialyzer reprocessing using Renalin and glutaraldehyde also has been reported (198). However, a direct causative link between these germicides and increased patient mortality remains to be established. As a consequence, the FDA has instructed dialysis units to review their manual and automated reuse procedures carefully and to ensure meticulous adherence to manufacturer instructions.

In summary, water treatment is a vital aspect of hemodialysis in which knowledge and technical skills are of utmost importance. Each component of a WTS brings with it its own risks and requirements for safe and proper use as well as for monitoring and surveillance. Monitoring membrane integrity is as important as meeting the AAMI Standards for bacterial and endotoxin levels of water used to prepare disinfectant and rinse hemodialyzers. High-level disinfection is a requirement for safe dialyzer reuse to ensure adequate disinfection of nontuberculous mycobacteria.

The pathogenesis of febrile reactions remains controversial. The weight of evidence, however, favors the transit of endotoxin fragments across dialysis membranes to induce mononuclear cell cytokine production. Finally, bacterial contamination in dialysate may be underestimated when routine bacteriologic methods are used (Trypticase Soy Agar). Similarly, because of LAL-negative pyrogens, the LAL assay may not be adequate for monitoring the dialysate pyrogen level. The lack of sensitivity of these tests may partially explain the controversies surrounding the pathogenesis of PRs.

ACKNOWLEDGMENT

The excellent secretarial assistance of Nadine Cline is greatly appreciated.

REFERENCES

1. Ono T, Kataoka H, Kunimoto T: Quantitative analysis on the removal of b2-microglobulin from chronic dialysis patients. *Blood Purif* 4:212–214, 1985.
2. Kuhle C, Fricke H, Weld E, Schiffl H: High-flux hemodialysis postpones clinical manifestation of dialysis-related amyloidosis. *Am J Nephrol* 16:484–488, 1996.
3. Mujais SK, and Ivanovich P: Membranes for extracorporeal therapy. In: *Replacement* of Renal Function by Dialysis. J Matier, editor, 3rd edition 1989.
4. Gohl H, Konstantin P: Membrane and filters for hemofiltration. In: LW Henderson, EA Quellhorst, CA Baldamus, MJ Lysaght, eds, *Hemofiltration*. Springer-Verlag, Berlin, p 41, 1986.
5. Leypoldt JK, Frigon RP, Henderson LW: Macromolecular charge affects hemofilter solute sieving. *Trans Am Soc Artif Intern Organs* 32:384–387, 1986.
6. Konstantin P, Bailey RM: Polycarbonate-polyether (PC-PE) flat sheet membrane: manufacture, structure and performance. *Blood Purif* 4:6–12, 1985.
7. Gohl H, Raff M, Harttig D, Deppisch R: PC-PE hollow-fiber membrane structure, performance characteristics, and manufacturing. *Blood Purif* 4:23–31, 1985.
8. Akizawa T, Kitaoka T, Koshikawa S, Watanabe T, Imamura K, Tsurumi T, Suma Y, Eiga S: Development of a regenerated cellulose non-complement activating membrane for hemodialysis. *Trans Am Soc Artif Intern Organs* 32:76–84, 1986.
9. Hildebrand U, Quellhorst E: Influence of various membranes on the coagulation system during dialysis. *Contrib Nephrol* 46:92–101, 1985.
10. Van Stone JC: Hemodialysis apparatus. In: JT Daugirdas, TS Ing, *Handbook of Dialysis*, 2nd ed, Little, Brown, Boston, p 29, 1988.
11. Kaufman AM, Frinak S, Godmere RO, Levin NW: Clinical experience with heat sterilization for reprocessing dialyzers. *ASAIO J* 38:M338–M340, 1992.
12. Sigdell Jan Erik: Operating characteristics of hollow-fiber dialyzers. In: AR Nissenson, RN Fine, DE Gentile, eds, *Clinical Dialysis*, 2nd ed. Appleton and Lange, San Mateo, CA, pp 106–107, 1990.
13. Hakim RM: Clinical implications of hemodialysis membrane biocompatibility. *Kidney Int* 44:484–494, 1993.
14. Arnout MA, Hakim RM, Todd RF, Dana N, Colten HR: Increased expression of an adhesion promoting surface glycoprotein in the granulocytopenia of hemodialysis. *N Engl J Med* 312:457–462, 1985.
15. Dinarello CA: Cytokines and biocompatibility. *Blood Purif* 8:208–213, 1990.
16. Strasser T, Schiffl H: Generation of leukotriene B4 by hemodialyzer membranes: a novel index of biocompatibility. *Klin Wochenschr* 69:808–812, 1991.
17. Craddock PR, Fehr J, Delmasso AP, Brigham KL, Jacob HS: Hemodialysis leukopenia: pulmonary vascular leukostasis resulting from complement activation by dialyzer cellophane membranes. *J Clin Invest* 59:878–888, 1977.
18. Rault RB, Silver MR: Severe reactions during hemodialysis. *Am J Kidney Dis* 5:128–135, 1985.
19. Walker JF, Lindsay RM, Peters SD, Sibbalb WJ, Linton AL: A sheep model to examine the cardiopulmonary maniestations of blood dialyzer interactions. *Am Soc Artif Intern Organs* 6:123–130, 1983.
20. Hakim RM, Breillatt J, Lazarus JM, Port FK: Complement activation and hypersensitivity reactions to dialysis membranes. *N Engl J Med* 311:878–882, 1984.
21. Daugirdas JT, Ing TS: First use reactions during hemodialysis: a definition of subtypes. *Kidney Int* 33 (Suppl 24):S37–S43, 1988.
22. Pegues DA, Beck-Sague CM, Woollen SW, Greenspan B, Burns SM, Bland LA, Arduino MJ, Favero MS, Mackow RC,

Jarvis WR: Anaphylactoid reactions associated with reuse of hollow-fiber hemodialyzers and ACE inhibitors. *Kidney Int* 42:1232–1237, 1992.

23. Hakim RM, Fearon DT, Lazarus JM: Biocompatibility of dialysis membranes: effects of chronic complement activation. *Kidney Int* 26:194–210, 1984.

24. Himmelfarb J, Lazarus M, Hakim R: Reactive oxygen species production by monocytes and polymorphonuclear leukocytes during dialysis. *Am J Kidney Dis* 3:271–276, 1991.

25. Arora N, Lambrou FH, Stewart MW, Vidrine-Parks L, Sandroni S: Sudden blindness associated with central nervous symptoms in a hemodialysis patient. *Nephron* 59:490–492, 1991.

26. Davenport A, Williams AJ: The effect of dialyzer reuse on peak expiratory flow rate. *Respir Med* 84:17–21, 1990.

27. Stone WJ, Hakim RM: b2m amyloidosis in long-term hemodialysis patients. *Am J Nephrol* 9:177–183, 1989.

28. Brunner FP, Brynger H, Ehrich JHH: Case control study on dialysis arthropathy: the influence of two different dialysis membranes:data from the EDTA registry. *Nephrol Dial Transplant* 5:432–436, 1990.

29. van Ypersele de Strihou C, Jadoul M, Malghem J, Maldague B, Jamart J: Effect of dialysis membrane and patient's age on signs of dialysis-related amyloidosis. *Kidney Int* 39:1012–1019, 1991.

30. Chanard J, Bindi P, Lavand S: Carpal tunnel syndrome and type of dialysis membrane. *Br J Med* 298:867–868, 1989.

31. Jahn B, Betz M, Deppisch R, Janssen O, Hansch GM, Ritz E: Stimulation of b2m synthesis in lymphocytes after exposure to cuprophane dialyzer membranes. *Kidney Int* 405:285–290, 1991.

32. Lemke RP, Hample H, Lobech H: Lysine-specific cleavage of b2-m in amyloid deposits associated with hemodialysis. *Kidney Int* 36:675–681, 1989.

33. DiRaimondo CR, Pollak VE: b2m kinetics in maintenance hemodialysis: a comparison of conventional and high-flux dialyzers and the effects of dialyzer reuse. *Am J Kidney Dis* 5:390–395, 1989.

34. Conger JD: Does hemodialysis delay recovery from acute renal failure? *Semin Dial* 3:146–148, 1990.

35. Solez K, Morel-Moroger L, Sraer JD: The morphology of "acute tubular necrosis in man." *Medicine* (Baltimore) 58:362–376, 1979.

36. Badr KF, Schreiner GF, Wasserman M, Ichikawa I: Preservation of the glomerular capillary ultrafiltration coefficient during rat nephrotoxic serum nephritis by a specific leukotriene D4 receptor antagonist. *J Clin Invest* 81:1702–1709, 1988.

37. Linas SL, Whittenburg D, Parsons P, Repine JE: Mild renal ischemia activates primed neutrophils to cause acute renal failure. *Kidney Int* 42:610–616, 1992.

38. Schulman G, Fogo A, Gung A, Badr K, Hakim R: Complement activation retards resolution of acute ischemic renal failure in the rat. *Kidney Int* 40:1069–1074, 1991.

39. Hornberger JC, Chernew M, Petersen J, Garber AM: A multivariate analysis of mortality and hospital admissions with high-flux dialysis. *J Am Soc Nephrol* 3:1227–1237, 1993.

40. Zaoui P, Hakim RM: Natural killer cell function in hemodialysis patients: effect of the dialysis membrane. *Kidney Int* 43:1298–1305, 1993.

41. Degiannis D, Czarnecki M, Donati D: Normal T lymphocyte function in patients with end stage renal disease hemodialyzed with polysulfone membranes. *Am J Nephrol* 10:276–282, 1990.

42. Donati D, Degiannis D, Coates N, Raskova J, Raska K Jr: Mixed lymphocyte reaction-induced release of soluble IL-2 receptor. *Transplantation* 51:518–523, 1991.

43. Guiterrez A, Alvestrand A, Wahren J, Bergstrom J: Effect of in vivo contact between blood and dialysis membranes on protein catabolism in humans. *Kidney Int* 38:487–494, 1990.

44. Guiterrez A, Alvestrand A, Bergstrom J: Membrane selection and muscle protein catabolism. *Kidney Int* 42:S86–S90, 1992.

45. Lindsay RM, Spanner EA, Heidenheim P, Kortas C, Blake PG: PCR, Kt/V and membrane. *Kidney Int* 43 (Suppl 41):S268–S273, 1993.

46. Chanard J, Brunois JP, Melin JP, Lavaud S, Toupance O: Long term results of dialysis therapy with a highly permeable membrane. *Artif Organs* 6:262–266, 1982.

47. Van Stone JC: Hemodialysis apparatus. In: JT Daugirdas, TS Ing, ed, *Handbook of Dialysis*, 3rd ed. Little, Brown, Boston, p 29, 1993.

48. Mendelssohn S, Swartz CD, Yudis M, Onesti G, Ramirez O, Brest AN: High glucose concentration dialysate in chronic hemodialysis. *Trans ASAIO* 13:249–253, 1967.

49. Rosborough DC, Van Stone JC: Dialysate glucose. *Semin Dial* 6:260–263, 1993.

50. Ward RA, Wathen RL, Williams TE, Harding GB: Hemodialysate composition and intradialytic metabolic, acid–base, and potassium changes. *Kidney Int* 32:129–35, 1987.

51. Wathen RA, Keshairah P, Hommeyer P, Cadwell K, Comty CM: The metabolic effects of hemodialysis with and without glucose in the dialysate. *Am J Clin Nutr* 31:1870–1875, 1978.

52. Grajower MM, Walter L, Albin J: Hypoglycemia in chronic hemodialysis patients: association with progranolol use. *Nephron* 26:126–129, 1980.

53. Uraemic hypoglycaemia. *Lancet* 1:660–661, 1986.

54. Ganda OP, Aoki TT, Soeldner JS, Morrison RS, Cahill GF Jr: Hormone-fuel concentrations in anephric subjects: effects of hemodialysis (with special reference to amino acids). *J Clin Invest* 57:1403–1411, 1976.

55. Koppel JD, Swendseid ME, Shinaberger JH, Umezawa CY: The free and bound amino acids removed by hemodialysis. *Trans ASAIO* 19:309–303, 1973.

56. Ward RA, Shirlow MJ, Hayes JM, Chapman GV, Farrel PC: Protein catabolism during hemodialysis. *Am J Clin Nutr* 32:2443–2449, 1979.

57. Hubner W, Sieberth HG, Diemer A, Finke K, Prange E: Effects of regular hemodialysis with glucose and glucose free dialysate on hyperlipemia. *Proc EDTA* 8:174–181, 1971.

58. Ramirez G, Butcher DE, Morrison AO: Glucose concentration in the dialysate and lipid abnormalities in chronic hemodialysis patients. *Int J Artif Organs* 10:31–36, 1987.

59. Ramirez G, Bercaw BL, Butcher DE, Mathis HL, Brueggemeyer C, Newton JL: The role of glucose in hemodialysis: the effect of glucose free dialysate. *Am J Kidney Dis* 7:413–420, 1986.

60. Daugirdas JT: Dialysis hypotension: a hemodynamic analysis. *Kidney Int* 39:233–246, 1991.

61. de Vries PM: Plasma volume changes during hemodialysis. *Semin Dial* 5:42–47, 1992.

62. Sherman RA: The pathophysiologic basis for hemodialysis-related hypotension. *Semin Dial* 1:136–142, 1988.

63. Palmer BF: The effect of dialysate composition on systemic hemodynamics. *Semin Dialy* 5:54–60, 1992.

64. Kinet JP, Soyeur D, Ballard N, Saint-Remy M, Collilgnon P,

Godon J-P: Hemodynamic study of hypotension during hemodialysis. *Kidney Int* 21:868–876, 1982.

65. Rouby JJ, Rottembourg J, Durande JP, Basset JY, Doogoulet P, Glaser P, Legrain M: Hemodynamic changes induced by regular hemodialysis and sequential ultrafiltration hemodialysis: a comparative study. *Kidney Int* 17:808–810, 1980.

66. Wehle B, Asaba H, Castenfors J, Furst P, Gunnaroson B, Shaldon S, Bergstrom J: Hemodynamic changes during sequential ultrafiltration and dialysis. *Kidney Int* 15:411–418, 1979.

67. Baldamus CA, Ernst W, Frei U, Koch KM: Sympathetic and hemodynamic response to volume removal during different forms of renal replacement therapy. *Nephron* 31:324–332, 1982.

68. Petitclerc T, Drueke T, Man N, Funck-Brentano JL: Cardiovascular stability on hemodialysis. *Adv Nephrol* 16:351–370, 1987.

69. Raja R, Henriquez M, Kramer M, Rosenbaum JL: Intradialytic hypotension—role of osmolar changes and acetate influx. *Artif Organs* 9:17–21, 1985.

70. Henrich WL, Woodard TD, Blachley JD, Gomez-Sanches C, Pettinger W, Cronin RE: Role of osmolality in blood pressure stability after dialysis and ultrafiltration. *Kidney Int* 18:480–488, 1980.

71. Dumler F, Grondin G, Levin NW: Sequential high/low sodium hemodialysis: an alternative to ultrafiltration. *Trans ASAIO* 25:351–353, 1979.

72. Daugirdas JT, Al-Kudsi RR, Ing TS, Norusis MJ: A double-blind evaluation of sodium gradient hemodialysis. *Am J Nephrol* 5:163–168, 1985.

73. Raja R, Kramer M, Barber K, Chen S: Sequential changes in dialysate sodium (D_{Na}) during hemodialysis. *Trans ASAIO* 24:649–651, 1983.

74. Bedichek E, Kirschbaum B, Sica D: Comparison of the hemodynamic and hormonal effects of hemodialysis using programmable vs constant sodium dialysate (abstract). *J Am Soc Nephrol* 3:354, 1992.

75. Heineken FS, Evans MC, Keen ML: Intercompartmental fluid shifts in hemodialysis patients. *Biotechnol Prog* 3:69, 1987.

76. Star RA, Hootkins R, Thompson JR, Pool T, Toto RD: Variability and stability of two pool urea mass transfer coefficient (abstract). *J Am Soc Nephrol* 3:395, 1992.

77. Tokars JI, Alter MJ, Faverso MS: U.S. Department of Health and Human Services, Centers for Disease Control and Prevention: National surveillance of dialysis-associated diseases in the United States, 1992. USDHHS, 1992.

78. Leunissen KML, Hoorntje SJ, Fiers HA, Dekkers WT, Mulder AW: Acetate versus bicarbonate hemodialysis in critically ill patients. *Nephron* 42:146–151, 1986.

79. Graefe U, Milutenovich J, Follette WC, Vizzo JE, Babb AL, Scribner BH: Less dialysis induced morbidity and vascular instability with bicarbonate in dialysate. *Ann Intern Med* 88:332–336, 1978.

80. Vincent JL, Vanherweghem JL, Degante JP, Berre J, Dufaye P, Kahn RJ: Acetate induced myocardial depression during hemodialysis for acute renal failure. *Kidney Int* 22:653–657, 1982.

81. Novello A, Kelsch RC, Easterling RE: Acetate intolerance during hemodialysis. *Clin Nephrol* 5:29–32, 1976.

82. Hakim RM, Ponzer M-A, Tilton D, Lazarus JM, Gottlieb MN: Effects of acetate and bicarbonate dialysate in stable chronic dialysis patients. *Kidney Int* 28:535–540, 1985.

83. Tolchin N, Roberts JL, Hayashi J, Lewis EJ: Metabolic consequences of high mass-transfer hemodialysis. *Kidney Int* 11:306, 1977.

84. Henrich WL: Hemodynamic instability during hemodialysis. *Kidney Int* 30:605–612, 1986.

85. Lonnemann G, Bingel M, Koch KM, Shaldon S, Dinarello CA: Plasma interleukin-1 activity in humans undergoing hemodialysis with regenerated cellulosic membranes. *Lymphokine Res* 6:63–70, 1987.

86. Garella S, Chang BS: Hemodialysis-associated hypoxemia. *Am J Nephrol* 4:273–279, 1984.

87. Ross EA, Nissenson AR: Dialysis-associated hypoxemia: insights into pathophysiology and prevention. *Semin Dial* 1:33–39, 1988.

88. Wolff J, Pendersen T, Rossen M, Cleeman-Rasmussen K: Effects of acetate and bicarbonate dialysis on cardiac performance, transmural myocardial perfusion and acid–base balance. *Int J Artif Organs* 9:105–110, 1986.

89. Vaziri ND, Wilson A, Mukai D, Daruish R, Rutz A, Hyatt J, Moreno C: Dialysis hypoxemia—role for dialyzer membrane and dialysate delivery system. *Am J Med* 77:828–833, 1984.

90. Henrich WL, Woodard TD, Meyer BD, Chappell TR, Rubin L: High sodium bicarbonate and acetate hemodialysis: double blind crossover comparison of hemodynamic and ventilatory effects. *Kidney Int* 24:240–245, 1983.

91. Velez RL, Woodard TD, Henrich WL: Acetate and bicarbonate hemodialysis in patients with and without autonomic dysfunction. *Kidney Int* 26:59–65, 1984.

92. Mehta BR, Fischer D, Ahmad M, Dubose TD: Effects of acetate and bicarbonate hemodialysis on cardiac function in chronic dialysis patients. *Kidney Int* 24:782–787, 1983.

93. Vinay P, Prud'homme M, Vinet B, Cournoyer G, Degouet P, Ceville M, Gougoux A, St-Louis G, Lapierre L, Piette Y: Acetate metabolism and bicarbonate generation during hemodialysis: 10 years of observation. *Kidney Int* 31:1194–1204, 1987.

94. Feinfeld DA, Sherwood LM: Parathyroid hormone and $1,225(OH)_2D_3$ in chronic renal failure. *Kidney Int* 33:1049–1058, 1988.

95. Felsenfeld AJ, Rodriguez M, Dunlay R, Llach F: A comparison of parathyroid gland function in hemodialysis patients with different forms of renal osteodystrophy. *Nephrol Dial Transplant* 6:244–251, 1991.

96. Wing AJ: Optimum calcium concentration of dialysis fluid for maintenance haemodialysis. *Br Med J* 4:145, 1968.

97. Johnson WJ, Goldsmith RS, Beabout JW: Prevention and reversal of secondary hyperparathyroidism in patients maintained by hemodialysis. *Am J Med* 56:827–830, 1974.

98. Maynard JC, Cruz C, Kleerekoper M, Levin NW: Blood pressure response to changes in serum ionized calcium during hemodialysis. *Ann Intern Med* 104:358–361, 1986.

99. Sherman RA, Bialy GB, Gazinski B, Bernholc AS, Eisinger RP: The effect of dialysate calcium levels on blood pressure during hemodialysis. *Am J Kidney Dis* 8:244–247, 1986.

100. Fellner SK, Lang RM, Neumann A, Spencer KT, Bushinsky DA, Borow KM: Physiological mechanisms for calcium-induced changes in systemic arterial pressure in stable dialysis patients. *Hypertension* 13:213–218, 1989.

101. Henrich WL, Hunt JM, Nixon JV: Increased ionized calcium and left ventricular contractility during hemodialysis. *N Engl J Med* 310:19–23, 1984.

102. Lang RB, Fellner SK, Neuman A, Bushinsky DA, Borow KM: Left ventricular contractility varies directly with blood ionized calcium. *Ann Intern Med* 108:524–529, 1988.

103. Morton AR, Hercz G, Coburn JW: Control of hyperphosphatemia in chronic renal failure. *Semin Dial* 3:219–223, 1990.

104. Mai ML, Emmett M, Shelkh MS, et al.: Calcium acetate, an effective phosphorus binder in patients with renal failure. *Kidney Int* 36:690–695, 1989.

105. Coburn JW: Use of oral and parenteral calcitriol in the treatment of renal osteodystrophy. *Kidney Int* 38 (Suppl 29):S54–S-61, 1990.

106. Slatopolsky E, Weerts C, Lopez-Hilker S: Calcium carbonate as a phosphate binder in patients with chronic renal failure undergoing dialysis. *N Engl J Med* 315:157–161, 1986.

107. Slatopolsky E, Weerts C, Norwood K, et al.: Long-term effects of calcium carbonate and 2.5 mEq/L calcium dialysate on mineral metabolism. *Kidney Int* 36:897–903, 1989.

108. Sawyer N, Noonan K, Altmann P, Marsh F, Cunningham J: High-dose calcium carbonate with stepwise reduction in dialysate calcium concentration: effective phosphate control and aluminum avoidance in hemodialysis patients. *Nephrol Dial Transpl* 4:105–109, 1989.

109. Van der Merwe WM, Rodger RSC, Grant AC: Low calcium dialysate and high-dose oral calcetriol in the treatment of secondary hyperparathyroidism in haemodialysis patients. *Nephrol Dial Transplant* 5:874–877, 1990.

110. Ketchersid TL, Van Stone JC: Dialysate potassium. *Semin Dial* 4:46–51, 1991.

111. Spital A, Sterns RH: Potassium homeostasis in dialysis patients. *Semin Dial* 1:14–20, 1988.

112. Sherman RA, Hwang ER, Bernholz AS, Eisinger RP: Variability in potassium removal by hemodialysis. *Am J Nephrol* 6:284–288, 1986.

113. Feig PU, Shook A, Sterns RH: Effect of potassium removal during hemodialysis on the plasma potassium concentration. *Nephron* 27:25–30, 1981.

114. Hou S, McElroy PA, Nootens J, Beach M: Safety and efficacy of low-potassium dialysate. *Am J Kidney Dis* 13:137–143, 1989.

115. Morgan AG, Burkinshaw L, Robinson PJA, Rosen SM: Potassium balance and acid–base changes in patients undergoing regular hemodialysis therapy. *Br Med J* 1:779–783, 1970.

117. Morrison G, Michelson EL, Brown S, Morganroth J: Mechanism and prevention of cardiac arrhythmias in chronic hemodialysis patients. *Kidney Int* 17:811–819, 1980.

118. Wiegand CF, Davin TD, Raij LF, Kjellstrand CM: Severe hypokalemia induced by hemodialysis. *Arch Intern Med* 141:167–170, 1981.

119. Tokars JI, Alter MJ, Favero MS, Moyer LA, Bland LA: National surveillance of hemodialysis-associated diseases in the United States, 1990. *Trans ASAIO* 39:71–80, 1993.

120. Alter MJ, Favero MS, Moyer LA, Bland LA: National surveillance of dialysis-associated diseases in the United States, 1989. *Trans ASAIO* 37:97–109, 1991.

121. Dunea G, Mahurkas SD, Mamdani B, Smith EC: Role of aluminum in dialysis dementia. *Ann Intern Med* 88:502–504, 1978.

122. Coburn JW, Norros KC, Sherrard DJ, Bia M, Dach F, Alfrey A, Slatopolsky E: Toxic effects of aluminum in end-stage renal disease: discussion of a case. *Am J Kidney Dis* 12:171–184, 1988.

123. Llach F, Felsenfeld AJ, Coleman MD, Keveney JJ Jr, Pederson JA, Medlock R: The natural course of dialysis osteomalacia. *Kidney Int* 29 (Suppl 18):S74–S79, 1986.

124. Centers for Disease Control: Dialysis dementia from aluminum. *Epidemic Investigation Report EPI 81-39-2*, June 10, 1982. CDC, Atlanta, 1982.

125. Topple MA, Bland LA, Favero MS, Jarvis WR: Investigation of hemolytic anemia after chloramine exposure in a dialysis center (letter). *Trans ASAIO* 34:1060, 1988.

126. Yawata Y, Kjillstrand C, Buselmeier T, Howe R, Jacob H: Hemolysis in dialyzed patients: tap water-induced red blood cell metabolic deficiency. *Trans ASAIO* 18:301–304, 1992.

127. Neilan BA, Ehlers SM, Kolpin CF, Eaton JW: Prevention of chloramine-induced hemolysis in dialyzed patients. *Clin Nephrol* 10:105–108, 1978.

128. Gordon SM, Drachman J, Bland LA, Reid MH, Favero M, Jarvis WR: Epidemic hypotension in a dialysis center caused by sodium azide. *Kidney Int* 37:110–115, 1990.

129. Anderson R, Beard JH, Sorley D: Fluoride intoxication in a dialysis unit. *Maryland MMWR* 29:134–136, 1980.

130. Lough J, Noonan R, Gagnon R, Kaye M: Effects of fluoride on bone in chronic renal failure. *Arch Pathol* 99:484–487, 1975.

131. National News. Dialysis patients in Chicago die from fluoride poisoning; FDA issues safety alert. *Contemp Dial Nephrol* (Nov): 10–11, 1993.

132. Freeman RM, Lawton RL, Chamberlain MA: Hard-water syndrome. *N Engl J Med* 276:1113–1118, 1967.

133. Evans DB, Slapak M: Pancreatitis in the hard water syndrome. *Br Med J* 3:748, 1975.

134. Carlson DJ, Shapiro FL: Methemoglobinemia from well water nitrates: a complication of home dialysis. *Ann Intern Med* 73:757–759, 1970.

135. Manzler AD, Schreiner CW: Copper-induced acute hemolytic anemia. A new complication of hemodialysis. *Ann Intern Med* 73:409–412, 1970.

136. Matter BJ, Pederson J, Psimenos G, Lindeman RD: Lethal copper intoxication in hemodialysis. *Trans ASAIO* 15:309–315, 1969.

137. Gallery EDM, Blomfield J, Dixon SR: Acute zinc toxicity in haemodialysis. *Br Med J* 4:33, 1973.

138. Centers for Disease Control. Formaldehyde intoxication associated with hemodialysis—California. *Epidemic Investigation Report EPI 81-73-2*, May 7, 1984. CDC, Atlanta, 1984.

139. Orringer EP, Mattern WD: Formaldehyde-induced hemolysis during chronic hemodialysis. *N Engl J Med* 294:1416–1420, 1976.

140. Nickey WA, Chinitz VL, Kim KE, Onesti G, Swartz C: Hypernatremia from water softener and malfunction during home dialysis. *JAMA* 214:915–916, 1976.

141. Vlchek DL: Staying tuned in to the high-tech world. Part 3: Water treatment update. *Dial Transplant* 19:119–124, 1990.

142. Vlchek DL: Monitoring a hemodialysis water treatment system. In: *AAMI Standards and Recommended Practices. Vol. 3: Dialysis.* American National Standards, Arlington, VA, pp 267–277, 1993.

143. Johnson WJ, Taves DR: Exposure to excessive fluoride during hemodialysis. *Kidney Int* 5:451–454, 1974.

144. Association for the Advancement of Medical Instrumentation. In: *AAMI Standards and Recommended Practices. Vol. 3: Dialysis.* American National Standards, Arlington, VA, pp 1–332, 1993.

145. Favero MS, Petersen NJ, Carson LA, Bond WW, Hindman SH: Gram negative water bacteria in hemodialysis systems. *Health Lab Sci* 12:321–334, 1975.

146. Bland LA, Favero MS: Microbiologic aspects of hemodialysis systems. In: *AAMI Standerds and Recommended Practices. Vol. 3: Dialysis*. American National Standards, Arlington, VA, pp 257–265, 1993.

147. Carson LA, Bland LA, Cusick LB, Favero MS, Bolan GA, Reingold AL, Good RC: Prevalence of non-tuberculous mycobacterial in water supplies of hemodialysis centers. *Appl Environ Microbiol* 54(12): 3122–3125, 1988.

148. Lowry P, Beck-Sague CM, Bland LE, Aguero SM, Ardiuno MJ, Minuth AN, Murray RA, Swenson JM, Jarvis WR: *Mycobacterium Chelones* infections among patients receiving high-flux dialysis in a hemodialysis unit in California. *J Infect Dis* 161:85–90, 1990.

149. Bolan G, Reingold AL, Carson LA, Silcox VA, Woodley CL, Hayes PS, Hightower AW, McFarland L, Brown J, Petersen NJ, Favero MS, Good RC, Browne CV: Infestious with *Mycobactrium Chelonei* in patients receiving dialysis and using processed hemodialyzers. *J Infect Dis* 152:1013–1019, 1985.

150. Carson La, Petersen NJ, Favero MS, Aguero SM: Growth characteristics of Atypi cal mycobacteria in water and their comparative resistance to disinfectants. *Appl Environ Microbiol* 36:839–846, 1978.

151. Favero MS: Distinguishing between high-level disinfection, reprocessing, and sterilization. IN: AAMI, *Reuse of Disposables: Implications for Quality Health Care and Cost Containment*. Technical Assessment Report No. 6, Arlington, VA, pp 19–20, 1983.

152. Favero MS, Bland LA: Microbiologic principles applied to reprocessing hemodialyzers. In: N Deane, RJ Wineman, JA Bemis, eds, *Guide to Reprocessing of Hemodialyzers*. Martinus Nijhoff, Boston, pp 63–73, 1986.

153. Gordon SM, Oettinger CW, Bland LA, Oliver JC, Arduino MJ, Aguero SM, McAllister SK, Favero MS, Jarvis WR: Pyrogenic reactions in patients receiving conventional, high-efficiency, or high-flux hemodialysis treatments with bicarbonate dialysate containing high concentrations of bacteria and endotoxin. *J Am Soc Nephrol* 2:1436–1444, 1992.

154. Favero MS, Petersen NJ, Boyer KM, Carson LA, Bond WW: Microbial contamination of renal dialysis systems and associated health risks. *Trans ASAIO* 20:175–183, 1974.

155. Klein E, Pass T, Harding GB, Wright R, Millon C: Microbial and endotoxin contamination in water and dialysate in the central United States. *Artif Organs* 14:85–94, 1990.

156. Bland LA, Ridgeway MR, Aguero SM, Carson LA, Favero MS: Potential bacteriologic and endotoxin hazards associated with liquid bicarbonate concentrate. *Trans ASAIO* 33:542–545, 1987.

157. Pegues DA, Oettinger CW, Bland LA, Oliver JC, Arduino MJ, Aguero SM, McAllister SK, Gordon SM, Favero MS, Jarvis WR: A prospective study of pyrogenic reactions in hemodialysis patients using bicarbonate dialysis fluids filtered to remove bacteria and endotoxin. *J Am Soc Nephrol* 2:1002–1007, 1992.

158. Centers for Disease Control: Clusters of bacteremia and pyrogenic reactions in hemodialysis patients—Georgia. *Epidemic Investigation Report EPI 86-65-2*, April 22, 1987. CDC, Atlanta, 1987.

159. Centers for Disease Control: Bacteremia associated with re-use of disposble hollow-fiber hemodialyzers. *MMWR* 35:417–

418, 1986.

160. Centers for Disease Control: Pyrogenic reactions in patients undergoing high-flux hemodialysis—California. *Epidemic Investigation Report EPI 86-80-2*, June 1, 1987. CDC, Atlanta, 1987.

161. Alter MJ, Favero MS, Miller JK, Coleman PJ, Bland LA: Reuse of hemodialyzers. Results of nationwide surveillance for adverse effects. *JAMA* 260:2073–2076, 1988.

162. Bland LA, Favero MS, Oxborrow GS, Agnero SM, Seavy BP, Danielson JW: Effect of chemical germicides on the integrity of hemodialyzer membranes. *Trans ASAIO* 34:172–175, 1988.

163. Jenkins SR, Lin FUC, Lin RS, Israel I, Petersen NJ: Pyrogenic reactions and pseudomonas bacteremias in a hemodialysis center. *Dial Transplant* 16:192–197, 1987.

164. Oberle MW, Favero MS, Carson LA, Medina MS, Ramirez-Puente M, Perez-Figueroa S: Fatal endotoxemia in dialysis patients at a summer camp. *Dial Transplant* 9:549–550, 1980.

165. Bolan G, Reingold AL, Carson LA, Silcox VA, Woodley CL, Hayes PS, Hightower AW, McFarland L, Brown J, Peterson NJ, Favero MS, Good RC, Browne CV: Infections with Mycobactreium chelonia in patients receiving dialysis and using processed hemodialyzers. *J Infect Dis* 152:1013–1019, 1985.

166. Bland LA, Favero MS: Microbiologic and endotoxin considerations in hemodialyzer reprocessing. In: *AAMI Standards and Recommended Practices. Vol. 3: Dialysis*. American National Standards, Arlington, VA, pp 45–52, 1993.

167. Gazenfield-Grazit E, Eliabou HE: Endotoxin antibodies in patients on maintenance hemodialysis. *Israel J Med Sci* 5:1032–1035, 1969.

168. Jones DM, Tobin BM, Harlow GR, Ralston AJ: Antibody production in patients on regular hemodialysis to organisms present in dialysate. *Proc Eur Dial Transplant Assoc* 9:575–576, 1972.

169. Hindman SH, Favero MS, Carson LA, Petersen NJ, Schonberger LB, Solanto JT: Pyrogenic reactions during haemodialysis caused by entramural endotoxin. *Lancet* 2:732–734, 1975.

170. Raij L, Shapiro FL, Michael AF: Endotoxemia in febrile reactions during hemodialysis. *Kidney Int* 4:57–60, 1973.

171. Passavanti G, Buongiorno E, De Fino G, Fumarola D, Coratelli P: The permeability of dialytic membranes to endotoxins: clinical and experimental findings. *Int J Artif Organs* 12:505–508, 1989.

172. Dinarello CA: Interleukin-1 and its biologically related cytokines. *Adv Immunol* 44:153–205, 1989.

173. Loppnon H, Brade H, Durbaum I, Dinarello CA, Kusumoto S, Rictschel ET, Flad HO: IL-1 induction-capacity of defined lipopolysaccharide partial structures. *J Immunol* 142:3229–3238, 1989.

174. Duff GW, Atkins E: The detection of endotoxin by in-vitro production of endogenous pyrogen: comparison with limulus amebocyte lysate gelation. *J Immunol Methods* 52:323–331, 1982.

175. Lonnemann G, Bingel M, Floege J, Koch KM, Shaldon S, Dinarello CA: Detection of endotoxin-like interleukin-1-inducing activity during in vitro dialysis. *Kidney Int* 33:29–35, 1988.

176. Lonnemann G: Dialysate bacteriological quality and the permeability of dialyzer membranes to pyrogenes. *Kidney Int* 43(Suppl 41):S195–S200, 1993.

177. Favero MS, Port FK, Bernick JJ: In vivo studies of dialysis related endotoxemia and bacteremia. *Nephron* 27:307–312, 1981.
178. Klinkman H, Falkenhagen D, Smollich BP: Investigation of permeability of highly permeable polysulfone membranes for pyrogens. *Contrib Nephrol* 46:174–183, 1985.
179. Bingel M, Lonnemann G, Sheldon S, Koch KM, Dinarello CA: Human interleukin-1 production during hemodialysis. *Nephron* 43:161–163, 1986.
180. Lonnemann G, Endress S, Van Der Meer JWM, Cannon JG, Koch KM, Dinarello CA: Differences in the synthesis and kinetics of release of interleukin-1α, interleukin-1β, and tumor necrosis factor from human mononuclear cells. *Eur J Immunol* 19:1531–1536, 1987.
181. Hakim RM, Breillat J, Lazarus JM, Port FK: Complement activation and hypersensitivity reactions to dialysis membranes. *N Engl J Med* 311:878–882, 1984.
182. Cavallon J-M, Fitting C, Haeffner-Cavaillon N: Recombinant C5a enhances interleukin-1 and tumor necrosis factor release by lipopolysaccharide-stimulated monocytes and macrophages. *Eur J Immunol* 20:253–257, 1990.
183. Schindler R, Gelfand JA, Dinarello CA: Recombinant C5a stimulates transcription rather than translation of interleukin-1 (IL-1) and tumor necrosis factor: translational signal provided by lipopolysaccharide or IL-1 itself. *Blood* 76:1631–1638, 1990.
184. Urena P, Herbelin A, Zingraff J, Lair M, Man NK, Descamps-Latscha B, Drucke T: Permeability of cellulosic and non-cellulosic membranes to endotoxins subunits and cytokine production during in-vitro haemodialysis. *Nephrol Dial Transplant* 7:16–28, 1992.
185. Heberlin A, Urena P, Man NK, Drueke T, Descamp-Latscha B: In vitro studies of endotoxin transfer across cellulosic and non-cellulosic dialysis membranes. Part II. Interleukin-1 production. *Contrib Nephrol* 74:79–85, 1989.
186. Dinarello CA, Koch KM, Shaldon S: Interleukin 1 and its relevance to patients treated with hemodialysis. *Kidney Int* 33 (Suppl 24):S21–S26, 1988.
187. Bingel M, Lonnemann G, Shaldon S, Koch KM, Dinarello CA: Human interleukin-1 production during hemodialysis. *Nephron* 43:161–163, 1986.
188. Haeffner-Cavaillon N, Cavaillon JM, Ciancioni C, Bacle F, Delons S, Kazatchkine MD: In vivo induction of interleukin-1 during hemodialysis. *Kidney Int* 35:1212–1218, 1989.
189. Schindler R, Lonnemann G, Shaldon S, Koch KM, Dinarello CA: Transcription, not synthesis, of interleukin-1 and tumor necrosis factor by complement. *Kidney Int* 37:85–93, 1990.
190. Pearson FC, Bohan JLW, Brunzer G: Comparison of chemical analysis of hollow-fiber dialyzer extracts. *J Artif Organs* 8:291–298, 1984.
191. Harding GB, Pass T, Million C, Wright R, DeJarnette J, Klein E: Bacterial contamination of haemodialysis center water and dialysate: are current assays adequate? *Artif Organs* 13:155–169, 1989.
192. Gould MJ: Performing the LAL gel-clot test in facilities. *Nephrol News Issues* 2911:26–29, 1988.
193. Hakim RM, Friedrich RA, Lowrie EG: Formaldehyde kinetics in reused dialyzers. *Kidney Int* 28:936–943, 1985.
194. Kaufman AM, Frinak S, Godmere RO, Levin NW: Clinical experience with heat sterilization for reprocessing dialyzers. *ASAIO J* 38:M338–M340, 1992.
195. Vanholder R, NoensL, Eng RDS, Ringoior S: Development of anti-N-like antibodies during formaldehyde reuse in spite of adequate predialysis rinsing. *Am J Kidney Dis* 11:477–480, 1988.
196. Pegues DA, Beck-Sague CM, Woollen SW, Reeenspan B, Burns SM, Bland LA, Ardeuno MJ, Favero MS, Mackow RC, Jarvis WR: Anaphylactoid reactions associated with reuse of hollow-fiber hemodialyzer and ACE inhibitor. *Kidney Int* 42:1232–1237, 1992.
197. Schmitter L, Sweet S: Anaphylactic reactions with the addition of hypochlorite to reuse in patients maintained on reprocessed polysulfone hemodialyzers and ACE inhibitors. Paper presented at the annual meetings of the American Society of Artificial Internal Organs, New Orleans, April 1993.
198. U.S. Department of Health and Human Services, Food and Drug Administration: *Tlk Paper T92-46*, October 13, 1992.

CHAPTER 61

Membrane Biocompatibility

DANIEL F. WALTON & ALFRED K. CHEUNG

INTRODUCTION

In the past, the topic of dialysis membrane biocompatibility had been viewed by some dialysis personnel to be limited to intradialytic anaphylactoid reactions. In contrast, bioengineers considered biocompatibility to encompass any interactions between biomaterial and the body (1). Besides leukopenia and complement activation, investigative efforts in recent years have focused on neutrophil function and peripheral blood mononuclear cells due to their potential effects on long-term clinical outcome. Thrombogenesis is an area that has received relatively little attention in the last 15 years. However, it has become increasingly clear that cellular and noncellular constituents of blood as well as the vascular endothelium interact in a complex manner, such that these systems (e.g., coagulation and complement cascades) cannot be considered in an isolated manner. This chapter will start from the standpoint of clinical disorders that are related to dialysis membrane biocompatibility. The pathophysiology that may explain these individual entities and the general mechanisms of bioincompatibility will be briefly discussed.

VARIOUS COMPONENTS IN THE HEMODIALYSIS CIRCUIT THAT AFFECT BIOCOMPATIBILITY

The dialysis membrane constitutes the largest surface area in the extracorporeal circuit and is therefore expected to have the greatest impact on biocompatibility. However, many other components in the circuit have influence on the patient as well. Dialysis needle size can affect the shearing of blood cells (2). Dialysis tubings, which are primarily made of synthetic polymers, have their own biocompatibility characteristics. Particulates can be dislodged from the dialysis tubings and dialyzers into the bloodstream, a process known as spallation. For example, spallation of silicone has resulted in granulomatous hepatitis (3), while spallation of polyvinylchloride has been reported to cause dermatitis (4). With the improvement in design of dialysis tubings and blood pumps, reports of problems associated with spallation are nowadays rare. Examination of the effluents from the blood compartment of hemodialyzers, however, continues to show significant numbers of particles (5). These particles are usually small (less than 5 µm in diameter), and most of them can be removed by rinsing with 0.5 L of fluid. It is unclear whether more particles could be eluted from the dialyzers during multiple reuses. The structure of these particles and their clinical significance are also unknown.

Leaching of residual sterilants and cleansing agents from the dialyzers into the body can cause direct noxious (6) or allergic (7,8) reactions. Although this is not strictly a biocompatibility issue, chemical contamination or incorrect composition of dialysate, such as high chloramine (9), aluminum, or calcium or low sodium concentrations, can be detrimental.

MATERIALS FOR HEMODIALYSIS MEMBRANES

Low flux hemodialysis membranes refer to those that have small pore sizes, and therefore, relatively low ultrafiltration coefficients and low clearances of larger solutes (*middle molecules*). These membranes are sometimes called *conventional* membranes. Increasing their surface area improves their clearances of both small (e.g., urea) and larger solutes; these larger-surface-area membranes are known as *high-efficiency* membranes. *High-flux* membranes have large pores that permit high ultrafiltration rates and clearances of larger solutes. In general, they also clear small solutes efficiently.

Materials for the manufacturing of hemodialysis membranes fall into two general categories: cellulose derivatives and synthetic polymers (10). Cellulose is part of the cell wall matrix from plants. Cuprophan® membrane (Akzo), the original membrane employed for hemodialysis, is regenerated from cellulose using the cuprammonium process. This membrane is still widely used around the world, despite some loss in popularity in the last decade. It is sometimes referred to generically as *cuprophan* or *cuprophane*. Since all cellulosic dialysis membranes are regenerated from cellulose by one method or another, the term *regenerated cellulose* is nonspecific and theoretically encompasses all such membranes. Another commonly used regenerated cellulosic membrane is cellulose acetate, which has most of the surface hydroxyl groups of cellulose replaced by acetyl residues. It is relatively inexpensive, as is cuprophan, and it induces less complement activation and leukopenia than does cuprophan (11–13). Hemophan® (Akzo) has been commercially available for approximately 10 years. Despite the fact that only approximately 1% of the surface hydroxyl groups have been replaced by DEAE moieties, this membrane is associated with far less complement activation and leukopenia compared to cuprophan (14–16). The more recent cellulosic membranes on the market are cellulose diacetate (Althin) and cellulose triacetate (Toyoba), which are available as high-flux dialyzers.

Synthetic polymers used to fabricate dialysis membranes include polyacrylonitrile (PAN), polysulfone, polymethylmethacrylate (PMMA), and polycarbonate. In general, the surfaces of most synthetic membranes are hydrophobic and have large capacities to adsorb proteins. In addition, the PAN membrane from Cobe/Gambro/Hospal (AN69) is a copolymer of acrylonitrile and methallyl sulfonate. Due to the negative charge of the sulfonate moiety, the AN69 membrane has a high affinity for anaphylatoxins (17,18) and the contact protein factor XII (19,20). Binding of these specific proteins has implications from the biocompatibility standpoint, as will be discussed below.

Most cellulosic membranes are low flux and are considered by many to be bioincompatible, while most synthetic membranes are high-flux and are in general considered to be biocompatible. There are, however, many exceptions to these generalizations. Given a certain material, the porosity of the membranes can vary greatly depending on the manufacturing process. For example, the commercial cellulose diacetate (Althin) and cellulose triacetate (Toyoba) membranes are high flux. PMMA membranes (Toray) and polysulfone membranes (Fresenius) can be either low flux or high flux. Biocompatibility characteristics also vary among membranes of either categories, depending on the criteria applied to evaluate the membranes. For example, PMMA activates complement relatively poorly (12), but it has been shown to induce greater neutrophil degranulation than cuprophan membrane (21–23). The AN69 membrane does not induce significant leukopenia (24), but it has been associated with activation of contact proteins and acute anaphylactoid reactions (19,20,25–28).

It is apparent from these discussions that not all cellulosic membranes are the same; likewise, all synthetic membranes should not be considered the same. Failure to recognize their differences may lead to misinterpretation of experimental results. Clinical outcome is likely influenced by many biocompatibility factors. For example, if a membrane activates complement less than cuprophan does, but is associated with more intense activation of the contact proteins, the overall clinical outcome associated with this particular membrane may or may not be superior to that associated with cuprophan. This does not imply that dialysis membrane biocompatibility is unimportant, but rather suggests that the determination of the biocompatibility of a membrane may require multiple laboratory criteria and that continued efforts to improve biocompatibility should be made.

MECHANISMS OF MEMBRANE BIOINCOMPATIBILITY

Bioincompatibility of dialysis membranes is often initiated by the transformation of plasma proteins or activation of blood cells (1). Two plasma protein systems are of particular relevance to hemodialysis: the complement system and the intrinsic pathway of coagulation. Cuprophan membrane is the prototypic complement activator among the dialysis membranes, while the synthetic polymers are, in general, weak activators. Regardless of their composition and structure, however, all clinically used dialysis membranes have been shown to activate complement (11–18,24,29). While evidence strongly indicates that complement activation associated with cuprophan and cellulose acetate membranes occurs via the alternative pathway (13,24,30), the mechanism(s) by which complement activation occurs on the surface of other dialysis membranes is less certain.

Activation of complement by cuprophan membrane results in the formation of anaphylatoxins C3a and C5a (12,24). In addition, other biologically active fragments of C3, such as C3b and iC3b (31,32), as well as the terminal complement complex (C5b-9) (33), are generated. These complement products exert their biological effects by binding to nonhematogenous tissues (e.g., pulmonary arteriolar or bronchial smooth muscles (34,35)) or by modulation of peripheral leukocyte functions (36). The spasmogenic properties of C3a and C5a are markedly diminished when they are converted to their respective desArginine derivatives by serum carboxypeptidase N as a normal control mechanism (37). Plasma carboxypeptidase activities, however, have been shown to diminish during hemodialysis (38), which allows the anaphylatoxins to exert their spasmogenic effects. In addition, $C3a_{desArg}$ and $C5a_{desArg}$ retain leukocyte-modulating activities (36,39). Since the commonly used radioimmunoassays (RIAs) do not distinguish between the uncleaved anaphylatoxins and their desArginine derivatives, the functional activities of the $C3a_{desArg}$ and $C5a_{desArg}$ in the plasma during hemodialysis are usually unknown. $C3a_{desArg}$ and $C5a_{desArg}$ are relatively small peptides (approximately 9–11 kDa) and should therefore be readily transported across high-flux membranes. In addition, these cationic peptides tend to bind to anionic surfaces, such as the AN69 membrane (17,18). Therefore, plasma $C3a_{desArg}$ and $C5a_{desArg}$ levels may not accurately reflect the complement activation potentials of these membranes. Although their immunoassays are also available, the other active complement fragments, such as iC3b and C5b-9, are seldom assessed in the hemodialysis setting.

The contact proteins were of interest primarily due to their potential role in initiating clotting in the hemodialysis circuit. In recent years, the focus on these proteins has been directed to their participation in the generation of kinins, which have been incriminated in the pathogenesis of certain anaphylactoid reactions associated with hemodialysis treatments (25–28). The four contact proteins—factor XII (Hageman factor), high-molecular-weight kininogen, prekallikrein, and factor XI—are components of the intrinsic pathway of coagulation (40). Activation of the contact proteins is initiated by the binding of factor XII to a surface and its autocleavage, followed by the binding and activation of the other contact proteins. Anionic surfaces, such as glass, favor the binding of factor XII (40–42). Detection of contact protein activation in plasma samples obtained during hemodialysis had been difficult due to the binding of the activated proteins to the dialysis membrane surface and the relatively low sensitivity of most available assays. Recent studies have demonstrated the generation of kinins from kininogen when plasma was exposed to dialysis membranes in vitro (20) and during clinical dialysis (28). The generation in the presence of the AN69 membrane was far greater than that in the presence of the cuprophan membrane, presumably due to the anionic domains on the AN69 surface.

Hemolysis can be induced by improper preparation of the dialysate, such as overheating, hypotonicity from erroneous proportioning of the concentrate, and contamination with chloramine (9). Exposure of blood to formaldehyde has led to the formation of anti-N antibodies, which cause lysis of erythrocytes at low temperatures (43). A mechanism of hemolysis related to membrane bioincompatibility has also been postulated. Activation of the terminal components of complement by cuprophan membrane results in the formation of the membrane attack complex (C5b-9) (33). These complexes are known to induce cytolysis when they are generated on susceptible cell surfaces (44). The presence of C5b-9 has been demonstrated on erythrocyte fragments during cardiopulmonary bypass (45). Whether activation of the terminal complement components causes increased fragility or lysis of erythrocytes during clinical hemodialysis is unclear.

Neutrophils (12,21–24,46–48), monocytes (49–51), T lymphocytes (52), B lymphocytes (53), and natural killer cells (54) have all been shown to be activated during hemodialysis. While activation of neutrophils (32) and monocytes (55,56) is likely attributed in part to complement activation, the mechanisms of activation of the other leukocytes are less certain. Activation of leukocytes during hemodialysis has two general consequences. First, it leads to intradialytic release of cellular products, many of which are proinflammatory and mediate tissue injury. Second, the

activated cells lose their responsiveness to further stimuli, a phenomenon sometimes referred to as *deactivation*.

More detailed accounts of the scientific basis and methods for assessment of hemodialysis membrane biocompatibility can be found in other publications (57).

THROMBOSIS IN THE HEMODIALYSIS CIRCUIT

Activation of platelets and clotting proteins is a classical bioincompatibility event; it occurs as a result of interactions between the dialyzer (and, to a lesser extent, the dialysis tubings) and the clotting elements in the blood. The result is of clinical importance, namely, gross thrombosis inside the dialyzer and other components of the extracorporeal circuit. Microthrombosis in the hollow fibers decreases the dialyzer efficiency and the number of times that the dialyzer can be reused. Although clotting can largely be counteracted by the use of anticoagulants, anticoagulants predispose the patients to bleeding, especially in susceptible individuals such as those with peptic ulcer disease and the postoperative patients. Therefore, minimizing the thrombogenecity of dialysis membranes would be beneficial. In addition, activated platelets, coagulation factors, and fibrinolytic proteins interact with other blood constituents such as leukocytes; preventing their activation is desirable.

A number of studies have compared the propensity of different membranes to induce clotting. For example, cuprophan has been shown to activate platelets more than PMMA (58) and polycarbonate (59) membranes. Polyacylonitrile membranes have been reported to activate more contact proteins than cuprophan (20,28) and more clotting factors than cellulose acetate (60). At present, there are no convincing data to allow for definitive ranking of commercially available dialysis membranes according to their thrombogenic potential. This difficulty is further complicated by the many other factors that influence clotting during hemodialysis, for example, the geometry of the dialyzer blood compartment, cannulae, tubings and blood chambers, blood flow rate, the type and amount of anticoagulant employed, and the ultrafiltration rate. The individual patient's hematocrit, the amount and functional state of the platelets, coagulation proteins, fibrinolytic proteins, metabolism of exogenous anticoagulant, reactivity of the endothelium, and stenosis in the arteriovenous fistula also have substantial effects.

Intradialytic alterations in platelets and clotting factors may affect the interdialytic periods and impact on long-term morbidity as well. Platelets after dialysis using cuprophan membrane have been reported to become relatively resistant to collagen-induced aggregation (59,61). On the other hand, one study has shown that patients chronically dialyzed with cuprophan membrane suffered more thrombosis in their vascular accesses and lower extremities than those dialyzed with AN69 membrane (62). The study was retrospective, and there were overlaps in the patient population between the two groups. This interesting finding has not been confirmed by other investigators, and the explanation is not apparent.

ANAPHYLACTOID REACTIONS

The terms *anaphylactoid reactions, hypersensitivity reactions,* and *dialyzer reactions* refer to a spectrum of acute reactions occuring during hemodialysis with signs and symptoms resembling those of anaphylaxis. By definition, they do not include those reactions caused by hypovolemia or rapid changes in serum electrolytes and osmolality. Impurities in the dialysate may or may not be included. For example, chloramine contaminating the dialysate is excluded, while bacterial and endotoxin contaminations are often included in the discussions, probably because their effects on complement and monocytes are similar to some of the effects of the dialysis membranes themselves.

Some of these reactions have been called *first-use syndrome* because they were described primarily in patients using new dialyzers 10–15 years ago (63–68). Cuprophan hollow-fiber dialyzers were most frequently incriminated at that time, although cuprophan plate dialyzers and synthetic membrane dialyzers were also implicated. Reactions also occur with reused dialyzers (65,69). Under these circumstances, the terms *anaphylactoid reactions* or simply *dialyzer reactions* would be more appropriate descriptions than *first-use syndrome.*

The clinical manifestations of these reactions vary. They include various combinations of coughing, sneezing, wheezing, choking, respiratory distress, chest pain, back pain, angioedema, and hypotension or hypertension. The severity of the reactions also varies greatly. Some are minor and do not require intervention, while some have resulted in death. Several different classifications of these reactions have been proposed (63–65), but none has been adopted as standard terminology.

Several pathogenic mechanisms have been proposed for these reactions. Each has a scientific basis and epidemiologic evidence to support its role. Most investigators agree that some of these reactions are due to ethyleneoxide (ETO), a sterilant commonly employed in the manufacturing of dialyzers. ETO produces toxic effect through the generation of a derivative, 2-chloroethanol (6). Alternatively, it serves as a hapten and combines with a serum protein such as albumin to elicit an antibody response (8,66,67,70). IgE antibodies directed against ETO have been detected in some dialysis patients with anaphylactoid reactions. However, some dialysis patients who have not suffered from these reactions and some dialysis unit personnel have also been found to have antibodies against ETO (70). The presence of anti-ETO antibody is therefore nonspecific, and the test is not often used in the differential diagnosis of specific cases of dialysis-induced anaphylactoid reactions. Removal of residual ETO from

the dialyzers is obviously important in eliminating ETO-induced reactions. Part of the ETO can be eliminated from new dialyzers by rinsing with saline. This may explain why treating a new dialyzer with the reuse procedure prior to use sometimes alleviates symptoms. However, the potting compound polyurethane (used to hold the fibers together at the ends of the dialyzer) has been shown to be a reservoir for ETO (71), and dissipation of ETO may continue for weeks. It is, therefore, conceivable that substantial amounts of ETO can be leached from the dialyzer and may account for some of the reactions occuring during reuse. Although these reactions are sometimes called *hypersensitivity reactions,* it is unclear whether these patients are indeed hypersensitive to ETO or have simply received a larger dose of ETO when they experience these reactions, since the amount of ETO that actually leaches into the blood stream is not measured. Other chemicals in the dialyzers, such as isocyanate and isopropyl myristate, potentially cause allergic reaction as well, but evidence supporting their pathogenicity in the dialysis patients is weak.

Anaphylatoxins C3a and C5a generated during hemodialysis have also been incriminated (12). The biological activities of these anaphylatoxins in vitro (34,36,37) and in animals (34,35,72,73), as well as studies in other clinical settings (74,75), suggest that they play a role in dialysis-induced anaphylactoid reactions. In one study, peak plasma $C3a_{desArg}$ levels during hemodialysis using new cuprophan membranes were higher in patients who developed recurrent reactions (as manifested by respiratory symptoms, chest and back pain, flushing, and/or angioedema) than in those who did not (12). Data on the relationship between plasma $C3a_{desArg}$ levels and mild to moderate intradialytic symptoms are conflicting. Some have found that clinical dialysis using cuprophan membrane was associated with higher plasma $C3a_{desArg}$ levels than dialysis using cellulose acetate membrane. Accordingly, intradialytic symptom scores were higher with cuprophan (11). Using cellulosic membrane dialyzers processed with various reuse methods (formaldehyde, peracetic acid, and/or bleach), another study has found a linear correlation between symptom scores and plasma $C3a_{desArg}$ levels (76). In contrast, a recent multicenter trial on acute intradialytic hypotension and symptoms did not observe differences between cuprophan membrane (a potent complement activator) and polysulfone membrane (a weak complement activator) (77). Another clinical trial also failed to find differences between high-efficiency cuprophan and AN69 membranes (78). In this context, it is worthwhile to reiterate that plasma $C3a_{desArg}$ levels underestimate the complement-activating potential of AN69 membrane due to binding of the complement fragments to the membrane surface (17,18).

More recently, anaphylactoid reactions associated with AN69 membrane have been described by several groups of investigators (25–28). Many of these patients were also taking angiotensen-converting enzyme (ACE) inhibitors.

As discussed above, the anionic sulfonate domains on the AN69 membrane favors the binding and activation of factor XII and the subsequent generation of kinins from kininogen. In addition to catalyzing the conversion of angiotensin I to angiotensin II, ACE also functions as a kininase that inactivates bradykinin. The presence of an ACE inhibitor therefore allows the accumulation of bradykinin, which is generated as a result of blood contact with AN69 membrane. Activated factor XII increases vascular permeability (40). The proinflammatory properties of bradykinin have been well described and include increasing vascular permeability, stimulating smooth muscle contraction, diminishing arterial resistance, enhancing intestinal motility, and inducing pain (40). Exposure of sheep to AN69 membrane and an ACE inhibitor resulted in high plasma bradykinin levels and anaphylactoid reactions with hypotension (79). A recent clinical study showed that substantially more bradykinin was generated during hemodialysis using AN69 membrane even in the absence of ACE inhibitors, compared to cuprophan, Hemophan, or polysulfone membranes. Patients who experienced anaphylactoid reactions while dialyzed with AN69 membrane with or without ACE inhibitors had markedly elevated bradykinin levels (28). The relative inability of AN69 membrane to induce leukopenia but its high propensity to activate the contact proteins is a clear example of variations in biocompatibility for a given membrane, depending on the criteria employed.

A cluster of anaphylactoid reactions has recently been reported with polysulfone membrane dialyzers (69). This membrane activates complement poorly (29,77) and does not have a theoretical basis to activate contact proteins vigorously. Most of the patients in that report were taking ACE inhibitors. Investigation of these cases led to the conclusion that reuse might have been responsible for the reactions, since they disappeared after reuse was stopped, despite the continued administration of ACE inhibitors. Although peracetic acid was used as the sterilant in that specific dialysis unit, it is likely that other sterilants employed for reuse processing can cause similar problems. Systemic exposure to high concentrations of peracetic acid, formaldehyde, glutaraldehyde, and hypochlorite (bleach) can certainly be fatal without eliciting an antibody response.

When reactions occur during hemodialysis using high-flux membranes, back-diffusion or back-filtration of endotoxins from the dialysate to the blood compartment is an additional concern, particularly if fever and rigors are prominent features of the reactions. Dialysates, especially those containing bicarbonate as buffer, are frequently contaminated by bacteria and endotoxins (80,81). There had been controversies over the issue of whether endotoxins can cross the hemodialysis membranes. An earlier study failed to demonstrate the transfer of endotoxins across polysulfone membranes, using limulus amebocyte lysate (LAL) assay to detect the endotoxins (82). In contrast, recent studies using radiolabeled lipopolysaccharides (part of endotoxin) (83) or induction of cytokine production as the assay (84,85) have clearly demonstrated the transfer of endotoxins or endotoxin fragments across both high-flux and low-flux membranes. Endotoxins and some of their fragments are potent activators of monocytes. Interleukin-1β (IL-β) and tumor necrosis factor-α (TNF-α) released from activated monocytes produce fever and many other proinflammatory responses (49). These cytokines presumably account for some pyrogenic reactions occurring during and after hemodialysis.

Recent studies from the U.S. Centers for Disease Control, however, showed that the incidence of pyrogenic reactions (rigors and/or oral temperature $\leq 37.8°C$ without antecedent infection) was low (0.12%) during hemodialysis using high-flux polysulfone membrane and was not statistically greater than that observed with dialysis using low-flux cellulose acetate membrane (0.05%) (80,81). This low incidence was observed despite heavily contaminated bicarbonate dialysate. The two patients who experienced pyrogenic reactions in the study, however, had plasma levels of TNF-α that were more than 100 times higher than controls (80), suggesting that cytokines released from monocytes mediated those particular reactions. It should also be noted that some synthetic membranes, including polysulfone, have been shown to adsorb endotoxin fragments, thus preventing their transport across the membrane (86–88). The lack of a statistically significant difference in the incidence of pyrogenic reactions between high-flux synthetic membranes and low-flux cellulosic membranes can be further explained by the ability of the latter to induce cytokine production by activating complement (39,56).

Identification of the specific etiologic agent in individual cases of anaphylactoid reactions is often difficult. The severity of the reaction is usually not helpful, since the severity probably depends at least as much on the dose as on the nature of the offending agent. Complement activation and the subsequent accumulation of anaphylatoxins in the plasma occur gradually during the initial 10–15 minutes of hemodialysis (12,24), in contrast to ETO, which is already stored in the dialyzers and may be infused into the patient as a bolus at the beginning of the dialysis session. Therefore, an anaphylactoid reaction occurring within the first 1 or 2 minutes is unlikely to be related to complement activation. Prominent fever and rigors raise the possibility of dialysate contaminated with endotoxins, but bacteremia from other sources (e.g., dialysis catheter entry sites) should also be considered.

Treatments for dialysis-induced anaphylactoid reactions are largely symptomatic. For severe acute reactions, dialysis must be aborted immediately, and the blood in the extracorporeal circuit should be discarded instead of being returned to the patient. Epinephrine, corticosteroids, and antihistamines all have a theoretical basis for treating these reactions. Hemodynamic support using volume expansion and pressors as well as respiratory supports should be instituted as necessary.

Preventive measures for anaphylactoid reactions are often empirical unless the etiology of the specific cases can be determined. These measures include more intense rinsing of the dialyzers before use (e.g., 2 L saline through the blood compartment and extensive rinsing of the dialysate compartment with dialysate) in order to remove ETO and other soluble or insoluble contaminants. Reused dialyzers must be thoroughly rinsed to eliminate the sterilants. One may consider switching from an ETO-sterilized dialyzer to one that is sterilized by radiation or heat, or changing from a membrane with strong complement-activating potential (e.g., cuprophan) to a weaker complement activator (e.g., Hemophan or polysulfone). If reactions occur with AN69 membrane while the patient is taking an ACE inhibitor, one or both of these potential offenders should be discontinued. Switching dialysis tubings and the type of heparin is sometimes useful. Mild allergic symptoms, such as sneezing and pruritis, in certain patients can be prevented by prophylactic administration of antihistamines immediately prior to the dialysis session. If recurrent pyrogenic reactions occur, bacterial counts and endotoxin concentrations in the water or dialysate should be determined. Bacterial and endotoxin contamination can be decreased by limiting the storage time of dialysate and passing the dialysate through a hemofilter (86–89).

HEMODIALYSIS-INDUCED HYPOXEMIA

A decrease of 10–12 mmHg in systemic arterial partial oxygen tension is occasionally observed during hemodialysis (90–92). The decrease is most rapid during the first hour of treatment. This degree of hypoxemia usually goes unnoticed in relatively healthy patients, but it may contribute to intradialytic symptoms in other patients, particularly in those with underlying cardiac or pulmonary diseases. The etiologies of dialysis-induced hypoxemia have been extensively studied. No new information has been presented in recent years that would significantly change the concepts of its pathogenesis. There is no question that the loss of carbon dioxide from diffusion into the acetate dialysate (90) or metabolism of acetate (91) is a major contributing factor. Hypocapnea leads to hypoventilation and consequently hypoxemia.

There is also substantial evidence supporting the role of membrane bioincompatibility, especially during the first hour of the dialysis treatment:

1. Patients on mechanical ventilators with constant minute volume, and therefore no hypoventilation, still developed hypoxemia during hemodialysis (92)
2. Impairment in various parameters of pulmonary gas exchange has been well documented during hemodialysis (93–99), which cannot be explained by hypoventilation alone
3. Infusion of plasma that has been treated with cuprophan membrane into experimental animals (72,93) or humans (97) produces hypoxemia

4. Sham hemodialysis without dialysate in normal human produces hypoxemia (100)
5. Dialysis with cuprophan membrane was associated with a larger decrease in diffusion capacity than with PAN membrane (101)
6. The degree of intradialytic peripheral leukopenia has been correlated with the degree of hypoxemia (102)
7. Replacement of cellulosic membranes by PMMA or PAN membranes ameliorated the hypoxemia (94,95,103)
8. Replacement of acetate by bicarbonate dialysate during cuprophan dialysis does not necessarily abolish the hypoxemia, but dialysis with the combination of reused cuprophan membrane and bicarbonate dialysate did (101,102,104)

These data clearly demonstrate that membrane bioincompatibility plays a role in the development of dialysis-induced hypoxemia, although its role is smaller than that of acetate dialysate. The bioincompatible effect appears to be mediated by anaphylatoxins and arachidonic acid metabolites (34,72).

Pulmonary hypertension can also occur during clinical hemodialysis (105) and sham hemodialysis (106) in uremic patients using cuprophan membrane. The etiology is also likely to be complement activation and the subsequent release of thromboxanes from the lungs (107).

IMPAIRED IMMUNITY AS A RESULT OF MEMBRANE BIOINCOMPATIBILITY

Infections are common among hemodialysis patients. These infectious agents include the common bacteria (e.g., staphalococcus) and viruses (e.g., hepatitis C) as well as opportunistic microorganisms (e.g., tuberculosis). Anatomical abnormalities undoubtedly play an important role in some of these infections. For example, permanent or temporary vascular accesses are prone to invasion by gram-positive and gram-negative bacteria, which often lead to bacteremia. It is also clear that hemodialysis patients have multiple functional defects in their leukocytes. In nonuremic subjects, abnormalities in neutrophils (as in chronic granulomatous disease or integrin deficiency) (108) and T lymphocytes (as in human immunodeficiency virus infection) are associated with high infection rates. It is conceivable that leukocyte abnormalities in dialysis patients also render them inherently more susceptible to infection.

Abnormalities in neutrophils (109), T lymphocytes (52,110), monocytes (111), and natural killer cells (54) have all been demonstrated in hemodialysis patients. Many early studies failed to distinguish the effects of uremia from those of hemodialysis on leukocyte function. A recent clinical study showed that both uremia and the hemodialysis procedure itself have separate, and perhaps additive, negative effects on neutrophils (109). The basic common theme for the various types of leukocytes is that, after the cells have been activated as a result of blood–membrane interactions during hemodialysis, they become deactivated or relatively unresponsive to subsequent stimuli such as infectious agents. This hyporesponsiveness may be the consequence of alterations in cell surface receptors, signal transduction mechanisms, and/or depletion of the intracellular machineries that are necessary for proper function.

Neutrophils are activated by both complement-dependent and complement-independent mechanisms during hemodialysis using cuprophan membrane (21–23,32). As a result, they aggregate (93) and release oxygen radicals (46) and intragranular enzymes (21–23), which can damage plasma proteins (112,113), lipids (114), and perhaps solid tissues in the lungs (115) and kidneys (116). Neutrophils obtained during dialysis using cuprophan membrane failed to release oxygen radicals normally when stimulated in vitro (46). Intradialytic activation also leads to alterations in the expression of surface receptors, such as C5a receptor (117), MAC-1 (CR3) (47,48), and LAM-1 (48), which diminish the ability of the neutrophils to respond to chemotactic stimuli and attach to endothelial cells at the sites of inflammation. Recent clinical studies have shown that dialysis membranes vary in their abilities to induce neutrophil deactivation. Vanholder et al. studied glucose metabolism and oxygen radical production by leukocytes in a whole-blood system upon challenge with phagocytic stimuli such as zymosan and latex particles (109). In a cross-sectional study, they found that leukocyte metabolism remained relatively normal throughout the course of progressive chronic renal failure until the serum creatinine concentrations exceeded 6.0 mg/dL. Thereafter, metabolism decreased by approximately 20%–55%. Fifteen new patients with end-stage renal disease were prospectively randomized into two groups dialyzed with cuprophan and low-flux polysulfone membrane, respectively (109). Both groups suffered further deterioration of phagocytic metabolism upon initiation of chronic hemodialysis. However, the cuprophan group was affected more severely. Limited information in the same study indicated that the cuprophan group also had more frequent septic episodes than the polysulfone group ($p = °$) over a 20-week observation period. In a larger-scale but retrospective and nonrandomized study, patients chronically dialyzed with high-flux polysulfone membrane had lower hospitalization rates for infectious complications than those chronically dialyzed with conventional cellulosic membranes (118).

Intradialytic T-lymphocyte activation has been studied using cell surface interleukin-2 receptor (IL-2R) as a marker. When T cells are activated, IL-2 is released from the cell, and the expression of its receptor (IL-2R) on the cell surface is increased. Binding of IL-2 to its receptor is necessary for cell proliferation and development of functionally active effector T cells. Upregulation of cell-surface IL-2R is therefore indicative of T-cell activation. Hemodialysis using cuprophan membrane has been found to be associated with greater expression of IL-2R on T lymphocytes, compared to dialysis using PMMA membrane (52). When the cells were subsequently stimulated in vitro using phytohemagglutinin, those that had been exposed to cuprophan responded poorly. In another study, in vitro proliferation of T lymphocytes obtained from patients chronically dialyzed with polysulfone membrane was found to be normal, whereas proliferation of cells from patients chronically dialyzed with cuprophan membrane was impaired (110). The mechanisms by which T cells are activated during cuprophan dialysis are unclear, but may be related to the ability of the membrane to activate complement (52) and monocytes (119). Theoretically, abnormal T-cell function may be responsible in part for the cutaneous anergy, increased viral infection, abnormal antibody response to vaccines, prolonged clinical course of tuberculosis, and other infectious complications seen in the hemodialysis patients. Whether the choice of dialysis membrane indeed has an impact on these disorders has not been determined in controlled studies. Other factors, such as the administration of recombinant erythropoietin (120), may also play a role in modulating T-cell function in hemodialysis patients.

As discussed above, monocytes are often activated as a result of hemodialysis (49–51). Anaphylatoxins generated as a result of complement activation and endotoxins (and their fragments) (39,49) are two major factors that promote monocyte activation in this setting. Activated monocytes release IL-1β, IL-6, and TNF-α, which are potent proinflammatory, catabolic, and immunoregulatory proteins (49). Acute release of large amounts of these cytokines may cause intradialytic pyrogenic reactions. Based on experimental evidence, it has also been suggested that peripheral monocytes in hemodialysis patients are in a chronically low-grade activated state (49). The release of cytokines from these cells on a continuous or intermittent basis has been postulated to be responsible for an array of medical problems encountered by dialysis patients. Definitive evidence supporting this hypothesis (*cytokine hypothesis* or *monokine hypothesis*) is pending. Perhaps because of their chronically activated state, monocytes from patients repeatedly dialyzed with cuprophan membrane have been shown to release cytokines poorly in response to stimuli in vitro (111). Since monocytes are important in the presentation of antigens and activation of lymphocytes, defective cytokine production may also contribute to the immunodeficiency state seen in dialysis patients.

Natural killer cells are normal peripheral leukocytes with cytotoxic activity against tumor cells, microorganisms, infected cells, and transplanted tissues. Natural killer cells obtained after in vitro (121) or clinical (54) exposure to cuprophan membrane were found to exhibit diminished cytotoxicity. It has been reported that ESRD patients have an increased incidence of malignancy (122). Whether this increased malignancy is related in part to dialysis-membrane-induced dysfunction of their natural killer cells has not been studied.

Information on B lymphocytes in hemodialysis is very limited. Using soluble CD23 as a marker of activation, B lymphocytes have been found to be activated during clinical dialysis using cuprophan, cellulose acetate, or polysulfone membranes, but not with AN69 membrane (53). The mechanisms of dialysis-induced B-cell activation and its clinical implications are at present unknown.

DIALYSIS MEMBRANES AFFECTING RENAL FUNCTION

Cuprophan membrane activates complement and neutrophils. As a result, the neutrophils release oxygen radicals and intragranular proteolytic enzymes (21–23,46). It has been shown that complement-mediated release of oxygen radicals from neutrophils can induce lung injury (115). It therefore seems reasonable to postulate that neutrophils activated by complement during hemodialysis can also cause damage to kidneys with either acute or chronic failure. When rats with ischemic acute renal failure were exposed to cuprophan-activated plasma, their renal function recovered at a slower rate as compared to rats that had been exposed to AN69 membrane-treated plasma (116). Examination of the kidneys from the cuprophan group revealed infiltration of neutrophils in the glomeruli. The effect of cuprophan-activated plasma on renal function could be reproduced by substitution with zymosan-activated plasma, suggesting that the effect of cuprophan was mediated by complement activation. Recent studies in patients with acute renal failure showed that dialysis using cuprophan membrane was associated with lower rates of recovery of renal function, more days requiring hemodialysis, and higher mortality compared to those dialyzed with PMMA membrane (123).

Dialysis-membrane bioincompatibility may also have an effect on kidneys with chronic failure. A preliminary study in partially nephrectomized rats showed that glomerular filtration rates were better preserved after exposure to PAN membrane than to cuprophan membrane (124). Clinical data are currently unavailable.

β₂-MICROGLOBULIN ASSOCIATED AMYLOID DISEASE

β_2-microglobulin (β_2MG) has been recognized as a major component of the AH (amyloidosis of hemodialysis) deposit in chronic dialysis patients (125,126). β_2MG is the light chain of the major histocompatibility antigen (MHC) complex present on the surface of nucleated cells. The pathogenesis of this disease has not been precisely defined, but high concentrations of β_2MG in plasma (127–130) and structural modifications of the protein (131–133) presumably play a role. If the tissue deposition of β_2MG occurs only due to accumulation of the protein in plasma as a result of chronic renal failure, it should not be considered a

biocompatibility issue. The ability of high-flux membranes to remove β_2MG is an issue of dialysis efficiency and likewise should not be considered to be a biocompatibility issue. On the other hand, if the dialysis membrane promotes the cellular release of β_2MG into plasma (134), alters the structure of the protein (131) such that its deposition is favored, or participates in the destruction of the tissues around the β_2MG deposits (135), then β_2MG would become a biocompatibility issue.

There is evidence supporting the thesis that membrane bioincompatibility affects cellular generation and/or release of β_2MG. The effect is dependent on the type of dialysis membrane used. When peripheral-blood mononuclear cells were incubated with cuprophan in the presence of plasma, more β_2MG was released compared to incubation with PMMA and AN69 (134). Stimulation of the cells with C5a or IL-1β also enhanced β_2MG release. These in vitro data suggest that cuprophan membrane induces β_2MG release from peripheral mononuclear cells by activating complement and monocytes. It would also seem reasonable to postulate that clinical dialysis using cuprophan membrane increases the plasma concentrations of β_2MG. Information on this issue is conflicting. Some investigators have presented data suggesting that the apparent increase in plasma β_2MG concentrations during cuprophan dialysis can be attributed to hemoconcentration as a result of ultrafiltration during the treatment (127,128). Others have argued that, even when fluid removal had been taken into account, there was still a 3%–15% increase in plasma β_2MG levels (129,130). A 15% (or ~6mg/L) increment from predialysis levels of 30–40mg/L might not appear to be very substantial, but it probably reflects significant perturbations of the cells that release the protein, considering that the plasma concentrations in normal human are only about 1mg/L.

Estimation of the appearance (synthetic) rate of β_2MG using radiolabeled β_2MG turnover techniques is another approach to address this issue. Two studies have shown that β_2MG appearance rates in patients dialyzed with cuprophan were 30%–50% higher than those in normal subjects, but the differences did not reach statistical significance (136,137). The β_2MG appearance rates in patients chronically dialyzed with AN69 were reported to be normal and lower than the values for patients chronically dialyzed with cuprophan membrane. The differences between AN69 and cuprophan were also statistically insignificant (137). Taken together, these observations and the aforementioned incubation studies suggest that dialysis membrane bioincompatibility can increase β_2MG release from peripheral leukocytes. The magnitude of this increase is, however, relatively small compared to the amounts that can be removed by high-flux membranes via transport and/ or adsorption (corresponding to a 10–25mg/L or 20%–60% decrease in plasma concentrations during one session of dialysis (138,139)). In other words, the major difference between the effects of high-flux synthetic and cuprophan membrane on plasma β_2MG levels resides primarily in the ability of the former to remove the protein, and to a lesser extent in the ability of the latter to enhance its generation.

In addition to enhancing the release of β_2MG, membrane bioincompatibility potentially contributes to AH amyloid disease either by altering the structure of β_2MG and thereby favoring its deposition in tissues or by potentiating the local destructive effects of the amyloid fibrils. β_2MG molecules, which are smaller and more acidic than the native protein, have been found in amyloid fibrils and sera from uremic patients (132). Activated neutrophils release oxygen radicals and proteases that are capable of cleaving or damaging proteins. It has been postulated that neutrophils activated during hemodialysis could alter β_2MG in a manner that would promote its deposition in tissues. Monocytes activated during dialysis release cytokines, which are known to have bone resorptive properties (140) and could therefore contribute to the local inflammatory and destructive process. This hypothesis is supported by the demonstration of macrophages that stained positively for IL-1β and TNF-α in bone tissues from uremic patients afflicted by β_2MG deposits (135).

Given the effects of cuprophan membrane on plasma levels and perhaps on structural alterations of β_2MG and the ability of high-flux synthetic membranes to remove β_2MG, one would expect that patients chronically dialyzed with high-flux membranes suffer from less β_2MG amyloid disease than those dialyzed with cuprophan membrane. Several studies have, in fact, shown that patients chronically dialyzed with AN69 membrane developed fewer bone cysts and required less decompresssion surgery for carpal tunnel syndrome than those chronically dialyzed with cuprophan membrane (141–143). Although these studies were retrospective, contained overlaps between the study groups, and did not obtain histologic confirmation for β_2MG uniformly, they nonetheless suggest that certain high-flux synthetic membranes may postpone the development of β_2MG amyloid disease compared to conventional low-flux cellulosic membranes.

PROTEIN CATABOLISM INDUCED BY MEMBRANE BIOINCOMPATIBILITY

The release of proteolytic enzymes and oxygen radicals from activated neutrophils and cytokines from activated monocytes suggest that membrane bioincompatibility may alter proteins and lipids in blood and other tissues as well. The neutrophil product elastase cleaves a variety of human body proteins (144). After it is released into plasma, elastase is complexed to the α_1-proteinase inhibitor, which limits its biological activity. However, it has also been demonstrated that oxygen radicals potentiate the effect of elastase on protein degradation, even in the presence of the inhibitor (145). The simultaneous release of both intragranular enzymes (21–23) and oxygen radicals (46) from neutrophils during hemodialysis could therefore result in plasma protein damage (112,113).

Using the release of free amino acids as an indicator, sham hemodialysis in normal humans using cuprophan membrane has been shown to induce more protein catabolism than dialysis using AN69 membrane (146). The enhanced release occurred almost 3 hours after the dialysis procedure had been completed, and could be partially inhibited by a cyclooxygenase inhibitor. Since IL-1β-induced protein degradation is mediated by prostaglandin E_2, these data are compatible with the hypothesis that cytokine release as a result of membrane bioincompatibility causes protein catabolism. Both in vitro (147) and clinical (51) data on the ability of AN69 membrane to induce cytokine production, however, do not support this mechanism. A recent study using a radiolabeled leucine turnover technique found no net release of free amino acids from tissues during and 4 hours after clinical dialysis using cuprophan membrane (148). The effect of hemodialysis membrane on protein catabolism remains unsettled at present.

MORTALITY RATES ASSOCIATED WITH DIFFERENT DIALYSIS MEMBRANES

Data on the effects of various dialysis membranes on patient mortality rates are very limited. In a recent retrospective study, 146 patients chronically dialyzed with conventional cellulosic dialysis membranes were compared to 107 patients chronically dialyzed with high-flux polysulfone membrane (118). In the high-flux group, 84% of the patients had previously employed conventional membranes for at least 1 month prior to switching to high-flux membranes. Annual mortality was 7% for the high-flux group versus 20% for the conventional group. In addition, the rate of hospitalization for infection and vascular access surgery was lower in the high-flux group, although there was no difference in overall hospitalization rates between the two groups. It should be noted, however, that the mean dose of dialysis, as determined by the KT/V of urea, between the two groups was different (1.14 for high-flux versus 1.04 for conventional), which could also have influenced the outcome.

ROLE OF MIDDLE-MOLECULE CLEARANCE AND REUSE ON CLINICAL OUTCOME

Although the numerous cellular and noncellular bioincompatible events occurring as a result of blood-dialysis membrane interactions suggest that they may have an impact on long-term patient outcome, definitive evidence is lacking at present. Large-scale, long-term, well-controlled, and prospective clinical trials are necessary to examine this hypothesis. Current clinical trials conducted in both the U.S. and Europe may provide some answers. From the biocompatibility standpoint, there are several difficulties in the design of these studies and the interpretation of their results. First, biocompatibility of dialysis membranes is not absolute; it varies depending on the criteria employed to examine the membranes. For example, cuprophan membrane is a potent activator of complement but a relatively weak activator of the contact proteins. In contrast, the AN69 membrane has high kinin-generating activities but is sometimes classified as biocompatible based on its lack of ability to induce leukopenia. Comparisons between biocompatible and bioincompatible membranes using these membranes as models may be problematic.

Second, many cellulosic membranes differ from many synthetic membranes not only in the biomaterials but also in the pore sizes of the membranes that permit or retard the transport of larger solutes (middle molecules). *Middle molecules* are defined herein as molecules that accumulate as a result of renal failure, are more effectively removed by high-flux hemodialysis membranes or the peritoneal membrane than by low-flux hemodialysis membranes due to size (and/or charge), and have potential deleterious effects when present in high concentrations in the body. Some of the middle molecules and candidates that have been identified from uremic plasma include parathormone, β_2MG or glycosylated β_2MG (133), peptides that inhibit granulocyte metabolism and function (149), advanced glycosylation end products that contribute to organ damage in diabetes mellitus (150), delta sleep-inducing peptide, and opioid peptides (151). Besides the other problems associated with their designs, many published studies so far have compared low-flux conventional cellulosic membranes with high-flux synthetic membranes. Theoretically, the removal of middle molecules by high-flux hemodialysis would also have beneficial effects on the patients. Studies using membranes with different biocompatibility characteristics but similar solute clearance profiles and membranes with different clearance profiles but similar biocompatibility characteristics will be necessary to separate the effects of these two factors. Complicating the issue is the interrelationships between these two factors. For example, anaphylatoxins generated as a result of blood–membrane interactions may be removed by high-flux dialysis membranes due to their relatively low molecular weights ($M_r \sim 10\,kDa$). Therefore, the porosity of a dialysis membrane may improve its biocompatibility.

Finally, although reuse of cuprophan membrane with formaldehyde as sterilant is associated with improved biocompatibility based on certain criteria (48,76,152), the effects of reuse on biocompatibility (and on clearances of middle molecules and larger proteins such as albumin (153)) of many other types of dialysis membranes have not been systematically examined. Cautions should be exercised when one projects the results from cuprophan membrane and formaldehyde to other membranes without experimental verification, especially when other reuse sterilants are employed. The types of sterilants employed, by themselves, may also have an impact on the long-term outcome. Clinical studies comparing biocompatibility of different dialysis membranes must take these caveats into account.

The current choice of hemodialyzers in the U.S. is primarily dictated by the clearance of urea (mass transfer-area coefficient or K_oA) of the dialyzers. Biocompatibility and middle-molecule (e.g., β_2MG) clearances are also important considerations. Until more definitive evidence of the long-term clinical effects of these two factors and more information on reuse become available, the expense of employing high-flux synthetic membrane dialyzers will continue to be a deterrent to their widespread use around the world.

ACKNOWLEDGMENT

The authors acknowledge support from the National Institute of Health (DK-45575), the U.S. Department of Veterans Affairs, and the Division of Nephrology and Hypertension, University of Utah School of Medicine.

REFERENCES

1. Leonard EF: Dialysis membranes. *Proc EDTA-ERA* 21:99–109, 1984.
2. Leonard EF, Van Vooren C, Hauglustaine D, Haumont S: Shear-induced formation of aggregates during hemodialysis. *Contr Nephrol* 36:34–45, 1983.
3. Altmann P, Dodd S, Williams A, Marsh F, Cunningham J: Silicone-induced hypercalcaemia in haemodialysis patients. *Nephrol Dial Transplant* 2:26–29, 1987.
4. Bommer J, Ritz E, Andrassy K: Necrotizing dermatitis resulting from hemodialysis with polyvinylchloride tubing. *Ann Intern Med* 91:869–870, 1979.
5. Hoenich NA, Thompson J, McCabe J, Appleton DR: Particle release from haemodialyzers. *Int J Artif Organs* 13:803–808, 1990.
6. Gutch CF, Eskelson CD, Ziegler E, Ogden DA: 2-chloroethanol as a toxic residue in dialysis supplies sterilized with ethylene oxide. *Dial Transplant* 5:21–25, 1976.
7. Röckel A, Klinke B, Hertel J, Baur X, Thiel Cl, Abdelhamid S, Fiegel P, Walb D: Allergy to dialysis materials. *Nephrol Dial Transplant* 4:646–652, 1989.
8. Bousquet J, Maurice F, Rivory JP, Skassa-Brociek W, Florence P, Chouzenoux R, Mion C, Michel FB: Allergy in long-term hemodialysis: II. Allergic and atopic patterns of a population of patients undergoing long-term hemodialysis. *J Allergy Clin Immunol* 81:605–610, 1988.
9. Tipple MA, Shusterman N, Bland LA, McCarthy MA, Favero MS, Arduino MJ, Reid MH, Jarvis WR: Illness in hemodialysis patients after exposure to chloramine contaminated dialysate. *Trans Am Soc Artif Intern Organs* 37:588–591, 1991.
10. Lyman DJ: Membranes. In: W Drukker, FM Parsons, JF Maher, eds, *Replacement of Renal function by Dialysis.* Martinus Nijhoff Publishers, Boston, pp 97–105, 1983.
11. Ivanovich P, Chenoweth DE, Schmidt R, Klinkmann H, Boxer LA, Jacob HS, Hammerschmidt DE: Symptoms and activation of granulocytes and complement with two dialysis membranes. *Kidney Int* 24:758–763, 1983.

12. Hakim RM, Breillatt J, Lazarus JM, Port FK: Complement activation and hypersensitivity reactions to dialysis membranes. *N Engl J Med* 311:878–882, 1984.

13. Cheung AK, Parker CJ, Wilcox L, Janatova J: Activation of the alternative pathway of complement by hemodialysis membranes. *Kidney Int* 36:257–265, 1989.

14. Henne W, Duenweg G, Bandel W: A new cellulose membrane generation for hemodialysis and hemofiltration. *Artif Organs* 3 (Suppl):466–469, 1979.

15. Spencer PC, Schmidt B, Samtleben W, Bosch T, Gurland HJ: Ex vivo model of hemodialysis membrane biocompatibility. *Trans Am Soc Artif Intern Organs* 31:495–498, 1985.

16. Falkenhagen D, Bosch T, Brown GS, Schmidt B, Holtz M, Maurmeister U, Gurland H, Klinkman H: A clinical study on different cellulosic dialysis membranes. *Nephrol Dial Transplant* 2:537–545, 1987.

17. Cheung AK, Chenoweth DE, Otsuka D, Henderson LW: Compartmental distribution of complement activation products in artificial kidneys. *Kidney Int* 30:74–80, 1986.

18. Cheung AK, Parker CJ, Wilcox L, Janatova J: Activation of complement by hemodialysis membranes: polyacrylonitrile binds more C3a than cuprophan. *Kidney Int* 37:1055–1059, 1990.

19. Schulman G, Hakim R, Arias R, Silverberg M, Kaplan A, Arbeit L: Bradykinin generation by dialysis membranes: possible role in anaphylactic reaction. *J Am Soc Nephrol* 3:1563–1569, 1993.

20. Lemke HD, Fink E: Accumulation of bradykinin formed by the AN69- or PAN 17DX-membrane is due to the presence of an ACE-inhibitor in vitro. *J Am Soc Nephrol* 3:376(A), 1992.

21. Hörl WH, Riegel W, Schollmeyer P, Rautenberg W, Neumann S: Different complement and granulocyte activation in patients dialyzed with PMMA dialyzers. *Clin Nephrol* 25:304–307, 1986.

22. Hörl WH, Schaefer RM, Heidland A: Effect of different dialyzers on proteinases and proteinase inhibitors during hemodialysis. *Am J Nephrol* 5:320–326, 1985.

23. Hörl WH, Steinhauer HB, Riegel W, Schollmeyer P, Schäfer RM, Heidland A: Effect of different dialyzer membranes on plasma levels of granulocyte elastase. *Kidney Int* 33 (Suppl):S90–S91, 1988.

24. Chenoweth DE, Cheung AK, Henderson LW: Anaphylatoxin formation during hemodialysis: effects of different dialyzer membranes. *Kidney Int* 24:764–769, 1983.

25. Tielemans C, Madhoun P, Lenaers M, Schandene L, Goldman M, Vanherweghem JL: Anaphylactoid reactions during hemodialysis on AN69 membranes in patients receiving ACE inhibitors. *Kidney Int* 38:982–984, 1990.

26. Tielemans C, Goldman M, Vanherweghem J: Immediate hypersensitivity reactions and hemodialysis. *Adv Nephrol* 22:401–416, 1993.

27. Parnes EL, Shapiro WB: Anaphylactoid reactions in hemodialysis patients treated with AN69 dialyzers. *Kidney Int* 40:1148–1152, 1991.

28. Verresen L, Fink E, Lemke H-D, Vanrenterghem Y: Bradykinin is a mediator of anaphylactoid reactions during hemodialysis with AN69 membranes. *Kidney Int* 45:1497–1503, 1994.

29. Smeby LC, Widerøe TE, Balstad T, Jørstad S: Biocompatibility aspects of cellophane, cellulose acetate, polyacrylonitrile, polysulfone and polycarbonate hemodialyzers. *Blood Purif* 4:93–101, 1986.

30. Cheung AK, Parker CJ, Janatova J: Analysis of the complement C3 fragments associated with hemodialysis membranes. *Kidney Int* 35:576–588, 1989.

31. Cheung AK, Hohnholt M, Gilson J: Adherence of neutrophils to hemodialysis membranes: role of complement receptors. *Kidney Int* 40:1123–1133, 1991.

32. Cheung AK, Parker CJ, Hohnholt M: β_2 integrins are required for neutrophil degranulation induced by hemodialysis membranes. *Kidney Int* 43:649–660, 1993.

33. Deppisch R, Schmitt V, Bommer J, Hansch GM, Ritz E, Rauterberg EW: Fluid phase generation of terminal complement complex as a novel index of bioincompatibility. *Kidney Int* 7:696–706, 1990.

34. Stimler-Gerard NP: Immunopharmacology of anaphylatoxin-induced bronchoconstrictor responses. *Complement* 3:137–151, 1986.

35. Cheung AK, Parker CJ, Wilcox L: Effects of two types of cobra venom factor on porcine complement activation and pulmonary artery pressure. *Clin Exp Immunol* 78:299–306, 1989.

36. Goldstein IM: Complement: biologically active products. In: JI Gallin, IM Goldstein, R Snyderman, eds, *Inflammation: Basic Principles and Clinical Correlates*. Raven Press, New York, pp 55–74, 1988.

37. Hugli TE: The structural basis for anaphylatoxin and chemotactic functions of C3a, C4a, and C5a. *CRC Crit Rev Immunol* 2:321–366, 1981.

38. McCormick JR, Kreutzer DL, Keating HJ, Hupp J, Despins A, Moore M: Alterations in activities of anaphylatoxin inactivator and chemotactic factor inactivator during hemodialysis. *Am J Pathol* 109:282–287, 1982.

39. Haeffner-Cavaillon N, Cavaillon J-M, Laude M, Kazatchkine M: C3a(C3a$_{desArg}$) induces production and release of interleukin 1 by cultured human monocytes. *J Immunol* 139:794–799, 1987.

40. Kozin F, Cochrane CG: The contact activation system of plasma: biochemistry and pathophysiology. In: JI Gallin, IM Goldstein, R Snyderman, eds, *Inflammation: Basic Principles and Clinical Correlates*. Raven Press, New York, pp 101–120, 1988.

41. Vroman L, Adams AL, Klings M: Interactions among human blood proteins at interfaces. *Fed Proc* 30:1494–1502, 1971.

42. Salzman EW: Role of platelets in blood-surface interactions. *Fed Proc* 30:1503–1508, 1971.

43. Lewis KJ, Dewar PJ, Ward MK, Kerr DNS: Formation of anti-N-like antibodies in dialysis patients: effect of different methods of dialyzer rinsing to remove formaldehyde. *Clin Nephrol* 15:39–43, 1981.

44. Müller-Eberhard HJ: Complement: chemistry and pathways In: JI Gallin, IM Goldstein, R Snyderman, eds, *Inflammation: Basic Principles and Clinical Correlates*. Raven Press, New York, pp 21–54, 1988.

45. Salama A, Hugo F, Heinrich D, Hoge R, Muller R, Kiefel V, Mueller-Eckhardt C: Deposition of terminal C5b-9 complement complexes on erythrocytes and leukocytes during cardiopulmonary bypass. *N Engl J Med* 318:408–414, 1988.

46. Himmelfarb J, Lazarus JM, Hakim RM: Reactive oxygen species production by monocytes and polymorphonuclear leukocytes during dialysis. *Am J Kidney Dis* 17:271–276, 1991.

47. Arnaout MA, Hakim RM, Todd RF, Dana N, Colten HR:

Increased expression of an adhesion-promoting surface glycoprotein in the granulocytopenia of hemodialysis. *N Engl J Med* 312:457–462, 1985.

48. Himmelfarb J, Zaoui P, Hakim R, Holbrook D: Modulation of granulocyte LAM-1 and MAC-1 during dialysis: a prospective, randomized controlled trial. *Kidney Int* 41:388–395, 1992.

49. Dinarello C: Cytokines: agents provocateurs in hemodialysis? *Kidney Int* 41:683–694, 1992.

50. Luger A, Kovarik J, Stummvoll H-K, Urbanska A, Luger TA: Blood-membrane interaction in hemodialysis leads to increased cytokine production. *Kidney Int* 32:84–88, 1987.

51. Haeffner-Cavaillon N, Cavaillon J-M, Ciancioni C, Bacle F, Delons S, Katzatchkine MD: In vivo induction of interleukin-1 during hemodialysis. *Kidney Int* 35:1212–1218, 1989.

52. Zaoui P, Green W, Hakim RM: Hemodialysis with cuprophane membrane modulates interleukin-2 receptor expression. *Kidney Int* 39:1020–1026, 1991.

53. Descamps-Latscha B, Herbelin A, Nguyen AT, de Groote D, Chauveau P, Verger C, Jungers P, Zingraff J: Soluble CD23 as an effector of immune dysregulation in chronic uremia and dialysis. *Kidney Int* 43:878–884, 1993.

54. Zaoui P, Hakim RM: Natural killer-cell function in hemodialysis patients: effect of the dialysis membrane. *Kidney Int* 43:1298–1305, 1993.

55. Schindler R, Gelfand JA, Dinarello CA: Recombinant C5a stimulates transcription rather than translation of IL-1 and TNF: priming of mononuclear cells with recombinant C5a enhances cytokine synthesis induced by LPS, IL-1 or PMA. *Blood* 76:1631–1635, 1990.

56. Schindler R, Lonnemann G, Shaldon S, Koch K-M, Dinarello CA: Transcription, not synthesis, of interleukin-1 and tumor necrosis factor by complement. *Kidney Int* 37:85–93, 1990.

57. Proceedings, Consensus Conference on Biocompatibility. *Nephrol Dial Transplant*, 9(suppl 2), 1994.

58. Hakim RM, Schafer AI: Hemodialysis-associated platelet activation and thrombocytopenia: *Am J Med* 78:575–580, 1985.

59. Sreeharan N, Crow MJ, Salter MCP, Donaldson DR, Rajah SM, Davison AM: Membrane effect on platelet function during hemodialysis: a comparison of cuprophan and polycarbonate. *Artif Organs* 6:324–327, 1982.

60. Moll S, De Moerloose P, Reber G, Schifferli J, Leski M: Comparison of two hemodialysis membranes, polyacrilotrile and cellulose acetate, on complement and coagulation systems. *Int J Artif Organs* 13:273–279, 1990.

61. Pavlopoulou G, Perzanowski C, Hakim RM, Lazarus JM: Platelet aggregation studies during dialysis. *Kidney Int* 29:221(A), 1986.

62. Simon P, Ang KS, Cam G: Enhanced platelet aggregation and membrane biocompatibility: possible influence on thrombosis and embolism in hemodialysis patients. *Nephron* 45:172–173, 1987.

63. Henderson LW, Cheung AK, Chenoweth DE: Choosing a membrane. *Am J Kidney Dis* 3:5–20, 1983.

64. Daugirdas JT, Ing TS: First-use reactions during hemodialysis: a definition of subtypes. *Kidney Int* 33:S37–S43, 1988.

65. Villarroel F, Ciarkowski AA: A survey on hypersensitivity reactions in hemodialysis. *Artif Organs* 9:231–238, 1985.

66. Nicholls AJ, Platts MM: Anaphylactoid reactions during haemodialysis are due to ethylene oxide hypersensitivity.

Proc Eur Dial Transplant Assoc 121:173–177, 1984.

67. Poothullil J, Shimizu A, Day RP, Dolovich J: Anaphylaxis from the product(s) of ethylene oxide gas. *Ann Intern Med* 82:58–60, 1975.

68. Rault R, Silver MR: Severe reactions during hemodialysis. *Am J Kidney Dis* 5:128–131, 1985.

69. Pegues DA, Beck-Sague CM, Woollen SW, Greenspan B, Burns SM, Bland LA, Arduino MJ, Favero MS, Mackow RC, Jarvis WR: Anaphylactoid reactions associated with reuse of hollow-fiber hemodialyzers and ACE inhibitors. *Kidney Int* 42:1232–1237, 1992.

70. Bommer J, Wilhelms OH, Barth HP, Schindele H, Ritz E: Anaphylactoid reactions in dialysis patients: role of ethylene-oxide. *Lancet* 2:1382–1385, 1985.

71. Lee FF, Durning CJ, Leonard EF: Urethanes as ethylene oxide reservoirs in hollow-fiber dialyzers. *Trans Am Soc Artif Intern Organs* 31:526–533, 1985.

72. Cheung AK, LeWinter M, Chenoweth DE, Lew W, Henderson LW: Cardiopulmonary effects of cuprophane-activated plasma in the swine: role of complement activation products. *Kidney Int* 29:799–806, 1986.

73. del Balzo UH, Levi R, Polley MJ: Cardiac dysfunction caused by purified human C3a anaphylatoxin. *Proc Natl Acad Sci USA* 82:886–890, 1985.

74. Vogt W: Anaphylatoxins: possible roles in disease. *Complement* 3:177–188, 1986.

75. Westaby S, Dawson P, Turner MW, Pridie RB: Angiography and complement activation: evidence for generation of C3a anaphylatoxin by intravascular contrast agents. *Cardiovasc Res* 19:85–88, 1985.

76. Dumler F, Zasuwa G, Levin NW: Effect of dialyzer reprocessing methods on complement activation and hemodialyzer-related symptoms. *Artif Organs* 11:128–131, 1987.

77. Bergamo Collaborative Dialysis Study Group: Acute intradialytic well-being: results of a clinical trial comparing polysulfone with cuprophan. *Kidney Int* 40:714–719, 1991.

78. Collins DM, Lambert MB, Tannenbaum JS, Oliverio M, Schwab SJ: Tolerance of hemodialysis: a randomized prospective trial of high-flux versus conventional high-efficiency hemodialysis. *J Am Soc Nephrol* 4:148–154, 1993.

79. Lemke HD, Eisenhauer T, Krieter D, Fink E, Shimamoto K, Verresen L: Generation of bradykinin, hypotension and anaphylactoid shock during hemodialysis. *J Am Soc Nephrol* 4:362(A), 1993.

80. Powell AC, Bland LA, Oettinger CW, McAllister SK, Oliver JC, Arduino MJ, Favero MS: Lack of plasma interleukin-1β or tumor necrosis factor—an elevation during unfavorable hemodialysis conditions. *J Am Soc Nephrol* 2:1007–1013, 1991.

81. Gordon SM, Oettinger CW, Bland LA, Oliver JC, Arduino MJ, Aguero SM, McAllister SK, Favero MS, Jarvis WR: Pyrogenic reactions in patients receiving conventional, high-efficiency, or high-flux hemodialysis treatments with bicarbonate dialysate containing high concentrations of bacteria and endotoxin. *J Am Soc Nephrol* 2:1436–1444, 1992.

82. Bommer J, Becker KP, Urbaschek R, Ritz E, Urbaschek B: No evidence for endotoxin transfer across high flux polysulfone membranes. *Clin Nephrol* 27:278–282, 1987.

83. Laude-Sharp M, Caroff M, Simard L, Pusineri C, Kazatchkine MD, Haeffner-Cavaillon: Induction of IL-1 during hemodialysis: transmembrane passage of intact endotoxins (LPS). *Kidney Int* 38:1089–1094, 1990.

84. Bingel M, Lonnemann G, Shaldon S, Koch KM, Dinarello CA: Human interleukin-1 production during hemodialysis. *Nephron* 43:161–163, 1986.

85. Lonnemann G, Bingel M, Flöege J, Koch KM, Shaldon S, Dinarello CA: Detection of endotoxin-like interleukin-1-inducting activity during in vitro dialysis. *Kidney Int* 33:29–35, 1988.

86. Dinarrello CA, Lonnemann G, Maxwell R, Shaldon S: Ultrafiltration to reject human interleukin-1 inducing substances derived from bacterial cultures. *J Clin Microbiol* 25:1233–1238, 1987.

87. Lonnemann G, Behme TC, Lenzner B, Flöege J, Schulze M, Colton CK, Koch KM, Shaldon S: Permeability of dialyzer membranes to TNFα-inducing substances derived from water bacteria. *Kidney Int* 42:61–68, 1992.

88. Schindler R, Dinarello CA: A method for removing interleukin-1 and tumor necrosis factor inducing substances from bacterial cultures by ultrafiltration with polysulfone. *J Immunol Methods* 116:159–165, 1989.

89. Pegues DA, Oettinger AW, Bland LA, Oliver JC, Arduino MJ, Aguero SM, McAllister SK, Gordon SM, Favero MS, Jarvis WR: A prospective study of pyrogenic reactions in hemodialysis patients using bicarbonate dialysis fluids flitered to remove bacteria and endotoxin. *J Am Soc Nephrol* 4:1002–1007, 1992.

90. Dolan MJ, Whipp BJ, Davidson WD, Weitzman RE, Wasserman K: Hypopnea associated with acetate hemodialysis: carbon-dioxide-flow dependent ventilation. *N Engl J Med* 305:72–75, 1981.

91. Oh MS, Uribarri J, Del Monte ML, Heneghan WF, Kee CS, Friedman EA: A mechanism of hypoxemia during hemodialysis. *Am J Nephrol* 5:366–371, 1985.

92. Jones RH, Broadfield JB, Parsons V: Arterial hypoxemia during hemodialysis for acute renal failure in mechanically ventilated patients: observations and mechanisms. *Clin Nephrol* 14:18–22, 1980.

93. Craddock PR, Fehr J, Brigham KL, Kronenberg RS, Jacob HS: Complement and leukocyte-mediated pulmonary dysfunction in hemodialysis. *N Engl J Med* 296:769–774, 1977.

94. DeBacker WA, Verpooten GA, Borgonjon DJ, Vermeire PA, Lins RR, De Broe ME: Hypoxemia during hemodialysis: effects of different membranes and dialysate compositions. *Kidney Int* 23:738–743, 1983.

95. Hakim RM, Lowrie EG: Hemodialysis-associated neutropenia and hypoxemia: the effect of dialyzer membrane materials. *Nephron* 32:32–39, 1982.

96. Mahajan S. Gardiner H, DeTar B, Desai S, Muller B, Johnson N, Briggs W, McDonald F: Relationship between pulmonary functions and hemodialysis induced leukopenia. *Trans Am Soc Artif Intern Organs* 23:411–415, 1977.

97. Graf H, Stummvoll HK, Haber P, Kovarik J: Pathophysiology of dialysis related hypoxaemia. *Proc Eur Dial Transplant Assoc* 17:155–161, 1980.

98. Morrison JT, Wilson AF, Vaziri ND, Brunsting L, Davis J: Determination of pulmonary tissue volume, pulmonary capillary blood flow and diffusing capacity of the lung before and after hemodialysis. *Int J Artif Organs* 3:259–262, 1980.

99. De Backer WA, Verpooten GA, Borgonjon DJ, Vermeire PA, Lins RR, De Broe ME: Hypoxemia during hemodialysis: effects of different membranes and dialysate composition. *Contrib Nephrol* 37:134–141, 1984.

100. Bergström J, Danielsson A, Freyschuss U: Dialysis, ultrafiltration and sham dialysis in normal subjects. *Kidney Int* 27:157(A), 1984.

101. Fawcett S, Hoenich NA, Laker MF, Schorr W, Ward MK, Kerr DNS: Haemodialysis-induced respiratory changes. *Nephrol Dial Transplant* 2:161–168, 1987.

102. Abu-Hamdan DK, Desai SG, Mahajan SK, Muller BF, Briggs WA, Lynne-Davies P, McDonald FD: Hypoxemia during hemodialysis using acetate versus bicarbonate dialysate. *Am J Nephrol* 4: 248–253, 1984.

103. Vaziri ND, Barton CH, Warner A, Toohey J, Lintner C, Hung E, Mullin P, Samiminia B, O'Donnell M, Mallot K: Comparison of four dialyzer–dialysate combinations: effects on blood gases, cell counts, complement contact factors and fibrinolytic system. *Contrib Nephrol* 37:111–119, 1984.

104. Vanholder RC, Pauwels RA, Vandenbogaerde JF, Lamont HH, Van Der Straeten ME, Ringoir SM: Cuprophan reuse and intradialytic changes of lung diffusion capacity and blood gasses. *Kidney Int* 32:117–122, 1987.

105. Agar JW, Hull JD, Kaplan M, Pletka PG: Acute cardiopulmonary decompensation and complement activation during hemodialysis. *Ann Intern Med* 90:792–793, 1979.

106. Schohn DC, Jahn HA, Eber M, Hauptmann G: Biocompatibility and hemodynamic studies during polycarbonate versus cuprophan membrane dialysis. *Blood Purif* 4:102–111, 1986.

107. Cheung AK, Baranowski RL, Wayman AL: The role of thromboxane in cuprophan-induced pulmonary hypertension. *Kidney Int* 31:1072–1079, 1987.

108. Gallin JI: Phagocytic cells: disorders of function. In: JI Gallin, IM Goldstein, R Snyderman, eds, *Inflammation: Basic Principles and Clinical Correlates*. Raven Press, New York, pp 493–511, 1988.

109. Vanholder R, Ringoir S, Dhondt A, Hakim R: Phagocytosis in uremic and hemodialysis patients: a prospective and cross sectional study. *Kidney Int* 39:320–327, 1991.

110. Degiannis D, Czarnecki M, Donati D, Homer L, Eisinger RP, Raska K, Raskova J: Normal T lymphocyte function in patients with end-stage renal disease hemodialyzed with "high-flux" polysulfone membranes. *Am J Nephrol* 10:276–282, 1990.

111. Zaoui P, Hakim RM: The effects of the dialysis membrane on cytokine release. *J Am Soc Nephrol* 4:1711–1718, 1994.

112. Hörl WH, Heidland A: Evidence for the participation of granulocyte proteinases on intradialytic catabolism. *Clin Nephrol* 21:314–322, 1984.

113. Heidland A, Hörl WH, Heller N, Heine H, Neumann S, Heidbreder E: Proteolytic enzymes and catabolism: enhanced release of granulocyte proteinases in uremic intoxication and during hemodialysis. *Kidney Int* 24 (Suppl):S27–S36, 1983.

114. Maher ER, Wickens DG, Griffin JFA, Kyle P, Curtis JR, Dormandy TL: Increased free-radical activity during haemodialysis? *Nephrol Dial Transplant* 2:169–171, 1987.

115. Till GO, Johnson KJ, Kunke R, Ward PA: Intravascular activation of complement and acute lung injury. *J Clin Invest* 69:1126–1135, 1982.

116. Schulman G, Fogo A, Gung A, Badr K, Hakim R: Complement activation retards resolution of acute ischemic renal failure in the rat. *Kidney Int* 40:1069–1074, 1991.

117. Skubitz KM, Craddock PR: Reversal of hemodialysis granulocytopenia and pulmonary leukostasis: a clinical manifestation of selective down-regulation of granulocyte responses to $C5a_{desarg}$. *J Clin Invest* 67:1383–1391, 1981.

118. Hornberger JC, Chernew M, Petersen J, Garber AM: A

multivariate analysis of mortality and hospital admissions with high-flux dialysis. *J Am Soc Nephrol* 3:1227–1237, 1992.

119. Meuer SC, Hauer M, Kurz P, Meyer zum Büschenfelde KH, Köhler H: Selective blockade of the antigen-receptor-mediated pathway of T cell activation in patients with impaired immune responses. *J Clin Invest* 80:743–749, 1987.

120. Sennesael JJ, Van der Niepen P, Verbeelen DL: Treatment with recombinant human erythropoietin increases antibody titers after hepatitis B vaccination in dialysis patients. *Kidney Int* 40:121–128, 1991.

121. Kay NE, Raij L: Differential effect of hemodialysis membranes on human lymphocyte natural killer function. *Artif Organs* 11:165–167, 1987.

122. Port FK, Ragheb NE, Schwartz AG, Hawthorne VM: Neoplasms in dialysis patients: a population-based study. *Am J Kidney Dis* 14:119–123, 1989.

123. Hakim RM, Wingard RL, Parker RA: Effect of the dialysis membrane in the treatement of patients with acute renal failure. *N Engl J Med* 331:1338–1374, 1994.

124. Gung A, Schulman G, Hakim R: Hemodialysis membrane choice influences maintenance of residual renal function (RRF) in an animal model. *J Am Soc Nephrol* 2:327(A), 1991.

125. Gorevic PD, Casey TT, Stone WJ: Beta-2 microglobulin is an amyloidogenic protein in man.*J Clin Invest* 76:2425–2429, 1985.

126. Gejyo F, Odani S, Yamada T, Honma N, Saito H, Suzuki Y, Nakagawa Y, Kobayashi H, Maruyama Y, Hirasawa Y, Suzuki M, Arakawa M: β_2-microglobulin: a new form of amyloid proteins associated with chronic hemodialysis.*Kidney Int* 30:385–390, 1986.

127. Bergström J, Wehle B: No change in corrected β_2-microglobulin concentration after cuprophane haemodialysis. *Lancet* 1:629, 1987.

128. Flöege J, Granolleras C, Merscher S, Eisenbach GM, Deschodt G, Colton CK, Shaldon S, Koch KM: Is the rise in plasma beta-2-microglobulin seen during hemodialysis meaningful? *Nephron* 51:6–12, 1989.

129. Flöege J, Granolleras C, Koch KM, Shaldon S: Which membrane? Should beta-2-microglobulin decide on the choice of today's hemodialysis membrane? *Nephron* 50:177–181, 1988.

130. Ritz E, Bommer J: Beta-2-microglobulin-derived amyloid-problems and perspectives.*Blood Purif* 6:61–68, 1988.

131. Linke RP, Hampl H, Lobeck H: Lysine-specific cleavage of β_2-microglobulin in amyloid deposits associated with hemodialysis. *Kidney Int* 36:675–681, 1989.

132. Ogawa H, Saito A, Ono M, Oda O, Nakajima M, Chung TG: Novel β_2-microglobulin and its amyloidogenic predisposition in patients on haemodialysis. *Nephrol Dial Transplant* 4 (Suppl):14–18, 1989.

133. Miyata T, Oda O, Inagi R: β_2-microglobulin modified with advanced glycation end products is a major component of hemodialysis-associated amyloidosis. *J Clin Invest* 92:1243–1252, 1993.

134. Zaoui PM, Stone WJ, Hakim RM: Effects of dialysis membranes on beta$_2$-microglobulin. *Kidney Int* 38:962–968, 1990.

135. Ohashi K, Hara M, Kawai R, Ogura Y, Honda K, Nihei H, Mimura N:. Cervical discs are most susceptible to beta$_2$-microglobulin amyloid deposition in the vertebral column. *Kidney Int* 41:1646–1652, 1992.

136. Flöege J, Bartsch A, Schulze M, Shaldon S, Koch KM, Smeby

LC: Clearance and synthesis rates of β_2-microglobulin in patients undergoing hemodialysis and in normal subjects. *J Lab Clin Med* 118:153–165, 1991.

137. Vincent C, Chanard J, Caudwell V, Lavaud S, Wong T, Revillard J: Kinetics of ^{125}I-β_2-microglobulin turnover in dialyzed patients. *Kidney Int* 42:1434–1443, 1992.

138. Flöege J, Granolleras C, Bingel M, Deschodt G, Branger B, Oules R, Koch KM, Shaldon S: β_2-microglobulin kinetics during haemodialysis and haemofiltration. *Nephrol Dial Transplant* 1:223–228, 1987.

139. Jørstad S, Smeby LC, Balstad T, Widerøe TE: Removal, generation and adsorption of beta-2–microglobulin during hemofiltration with five different membranes. *Blood Purif* 6:96–105, 1988.

140. Dinarello CA: Interleukin-1 and its biologically related cytokines. *Adv Immunol* 44:153–205, 1989.

141. Chanard J, Bindi P, Lavaud S, Toupance O, Maheut H, Lacour F: Carpal tunnel syndrome and type of dialysis membrane. *Br Med J* 867–868, 1989.

142. van Ypersele de Strihou C, Jadoul M, Malghem J, Maldague B, Jamart J: Effect of dialysis membrane and patient's age on signs of dialysis-related amyloidosis. *Kidney Int* 39:1012–1019, 1991.

143. Miura Y, Ishiyama T, Inomata A, Takeda T, Senma S, Okuyama K, Suzuki Y: Radiolucent bone cysts and the type of dialysis membrane used in patients undergoing long-term hemodialysis. *Nephron* 60:268–273, 1992.

144. Elsbach P, Weiss J: Phagocytic cells: oxygen-independent antimicrobial systems. In: JI Gallin, IM Goldstein, R Snyderman, eds, *Inflammation: Basic Principles and Clinical Correlates*. Raven Press, New York, pp 445–470, 1988.

145. Weiss SJ, Regiani S: Neutrophils degrade subendothelial matrices in the presence of alpha-1-proteinase inhibitor: cooperative use of lysosomal proteinases and oxygen metabolites. *J Clin Invest* 73:1297–1303, 1984.

146. Gutierrez A, Alvestrand A, Wahren J, Bergström J: Effect of in vivo contact between blood and dialysis membranes on protein catabolism in humans. *Kidney Int* 38:487–494, 1990.

147. Lonnemann G, Koch KM, Shaldon S: Studies on the ability of hemodialysis membranes to induce, bind, and clear human interleukin-1. *J Lab Clin Med* 112:76–86, 1988.

148. Lim VS, Bier DM, Flanigan MJ, Sum-Ping ST: The effect of hemodialysis on protein metabolism: a leucine kinetic study. *J Clin Invest* 91:2419–2436, 1993.

149. Haag-Weber, M, Hörl WH: Uremia and infection: mechanisms of impaired cellular host defense. *Nephron* 63:125–131, 1993.

150. Makita Z, Radoff S, Rayfield EJ, Yang Z, Skolnik E, Delaney V, Friedman EA, Cerami A, Vlassara H: Advanced glycosylation end products in patients with diabetic nephropathy. *N Engl J Med* 325:836–842, 1991.

151. Hegbrant J, Thysell H, Ekman R: Elevated plasma levels of opioid peptides and delta sleep-inducing peptide but not of corticotropin-releasing hormone in patients receiving chronic hemodialysis. *Blood Purif* 9:188–194, 1991.

152. Chenoweth DE, Cheung AK, Ward DM, Henderson LW: Anaphylatoxin formation during hemodialysis: comparison of new and reused dialyzers. *Kidney Int* 24:770–774, 1983.

153. Kaplan AA, Halley SE, Lapkin RA, Graeber CW, Graeber CA: Dialysate protein losses with bleach processedd polysulphone dialyzers. *Kidney Int* 47:573–578, 1995.

CHAPTER 62

Hemodialysis, Ultrafiltration, and Hemofiltration

RAYMOND C. VANHOLDER, ANN A. VAN LOO & SEVERIN M. RINGOIR

INTRODUCTION

The treatment of end-stage renal failure by extracorporeal circulatory support is a well-recognized and widely practiced therapeutic option. If this option is not applied, a progressive deterioration of clinical condition will finally result in undernourishment, enhanced morbidity, coma, and death; these events are largely attributed to the accumulation of uremic retention solutes that in health are eliminated by the functioning kidneys. Hemodialysis and related strategies (hemofiltration, hemodiafiltration) are today the most widely used methods of extracorporeal circulatory support in end-stage renal failure; a number of improvements have been made over the past decades by the introduction of more biocompatible membranes, bicarbonate buffering of the dialysis fluid, measures to estimate and to improve the adequacy of dialysis, and the availability of various alternative access methods.

Despite the widespread use of dialysis techniques for the treatment of both chronic and acute renal failure, dialysed patients continue to exhibit metabolic derangements related to a mixture of deficiencies as well as to the incomplete removal of nitrogenous and other metabolites that are retained as a consequence of renal failure. These shortcomings of hemodialysis therapy have led to the development and clinical application of alternative concepts of extracorporeal blood purification such as continuous arteriovenous hemofiltration (CAVH), continuous venovenous hemofiltration (CVVH), continuous ambulatory peritoneal dialysis (CAPD), and plasma exchange and hemoperfusion. The purpose of this chapter is to review the available strategies, to examine their relationship to each other, and to focus on specific aspects relating to their clinical use. Emphasis will be on diverse aspects of extracorporeal blood purification, with the exception of CAPD, which will be covered in specific chapters.

ACCESS METHODS FOR EXTRACORPOREAL THERAPY

The need for adequate and reliable vascular access remains one of the major problems in extracorporeal blood purification therapy, since in case of hemodialysis or related strategies, adequate contact with the bloodstream must be obtained and a substantial blood flow achieved to allow the therapeutic technique to be performed. Within this context, a number of solutions have been proposed, some suitable for short-term acute use and others intended for long-term chronic use.

Temporary access techniques

Acute vascular access was historically first obtained by the creation of external arteriovenous shunts (1). This technique necessitates surgical intervention, makes reintervention necessary in the case of thrombosis, and can be the cause of the loss of one or more vessels that could be useful for subsequent creation of endogenous arteriovenous fistulae. Alternative temporary access procedures include the placement of catheters in the femoral (2–4), internal jugular (5), or subclavian (6,7) positions. Although large population studies show that these techniques have a low complication rate when properly performed (8,9), especially with the subclavian insertion site, a number of acute complications such as hemothorax or pneumothorax (10–14), as well as central venous thrombosis (15,16), have been described. In addition, subclavian catheters also remain a major point of concern if they remain in place for prolonged periods, due to a high prevalence of postcatheterization vein stenosis (17–20). Especially if they are applied at the same side of an arteriovenous fistula, or if an arteriovenous fistula is created ipsilaterally later on, this will result in painful swelling of the limb and inadequate dialysis related to blood recirculation (19,20).

Central venous catheters are available either in a single- or two-lumen version (Figure 1). The latter are conceived to allow a better adequacy of dialysis by the reduction of recirculation in the absence of a common trajectory for the blood entering and leaving the hemodialyzer. They are at the same time, however, characterized by a higher blood flow resistance and subsequent lower blood flow, thereby limiting solute exchange and counterbalancing the gain in efficacy resulting from the decrease in recirculation (21).

Suki, WN and Massry SG (eds), Suki and Massry's Therapy of Renal Diseases and Related Disorders, Third Edition. ISBN 978-1-4757-6634-9.
©*1998, Kluwer Academic Publishers, Boston/Dordrecht/London. All rights reserved.*

Long-term access techniques

The Cimino–Brescia fistula, introduced in 1966, remains the most widely used method of long-term vascular access (22), whereby an artery is surgically connected to a vein to allow the creation of a large-capacitance vessel. The latter is necessary because hemodialysis necessitates the possibility of creating high blood flows without the collapse of the access. This type of fistula is most currently established at the wrist between the cephalic vein and the radial artery. Long-term access can be achieved only if the fistula is established well before the patient needs to use it, in order to allow the vasculature to enlarge before the needles are inserted for extracorporeal therapy. Clearly, such access requires the availability of an adequate vascular system. In the absence of such a system (e.g., in the case of diabetes mellitus, atheromatosis, or vasculitis), a number of artificial alternate solutions have been described, such as the implantation of exogenous polymeric materials (Gore-Tex or PTFE) (23), bovine grafts (24), or specially prepared cadaveric or umbilical veins (25). More recently, central vein catheters have become available for prolonged use. They are characterized by a larger bore size and a softer physical structure than the indwelling catheters for temporary use. These catheters can be inserted either surgically (modified Hickman–Broviac catheter type for dialysis use), with specific usefulness in infants, children, and the elderly (26,27), or by the classical blind techniques for catheter insertion. Proper studies to compare the complication profile of the two approaches are lacking today. Overall, both approaches may carry a lower risk of thrombotic and infectious complications per unit of time in comparison to the temporary indwelling intravenous catheters (27). Nevertheless, any access method based on foreign (polymeric) material will always remain more prone to complications than the classical endogenous arteriovenous fistula.

HEMODIALYSIS

Hemodialysis relies upon the use of a hemodialyzer containing a semipermeable membrane, whereby blood flows on one side while the other side is bathed by a fast-flowing isotonic electrolyte solution (dialysate) (Figure 2). Transfer of toxins then occurs through the pores of the membrane, mainly according to the laws of osmotic gradient diffusion. Until recently, the formats of the membrane were mostly either flat sheet or hollow fiber (Figure 3). With time, hollow-fiber (capillary) dialyzers became the most popular approach.

Metabolites, elevated as a consequence of renal insufficiency, diffuse across the membrane and are carried to

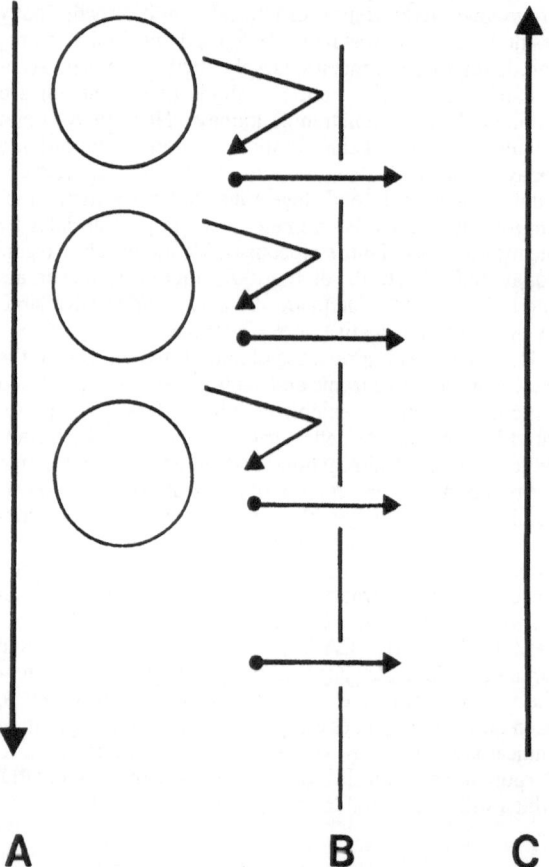

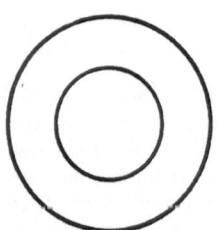 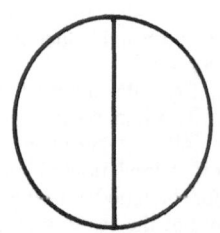

Figure 1. Configurations of two types of two-lumen central vein catheter are shown in transverse section. Left: double-lumen catheter (coaxial type); right: dual-lumen catheter (double-D shaped). For the same diameter and blood flow as a single-lumen catheter, resistance in the two-lumen catheters will be higher.

Figure 2. Principles of dialysis. On one side of a semipermeable membrane (B), blood (A) is flowing, containing formed elements (blood cells and proteins—large circles) and smaller solutes (dots). On the other side of the membrane, there is a countercurrent flow of dialysate (C). Whereas the formed elements are reflected (bent arrows), a shift of solutes from A to C occurs (straight arrows) according to the laws of diffusion.

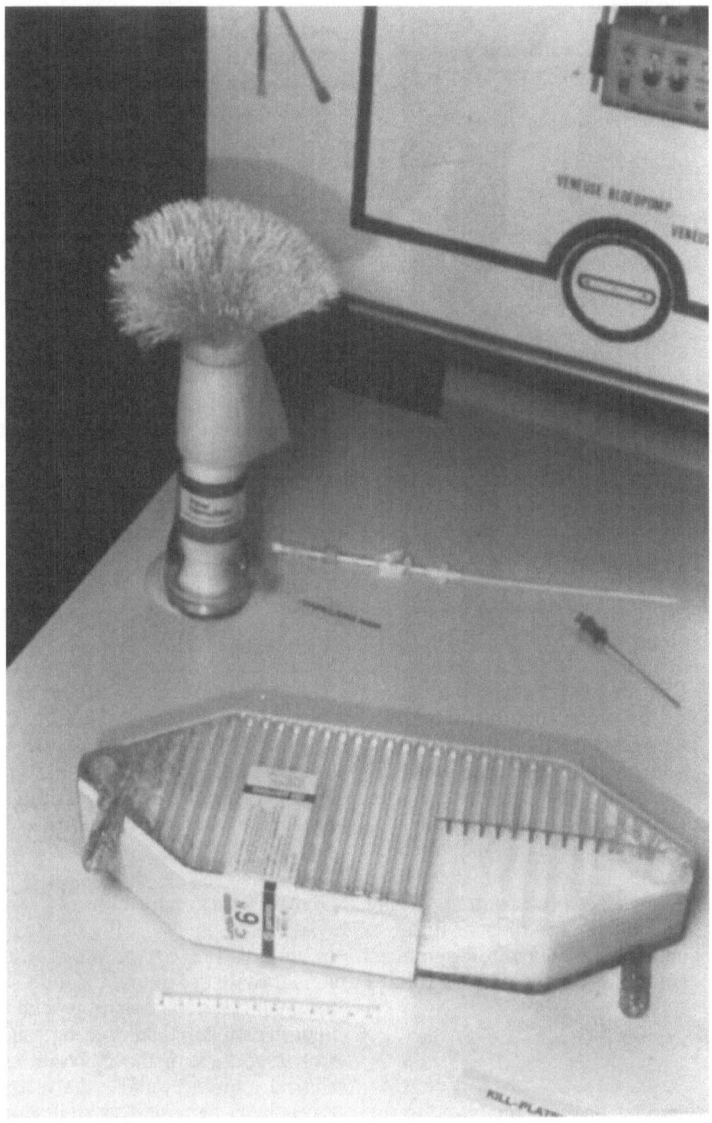

Figure 3. Two different formats of hemodialyzers: flat sheet (front) and capillary (back). The housing of the dialyzers has been partially removed to disclose the interior aspect and geometric arrangement of the membrane.

waste (Figure 2). Formed elements (blood cells, proteins) are prevented from passing across the membrane by their size. Fluid retained as a consequence of oliguria is removed principally by the application of a hydrostatic pressure across the semipermeable membrane, either positive at the blood side or negative at the dialysate side (ultrafiltration). This ultrafiltration carries away an extra amount of solutes by convection and adds to the efficacy of dialysis.

A wide variety of hemodialyzers, suitable for use for small children up to large adults, is available for clinical use. These hemodialyzers offer a range of solute- and water-removal efficiencies depending upon their size and type of membrane. The choice is a complex decision that is dependent not only upon functional performance but also on biocompatibility and economic as well as other considerations. This chapter will not discuss the criteria of choice

Table 1. Requirements of an ideal dialyzer

High clearance of small- and middle-molecular-weight solutes
Maintenance of efficacy throughout the dialysis session
Negligible loss of vital solutes
Absence of uptake of impurities across the semipermeable
  membrane
Appropriate range of ultrafiltration
Low blood volume contained within the device
Good washback characteristics
High reliability
Biocompatible membrane and construction
Low weight, transparency
Low cost

in detail, but the requirements of an ideal hemodialysis are summarized in table 1 in order to give the reader a yardstick of comparison against which potential choices may be matched. In common with other modes of extracorporeal therapy, safety precautions during hemodialysis are mandatory, and consequently both the blood and the dialysate circuits incorporate a variety of safety devices. These include the monitoring of the pressure in the extracorporeal blood circuit, the composition and temperature of the dialysis fluid, the monitoring for the presence of free hemoglobin in case of rupture of the semipermeable membranes, and devices for the detection and the prevention of air embolisms. Blood flow through the extracorporeal circuit is maintained by the use of one or more blood pumps that are linked to the above safety and monitoring devices, ensuring arrest of blood flow in the event of a malfunction. More recent options offer the possibility of alternating ultrafiltration rate and dialysate electrolyte contents during the course of the dialysis session, and in the near future it can be expected that the possibility will be offered to measure on-line dialysate concentration of at least some solutes (e.g., urea) (28).

Dialysis fluid

Hemodialysis relies on the diffusion from the blood to the dialysis fluid of metabolites with an elevated concentration as a consequence of renal insufficiency. The dialysis fluid is obtained by the mixing of a commercially available concentrate of electrolyte and buffer solution with treated tap water by a proportionating system designed either for use by a single patient or for batch production suitable for multiple patient use.

One of the major problems with dialysate is its contamination with bacteria, mostly pseudomonads, which became a pitfall essentially from the moment that the technical possibility was offered of preparing dialysate with bicarbonate as a buffer; inadequately purified bicarbonate concentrate currently contains bacterial contaminants (29), since alkaline bicarbonate is more prone to bacterial infec-

tion than the acidic acetate concentrate. These bacteria in turn release pyrogens, such as endotoxins (lipopolysaccharides, or LPSs), endotoxin fragments, and other compounds enhancing cytokine release from mononuclear leukocytes, that may cross the transmembrane barrier of the dialyzer (30).

Dialysate concentrate was originally prepared in the hospital, but later it became possible to purchase industrially manufactured concentrates. These, however, were originally available in containers that offered no guarantee of absence of bacteria or pyrogens. More recently, sterile and pyrogen-free dialysate concentrate became available in plastic bags. However, the other constituent of dialysate, namely, tap water, should be sterile as well, which was certainly not guaranteed with the older water preparation systems. The newer reverse osmosis (RO) systems make this option possible if the technique is applied properly, together with an architectural design of water distribution systems that avoids dead spaces and trapping. This necessitates regular control of the final dialysate in order to check on sterility, systematic replacement of RO columns at preset time points before bacteria can grow through the system, and immediate decontamination of the conduits beyond the RO system if bacteria are cultured in the circuit water. According to the Association for the Advancement of Medical Instrumentation (AAMI), preset standard levels of 200 colony-forming units (CFU)/mL in purified tap water and 2000 CFU/mL in dialysate should not be exceeded (31,32), but ideally, no bacterial growth should be present. Bacterial cultures should be performed on the appropriate culture media as well, at room temperature and at 37°C (29,33).

Dialysis fluid composition

In theory, the composition of dialysis fluid should be similar to that of interstitial fluid, with a suitable correction for the protein fraction. In practice, considerable variations in both cation and anion composition may occur. The electrolyte content of the dialysate can be important for the clinical tolerance, and a dialysate containing low sodium levels is, in general, less well supported, especially in the hemodynamically labile patients (34). A specific series of problems is related to the composition of the buffer and especially to the presence of unphysiologic anionic components (35). Dialysis was first performed with bicarbonate as a buffer; however, the advent of early single-patient proportionating systems meant that, for chemical reasons, bicarbonate-based dialysis fluid could not be produced in batch in the presence of calcium in the concentrate, since the formation of calciumcarbonate precipitate was unavoidable, and the addition of calcium to the dialysate is essential for the attainment of a positive calcium balance and the prevention of bone decalcification. For these reasons, Mion proposed in 1964 to use acetate as an alternative buffer (36). By the early 1970s, it became possible to mix bicarbonate and calcium without precipitation, and this led to the more widespread use of bicarbonate-based dialysis fluid. A further interest in the return to bicarbonate buffering from the more commonly used acetate buffer arose with the introduction of high-efficiency dialyzers and shorter dialysis times: a more rapid exchange of dialysate contents towards the blood resulted in a more pronounced clinical instability for dialysis patients subject to acetate dialysis (37). These problems were markedly reduced by the introduction of bicarbonate dialysate.

Clinical problems related to buffer composition

In general, it can be proclaimed that too little attention is paid to the correct physiological anion content in dialysate and that this neglect carries a serious morbidity (35). A number of clinical studies have demonstrated that patients on acetate- based dialysis treatment are prone to hemodynamic problems (34,38,39). There is, however, no universal agreement on this observation, partly due to differences in the efficiency of the dialyzers used in the studies and to the patient's cardiovascular status (40,41). One may state that with acetate dialysis hemodynamic instability will occur, unless the possibility exists for the patient's cardiovascular system to correct for this disadvantage by increasing cardiac output. Acetate hemodialysis is also associated with a marked hypoxemia, resulting from the loss of CO_2 from the blood across the membrane into the dialysate (42,43), which decreases the impulse to breathe, and hence the respiratory volume. This is a specific danger in patients who are already at the borderline of hypoxemia, e.g., as a consequence of chronic cardiopulmonary disease. In addition, acetate dialysis will result in an irregular respiratory pattern (44). In contrast, these aspects of dialysis therapy may be prevented or at least ameliorated by the use of bicarbonate buffering. There is also the possibility that acetate may be metabolized into lactate, may be incorporated into lipids and be responsible for the hyperlipidemia observed in dialysed patients (45), and may contribute to the cardiovascular problems of patients treated by long-term hemodialysis. The data presented in support of this hypothesis are, however, not convincing. Morin et al. (46) failed to demonstrate significant differences in the serum lipid profiles of patients on acetate- or bicarbonate-based dialysis fluid.

Acetate may interfere with the buffering mechanism not only in the extracellular fluid but also in the bone. This finding may be of importance in chronic acidosis, when calcium phosphate and calcium carbonate crystals from the bone dissolve, releasing their respective ions, which then act as a buffering agent. Since calcium carbonate is one of the major components of bone, loss of the bone buffering capacity may at the same time precipitate osteomalacia.

The use of bicarbonate as a buffer allows a quick correction of acid–base disturbances in uremic patients.

It is conceivable that bicarbonate is preferable to acetate as a dialysate buffer, but there remains a risk of overshooting and excess delivery of bicarbonate, which is especially threatening to patients with already increased blood CO_2 contents (e.g., in chronic hypercapnia).

It should not be forgotten that dialysate may also increase morbidity through the presence of undesired contaminants, e.g., ions (aluminum), bacteria, or bacterial products such as exotoxins and endotoxins.

SEQUENTIAL ULTRAFILTRATION AND HEMODIALYSIS

In conventional hemodialysis, fluid removal is sustained during the period of treatment to rid the patient of excess of water and extracellular electrolytes. Bergström et al. (47) showed that by introducing a period of ultrafiltration without dialysate flow in the dialysis schedule, i.e., separating the processes of ultrafiltration and dialysis, it was possible to remove up to 3 L/hr of fluid from an overhydrated patient without adverse effects. The absence of hypotension or muscle cramps during the period of ultrafiltration appeared to be related to the absence of osmolality changes. Sequential ultrafiltration and dialysis may be performed in a number of different ways: the simplest is by the application of a positive pressure on the blood side or a negative pressure on the dialysate side in the absence of dialysate flowing through the dialyzer. One hour or more of ultrafiltration is then followed by 3–4 hours of hemodialysis. Since the advent of bicarbonate dialysate and the subsequent decrease in risk for hemodynamic instability, and with the availability of hemofilters and high-flux hemodialyzers, sequential ultrafiltration and hemodialysis remain of interest mainly to those with access only to conventional hemodialyzers and/or acetate dialysate. This strategy is then reserved for patients with severe hemodynamic instability and the necessity of removing substantial quantities of excess water, i.e., in acute renal failure patients with sepsis or preload cardiac failure or in the presence of contraindications for more continuous alternatives such as CAVH, CVVH, or CAPD. In spite of the relative simplicity of the procedure, the treatment time is prolonged due to the necessity to sequence ultrafiltration and hemodialysis. Furthermore, there is a danger of imbalance in the electrolytes, e.g., hypercalcemia. In the treatment of chronic renal failure, sequential ultrafiltration and dialysis should only be used on selected patients or in special situations. They may be considered for patients who develop symptomatic hypotension during hemodialysis, patients whose interdialytic weight gain is excessive, or patients with cardiovascular disease or myocardial insufficiency who are intolerant of conventional hemodialysis. In addition, it may also be useful in controlling volume-related hypertension in the early stage of dialysis treatment.

HEMOFILTRATION

During conventional dialysis, the principal method of solute removal is by diffusion, which is augmented to a lesser extent by convective mass transport (ultrafiltration). In hemofiltration, the ultrafiltrate flow through highly permeable membranes is augmented by increasing transmembrane pressure and hydraulic permeability with absence of dialysate flow; ultrafiltrative fluid losses are replaced by a substitution fluid, which is most often a modified Ringer lactate solution. The administration may take place either before (predilution) or after (postdilution) the hemofilter. Predilution requires substantially more substitution fluid than postdilution. As a consequence, postdilution has been historically the more widely used technique. However, predilution became a more valuable alternative in patients with higher red blood cell counts and hence increased blood viscosity, as a consequence of the current use of erythropoietin for the treatment of renal anemia; this enhances the risk of clogging in the filter capillaries, especially in the distal parts of the filters where the filtered volume of water extracted from the blood is high. This risk may be reduced by the application of predilution. Predilution may add extra efficacy in the continuous variants of hemofiltration (CAVH/CVVH) (48), since clogging and clotting of the filters is prevented.

The total volume of exchange for classical hemofiltration ranges from 20 to 40 L/treatment; the treatment is typically carried out in three-times-weekly sessions lasting 4–5 hours. The equipment for hemofiltration consists of the extracorporeal blood circuit, which has a geometric organization roughly analogous to that used in hemodialysis. Ultrafiltration across the hemofilter is achieved by the exertion of a hydrostatic pressure gradient across the membrane, resulting in the transfer of plasma water and solutes. In contrast to the complex hydraulic system required for hemodialysis, the hydraulic circuit to achieve this result in hemofiltration is markedly simpler. In general, a roller

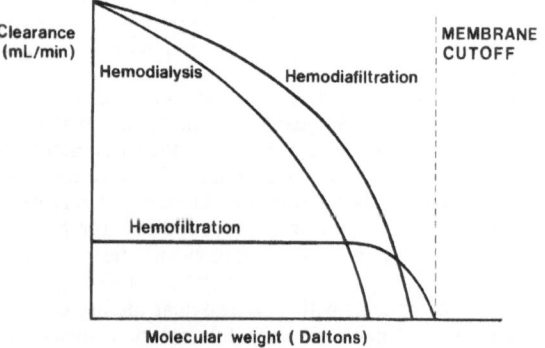

Figure 4. Comparative solute removal rate by hemodialysis, hemofiltration, and hemodiafiltration.

pump creates the negative pressure in the dialysate compartment and carries the ultrafiltrate from the hemofilter through a disposable tubing set to a collection canister. Alternatively, a similar aim can be pursued by imposing a positive pressure in the blood compartment, such as with single needle/cannula dialysis of the pressure-pressure type (see Single Needle/Cannula/Catheter Dialysis below). A negative pressure monitor in the circuit prevents the pressure limits from being exceeded, and the circuit also contains a blood-leak detector that stops the extracorporeal blood flow in the event of a membrane rupture. In a separate circuit, substitution fluid is delivered into the extracorporeal circuit by a separate roller pump. Due to the large volume of fluid exchange during each treatment, an accurate balancing and monitoring system is used that generally is microprocessor operated and that balances the amount of fluid removed from the circuit with that infused. The removal of low-molecular-weight substances such as urea and creatinine with this strategy is less effective than with hemodialysis (Figure 4), due to the lack of diffusion, unless extremely large exchange volumes are pursued. In contrast, however, hemofiltration is considerably more effective in removing substances of the higher molecular weight, due to the larger pore size of the membranes necessary to allow enough plasma water to be carried away. A further advantage is the absence of dialysate, which avoids the entrance into the body of dialysate contaminants such as aluminum, endotoxins, or pyrogens. This is probably one of the reasons for the better hemodynamic stability and clinical tolerance that has been described for hemofiltration during the early days of its application (49). With the current possibilities of producing clean dialysate, this advantage has become less important.

Treatment of chronic renal failure by long-term hemofiltration was first described in 1973 (50). By 1984, statistical returns from the EDTA-ERA Registry (51) showed that 1740 patients representing 2.4% of the European treatment group used this method of treatment, but this incidence had again decreased to 1.8% in 1991 (52). To our knowledge, no records are available for the U.S.A. regarding the number of hemofiltration procedures performed, but the clinical use of hemofiltration has been described by several workers (53,54). The need for special equipment to allow hemofiltration to be performed safely, together with the high cost of replacement fluid (unless the fluid is manufactured on site), has limited the use of this technique to patients with vascular instability episodes or hypertension or hypotension between treatments, as well as to those patients with autonomic insufficiency. In addition, it has also been used successfully in the treatment of acute renal failure (55). If a sufficient number of purification and safety measures are taken, ultrafiltrative losses may be replaced by reabsorption of fluid from the dialysate to the blood side (56) (so-called *on-line reinfusion*); this process results from the subtle interplay between hydrostatic pressures on the blood and dialysate sides and the negative pressure exerted at the exit of the dialyzer by the colloid osmotic effect of increased blood protein concentrations. These measures allow a reduction of cost, but although an optimum quality of fluid entering the bloodstream can be achieved, the substitution fluid delivered can no longer be submitted to the rigid pharmacological quality control that is currently imposed.

One major remaining concern about hemofiltration is related to the fact that essentially larger molecules are removed and that small-molecule removal is disappointing unless huge volumes are ultrafiltered and substituted. Hemofiltration was developed during a period of emphasis on the role of middle-molecule compounds in the pathophysiology of the uremic syndrome. With the later advent of emphasis on small molecular compounds as indicators of adequate solute removal, hemofiltration often turned out to be unsatisfactory. Hemodiafiltration, coupling the principles and the removal characteristics of both conventional hemodialysis and hemofiltration, is more appropriate in this context. A more common use of hemofiltration may be found in its continuous application for intensive care patients (CAVH/CVVH).

HEMODIAFILTRATION

Hemodiafiltration combines the characteristics of conventional hemodialysis with hemofiltration. The combination of the two methods allows an increased clearance rate for both middle and small molecules compared to the use of only one of the two strategies. Low-molecular-weight substances are removed predominantly by diffusion, whereas larger molecules are removed by convection. This strategy may have a beneficial effect, not only on removal of molecules with a higher molecular weight but also on removal of smaller molecules with substantial protein binding: the latter are characterized by a behavior similar to that of larger molecules, their protein binding being a source of resistance to their removal. At least for small protein-bound compounds, such as hippuric acid and indoxyl sulfate, superior removal by hemodiafiltration has been demonstrated compared to conventional hemodialysis (57). In contrast to hemofiltration, during hemodiafiltration only 8–15 L of replacement solution is used, which is infused into the venous return of the extracorporeal circuit. In general, an isotonic saline solution containing lactate as a buffer is used as a substitution fluid.

Acetate-free biofiltration is a specific variant of hemodiafiltration in which dialysate without buffer is used, together with bicarbonate in the postdilution reinfusate (58); the rationale behind this strategy is to pursue hemodynamic stability with dialysate that is not contaminated by germs and/or endotoxins. In paired hemofiltration/hemodialysis, two filters are coupled in series, whereas dry ultrafiltration is performed with one filter and hemodialysis by the other (Figure 5) (59). In general, the net results of this strategy are similar to those of classical hemodiafiltration. One of the advantages, however, could be the easy, con-

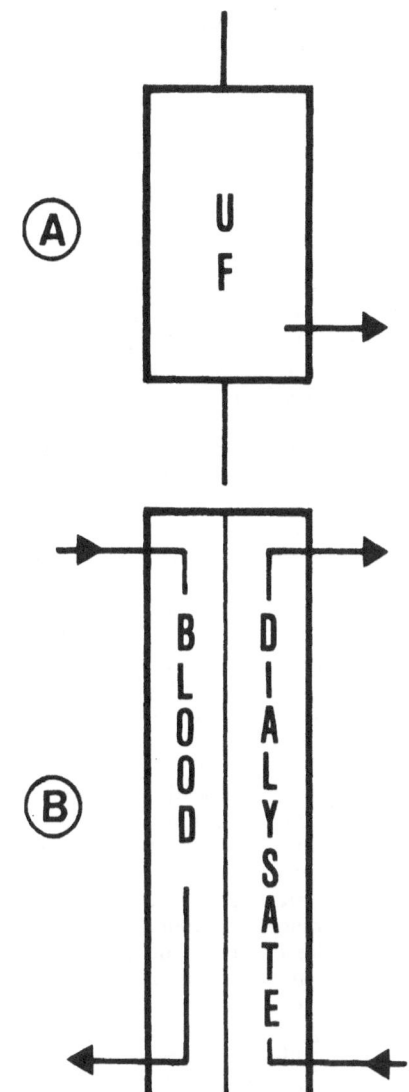

Figure 5. Diagrammatic illustration of the setup for paired filtration–dialysis: the first device (A) is used for dry ultrafiltration (UF), and the second device is used for conventional hemodialysis according to the classical countercurrent principle.

tinuous on-line measurement of concentration of uremic retention solutes, such as urea, in the ultrafiltrate, given the hypothesis that the concentration in the blood and the ultrafiltrate were the same. This measurement necessitates, of course, the availability of adequate sensors to allow continuous kinetic modeling for the estimation of dialysis adequacy.

CONTINUOUS ARTERIOVENOUS HEMOFILTRATION (CAVH)

In continuous arteriovenous hemofiltration, fluid, electrolytes, and small- and middle-molecule-sized solutes are removed from the patient by ultrafiltration for an extended period, ranging from several hours to days. Simultaneously, the blood volume is reconstituted by the administration of a fluid with an electrolyte composition comparable to that of normal plasma, except in the case of fluid overload, where gradual ultrafiltration is pursued. The process of gradual fluid removal allows for much larger quantities of ultrafiltration than an intermittent procedure. The process relies on a small filter containing a highly permeable membrane, and the patient's arterial-to-venous pressure gradient is usually sufficient to provide circulation through the extracorporeal circuit. One of the consequences, of course, is that the ultrafiltered volume and hence overall efficacy are dependent on this pressure gradient, and therefore efficacy is lost in patients with hypotension, shock, and/or severe low-output cardiac failure.

Continuous arteriovenous hemofiltration has seen wide acceptance as a mode of treatment in patients with acute renal failure. CAVH is ideally suited for such patients who are hemodynamically unstable or who have a contraindication for the use of peritoneal dialysis. Patients with multiple organ failure or patients with traumatic injuries and acute renal failure are considered ideal candidates for CAVH, if there are no contraindications for continuous anticoagulation. In the case of bleeding tendency, locoregional heparinization may be a solution, whereby heparin introduced at the inlet of the filter is neutralized at the outlet by proportionate doses of protamine. Only the presence of active bleeding is a contraindication for the use of CAVH, due to the drawbacks of continuous anticoagulation. CAVH may be used advantageously for initial dehydration in the cases of diuretic-resistant cardiac insufficiency. Adult respiratory distress syndrome (ARDS), a complication frequently accompanying acute renal failure, is considered another indication for the application of continuous hemofiltration because oxygenation is improved only when dehydration of the patient is performed simultaneously with PEEP respiration.

Several improvements have been made to enhance the efficacy of this treatment modality. Among those are continuous arteriovenous hemodialysis (CAVHD), in which a dialysate solution is passed at low flow through the dialysate compartment; this strategy allows a better removal of low-molecular-weight compounds, such as urea and potassium (60). Another alternative is continuous venovenous hemofiltration (CVVH), in which both access catheters are positioned intravenously (e.g., femorofemoral), the necessary flow and transmembrane pressure being delivered by a pump system at low flow speeds (61). The advantage of this alternative is that even at low arterial blood pressure, as is frequently seen in intensive care patients, a sufficient blood flow and transmembrane pressure can be obtained. This makes treatment more efficient and prevents clogging of the filter, incidentally reducing the need for frequent replacement of the filter. On the other hand, it should be kept in mind that CAVH originally was developed as a simple means of treating patients and that each pump, detector, or sensor that is added reintroduces some of the complex technicalities of classical hemodialysis.

The major advantage of all continuous techniques remains their slow but continuous capacity to remove water, which allows a much more efficient total volume of ultrafiltration than conventional dialysis techniques.

PLASMA SEPARATION

The separation of plasma from cells may be achieved either by centrifugation or by filtration through membranes (62). There is little difference in the therapeutic effects of plasmafiltration through membranes and cell centrifugation, and the choice of technique is dictated by the facilities available. When plasma separators are used, an extracorporeal circuit comparable to that of hemodialysis or hemofiltration may be used. Plasma separation is used in the treatment of disorders provoked by plasma components such as immunoglobulins, immune complexes,

Table 2. Disease states in which plasmapheresis has been used as a therapeutic modality

Amanita phalloides intoxication
ANCA+ vasculitis
Antiglomerular basement membrane glomerulonephritis
Autoimmune hemophilia
Cryoglobulinemia
Goodpasture's syndrome
Guillain–Barré syndrome
Hemolysis
Hemolytic uremic syndrome
Hepatic failure
Hyperlipidemia
Hyperviscosity syndrome
Incompatible transfusion
Lupus erythematodes disseminatus
Mixed connective tissue disease
Multiple myeloma
Multiple sclerosis
Myasthenia gravis
Overlap syndrome (Goodpasture's/ANCA+ vasculitis)
Paraproteinemia
Periarteritis nodosa (macroscopic)
Periarteritis nodosa (microscopic)
Rheumatoid arthritis
Thrombotic thrombocytopenic purpura
Thyreotoxicosis
Transplant rejection (vascular)
Wegener's granulomatosis

and substances with a strong protein binding, e.g., in rapidly progressive glomerulonephritis, severe lupus erythematodes disseminatus, intoxication with amanita phalloides, or thyreotoxicosis (Table 2). The pathogenic proteins/immune complexes are then eliminated through the large pores of the plasmafilter and are replaced by a solution containing normal proteins (plasma, or solutions containing plasmatic proteins or albumin). A recent advance has been the development of adsorption columns that eliminate from the plasma only specific target molecules, after which the purified plasma can be reinfused without the necessity of replacing wasted plasma by expensive fresh plasma or colloid solutions. At present, these specific adsorption systems are used for the removal of immunoglobulins (e.g., Protein A columns for hypersensitized transplant candidates), cholesterol, or cryoglobulins. A potential advantage of such systems is the decreased risk of infection (hepatitis, HIV) and allergy by obviating the need to administer foreign blood products as a substitution for removed plasma. A drawback is the high cost of the adsorption columns.

HEMOPERFUSION

Direct contact between blood and sorbent systems is pursued in hemoperfusion. Most clinically available sorbent systems use activated carbons (charcoals), ion exchange resins, or nonionic macroporous resins. The sorbents are generally contained within cartridges or columns. Such devices may be used not only in the treatment of uremia but also, and most frequently, in the treatment of drug intoxication and hepatic encephalopathy. Hemoperfusion alone, however, is not sufficient for the control of symptoms or removal of water in uremic subjects, and consequently, composite devices combining a charcoal column with a hemodialyzer have been developed. The original idea for the use of hemoperfusion columns in the treatment of end-stage renal disease (63) has largely been abandoned, perhaps incorrectly, since these columns may remove a large amount of organic acids that are considered today to be potential uremic toxins. Once the causative factors of the uremic syndrome are better known, more specific adsorption systems may be developed in order to enhance the removal of well-defined compounds responsible for specific clinical or biochemical disturbances.

SPECIFIC ASPECTS OF EXTRACORPOREAL THERAPY

Single-needle/cannula/catheter dialysis

As stated earlier, the current access method for extracorporeal therapy is through the use of two needles, cannulas, or catheters to gain access to the patient's circulation and to facilitate the return of blood from the extracorporeal

circuit. Since 1972, it has been possible to perform extracorporeal procedures such as dialysis through the insertion of a single needle, a technique known as *single-needle dialysis* (64). Although vascular access is more often obtained by plastic cannulas or catheters than by real "needles"—the latter terminology suggesting a metallic structure of the access devices—we will use the current term *single-needle dialysis* in the following discussion. This method of access is more comfortable and acceptable for the patient, but even so, it has not become as widespread as might have been expected. The reluctance to adopt this technique routinely may be attributed to a belief that single-needle dialysis is inadequate. This prejudice is based on the poor clinical experience obtained with the older single-needle systems (65), which resulted in low blood flows and high recirculation rates during clinical use. Furthermore, in the past, such a technique of vascular access has been preferentially used in patients with poor fistulae in whom it was not possible to insert two access catheters or needles. Data obtained in groups of patients treated by single-needle techniques operating on a pressure–pressure basis, as first described in 1973 by Van Waeleghem et al. (66), have demonstrated that the adequacy of this type of dialysis when estimated by clearance measurements as well as urea kinetics is similar to conventional two-needle dialysis (67); patient mortality and morbidity were also equivalent to those of the more conventional method. An additional benefit of the single-needle system for patients may be the possibility of achieving ultrafiltration control without the newer proportionating systems (68). This advantage becomes less significant, however, when recent hardware is used, through which ultrafiltration control is currently available even for the two-needle approach.

The single-needle technique may be especially useful in the treatment of acute conditions, such as acute renal failure, fluid overload, or intoxication, in which a single catheter can be inserted intravenously (16), thereby reducing the risk of traumatic complications due to catheter insertion by a factor two. Since puncture of a classical arteriovenous access fistula occurs only once, the risk of damage to the fistula is also reduced; better fistula survivals have been described with the single-needle technique, which may be especially useful in pediatric hemodialysis.

Uremic toxin removal

The uremic syndrome has many characteristics in common with the clinical picture arising from ingestion of exogenous toxins (69). The main difference is that, in the uremic syndrome, a major portion of the responsible toxins are formed in the body itself due to metabolic breakdown of food and other ingested substances. It has long been recognized that the uremic syndrome affects multiple organ systems, particularly neurological, cardiovascular, hematological, and gastrointestinal systems (70). On the other hand, it has also been demonstrated that uremic biological fluids such as serum or ultrafiltrate of serum may affect several biological functions and that these disturbances may be dose related (71). The most important systems in this context are the immunological systems, especially phagocytosis and phagocytic functional capacity (72–75), the production and fragility of red blood cells (76–81), heart cell contractility (82,83), glucose metabolism and the response to insulin (84–86), drug protein binding as well as the protein binding of other (uremic) solutes (87–92), nerve conduction (93), production and degradation of calcitriol (94–96), and hepatic functional capacity (97). It is well recognized that numerous substances are retained during uremia and that many of these are partially removed by extracorporeal therapy; however, the link between the uremic symptoms and the inhibitory effects on biological systems on the one hand and the responsible retained solutes on the other is less clear. Since symptomatic improvement can be obtained by starting dialysis or imposing a protein-restrictive diet, solute retention is unquestionably one of the main causative aspects of the uremic syndrome. Due to our incomplete knowledge about the causative factors, however, our therapeutic measures for reducing solute concentration should be considered to be aspecific and imprecise. The possibility may well exist that a single substance is not toxic in isolation but becomes toxic only when it is mixed with other substances that are retained. One of the major problems in this identification has been the incomplete recognition of metabolites re-

Table 3. Uremic retention solutes classified according to their toxicity

Compounds with no proven or only minor toxicity
  Urea
  Creatinine
  Pseudouridine
  P-OH hippuric acid
  Phenylacetylglutamine
Classical "uremic toxins"
  Myoinositol
  Uric acid
  Organic phosphates
  Peptides
  Parathormone
  Guanidines
  Polyamines
  Phenols
  Indoles
Recently recognized "uremic toxins"
  Xanthine
  Hypoxanthine
  Dimethylarginine
  β_2-microglobulin
  Indoxyl sulfate
  Hippuric acid
  3-carboxy-4-methyl-5-propyl-2-furanpropionic acid (CMPF)
  Organic chloramines

tained, as well as the technical difficulties in isolating substances responsible for biological changes. Until approximately 10 years ago, the most commonly used separation technique was gel chromatography; however, one of its major pitfalls was an incomplete separation of uremic substances, in addition to the presence of sugar and salt in the eluate, which could alter biological functions in in vitro setups (98,99). Recently, HPLC has been used as an alternative separation technique that allows better separation with less chance for the presence of interfering factors (100,101).

In the light of these difficulties relating to the technique of separation and identification, only a restricted list of metabolites have been recognized as having a truly toxic effect (Table 3). One substance that has been classically considered to be a uremic toxin is urea, although most of its side effects are known to occur only at high concentrations rarely seen today in renal failure (102,103). Methylguanidine has also been shown to have adverse effects, principally on nerve function (104,105). Parathormone, oversecreted in the majority of renal failure patients due to an inappropriate homeostatic action of the parathyroids in relation to hypocalcemia, hypovitaminosis D, reduced sensibility to vitamin D, and hyperphosphatemia, interferes with many biological functions (78,80). It should be admitted, however, that with the advent of intensive $1,25\alpha(OH)_2VitD_3$ therapy, the incidence and severity of hyperparathyroidism has been reduced (106). Among the more recently identified uremic toxins, indoxyl sulphate and hippuric acid are known to interfere with drug protein binding (89,90). β_2-microglobulin has been shown to accumulate in uremic patients (107) and has been linked to the development of amyloidosis, which occurs after several years of dialysis therapy (108–110). Several other new uremic metabolites have been added to this list recently, including 3-carboxy-4-methyl-5-propyl-2-furanpropionic acid, the purines xanthine and hypoxanthine, and various peptides (95,111,112).

Metabolites with a wide range of molecular weights are thus retained as a consequence of renal insufficiency and are inadequately removed by replacement renal therapy. A few years ago, there was a tendency to attribute at least part of the uremic toxicity to the retention of so-called *middle molecules*, whose molecular weight lies between 500 and 10,000 daltons (99). A number of investigations were started in an attempt to identify the substances responsible and to define their toxicity. The findings of the resulting studies were conflicting; despite extensive evaluations, only a few distinct substances were isolated (113–115), and the toxicity of these compounds remains a matter of debate. Many of these substances have molecular weights below 500 daltons. It is therefore probable that some molecules behave like middle molecules during dialysis and chromatography, although their molecular weight is lower than would be expected from their intradialytic behavior. The reasons for this specific behavior may be protein binding, electrostatic charge, hydrophobicity, and/or steric configuration, all of which impose additional resistance to the diffusive and convective removal of compounds through dialyzer pores (116). A number of the so-called middle molecular compounds originally identified turned out to be glucuronides of orthohydroxyhippuric acid, a major metabolite of aspirin (117). Consequently, the middle-molecule hypothesis was abandoned when emphasis shifted to the toxicity of smaller molecules; however, it may make a comeback in the near future, given the substantial number of middle-molecule-like substances that accumulate in uremia and behave like middle molecules due to their physical and chemical characteristics (118). In addition, β_2-microglobulin, parathormone, and several peptides are substances in the middle-molecular weight range whose toxicity has been demonstrated (118). The knowledge about the characteristics of these compounds may have important implications for the concept of dialysis treatment, since removal of such compounds may be rather disappointing with conventional hemodialysis.

As a matter of fact, the adequacy of dialysis is today virtually uniquely defined on the basis of the kinetic behavior of small water-soluble compounds such as urea, the latter being a compound with debatable toxicity. Nevertheless, the importance of urea kinetics has been emphasized by the studies of the American National Cooperative Dialysis Study (NCDS), which showed urea to be an adequate parameter of dialysis efficiency and a predictor of dialytic morbidity (119). Urea, however, can only be considered to be an indirect indicator; furthermore, it should be stressed that the data presented in the National Cooperative Study were obtained with hemodialyzers containing cellulose-based (cuprophan) membranes and not with the newer devices that have been recently introduced into clinical practice; the latter contain synthetic membranes that not only are more porous to middle molecules but also offer an improved biocompatibility. If middle molecules and/or middle-molecule-like substances are accepted to exert toxicity—and there is progressively more evidence to support this point (118)—then it can be accepted that the intradialytic behavior of urea is barely representative for these and many other compounds (57). Therefore, there is an urgent need for alternative markers that are more representative for middle molecules and middle-molecule-like substances. Potential candidates today are hippuric accid and β_2-microglobulin. Another problem related to urea kinetic modeling is that most bedside methods are theoretically based on a single-compartment behavior of urea, whereas it is clear that urea follows at least two pool kinetics even during low-flux conventional dialysis. A fortiori, most other retention solutes, which have a less straightforward kinetic behavior than urea, will demonstrate even more complex intradialytic and interdialytic concentration patterns.

It cannot be denied that uremic toxicity is a multifactorial problem, and our knowledge of it, at present, is characterized by multiple flaws and blind spots. Until our knowledge becomes less scanty, an overall solute elimination should be pursued that encompasses as wide a molecular-weight range as possible. The most ideal (but at this moment unattainable) aim is to obtain postdialysis serum profiles in uremia that are comparable to normal serum profiles. In this respect, however, it should be recognized that such an overstressed removal may result in the elimination not only of toxins but also of useful compounds such as trace elements, growth hormones, etc.

Reuse of hemodialyzers

The initial motivation for reuse of hemodialyzers was economics and convenience. Later on, it appeared that an improved biocompatibility may exist for reused dialyzers as compared with new dialyzers (120,121). This better biocompatibility is mainly related to the fixation of blood proteins to the surface of less-biocompatible membranes such as cuprophane—hence attenuating their capacity to activate complement (122)—and to a reduction of severe allergic reactions through a better and more consistent rinsing of dialyzers (120).

The technique of reuse, in which hemodialyzers are used for multiple dialyses of the same patient, may be subdivided into four distinct steps: first the rinsing of the dialyzer at the termination of dialysis, followed by cleaning, then sterilization to allow its storage between uses, and finally the preparation of the dialyzer prior to subsequent use. The technique may be carried out manually or automatically using equipment designed specifically for this purpose. Several different sterilants are available for reuse, and until recently the most popular one was formaldehyde (123). It was frequently used at a 2% concentration, although sterilization may be incomplete under these conditions and contamination by non tuberculous microbacteria has been reported (123). A 4% concentration may be more appropriate, but it will become more difficult to remove the formaldehyde from the dialyzer before dialysis, since remnant concentrations will remain too high even after thorough rinsing. The use of formaldehyde as a sterilant for hemodialyzers poses risks not only to patients but also to staff. Occupational exposure to formaldehyde may be associated with respiratory tract and eye irritation. Prolonged handling of formaldehyde by staff and patients is associated with contact dermatitis and asthma (124–126). A more serious concern is its carcinogenicity or cocarcinogenicity. Animals exposed to atmospheric levels of 6 and 15 ppm over an 18-month period have developed nasal squamous cell carcinomas. A spillage of 1 mL of 37% formalin in a $3 \times 4 \times 7$-meter room will, if the formalin is completely volatile, produce vapors of about 3.6 ppm. An additional potential hazard in patients receiving regular dialysis treatment in which the dialyzer has been exposed to formalin is the increased presence of anti-N-like antibodies (127); this, in turn, may result in hemolytic anemia (128,129). The reduction of formaldehyde concentrations in the venous effluent of the dialyzer to below 3 ppm has been recommended to avoid this problem (128), although in our own experience, target concentrations of below 1 ppm have still resulted in the anti-N-like antibody development (130). Alternative sterilants that may be more suitable than formalin are peracetic acid (131) and glutaraldehyde (132). With glutaraldehyde, the structural degradation of some specific dialyzer membranes was reported, resulting in dialyzer dysfunction not detectable by standard reuse validation procedures (133). Sodium hypochlorite has also been used as a sterilant (134); it breaks down the protein layer on the membrane surface instead of fixing it, so there is no gain in biocompatibility when using this agent (135). Sodium hypochlorite is especially suitable for the reuse of primarily biocompatible synthetic membranes such as polyacrylonitrile (136), since it does not structurally weaken such membranes—in contrast to cellulose-based membranes, where repeated exposure to sodium hypochlorite reduces the membrane strength and leads to blood leak during use.

The issues surrounding reuse of hemodialyzers are complex and involve medical, ethical, social, and financial considerations. At present, few codes of practice exist concerning reuse of devices intended for single use. That such codes are nevertheless needed is illustrated by recent reports of bacteremia and pyrogenic reactions due to failure of alarm systems that should have indicated problems with the reuse procedure (137,138). In spite of intensive quality control and built-in systems to measure parameters related to dialysis efficacy (such as fiber volume), the loss of solute removal capacity may occur and remain unrecognized (133). In general, it can be concluded that, despite a hint of better biocompatibilty, the hazards of reuse remain important and may even outweigh the possible benefits.

Biocompatibility

Biocompatibility may be defined as the absence of a reaction when the body or part of the body is brought in contact with a foreign chemical structure or device (139). Perfect biocompatibility probably does not exist; a certain degree of reactions cannot be avoided in any given condition. Biocompatibility problems have been observed with all types of artificial organs. The biocompatibility of hemodialysis has been extensively studied, since patients receiving this type of therapy are exposed to foreign materials regularly over a period of several years.

The exposure of blood to the membrane contained within the hemodialyzer may be associated with a rapid, transient *fall in white cell count*, activation of the complement system, and a fall in arterial blood oxygenation. The fall in white cell counts occurs during the first hour of treatment. Its duration is short, with the nadir being reached 10–20 minutes after the commencement of treatment. This is followed by a gradual return to pretreatment levels by the end of the first hour. Differential counts performed during the phenomenon indicate that the leukopenia is mainly due to a fall in polymorphonuclear

Table 4. Evolution of total leukocyte counts and leukocyte differentiation during cuprophan hemodialysis ($10^3/mm^3$).[a]

	Before	15 min	60 min	240 min
Total WBC	6.38 ± 1.43	1.36 ± 3.34[b]	5.54 ± 2.01	6.60 ± 2.73
Granulocytes	2.98 ± 0.95	0.19 ± 0.19[b]	3.20 ± 1.80	3.80 ± 2.18
Monocytes	1.05 ± 0.33	0.07 ± 0.06[b]	0.51 ± 0.29[b]	1.08 ± 0.47
Lymphocytes	1.94 ± 0.61	0.96 ± 0.27[b]	1.46 ± 0.60[a]	1.28 ± 0.40[b]

[a] $p < 0.05$ vs. before.
[b] $p < 0.01$.
WBC, white blood cells.

and monocytic phagocytes, whereas the fall in lymphocytes is less pronounced, even if more prolonged (Table 4). *Activation of the complement system* also occurs and may be demonstrated by a fall in indices such as total complement activity of serum (CH 50) or by falls in the concentration of complement components such as C3 and Factor B, although study of these factors, which were developed years ago, often gave rise to contradictory results. A more sensitive illustration of this problem can be obtained by more recently developed test methods such as the determination of concentration of the stable metabolites of the anaphylatoxins C5a and C3a ($C5a_{desArginin}$ and $C3a_{desArginin}$). The concentration of the latter parameters is increased in the presence of activation of the alternate complement pathway.

Also, even more recently, a marked deviation in the concentration of a further element in the alternate complement cascade was demonstrated by the measurement of C5b-9 complex after reaction with plasmatic S-protein (SC5b-9 or terminal complement complex (TCC)), which was suggested to be a sensitive index of biocompatibility (140). Both the fall in leukocyte count and the complement activation preferentially occur during treatment with dialyzers containing cuprophane or cellulose diacetate membranes. This subsequently results in activation of leukocytes, with release in the tissues of free radical species (73). Craddock and coworkers (141,142) demonstrated that this activation was a direct consequence of blood–membrane contact. They based their hypothesis on the fact that polysaccharides, which are similar in structure to cellulose, are capable of activating complement by the alternative pathway, with depletion of both C3a and Factor B. In addition, they showed that after contact between plasma and membrane, the released C5a acts as a granulocyte aggregant that increases the stickiness of the leukocytes and causes them to adhere to the first vascular surface with which they come into contact after passing through the hemodialyzer, namely, the pulmonary capillaries. Patients receiving dialysis treatment with cuprophane experience a fall in arterial oxygen tension (PaO_2), resulting from a fall in lung diffusion capacity (DLCO) (122). This fall occurs over the same time span as leukopenia and ranges between 5% and 25% (Figure 6). The onset of hypoxia is rapid, but unlike leukopenia, it may persist throughout treatment,

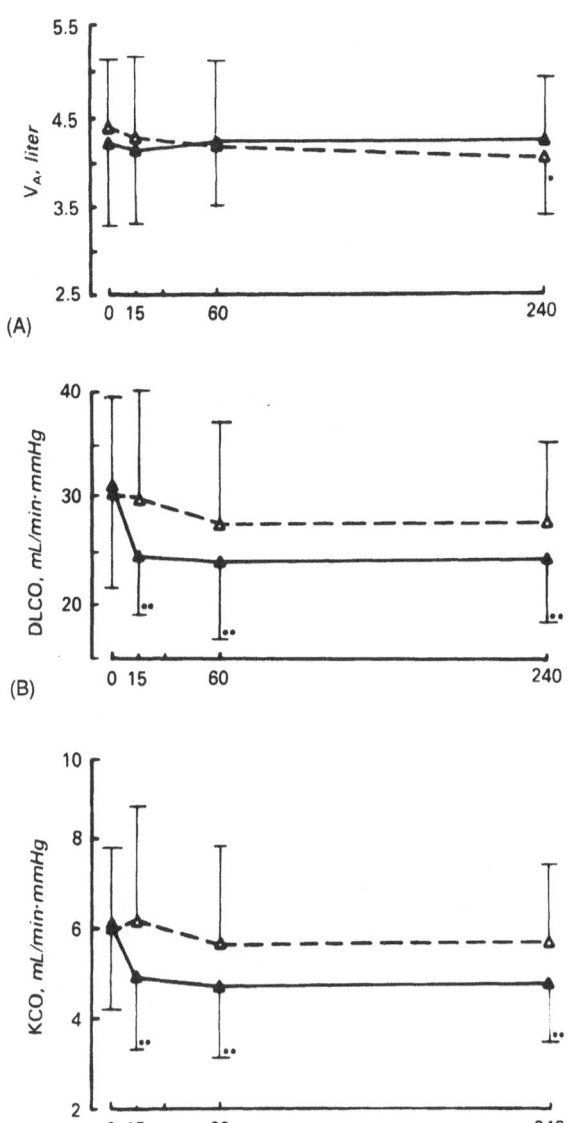

Figure 6. (**A**) Alv vol (V$_A$) (**B**) lung diffusion capacity (DLCO), and (**C**) transfer factor (KCO) before and after 15, 60, and 240 minutes of first-use (full line) and third-reuse (dotted line) cuprophan dialysis. **: $p < 0.01$ vs. predialysis. Both DLCO and KCO curves were significantly different by variance analysis ($p < 0.001$); for V$_A$, no differences were found. Reproduced with permission from Vanholder et al. (122).

with the arterial oxygen tension not returning to predialysis levels until the termination of dialysis (122). All these events might be prevented or at least attenuated when dialysis membranes with a lower complement-activating

capacity are used (43). Craddock et al., in their studies, demonstrated that leukopenia was associated with changes in pulmonary function that manifested as a rise of intrapulmonary arterial pressure and an increase in lymph effluent from the lungs, a consequence of endothelial leakage when plasma incubated with cellophane was injected into animals. Based on their findings, these authors concluded that the most probable sequence of events was complement activation leading to neutrophil aggregation in the lungs, which resulted in impaired oxygen transport across the lungs, leading to hypoxia (142). Several studies revealed a relationship between intradialytic leukopenia and complement activation, on the one hand, and pulmonary function—more precisely, lung diffusion capacity—on the other (43,122). A further change of cardiovascular and pulmonary hemodynamics was also demonstrated after injection of cuprophan-activated serum into swine, and this effect was related to thromboxane release (143). It cannot be denied, however, that other mechanisms may also play a role in the development of intradialytic hypoxia (144,145), such as the loss of CO_2 through the dialyzer, which results from dialysis against acetate-containing dialysate.

On the basis of these differences in the capacity for leukocyte and complement activation, the membranes currently used in hemodialyzers may be divided into two categories: those that are based on cellulose and those that are synthetic copolymers. Leukopenia induced by synthetic membranes is significantly lower than that induced by cellulose membranes, although a new generation of cellulose-based membranes with modified structure has been introduced into clinical use: in such membranes, the magnitude of leukopenia induced is comparable with that induced by synthetic membranes (146,147). In common with the (albeit minor) leukopenia, complement activation is also induced for synthetic membranes when measurements using the recently developed radioimmunoassays for anaphylatoxins C3a and C5a and their desArg derivates are used, but this effect is markedly less pronounced in comparison with cuprophane and cellulose diacetate.

The implications of these phenomena and their long-term consequences on the immune system are far from clear. Leukopenia may be associated with *functional changes in neutrophils* such as chemotaxis, phagocytability, decreased random mobility, and increased adherence. Although phagocytic function is generally depressed in dialysis patients (72), Nguyen et al. demonstrated that baseline (resting-state) phagocytic activity increased during cuprophan dialysis, in contrast to dialysis with polyacrylonitrile membranes (73). However, once this activation has occurred and the phagocytic leukocytes are confronted with an additional bacterial or other challenge, the response is blunted acutely during dialysis with dialyzers that activate basic leukocyte activity. This phenomenon has been corroborated repeatedly in the literature (75,148–150) and culminates after 15 minutes of dialysis, shortly after the bloodstream has been exposed to the external world, at the connection of the dialyzer with the vascular access. The question that then arises is whether the currently observed predialysis depression of phagocytic systems can be attributed to a kind of exhaustion of the phagocytic system due to its repeated intradialytic stimulation. In any case, phagocytic function may be more depressed in dialysed than in nondialysed renal patients (151). Furthermore, Henderson et al. showed that a decrease in phagocytic mobility occurred after contact of white blood cells with cellulose acetate, whereas this reaction remained absent after contact with a more biocompatible membrane (152). Later it was demonstrated by the authors that repeated dialysis with complement-activating cuprophane resulted in a more profound decrease of polymorphonuclear functional capacity than that observed in dialysis with lesser-complement-activating polysulfone, especially during the first weeks after the start of hemodialysis. This finding points to a chronic deleterious effect on immune function by recurrent complement activation (75). Patients treated with dialysis for prolonged time periods, however, showed a gradual but progressive improvement of polymorphonuclear function (153). The factors playing a role in these events remain largely unidentified, but the possibility should be considered that organic chloramines are produced as free radical species, especially during dialysis with complement- activating dialyzers; these organic chloramines may then have a greater longevity and an easier penetrance in the cell membrane than anorganic chloramines, hence increasing their cellular toxicity.

Dialysis may be related to the release and accumulation of another group of important immunoactive humoral compounds, the *cytokines* (154). Cytokine release has been related to the complement-activating nature of the membranes, to their ability to induce, bind, and clear cytokines, to dialysate contamination by pyrogens and endotoxins, and to the use of acetate as a dialysate buffer (155,156). Cytokines are stimulants of immune function, and therefore the finding of their enhanced release may seem in contradiction with the currently found immune depression of dialyzed patients. This apparent contradiction may be related to the simultaneous accumulation of naturally occurring cytokine antagonists in the blood of dialysed patients (157). This issue, however, needs further elucidation.

The clinical implications of repeated complement activation have received little attention. The possibility exists that the difference between synthetic- and cellulose-based membranes may exert an important influence on *cardiovascular function* (143). Studies by Chanard et al. (158) and Kant et al. (159) have demonstrated markedly less intradialytic morbidity when more biocompatible membranes are used. Especially in specific groups of patients, such as the elderly, patients who have experienced hypersensitivity or allergic reactions with cellulose-based membranes, and those with coexisting cardiovascular and pulmonary complications, the use of more biocompatible synthetic membranes in conjunction with bicarbonate-based dialysis appears to be preferable.

A substantial depression of immune function should logically result in a higher *susceptibility for infectious disease*. At this time, however, there are only a few retrospective studies about this issue available; they point to a higher infectious morbidity and mortality of patients treated with cellulosic membranes (without further specification about the nature of the membranes used, i.e., whether these are cuprophane, cellulose diacetate, or other cellulosic membranes) (160,161). Results of more focused and preferentially prospective studies most be awaited before this problem can be clarified definitively.

Recent data point to a slower recovery from acute tubular necrosis in animals and patients treated with dialyzers containing cuprophane membranes (162,163) in comparison to other, more biocompatible membranes; this finding is attributed to the capacity of cuprophan to activate leukocytes and generate free radical species, activated neutrophils being known to be especially deleterious for ischemic kidneys (164). Catabolic effects due to protein breakdown may also be more pronounced during treatment with complement-activating dialyzers (165). *Dialysis-related amyloidosis* becomes essentially manifest after prolonged dialysis treatment and results in the carpal tunnel syndrome and deposition of amyloid loaded cysts in bones and tendons (166). The polymer composing this amyloid is essentially built up by β_2-microglobulin, a compound progressively accumulated during the progress of renal disease and its treatment by dialysis (167). The nature of the dialysis membrane may affect β_2-microglobulin concentration in two ways: 1) removal by diffusion, convection, and/or adsorption may be different from dialyzer to dialyzer, and removal may be reduced to zero in small-pore dialyzers, resulting even in a rise in concentration due to concomitant ultrafiltration of blood water (168)—an effect that is by no means related to the biocompatibility of the dialyzer; and 2) release from leukocytic cells may be influenced by the repeated inflammatory state of dialysis, imposed by membrane incompatibility on the one hand and dialysate contamination by pyrogens and endotoxins on the other, thus stimulating monocytes to releasing more β_2-microglobulin (169). The incidence of dialysis-related amyloidosis was shown by van Ypersele et al. to be attenuated and postponed by dialysis with large-pore AN69 as compared to cuprophane, whereas older age enhanced the chance to develop the disease (170). Whether this beneficial effect of AN69 is related to differences in removal, leukocyte activation, or both has not been demonstrated.

Allergic reactions have also been described, especially when a new brand of dialyzer was started or restarted after temporary withdrawal (first-use syndrome) (171). Some of these allergic events may have a dramatic and even fatal character. In addition to such events, a more protracted, less severe, repeated type of allergic reaction has been described. Clinical manifestations are variable and include nausea, weakness, burning sensation, dyspnea, hypotension, cardiopulmonary arrest, angioedema, flushing, urticaria, rhinorrhea, lacrimation, itching, and abdominal cramps (172,173). The occurrence of these phenomena is more frequent in patients treated with capillary dialyzers that have been gas sterilized with ethylene oxide (172), possibly due to a preferential accumulation of ethylene oxide in the polyurethane potting material used in the housing of the capillary bundle. Ethylene oxide allergy may develop in a substantial fraction of patients routinely subjected to extracorporeal therapy and is characterized by positive radioimmunoabsorbent (RAST) tests (174). Adequate prerinsing or rinsing by using the sterilization procedure of reuse has been demonstrated to attenuate these phenomena. Furthermore, a shift to disposable dialyzers sterilized by alternative methods, such as gamma rays or steam, may have a beneficial influence on the incidence of allergic reactions.

Hakim and colleagues investigated the complement activation in patients with and without first-use syndrome who used cuprophan-containing hemodialyzers (175). These authors demonstrated an association between level of complement activation as measured by C3a and adverse allergic reactions experienced during treatment. Since such allergic reactions may result from other causes as well, their dependence on a single cause is speculative.

Recently, a severe and specific type of allergic reaction was described with respect to the dialysis with AN69 dialyzers of patients treated for hypertension with angiotensin-converting enzyme (ACE) inhibitors (176–177). These reactions are probably induced by an enhanced generation of bradykinin due to blood contact with the highly negative charge of the AN69 dialyzer, combined with a blockade of bradykinin breakdown by ACE inhibition (178).

Dialysate may be a source of biocompatibility problems due to use of acetate buffer, resulting in hypoventilation and hemodynamic changes (37–40,43); the presence of aluminum, resulting in osteomalacia and encephalopathy (179,180); and the transfer of bacterial contaminants such as endotoxins and endotoxin fragments, resulting in cytokine release and a chronic inflammatory state (154,181). Transfer of endotoxins or endotoxin fragments from dialysate to blood may be induced by various factors such as the chemical and geometric composition of the dialyzer membrane and the interplay of hydraulic pressures in relation to the dialysis strategy used (182). The primary cause, however, remains the contamination of the dialysate.

Coagulation

Contact of blood with surfaces other than the vascular wall triggers coagulation. This process is dependent not only upon the chemical characteristics of the contact surface, such as charge and structure, but also on the geometrical structure and shear-generating capacity of the surface or material in contact with the blood (183,184). Extracorporeal therapy may trigger coagulation not only by membrane contact but also by blood contact with components of the extracorporeal circuit. In vitro data on the degree of coagulability due to different materials is conflicting; in vivo results, however, show no clear-cut differences between membranes (185), probably due to the clotting-generating effect of extramembrane factors such as shear stress and contact with tubings. Different polymers have been developed in an attempt to minimize coagulability, and polyurethane is probably one of the polymers used for this purpose. Polyurethane is used in the manufacturing of indwelling catheters. The use of softer materials, such as silicone in large-bore catheters for permanent insertion (Hickman), also is characterized by less capacity to induce clotting events. The incorporation of heparin or other anticoagulants into the polymer structures and other contact surfaces is an appealing alternative to the routine administration of anticoagulants during therapy but is only at the experimental stage at present. Up to now, the commercial availability remains low, probably due to cost and a progressive loss of the anticoagulant from the surface.

During extracorporeal therapy, it is therefore necessary to administer an anticoagulant to prevent clotting in the extracorporeal circuit. Intravenously administered heparin is widely used for this purpose. If the level of anticoagulation is too low, clotting of the circuit can occur, while in excessive anticoagulation there is an increased risk of patient bleeding after therapy. The goal of heparinization is to achieve a uniform, adequate level of anticoagulation, and the dose of heparin required may vary considerably from patient to patient. To overcome these difficulties, kinetic modeling techniques may be used to calculate heparin requirements for an individual patient.

Heparin is an aspecific anticoagulant affecting several coagulation factors other than the necessary prothrombin–thrombin pathway; at the same time, heparin also binds to a number of plasma proteins, such as platelet factor 4 (PF4), which reduces heparin bioavailability at low concentrations (186). Adverse effects such as osteoporosis, liver cell dysfunction, skin reactions, and thrombocytopenia have been described (187). In patients with a risk of complications associated with heparin use, prostacyclin has been proposed as an alternative (188,189). Prostacyclin is expensive for routine use and may cause hemodynamic side effects. Low-molecular-weight heparin is another alternative that has been available for about 10 years (190) and that has gained a progressively more important use. The tendency toward hyperlipidemia and intestinal blood losses would be less important than with regular heparin (191), possibly due to the fact that low-molecular-weight heparin gives rise to a more specific inhibition of the prothrombin–thrombin axis. Hirudin is considered to be another future alternative and has the advantage of being the most specific antithrombin available at present, but its drawbacks are its slow half-life in end-stage renal failure and its lack of an antidote (192). In the case of hirudin anticoagulation, clotting risk can be predicted from the activated clotting time (192).

Leaching of toxic substances

Elution of toxic substances from components of the extra-corporeal circuit is a well-recognized complication of extracorporeal therapy. Substances released during extracorporeal therapy include the spallation of silicone from blood tubings (193); the degree of spallation has been shown to correlate with duration of dialysis, with the weight of the reticuloendothelial system organs at autopsy, and with functional liver disturbances (194). The intravenous injection of silicone into rats caused an increase in prostaglandin E_2 and thromboxane release from the spleen into the blood (195). The magnitude of spallation may be modified by careful attention to the occlusion pressure of the peristaltic blood pumps used in extracorporeal circulation (196–198). Other materials that have been shown to be released from extracorporeal circuits include the plasticizers, which are used for softening tubings and fluid bags so as to allow blood propulsation by roller pumps and maintenance of vacuum during the substitution fluid administration. The most commonly used plasticizer is di(-2-ethylhexyl)-phthalate (DEHP), which may represent up to 40% of the dry weight of polyvinylchloride (PVC). DEHP is released during extracorporeal therapy and may accumulate in the body and cause liver damage (199). Ethylene oxide is commonly used for sterilization of devices and may slowly release into the blood, especially after inadequate rinsing of the extracorporeal circuit (200).

WHEN TO START TREATMENT?

The most appropriate moment to start renal replacement therapy depends upon the indication and the treatment modality.

In acute renal failure, especially when the established phase has been reached, hemodialysis or related techniques should be started early; a serum BUN of 1 g/L or more is currently accepted as the lower limit at which to commence treatment (201). Exceptions to this rule are patients with overt prerenal failure where renal function may recover after rehydration (especially in the case of reversible forward failure such as follows cardiac or cardiovascular surgery) and patients with gastrointestinal bleeding. The rule to maintain a low serum urea in acute renal failure (especially in relation to ischemia and sepsis) is related to the fact that the concentration of serum urea is increased in relation to not only renal failure but also catabolic conditions, whereby an extra load of toxins due to protein breakdown may be released into the bloodstream. Sudden and important shifts in urea concentration may enhance the risk of gastrointestinal bleeding.

Dialysis should be started even earlier in the case of total anuria, fluid overload, hyperkalemia, and/or acidosis.

Hemodialysis for chronic renal failure without complications is generally started at a creatinine clearance of 5 mL/min (202), although some groups start earlier (203); in the latter studies, survival is noted to be better with an early start of dialysis, although some of the results leading to this conclusion may be affected by methodological bias. Dialysis should be started earlier in diabetic patients or in those suffering from severe hypertension, and here a 10-mL/min glomerular filtration rate may be considered the minimum at which to initiate therapy (202). It should be stressed that if hemodialysis is planned in diabetics, fistula creation should be started early, e.g., at a glomerular filtration rate of 18–20 mL/min or a creatinine level of 4 mg/100 mL due to the risk of fistula thrombosis and other fistula problems in this group of patients. In our department, we start dialysis at a clearance of 15 mL/min for diabetics and 10 mL/min for hypertensives, fistula creation being planned a little earlier. Plasma separation or plasmapheresis remains a controversial issue in many respects and should only be used in life-threatening situations, if its benefit is proven (204,205).

WHICH TREATMENT MODALITY?

The wide range of therapies currently available makes it difficult to reach a consensus regarding specific advantages and disadvantages.

Conventional dialysis with acetate has lost its attraction during recent years and is being replaced more and more by bicarbonate-based dialysis, which may be considered as the method of choice especially for acute renal failure patients, as well as for those with cardiovascular instability and for the older age group. However, a particular drawback of bicarbonate dialysate is its higher risk of bacterial contamination, with transfer of pyrogens and cytokine inducing substances into the bloodstream. This situation can only be avoided through the use of pyrogen-free water (reverse osmosis) and sterile, pyrogen-free concentrate (based on pharmacological purity rules) for the preparation of dialysate.

The question of whether one should use a more biocompatible membrane remains partially unanswered at present. Especially jeopardized in this context are acute renal failure patients, the elderly, patients with cardiovascular and pulmonary dysfunction, patients in whom dialysis is planned for a prolonged period of years, and patients with sepsis or at risk for infectious disease. Sequential ultrafiltration and dialysis may be useful for patients with a high interdialytic weight gain, especially those that are hemodynamically labile, but the introduction of bicarbonate dialysate and better proportionating systems for ultrafiltration control has made this option less necessary. Hemofiltration or hemodiafiltration may also be of help in patients with problematic hemodynamics, although the availability of bicarbonate or a variable sodium during dialysis may also resolve these problems. The use of hemodiafiltration may turn out to be superior due to a better elimination of uremic toxins such as organic acids and protein-bound compounds, as well as preferential use of more biocompatible dialysis membranes in this strategy. Continuous arteriovenous hemofiltration (CAVH) is a technique that may be useful for acute renal failure patients, especially hemodynamically labile patients and those with a severe fluid overload that cannot be removed easily through intermittent dialytic treatment.

Accepted indications for the use of plasma separation include Goodpasture's syndrome, rapidly progressive glomerulonephritis, hyperviscosity syndrome, thyrotoxic crisis, thrombotic thrombocytopenic purpura, intoxication with digitalis or amanita phalloides, and Guillain–Barré syndrome (204,205). For other kidney-related diseases such as lupus erythematodes disseminatus or ANCA+ vasculitis, other treatments such as enforced immune suppression must be considered first and maintained even after the start of plasma separation.

The use of hemoperfusion may be useful in the treatment of severely drug-intoxicated patients, and still remains an underrated alternative means to add toxin elimination to the classical diffusive process of conventional hemodialysis.

CONCLUSIONS

The spectrum of available therapeutic modalities for the treatment of acute and chronic end-stage renal failure is changing continuously. Whereas originally only diffusive hemodialysis was offered, with time several other alternatives such as hemofiltration, hemodiafiltration, and hemoperfusion have become available. Traditionally, these modalities are offered on an intermittent schedule, but recently, the possibility of pursuing such strategies on a continuous basis has also been offered, especially in the gravely ill intensive care patient.

Although the ideal to be pursued is continuous treatment, through which blood and tissue concentrations mimic those found in the healthy population, the application of this option is certainly hampered by the difficulty of maintaining adequate vascular access for prolonged periods of time in ambulatory patients. Consequently, the mainstay of treatment in this population is still intermittent, which partially reduces solute elimination.

Unfortunately, the main purpose of dialysis has so far been the elimination of water-soluble compounds, whereas efficiency estimations continue to be based on the removal pattern of urea, a water-soluble and barely toxic compound. More attention should be paid to the concentration and elimination pattern of a number of larger, protein-bound and/or hydrophobic compounds, among which a number of true uremic toxins can be found.

REFERENCES

1. Hegstrom RM, Quinton WE, Dillard DH, Cole JJ, Scribner BH: One year's experience with the use of indwelling teflon cannulas and bypass. *Trans Am Soc Artif Intern Organs* 7:47, 1961.
2. Shaldon S, Chiandussi L, Higgs B: Haemodialysis by percutaneous catheterisation of the femoral artery and vein with regional heparinisation. *Lancet* 2:857, 1961.
3. Shaldon S, Rae AI, Rosen SM, Silva H, Oakley J: Refrigerated femoral venous–venous haemodialysis with coil preservation for rehabilitation of terminal uraemic patients. *Lancet* 1:1716, 1963.
4. Fuchs HJ, Jenett G, Klehr V, Richter G, Wilbrandt R, Frotscher U: Die perkutane Punktion der Vena Femoralis zur Hamodialysebehandlung. *Dtsch Med Wochenschr* 102:1280, 1977.
5. Bambauer R, Jutzler GA: Jugularis-Interna-Punktion zur Shaldon-Ka theterisierung. Ein neuer Zugang fur akute Hämodialysen. *Nieren Hoch druckkrankheiten* 3:109, 1980.
6. Uldall PR, Dyck RF, Woods F, Merchant N, Martin GS, Cardella CJ, Sutton D, Deveber GA: A subclavian cannula for temporary vascular access for hemodialysis or plasmapheresis. *Dial Transplant* 8:963, 1979.
7. De Cubber A, De Wolf C, Lameire N, Schurgers M, Ringoir S: Single needle hemodialysis with the double headpump via the subclavian vein. *Dial Transplant* 7:1261, 1978.
8. Vanholder R, Lameire N, Verbanck J, Van Rattinghe R, Kunnen H, Ringoir S: Complications of subclavian hemodialysis: a 5 year prospective study in 257 consecutive patients. *Int J Artif Organs* 5:297, 1982.
9. Vanholder R, Hoenich N, Ringoir S: Morbidity and mortality of central venous catheter hemodialysis: a review of 10 years' experience. *Nephron* 47:274, 1987.
10. Fine A, Churchill D, Gault H, Mathieson G: Fatality due to subclavian dialysis catheter. *Nephron* 29:99, 1981.
11. Merrill RH, Raab SO: Dialysis catheter-induced pericardial tamponade. *Arch Intern Med* 142:1751, 1982.
12. Barton BR, Hermann G, Weill R: Cardiothoracic emergencies associated with subclavian hemodialysis catheters. *JAMA* 250:2660, 1983.
13. Vaziri ND, Maksy M, Lewis M, Martin D, Edwards K: Massive mediastinal hematoma caused by a double-lumen subclavian catheter. *Artif Organs* 8:223, 1984.
14. Ducatman BS, Mac Michan JC, Edwards MD: Catheter-induced lesions of the right side of the heart. A one year prospective study of 141 autopsies. *JAMA* 253:791, 1985.
15. Ratcliffe PJ, Oliver DO: Massive thrombosis around subclavian cannulas used for hemodialysis. *Lancet* 1:1472, 1982.
16. Cheung AK, Gregory MC: Subclavian vein thrombosis in hemodialysis patients. *Trans Am Soc Artif Intern Organs* 31:131, 1985.
17. Vanherweghem JL, Yassine T, Goldman M, Vandenbosch G, Delcour C, Struyven J, Kinnaert P: Subclavian vein thrombosis: a frequent complication of subclavian vein cannulation for hemodialysis. *Clin Nephrol* 26:235, 1986.
18. Spinowitz BS, Galler MG, Golden RA, Rascoff JH, Schechter L, Held B, Charytan C: Subclavian vein stenosis as a complication of subclavian catheterization for hemodialysis. *Arch Intern Med* 147:305, 1987.
19. Schwab SJ, Quarles D, Middleton JP, Cohan RH, Saeed M, Dennis V: Hemodialysis-associated subclavian vein stenosis. *Kidney Int* 33:1156, 1988.

20. De Moor B, Vanholder R, Ringoir S: Subclavian vein hemodialysis catheters: advantages and disadvantages. *Artif Organs* 18:293, 1994.

21. Uldall PR, Joy C, Merchant N: Further experience with double lumen subclavian cannula for hemodialysis. *Trans Am Soc Artif Intern Organs* 28:71, 1982.

22. Brescia MJ, Cimino JE, Appel K, Hurwich BJ: Chronic hemodialysls using venipuncture and a surgically created arteriovenous fistula. *N Engl J Med* 275:1089, 1966.

23. Tellis VA, Kohnberg WJ, Bhat DJ, Driscoll B, Veith FJ: Expanded polytetrafluoroethylene graft fistula for chronic hemodialysis. *Ann Surg* 189:101, 1979.

24. Knutson R, Wathen R, Comty CM, Shapiro FL: Bovine carotid artery grafts as blood access devices. *Proc EDTA* 10:229, 1973.

25. Zerbino VR, Tice DA: Successful use of preserved allograft vein for chronic hemodialysis. *Nephron* 10:61, 1973.

26. Mahan JD, Mauer SM, Nevins TE: The Hickman catheter: a new hemodialysis access device for infants and small children. *Kidney Int* 24:694, 1983.

27. De Meester J, Vanholder R, De Roose J, Ringoir S: Catheter and technique survival with permanent single-lumen dialysis catheters. *Nephrol Dial Transplant* 9:478, 1994.

28. Garred LJ, St Amour N, McCready W, Canaud B: Urea Kinetic modeling with a prototype urea sensor in the spent dialysate stream. *Abstracts of the 1993 ASAIO Meeting*, p 80 1993.

29. Ebben JP, Hirsch DN, Luehmann DA, Collins AJ, Keshaviah PR: Microbiologic contamination of liquid bicarbonate concentrate for hemodialysis. *Trans Am Soc Artif Intern Organs* 33:269, 1987.

30. Laude-Sharp M, Caroff M, Simard L, Pusineri C, Kazatchkine MD, Haeffner-Cavaillon N: Induction of IL-1 during hemodialysis: transmembrane passage of intact endotoxins (LPS). *Kidney Int* 38:1089, 1990.

31. Bolon G, Reingold AL, Carson LA, Solcox VA, Woodley CL, Hayes PS, Hightower AW, McFarland L, Brown JW, Petersen NJ, Favero MS, Good RC, Broome CV: Infections with Mycobacterium chelonei in patients receiving dialysis and using processed hemodialyzers. *J Infect Dis* 152:1013, 1985.

32. Gordon SM, Tipple M, Jarvis WR: Pyrogenic reactions associated with the reuse of disposable hollow-fiber hemodialyzers. *JAMA* 260:2077, 1988.

33. Bommer J, Ritz E: Water quality—a neglected problem in hemodialysis. *Nephron* 46:1, 1987.

34. Wehle B, Asaba H, Castenfors J, Fürst P, Grahn A, Gunnarson B, Shaldon S, Bergström J: The influence of dialysis fluid composition on the blood pressure response during dialysis. *Clin Nephrol* 10:62, 1978.

35. Veech RL: The untoward effects of the anions of dialysis fluids. *Kidney Int* 34:587, 1988.

36. Mion CM, Hegstrom RM, Boen ST, Scribner BH: Substitution of sodium acetate for sodium bicarbonate in the bath fluid for hemodialysis. *Trans Am Soc Artif Intern Organs* 10:110, 1964.

37. Graefe U, Milutinovich J, Follette WC, Vizzo JE, Babb AL, Scribner BH: Less dialysis-induced morbidity and vascular instability with bicarbonate in dialysate. *Ann Intern Med* 88:332, 1978.

38. Aizawa Y, Ohmori T, Imai K, Nara Y, Matsuoka M, Hirasawa Y: Depressant action of acetate upon the human cardiovascular system. *Clin Nephrol* 8:477, 1977.

39. Leenen FHH, Buda AJ, Smith DL, Farrel S, Levine DZ, Uldall PR: Hemodynamic changes during acetate and bicarbonate hemodialysis. *Artif Organs* 8:411, 1984.

40. Borges HF, Fryd DS, Rosa AA, Kjellstrand CM: Hypotension during acetate and bicarbonate dialysis in patients with acute renal failure. *Am J Nephrol* 1:24, 1981.

41. Vanholder R, Piron M, Ringoir S: Absence of a beneficial hemodynamic effect of bicarbonate versus acetate haemodialysis. *Proc EDTA-ERA* 21:195, 1984.

42. Dolan MJ, Whipp BJ, Davidson WD, Weitzman RE, Wasserman K: Hypopnea associated with acetate hemodialysis: carbondioxide flow-dependent ventilation. *N Engl J Med* 305:72, 1981.

43. De Backer WA, Verpooten GA, Borgonjon DJ, Vermeire PA, Lins RR, De Broe ME: Hypoxemia during hemodialysis: effects of different membranes and dialysate compositions. *Kidney Int* 23:738, 1983.

44. De Backer WA, Heyrman RM, Wittesaele WM, Van Waeleghem JP, Vermeire PA, De Broe ME: Ventilation and breathing patterns during hemodialysis-induced carbon dioxide unloading. *Am Rev Respir Dis* 136:406, 1987.

45. Novello AC, Kjellstrand CM: Is bicarbonate dialysis better than acetate dialysis. *ASAIO J* 6:103, 1983.

46. Morin RJ, Srikantaiah MV, Woodley Z, Davidson WD: Effect of hemodialysis with acetate vs. bicarbonate on plasma lipid and lipoprotein levels in uremic patients. *J Dial* 4:9, 1980.

47. Bergström J, Asaba H, Fürst P, Oules R: Dialysis, ultrafiltration and blood pressure. *Proc EDTA* 13:293, 1976.

48. Pallone TL, Petersen J: Continuous arteriovenous hemofiltration: an in vitro simulation and mathematical model. *Kidney Int* 33:685, 1988.

49. Baldamus CA, Pollok M: Ultrafiltration and hemofiltration: practical applications. In: JF Maher, ed, *Replacement of Renal Function by Dialysis*. Kluwer Academic Publishers, Dordrecht, pp 327–346, 1989.

50. Henderson LW, Livoti LG, Ford CA, Kelly AB, Lysaght MJ: Clinical experience with intermittent hemofiltration. *Trans Am Soc Artif Intern Organs* 19:119, 1973.

51. Brunner FP, Broyer M, Brynger H, Challah S, Fassbinder W, Oules R, Rizzoni G, Selwood NH, Wing AJ: Combined report on regular dialysis and transplantation in Europe, XV, 1984. *Proc EDTA* 22:5, 1985.

52. Raine AEG, Margreiter R, Brunner FP, Ehrich JHH, Geerlings W, Landais P, Loirat C, Mallick NP, Selwood NH, Tufveson G, Valderrabano F: Report on management of renal failure in Europe, XXII, 1991. *Nephrol Dial Transplant* 2:7, 1992.

53. Bosch JP, Lauer A, Glabman S: Mortality and morbidity associated with hemofiltration. *ASAIO J* 8:28, 1985.

54. Collins AJ, Keshaviah P, Ilstrup KM, Shapiro F: Clinical comparison of hemodialysis and hemofiltration. *Kidney Int* 28:S18, 1985.

55. Hakim M, Wheeldon D, Bethune DW, Milstein BB, English TAH, Wallwork J: Haemodialysis and haemofiltration on cardiopulmonary bypass. *Thorax* 40:101, 1985.

56. Canaud B, Nguyen QV, Argiles A, Polito C, Polaschegg HD, Mion C: Hemodiafiltration using dialysate as substitution fluid. *Artif Organs* 11:188, 1987.

57. Vanholder RC, De Smet RV, Ringoir SM: Assessment of urea and other uremic markers for quantification of dialysis efficacy. *Clin Chem* 38:1429, 1992.

58. Albertazzi A, Palmieri PF, Mastrangelo E: Efficacy and tol-

erance of acetate free biofiltration: a central Italian multicenter study. *Kidney Int* 43:S188, 1993.

59. Botella J, Ghezzi P, Sanz-Moreno C, Milan M, Conz P, La Greca G, Ronco C: Multicentric study on paired filtration dialysis as a short, highly efficient dialysis technique. *Nephrol Dial Transplant* 6:715,1991.

60. Sigler MH, Teehan BP: Solute transport in continuous hemodialysis: a new treatment for acute renal failure. *Kidney Int* 32:562, 1987.

61. Tam PYW, Huraib S, Mahan B, LeBlanc D, Lunski CA, Holtzer C, Doyle CE, Vas SI, Uldall PR: Slow continuous hemodialysis for the management of complicated acute renal failure in an intensive care unit. *Clin Nephrol* 30:79, 1988.

62. Kambic HE, Nosé Y: Plasmapheresis: historical perspective, therapeutic applications, and new frontiers. *Artif Organs* 17:850, 1993.

63. Yatzidis H, Yulis G, Digenis P: Hemocarboperfusion–hemodialysis treatment in terminal renal failure. *Kidney Int* 10:S312, 1976.

64. Kopp KF, Gutch CF, Kolff WJ: Single needle dialysis. *Trans Am Soc Artif Intern Organs* 18:75 1972.

65. Beretta-Piccoli C, Golder S, Weidmann P, Descoeudres C: Einnadelhämodialyse. *Schweiz Med Wochenschr* 105:289, 1975.

66. Van Waeleghem JP, Boone L, Ringoir S: New technique on the one needle system during haemodialysis. *Eur Dial Transplant Nurses Assoc* 1:10, 1973.

67. Vanholder R, Hoenich NA, Ringoir S: Adequacy studies of fistula single needle dialysis. *Am J Kidney Dis* 10:417, 1987.

68. Vanholder R, Hoenich N, Piron M, Billiouw JM, Ringoir S: Haemodialysis in a single and a two needle vascular access system: a comparative study. *Proc EDTA* 20:176, 1983.

69. Knochel JP: Pathogenesis of the uremic syndrome. *Postgrad Med* 64:88, 1978.

70. Teschan PE: The presentation of the patient with chronic renal failure. In: WJ Stone, PL Rabin, eds, *End Stage Renal Disease*. Academic Press, New York, pp 31–56, 1983.

71. Vanholder R, Schoots A, Ringoir S: Uraemic toxicity. In: JF Maher, ed, *Replacement of Renal Function by Dialysis*. Kluwer Academic, Dordrecht, pp 4–19, 1989.

72. Ritchey EE, Wallin JD, Sham SV: Chemiluminescence and superoxide anion production by leucocytes from chronic hemodialysis patients. *Kidney Int* 19:349, 1981.

73. Nguyen AT, Lethias C, Zingraff J, Herbelin A, Naret C, Descamps-Latscha B: Hemodialysis membrane-induced activation of phagocyte oxidative metabolism detected in vivo and in vitro within microamounts of whole blood. *Kidney Int* 28:158, 1985.

74. Ringoir S, Van Looy L, Van de Heyning P, Leroux-Roels G: Impairment of phagocytic activity of macrophages as studied by the skin window test in patients on regular hemodialysis treatment. *Clin Nephrol* 4:234, 1975.

75. Vanholder R, Ringoir S, Dhondt A, Hakim R: Phagocytosis in uremic and hemodialysis patients: a prospective and cross sectional study. *Kidney Int* 39:320, 1991.

76. Ota K, Sanaka T, Agishi T, Nakajima O: Influence of uremic middle molecules on blood cells. *Artif Organs* 4:113, 1980.

77. Wallner SF, Vautrin RM: The anemia of chronic renal failure: studies of the effect of organic solvent extraction of serum. *J Lab Clin Med* 92:363, 1978.

78. Meytes D, Bogin E, Ma A, Dukes PP, Massry SG: Effect of parathyroid hormone on erythropoiesis. *J Clin Invest* 67:1263, 1981.

79. Delwiche F, Segal GM, Eschbach JW, Adamson JW: Hematopoietic inhibitors in chronic renal failure: lack of in vitro specifity. *Kidney Int* 29:641, 1986.

80. Bogin E, Massry SG, Levi J, Djaldetti M, Bristol G, Smith J: Effect of parathyroid hormone on osmotic fragility of human erythrocytes. *J Clin Invest* 69:1017, 1982.

81. Malachi T, Bogin E, Gafter U, Levi J: Parathyroid hormone effect on the fragility of human young and old red blood cells in uremia. *Nephron* 42:52, 1986.

82. Bogin E, Massry SG, Harary I: Effect of parathyroid hormone on rat heart cells. *J Clin Invest* 67:1215, 1981.

83. Mann JFE, Jakobs KH, Riedel J, Ritz E: Reduced chronotropic responsiveness of the heart in experimental uremia. *Am J Physiol* 250 (*Heart Circ Physiol* 19): H846, 1986.

84. Defronzo RA, Smith D, Alvestrand A: Insulin action in uremia. *Kidney Int* 24:S102, 1983.

85. Dzurik R, Spustova V, Gerykova M: Pathogenesis and consequences of the alteration of glucose metabolism in renal insufficiency. In: S Massry, R Vanholder, S Ringoir, eds, *Uremic Toxins*. Plenum Press, New York, pp 105–109, 1987.

86. Lockwood DH, Hayes GR, MacCaleb ML: The insulin-resistance inducing factor associated with uremia. In: S Massry, R Vanholder, S Ringoir, eds, *Uremic Toxins*. Plenum Press, New York, pp 97–104, 1987.

87. Reidenberg MM, Odar-Cederlof I, Van Bahr C, Borga O, Sjoqvist F: Protein binding of diphenylhydantoin and desmethylimipramine in plasma from patients with poor renal function. *N Engl J Med* 285:264, 1971.

88. Depner TA, Gulyassy PF: Plasma protein binding in uremia: extraction and characterisation of an inhibitor. *Kidney Int* 18:86, 1980.

89. Gulyassy PF, Bottini AT, Stanfel LA, Jarrard EA, Depner TA: Isolation and chemical identification of inhibitors of plasma ligand binding. *Kidney Int* 30:391, 1986.

90. Mac Namara PJ, Lalka D, Gibaldi M: Endogenous accumulation products and serum protein binding in uremia. *J Lab Clin Med* 98:730, 1981.

91. Vanholder R, Van Landschoot N, De Smet R, Schoots A, Ringoir S: Drug protein binding in chronic renal failure: evaluation of nine drugs. *Kidney Int* 33:906, 1988.

92. Vanholder R, Hoefliger N, De Smet R, Ringoir S: Extraction of protein bound ligands from azotemic sera: comparison of 12 deproteinization methods. *Kidney Int* 41:1707, 1992.

93. Funck-Brentano JL, Boudet J, Sausse A, Cueille G, Man NK: In vitro sural nerve test for the evaluation of middle molecule neurotoxicity in uraemia. In: TH Frost, ed, *Technical Aspects of Renal Dialysis*. Pitman Medical, Tunbridge Wells, U.K., pp 256–263, 1978.

94. Hsu CH, Vanholder R, Patel S, De Smet R, Sandra P, Ringoir SMG: Subfractions of uremic plasma ultrafiltrate inhibit calcitriol metabolism. *Kidney Int* 40:868, 1991.

95. Hsu CH, Patel SR, Young EW, Vanholder R: Effects of purine derivatives on calcitriol metabolism in rats. *Am J Physiol* 260:F596, 1991.

96. Hsu CH, Patel SR, Vanholder R: Mechanism of decreased intestinal calcitriol receptor concentration in renal failure. *Am J Physiol* 264:F662, 1993.

97. Abreo K, Sella M, De Smet R, Vogeleere P, Ringoir S: Uremic extracts enhance the uptake and toxicity of aluminum (A1) in cultured mouse hepatocytes (abstract). *J Am Soc Nephrol* 4:763, 1993.

98. Schoots AC, Mikkers FEP, Claessens HA, De Smet R, Van Landschoot N, Ringoir S: Characterization of uremic "middle molecular" fractions by gas chromatography, mass spectrometry, isotachophoresis and liquid chromatography. *Clin Chem* 28:45, 1982.

99. Schoots A, Mikkers F, Cramers C, De Smet R, Ringoir S: Uremic toxins and the elusive middle molecules. *Nephron* 38:1, 1984.

100. Schoots AC, Homan HR, Gladdines MM, Cramers C, De Smet R, Ringoir S: Screening of UV-absorbing solutes in uremic serum by reversed phase HPLC—change of blood levels in different therapies. *Clin Chim Acta* 146:37, 1985.

101. Schoots A, Vanholder R, De Smet R, Cramers C, Ringoir S: Hippurate and an unknown compound as indicators of residual renal function in dialysed patients. In: LC Smeby, S Jorstad, TE Wideroe, eds, *Immune and Metabolic Aspects of Therapeutic Blood Purification Systems.* Karger, Basel, pp 240–245, 1986.

102. Sargent JA, Gotch FA: Mathematic modeling of dialysis therapy. *Kidney Int* 18:2, 1980.

103. Scheuer J, Stezoski SW: The effects of uremic compounds on cardiac funtion and metabolism. *J Mol Cell Cardiol* 5:287, 1973.

104. Giovannetti S, Balestri PL, Barsotti G: Methylguanidine in uremia. *Arch Intern Med* 131:709, 1973.

105. Giovannetti S, Barsotti G: Uremic intoxication. *Nephron* 14:123, 1975.

106. Nordal KP, Dahl E: Low dose calcitriol versus placebo in patients with predialysis chronic renal failure. *J Clin Endocrinol Metab* 5:929, 1988.

107. Vincent C, Revillard JP, Galland M, Traeger J: Serum beta 2-microglobulin in hemodialyzed patients. *Nephron* 21:260, 1978.

108. Shirahama T, Skinner M, Cohen AS, Gejyo F, Arakawa M, Suzuki M, Hirasawa Y: Histochemical and immunohistochemical characterization of amyloid associated with chronic hemodialysis as beta 2-microglobulin. *Lab Invest* 53:705, 1985.

109. Gejyo F, Odani S, Yamada T, Honma N, Saito H, Suzuki Y, Nakagawa U, Kobayashi H, Maruyama Y, Hirasawa Y, Suzuki M, Arakawa M: Beta 2-microglobulin: a new form of amyloid protein associated with chronic hemodialysis. *Kidney Int* 30:385, 1986.

110. Vandenbroucke JM, Jadoul M, Maldague B, Huaux JP, Noel H, van Ypersele de Strihou C: Possible role of dialysis membrane characteristics in amyloid osteo-arthropathy. *Lancet* 1:1210, 1986.

111. Niwa T, Yazawa T, Kodama T, Uehara Y, Maeda K, Yamada K: Efficient removal of albumin-bound furancarboxylic acid, an inhibitor of erythropoiesis, by continuous ambulatory peritoneal dialysis. *Nephron* 56:241, 1990.

112. Niwa T, Fujishiro T, Uema K, Tsuzuki T, Tominaga Y, Emoto Y, Miyazaki T, Maeda K: Effect of hemodialysis on plasma levels of vasoactive peptides: endothelin, calcitonin-gene related peptide and human atrial natriuretic peptide. *Nephron* 64:552, 1993.

113. Zimmerman L, Fürst P, Bergström J, Jornvall H: A new glycine containing compound with a blocked amino group from uremic body fluids. *Clin Nephrol* 14:109, 1980.

114. Cueille G: Mise en évidence et évaluation des "moyennes molecules" de la taille de la vitamine B12 présents dans les liquides biologiques de sujets normaux et de patients urémiques. *J Chromatogr* 146:55, 1978.

115. Cueille G, Man NK, Farges JP, Funck-Brentano JL: Characterization of sub-peak b4.2 middle molecule. *Artif Organs* 4:28, 1980.

116. Vanholder R, Ringoir S: Adequacy of dialysis: a critical analysis. *Kidney Int* 42:540, 1992.

117. Asaba H, Zimmerman L, Bergström J: On drug artifacts in middle molecule analysis. *Nephron* 39:73, 1985.

118. Vanholder R, De Smet R, Hsu C, Vogeleere P, Ringoir S: Uremic toxicity: the middle molecule hypothesis revisited. *Semin Nephrol*, in press.

119. Lowrie EG, Laird NM, Parker TF, Sargent JA: Effect of the hemodialysis prescription on patient morbidity. *New Engl J Med* 305:1176, 1980.

120. Vanholder R, Ringoir S: Influence of reuse and of reuse sterilants on the first-use syndrome. *Artif Organs* 11:137, 1987.

121. Vanholder R: Biocompatibility issues in hemodialysis. *Clin Materials* 10:87, 1992.

122. Vanholder RC, Pauwels RA, Vandenbogaerde JF, Lamont HH, Van Der Straeten ME, Ringoir SM: Cuprophan reuse and intradialytic changes of lung diffusion capacity and blood gasses. *Kidney Int* 32:117, 1987.

123. Bland L, Alter M, Favero M, Carson L, Cusick L: Hemodialyzer reuse: practices in the United States and implication for infection control. *Trans Am Soc Artif Intern Organs* 31:556, 1985.

124. Sakula A: Formalin asthma in hospital laboratory staff. *Lancet* 2:816, 1975.

125. Porter JAH: Acute respiratory distress following formalin inhalation. *Lancet* 2:603, 1975.

126. Hendrick DJ, Lane DJ: Formalin asthma in hospital staff. *Br Med J* 1:607, 1975.

127. Lewis KJ, Dewar PJ, Ward MK, Kerr DNS: Formation of anti-N-like antibodies in dialysis patients: effects of different methods of dialyzer rinsing to remove formaldehyde. *Clin Nephrol* 15:39, 1981.

128. Koch KM, Frei U, Fassbinder W: Hemolysis and anemia in anti-N-like antibody positive hemodialysis patients. *Trans Am Soc Artif Intern Organs* 24:709, 1978.

129. Fassbinder W, Koch KM: A specific immunohaemolytic anaemia induced by formaldehyde sterilisation of dialyzers. *Contrib Nephrol* 36:51, 1983.

130. Vanholder R, Noens L, De Smet R, Ringoir S: Development of anti-N-like antibodies during formaldehyde reuse in spite of adequate pre-dailysis rinsing. *Am J Kidney Dis* 11:477, 1988.

131. Berkseth R, Luehmann D, Mac Micael C, Keshaviah P, Kjellstrand C: Peracetic acid for reuse of hemodialyzers: clinical studies. *Trans Am Soc Artif Organs* 30:270, 1984.

132. Petersen NJ, Carson LA, Doto IL, Aguero SM, Favero MS: Microbiologic evaluation of a new glutaraldehyde-based disinfectant for hemodialysis systems. *Trans Am Soc Artif Intern Organs* 28:287, 1982.

133. Delmez JA, Weerts CA, Hasamear PD, Windus DW: Severe dialyzer dysfunction undetectable by standard reprocessing validation tests. *Kidney Int* 36:478, 1989.

134. Rancourt M, Senger K, De Oreo P: Cellulosic membrane induced leukopenia after reprocessing with sodium hypochlorite. *Trans Am Soc Artif Intern Organs* 30:49, 1984.

135. Hoenich NA, Johnston SRD, Woffindin C, Kerr DNS: Haemodialys leucopenia: the role of membrane type and reuse. *Contrib Nephrol* 37:120, 1984.

136. Hoenich NA, Kerr DNS, Ward MK, Aljama P, Sussman M: Two special properties of polyamylonitrile membrane—suitability for reuse and biocompatibility. *Contemp Dial* 1:31, 1984.

137. Gordon SM, Tipple M, Jarvis WR: Pyrogenic reactions associated with the reuse of disposable hollow-fiber hemodialyzers. *JAMA* 260:2077, 1988.

138. Vanholder R, Vanhaecke E, Ringoir S: Pseudomonas septicemia due to deficient disinfectant mixing during reuse. *Int J Artif Organs* 15:19, 1992.

139. Ringoir S, Vanholder R: An introduction to biocompatibility. *Artif Organs* 10:20, 1986.

140. Deppisch R, Schmitt V, Bommer J, Hänsch GM, Ritz E, Rauterberg EW: Fluid phase generation of terminal complement complex as a novel index of bioincompatibility. *Kidney Int* 37:696, 1990.

141. Jacob HS, Craddock PR, Hammerschmidt DE, Moldow CF: Complement-induced granulocyte aggregation. An unsuspected mechanism of disease. *N Engl J Med* 302:789, 1980.

142. Craddock PR, Fehr J, Dalmasso AP, Brigham KL, Jacob HS: Hemodialysis leukopenia. Pulmonary vascular leukostasis resulting from complement activation by dialyzer cellophane membranes. *J Clin Invest* 59:879, 1977.

143. Cheung AK, Baranowski RL, Wayman AL: The role of thromboxane in cuprophane-induced pulmonary hypertension. *Kidney Int* 32:1072, 1987.

144. Eiser AR: Pulmonary gas exchange during haemodialysis and peritoneal dialysis: interaction between respiration and metabolism. *Am J Kidney Dis* 6:131, 1985.

145. Nissenson AR, Kraut JA, Shinaberger JA: Dialysis associated hypoxemia. Pathogenesis and prevention. *ASAIO J* 7:1, 1984.

146. Mahiout A, Meinhold H, Kessel M, Schulze H, Baurmeister U: Dialyzer membranes: effect of surface area and chemical modification of cellulose on complement and platelet activation. *Artif Organs* 11:149, 1987.

147. Akizawa T, Kitaoka T, Koshikawa S, Watanabe T, Imamura K, Tsurumi T, Suma Y, Eiga S: Development of a regenerated cellulose non-complement activating membrane for hemodialysis. *Trans Am Soc Artif Intern Organs* 32:76, 1986.

148. Himmelfarb J, Lazarus JM, Hakim R: Reactive oxygen species production by monocytes and polymorphonuclear leukocytes during dialysis. *Am J Kidney Dis* 17:271, 1991.

149. Vanholder R, Ringoir S: Infectious morbidity and defects of phagocytic function in end-stage renal disease. *J Am Soc Nephrol* 3:1541, 1993.

150. Vanholder R, Dell'Aquila R, Jacobs V, Dhondt A, Veys N, Waterloos MA, Van Landschoot N, Van Biesen W, Ringoir S: Depressed phagocytosis in hemodialyzed patients: in vivo and in vitro mechanisms. *Nephron* 63:409, 1993.

151. Hallgren R, Fjellstrom KE, Hakanson L, Venge P: Kinetic studies of phagocytosis II. The serum-independent uptake of IgG-coated particles by polymorphonuclear leukocytes from uremic patients on regular dialysis treatment. *J Lab Clin Med* 94:277, 1979.

152. Henderson LW, Miller ME, Hamilton RW, Norman ME: Hemodialysis leukopenia and polymorph random mobility—a possible correlation. *J Lab Clin Med* 85:191, 1975.

153. Vanholder R, Van Biesen W, Ringoir S: Contributing factors to the inhibition of phagocytosis in hemodialyzed patients. *Kidney Int* 44:208, 1993.

154. Lonnemann G, Bingel M, Floege J, Koch KM, Shaldon S,

Dinarello CA: Detection of endotoxin-like interleukin-1 inducing activity during in vitro dialysis. *Kidney Int* 33:29, 1988.

155. Bingel M, Lonnemann G, Koch KM, Dinarello CA, Shaldon S: Plasma interleukin-1 activity during hemodialysis: the influence of dialysis membranes. *Nephron* 50:273, 1988.

156. Lonnemann G, Koch KM, Shaldon S, Dinarello CA: Studies on the ability of hemodialysis membranes to induce, bind and clear human interleukin-1. *J Lab Clin Med* 112:76, 1988.

157. Dinarello CA: Interleukin-1 and tumor necrosis factor and their naturally occurring antagonists during hemodialysis. *Kidney Int* 42:S68, 1992.

158. Chanard J, Brunois JP, Melin JP, Lavaud S, Toupance O: Longterm results of dialysis therapy with a highly permeable membrane. *Artif Organs* 6:261, 1982.

159. Kant KS, Pollak VE, Cathey M, Goetz D, Berlin R: Multiple use of dialyzers: safety and efficacy. *Kidney Int* 19:728, 1981.

160. Levin NW, Zasuwa G, Dumler F: Effect of membrane type on causes of death in hemodialysis patients (abstract). *J Am Soc Nephrol* 2:335, 1991.

161. Hornberger JC, Chernew M, Petersen J, Garber AM: A multivariate analysis of mortality and hospital admissions with high-flux dialysis. *J Am Soc Nephrol* 3:1227, 1992.

162. Schulman G, Fogo A, Gung A, Badr K, Hakim R: Complement activation retards resolution of acute ischemic renal failure in the rat. *Kidney Int* 40:1069, 1991.

163. Hakim RM, Wingard RL, Lawrence P, Parker RA, Schulman G: Use of biocompatible membranes improves outcome and recovery from acute renal failure (abstract). *J Am Soc Nephrol* 3:367, 1992.

164. Linas SL, Whittenburg D, Parsons P, Repine JE: Mild renal ischemia activates primed neutrophils to cause acute renal failure. *Kidney Int* 42:610, 1992.

165. Guitterez A, Alvestrand A, Wahren J, Bergström J: Effect of in vivo contact between blood and dialysis membranes on protein catabolism in humans. *Kidney Int* 38:487, 1990.

166. Koch KM: Dialysis-related amyloidosis. *Kidney Int* 41:1416, 1992.

167. Vincent C, Revillard JP, Galland M, Traeger J: Serum β_2-microglobulin in hemodialyzed patients. *Nephron*, 21:260, 1978.

168. Vanholder RC, Ringoir SM: Intradialytic body weight changes and dialyzer pore size as main contributing factors to the evolution of beta-2-microglobulin in dialysis. *Blood Purif* 8:32, 1990.

169. Zaoui P, Stone WJ, Hakim RM: Effects of dialysis membranes on β_2m production and cellular expression. *Kidney Int* 38:962, 1990.

170. van Ypersele de Strihou C, Jadoul M, Malghem J, Maldague B, Jamart J: Effect of dialysis membrane and patient's age on signs of dialysis-related amyloidosis. *Kidney Int* 39:1012, 1991.

171. Villaroel F, Ciarkowski AA: A survey of hypersensitivity reactions in hemodialysis. *Artif Organs* 11:137, 1985.

172. Popli S, Ing TS, Daugirdas JT, Kheirbek AO, Viol GW, Vilbar RM, Ghandi VC: Severe reactions to cuprophan capillary dialyzers. *Artif Organs* 6:312, 1982.

173. Daugirdas JT, Ing TS: First-use reactions during hemodialysis: a definition of subtypes. *Kidney Int* 33:S37, 1988.

174. Marshall C, Shimizu A, Smith EKM, Dolovich J: Ethylene oxide allergy in a dialysis center: prevalence in hemodialysis and peritoneal dialysis populations. *Clin Nephrol* 21:346, 1984.

175. Hakim RM, Breilatt J, Lazarus JM, Port FK: Complement activation and hypersensitivity reactions to dialysis membranes. *N Engl J Med* 311:878, 1984.

176. Verresen L, Waer M, Vanrenterghem Y, Michielsen P: Angiotensin-converting-enzyme inhibitors and anaphylactoid reactions to high-flux membrane dialysis. *Lancet* 336:1360, 1990.

177. Tielemans C, Madhoun P, Lenaers M, Schandene L, Goldman M, Vanherweghem JL: Anaphylactoid reactions during hemodialysis on AN69 membranes in patients receiving ACE inhibitors. *Kidney Int* 38:982, 1990.

178. Schulman G, Hakim RM, Arias R, Silverberg M, Kaplan AP, Arbeit L: Bradykinin generation by dialysis membranes: possible role in anaphylactoid reaction. *J Am Soc Nephrol* 3:1563, 1993.

179. Alfrey AC, Legendre GR, Kaehny WD: The dialysis encephalopathy syndrome. Possible aluminum intoxication. *N Engl J Med* 294:184, 1976.

180. Drüeke T: Dialysis osteomalacy and aluminum intoxication. *Nephron* 26:207, 1980.

181. Haeffner-Cavaillon N, Cavaillon JM, Cianconi C, Bacle F, Delons S, Kazatchkine M: In vivo induction of interleukin-1 during hemodialysis. *Kidney Int* 35:1212, 1989.

182. Vanholder R, Van Haecke E, Veys N, Ringoir S: Endotoxin transfer through dialysis membranes: small- versus large-pore membranes. *Nephrol Dial Transplant* 7:333, 1992.

183. Klinkmann H, Wolf H, Schmidt E: Definition of biocompatibility. *Contrib Nephrol* 37:70, 1984.

184. Lyman DJ, Knutson K, Mc Neil L B, Shibatani K: The effects of chemical structure and surface properties of synthetic polymers on the coagulation of blood. IV. The relation between polymer morphology and protein absorption. *Trans Am Soc Artif Intern Organs* 21:49, 1975.

185. Gasparotto ML, Bertoli M, Vertolli U, Ruffatti A, Stoppa ML, Di Landro D, Romagnoli GF: Biocompatibility of various dialysis membranes as assessed by coagulation assay. *Contrib Nephrol* 37:96, 1984.

186. Hirsh J, Dalen JE, Deykin D, Poller L: Heparin: mechanism of action, pharmacokinetics, dosing considerations, monitoring, efficacy, and safety. *Chest* 102:337S, 1992.

187. Freedman MD: Pharmacodynamics, clinical indications, and adverse effects of heparin. *J Clin Pharmacol* 32:584, 1992.

188. Rylance PB, Gordge MP, Ireland H, Lane DA, Weston MJ: Haemodialysis with prostacyclin (epoprostenol) alone. *Proc EDTA-ERA* 21:281, 1984.

189. Camici M, Evangelisti L: Prostacyclin and heparin during haemodialysis. Comparative effects. *Life Support Systems* 4:205, 1986.

190. Renaud H, Moriniére P, Dieval J, Abdull-Massin Z, Dkhissi H, Toutlemonde F, Delobel J, Fournier A: Low molecular weight heparin in haemodialysis and haemofiltration—comparison with unfractioned heparin. *Proc EDTA-ERA* 21:276, 1984.

191. Schrader J, Stibbe W, Armstrong VW, Kandt M, Muche R, Köstering H, Seidel D, Scheler F: Comparison of low molecular weight heparin to standard heparin in hemodialysis/hemofiltration. *Kidney Int* 33:890, 1988.

192. Vanholder R, Camez A, Veys N, Soria J, Mirshahi MC, Soria C, Ringoir S: Recombinant hirudin: a specific thrombin inhibiting anticoagulant for haemodialysis. *Kidney Int* 45:1754, 1994.

193. Leong ASY, Disney APS, Gove DW: Spallation and migration of silicone from blood-pump tubing in patients on hemodialysis. *N Engl J Med* 306:135, 1982.

194. Bommer J, Waldherr R, Ritz E: Silicone storage disease in longterm hemodialysis patients. *Contrib Nephrol* 36:115, 1983.

195. Bommer J, Gemsa D, Waldherr R, Kessler J, Ritz E: Plastic filing from dialysis tubing induces prostanoid release from macrophages. *Kidney Int* 26:331, 1984.

196. Bommer J, Pernicka E, Kessler J, Ritz E: Reduction of silicone particle release during haemodialysis. *Proc EDTA-ERA* 21:287, 1984.

197. Barron D, Harbottle S, Hoenich NA, Morley AR, Appleton D, McCabe JF: Particle spallation induced by blood pumps in hemodialysis tubing sets. *Artif Organs* 10:226, 1986.

198. Morley AR, Barron D, Thompson P, Hoenich NA, Harbottle S, Kerr DNS: Surface alterations in dialysis roller pump inserts: a scanning electron microscopy study. *J Biomed Eng* 8:255, 1986.

199. Kevy S, Jacobson M: Hepatic effects of the leaching of phthalate ester plasticizer and silicon. *Contrib Nephrol* 36:82, 1983.

200. Dolovich J, Marshal L CP, Smith EKM, Shimizu A, Pearson FC, Sugona MA, Lee W: Allergy to ethylene oxide in chronic hemodialysis patients. *Artif Organs* 8:334, 1984.

201. NG RCK, Suki WN: Treatment of acute renal failure. In: BM Brenner, JH Stein, eds, *Treatment of Acute Renal Failure*. Churchill Livingstone, New York, pp 229–273, 1980.

202. Delano BG: Regular dialysis treatment (RDT). In: JF Maher, ed, *Replacement of Renal Function by Dialysis*. Kluwer Academic Publishers, Dordrecht, pp 669–685, 1989.

203. Bonomini V, Albertazzi A, Vangelista A, Bartolotti GC, Stefoni S, Scolari MP: Residual renal function and effective rehabilitation in chronic dialysis. *Nephron* 16:89, 1976.

204. Kiprov DD: An overview of therapeutic apheresis. *Dial Transplant* 14:195, 1985.

205. Gurland HJ, Lysaght MJ, Samtleben W: Immunomodulation: clinical aspects. *Artif Organs* 10:122, 1986.

CHAPTER 63

Use of Drugs in Uremia and Dialysis

D. CRAIG BRATER

INTRODUCTION

A host of drugs are eliminated by the kidney and thereby require dose adjustment in patients with renal insufficiency (1–5). In addition, some drugs that themselves are not dependent upon the kidney for excretion are converted in the liver to active metabolites that accumulate in patients with diminished renal function (6,7). Examples include N-acetyl procainamide and normeperidine, the metabolites of procainamide and meperidine, respectively. These compounds can accumulate to toxic concentrations in patients with renal insufficiency. To avoid toxicity from either parent drug or active metabolites, doses of many drugs must be adjusted downward in patients with decreased renal function. The precision required in this dose adjustment is not always great and depends upon the therapeutic index of individual drugs. For example, penicillins and cephalosporin antibiotics have wide margins of safety. Many antibiotics in these classes are administered in smaller doses to patients with severe renal insufficiency, but this administration does not require the same degree of precision as dose adjustment with drugs having narrow therapeutic indices, such as aminoglycoside antibiotics. With the latter, serum concentrations are measured to assure attainment of therapeutic yet nontoxic levels (8).

In addition to drug accumulation due to compromised elimination pathways, the patient treated with hemodialysis or peritoneal dialysis presents an additional challenge. A drug may be removed by the dialysis procedure itself, thereby requiring compensatory dose supplementation, the extent of which is a function of the amount of drug removed (1). The ability of dialysis to remove drugs is influenced by factors such as the binding of drug to protein, which limits dialyzability, molecular size, etc. These factors are highly variable among drugs, even those in the same chemical class, rendering a priori predictions impossible. As a result, one must rely on experimental data in appropriate patient populations to guide therapy. In addition, for drugs with narrow therapeutic indices, drug serum concentrations can be measured to guide therapy.

This chapter will first discuss principles of drug dosing that will serve as a framework for dosing-regimen adjustment in patients with renal insufficiency. Subsequently, dosing guidelines for patients with various degrees of renal dysfunction, including dialysis, will be offerred. The objective of the chapter, then, is to provide both a conceptual framework and specific recommendations for treating patients with renal disease.

PRINCIPLES OF DOSE ADJUSTMENT IN PATIENTS WITH RENAL DISEASE

Loading dose

The use of some drugs entails a *loading dose strategy* in which an initial dose larger than the maintenance dose is administered in order to rapidly attain therapeutic drug concentrations (9–11). This approach is usually employed in therapeutic settings in which an effective drug concentration is needed quickly. Examples include the use of lidocaine, digoxin, and aminoglycoside antibiotics. The loading dose needed is a function of the volume of distribution (V_d) of the drug and the target blood concentration to initially be attained ($C_{initial}$):

$$\text{Loading Dose} = (C_{initial}) \ (V_d).$$

For example, if the V_d for an aminoglycoside antibiotic is 0.25 L/kg and the desired peak serum concentration is 8 mg/L, the necessary loading dose can be calculated as follows:

$$\text{Loading Dose} = (8 \text{ mg/L}) \ (0.25 \text{ L/kg})$$
$$= 2 \text{ mg/kg}.$$

It is customary for clinicians to think in terms of the loading dose itself as opposed to calculating it from values for V_d and the desired concentration. Such an approach can be hazardous, particularly in settings where the patient's disease may influence V_d and thereby mandate a change in the loading dose. For example, if the V_d of a drug in a patient with renal insufficiency was one half that in a patient with normal renal function, and the patient with renal

Suki, WN and Massry SG (eds), Suki and Massry's Therapy of Renal Diseases and Related Disorders, Third Edition. ISBN 978-1-4757-6634-9.

Table 1. Drugs for which the volume of distribution is affected by renal disease[a]

Drug	Normal renal function	V_d (L/kg) ESRD
Analgesics		
Codeine	3.5–6.0	7.3
Salicylate	0.15	Increase (no change)[b]
Anesthetics and drugs used during anesthesia		
Thiopental	1.9 (12)	3.0 (12)
Anti-inflammatory agents		
Azapropazone	0.15–0.25	No change (decrease)
Oxaprozin	0.15–0.25	(decrease)
Antianxiety agents		
Oxazepam	1.0	Increase (no change)
Anticoagulants, antifibrinolytics, and antiplatelet agents		
Sulfinpyrazone	0.06	Increase (no change)
Warfarin	0.14	Increase (no change)
Anticonvulsants		
Phenytoin	0.6	Increase (no change)
Valproate	0.19	Increase (no change)
Antihistamines		
Roxatidine	3.2	2.0
Antimicrobial agents/antibacterials		
Cephalosporins		
Cefazolin	0.11–0.14	0.17
Cefoxitin	0.27	Increase
Macrolide antibiotics		
Erythromycin	0.8	1.2
Penicillins		
Azlocillin	0.18	0.3
Timocillin	0.15–0.24	Increase (no change)
Quinolones		
Norfloxacin	3.2	1.7
Antifungals		
Miconazole	21	Decrease
Bronchodilators		
Albuterol	2.0–2.5	0.8
Cardiovascular agents		
Antiarrhythmics		
Disopyramide	0.91	Decrease
Encainide	5.7	Decrease
Blood lipid lowering agents		
Acifran	0.5	(Decrease to 1/3 normal)
Clofibrate	0.14	Increase (no change)
Cardiac inotropes		
Digitoxin	0.73	Increase (no change)
Digoxin	$V_d = 3.84 + 0.0446\,Cl_{Cr}$	
Miscellaneous		
Bendazac	0.18	Increase (no change)

[a] V_d, volume of distribution; ESRD, end-stage renal disease; Cl_{Cr}, creatinine clearance.
[b] Values in parentheses indicate data for unbound drug.

disease received a 'standard' loading dose, the resulting initial concentration would be twice that expected, with a consequent risk of toxicity. To illustrate using the previous example, if the 'normal' loading dose of 2 mg/kg were administered to a patient whose V_d was 0.125 L/kg (i.e., half the usual value), then a concentration of 16 mg/L would result:

$$2 \text{ mg/kg} = (C_{initial}) \quad (0.125 \text{ L/kg}),$$
$$C_{initial} = 2 \text{ mg/g} + 0.125 \text{ L/g}$$
$$= 16 \text{ mg/L}.$$

If this scenario occurred with an aminoglycoside antibiotic, serious ototoxicity and/or nephrotoxicity could result.

It should be clear from this example that clinicians need to be alert to changes that occur in the V_d of drugs. Table 1 lists drugs in which a change in V_d has been documented in patients with renal disorders. If a loading dose strategy is used in such patients, the dose to be administered can be calculated as shown previously if the desired concentration is known. Alternatively, if the clinician knows the usual loading dose, the data in Table 1 can be used to calculate a modified dose:

$$\frac{\text{Usual Loading Dose}}{\text{Modified Loading Dose}} = \frac{\text{Normal } V_d}{\text{Patient's } V_d},$$

or

$$\text{Modified Loading Dose} = \frac{\text{Patient's } V_d}{\text{Normal } V_d}(\text{Usual Loading Dose}).$$

The direct proportionality between the loading dose and V_d should make such dose adjustments easy and routine. Unfortunately, the need for altering the loading dose is often ignored.

Another caution that needs emphasis concerning loading doses and V_d is the influence of changes in drug protein binding. When V_d is determined experimentally in pharmacokinetic studies, the total concentration of drug in serum is usually used as a reference point. For drugs that are highly protein bound, assessing V_d (or other pharmacokinetic parameters) solely in terms of total drug concentrations can be misleading (12). For example, consider a drug that is 90% protein bound and has an initial total serum concentration of 10 mg/L; therefore, this value constitutes 9 mg/L of protein-bound drug but only 1 mg/L of unbound, free drug. It is the latter that is able to gain access to tissues and is active. If a loading dose of 100 mg is needed to attain this concentration of 10 mg/L, one can calculate the V_d for both total and unbound drug:

$$V_d = \frac{\text{Loading Dose}}{C_{initial}},$$

$$V_d \text{ (total)} = \frac{100 \text{ mg}}{10 \text{mg/L}} \quad V_d \text{ (free)} = \frac{100 \text{ mg}}{1 \text{mg/L}}$$
$$= 10 \text{ L}, \qquad\qquad = 100 \text{ L}.$$

In patients with renal insufficiency, the protein binding of many drugs is decreased (13). This finding is particularly true of acidic drugs bound to serum albumin, in which accumulated endogenous organic acids can displace the drug from binding sites (14). In the preceding example, such a scenario could manifest in two different fashions.

For drugs like phenytoin, valproate, and warfarin, all of which are highly protein bound, a decrease in binding to albumin might be expected to cause an increase in the unbound concentration and thereby to result in increased effect. However, the increased free drug is also readily available for metabolism of these drugs by the liver such that the unbound concentration is no different than in patients with normal renal function (12,13). In other words, using the example outlined above, in patients with normal renal function, a total serum concentration of 10 mg/L may yield 1 mg/L of free drug; in contrast, in a patient with end-stage renal disease (ESRD), a total concentration of 5 mg/L may result in the same free concentration:

	Bound	+ Free	= Total	% Bound
Normal renal function	9	+ 1	= 10 mg/L	90%
ESRD	4	+ 1	= 5mg/L	80%

From this information, one can examine the various volumes of distribution that might be calculated:

Normal renal function
$$V_d(\text{total}) = \frac{100 \text{ mg}}{10 \text{ mg/L}} \qquad V_d(\text{free}) = \frac{100 \text{ mg}}{1 \text{ mg/L}}$$
$$= 10 \text{ L} \qquad\qquad = 100 \text{ L}$$

ESRD
$$V_d(\text{total}) = \frac{100 \text{ mg}}{5 \text{ mg/L}} \qquad V_d(\text{free}) = \frac{100 \text{ mg}}{1 \text{ mg/L}}$$
$$= 20 \text{ L} \qquad\qquad = 100 \text{ L}$$

If one calculated V_d in the patient with ESRD using total drug concentration, the conclusion would be that such patients had twice as great a V_d as subjects with normal renal function (20 L vs. 10 L). If one then used these data to calculate a loading dose in a patient with ESRD, a dose twice that in patients with normal renal function would be recommended. However, since it is the free, unbound drug that is pharmacologically active, it is the V_d of this component of the total drug concentration that is therapeutically relevant. As should be apparent, in the example chosen, this V_d was the same in both patients, namely, 100 L. Thus, in terms of unbound drug concentration, if the V_d from total drug concentration were used to guide therapy and the loading dose were doubled to 200 mg, the free concentration would double and might lead to toxicity:

$$C_{initial}(\text{free}) = \frac{\text{Loading Dose}}{V_d}$$
$$= \frac{200 \text{ mg}}{100 \text{ L}}$$
$$= 2 \text{ mg/L}.$$

Early studies with phenytoin reported an increase in the V_d in patients with renal insufficiency (13). As our knowledge in this area increased, it became clear that the scenario exemplified above was applicable to phenytoin: namely, decreased protein binding occurred and the free drug concentration, and therefore V_d of the free drug, was unchanged. Until this was discovered, misleading data led to inappropriate dosing recommendations for phenytoin. Clinicians should be alert to this potential problem as they read the proliferating medical literature dealing with disposition of drugs in patients with renal diseases. For acidic drugs that are highly protein bound (> 90%), V_d and other pharmacokinetic parameters expressed as total drug concentration may be misleading, and the reader should search for data concerning unbound drug concentrations.

Another misleading scenario that is the converse of that discussed above can also occur. In the preceeding example, V_d calculated from total serum concentrations led to a misleading conclusion that a modification of the loading dose was needed. With some drugs (e.g., nonsteroidal anti-inflammatory drugs (NSAIDs)), V_d for total drug appears normal (implying no change in loading dose), whereas the V_d for free drug is altered, mandating a change (15).

For example, this situation might occur if a drug is displaced from protein binding but the increased free drug concentration is not eliminated and remains elevated:

	Bound	+	Free	=	Total	% Bound
Normal renal function	9	+	1	=	10 mg/L	90%
ESRD	8	+	2	=	10 mg/L	80%

Note that the percent binding in patients with ESRD is identical to that in the previous example, namely, 80%. However, in this example, the free drug concentration is doubled to 2 mg/L. Again, one can calculate V_d's for both total and unbound drug:

Normal renal function
$$V_d(\text{total}) = \frac{100\,\text{mg}}{10\,\text{mg/L}} \qquad V_d(\text{free}) = \frac{100\,\text{mg}}{1\,\text{mg/L}}$$
$$= 10\,\text{L} \qquad = 100\,\text{L}$$

ESRD
$$V_d(\text{total}) = \frac{100\,\text{mg}}{10\,\text{mg/L}} \qquad V_d(\text{free}) = \frac{100\,\text{mg}}{2\,\text{mg/L}}$$
$$= 10\,\text{L} \qquad = 50\,\text{L}$$

The misleading conclusion in this setting from values related to total drug concentration would be that no change in loading dose is indicated. In contrast, if assessed as free concentration, it is apparent that V_d in patients with ESRD is half that in patients with normal renal function. If the loading dose given to the patient with ESRD were not decreased proportionally, then an elevated free drug concentration could cause toxicity.

These examples are meant to emphasize the importance of assessment of V_d (and other pharmacokinetic parameters) in terms of free drug concentration. It should be clear that basing conclusions about loading dose adjustment on the total drug concentration can be misleading; sometimes a clinician might erroneously assume no change is needed and with other drugs incorrectly assume that a

modified loading dose is needed. Table 1 presents pertinent data for available free drug concentrations. Unfortunately, in the case of many drugs, the experimental design of studies has been flawed, and free drug concentrations have not been measured. In this case, the clinician must be aware of the potential pitfalls illustrated above. A recognition of the problems inherent in the extant data should result in cautious dosing and close assessment of the patient.

Maintenance dose

As the name implies, a *maintenance dose* is administered to maintain desired drug concentrations at steady state (9–11). This dose is determined by the desired average steady-state drug concentration, C_{average}, and the clearance (Cl) of the drug from the body:

Maintenance Dose = (C_{average}) (Cl).

Note the similarity between this relationship and that for loading dose. This relationship is easy to derive and is a function of the definition of steady state; namely, at steady state, the rate of drug entering the body must equal the rate being removed. In turn,

Rate In = Administration Rate = Maintenance Dosing Rate
and
Rate Out = (C_{average}) (Cl).

Determination of the maintenance dosing rate is dependent upon the route of administration. For example, if a drug is administered as a continuous intravenous infusion, the maintenance dosing rate is the infusion rate of the drug. If a drug is administered as separate, intermittent intravenous doses, the dosing rate is expressed as

Dosing Rate = (Individual Dose)/Dosing Interval.

Lastly, if a drug is administered by mouth, one must incorporate a term that accounts for incomplete bioavailability, the fraction of dose absorbed (F). In this circumstance, the maintenance dosing rate becomes

Dosing Rate = (F) (Individual Dose)/Dosing Interval.

Hence, depending on the route of administration, any of the following relationships may apply:

Infusion Rate = (C_{average}) (Cl),

Dose/Dosing Interval = (C_{average}) (Cl),

F × Dose/Dosing Interval = (C_{average}) (Cl).

It should be apparent from these relationships that a change in clearance mandates a proportional change in the rate of drug administration if the average drug concentration is to remain the same. In patients with renal insufficiency, the clearance of drugs is often diminished and, consequently, maintenance doses must be adjusted. In a subsequent section, specific guidelines will be offered for maintenance doses of a variety of drugs; these recommendations derive from studies that quantify the effect of renal insufficiency on the clearance of these drugs.

When analyzing published literature concerning the clearance of a drug and whether or not a clinical condition mandates a change in the maintenance dose, the caveats discussed in detail above concerning the influence of protein binding on V_d are also applicable to clearance (12,13). Hence, if changes in binding occur, clearance calculations based on total drug concentration can be misleading, and one should seek data relevant to unbound drug. The recommendations that follow are based on free drug concentrations when data are available; unfortunately, for many drugs this information does not exist.

Half-life

The half-life (t_2^1) of a drug refers to the time required for its serum concentration to decrease by half. The rate of elimination of most drugs (exceptions being phenytoin and salicylate) is independent of drug serum concentration and is referred to as being linear. This also means that the t_2^1 is independent of serum concentration; therefore, the time for a drug's concentration to decrease from 100 to 50 units of concentration is the same time it takes to decrease from 10 to 5 units.

Many clinicians use t_2^1 synonymously with clearance of a drug. In so doing, they presume that an increase in t_2^1 indicates a decrease in clearance that thereby requires a compensatory decrease in the maintenance dose. This popular misconception can lead to errors in dose adjustment in patients with renal insufficiency. As opposed to being solely a reflection of drug clearance, t_2^1 is a function of both V_d and Cl:

$$t_2^1 = 0.693 \ V_d/Cl.$$

Hence, a change in t_2^1 can reflect either a change in V_d, a change in Cl, or a change in both. The correct dosing regimen adjustment that must be made depends on whether an alteration in V_d or in Cl is responsible for the change in t_2^1. If t_2^1 increases solely due to an increase in V_d, then the loading dose should be increased but the maintenance dose should remain unchanged. If one incorrectly assumed that t_2^1 increased because Cl decreased and therefore administered a 'normal' loading dose and a diminished maintenance dose, the result would be that the loading dose, which is too small, would not attain the desired initial concentration, and the inappropriately diminished maintenance dose would maintain a lower drug concentration than desired. The result could be lack of efficacy.

A good example of this potential scenario is the use of digoxin in patients with renal insufficiency. In patients with mild to moderate renal insufficiency, the V_d of digoxin is approximately the same as in patients with normal renal function, while Cl may be about one half to two thirds normal (16). In such patients, the prolonged t_2^1 is inversely proportional to the diminished Cl. In patients with severe

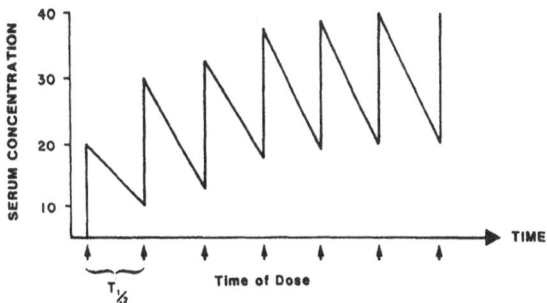

Figure 1. Schematic illustrating that 4 to 5 times the half-life (t_2^1) are needed to reach steady-state serum concentrations of a drug. Arrows represent the time of dosing; the drug is administered every t_2^1.

renal insufficiency, however, V_d is decreased to one half to two thirds normal and Cl is decreased even more, to about one third normal (16,17). In this setting, t_2^1 is influenced by both parameters, and although the half-life is prolonged compared to patients with normal renal function, it is little different than in the patient with mild to moderate renal insufficiency. In the patient with severe renal insufficiency, if the change in t_2^1 were erroneously presumed to quantitatively reflect the decrease in digoxin clearance and thereby maintenance dose, a serious dosing error would occur. Since no downward adjustment in loading dose would be made, the initial concentration would be higher than desired; in addition, the needed decrease in maintenance dose would be underestimated, so the patient's steady-state serum concentration would be maintained at a higher concentration than desired. The hazards of such an error are obvious.

One must realize the limitations of using t_2^1 to predict needed dosing adjustments and instead must dissect it into its component parts of V_d and Cl. Of what use, then, is t_2^1? Knowing t_2^1 allows one to determine the time necessary for serum drug concentrations to reach steady state. As illustrated in Figure 1, steady state is reached after administering a drug for 4 to 5 times the t_2^1. If necessary, this delay in attaining plateau drug concentrations can be avoided by giving a loading dose designed to attain the desired drug concentration quickly; this concentration can then be maintained.

It is important to remember that the concept of attainment of steady state applies to any change in dose, not just starting therapy. For example, if a maintenance dose is doubled, 4 to 5 times the t_2^1 is required for the serum concentration to reach the new plateau. Similarly, if the maintenance does is decreased, 4 to 5 times t_2^1 must elapse for the new, lower steady-state concentration to be reached. Lastly, if drug is stopped altogether, 4 to 5 times the t_2^1 is needed for concentrations to become negligible.

In summary, half-life should be used to predict the time necessary for a drug to reach steady-state concentrations. It is a hybrid value influenced by both V_d and Cl and as such provides no direct information about loading or maintenance dose.

Dosing regimens

When renal dysfunction dictates a need to modify the dosing regimen, several options are available. Changes in loading dose simply entail giving a larger or smaller dose depending on whether V_d is increased or decreased. It must be emphasized that one is often uncertain as to the need to modify a loading dose. In such cases, one should first decide whether or not a loading dose strategy is actually necessary. If it is, one should err on the side of caution and administer a smaller loading dose than usual. If monitoring of clinical endpoints and/or serum drug concentrations shows the dose to have been too low, a supplementary dose can be given. In contrast, if too large a dose is administered, the clinician may be faced with iatrogenic drug toxicity and the need for remedial measures until the drug concentration diminishes.

To adjust maintenance doses of a drug, several strategies can be employed. The primary objective is to maintain the same average drug concentration as would occur if the patient did not have renal disease. Because the majority of drugs obey linear or first-order elimination kinetics, the change in clearance can be compensated for by a proportional change in the dosing rate:

$$\frac{\text{Usual Maintenance Dose}}{\text{Modified Maintenance}} = \frac{\text{Usual Clearance}}{\text{Patient's Clearance}}$$

or

$$\begin{array}{l}\text{Modified} \\ \text{Maintenance} \\ \text{Dose}\end{array} = \frac{\text{Patient's Clearance}}{\text{Usual Clearance}}\left(\begin{array}{l}\text{Usual Maintenance} \\ \text{Dose}\end{array}\right)$$

Hence, if the clearance of a drug in a patient with renal insufficiency is half the 'normal' value, then the patient's maintenance dose should be one half that usually administered. Such dose modifications will keep the average steady-state drug concentration in the patient with renal disease the same as in those with normal renal function.

If a patient is receiving a drug by continuous intravenous infusion, maintenance dose modification simply requires a modified infusion rate. If, however, the patient is receiving intermittent doses, a reduction of the total dose being administered can be accomplished in three different fashions:

1. Decreasing each individual dose and maintaining the same dosing frequency; this approach is often referred to as the *variable dose method*
2. Maintaining the same individual dose but administering each dose less frequently; this approach is called the *variable frequency* (or interval) *method*
3. Modifying both individual doses and the frequency of their administration, which is a combination method

All three methods attain the same average drug concentration. For example, if a drug is administered to a patient

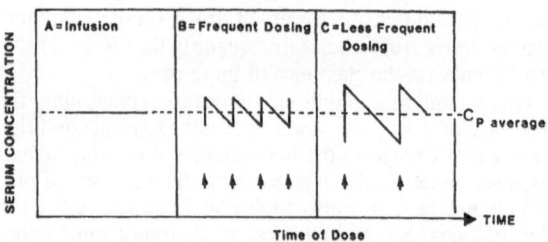

Figure 2. Illustration of three different dosing regimens. The total amount of drug administered is the same in all three, so the average drug concentration, $C_{p\,average}$, is identical. The regimen with least frequent administration of large doses results in the greatest difference between peak and trough concentrations.

with normal renal function at a dose of 500 mg every 12 hours, and one wished to administer half as much drug to a patient with renal insufficiency, viable options according to the above include

1. 250 mg every 12 hours
2. 500 mg every 24 hours
3. 375 mg every 18 hours

Over a course of therapy, the total amount of drug administered with each of these regimens is the same, and it is half the amount in patients with normal renal function. These regimens differ, however, in the profile of serum drug concentrations. Regimens with closer dosing frequencies and smaller individual doses result in less difference between peak and trough drug concentrations (Figure 2).

It is unclear which of these options is best to employ. For aminoglycoside antibiotics, an extensive literature has evolved that includes derivations of numerous dosing nomograms employing all three options (18,19). As is apparent from Figure 2, modifying only the individual dose and maintaining the same frequency results in lower peak and higher trough concentrations than in alternative methods. With aminoglycosides in particular, the elevated trough concentrations likely increase the risk of toxicity, while in some patients the peak may be so low as to be subtherapeutic. In contrast, regimens that diminish the total dose of a drug solely by decreasing the frequency of administration (increasing the dosing interval) may result in long periods of time with subtherapeutic serum drug concentrations. For these reasons, the present author recommends a combination approach to dose adjustment. For aminoglycosides, for example, the method of Sarubbi and Hull seems best (20). They suggest that a variable frequency method be used with these antibiotics, with the limitation that the dosing interval never be longer than 24 hours. When this time point is reached, they suggest switching to a variable dose method; hence, in patients with severe renal insufficiency, the dosing interval would be 24 hours and individual doses would also be smaller than usual.

Some may wonder about administering a single large

daily dose of aminoglycoside antibiotic, as has been reported to patients with normal renal function (21–23). However, to date, this method of dosing has not been investigated in patients with renal insufficiency and should not be used.

There is no general rule that can be applied to determine maximum length of a dosing interval. Twenty-four hours seems a reasonable rule of thumb. Clinicians should realize the different options available and try to correlate these options with individual therapeutic settings. For example, if a patient is not responding to a drug, the clinician should realize that a possible explanation is an inappropriate dosing regimen. Similarly, signs of toxicity shortly after administration of an individual dose may indicate a need to give the drug more frequently in smaller doses to optimize the dosing regimen in an individual patient. Just the recognition of these possibilities can help in tailoring therapy to individual patients, whereas ignorance of these possibilities can lead to inadequate therapeutics.

Dialysis

Patients with end-stage renal disease (ESRD) treated with hemodialysis (including hemofiltration) or chronic ambulatory peritoneal dialysis (CAPD) have a unique additional mechanism by which drugs can be eliminated from the body (24,25). If substantial elimination by these routes occurs, the dosing regimen must be modified. In patients maintained on hemodialysis, this modification is most easily accomplished through the administration of a supplemental dose of drug at the completion of the dialysis session. The dose given is equal to the amount of drug removed during the hemodialysis procedure.

With CAPD, there is a more or less continual process of drug removal. In this setting, the patient's total clearance of a drug is equal to clearance relative to the patient's residual level of renal function plus clearance via CAPD. The clinician simply adjusts the dosing regimen (either individual dose, dosing interval, or both) upwards in proportion to the added increment in clearance from CAPD.

It is not infrequent for clinicians to encounter a setting where they are administering a drug to a patient receiving dialysis and are unable to find any information about dialytic removal of the agent. In this setting, the clinician can often gain insight into the dialyzability of a drug by examining some of its pharmacokinetic parameters. One limitation to removal by dialysis is molecular size. If a drug is too large to pass across the dialysis membrane (including the peritoneum), it will not be removed by dialysis. This consideration, for example, applies to vancomycin and amphotericin. Drugs that are highly bound to serum proteins have restricted access to the dialysis membrane, since only free, unbound drug can cross this barrier. Hence, if a drug is bound in excess of 90%, it is unlikely that dialysis will contribute appreciably to its elimination. Water-soluble drugs are more readily dialyzed; in turn, one clue

that a drug is water soluble is the fact that such drugs are usually eliminated predominantly by the kidney as unchanged drug. Lastly, drugs with large volumes of distribution have minimal dialyzability. Conceptually, one can think of such drugs as having only a small portion in the vascular space and a predominant portion in peripheral tissues. The drug in the vascular space can be removed, but once dialysis ends, the large amount of drug in the tissues can refill the vascular compartment; the dialysis procedure thereby removes only an insignificant quantity of the total amount of drug in the body.

Specific examples can be used to illustrate these principles. Aminoglycoside antibiotics are water soluble and are eliminated primarily by the kidney (100% of the dose is normally excreted unchanged in the urine); they have negligible protein binding, and they have small volumes of distribution ($0.25 \, L/g$). These drugs are removed by dialysis procedures in sufficient quantities to require dose supplementation. In contrast, cefonicid has a small V_d ($0.10 \, L/g$) but is highly bound to serum proteins (98%) and thereby is not removed by hemodialysis or CAPD. Cefadroxil, on the other hand, though having a somewhat larger V_d than cefonicid ($0.30 \, L/g$), is only 16% bound to serum proteins. Hemodialysis is sufficient with this cephalosporin to require a supplemental dose. Lastly, drugs such as phenothiazines and tricyclic antidepressants, which have very large V_d's ($>10 \, L/g$), are not eliminated by dialysis even if they are negligibly bound to serum proteins.

Gwilt and Perrier have examined in detail the relationship between dialyzability, protein binding, and V_d (26) and have quantified the general relationships discussed above. If the percent of free drug in serum divided by V_d (expressed in L/g) is greater than 80, 6 hours of hemodialysis will in general remove 20%–50% of the body burden of the drug and thereby will require a supplemental dose at the end of the procedure. In contrast, if this ratio is less than 20, in general less than 10% of a drug will be removed, and no supplemental dosing will be necessary. As with any generalization, there are exceptions to the above concepts; however, when specific information concerning removal by dialysis is lacking, these relationships can be used as a starting point for therapeutic decisions, with further refinements based on clinical endpoints and/or measured serum drug concentrations.

Table 2 lists the amount of a drug removed by dialysis (as a percentage of a "normal" dose in a patient with normal renal function). This value allows calculation of the increment in dosing that must be given to compensate for removal by dialysis. Table 2 does not include removal of drugs by hemoperfusion, hemofiltration, or hemodiafiltration. Hemoperfusion is applicable to toxicologic settings and is outside the scope of this chapter.

For hemofiltration, one should remember that hemofiltration removes unbound drug in the serum. The amount removed (and thereby the dose increment needed) can be calculated as

Table 2. Dialyzability of drugs: percent of a normal dose removed by one session of hemodialysis or 24 hours of CAPD[a]

Drug	Hemodialysis	CAPD	Drug	Hemodialysis	CAPD
Analgesics			**Carbapenems**		
Meperidine	Negligible	Negligible	Imipenem	80%–90%	Negligible
Methadone	Negligible (<1%)	Negligible (<1%)	**Cephalosporins**		
			Cefaclor	33%	
Propoxyphene	Negligible	Negligible	Cefadroxil	50%	
Salicylates	Negligible Considerable in overdose settings	Negligible	Cefamandole	50%	Negligible (5%)
			Cefazolin	50%	20%
			Cefipime	40%–70%	26%
Anesthetics and drugs used during anesthesia			Cefixime	Negligible (1.6%)	Negligible
Gallamine	Considerable	Considerable	Cefmenoxime	16%–51%	Negligible (<10%)
Antianxiety agents, sedatives, and hypnotics			Cefmetazole	60%	
			Cefodizime	50%	Negligible (15%)
Buspirone	Negligible		Cefonicid	Negligible	Negligible (6.5%)
Chloral Hydrate	Negligible				
Ethchlorvynol	Negligible		Cefoperazone	Negligible	Negligible
Glutethimide	Negligible		Ceforanide	20%–50%	
Meprobamate	Negligible		Cefotaxime	60%	Negligible (5%)
Methaqualone	Negligible		Cefotetan	Negligible (5%–9%)	
Oxazepam	Negligible				
Phenobarbital	Negligible		Cefotiam	30%–40%	
Zopiclone	Negligible		Cefoxitin	50%	Negligible
Anticholinergics and cholinergics			Cefpirome	50%	Negligible (12%)
Cisapride	Negligible		Cefpodoxime	50%	
Metoclopramide	Negligible		Cefprozil	55%	
Pirenzipine	11–15%		Cefroxadine	50%	
			Cefsulodin	60%	
Anticoagulants, antifibrinolytics, and antiplatelet agents			Ceftazidime	50%	Negligible (16%)
Warfarin	Negligible	Negligible	Ceftizoxime	50%	Negligible
			Ceftriaxone	40%	Negligible (4.5%)
Anticonvulsants			Cefuroxime		20%
Gabapentin	50%		Cephacetrile	50%	
Phenytoin	Negligible	Negligible	Cephalexin	50%	Negligible
Primidone	30%		Cephalothin	50%	
Valproic Acid	Negligible (1%)	Negligible	Cephapirin	20%	
			Macrolide antibiotics		
Antihistamines		Negligible (9%)	Clindamycin	Negligible	Negligible
Cetirizine			Lincomycin	Negligible	Negligible
Cimetidine	10%–20%	Negligible	**Monobactams**		
Famotidine	Negligible	Negligible	Aztreonam	40%	Negligible
Nizatidine	Negligible (10%)		Carumonam	51%	
			Moxalactam	30%–50%	Negligible (15%–20%)
Ranitidine	50%–60%	Negligible (<1%)	**Penicillins**		
			Amdinocillin	32%–70%	Negligible (<4%)
Anti-inflammatory agents					
Azapropazone	Negligible	Negligible	Amoxicillin	30%	
Oxaprozin	Negligible	Negligible	Ampicillin	40%	
Penicillamine	30%		Azlocillin	30%–45%	
Sulindac	Negligible		Carbenicillin	50%	
			Cloxacillin	Negligible	
Antimicrobial agents/ antibacterials			Dicloxacillin	Negligible	
			Methicillin	Negligible	
Aminoglycosides	50%	20%–25%	Mezlocillin	20%–25%	Negligible
Spectinomycin	50%				

Table 2. (continued)

Drug	Hemodialysis	CAPD	Drug	Hemodialysis	CAPD
Nafcillin	Negligible		Antineoplastics and antimetabolites		
Oxacillin	Negligible		Cyclophosphamide	30%–60%	
Penicillin	50%		Etoposide	Negligible	
Piperacillin	30%–50%	Negligible (6%)	Methotrexate	Negligible	
Temocillin	50%	Negligible	Antiulcer agents and antacids		
Ticarcillin	50%	Negligible	Omeprazole	Negligible	
Polymyxins					
Colistin	Negligible	Negligible	Bronchodilators		
Quinolones			Dyphylline	28%	
Ciprofloxacin	Negligible (2%)	Negligible (0.4%–1.6%)	Theophylline	40%	
Enoxacin	Negligible		Cardiovascular agents		
Fleroxacin	Negligible (3%–7%)	Negligible (10%)	Antianginal agents		
Lomefloxacin	Negligible		Diltiazem		Negligible (<0.1%)
Norfloxacin	Negligible		Felodidine	Negligible	
Ofloxacin	Negligible (15%–25%)	Negligible (4%–6%)	Isradipine	Negligible	
Temafloxacin	Negligible (9.4%)		Nifedipine	Negligible (<1%)	Negligible
Sulfonamides			Antiarrhythmics		
Sulfamethoxazole	50%	Negligible (8%)	N-acetylprocainamide	50%	Negligible
Trimethorprim	50%	Negligible (7%)	Amiodarone	Negligible	
Tetracyclines			Bretylium	Negligible	
Doxycycline	Negligible	Negligible	Cibenzoline	Negligible	
Minocycline	Negligible	Negligible	Disopyramide	Negligible (2%–4%)	
Vancomycin	Negligible	Negligible (15%–20%)	Flecainide	Negligible (1%)	Negligible
Teicoplanin	Negligible	Negligible (5%)	Lorcainide	Negligible (8%–12%)	
Antifungals			Mexiletine	Negligible	Negligible
Amphotericin B	Negligible		Procainamide	Negligible	Negligible
Fluconazole	40%	Negligible (18%)	Propafenone	Negligible	
Flucytosine	50%		Quinidine	Negligible (<1%)	
Itraconazole	Negligible	Negligible	Sotalol	40%–57%	
Ketoconazole	Negligible	Negligible	Tocainide	25%	Negligible (2%)
Miconazole	Negligible	Negligible	Antihypertensives		
Antimalarials			Acebutolol	Negligible	
Chloroquine	Negligible		Atenolol	50%	
Quinine	Negligible		Captopril	35%–40%	Negligible (<1%)
Antiparasitics			Cilazapril	Negligible (14%)	
Metronidazole	45%	Negligible	Clonidine	Negligible	
Ornidazole	42%	Negligible (6%)	Diazoxide	Negligible	
Tinidazole	40%		Doxazosin	Negligible	
Antituberculous Agents			Enalapril	50%	
Ethambutol	35%–50%		Esmolol	Negligible	Negligible
Isoniazid	75%		Fosinopril		Negligible (2%)
Para-aminosalicylic acid	50%		Guanfacine	Negligible	
Antiviral Agents			Ketansirin	Negligible	
Acyclovir	60%	Negligible (<10%)	Labetalol	Negligible (2%–5%)	Negligible (0.14%)
Amantadine	Negligible		Lisinopril	50%–60%	
Ganciclovir	Negligible		Metoprolol	Negligible	
Ribavirin	Negligible (8%)		Minoxidil	24%–43%	
Vidarabine	50%				
Zidovudine	Negligible	Negligible			

Table 2. (continued)

Drug	Hemodialysis	CAPD	Drug	Hemodialysis	CAPD
Nadolol	50%		Hypouricemic agents		
Perindopril	55%		Allopurinol (oxipurinol)	40%	
Quinapril		Negligible (2.6%)	Psychotherapeutic agents		
			Lithium	Considerable	Considerable
Urapadil	Negligible (6.5%)		Steroids		
Cardiac inotropes			Prednisone	Negligible	
Digoxin	Negligible	Negligible (8%)	Miscellaneous		
Lipid lowering agents			Cyclosporine	Negligible	
Bezafibrate		Negligible (1.6%)	Sulbactam		Negligible
			Tazobactam	40%	Negligible (11%)
Gemfibrozil	Negligible				

[a] For removal by hemofiltration, see text.

$$\text{Amount Removed (mg)} = \frac{\left(\begin{array}{c}\text{Serum Concentration} \\ \text{(mg/L)}\end{array}\right)\left(\begin{array}{c}\text{Unbound} \\ \text{Fraction}\end{array}\right)}{\left(\begin{array}{c}\text{Ultrafiltration} \\ \text{Rate (L/min)}\end{array}\right)\left(\begin{array}{c}\text{Time of Procedure} \\ \text{(min)}\end{array}\right)}.$$

The ultrafiltration rate and the duration of the hemofiltration procedure are known. The unbound fraction can be found in the tables, namely,

Unbound Fraction = (100 − % Bound)/100.

Serum concentration can be directly measured for many drugs. Alternatively, the average concentration at steady state can be reasonably estimated as follows:

$$\frac{\text{Average}}{\text{Concentration}} = \frac{\text{Dosing Rate (mg/min)}}{\text{Clearance in (mL/min)}}$$
(mg/L)

Dosing rate is the infusion rate for a drug given by continuous I.V. infusion or the dose divided by the dosing interval if given intermittently.

Active metabolites

As noted in the introductory comments, even though many drugs are not themselves eliminated by renal routes, they are converted by the liver to active metabolites that depend on the kidney for excretion. Hence, in patients with renal disease, the metabolite can accumulate, causing its own pharmacologic effect(s) (6,7). For example, meperidine is converted to normeperidine, which is not an analgesic like the parent drug but rather is a central nervous system stimulant. It is excreted by the kidney and accumulates in patients with renal insufficiency. Even in elderly patients with mild decrements in renal function, this metabolite can reach sufficient concentrations to cause seizures. Its use in patients with renal

compromise requires lower doses of meperidine (which may limit its efficacy). A better alternative is to use another analgesic, such as morphine, for which the parent drug and metabolite(s) do not depend on the kidney for elimination.

Procainamide is another good example of the difficulties engendered in constructing dosing regimens when an active metabolite is formed. Procainamide is a Type IC antiarrhythmic agent that is metabolized by the liver to N-acetylprocainamide (NAPA), a drug with a different spectrum of antiarrhythmic effect (Type III) than procainamide. In patients with normal renal function, procainamide concentrations exceed those of NAPA, and the latter has negligible pharmacologic effects. As such, dosing regimens are aimed at maintaining therapeutic concentrations of the parent drug. In patients with renal insufficiency, NAPA accumulates and often reaches concentrations exceeding those of procainamide. In this circumstance, the patient essentially has circulating pharmacologic (and perhaps toxic) concentrations of two different antiarrhythmics. Designing a dosing regimen that will precisely maintain the desired concentrations of each is virtually impossible. Hence, therapy can be hazardous, and alternative drugs should be sought.

Table 3 lists drugs that are converted to active metabolites that in turn are eliminated by the kidney. It is important to emphasize that numerous other drugs are metabolized to active compounds that are eliminated by other routes (e.g., many benzodiazepines); for these drugs there is no need for dose adjustment in patients with renal disease. For these drugs listed in Table 3, the degree of accumulation of active metabolite is difficult to predict, and therefore precise dosing guidelines are not possible. If these drugs are used in patients with renal insufficiency, caution is mandatory, and clinical endpoints of drug and metabolite effect must be monitored closely. Whenever possible, it would seem prudent to use alternative therapeutic agents.

Table 3. Drugs with active metabolites dependent on the kidney for elimination

Drug	Active metabolite	Drug	Active metabolite
Analgesics		Antineoplastics and	
Meperidine	Normeperidine	antimetabolites	
Morphine	Morphine-6-glucuronide	Cyclophosphamide	4-Hydroxycyclophosphamide
Propoxyphene	Norpropoxyphene		Aldophosphamide
Anesthetics and drugs used		Antispasticity agents	
during anesthesia		Dantrolene	Hydroxy and amino
Pancuronium	3-OH pancuronium		metabolites
Antianxiety agents, sedatives,		Cardiovascular agents	
and hypnotics		Antiarrhythmics	
Buspirone	1-(2-Pyrimidinyl)-piperazine	Disopyramide	Mono-N-desisopropyl-
Anticoagulants, antifibrinolytics,			disopyramide (MND)
and antiplatelet agents		Encainide	O-desmethylencainide
Sulfinpyrazone	Thioether metabolite		(ODE)
Anticonvulsants			3-Methoxy-ODE (MODE)
Primidone	Phenylethylmalonamide	Flecainide	Meta-O-dealkylflecainide
Valproic acid	Not identified	Procainamide	N-acetylprocainamide
Antihistamines			(NAPA)
Cimetidine	Cimetidine sulfoxide	Antihypertensives	
Hydroxyzine	Cetirizine	Acebutolol	N-acetylacebutolol
Nizatidine	N_2-monodesmethylnizatidine		(diacetolol)
Antimicrobial agents/		Captopril	Mixed disulfides with
antibacterials			endogenous thiols
Cephalosporins		Delapril	Two active metabolites
Cefotaxime	Desacetylcefotaxime		designated M1 & M3
Cefoxitin	Decarbamoylcefoxitin	Methyldopa	Methyldopamine
Cephalothin	Desacetylcephalothin	Metoprolol	α-hydroxymetoprolol
Cephapirin	Desacetylcephapirin	Nitroprusside	Thiocyanate
Macrolides		Blood lipid lowering agents	
Clarithromycin	14-hydroxy (R)-	Clofibrate	Parachlorophenoxyisobutyric
	clarithromycin		acid (CPIB)
Quinolones		Lovastatin	Numerous
Ciprofloxacin	Four different metabolites	Cardiac inotropes	
Enoxacin	3-Oxoenoxacin	Digitoxin	Digoxin
Fleroxacin	N-demethylfleroxacin	Enoximone	Piroximone
Norfloxacin	Six different metabolites	Flosequinan	7-Fluoro-1-methyl-3-
Pefloxacin	N-desmethylpefloxacin and		methylsulfinyl-4-
	norfloxacin		quinolone
Sulfonamides		Diuretics	
Sulfamethoxazole	Acetyl metabolite	Triamterene	Sulfuric ester of
Sulfisoxazole	Acetyl metabolite		hydroxytriamterene
Antifungals		Hypoglycemic agents	
Itraconazole	Hydroxyitraconazole	Acetohexamide	Hydroxyhexamide
Antiparasitics		Tolbutamide	Hydroxytolbutamide
Metronidazole	Hydroxymetabolite		Carboxytolbutamide
Antiviral agents		Hypouricemic agents	
Vidarabine	Hypoxanthine arabinoside	Allopurinol	Oxipurinol

DOSING RECOMMENDATIONS IN PATIENTS WITH VARIOUS DEGREES OF RENAL INSUFFICIENCY

When renal insufficiency affects the volume of distribution of a drug (as previously listed in Table 1 and discussed above), the loading dose must be modified. More commonly, one needs to compensate for decreased clearance of drugs by adjusting the maintenance dose. The principles for doing so have been discussed above, the most important of which is the proportionality that exists between clearance, dose, and steady-state serum drug concentration. Hence, a clearance that is half of normal can be compensated for by decreasing the dose to one half normal.

Table 4. Dosing recommendations in patients with renal insufficiency (relative to normal dose)

Drug	Creatinine clearance (mL/min) >50	20–50	<20	Drug	Creatinine clearance (mL/min) >50	20–50	<20
Analgesics				Cefepime	2/3	1/5	1/8
Codeine			1/2	Cefetamet	1/2	1/4	1/8
Tramadol			1/2	Cefixime		1/2	1/3
Anesthetics and drugs used				Cefmenoxime	1/2	1/4	1/6
during anesthesia				Cefmetazole	2/3	1/2	1/3
Alcuronium			1/3	Cefodizime			1/2
Doxacurium			1/2	Cefonicid	1/2	1/5	1/10
Gallamine			1/8	Ceforanide	1/2	1/3	1/5
Metocurine			1/2	Cefotaxime		1/2	1/4
Pancuronium			1/5	Cefotetan	1/2	1/4	1/10
Pipecuronium			1/2	Cefotiam		3/4	1/2
D-Tubocurarine			1/2	Cefoxitin	1/2	1/4	1/6
Anti-inflammatory agents				Cefpirome		1/2	1/4
Azapropazone	1/2	1/5	1/10	Cefpodoxime		1/4	1/8
Diflunisal			1/2	Cefprodoxime	1/2	1/3	1/5
Indobufen		1/2	1/3	Cefprozil			1/2
Ketoprofen			1/2	Cefroxadine		1/2	1/4
Ketorolac			2/3	Cefsulodin	1/2	1/4	1/10
Oxaprozin			1/2	Ceftazidime	1/2	1/5	1/10
Ximoprofen		1/2	1/3	Ceftizoxime	1/2	1/4	1/10
Anticholinergics and cholinergics				Cefuroxime		1/2	1/4
Metoclopramide		1/2	1/4	Cephacetrile	1/2	1/4	1/10
Neostigmine		1/2	1/3	Cephalexin		1/3	1/10
Pirenzipine			1/2	Cephalothin	2/3	1/2	1/6
Pyridostigmine	1/2	1/3	1/5	Cephapirin		1/2	1/3
Anticoagulants, antifibrinolytics,				Cephradine		1/3	1/10
and antiplatelet agents				Loracarbef	1/2	1/4	1/10
Iloprost			1/2	**Chloramphenicol and**			
Low-molecular-weight				**thiamphenicol**			
heparins			1/2	Thiamphenicol	1/2	1/3	1/10
Sulotroban	1/2	1/5	1/20	**Macrolide antibiotics**			
Tranexamic Acid	1/2	1/4	1/8	Clarithromycin			1/3
Anticonvulsants				Lincomycin		1/2	1/3
Gabapentin	1/2	1/4	1/10	Roxithromycin			1/2
Vigabatrin		1/2	1/4	**Monobactams**			
Antihistamines				Aztreonam	1/2	1/3	1/4
Cimetidine		1/2	1/6	Carumonam	2/3	1/3	1/6
Cetirizine			1/3	Moxalactam	1/2	1/3	1/10
Famotidine	1/2	1/3	1/5	**Penicillins**			
Nizatidine	1/2	1/4	1/4	Amdinocillin		1/2	1/4
Ranitidine	1/2	1/3	1/4	Amoxicillin		1/2	1/6
Roxatidine	3/4	1/2	1/4	Ampicillin	1/2	1/4	1/10
Antimicrobial agents/				Azlocillin		1/2	1/4
antibacterials				Carbenicillin	1/3	1/5	1/10
Aminoglycosides	1/3	1/2	1/4	Methicilin		1/2	1/4
Carbapenems				Mezlocillin	1/2	1/4	1/8
Imipenem		1/2	1/4	Penicillin		1/5	1/8
Meropenem		1/2	1/3	Piperacillin		1/2	1/3
Cephalosporins				Ticarcillin	1/2	1/3	1/4
Cefaclor		1/2	1/4	Timocillin		1/2	1/4
Cefadroxil	1/2	1/4	1/8	**Polymyxins**			
Cefamandole	1/2	1/3	1/4	Colistin	1/2	1/3	1/6
Cefazolin	1/2	1/4	1/6	**Quinolones**			
				Ciprofloxacin			1/2
				Enoxacin	1/2	1/3	1/4
				Fleroxacin	3/4	1/2	1/3

Table 4. (continued)

Drug	Creatinine clearance (mL/min)			Drug	Creatinine clearance (mL/min)		
	>50	20–50	<20		>50	20–50	<20
Lomefloxacin			1/6	Antihypertensives			
Norfloxacin			1/2	Acebutolol		1/2	1/3
Ofloxacin			1/2	Atenolol		1/2	1/4
Temafloxacin	3/4	1/2	1/4	Betaxolol			1/2
Sulfonamides				Benazepril			1/4
Sulfamethoxazole			1/2	Bisoprolol		1/2	1/3
Sulfisoxazole	3/4	1/2	1/4	Captopril	1/2	1/6	1/12
Trimethoprim			1/2	Carteolol		1/2	1/4
Tetracyclines				Cetamolol			1/3
Tetracycline		1/3	1/10	Cilazapril	3/4	1/2	1/4
Vancomycin-like agents				Clonidine		1/2	1/3
Teicoplanin		1/2	1/3	Delapril			1/3
Vancomycin	2/3	1/2	1/10	Diazoxide		2/3	1/2
				Enalapril		1/3	1/5
Antifungals				Fosinopril			1/2
Fluconazole		1/2	1/3	Guanadrel	1/2	1/5	1/10
Flucytosine	1/2	1/3	1/4	Lisinopril		1/2	1/4
Miconazole			1/3	Methyldopa			1/2
Terbinafine			1/2	Metoprolol			1/2
				Minoxidil			1/2
Antimalarials				Moxonidine			1/3
Chloroquine	1/2	1/5	1/10	Nadolol	3/4	1/2	1/4
				Pentopril		Avoid	
Antituberculous agents				Perindopril			1/10
Ethambutol		1/2	1/3	Quinapril	1/2	1/4	1/8
Isoniazid			1/2	Ramipril		2/3	1/3
				Rilmenidine	2/3	1/3	1/5
Antiviral agents				Temocapril			1/2
Acyclovir		1/2	1/5	Trandolapril			1/3
Amantadine	1/2	1/5	1/10	Blood lipid lowering agents			
Didanosine			1/3	Acifran			1/4
Ganciclovir	1/2	1/5	1/10	Bezafibrate	2/3	1/3	1/6
Rimantadine			1/2	Ciprofibrate			1/2
Zalcitabine		1/2	1/4	Clofibrate	1/2	1/4	1/10
Zidovudine			1/2	Fenofibrate			1/6
				Lovastatin			1/2
Antineoplastic agents				Cardiac inotropes			
Bleomycin			1/2	Digoxin	1/2	1/3	1/5
Carboplatin		1/2	1/3	Flosequinan			1/3
Etoposide		1/2	1/3	Milrinone			1/10
Methotrexate		Undefined					
Pentostatin			1/2	Hypoglycemic agents			
				Chlorpropamide		Avoid	
Bronchodilators				Tolrestat			1/2
Albuterol			1/3				
Dyphylline		Undefined		Hypouricemic agents			
				Allopurinol	2/3	1/3	1/6
Cardiovascular agents				Colchicine			1/2
Antianginal agents							
Isradipine			1/4	Psychotherapeutic agents			
Antiarrhythmics				Remoxipride			1/2
N-acetylprocainamide (NAPA)		1/2	1/4	Sulpiride	2/3	1/2	1/4
Bretylium			1/5				
Cibenzoline		1/2	1/3	Miscellaneous			
Disopyramide		1/2	1/5	Dextran 40			1/4
Encainide		1/2	1/4	EDTA		1/2	1/4
Flecainide			1/3	Sulbactam			1/5
Procainamide		(See NAPA)		Tazobactam			1/4
Sotalol		1/3	1/8				
Tocainide		3/4	1/2				

Different strategies for dose adjustment have also been discussed; the clinician can change each individual dose, the interval between them, or both. Which strategy to use depends on the drug and the individual patient, but a reasonable starting point for most drugs is to lengthen the interval until a maximum of 24 hours is reached, after which further modification of the individual dose is appropriate.

Table 4 offers recommendations for modification of the maintenance dose in patients with various degrees of renal insufficiency. It must be emphasized that these guidelines should serve only as starting points of therapy. Subsequent dosing requires tailoring the regimen to each individual patient, which in turn must be based on clinical endpoints and/or measurement of serum concentrations of drugs.

REFERENCES

1. Brater DC: *Pocket Manual of Drug Use in Clinical Medicine*, 6th ed. Improved Therapeutics, Inc., Indianapolis, IN, 1993.
2. Brater DC: The pharmacological role of the kidney. *Drugs* 19:31–48, 1980.
3. Bjornsson TD: Nomogram for drug dosage adjustment in patients with renal failure. *Clin Pharmacokinet* 11:164–170, 1986.
4. Bennett WM, Muther RS, Parker RA, Feig P, Morrison G, Golper TA, Singer I: Drug therapy in renal failure: dosing guidelines for adults. Part I: Antimicrobial agents, analgesics. *Ann Intern Med* 93:62–89, 1980.
5. Bennett WM, Muther RS, Parker RA, Feig P, Morrison G, Golper TA, Winger I: Drug therapy in renal failure: dosing guidelines for adults. Part II: Sedatives, hypnotics, and tranquilizers; cardiovascular, antihypertensive, and diuretic agents; miscellaneous agents. *Ann Intern Med* 93:286–325, 1980.
6. Drayer DE: Pharmacologically active drug metabolites: therapeutic and toxic activities, plasma and urine data in man, accumulation in renal failure. *Clin Pharmacokinet* 1:426–443, 1976.
7. Verbeeck RK, Branch RA, Wilkinson GR: Drug metabolites in renal failure: pharmacokinetic and clinical implications. *Clin Pharmacokinet* 6:329–345, 1981.
8. Koch-Weser J: Serum drug concentrations as therapeutic guides. *N Engl J Med* 287:227–231, 1972.
9. Grenblatt DJ, Koch-Weser J: Clinical pharmacokinetics. *N Engl J Med* 293:702–705, 964–970, 1975.
10. Gibaldi M, Levy G: Pharmacokinetics in clinical practice. I. Concepts. *JAMA* 235:1864–1867, 1976.
11. Gibaldi M, Levy G: Pharmacokinetics in clinical practice. 2. Applications. *JAMA* 235:1987–1992, 1976.
12. Oie S: Drug distribution and binding. *J Clin Pharmacol* 26:583–586, 1986.
13. Reidenberg MM, Drayer DE: Alteration of drug–protein binding in renal disease. *Clin Pharmacokinet* 9:18–26, 1984.
14. Gulyassy PF, Bottini AT, Stanfel IA, Jarrard EA, Depner TA: Isolation and chemical identification of inhibitors of plasma ligand binding. *Kidney Int* 30:391–398, 1986.
15. Anttila M, Haataja M, Kasanen A: Pharmacokinetics of naproxen in subjects with normal and impaired renal function. *Eur J Clin Pharmacol* 18:263–268, 1980.
16. Sheiner LB, Rosenberg BG, Marathe VV: Estimation of population characteristics of pharmacokinetic parameters from routine clinical data. *J Pharmacokinet Biopharm* 5:445–479, 1977.
17. Gault MH, Churchill DN, Kalra J: Loading dose of digoxin in renal failure. *Br J Clin Pharmacol* 9:593–597, 1980.
18. Burton ME, Vasko MR, Brater DC: Comparison of drug dosing methods. *Clin Pharmacokinet* 10:1–37, 1985.
19. Chennavasin P, Brater DC: Nomograms for drug use in renal disease. *Clin Pharmacokinet* 6:193–214, 1981.
20. Hull JH, Sarubbi FA: Gentamicin serum concentrations: pharmacokinetic predictions. *Ann Intern Med* 85:183–189, 1976.
21. Prins JM, Büller HR, Kuijper EJ, Tange RA, Speelman P: Once versus thrice daily gentamicin in patients with serious infections. *Lancet* 341:335–339, 1993.
22. Gilbert DN: Once-daily aminoglycoside therapy. *Antimicrob Agents Chemother* 35:399–405, 1991.
23. The International Antimicrobial Therapy Cooperative Group of the European Organization for Research and Treatment of Cancer: Efficacy and toxicity of single daily doses of amikacin and ceftriaxone versus multiple daily doses of amikacin and ceftazidime for infection in patients with cancer and granulocytopenia. *Ann Intern Med* 119:584–593, 1993.
24. Gibson TP, Nelson HA: Drug kinetics and artificial kidneys. *Clin Pharmacokinet* 2:403–426, 1977.
25. Chrsitopher TG, Blair AD, Forrey AW, Cutler RE: Hemodialyzer clearances of gentamicin, kanamycin, tobramycin, amikacin, ethambutol, procainamide, and flucytosine, with a technique for planning therapy. *J Pharmacokinet Biopharm* 4:427–441, 1976.
26. Gwilt PR, Perrier D: Plasma protein binding and distribution characteristics of drugs as indices of their hemodialyzability. *Clin Pharmacol Ther* 24:154–161, 1978.

CHAPTER 64

Donor and Recipient Selection

STUART M. FLECHNER

INTRODUCTION

Kidney transplantation has evolved from an experiment to the preferred form of replacement therapy for the majority of patients suffering from end-stage renal disease (ESRD) (1,2). During the 1980s, the number of transplants performed in the United States increased yearly, but has now plateaued at about 10,000 cases per year due primarily to the current ceiling of available cadaveric organs (3,4). This fact, coupled with an ever-increasing number of new patients maintained on dialysis, has made transplantation available to no more than 5% of the current ESRD population. As reported to the Health Care Financing Administration by January 1, 1992, there were 180,000 patients receiving dialysis therapy of all types in the United States (5). In the previous year, 10,052 received kidney transplants—7667 from cadaveric donors and 2385 from living donors—which left an additional 18,314 patients on active waiting lists for a donor kidney (6). It has also been estimated that an additional 10,000–20,000 ESRD patients would elect to receive a kidney transplant if they received further education and information and if the available pool of cadaveric kidneys were expanded.

The increasing demand for transplantation is a natural trend that parallels the diminished morbidity and mortality experienced by today's recipients as compared to the earlier generations of transplanted patients (7–9). These results, coupled with improved graft survival, have encouraged more and more patients to seek the transplant option. At the same time, improved results have expanded the pool of potential recipients for which transplantation can be safely performed. Absolute criteria that previously rendered a patient too old, too young, too small, too debilitated, or too atherosclerotic or diabetic have been liberalized or even eliminated by most transplant centers (10). The primary indication for transplantation today is the patient-driven desire to return to preillness levels of activity, well-being, self-image, employment status, and sexual performance. While not a cure for renal failure, a well-functioning renal allograft comes closest to achieving these goals (1,11–13). However, the proper evaluation of every potential recipient and donor is of critical importance to ensure the best clinical outcome and the best utilization of a limited resource.

INDICATIONS FOR TRANSPLANTATION

The option of renal transplantation should be entertained by any patient with permanent renal failure, even though not every patient would be medically suitable nor would desire a surgical form of therapy. In addition, the unique risks and responsibilities required of an individual receiving chronic immunosuppression would not be appropriate for all. Nevertheless, a complete discussion of treatment options at the onset of renal failure permits maximal patient involvement in treatment planning. A candid presentation of treatment options may relieve anxiety among individuals who feel a loss of control over their own destiny (14). Such feelings are not uncommon among patients who are diagnosed with a lifelong chronic illness.

Nephrologists and transplant surgeons often debate the merits of kidney transplantation versus those of chronic dialysis for ESRD therapy. It is more constructive, however, to consider renal transplantation and dialysis as complementary forms of replacement therapy, rather than as competing alternatives. In reality, most recipients have been dialyzed for months or years after the onset of ESRD, and most will return to dialysis either after a failed transplant while awaiting another kidney or permanently (15).

There is little controversy that patients with a functioning renal allograft enjoy increased exercise tolerance that permits increased physical activity, participation in sporting events, and travel (1,11–13,16). For many, increased libido, sexual performance, and the ability to have children are major contributors to an improved sense of well-being (17,18). In addition, many patients afflicted with persistent uremic symptoms such as chronic nausea, vomiting, hiccups, headaches, pruritus, leg cramps, belching, weakness, lassitude, loss of appetite, etc. while on dialysis experience dramatic relief with a functioning kidney transplant (19).

Suki, WN and Massry SG (eds), Suki and Massry's Therapy of Renal Diseases and Related Disorders, Third Edition. ISBN 978-1-4757-6634-9.

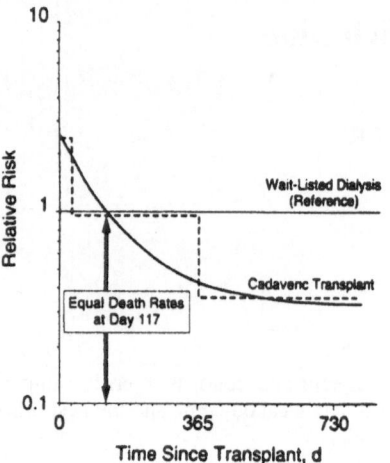

Figure 1. Relative risk of mortality for cadaveric transplant recipients over time after transplantation versus wait-listed dialysis patients. The continuous line describes an exponential decay in relative risk, while the interrupted line shows the relative risk for 0–30, 31–365, and more than 365 days. From Port et al. (27).

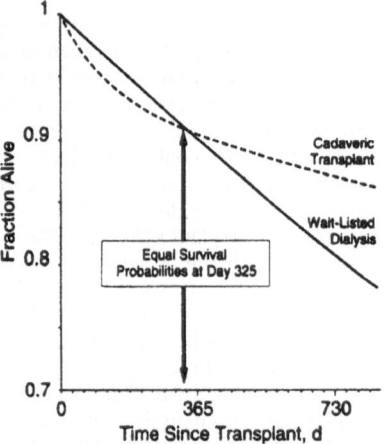

Figure 2. Adjusted actuarial survival probabilities for cadaveric transplant recipients and wait listed dialysis patients. From Port et al. (27).

Other uncontrollable uremic complications such as peripheral neuropathy, pleurisy, pericarditis, enteropathy, hyperparathyroidism, and (less commonly) anemia are also usually reversed when adequate renal function returns. These changes permit the majority of motivated recipients to return to the work force and to pursue educational goals that were sharply curtailed when the diagnosis of renal failure was made.

There remains lingering controversy as to the impact of transplantation on survival in ESRD patients as compared to survival with chronic dialysis. Since no prospective analysis of the question has been done in which the treatment option is truly randomized, the answer continues to be subjective. Most comparisons of survival between dialysis and transplantation are flawed due to poor case mix and uneven comorbidities (6,9,20,21). The common practice has been to select younger, healthier patients for transplantation and to triage older patients, many of whom have multiorgan system disease, to dialysis (21,22). In addition, many previous studies did not account for a time-to-treatment bias, which results from the time accrued on dialysis waiting for a cadaveric organ for transplant (20,23—25). Since the risk of dying on dialysis is relatively high during the first few months of ESRD therapy, it is survivors on dialysis who are actually transplanted (26). With these limitations in mind, and given attempts to control for comorbid conditions, a general consensus would be that 5-year survival is about the same for dialysis patients and recipients of cadaver renal transplants. Recipients who are fortunate enough to receive a kidney from a living relative would enjoy about a 10% increase in survival during this interval (20–26). The one determinant that favors transplantation in each category is the diagnosis of diabetes mellitus (23,27).

In an attempt to bypass some of the above confounding limitations, Port et al. looked at this question from a different perspective (27). They tracked the survival of all patients placed on cadaver waiting lists in Michigan between 1984 and 1989, with time 0 being date of listing, thus eliminating the question of selection bias for transplantation and including the time that recipients on dialysis await a transplant. They compared the relative risk of mortality (RR) between those transplanted and those remaining on the waiting list, adjusting for age, sex, race, and primary cause of ESRD. They found an initial increased mortality risk for transplantation, presumably due to surgery-related complications and heavy immunosuppression. However, by day 117 these risks equalized, and after day 325 a distinct survival advantage was observed for those who received transplants (RR, 0.36; $p < 0.001$) (Figures 1 and 2). This lower long-term risk was most pronounced (RR, O.25) among diabetic recipients ($p < 0.001$), but was not significant among patients with glomerulonephritis as the cause of ESRD.

The timing of renal transplantation may also have a significant impact on outcome. Some renal physicians advocate a mandatory period of dialysis prior to transplantation so that patients can "get used to" their diagnosis of ESRD. In some circumstances, this approach may be psychologically beneficial, especially when renal function has been waxing and waning or when the etiology of renal failure is uncertain. Clearly, transplantation should not be performed as an emergency, and patients who first present in florid uremia require acute dialysis and stabilization. However, among those with slowly progressing renal fail-

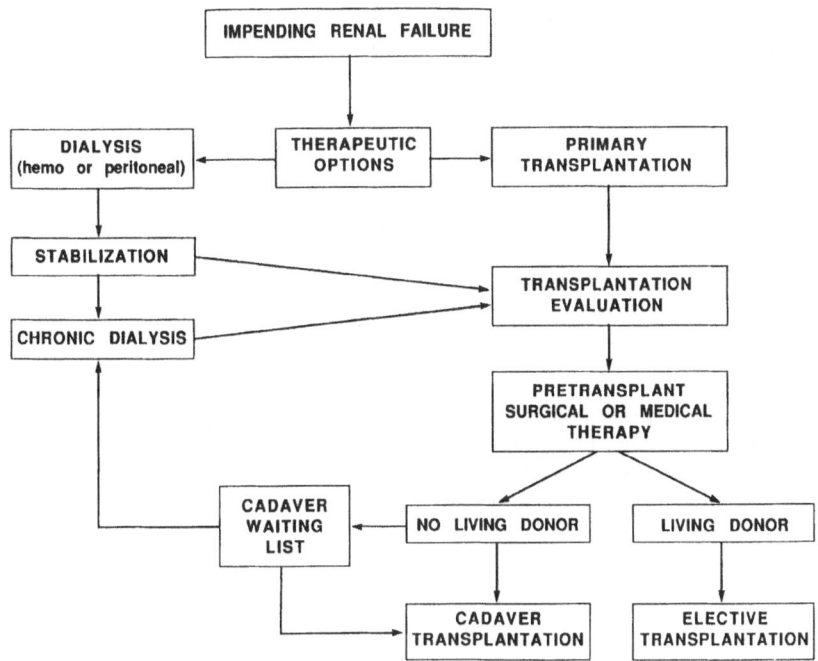

Figure 3. Patient options in end-stage renal disease.

ure, many highly motivated individuals have requested that the transplant be performed prior to the need for chronic dialysis (28,29). These patients see elective or preemptive transplantation as less disruptive to their lives, and they can avoid (or at least delay) the additional surgery required to create vascular access. Such an approach in carefully screened and selected patients can be taken successfully, especially when a living donor is available. Therefore, the patient with ESRD has several options to consider in the choice and timing of renal replacement therapy (Figure 3). Ultimately, though, the majority of transplant recipients will come from the pool of patients on chronic dialysis. They will be waiting for a cadaver kidney, a relatively diminishing resource. They will seek the option of transplantation because they want to feel better and return to a more normal life.

CONTRAINDICATIONS TO TRANSPLANTATION

The ever-increasing worldwide shortage of donor organs necessitates a strategy of donor allocation that provides for the best possible outcome among a given ESRD population (3,30–32). The altruism of donor families, which is the engine that drives organ donation, is dependent on the doctrine that needy recipients will have equitable access to organs and that recipient selection will be based on sound medical criteria. While it is beyond the scope of this chap-

ter to debate the socioeconomic, moral, psychosocial, ethical, and ultimately political ramifications of organ distribution, it remains an inherent responsibility of all transplant practitioners to ensure that the "gift" of organ donation is allocated wisely (33). It is therefore useful to identify those that are least likely to benefit from renal transplantation.

Simply put, the option of renal transplantation should not be entertained when the risks of the surgical procedure and the attendant lifelong use of immunosuppressive drugs outweigh the benefits of a functioning kidney. Each individual must be carefully evaluated for any coexisting medical or psychosocial problem that would lead to a poor outcome if left uncorrected (34). The following considerations should be part of the process of patient evaluation.

Chronological age has often been a barrier to transplantation, with arbitrary cutoffs established for upper and lower age ranges at many centers. While over a decade ago, the ideal candidate may have been between 15–45 years of age, improved transplant practice and delivery of immunosuppression have permitted the transplantation of small children of less than 10 kg in weight and older patients in their 60s and 70s. The physiological age of the patient is a more significant determinant of outcome (22,39). Such older candidates should be aggressively screened for active cardiovascular disease. Posttransplant myocardial infarction, stroke, and peripheral vascular disease remain the most common cause of morbidity and mortality in these patients, whether they are transplanted or remain on dialysis (40). Therefore, careful history and physical examination and the liberal use of noninvasive and invasive (angiography) studies, when indicated, best determine suitability for transplantation (41,42). The older age patient with atherosclerotic disease should have realistic goals regarding rehabilitation and physical activity. Those patients with severe, noncorrectable atherosclerotic disease and little expectation for physical rehabilitation are probably best served by chronic dialysis, regardless of their chronological age. On the other hand, those patients with identifiable atherosclerotic lesions should have these repaired by surgery and/or angioplasty prior to transplant (42,43).

Small children less than 20 kg in size have been considered high-risk patients due to the technical difficulties associated with dialysis and surgery in this group (44). In addition, many small babies with progressive uremia are severely malnourished and have somatic and neurological growth retardation. The wisdom of replacement therapy for uremic infants with severe cerebral impairment, and possibly with other nonrenal organ system anomalies, has been questioned (45). Clearly, such decisions should be carefully individualized and require the input of the parents and other social, ethical, religious, and legal support services where appropriate. Refinements in pediatric anesthesia, intensive care practice, and surgical technique have substantially improved transplant outcome, and size per se should no longer be considered an contraindication (46–48). While some have advocated the transplantation of small infants on an urgent basis, such a practice is rarely if ever indicated. Small uremic children can be safely stabilized with peritoneal dialysis (49). During this period of time, they can be nutritionally repleted. The use of small nasogastric tubes for enteral hyperalimentation during continuous peritoneal dialysis has been a major advance. Since many such children have willing parental donors, the once high-risk endeavor of transplanting small children can now proceed in an orderly, elective fashion.

Patients with metastatic malignancy should not be transplanted regardless of which organ system is involved. The use of continuous immunosuppressive therapy may exacerbate tumor growth and prevent a cure (50). A dilemma arises concerning the transplantation of patients who have been considered cured of a primary malignancy. It would appear that the incidence of tumor recurrence posttransplant is inversely proportional to the length of time after tumor excision (51). This point is best illustrated by the rates of tumor recurrence after the excision of a symptomatic renal cell carcinoma. If patients are transplanted within 12 months of nephrectomy, the recurrence rate is 48%; between 13 and 24 months, the rate drops to 20%; after 24 months, to 14%; and no recurrences reported if the interval is over 4 years. Interestingly, no recurrences of asymptomatic incidentally excised renal cancers have been

reported posttransplant (51). Using data reported to the Cincinnati Tumor Transplant Registry, Penn has suggested the following plan. It is prudent to wait 2 years after excision of most solid tumors to insure that a potential recipient remains free of disease. For aggressive cancers such as breast adenocarcinomas, colon cancer, soft tissue sarcomas, and melanomas, a 5-year cancer-free survival may be more appropriate. Transplantation can proceed more quickly for less aggressive cancers such as nonmelanoma skin cancer, bladder papillomas, and small solitary foci of well-differentiated malignancies (52). Such an approach should result in the reasonable goal of recurrences in under 10% of those subsequently transplanted and immunosuppressed.

Renal transplantation should be delayed or even avoided in patients with active infectious disease (53). Patients should be carefully screened to rule out bacterial, viral, fungal, and/or parasitic infections that can have life-threatening consequences under immunosuppressive therapy. All infectious illnesses should be properly diagnosed, treated with full courses of antibiotics and/or surgical drainage, and adequately monitored after therapy is complete (54,55). This approach also applies to a number of occult and at times asymptomatic infections such as sinus infections, dental abscesses, perirectal abscesses, vaginal discharges, nonhealing bone or osteomyelitis, chronic epididymitis or prostatitis, and infected vascular access grafts or peritoneal dialysis catheters (56). Chronic leukocytosis or eosinophilia should not be overlooked in a dialysis-dependent population. Newly uncovered cardiac murmurs should be thoroughly evaluated as well.

Patients with active tuberculosis (TB) should complete a full course of therapy prior to transplantation (57,58). This usually entails two-drug therapy for pulmonary TB and three-drug therapy for extrapulmonary TB. Patients with well-documented renal tuberculosis should have the effected renal unit removed, since drug delivery will be inadequate in tubercular nonfunctioning kidneys (59). Potential recipients with a well-documented but remote history of TB, or those with a strong likelihood of recent exposure, create a special problem. Skin testing may not be useful due to the high frequency of anergy in uremic patients. Such patients are probably best treated with prophylactic isoniazid posttransplant. However, possible hepatotoxicity and drug interactions due to isoniazid may complicate posttransplant management.

Current evidence suggests that ESRD patients infected with the human immunodeficiency virus should not be transplanted. The use of immunosuppression in these patients may increase their rate of demise, although graft function appears to be satisfactory (60,61). Patients with progressive liver disease such as cirrhosis and clinically active hepatitis should not undergo renal transplantation, since many will progress to end-stage liver disease (62–66). ESRD patients who are infected with the hepatitis B virus continue to be a high-risk group for renal transplantation.

Infected patients who are given immunosuppression have a decreased ability to clear the virus and are at greater risk to develop chronic active hepatitis, cirrhosis, and hepatomas, resulting in greater mortality (62–71). Many prior observations of hepatitis-B-positive transplanted patients were made in recipients given azathioprine and prednisone therapy (67,72). The question of possible azathioprine-induced liver injury has been raised. However, since many patients initially given cyclosporine also end up on azathioprine-containing triple therapy, this association will continue (73). Patients with only elevated liver transaminases need to be monitored, delaying transplantation until those fluctuations resolve. A liver biopsy may be helpful to identify those with chronic active hepatitis and/or cirrhosis. Previous reports have demonstrated that regardless of liver function test abnormalities, patients with histologic evidence of chronic active hepatitis or cirrhosis are at the greatest risk for progressive liver disease and death. However, since there are no prospective studies demonstrating that hepatitis-B antigen-positive patients have a greater life expectancy with dialysis vis-à-vis transplantation, each case must be carefully individualized, and potential recipients with hepatitis B should be apprised of their increased risk of progressive liver disease (66,74). Recent evidence suggests that this increased risk may not be the case for patients who are seropositive for the hepatitis C virus but who have no active disease (74–77). For those patients who were seropositive for hepatitis C but had normal liver function tests at the time of transplant, the 5-year outcomes were not different from those who were seronegative at the time of transplantation (78).

Noncompliance with the prescribed transplant regimen, most notably with immunosuppressive drugs, has become one of the leading causes of late graft loss (79). Noncompliance may be due to patient dissatisfaction with transplant outcome or specific side effects and complications due to these drugs. Some reports have pointed out several risk factors that can be identified prior to transplantation. A past record of medical noncompliance, hostility to the medical personnel, psychiatric disorders, a dysfunctional family unit, depression, lower socioeconomic status/lack of medical sophistication, and adolescence should alert the transplant team to the potential for noncompliance (80). This issue should be carefully screened during the pretransplant evaluation, preferably by the social service and/or psychological support staff. Patients who are incapable or unwilling to comply with the complex posttransplant regimen should not be transplanted unless a reasonable program of supervision can be implemented. A similar consideration should be made for potential recipients with a recent or current history of substance abuse. A period of observation, such as 6 months, with random drug screening should be implemented. This may require the assistance of drug counseling and rehabilitation personnel as well as coordination with the dialysis unit.

CAUSES OF ESRD LEADING TO TRANSPLANTATION

The diagnoses listed in Table 1 represent the leading causes of kidney disease that eventuate in the diagnosis of end-stage renal disease. This large spectrum includes both congenital and acquired renal disease and those diseases isolated to the kidney as well as those associated with systemic disease. With a few exceptions, patients with any

Table 1. Most common forms of chronic renal failure leading to renal transplantation

Glomerular disease
  Membranoproliferative glomerulonephritis
  Rapidly progressive glomerulonephritis
  Antiglomerular basement membrane disease
  Membranous nephropathy
  IgA nephropathy (Berger's)
  Focal segmental glomerulosclerosis
Diabetic nephropathy
Arteriolar nephrosclerosis
  Essential hypertension
  Malignant hypertension
  Bilateral renovascular disease
Interstitial disease
  Chronic pyelonephritis
  Analgesic nephropathy
  Toxic nephropathy
Congenital disorders
  Renal agenesis
  Renal dysplasia
  Posterior urethral valves
  Vesicoureteral reflux
  Prune-belly syndrome
  Ureteropelvic junction obstruction
Neurogenic bladder
  Congenital (meningomyelocele)
  Acquired
Hereditary diseases
  Polycystic kidney disease
  Medullary cystic disease
  Alport's syndrome
Nephrolithiases
  Infection stones
  Hyperoxaluria
  Cystinuria
Systemic diseases
  Lupus erythematosus
  Hemolytic uremic syndrome
  Amyloidosis
  Scleroderma
  Polyarteritis nodosa
  Henoch-Schonlein purpura
Infections
  Tuberculosis
  Schistosomiasis
Surgicalnephrectomy
  Trauma
  Renal malignancy

of these primary diagnoses have been successfully transplanted with either a living related or a cadaveric organ. When the practice of transplantation was in its early stages, the predominant recipient was a young male age 20–40 with some form of congenital nephropathy or glomerulonephritis. Now, however, the demographics of both the recipient population and those waiting for a transplant have changed. According to data on United States residents reported the Health Care Financing Administration at the end of 1991 (5), over 58% of the individuals on dialysis were over the age of 50, and 46% were female. In addition, nearly 37% of the transplants done that year were in individuals over age 44, and nearly 40% were female (6).

The predominant etiologies for renal failure in those patients receiving renal transplants have also changed. While all forms of glomerulonephritis are still the most frequent etiology (26%), diabetes is now the second most frequently encountered diagnosis (21%), followed by hypertension (14%), cystic disease of the kidney (8%), other causes (8%), urologic disorders (previously obstructive uropathy) (6%), cause unknown (7%), and missing information (9%). It is not unusual for patients to seek medical attention after their chronic renal failure is so far advanced that they have small shrunken kidneys. At such a late stage, it is often impossible to define the cause of renal failure—hence the "unknown etiology" category. Interestingly, over 11,000 new patients entering dialysis for the first time each year enter into this category.

As might be predicted, patients with primary glomerular diseases may develop recurrent disease in the transplant kidney. The rates of recurrence of membranoproliferative glomerulonephritis, focal sclerosis, IgA nephropathy, and antiglomerular basement membrane (anti-GBM) disease have been reported to be as high as 50% on posttransplant biopsies (81–85). However, the continuous use of immunosuppressive drugs may significantly retard the progression of recurrent disease, and actual graft loss from recurrent disease occurs in only a few percent of patients (86). A rapid recurrence of focal segmental sclerosis has been reported, with heavy proteinuria and the nephrotic syndrome occurring as early as several weeks posttransplant (87). Anecdotal reports of the use of increased immunosuppression and plasma exchange have slowed this progression in some patients (88,89). De novo disease such as membranous nephropathy has also been reported (90,91). While the fear of recurrent disease should not alter the decision to proceed with transplantation, the timing of the transplant should be considered carefully. Patients with a very rapid and aggressive course to renal failure, such as those with focal segmental sclerosis, rapidly progressive crescentic glomerulonephritis, or high titers and anti-GBM or circulating immune complexes, should probably wait 6–12 months on dialysis until the disease is quiescent.

Insulin-dependent diabetics compose a steadily increasing percentage of the ESRD population. They now represent up to 30% of transplant recipients in many centers (92). Although transplantation is not a cure for diabetes, uremic diabetics often experience dramatic improvement in exercise tolerance, mobility, and well-being after renal transplantation. Much of this improvement is due to a reversal of uremic neuropathy, which often compounds the peripheral neuropathy of diabetes (93). Diabetics with severely compromised vision often experience a degree of rehabilitation similar to sighted patients and should not be excluded from transplantation (94). Unfortunately, progressive vasculopathy posttransplant continues, which leads to a higher frequency of myocardial infarction, stroke, and amputation than in the nondiabetic transplant population (95). For this reason, it is very important to screen diabetics for correctable coronary artery, carotid, and peripheral vascular lesions prior to transplantation. The improving results with simultaneous pancreas–kidney transplantation may provide an additional opportunity for selected patients to slow the progression of diabetic vasculopathy (96,97).

Arteriolar nephrosclerosis, often associated with malignant hypertension, is another frequent cause of renal failure. This disease represents the most common etiology leading to renal transplantation in young black males. While some patients have a dramatic improvement in blood pressure control with the onset of dialysis, others may require nephrectomy to prevent cardiovascular and cerebrovascular accidents. Newer classes of antihypertensive agents have made control of blood pressure in ESRD patients more predictable. It should be noted that control of blood pressure with medications may significantly improve renal function in previously untreated patients as well (98). Such patients should not be transplanted until irreversible renal failure has been established.

The transplantation of patients with metabolic, hereditary, and systemic diseases will be discussed in another chapter. Each group has some unique considerations in recipient preparation and posttransplant management. The transplantation of patients with a previous history of self-destructive behavior leading to renal failure, such as those with analgesic abuse nephropathy, intravenous drug use nephropathy, etc., must be carefully screened and evaluated. This often requires the input of various family, community, social service, and religious support systems (99,100).

PRETRANSPLANT EVALUATION OF THE POTENTIAL RECIPIENT

It is imperative that each potential recipient undergo a complete evaluation prior to transplantation by the team responsible for his or her surgery and immunosuppression. The majority of this evaluation can be done on an outpatient basis; in a few specific instances, some tests may require hospitalization to complete. The main purpose of this evaluation is to uncover any preexisting medical or psychosocial conditions that could lead to increased

Table 2. Pretransplant evaluation for potential recipients

General studies
  History and physical examination
  Pelvic examination, Pap smear
  Stool for occult blood
  Chest radiograph, electrocardiogram
Blood chemistry
  Electrolytes, blood urea nitrogen, creatinine
  Ca, PO$_4$, alkaline phosphatase, parathyroid hormone
  Bilirubin, SGOT, SGPT, LDH
  Amylase, uric acid
  Cholesterol, triglycerides
Hematologic studies
  Complete blood count and differential
  Platelets, prothrombin time, partial thromboplastin time
  Direct Coombs' test
  Cold agglutinins
Serology
  Cytomegalovirus, Epstein–Barr virus, herpes simplex virus,
    Venereal Disease Research Laboratory test
  Human immunodeficiency virus
  Hepatitis A, B, C
Urologic studies
  Urinalysis
  24-hour urine for creatinine clearance, protein
  Voiding cystourethrogram
Radiologic studies
  Ultrasonography of kidneys, liver
  Radiograph of mandible, sinuses
Cultures
  Urine, blood, nasal
Selected studies
  Pulmonary function tests
  Arterial blood gases
  Mammogram (age over 40)
  Barium enema/colonoscopy (age over 50)
  Upper GI endoscopy
  Cystoscopy
  Urodynamic studies
  Abdominal computed tomography
  Vascular Doppler studies
  Stress thallium/coronary angiography
  Echocardiogram
Immunologic studies
  Serum immunoglobulins
  Serum complement
  T-cell subsets
  Panel mixed lymphocyte culture (MLC)
  Spontaneous blastogenesis
  Skin testing, purified protein derivative, mumps, Candida,
    histoplasmosis
Tissue typing
  ABO and Rh
  HLA-A, -B, -Dr
  Anti-HLA cytotoxic antibody screen
  Donor-specific MLC

posttransplant morbidity or mortality. Any such condition, if identified, should be corrected prior to transplant surgery and the administration of immunosuppressive therapy. Such information also serves as a database from which possible complications can be compared to the pretransplant state and different treatment regimens can be evaluated. The absolute list of studies performed may vary from center to center based on different practice philosophies and the distribution of various groups of ESRD patients. For a number of reasons, there has been a tendency to streamline the transplant evaluation, especially when a particular complication has not been observed frequently. In addition, some recipients may wait several years to receive a cadaveric organ from the time they are initially evaluated. Whatever the circumstance, it is incumbent on all transplant practitioners to ensure that patients are thoroughly prepared and can therefore maximize their opportunity for a successful outcome (101). This preparation may require that some screening evaluations are repeated if transplant candidates find themselves waiting many years for a transplant. The following is a representative compilation of a complete pretransplant evaluation (see Table 2). Some tests may have been performed for other indications and may be substituted if current and up to date.

History

The initial history should address the onset of renal failure and its presentation. Hypertension, proteinuria, edema, fever, weight gain, etc. may have resolved or may remain active. The cause of the disease and any available biopsy material should be reviewed. Associated problems such as recurrent urinary tract infections or pyelonephritis, stone disease, or gross hematuria should be explored. If the patient still produces urine, voiding patterns should be ascertained in an effort to diagnose bladder outlet obstruction. Symptoms related to vascular disease should be elicited, specifically those of coronary or carotid artery disease and peripheral vascular disease. A careful gastrointestinal history is important to uncover gall bladder, pancreatic, liver, or peptic ulcer disease symptoms. The family history may uncover a pattern of cancer bleeding diatheses or inherited renal disease. Previous use of immunosuppressive drugs and any complications should be noted. The reasons for previous hospitalizations should be identified. The quantity and time of administration of blood products should be recorded.

Physical examination

The initial physical examination may reflect patient compliance with dialysis and with medical therapy. Fluid overload and edema may represent intentional noncompliance. The eyes may reveal lipid abnormalities or cataracts. The fundi can demonstrate the degree of diabetic retinopathy or nephrosclerosis with hypertension. The cardiac exam may reveal new murmurs that have an infectious origin. All major blood vessels from the carotids to the dorsalis pedis should be palpated and auscultated. Diminished pulses or bruits should be evaluated further. Sources of occult infections such as otitis, dental abscesses, genital or perirectal abscesses, and the lower extremities of diabetics should be carefully inspected. The presence of lymph adenopathy in the inguinal, cervical, and axillary regions should be identified. A pelvic exam in females should include a Pap smear if not done the previous year. The rectal exam should also screen for occult blood in the stool.

Laboratory tests

Blood chemistry and serology studies are important in order to uncover any abnormalities or exposure to infectious agents that could complicate the transplant procedure or subsequent immunosuppression. The goal should be normalize metabolic balance and nutrition for each potential recipient. Anemia should be corrected using both vitamin replacement and erythropoietin, with a target hemoglobin of about 10–11 grams (102,103). Patients found to have a positive VDRL should have confirmation by specific treponemal antibody studies followed by treatment with long-acting penicillin. All potential recipients should be tested for antibody to the HIV virus, using confidentiality procedures and Western blot confirmation as appropriate (104). Prior or current exposure to the cytomegalovirus, Epstein–Barr virus, herpes simplex virus, and those causing hepatitis A, B, or C should be ascertained (105).

Screening immunologic studies test for persistent immune activity, especially in those patients with an autoimmune etiology for kidney failure. These would include patients with systemic lupus erythematosus (SLE), rapidly progressive glomerulonephritis, focal sclerosis, and anti-GBM disease. Such patients who continue to exhibit low complement levels, high titers of anti-GBM antibody, or circulating immune complexes may recur, and therefore should wait a period of 6–12 months on dialysis prior to proceeding with transplantation. For those centers that use immune monitoring to follow transplant recipients, baseline studies such as T-cell subsets, panel MLC, and spontaneous blastogenesis may be useful in identifying strong immune responders. Skin testing to microbial recall antigens along with PPD can identify anergic patients and those at risk for certain infections posttransplant.

Patients with positive blood or urine cultures should be treated after the source of the infection is identified. Cultures should be repeated after treatment to ensure a complete response. In centers where methicillin-resistant *Staphylococcus aureus* is commonly identified, nasal cultures may be a useful way to identify carriers (107).

Urologic studies

Routine evaluation should include a urinalysis; urine culture; 24-hour urine collection for volume, creatinine

clearance, and protein excretion; and a voiding cystourethrogram. Some studies may be limited in patients with oligoanuria, and others may be required only for those with specific complaints. Patients with hematuria, filling defects, incontinence, significant prostatism, or a history of previous lower urinary tract pathology should be cystoscoped. Retrograde pyelograms may be required in certain patients. Selected urodynamic studies may be used for those with incontinence or suggestion of a neurogenic bladder. It should be noted that virtually all ESRD patients with a defunctionalized bladder (<200 cc/day urine output) demonstrate high voiding pressures, uninhibited contractions, and low flow rates. These findings invariably resolve when normal voided volume are restored after transplantation. Men over the age of 40 should have a PSA blood test to screen for occult prostate cancer (108).

Radiographic studies

In addition to the chest x-ray, ultrasound examination of the gall bladder, bile ducts, and pancreas should be done to rule out gall bladder disease. The native kidneys should be examined by ultrasound to rule out stones, tumors, acquired cystic disease, hydronephrosis, etc. An upper GI series or endoscopy is useful for those with a history of peptic ulcer disease or current symptoms, and a barium enema or colonoscopy is useful for older age patients (over 50) who may harbor diverticula or polyps or for those with occult blood in the stool. Plain films of the sinuses, mandible, and teeth often uncover small abscesses.

Selected studies

Patients with an extensive smoking history are instructed to stop prior to transplant. Such patients, and those with a history of frequent pulmonary infections, should undergo pulmonary function tests with blood gases. Reversible bronchospasm should be corrected if identified.

Coronary artery disease is a significant cause of morbidity and mortality posttransplant, especially in the older age population and in diabetics (95,109,110). These patients should be aggressively screened and evaluated for correctable lesions. Patients over 50 or any with cardiac symptoms should initially be screened with a treadmill or exercise-induced stress thallium scan (111). However, quite often noninvasive screening studies such as these fail to produce changes due to a less than maximal effort at heart rate, and are thus inconclusive (112,113). Therefore, in sedentary patients and especially in diabetics, a screening coronary angiogram is strongly recommended (114–116). Potential recipients with critical coronary artery lesions should have these repaired either by angioplasty or bypass surgery prior to transplantation (43,117). Using such a policy, several centers have demonstrated a reduction in death from myocardial infarction in this high-risk group 3–4 years posttransplant (114–116). Doppler studies are useful to screen for carotid and peripheral vascular lesions, especially in symptomatic patients or in those with audible bruits. These lesions should be carefully evaluated and corrected when identified.

SURGICAL PREPARATION FOR TRANSPLANTATION

The use of continuous chemical immunosuppression posttransplant increases the risks of complications for elective or emergency surgical procedures. For example, wound healing is impaired, sutured anastomoses have a greater tendency to leak, and wound hematomas are more likely. Otherwise minor pulmonary problems may also become more difficult to resolve in the immunosuppressed patient. For this reason, it is generally preferable to perform any necessary elective surgery prior to transplantation. This surgery would include more common procedures such as hernia repair, hemorrhoids, cosmetic surgery, skin biopsies, extensive dental work, and orthopedic procedures, etc. The following major surgical procedures may be required in order to prepare a recipient for transplantation and should also be completed and healed prior to the introduction of immunosuppressive drugs.

NEPHRECTOMY

Routine bilateral native nephrectomies are no longer considered a prerequisite for transplantation. The intended indication, removal of the stimulus that triggered immune-mediated renal injury, has been superseded by improved immunosuppression. Another common indication, hypertension, has been made much more manageable by the widespread introduction of new classes of antihypertensive agents. For dialysis-dependent patients, the retention of native kidneys has distinct advantages even if the kidneys are small and contracted; they contribute to red cell production and calcium homeostasis and provide an additional source of fluid and potassium elimination. There are a number of specific indications that remain for pre-transplant nephrectomy, which will be required in about 10%–15% of patients. These indications would include recurrent bacterial pyelonephritis, infected renal cysts, active stone passage, high-grade vesico ureteralreflux with residual urine, hypertension refractory to oral agents, renal tumors, and severe proteinuria causing malnutrition (usually greater than 10 g/24 hr). Occasionally, patients may have massive polycystic kidneys that cause abdominal symptoms or gross hematuria or become so large that they preclude placement of the graft in the iliac fossa. In patients with reflux, tuberculosis, hydronephrosis, or other ureteral pathology, a nephroureterectomy may be required.

Lower urinary tract dysfunction

The increased number of male patients over age 55 who elect the option of transplantation include many with symptoms of prostatism. Those who produce over a liter per day of urine should undergo standard evaluation and, if significantly obstructed, should undergo transurethral (electroresection or laser-assisted) prostatectomy. However, patients who produce small urine volumes are difficult to evaluate and have a propensity to develop bladder neck contractures and strictures after a resection (118). Such patients should await definitive management until urine volumes return to normal after transplantation. The role of pharmacotherapy for prostatic obstruction is currently evolving. Patients who develop retention posttransplant can be successfully managed by intermittent catheterization until definitive therapy is instituted. There is also a significant prevalence of prostatic carcinoma in the elderly male population. Screening with a digital rectal examination and a serum PSA should identify those most likely to harbor an occult carcinoma, which must be diagnosed and treated effectively before consideration for transplantation (108). Patients with urethral stricture disease should be treated by direct vision urethrotomy if possible. More complex reconstructions should be completely healed prior to transplant. If stricture patients produce small urine volumes, daily self-catheterization may be required to prevent recurrent stricture disease.

The adequacy of the bladder to both store and empty can usually be elicited by history and a voiding cystogram, although an occasional patient may need a more detailed urodynamic assessment. If unresolved, bladder filling, emptying, and continence can be reliably tested pre-transplant by the placement of a small percutaneous suprapubic tube and graduated saline irrigation (119). Patients with large flaccid bladders (some diabetics) that empty poorly can be managed posttransplant through the use of intermittent catheterization if their continence mechanism is intact (120). Most small defunctionalized bladders (even less than 50 cc) will dilate nicely after transplantation, even when anuria has been present for many years. However, a few may have contracted noncompliant and fibrosed bladders, most often secondary to tuberculosis, radiation, schistosomiasis, or severe interstitial cystitis. The bladders in such patients, as well as in those with total incontinence or high-pressure neurogenic bladders, are not suitable for transplantation and will require the use of intestinal segments (121,122). Some can be successfully managed by intestinal bladder augmentation, while many will require creation of an ileal conduit (123). In either case, the procedures should be completed at least 4–6 weeks prior to anticipated transplantation.

Splenectomy

Surgical removal of the spleen for the purpose of augmenting immunosuppression was once thought to be an integral component of pretransplant preparation, especially for those recipients undergoing retransplantation. Earlier reports of improved graft survival were no doubt the result of a greater tolerance for azathioprine in splenectomized patients (124). Leukopenia, which often limited the use of antiproliferative agents in patients with intact spleens, is now rarely observed in cyclosporine-treated recipients. In addition, splenectomized patients are known to have a greater long-term risk of sepsis, which has further diminished enthusiasm for the procedure (125). The rare patient may benefit from splenectomy if pancytopenia secondary to massive hypersplenism is present. In another setting, recipients of ABO mismatched kidneys can be salvaged by the combination of splenectomy, plasma pheresis, and antilymphocyte preparations (126).

Parathyroidectomy

The majority of ESRD patients suffer from secondary hyperparathyroidism, which can be medically managed and is readily reversible with a kidney transplant. However, a few develop tertiary hyperparathyroidism, often accompanied by peptic ulcer disease, metastatic calcification, itching, pancreatitis, and severe bone mineral reabsorption. Many of these patients have serum calcium levels at the upper limit of normal, but radioimmunoassay parathormone levels are elevated 10–100 times. These patients should undergo subtotal parathyroidectomy prior to transplantation.

Gastrointestinal disease

Transplant recipients with active peptic ulcer disease are at high risk for bleeding and/or perforation in the early postoperative period when doses of corticosteroids are highest (127,128). Therefore, patients with active disease, recurrent ulcers, and a history of significant bleeding requiring transfusion should have an acid-reducing procedure prior to transplant. The selective vagotomy has become the most popular approach. It is prudent to document complete healing by endoscopy prior to the introduction of immunosuppression. Patients with a history of peptic ulcer disease should remain on H-2 blockers posttransplant (129), although the use of these blockers may complicate cyclosporine nephrotoxicity (130).

The mortality associated with acute cholecystitis in transplant recipients has been reported to be up to 30%. Therefore, patients with active gall bladder disease as well as those with asymptomatic cholelithiases should undergo cholecystectomy prior to transplant (131). Laparoscopic techniques have revolutionized the management of this disease, permitting a more rapid recovery time (132). The laparoscopic approach has also been used successfully on ESRD patients undergoing peritoneal dialysis.

The presence of colon diverticula (usually patients over age 45) is of concern. Those patients with a well-documented history of diverticulitis should have a prophylactic colectomy (usually on the left side) if they are to be immunosuppressed. The mortality of posttransplant colon perforation has been reported to be as high as 50% (133,134). Those patients with scattered diverticula and no history of bowel symptoms need to be apprised of the possibility of perforation and its consequences. Although prophylactic colectomy in these patients seem hard to justify, the decision to proceed with transplantation should not be taken lightly. If possible, these patients should have the graft placed on the right side.

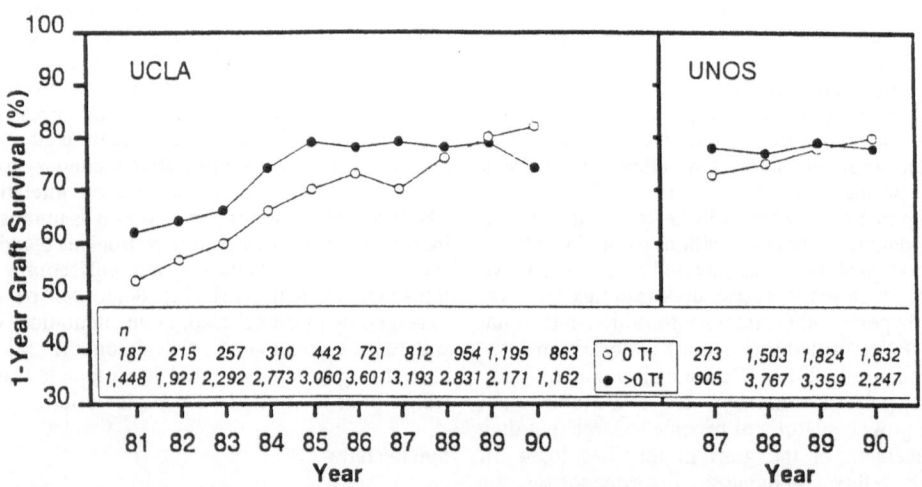

Figure 4. The effect of third-party blood transfusions on 1-year cadaveric graft survival. Results from the UNOS and UCLA data registries. From Terasaki PI, Cecka MJ, eds: *Clinical Transplants.* UCLA Tissue Typing Laboratory, Los Angeles, p 304, 1991.

Blood transfusions

Once thought a necessary component of recipient preparation, intentional third-party blood transfusions have fallen out of favor at most transplant centers. Results of a recently reported survey reveal that only 19% of U.S. transplant centers require preoperative blood transfusions prior to kidney transplantation (135). Previously cited advantages of transfusions included increased graft survival and fewer cases of accelerated graft loss, although the mechanisms responsible for these effects have never been conclusively explained (136). Some have attributed the effect to a "selecting out" of patients who develop broadly reacting cytotoxic antibodies due to the transfusions and subsequently are not transplanted. Others have reported the induction of nonspecific suppressor networks or enhancing antibodies as a theoretical basis for the transfusion effect (137,138). During the past few years, several changes have taken place that have curtailed the enthusiasm for routine transfusions. These have included the use of more potent immunosuppression (139), diminished transfusion requirements with the introduction of human recombinant erythropoietin (102), continued sensitization to disparate HLA phenotypes (140), and the fear of disease transmission (i.e., HIV, CMV, EBV, and hepatitis A, B, C) by blood products. The diminished frequency of pretransplant bilateral nephrectomy and splenectomy has also eliminated the frequent perioperative administration of blood products.

This reversal of previously standard transplant practice is supported by observations made in multicenter trials. In fact, it has now been demonstrated that, with the use of current cyclosporine-based immunosuppression, transfused recipients actually have inferior 1-year graft survival as compared to untransfused recipients of cadaveric kidneys (141) (Figure 4). Excellent patient and graft survival has also been accomplished in cyclosporine-treated untransfused recipients of live donor kidneys (142), although some groups continue to champion the use of donor-specific transfusions in this setting (143). If ESRD patients are to receive pretransplant blood transfusions for no other purpose than to improve graft survival, then it would seem prudent for each transplant center to demonstrate this advantage in its own particular environment. Otherwise, intentional transfusions may only sensitize certain individuals and diminish their opportunity to receive a transplanted organ.

SELECTION OF RENAL DONORS

Human renal allografts come from one of four sources. Healthy, willing, and highly motivated living relatives of the recipient such as siblings, parents, or children provide about 20% of the kidneys transplanted. More distant relatives such as aunts, uncles, grandparents, or cousins may also be suitable donors in certain circumstances. A second source of live donor kidneys is nonbiologically related individuals. A healthy spouse is the most likely representative of this group, but unusually motivated "friends" of the recipient have been used in highly selected circumstances. Currently, the largest number of donor kidneys comes from individuals who have suffered irreversible brain death and whose vital organs can be maintained for a limited period of time by artificial life-support systems. Such organs and tissues come from heartbeating, irreversible brain-dead individuals from whom the organs can be recovered with minimal warm ischemic injury. A fourth source of organs is patients who have suffered recent cardiac arrest and died. Such nonheartbeating organ donors sustain a period of warm ischemia to the kidneys and therefore do not provide a maximally protected organ. However, due to the generalized organ shortage, the possible inclusion of such organs in certain circumstances has been suggested. At the present time, xenograft kidneys have not been successfully transplanted in humans. There are certain advantages and disadvantages to the recipient from each donor source. The selection of the best donor for each recipient should be an individualized process, which often highlights the art of transplantation medicine as well as the science.

Living related donors

The use of living related donors (LRDs) in human renal transplantation has created a unique ethical dilemma for those involved with the daily care of transplant patients. In no other area in medicine is an otherwise healthy individual asked to subject himself or herself to the potential morbidity and mortality of major surgery for no apparent physical benefit. There are two basic reasons why LRD transplants are done, and each presents a variable degree of significance for a given donor–recipient pair. Firstly, LRD kidneys work better and last longer. This fact has been continuously observed using virtually all combinations of nonspecific chemical immunosuppression during the past 30 years (144). Secondly, there is a global shortage of suitable cadaver kidneys (2,3). Therefore, LRD transplantation will expedite the process for some recipients and may permit transplantation to be done in some patients who have been unable to secure a cross-match negative cadaver kidney after waiting an extended period of time. These benefits, which accrue solely to the recipient, must be balanced against the potential short-term and long-term harm to the donor.

Living related renal transplantation has been the clinical laboratory that validates the role of the major histocompatibility complex (MHC), on chromosome 6, in allograft rejection. While the importance of tissue typing in cadaver transplantation is debated, there is little question as to the impact of immune responses evoked by histoincompatibilities among family members. These differences appear to correlate directly with the eventual graft survival and clinical course of the recipient. Assuming that medical

Table 3. Donor selection by immunologic similarity

Monozygotic twins
HLA-identical siblings
Haploidentical siblings, parents, children, relatives
Less than haploidentical siblings, parents, children, relatives
Distant relatives
Unrelated living donors (spouse, etc.)
Cadaveric donors

and psychosocial parameters are equal, donors are selected based on their degree of histocompatibility. Table 3 provides, in descending order, the degree of tissue similarity among potential donors and suggests the order of preference for a specific recipient.

Tissue typing is done to identify the Class I (HLA A, B) and Class II (Dr) antigens present in each family member. Since each individual receives two alleles (one from each parent), a recipient has a 25% chance that a potential sibling donor is identical for each HLA antigen. In addition, there is a 50% chance that the potential sibling donor has inherited the same HLA antigens from one parent (called a haplotype). Since HLA antigens are inherited as a genetic region on chromosome 6 within a family, a specific haplotype may be found in more distant relatives as well. The tissue type between parents and children is almost always haploidentical, but aunts, uncles, grandparents, and cousins may also share a haplotype. The reason that matching among family members has such a powerful effect on outcome is that matching for the known HLA determinants within a family virtually assures compatibility for all the gene products of the entire MHC region. Tissue typing among unrelated individuals does not carry the certainty of linkage with other (as yet undetermined) products of the MHC. These differences and similarities will be further defined as current techniques in molecular biology using specific DNA probes help subclassify these MHC region gene products (145).

An additional MHC region gene product that can be identified is the HLA D-antigen. While this region can be subdivided into DP, DQ, and DR molecules, D-antigen identities can be identified using a mixed lymphocyte culture (MLC). HLA-identical siblings will share HLA D-antigens and will have a nonproliferative MLC reaction. The MLC test, which takes 6–7 days to assay, can be used to further stratify potential donors who have similar serologic HLA typing to a specific recipient. Diminished MLC responses between two individuals may signify similarity not only at the D-locus but also at other, as yet undetermined loci in the MHC region. Therefore, the strength of the MLC response should be coupled with tissue-typing information to select the most compatible potential donor among family members (146).

The first successful human renal transplant was performed between monozygotic twins without immunosuppression (147). Thirty such isografts have been done at the Brigham Hospital in Boston, and no recipient has experience graft rejection (148), thus validating the role of the MHC in human organ transplantation. The most common cause of graft loss in these recipients has been recurrence of glomerulonephritis in the graft or death from unrelated causes. Long-term graft survival in HLA-identical and haploidentical LRD transplants, as compiled by the UNOS Transplant Registry, appears in Figure 5. A clear difference between the LRD groups and cadaveric recipients has been observed consistently, using varying combinations of

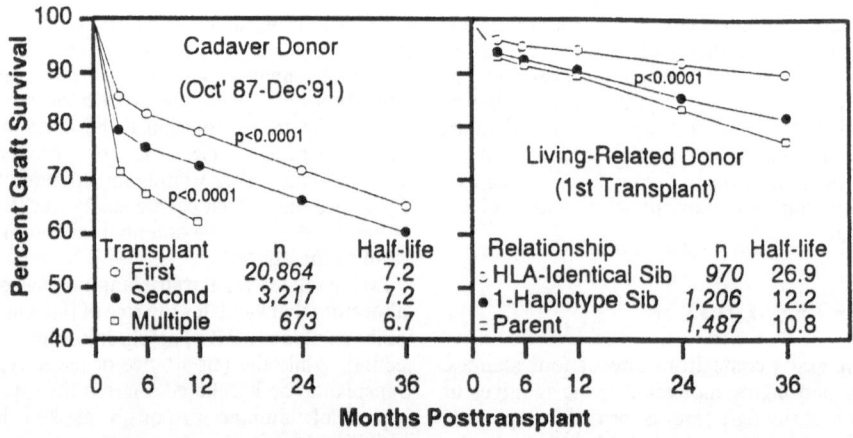

Figure 5. Overall graft survival rates for cadaveric and living related donor transplants. From the UNOS registry. From Terasaki PI, Cecka MJ, eds: *Clinical Transplants.* UCLA Tissue Typing Laboratory, Los Angeles, p 2, 1991.

immunosuppressive therapy. While these curves have been pushed upward and to the right since the introduction of cyclosporine, the powerful effect of histocompatibility remains. Since the advent of cyclosporine, rejection episodes occur in only about 10% of treated HLA-identical recipients, and graft loss is exceedingly rare (149). In addition, many of these patients can be treated with monodrug therapy and can avoid the long-term consequences of steroid therapy (142). The future introduction of newer immunosuppressive agents may further expand the number of recipients who may be adequately controlled with steroid-sparing therapy. Since the introduction of cyclosporine, many groups have reported over 90% 2–3-year graft survival for haploidentical live donor recipients (150,151), although the postoperative and long-term survival is not as favorable as in those fortunate enough to receive an HLA-identical kidney.

Prior to the introduction of cyclosporine-based immunosuppression, a marked improvement in HLA-nonidentical LRD transplants was observed if the recipient was given three pretransplant blood transfusions from the specific kidney donor (DST). As first reported by Cochrum et al., if such patients did not develop donor-specific cytotoxic antibodies to recipient T cells after the transfusions, graft survival of 90% at 1 year could be achieved with azathioprine and prednisone immunosuppression. While some centers have preferred this approach, up to 30% of recipients become sensitized from the DSTs and therefore cannot receive the intended donor kidney (153). This rate may be diminished with the simultaneous use of azathioprine during the DST treatment. Those who remain unsensitized can be transplanted without cyclosporine, thereby avoiding the potential for long-term drug nephrotoxicity. However, the incidence of acute rejection episodes exceeds 60% in DST-prepared patients, which may necessitate further courses of high-dose steroid therapy (153).

Despite the compelling arguments for the use of living donors, such procedures would not be done if significant morbidity or mortality were to be experienced by the donors. The concept of self-sacrifice and organ donation has been extensively examined by the medical, ethical, and legal professions. Postdonation analyses have consistently found that the donor experience was an overwhelmingly positive one, regardless of the outcome of the kidney in the recipient (154,155). The courts have found that donor altruism is an acceptable motivation to undergo nephrectomy. In fact, some courts have found that the donor will not only benefit psychologically and spiritually from the act of charity but also might even be psychologically harmed if prevented from donating when the life and well-being of a loved one is at stake (156). This argument is the basis for the use of potential donors who are legal minors. Life insurance companies have also considered the impact of renal donation. In a survey of over 60 major carriers, 97% responded that they would accept renal donors, assuming that the remaining renal function was normal. Half the companies felt that there is a minimal and temporary risk

to the donor (relating to the surgical procedure), and the other half did not feel there was any increased risk (157,158).

Clearly, renal donation is not an innocuous procedure, since all donors experience some degree of anxiety, physical pain, and disruption of their employment schedule, schooling, and home life. In addition, a degree of pressure and coercion can be present among family members that is not readily apparent to health care professionals. For these reasons, each donor must be given the opportunity to give their independent, informed consent to this decision. We have found that it is very important to counsel the spouse of the potential donor and to permit his or her input into the process as well. It is also helpful to allow the potential donor to determine the pace of the evaluation. Some may truly be undecided, and may require more time to evaluate their commitment or to want to opt out of the process. These complex social interactions make it very difficult to consider minors under age 18 as potential donors in all but the most unusual circumstances.

What then, is the potential risk to the potential renal donor? While the number of donor deaths worldwide is quite low, such deaths have occurred. It has been reported that the 5-year life expectancy of a unilaterally nephrectomized 35-year old healthy male donor will be 99.1% as compared with 99.3% for a matched control with two kidneys (159). Another estimate is that the mortality for donor nephrectomy is less than 0.1% (160). The long-term risk by actuarial methods has been calculated to equal that of commuting in a car 16 miles each working day. Fortunately, major postoperative complications such as life-threatening infections or cardiopulmonary events are rare. Minor complications such as atelectasis, urinary tract infection, phlebitis, urinary retention, etc. are reported to occur in 10%–20% of cases (161). A flurry of concern has been generated from the findings of Brenner et al. that rats who underwent renal ablation were subject to glomerular hyperfiltration in the remnant kidney (162). This process led to glomerular sclerosis and deterioration of renal function, which was related to protein intake and time. However, several studies of renal donors with over 20 years of follow-up failed to identify this problem in humans (162,164,165). Progressive renal deterioration is not observed, and the incidence of hypertension was consistent with that of the population at large. Some uninephrectomized donors did have an increased urinary protein excretion, the implications of which are presently unknown. In an interesting comparative report, adult kidney donors followed for over 20 years were compared to their siblings who did not donate for other than medical reasons (166). Both groups had similar renal function at the time of kidney donation. There was no evidence of progressive renal deterioration or other serious disorder in the donors compared with their siblings. Specifically, there was no significant difference in mean serum creatinine, creatinine clearance, blood urea nitrogen, blood pressure, or the numbers with proteinuria. Whether these findings will remain constant over 40–50 years of follow-up is certainly open to conjecture. Proper informed consent and risk appraisal should continue to be the cornerstone of the living donor evaluation.

Living unrelated donors

The utilization of kidneys from living unrelated individuals is a subject that raises the passions, both pro and con, of many in the transplant community. For some, it is the logical extension of the practice of transplantation; for others it is anathema to the principle *primum non nocere* (first do no harm). The impetus behind the use of living nonrelated donors comes from patients and physicians. Firstly, there has been an undeniable increase in the number of dialysis-dependent patients every year and a corresponding increase in the number of potential recipients awaiting a cadaveric transplant (Table 4). This trend, coupled with an insufficient quantity of available organ donors to meet the demand, creates pressure to explore all donor sources (3,167,168). Secondly, the bond between two individuals, such as husband and wife, is arguably as firm as that between blood relations. The same satisfaction in helping a loved one that is attributed to living related donation can be conveyed by spousal donation. In fact, the improved health and well-being of the recipient may provide more tangible benefits within a household than that obtained by more distant family members. Thirdly, as the results of transplantation continue to improved, the expectation for success with living unrelated donors has never been better. There is little question that the net histoincompatibility in these donor–recipient pairs is as great as that of cadaveric transplantation. However, the virtual elimination of donor ischemia, preservation injury, and the optimal condition of the recipient at the time of transplantation should potentiate the outcome (169). Indeed, 1-year patient and graft survival in excess of 90% has been reported by several centers (169–172). In the U.S., over 400 of these procedures have been done during the last year.

While the arguments for the use of living unrelated donors may appear cogent, they bypass an important reality, namely, that the number of kidneys available for transplantation is far less than the predicted number of potential organ donors that exist. Bart et al. have estimated that between 50 and 100 donors per million population in the United States could be realized each year (173). Currently only 10%–20% of this total is recovered. Therefore, some have argued, greater efforts in education and commitment to cadaveric organ procurement should be undertaken, rather than a reliance on living unrelated donors (174). The latter donors are considered to be merely a solution of expedience and convenience, since the living unrelated donor would be subject to the same risk and uncertain long-term consequences of kidney donation as the living related donor. Perhaps the greatest concern raised over this type of medical intervention is the possibility for

Table 4. Dialysis and transplantation in the united states

Year	Patients on dialysis at year's end	Size of waiting list	CAD TX	LRD TX	LUD TX
1986	112,209	—	7089	1887	—
1987	123,300	—	7002	1890	—
1988	134,456	13,943	7115	1761	56
1989	148,117	16,294	6982	1830	70
1990	165,353	17,883	7712	2001	90
1991	188,942	19,352	7667	2299	86

Source: UNOS 1993 Annual Report. OPTN and Scientific Registry.

Table 5. Pretransplant evaluation of potential living donor

I.   General studies
  a. History and physical exam
  b. Pelvic exam with Pap smear
  c. Stool for occult blood
  d. CXR, EKG
II. Blood chemistry
  a. BUN, creatinine, electrolytes
  b. Total protein, albumin, uric acid
  c. SGOT, SGPT, bilirubin, LDH
  d. Cholesterol, triglycerides, FBS
  e. Ca, PO_4, alkaline phosphatase
III. Hematologic studies
  a. CBC and differential
  b. PT, PTT, platelets
IV. Serology
  a. CMV, VDRL
  b. HIV, EBV
  c. Hepatitis A, B, C
V.   Tissue typing
  a. ABO type
  b. HLA A, B, C, Dr
VI. Urologic studies
  a. Urinalysis
  b. Urine culture
  c. 24-hour urine collection, creatine clearance, protein excretion
VII. Radiographic studies
  a. Excretory urogram
  b. Renal angiogram (standard or DSA)
VIII. Special studies
  a. Glucose tolerance test
  b. Anti islet cell antibodies (diabetic families)

exploitation and commercialization of living organ procurement. Precisely these considerations have made the sale and trafficking of human organs and tissue illegal in the United States (Public Law 98–507) and have been decried by virtually every transplantation organization (175,176).

In conclusion, the decision to use living unrelated donors is not a trivial one and should be carefully individualized by any transplant unit considering this approach. While clearly not a panacea for the global cadaveric organ shortage problem, this decision may have a role in highly selected circumstances. Those teams who wish to perform such procedures should make special efforts to ensure that proper informed consent has been obtained and that donor altruism is the predominant indication to proceed (177). Living unrelated transplantation will thus likely remain limited and should not interfere with the larger goal to expand cadaveric organ-procurement efforts.

Pretransplant evaluation of the potential living donor

The purpose of this pretransplant evaluation is to uncover any preexisting renal disease or predilection for renal disease in the potential donor (Table 5). These patients are also screened for risk factors that would preclude major surgery and general anesthesia. Not surprisingly, certain conditions may be identified that not only will lead to exclusion of the donor but also may require medical or surgical therapy for the donor's benefit. Therefore, prior to evaluation, every potential donor must be informed as to the nature of these studies and how the information will be used. It is important to maintain a strict doctor–patient relationship with donors and to accede to their request for confidentiality. In addition, it is important to identify any diseases that could be transmitted from the donor to the recipient by the transplanted kidney.

HISTORY AND PHYSICAL EXAMINATION

Potential donors should be adults, age 18 or over, who are competent to give their own informed consent for renal donation. It would be unusual for potential donors over age 65 to be suitable candidates (178). Donors should not have unexplained fevers, urinary tract infections, pyelonephritis, hematuria, or stone disease. Any history of urologic surgery should be documented. In general, donors with hypertension, diabetes, cardiovascular disease, or systemic illnesses involving the kidneys are excluded. Daily medications, nonprescription drug use, and allergies should be noted. The sexual history is also recorded. Donors should be reassured that donation will not alter present sexual performance (179).

LABORATORY TESTS

Screening chemistry and hematologic studies should be consistent with a normal physiologic state. Abnormalities such as elevated liver transaminases or prolonged coagulation profiles should be further evaluated. Serologic studies and cultures are necessary to identify present and/or past exposure to transmissible diseases. Donors with a previously unknown history of exposure to venereal disease should be completely treated prior to consideration for renal donation. Potential donors who are infected with hepatitis B or C or with human immunodeficiency virus should not donate organs or tissues (54,60). Donors with previous exposure to the cytomegalovirus may place recipients at increased risk for primary CMV disease, which will require appropriate prophylaxis (180).

Renal function studies are essential and should be performed in triplicate. While no absolute criteria have been established, renal donors should have a creatinine clearance in excess of 80 cc/min. We have seen several donors, usually thin, middle-aged females with a serum creatinine of 1.2–1.4 mg/dL, who have had a creatinine clearance under 60 cc/min. Such patients are excluded from donation. An inulin clearance or radionuclide determination of the glomerular filtration rate may be helpful in certain patients. The 24-hour urinary protein excretion should be less than 250 mg in adults. Patients with crystalluria on urinalysis require metabolic stone evaluation.

RADIOGRAPHIC STUDIES

The final piece in the donor evaluation confirms the anatomic integrity of the donor kidneys. An excretory urogram is performed initially to document two functioning renal units of generally normal size, shape, and position. Abnormalities, such as a solitary kidney, severe atrophy or scarring, stones, obstruction, horseshoe kidney, tumors, etc., would exclude renal donation. If the urogram is normal, an angiogram is done to identify the abdominal aorta and the number, position, and patency of renal vessels and to further delineate the renal parenchyma. The introduction of digital angiography techniques have been reported to be a useful and somewhat less invasive method of donor evaluation (181,182), but less accurate than standard catheter angiography.

Cadaver donors

The majority of renal transplant recipients will not have a willing family donor and must rely therefore on an organ from a cadaver. A well-functioning cadaveric kidney will provide the same opportunity for rehabilitation from ESRD as a live donor organ. However, a number of complicating factors in cadaveric transplantation arise from the fact that organ availability is both limited and a random event, which makes the surgical procedure nonelective in nature. Cadaver kidneys are preferably transplanted within 24 hours of recovery but can produce acceptable results with up to 48–60 hours of preservation. During this period of time, a previously evaluated and waiting recipient is identified and prepared for surgery. This preparation may include dialysis or metabolic adjustments for the recipient, as well as transport of the recipient or the kidney across the country. Unless initiated prior to organ recovery, a minimum period of 8–10 hours is usually required in order to tissue type the donor and perform specific crossmatch tests to screen out those with donor-directed cytotoxic antibody. The kidney is usually placed by using a weighted system encompassing ABO blood type, tissue type, length of time waiting, and possibly other medical or local factors (183).

CADAVER DONOR IDENTIFICATION

Potential renal donors generally come from individuals who have suffered irreversible head trauma, cerebral vascular accidents, or anoxic brain injury (184). Preferably, they should be between 5 and 60 years of age. There should be no history of systemic diseases that involve the kidneys, such as nephrolithiases, diabetes mellitus, hypertension (long-standing with drug therapy), autoimmune disease, etc. Patients with a history of malignant tumors other than localized brain or nonmelanoma skin cancer should not be used as organ donors. There should be no history of transmissible infectious disease or active untreated infection. It is best not to consider individuals with high-risk behavior for HIV disease, such as documented intravenous drug users, active homosexuals, hemophiliacs requiring blood transfusions, or those with known infected sexual partners (60,185). One of the great uncertainties associated with cadaver renal transplantation relates directly to the adequacy of the medical history of the cadaver donor. Many posttransplant recipient problems can be minimized or even avoided by an accurate donor history. This can be a special problem when the mortal injury occurs far from the patient's home. It is always important to obtain a medical history from someone who has had close recent contact with the individual, not merely a relative or friend.

Organs for transplantation cannot be removed until the surviving family gives specific permission for this act and brain death has been declared. The act of donation is therefore completely dependent upon the goodwill and altruism of the public at large. The use of a signed donor card on the back of a driver's license is not sufficient consent and has been of marginal value in increasing the donor supply. Interestingly, one of the greatest impediments to identifying donors and obtaining family consent has been delayed referral or nonreferral to local organ-procurement agencies by hospital personnel. It is hoped that increased local and national education policies as well as "required request' legislation will expand the pool of potential donors through greater public awareness (186).

DONOR MANAGEMENT

The process of organ procurement can only begin when an individual becomes brain dead and family consent is obtained. In most states, the diagnosis of brain death requires strict medical criteria to be met, and a signed declaration of death must be made by two physicians, neither of whom can be a member of the transplant team. Brain death remains a clinical diagnosis (Table 6) but can be supported by other objective tests (187). The absence of perfusion of

Table 6. Diagnosis of brain death

I. Clinical criteria
  a. Unresponsiveness to external stimuli pain, sound, light, noxious, ice water calorics
  b. Absence of spontaneous breathing
  c. No cranial nerve function
  d. Above findings present with body temperature over 90°F
  e. Absence of CNS depressant drugs
II. Clinical criteria can be supported by:
  a. Isoelectric electroencephalogram
  b. Lack of cerebral perfusion by angiogram or radiographic flow scan
  c. Absence of evoked potentials

the brain on isotopic cerebral blood flow scan is a useful confirmatory test due to its ease of performance and reliability (188). The absence of flow is not compatible with a return of brain function. It is important to make this diagnosis after ruling out hypothermia, metabolic encephalopathy, drug intoxication, and shock as confounding diagnoses.

Once declared brain dead and after family consent is obtained, the donor should be kept in a state as close to normal homeostasis as possible. Appropriate ventilatory support is required, and normothermia should be maintained. Maintenance of pulmonary care, nasogastric suction to prevent aspiration, lubrication and protection of the eyes, removal of all intravascular catheters placed without sterile technique, and monitoring of vital organ function with central venous and arterial pressure catheters and a Foley catheter are usually required. Blood transfusion is not routinely necessary, except in cases with ongoing hemorrhage. Quite often, donors are volume contracted and dehydrated (the appropriate management for brain injury), and must be resuscitated with fluids. Ringer's lactate is usually sufficient. Deterioration of brain function and loss of central neurohumoral regulatory control may result in severe systemic hypertension (Cushing's reflex) due to elevated circulating catecholamines and sympathetic activity. Beta blockers can be useful to protect the myocardium when this occurs. In some donors, brain herniation may result in bradycardia, hypotension, and diminished organ perfusion. Adequate systolic blood pressure, usually over 100 mmHg, is recommended. The use of vasopressors such as dopamine, which maintains renal blood flow, can be helpful. Urine output in adults should be maintained at over 1 mL/kg/hr. Frequently, donors may develop massive urine output (over 500 mL/hr) as a result of central diabetes insipidus due to low levels of circulating antidiuretic hormone from the destroyed hypothalamic pituitary axis. The resulting excessive free water loss can lead to hypokalemia, hypernatremia, hypocalcemia, and hypophosphatemia. This condition can be treated with exogenous vasopressin, which can be delivered as intranasal DDAVP.

The serum creatinine in a cadaver donor should be less than 2.0 mg/dL. A rising creatinine may be due to prolonged hypotension, which may cause irreversible renal ischemia. A rising serum creatinine, coupled with a markedly diminished urine output of under 30 cc/hr prior to removal of the kidneys, is associated with permanent renal injury. The maintenance of the donor prior to surgical nephrectomy is one of the most important factors contributing to immediate graft function after revascularization (189). Older donor kidneys, above age 60, are especially susceptible to adverse prerecovery donor function, and every effort should be made to normalize physiologic parameters in these patients. While no specific test can predict posttransplant organ viability and function, in recent years many have begun to rely on a pretransplant biopsy of the kidney as it is removed (190). The identification of sclerosed glomeruli, found in greater than 10%–20% of the biopsied specimens, has been associated with markedly diminished posttransplant function. This information may be useful when making the decision to use a donor with marginal characteristics, such as older age, hypertension, ischemic injury, etc.

KIDNEY PROCUREMENT

Cadaveric kidneys are usually removed in conjunction with the procurement of other solid organs such as the liver, pancreas, heart, and lungs. Techniques for multiple organ harvest have been developed that minimize warm ischemic injury (191). Cadaveric kidneys should be removed en bloc with the aorta and vena cava to prevent injury to renal units with multiple vessels. Once removed, the kidneys are flushed with a hypothermic (4°C) electrolyte solution that initially removes the blood and clotting factors from the donor. A number of perfusates are currently available, the most popular being Collin's solution and a perfusate developed at the University of Wisconsin (192). Each is hyperosmolar and mimics the in vivo intracellular sodium and potassium concentrations. An effective preservation solution should prevent the reperfusion injury initiated by oxygen-free radicals, provide adequate amounts of substrate for regenerating high-energy phosphate compounds (ATP) during reperfusion, prevent acidosis, and minimize the cellular swelling due to sodium, chloride, and water influx that occurs during anaerobic hypothermic ischemic (193). Ex vivo renal preservation and storage is hypothermic and is done by one of two methods. The majority of transplant centers in the United States now preserve kidneys using simple cold storage, with the organ immersed in the same flushing solution. An alternative preservation method utilizes continuous pulsatile perfusion with albumin or colloid solutions. The former method is simpler and cheaper and is therefore preferred for preservation up to 48 hours. The latter method may be beneficial if extended preservation up to 72 hours is to be anticipated.

THE MARGINAL DONOR

The continued shortage of cadaver kidneys to meet the needs of the ever-expanding number of waiting recipients has led to consideration of so-called *marginal* donors (194). The use of such kidneys remains controversial because they are more likely to result in inferior outcome and increased costs compared to so-called *optimal* donor kidneys. The use of marginal donor kidneys is often associated with increased rates of delayed graft function or even primary nonfunction, as well as greater numbers of grafts lost due to technical complications. Nevertheless, their use may be considered reasonable in certain selected circumstances, and they provide an increased source of organs to supply individuals who would otherwise not be transplanted. The potential recipient should always be informed and should participate in the decision to use a marginal donor kidney. Some examples of marginal donors include the following:

Donors at either end of the age spectrum, under age 5 and over age 60, have consistently produced graft survival rates 10%–20% lower than those achieved with kidneys in the ideal age range when analyzed in large multicenter registries (195–197). There have been individual centers, however, that have reported results comparable to those of normal-risk donors.

There are two important issues to consider in using the older-age kidney. Firstly, there is a well-known decrease in glomerular filtration rate (GFR) as the kidney ages. This fact, coupled with an increase in atherosclerosis with aging, will decrease the tolerance of the older kidney for preservation injury and may result in diminished graft function in the host (197). For this reason, it may also be harder to maintain good homeostasis in the aged donor with any degree of prerecovery injury. While not precise, the renal biopsy may be the only way to identify an older kidney as compromised (190). The second factor that contributes to a poor outcome is the increased incidence of delayed graft function observed in the older kidney (198). Delayed graft function has been associated with longer hospitalization, decreased ultimate level of renal function, decreased 1-year graft survival, and ultimately increased cost to the cadaver transplant recipient (199). Another concept is emerging from animal investigations demonstrating that there is an increase in MHC antigen expression in the vasculature and the tubular epithelium of the damaged graft (200,201). Therefore, the kidney with delayed graft function may be more susceptible to posttransplant rejection, which adds a further ischemic insult to the damaged kidney (202). In practice, if kidneys from older donors are used, efforts should be made to minimize ischemic times.

The small pediatric donor kidney, less than age 5, also represents an area of potential organ pool expansion that does not come without a unique set of risks. The use of small kidneys has long been associated with an increase in technical graft loss, especially vascular thrombosis of the small renal artery (203,204). Some have thought this outcome was due to hypermobility of the small kidney in the iliac fossa. Attempts at fixation and anticoagulation have yielded mixed results. While the small pediatric kidney placed into the adult will hypertrophy and grow, yielding a GFR that can exceed 50cc/min, there is some emerging evidence that these small kidneys may ultimately suffer from hyperfiltration injury with subsequent proteinuria and sclerosis. To avoid this possibility, the concept of transplanting two pediatric kidneys en bloc through the common aorta and vena cava of the donor is gaining popularity (205,206). While this permits only one recipient to receive kidneys from one donor, it would appear than an adequate renal mass can be delivered by this technique. Interestingly, the use of small pediatric kidneys in small children with renal failure has not been ideal; the high rate of technical graft loss and thrombosis has been just as prominent in small recipients. At the current time, most pediatric centers prefer the use of an adult cadaver donor kidney for the small child (207). It has been proffered that low perfusion pressures in small children coupled with high intrarenal resistance in ischemic small kidneys may result in intrarenal thrombosis.

With careful selection, cadaver kidneys in donors with systemic diseases of early onset may be suitable for transplantation. Two examples are donors with hypertension and those with diabetes. Kidneys from donors with recent-onset essential hypertension, under age 50, without systemic atherosclerosis have been successfully transplanted (208). Similarly, donors with a recent diagnosis of diabetes without other overt diabetic complications may also be suitable (209,210). In these instances, the renal biopsy is essential to rule out both long-standing hypertensive changes and microvascular disease. The absence of diabetic glomerulosclerosis on biopsy is also important. Of course, these kidneys should only be used with good historical documentation, excellent renal function, and good donor maintenance and physiology. The maintenance of normal glucose metabolism in the host has actually been shown to diminish some established diabetic renal lesions (210). Other examples of intrinsic renal disease such as polycystic kidney disease, renal artery dysplasias, and congenital obstructions have also been utilized in highly selected cases. It is incumbent upon the transplant team to inform the potential recipient of the donor status.

The development of formal brain death statutes has permitted cadaver transplantation to go forward in an orderly fashion. Donor identification and family consent is normally obtained in the window of time after brain death has occurred and cardiovascular function can be maintained. There continue to be a number of potential donors in whom sudden death and cardiovascular collapse occur shortly after or simultaneous with brain death. These so-called *nonheartbeating* donors could be the source of usable organs in certain circumstances. Theoretically, cannulas could be placed to cool the potential donor organs with perfusate shortly after cardiovascular function

ceases to prevent significant warm ischemia (211). The issue of proper informed family consent has always been paramount in donor identification in the United States, and becomes practically quite difficult in this setting (212). There are, however, occasional potential donors that are identified who have nonrecoverable brain injuries that do not meet brain death criteria. These individuals could be candidates for this approach. In Holland between 1981 and 1990, this approach was used to increase the donor pool by as much as 20% (213). As long as the organ shortage remains, this type of donor expansion should continue to be evaluated in the context of proper ethical considerations.

HLA MATCHING

The impact of donor and recipient HLA matching on allograft survival has been debated since the beginnings of clinical renal transplantation. Graft survival is multifactorial and depends on a number of characteristics of both the donor and the recipient. There is little debate that HLA matching is the most powerful determinant of graft survival among living-related kidney recipients, as previously discussed (142,144). However, merely matching HLA alleles in nonrelated individuals does not guarantee that an entire MHC region will be the same as it is between relatives. As is currently practiced, matching entails serological identification of HLA Class I (A, B) and Class II (Dr) loci on donor and recipient lymphocytes using a microcytotoxicity assay (214). Lymphocytes are incubated in antiserum that is specific for various HLA antigens. Complement-dependent cell lysis occurs when the antigen in question is present and can be microscopically visualized by adding a vital dye such as eosin. Since Class I antigens are present on all nucleated cells, typing for these antigens can be done on leukocyte-rich preparations from whole blood. Serotyping for Class II antigens is more difficult because the preparations must be enriched for B lymphocytes and monocytes. Prospective cadaveric matching at the HLA D locus, which requires the week-long MLC test is of course not possible (146).

A newer technique for analysis of HLA D types involves analysis of the DNA from test cells. The DNA can be amplified by the polymerase chain reaction or digested with various enzymes to form fragments that can be separated by electrophoresis. The fragments form profiles that are unique for the DNA sequences (215,216). An alternative form of molecular analysis involves DNA sequence-specific oligonucleotides that will anneal to specific portions of the DNA molecules. This technique promises to be rapid, sensitive, and specific for tissue typing, especially for Class II antigens (217).

Since 1987, a UNOS-stipulated policy has been in place that mandates the national sharing of cadaver kidneys matched for all six antigens (2 HLA A, B, Dr loci). In 1990, the policy was extended to include all phenotypically identical matches (no mismatches when less than six antigens are identified) (218). Enhanced graft survival for perfectly matched recipients was determined to outweigh all other claims on a donated organ and to justify the excess cost and effort for transport on a national level (219). Graft survival of 88% at 1 year has been excellent for 1004 of these mandatorily shared kidneys. During the same time, 22,188 recipients of mismatched cadaver kidneys enjoyed a 79% 1-year graft survival rate (220). Improved 1-year graft survival has not been consistently demonstrated with more than one HLA antigen mismatch, although some reports attribute greater reliability on B or Dr antigen identity (221).

The positive impact of matching has been reported to be lasting, resulting in longer half-lives (t 1/2) of kidney graft survival. The average t 1/2 for first cadaver kidneys is about 8.2 years, while that of zero-mismatched HLA A, B, Dr kidneys is extended to 19 years (222). All other A, B, Dr match grades (1–6) had t 1/2's that differ from each other by a standard deviation of only 1.6 years, thus having little impact. The majority of studies supporting the influence of tissue typing come from large multicenter data banks (UNOS, UCLA, CTS, registries) that represent several thousand patients. The advantages of such studies depend on large patient numbers, whereby small differences are statistically validated and a sufficient number of all match grades can be included. The disadvantages of these studies are the inclusion of centers with different patient demographics, patient selection, cross-match eligibility criteria, and immunosuppressive protocols, all of which influence transplant outcome (223). In addition, univariate analysis for tissue typing has been questioned due to the multifactorial influences on cadaver transplant outcome. Single-center reports that show little impact of tissue typing often employ consistent immunosuppression and clinical practice for all patient groups (224). However, they also usually include very few well-matched recipients, preventing statistical confirmation of small but significant differences.

Unfortunately, the extreme polymorphism of the HLA alleles makes it unlikely that two unrelated individuals will be very well matched. Indeed, even with a national waiting list of over 20,000 individuals, less than 5% will find a six-antigen matched organ. Apparently, even one Class I or Class II antigen mismatch will significantly diminish the matching effect (225,226). This outcome may be due to the ability of the immune system to recognize and target one antigen as effectively as several HLA antigens. Since the vast majority of cadaver recipients will receive a mismatched organ, a number of other factors may have just as a significant impact as HLA matching on transplant outcome. Many have questioned the expanded impact of HLA matching in the distribution algorithms for cadaveric transplantation that are currently employed by UNOS.

The tissue-typing debate is further complicated by several other factors. There is a question of accuracy of typing data using current methodologies. The collaborative transplant study group recently compared serologic and DNA typing for 3325 and 4076 recipients. Serologic typing of Dr was inaccurate for 25% of organ donors and 27.6% of recipients (227). Individual centers had discrepancy rates between 9.7% and 86.7%. Thus, the overall chance of an error in donor and recipient typing is about 46%. Similar findings on the error rate of Dr serotyping were reported by another group (228). With such a high error rate, some have questioned the use of matching as a major criterion for organ allocation. Perhaps the streamlining of typing using molecular analysis can eliminate these errors. However, further refinements and specificities in the tissue typing of a cadaver donor may actually increase the number of HLA alleles and decrease the chance of finding a very-well-matched donor–recipient pair. For this reason, further refinements in typing are being developed that try to group together Class I residues that represent certain cross-reacting groups of HLA antigens (cregs) and so-called "permissible" HLA Class II antigen mismatches (229).

National organ sharing and the transport of kidneys across the country must by necessity increase the length of time that organs are preserved. It has been consistently shown that preservation time is directly related to the incidence of delayed graft function posttransplant, and delayed graft function directly translates to decreased graft survival (230). Therefore, a balance must continually be reached between the goals of idealizing tissue matching and avoidance of increasing the likelihood of posttransplant delayed graft function. An unnecessary increase in the rate of posttransplant delayed graft function also increases cost due to the need for dialysis and increased length of stay (199).

A recent recognized problem resulting from allocation of kidneys based on HLA matching is the promotion of racial disparity in access to renal transplantation in the United States. Since only 8% of cadaveric kidneys come from black donors, and approximately 34% of waiting recipients are black, many wait up to two times as long for a cadaveric kidney (231). This wait is due to the fact that profound racial differences exist in HLA antigen expression. Blacks have less well-defined HLA antigen specificities than do whites, particularly at the Dr locus (232). Furthermore, HLA antigens are distributed differently among the races (233). For example, at the A locus, HLA-A1 is found in 23% of whites but in only 10% of blacks; conversely, HLA-A23 is much less common in whites (6%) than in blacks (22%). Therefore, the algorithm for organ distribution, which heavily weights HLA matching, appears to be discriminatory in certain areas of the country. This fact is confirmed by UNOS data, which call attention to the fact that blacks receive six-antigen-matched kidneys at one tenth the rate of whites (234,235). Interestingly, the improved graft survival enjoyed by six-antigen-matched Caucasian recipients is not duplicated when black recipients receive six-antigen-matched kidneys. Whether this fact is due to some intrinsic immune responsiveness in blacks or to the possible inaccuracies related to tissue typing is as yet unanswered. While all would support efforts at increasing the pool of black organ donors, it would appear that heavily weighting distribution algorithms toward HLA typing (other than perfectly matched kidneys) does create a disproportionately longer waiting time for black recipients.

The debate relating to the precise role of tissue matching in renal transplantation goes on. The clinical practice of kidney transplantation continuously evolves, and at the present time many regions of the country have established a variance with the organ-distribution algorithm based on tissue typing, in order to selectively weight other characteristics (236). As more and more elderly patients with atherosclerosis are requesting transplantation as an option, issues of 10- and 15-year survival become less realistic considerations due to the high incidence of cardiovascular demise in the elderly ESRD population. Many have come to realize that the impact of a national policy on the various local transplant waiting lists may have a variable outcome from one region of the country to another.

VIRAL INFECTIONS

Viral illnesses represent the most common identifiable cause of infectious morbidity in renal transplant recipients. The spectrum of disease is broad, ranging from self-limited skin eruptions to life-threatening sepsis and multiorgan system failure. By far the most common offenders are the herpes viruses: cytomegalovirus (CMV), Epstein–Barr virus (EBV), herpes simples virus (HSV), and varicella-zoster virus (VZV) (53,54). Each of these double-stranded DNA viruses share the property of latency, meaning they can exist in a dormant state within cells such as neural tissue, lymphocytes, and leukocytes. Since the activated T lymphocyte is usually required for viral clearance, it is not surprising that nonspecific immunosuppression causing T-cell dysfunction makes the host more vulnerable to viral proliferation. Recipients can experience primary infections due to new viral exposure or secondary infections due to reactivation of latent virus (237). Posttransplant immunosuppression and allograft rejection can lead to reactivation of latent virus. Primary infections are usually more severe and are associated with clinical symptoms.

CMV is the most frequently encountered viral illness, being observed in 50%–75% of transplant patients. Three epidemiological patterns of CMV infection are observed, each with a different rate of clinically overt disease. Primary CMV infection occurs when a seronegative recipient receives cells from a seropositive individual and reactivates the latent donor virus posttransplant. The source of infected cells is the donor kidney in over 90% of cases; however, blood transfusions from seropositive donors may cause up to 10% of cases (238). In over 60% of such (D-positive, R-negative) transplants, the recipient develops clinical symptoms of CMV disease (53). The second pattern involves posttransplant reactivation of latent virus already present in the seropositive host. In this group (D-positive or negative, R-positive), about 20% of patients will become clinically symptomatic. The term *CMV superinfection* is used to describe a seropositive recipient who receives a kidney from a seropositive donor (D-positive, R-positive) and reactivates the CMV virus of donor origin (238,239). It is currently not clear whether patients with CMV superinfection develop clinical symptoms at a higher rate than those with reactivation of virus of host origin. It is apparent that CMV seropositive recipients or those at risk for primary infection (D-positive, R-negative) are at greater risk for clinically symptomatic disease if they are given either polyclonal or monoclonal antilymphocyte preparations (55,240).

Although the frequencies may vary from center to center, only about 20% of recipients are CMV seronegative and receive a CMV seronegative kidney at the time of transplant (D-negative, R-negative). Therefore, the diagnosis of CMV infection should be considered during any febrile illness posttransplant, especially during the first 4 months. The symptoms associated with CMV disease include fever, leukopenia, thrombocytopenia, pneumonitis, hepatitis, gastrointestinal ulcers, and neurological disorders such as meningitis and encephalitis. The later stages of CMV disease may produce chorioretinitis. The treatment of CMV disease has improved dramatically with the introduction of the antiviral agents acyclovir, ganciclovir—which is more potent—and the passive immunity conferred by CMV hyperimmune globulin (241,242). Recent studies have demonstrated a dramatic reduction in overt CMV disease in the high-risk (D-positive, R-negative) population by using early prophylaxis with either short-term ganciclovir and hyperimmune globulin or a 3-month course of acyclovir (243). Diminished severity of reactivation disease has been reported for seropositive recipient who receive prophylaxis, but the ideal agent has yet to be identified. Diminished severity of disease for high-risk recipients can also be achieved by administering antiviral agents during and immediately after courses of high-dose antirejection therapy (55,244).

The EBV virus can also be transmitted from donor to host and can mimic the clinical syndrome caused by the CMV virus. While less ubiquitous than CMV, the EBV virus can be a more ominous pathogen due to its role in the pathogenesis of B-cell lymphoproliferative disease. The EBV virus normally replicates in the oropharynx but can be transmitted with the donor organ or blood products (245,246). During viral replication, B lymphocytes are infected via the C3 complement receptor on these cells. This is followed by immortalization of the B cells, a form of malignant transformation. While recent reports implicate the use of OKT3 in the development of EBV-related B-cell lymphoproliferation, the total accumulated dose of multidrug immunosuppression may have greater influence on EBV reactivation, increasing the opportunities for malignant transformation of EBV-infected B lymphocytes to occur (247). It is unclear whether antiviral prophylaxis will decrease the occurrence of EBV infection or reactivation in the transplant population.

The transmission of the HIV virus from a seropositive donor to the transplant recipient is extremely efficient (54,60,61). At the present time, it is UNOS policy not to transplant organs or tissues from HIV-positive donors, since some donors, especially those involved in severe trauma, may receive a large amount of blood products during their final hospitalization and can be rendered temporarily seronegative for HIV by exchange transfusion. It is therefore extremely important that HIV testing be done on serum samples obtained early during the hospitalization. In addition, there may be a window of a few months in which a newly infected donor does not generate a measurable titer of HIV antibody. For this reason, it is prudent not to use donors who demonstrate high-risk behavior for HIV infection. Currently, most centers do not transplant patients who are asymptomatic carriers of the HIV infection. Current evidence suggests that post-transplant immunosuppression will hasten progression to full-blown AIDS and will therefore increase mortality (60,61). This policy could be modulated if effective HIV therapies become available.

REFERENCES

1. Evans RW: The benefits of transplantation. Survival and quality of life. In: RW Evans, DL Manninen, F Dong, eds, *The National Cooperative Transplantation Study*. Battelle Research Center, Seattle, 1991.
2. Evans RW: Need, demand, and supply in kidney transplantation. A review of data and examination of the issues, and projections through the year 2000. *Semin Nephrol* 12:234–255, 1992.
3. Spital A: The shortage of organs for transplantation: Where do we go from here? *N Engl J Med* 325:1243–1246, 1991.
4. Evans RW, Orians CE, Ascher NL: The potential supply of organ donors: an assessment of the efficiency of organ procurement efforts in the United States. *JAMA* 267:239–246, 1992.
5. The United States Renal Data Systems: *1993 Annual Report. Prevalence of Reported ESRD Therapy.* The National Institutes of Health, Bethesda, MD, March 1993.
6. The United States Renal Data Systems: *1993 Annual Report. The Kidney Transplant Process.* The National Institutes of Health, Bethesda, MD, March 1993.
7. Cecka JM, Terasaki PI: The UNOS Scientific Registry. In: *Clinical Transplants 1993.* The University of California Press, Los Angeles, CA, pp 1–18, 1994.
8. Terasaki PI, Toyotome A, Mickey R, Iwaki Y, Cecka JM: Patient graft and functional survival rates. In: *Clinical Kidney Transplants.* University of California Press, Los Angeles, CA, pp 141–257, 1988.
9. Krakauer H, Grauman JS, McMullen MR, Creede CC: The recent U.S. experience in the treatment of ESRD by dialysis and transplantation. *N Engl J Med* 308:1558–1562, 1983.
10. Najarian JS, Matas AJ: The present and future of kidney transplantation. *Transplant Proc* 23:2075–2082, 1991.
11. Christiansen AJ, Holman JM, Turner CW: Quality of life in ESRD: influence of renal transplantation. *Clin Transplant* 3:46–53, 1989.
12. Flechner SM, Novick AC, Braun WE, et al.: Functional capacity and rehabilitation of recipients with a functioning renal allograft 10 years or more. *Transplantation* 35:572–576, 1983.
13. Simmons RG, Abress L, Andersen C. Rehabilitation after kidney transplantation. In: G Cerilli, ed, *Organ Transplantation and Replacement.* JB Lippincott, New York, pp 481–489, 1988.
14. Devins GM, Binik YM, Hutchinson TA: The emotional impact of ESRD: importance of patient's perceptions of intrusiveness and control. *Int J Psychiatry Med* 13:327–335, 1984.
15. Port FK: Worldwide demographics and future trends in ESRD. *Kidney Int* 43 (Suppl):51–57, 1993.
16. Hart LG, Evans RW: The functional status of ESRD patients as measured by the sickness impact profile. *J Chronic Dis* 40 (Suppl 1):117–130, 1987.
17. Armenti VT, Ahlswede KM, Jarrel B, et al.: National transplantation pregnancy registry: analysis at pregnancy outcome. *Transplant Proc* 25:1036–1037, 1993.
18. Davison JM: Dialysis, transplantation and pregnancy. *Am J Kidney Dis* 17:127–132, 1991.
19. Fox E, Peace K, Neale TJ, et al.: Quality of life for patients with ESRD. *Renal Failure* 13:31–35, 1991.
20. Vollmer WM, Wahl RW, Blagg CR: Survival with dialysis and transplantation in patients with ESRD. *N Engl J Med* 308:1553–1557, 1983.
21. Burton PR, Walls J: Selection adjusted comparison of life expectancy of patients on continuous ambulatory peritoneal dialysis, hemodialysis, and renal transplantation. *Lancet* 1:1115–1119, 1987.
22. Hutchinson TA, Thomas DC, MacFibbon B: Predicting survival in adults with ESRD: an age equivalency index. *Ann Intern Med* 96:417–424, 1982.
23. Garcia-Garcia G, Deddens JA, D'Achiardi-Rey R, et al.: Results of treatment in patients with ESRD: a multivariate analysis of risk factors and survival in 341 successive patients. *Am J Kidney Dis* 5:10–18, 1985.
24. Minetti L, Civati G, Brando B, et al.: A comparison between maintenance hemodialysis and transplantation in the treatment of ESRD. *Transplant Proc* 17 (Suppl 2):28–31, 1985.
25. Hutchinson TA, Thomas DC, Lemieux JC, Harvey CE: Prognostically controlled comparison of dialysis and renal transplantation. *Kidney Int* 26:44–51, 1984.
26. Weller JM, Port FK, Swartz RD, Ferguson CW, Williams GW: Analysis of survival of ESRD patients. *Kidney Int* 21:78–83, 1982.
27. Port FK, Wolfe RA, Mauger EA, Berling D, Jiang K: Comparison of survival probabilities for dialysis patients vs cadaveric renal transplant recipients. *JAMA* 270:1339–1343, 1993.
28. Flom LS, Riesman EM, Donovan JM, et al.: Favorable experience with preemptive renal transplantation in children. *Pediatr Nephol* 6:258–261, 1992.
29. Migliori RJ, Simmons R, Payne WD, et al.: Renal transplantation done safely without prior chronic dialysis therapy. *Transplantation* 43:51–55, 1987.
30. Engelhardt HT: Allocating scarce medical resources and the availability of organ transplantation. *N Engl J Med* 311:66–71, 1984.
31. Cohen B: Organ donor shortage: European situation and possible solutions. *Scand J Urol Nephrol* 92:77–80, 1985.

32. Organ Donors in the U.K.—getting the numbers right (editorial). *Lancet* 335:80–82, 1990.

33. Ubel PA, Arnold RM, Caplan A: Rationing failure. The ethical lessons of the retransplantation of scarce vital organs. *JAMA* 270:2469–2474, 1993.

34. Fryer JP, Matas AJ: How to identify the best candidates for kidney transplantation. *J Crit Illness* 9:362–374, 1994.

35. Cantarovich D, Baranger T, Tirouvanzian R, et al.: One hundred and five kidney transplants with cyclosporine in recipients over 60 years of age. *Transplant Proc* 25:1323–1324, 1993.

36. Pirsch J, Stratta RJ, Armbrust MJ, et al.: Cadaveric renal transplantation with cyclosporine in patients more than 60 years of age. *Transplantation* 47:259–263, 1989.

37. Schulak JA, Mayes JT, Johnston K, et al.: Kidney transplantation in patients age 60 years and older. *Surgery* 108:726–733, 1991.

38. Vivas CA, Hickey DP, Jordan M, et al.: Renal transplantation in patients 65 years or older. *J Urol* 147:990–993, 1992.

39. Mailloux LV, Bellucci AG, Wilkes BM, et al.: Mortality in dialysis patients: analysis of the causes of death. *Am J Kidney Dis* 18:326–335, 1991.

40. Horina JH, Holzer H, Reisinger EC, et al.: Elderly patients and chronic hemodialysis. *Lancet* 339:183–184, 1992.

41. Derfler K, Kletler K, Balcke P, et al.: Predictive value of thallium-201 dipyridamole myocardial stress scintigraphy in chronic hemodialysis patients and transplant recipients. *Clin Nephrol* 36:192–202, 1990.

42. Helderman JH: The role of cardiovascular disease in renal transplantation. In: M Garovoy, Guttmann, eds, *Renal Transplantation*. Churchill-Livingstone, New York, pp 209–232, 1986.

43. DeMeyer M, Wyns W, Dion R, et al.: Myocardial revascularization in patients on renal replacement therapy. *Clin Nephrol* 36:147–151, 1991.

44. Moel DI, Butt K: Renal transplantation in children less than two years of age. *J Pediatr* 99:535–539, 1981.

45. Fletcher JC: Moral problems and ethical issues in the management of children with chronic renal failure. In: *Proceedings of Conference on Chronic Renal Disease: Unique Problems of the Child with Renal Failure*. National Institutes of Health, Bethesda, MD, March 5–6, 1981.

46. McEnery PT, Stablein DM, Arbus G, et al.: Renal transplantation in children. Report of the North American Pediatric Renal Transplant Cooperative Study. *N Engl J Med* 326:1727–1732, 1992.

47. Conley SB, Flechner SM, Rose G, et al.: The use of cyclosporine in pediatric renal transplant recipients. *J Pediatr* 106:45–49, 1985.

48. Najarian JS, Frey DJ, Matas AJ, et al.: Renal transplantation in infants. *Ann Surg* 212:353–367, 1990.

49. Fine R: Peritoneal dialysis in children. *J Pediatr* 100:1–4, 1982.

50. Penn I: Leukemias and lymphomas associated with the use of cytotoxic and immunosuppressive drugs. *Cancer Res* 69:7–17, 1979.

51. Penn I: Renal transplantation in patients with pre-existing malignancies. *Transplant Proc* 15:1079–1082, 1983.

52. Penn I: The effect of immunosuppression on pre-existing cancers. *Transplantation* 55:742–747, 1993.

53. Rubin RH, Tolkhoff-Rubin NE: The impact of infection on the outcome of transplantation. *Transplant Proc* 23:2068–2074, 1991.

54. Rubin RH: Infectious disease complications of renal transplantation. *Kidney Int* 44:221–236, 1993.

55. Rubin RH, Tolkhoff-Rubin NE: Antimicrobial strategies in the case of organ transplant recipients. *Antimicrob Agents Chemother* 37:619–624, 1993.

56. Reyna J, Richardson J, Mattox D, et al.: Head and neck infection after renal transplantation. *JAMA* 247:3337–3339, 1982.

57. Coutts I, Jegarajah S, Stark TE: Tuberculosis in renal transplant patients. *Br J Dis Chest* 73:141–145, 1979.

58. Andrew OT, Schoenfield P, Hopewell PC, Humphreys M: Tuberculosis in patients with ESRD. *Am J Med* 68:59–65, 1980.

59. Flechner SM, Gow JG: Role of nephrectomy in treatment of the nonfunctioning unilateral tuberculous kidney. *J Urol* 123:822–825, 1980.

60. Erice A, Phame FS, Heussner RC, et al.: HIV infection in organ transplant recipients. *Rev Infect Dis* 13:537–540, 1991.

61. Keay S, Behrens MT, Klassen D, et al.: Impact of asymptomatic HIV infection on renal allograft recipients. *Transplant Proc* 25:1478–1480, 1993.

62. Parfrey PS, Forbes R, Hutchinson TA, et al.: The clinical and pathological course of hepatitis B liver disease in renal transplant recipients. *Transplantation* 37:461–465, 1984.

63. Parfrey PS, Forbes R, Hutchinson TA, et al.: The impact of renal transplantation on the course of hepatitis B liver disease. *Transplantation* 38:610–615, 1985.

64. Parfrey PS, Farge O, Forbes R, et al.: Chronic hepatitis in ESRD: comparison of HBsAg positive and HBsAg negative patients. *Kidney Int* 28:959–965, 1985.

65. Rao KV, Dasiske BL, Anderson WR: Variability in the morphology spectrum and clinical outcome of chronic liver disease in hepatitis B positive and B negative renal transplant recipients. *Transplantation* 51:391–394, 1991.

66. Katkow WN, Rubin RH: Liver disease in the organ transplant recipient: etiology, clinical impact, and clinical management. *Transplant Rev* 5:200–208, 1991.

67. Pirson Y, Alexandre G, Ypersele C: Long-term effect of HB antigenemia on patient survival after renal transplantation. *N Engl J Med* 296:194–198, 1977.

68. Weir MR, Kirkman RL, Strom TB, Tilney N: Liver disease in recipients of long functioning renal allografts. *Kidney Int* 28:839–845, 1985.

69. Harnett JD, Zeldis JB, Parfrey PS, et al.: Hepatitis B disease in dialysis and transplant patients. *Transplantation* 44:369–373, 1987.

70. Rao KV, Anderson RC: Long term results and complications in renal transplant recipients. Observations in the second decade. *Transplantation* 45:45–52, 1988.

71. Pol S, Debure A, Degott C, et al.: Chronic hepatitis in kidney allograft recipients. *Lancet* 335:878–880, 1990.

72. Weller IV, Bassendine M, Murray A, et al.: Effects of prednisolone/azathioprine in chronic hepatitis B viral infection. *Gut* 23:650–656, 1982.

73. Huang CC, Lai MK, Fong MT: Hepatitis B liver disease in cyclosporine treated renal allograft recipients. *Transplantation* 49:540–544, 1990.

74. Schweitzer EJ, Bartlett S, Keay S, et al.: Impact of hepatitis B or C infection on the practice of kidney transplantation in the U.S. *Transplant Proc* 25:1456–1457, 1993.

75. Roth D, Fernandez JA, Burke GW, et al.: Detection of antibody to hepatitis C virus in renal transplant recipients. *Transplantation* 51:396–401, 1991.

76. Huang CC, Liaw YF, Lai MM, et al.: The clinical outcome of hepatitis C virus antibody positive renal allograft recipients. *Transplantation* 53:763–769, 1992.

77. Orloff SL, Tomlanovitch S, Stock PG, et al.: Long-term outcome of kidney transplant patients with hepatitis C infection. *Proc Am Soc Transplanty Surgeons* 19:181, 1993.

78. Tesi RJ, Waller K, Morgan CJ, et al.: Transmission of hepatitis C by kidney transplantation—the risks. *Transplantation* 57:826–831, 1994.

79. Dunn J, Golden D, Van Baren CT, et al.: Causes of graft loss beyond two years in the cyclosporine era. *Transplantation* 49:349–353, 1990.

80. Delone P, Trollinger R, Fox N, et al.: Noncompliance in renal transplant recipients. Methods for recognition and intervention. *Transplant Proc* 21:3982–3984, 1989.

81. Artero M, Biava C, Amend W, et al.: Recurrent focal glomerulosclerosis. Natural history and response to therapy. *Am J Med* 92:375–383, 1992.

82. Berger J, Yaneva H, Nabarva B, et al.: Recurrence of mesangial deposition of IgA after renal transplantation. *Kidney Int* 7:232–241, 1975.

83. Goss JA, Cole BR, Jendrisak MD, et al.: Renal transplantation for systemic lupus erythematosus and recurrent lupus nephritis. *Transplantation* 52:805–810, 1991.

84. Matthew TH: Recurrence of disease following renal transplantation. *Am J Kidney Dis* 12:85–96, 1988.

85. McLean RH, Geiger H, Burke B, et al.: Recurrence of membranoproliferative GN following kidney transplantation. *Am J Med* 60:60–65, 1976.

86. Perez R, Matas AJ, Gillingham KJ, et al.: Lessons learned and future hopes: Three thousand renal transplants at the University of Minnesota. In: PI Terasaki, ed, *Clinical Transplants 1990.* UCLA Tissue Typing Laboratory, Los Angeles, 1991.

87. Ingulli E, Tejani A: Incidence, treatment, and outcome of recurrent focal segmental glomerulosclerosis posttransplantation in 42 allografts—a single center experience. *Transplantation* 51:401–405, 1991.

88. Dantal J, Bigot E, Bogers W, et al.: Effect of plasma protein adsorption on protein excretion in kidney transplant recipients with recurrent nephrotic syndrome. *N Engl J Med* 330:7–14, 1994.

89. Cochat P, Kassir A, Colon S, et al.: Recurrent nephrotic syndrome after transplantation: early treatment with plasma pheresis and cyclophosphamide. *Pediatr Nephrol* 7:50–54, 1993.

90. Schwartz A, Krause PH, Offerman G, et al.: Recurrent and de novo renal disease after kidney transplantation. *Am J Kidney Dis* 17:524–531, 1991.

91. Steinmuller DR, Stilmont M, Idelson B, et al.: De novo development of membranous nephropathy in cadaveric renal allografts. *Clin Nephrol* 9:210–218, 1978.

92. The United States Renal Data Systems: *1993 Annual Report Counts of Renal Transplants by Primary Disease Causing ESRD. F8.* National Institutes of Health, Bethesda, MD, March 1993.

93. Okiye S, Engen D, Sterioff S, et al.: Primary and secondary renal transplantation in diabetes. *JAMA* 249:492–495, 1983.

94. Haber W, Hoffken B, Freiling U, Ritz E: Professional training for the blind diabetic with nephropathy. *Diabetic Nephropathy* 4:88–92, 1985.

95. Lemmers MJ, Barry JM: Major role for arterial disease in morbidity and mortality after kidney transplantation in diabetes. *Diabetes Care* 14:295–301, 1991.

96. Kennedy WR, Navarro X, Goetz F, et al.: The effects of pancreas transplantation on diabetic neuropathy. *N Engl J Med* 322:1031–1037, 1990.

97. Nathan DM, Fogel H, Xiorman D, et al.: Long term metabolic and quality of life results with pancreatic renal transplantation. *Transplantation* 52:85–91, 1991.

98. Mamdani B: Recovery of prolonged renal failure in patients with accelerated hypertension. *N Engl J Med* 291:1343–1344, 1974.

99. Garcia LL, Agüeru AE, Cavalli J, et al.: Kidney transplantation: Absolute and relative psychological contraindications. *Transplant Proc* 23:1344–1345, 1991.

100. Wolcott D, Norquist G: Psychiatric aspects of kidney transplantation. In: G Darovitch, ed, *Handbook of Kidney Transplantation.* Little, Brown, Boston, pp 339–355, 1992.

101. Hunt J: Pretransplant evaluation and outcome. *Semin Nephrol* 12:227–223, 1992.

102. Eshbach J, Egrie JC, Downing MR, et al.: Correction of anemia of ESRD with recombinant human erythropoietin. *N Engl J Med* 316:73–78, 1987.

103. Ward HJ: Implications of recombinant erythropoietin therapy for renal transplantation. *Am J Nephrol* 10 (Suppl 2):44–52, 1990.

104. Kerman R, Flechner SM, Van Buren C, et al.: Investigation of HIV serology in a renal transplant population. *Transplantation* 43:241–248, 1987.

105. Rubin RH: Infection in the organ transplant patient. In: RH Rubin, LS Young, eds, *Clinical Approach to Infection in the Compromised Host,* 3rd ed. Plenum, New York, in press.

106. Kerman R: Immune monitoring considerations in transplantation. In: MW Flye, ed, *Principles of Organ Transplantation.* WB Saunders, Philadelphia, pp 135–154, 1989.

107. Aldridge KE: Methicillin resistent staph aureus. Clinical and laboratory features. *Infect Control* 6:461–465, 1985.

108. Catalona WJ, Smith DS, Ratliff T, et al.: Measurement of prostate specific antigen in serum as screening test for prostate cancer. *N Engl J Med* 324:1156–1161, 1991.

109. Weinrauch LA, D'Elia JA, Healy RW, et al.: Asymptomatic coronary artery disease in diabetic patients before renal transplantation. Relationship of findings to postoperative survival. *Ann Intern Med* 88:346–348, 1978.

110. Fischel RJ, Payne WD, Gillingham KJ, et al.: Long term outlook for renal transplant recipients with one year function. *Transplantation* 51:118–122, 1992.

111. American College of Physicians Health and Public Policy Committee: Efficacy of exercise thallium-201 scintigraphy in the diagnosis and prognosis of coronary artery disease. *Ann Intern Med* 113:703–704, 1990.

112. Holley JL, Fenton RA, Arthur RS: Thallium stress testing does not predict cardiovascular risk in diabetic patients with ESRD undergoing cadaver renal transplantation. *Am J Med* 90:563–570, 1991.

113. Marwick TH, Steinmuller DR, Underwood DA, et al.: Ineffectiveness of dipyridamole thallium imaging as a screening technique for coronary artery disease in patients with ESRD. *Transplantation* 49:100–102, 1989.

114. Braun WE, Phillips DF, Vidt D, et al.: Coronary artery disease in 100 diabetics with ESRD. *Transplant Proc* 16:603–607, 1984.

115. Lorber MI, Van Buren CT, Flechner SM, et al.: Pretransplant

coronary artery angiography for diabetic renal transplant recipients. *Transplant Proc* 19:1539–1541, 1987.

116. Manske C, Thomas W, Wang Y: Screening diabetic transplant candidates for coronary artery disease: identification of a low risk subgroup. *Kidney Int* 44:617–621, 1993.

117. Manske C, Wang Y, Wilson RF, et al.: Coronary revascularization in insulin dependent diabetics with chronic renal failure. *Lancet* 340:998–1002, 1992.

118. Bissada NK: Incidence of vesical neck contracture complicating prostatic resection in hemodialysis patients. *J Urol* 117:192–193, 1977.

119. Kogan S, Levitt S: Bladder evaluation in patients before undiversion in previously diverted urinary tracts.

120. Flechner SM, Conley SB, Brewer E, et al.: Intermittent clean catheterization. An alternative to diversion in continent transplant recipients. *J Urol* 130:878–881, 1983.

121. Nguyen DH, Reinberg Y, Gonzalez R, et al.: Outcome of renal transplantation after urinary diversion and enterocytoplasty. *J Urol* 144:1349–1351, 1990.

122. Thomalla JV, Mitchell M, Leapman S, et al.: Renal transplantation into the reconstructed bladder. *J Urol* 141:265–268, 1989.

123. Hatch DA, Belitsky P, Barry JM, et al.: Fate of renal allografts transplanted in patients with urinary diversion. *Transplantation* 56:838–842, 1993.

124. Fryd D, Sutherland D, Simmons R, et al.: Results of a prospective randomized study on the effect of splenectomy vs no splenectomy in renal transplantation. *Transplant Proc* 13:48–56, 1981.

125. Alexander JW, First M, Majeski J, et al.: The late adverse effect of splenectomy on patient survival following cadaver renal transplantation. *Transplantation* 37:467–470, 1984.

126. Alexandre EP, Squifflet JP, DeBruyere M, et al.: Splenectomy as a prerequisite for successful ABO incompatible renal transplantation. *Transplant Proc* 17:138–140, 1985.

127. Owens MC, Passaro E, Wilson SE, et al.: Treatment of peptic ulcer disease in the renal transplant patient. *Ann Surg* 186:19–21, 1979.

128. Stuart FP, Reckard C, Schulak J, et al.: Gastroduodenal complications in kidney transplant recipients. *Ann Surg* 194:339–345, 1981.

129. Klompmaker IJ, Sloof MJ, de Brnijn, et al.: Prophylaxis with ranitidine against peptic ulcer disease after liver transplantation. *Transplant Int* 1:209–212, 1988.

130. Jarowenko MV, Flechner SM, Van Buren C, et al.: Ranitidine, cimetidine, and the transplant kidney. *Transplantation* 42:311–312, 1986.

131. Lorber M, Van Buren CT, Flechner SM, et al.: Hepatobiliary complications of cyclosporine therapy in 466 renal transplant recipients. *Transplantation* 43:35–40, 1987.

132. An analysis of 1518 laparoscopic cholecystectomies. The Southern Surgeons Club. *N Engl J Med* 324:1073–1078, 1991.

133. Church IM, Fazio V, Braun WE, et al.: Perforation of the colon in renal homograft recipients. *Ann Surg* 203:69–74, 1986.

134. Guice K, Ratazzi L, Marchioro T: Colon perforation in renal transplant recipients. *Am J Surg* 138:43–48, 1979.

135. Ramos EL, Kasiske BL, Alexander SR, et al.: The evaluation of candidates for renal transplantation. Current practice of U.S. transplant centers. *Transplantation* 57:490–497, 1994.

136. Opelz G, Terasaki PI: Improvement in kidney graft survival with increased numbers of blood transfusions. *N Engl J Med* 299:799–803, 1978.

137. Singal DP, Joseph S, Szewczuk M: Possible mechanisms of the beneficial effect of pretransplant blood transfusions on renal allograft survival in man. *Transplant Proc* 14:316–318, 1982.

138. Fagnilli L, Singal O: Blood transfusions may induce anti-T cell receptor antibiotics in renal patients. *Transplant Proc* 14:319–322, 1982.

139. Groth C: There is no need to give blood transfusions for renal transplantation in the cyclosporine era. *Transplant Proc* 19:153–154, 1987.

140. Scornik JC, Ireland JE, Howard RI, et al.: Assessment of the risk for broad sensitization by blood transfusions. *Transplantation* 37:249–253, 1984.

141. Ahmed Z, Terasaki PI: Effects of transfusions. In: *Clinical Transplants 1992.* UCLA Tissue Typing Laboratory, Los Angeles, pp 305–312, 1992.

142. Flechner SM, Kerman RH, Van Buren CT, et al.: The use of cyclosporine in living related renal transplantation. *Transplantation* 38:685–690, 1984.

143. Cheigh JS, Suthanthrinan M, Fotino M, et al.: Minimal sensitization and excellent renal allograft outcome following DST with short course of cyclosporine. *Transplantation* 51:378–381, 1991.

144. Cecka MJ, Terasaki PI: The UNOS Scientific Transplant Registry. In: *Clinical Transplants 1993.* UCLA Tissue Typing Laboratory, Los Angeles, pp 1–18, 1994.

145. Opelz G, Mytilneos J, Scherer S, et al.: Survival of DNA HLA-Dr typed and matched cadaver kidney transplants. *Lancet* 338:461–463, 1991.

146. Cochrum KC, Salvatierra O, Belzer F: Correlation between MLC stimulation and graft survival in living related and cadaver transplants. *Ann Surg* 1801:617–622, 1974.

147. Murray J, Merrill J, Harrison J: Renal homotransplantation in identical twins. *Surg Forum* 6:432–435, 1955.

148. Tilney NL: Renal transplantation between identical twins: a review. *World J Surg* 10:381–388, 1986.

149. Flechner SM, Kerman RH, Van Buren CT, et al.: Does cyclosporine improve the results of HLA-identical renal transplantation? *Transplant Proc* 19:1485–1488, 1987.

150. Leivstad T, Albrechtsen D, Flatmark A, et al.: Renal transplants from HLA haploidentical living related donors. *Transplantation* 42:35–38, 1986.

151. Sommer BG, Ferguson RM: Mismatched living related renal transplantation. A prospective randomized study. *Surgery* 98:269–275, 1985.

152. Cochrum KC, Hanes D, Potter D, et al.: Donor specific blood transfusions in HLA-D disparate one haplotype related allografts. *Transplant Proc* 11:1903–1907, 1979.

153. Salvatierra O, Vincenti F, Amend W, et al.: Four year experience with donor specific blood transfusions. *Transplant Proc* 15:924–931, 1983.

154. Simmons RG: Long term reactions of renal recipients and donors. In: NB Levey, ed, *Psychonephrology: Psychologic Problems in Kidney Failure and Their Treatment.* Plenum Press, New York, pp 275–287, 1983.

155. Marshall J, Fellner C: Kidney donors revisited. *Am J Psychiatry* 134:575–576, 1977.

156. Madsen V: *Harrison (1957).* Massachusetts Supreme Judicial Court Equity number 68651.

157. Santiago EA, Simmons R, Kjellstrand C, et al.: Life insurance prospective for the living kidney donor. *Transplantation* 14:131–133, 1972.

158. Spital A: Life insurance for kidney donors, an update. *Trans-*

plantation 45:819–822, 1988.

159. Merrill JP: Moral problems of artificial and transplanted organs. *Ann Intern Med* 61:355–364, 1964.

160. Leary F, DeWeerd J: Living donor nephrectomy. *J Urol* 109:947–951, 1973.

161. Weiland D, Sutherland D, Chavers B, et al.: Information on 628 living related kidney donors at a single institution with long term follow up on 472 cases. *Transplant Proc* 16:5–7, 1984.

162. Brenner B, Meger T, Hostetter T: Dietary protein intake and the progressive nature of kidney disease. *N Engl J Med* 307:652–659, 1982.

163. Vincenti F, Amend W, Kaysen G, et al.: Long term renal function in kidney donors. *Transplantation* 36:626–629, 1984.

164. Dunn J, Nylander W, Ritchie R, et al.: Living related kidney donors. *Ann Surg* 203:637–642, 1986.

165. Robitaille P, Lortie L, Mongean J, et al.: Long term follow up of patients who underwent unilateral nephrectomy in childhood. *Lancet* 1:1297–1299, 1985.

166. Najarian JS, Chavers B, McHugh L, et al.: Twenty years or more of follow up of living kidney donors. *Lancet* 340:807–810, 1992.

167. Levery A, Hou S, Bash H: Sounding Board: Kidney transplantation from unrelated living donors. *N Engl J Med* 314:914–916, 1986.

168. Spital A: Unconventional living kidney donors—attitudes and use among transplant centers. *Transplantation* 48:243–245, 1989.

169. Kaufman D, Matas A, Arrazola L, et al.: Transplantation of kidneys from zero haplotype matched live donors and unrelated donors in the cyclosporine era. *Transplant Proc* 25:1530–1532, 1993.

170. Hiraga S, Tanaka K, Watanabe J, et al.: Unrelated living donor renal transplantation. *Transplant Proc* 24:1320–1322, 1992.

171. Pirsch J, D'Allessandro A, Sollinger H, et al.: Living unrelated renal transplantation at the University of Wisconsin. In: PI Terasaki, ed, *Clinical Transplants 1990*. UCLA Tissue Typing Laboratory, Los Angeles, 1991.

172. Wyner L, Novick AC, Streem S, et al.: Improved success of unliving related renal transplantation with cyclosporine. *J Urol* 149:706–709, 1993.

173. Bart KJ, Macon E, Humphreys A: Increasing the supply of cadaveric kidneys for transplantation. *Transplantation* 31:383–387, 1981.

174. Kries H: Why living related donors should not be used whenever possible. *Transplant Proc* 17:1510–1514, 1985.

175. Council of the Transplantation Society: Commercialization in transplantation. The problems and some guidelines for practice. *Lancet* 2:715–716, 1985.

176. Carpenter C, Ettenger R, Strom T: "Free market" approach to organ donation. *N Engl J Med* 310:395–396, 1984.

177. World Health Organization: Guiding principles on human organ transplantation. *Lancet* 337:1470–1471, 1991.

178. Askari A, Novick A, Braun W, et al.: The older living related donor. Prognosis for the donor and recipient. *J Urol* 129:779–780, 1980.

179. Buszta C, Steinmuller DR, Schreiber M, et al.: Pregnancy after donor nephrectomy. *Transplantation* 40:651–654, 1985.

180. Tolkoff-Rubin NE, Rubin RH: Clinical approach to viral and fungal infections in the renal transplant patient. *Semin Nephrol* 12:364–375, 1992.

181. Flechner SM, Sandler CM, Houston GK, et al.: 100 living related kidney donor evaluations using digital subtraction angiography. *Transplantation* 40:675–678, 1985.

182. Spencer W, Streem S, Geisinger MA, et al.: Outcome angiographic evaluation of living renal donors. *J Urol* 140:1364–1366, 1988.

183. Richmond, Va.: United network for organ sharing. *UNOS Update* 5:9, 1989.

184. Darby JM, Stein K, Grenuik A, et al.: Approach to management of the heartbeating "brain dead" organ donor. *JAMA* 261:2222–2226, 1989.

185. Rubin RH, Jenkins RL, Shaw BW, et al.: The acquired immunodeficiency syndrome and transplantation. *Transplantation* 44:1–4, 1987.

186. Phillips MG, ed: *Organ Procurement, Preservation, and Distribution in Transplantation*. UNOS, Richmond, VA, 1991.

187. Pallis C: Brainstem death. The evolution of a concept. In: PJ Morris, ed, *Kidney Transplantation. Principles and Practice*. Grune and Stratton, London, pp 101–127, 1984.

188. Schwartz J, Baxter J, Bull D: Radionuclide cerebral imaging confirming brain death. *JAMA* 249:246–247, 1983.

189. Lucas BA, Vaughn WK, Spees EK, et al.: Identification of donor factors predisposing to high discard rates of cadaveric kidneys and increased graft loss within one year post transplant. *Transplantation* 43:253–257, 1987.

190. Kaplan C, Posternak B, Shah H, et al.: Age related incidence of sclerotic glomeruli in human kidneys. *Am J Pathol* 80:227–234, 1975.

191. Starzl TE, Hakala TR, Shaw BW, et al.: A flexible procedure for multiple cadaveric organ procurement. *SGO* 158:223–230, 1984.

192. Ploeg R: Kidney preservation with the UW and and Euro-Collins solutions. *Transplantation* 49:281–284, 1990.

193. Southard JH, Van Gulik TM, Ametani MS, et al.: Important components of the UW solution. *Transplantation* 49:251–257, 1990.

194. Alexander JW: *Expanded Donor Criteria: Background and Suggestions for Kidney Donation*. Report of the UNOS Ad Hoc Donations Committee, Richmond, VA, 1992.

195. Yuge J, Cecka JM: Pediatric recipients and donors. In: PI Terasaki, ed, *Clinical Transplants 1990*. UCLA Tissue Typing Laboratory, Los Angeles, 1991.

196. Alexander JW, Vaughn WK: Use of "marginal donors" for organ transplantation. *Transplantation* 51:135, 1991.

197. Alexander JW, Bennett LE, Breen TJ: Effect of donor outcome of kidney transplantation: 2 year analysis of transplants reported to the UNOS Registry. *Transplantation* 57:871–876, 1994.

198. Preuschot L, Lobo C, Offerman G: Role of cold ischemic time and vascular rejection from elderly donors. *Transplant Proc* 23:1300–1303, 1991.

199. Rosenthal JT, Danovitch GM, Wilkinson A, et al.: The high cost of delayed graft function in cadaver renal transplantation. *Transplantation* 51:1115–1120, 1991.

200. Shackleton CR, Ettinger SL, McLoughlin MG, et al.: Effect of recovery from ischemic injury on class I and class II MHC antigen expression. *Transplantation* 49:641–645, 1990.

201. Wakabayashi H, Miyauchi A, Karasawa Y, et al.: Effect of warm ischemia on reperfusion injury on inducing major histocompatibility complex antigens. *Transplant Proc* 25:3205–3207, 1993.

202. Kuhan BD, Mickey R, Flechner SM, et al.: Multivariate

analysis of risk factors impacting on immediate and eventual graft survival in cyclosporine treated recipients. *Transplantation* 43:65–71, 1987.

203. Brown MW, Akyol AM, Bradley JA, et al.: Transplantation of cadaver kidneys from pediatric donors. *Clin Transplant* 2:87–90, 1988.

204. Creagh TA, McLean PA, Spencer S, et al.: Transplantation of kidneys from pediatric cadaver donors to adult recipients. *J Urol* 146:951–952, 1991.

205. Nghiem DD: En bloc transplantation of kidneys from donors weighing less than 15 kg into adult recipients. *J Urol* 145:14–16, 1991.

206. Darras F, Jordan M, Shapiro R, et al.: Transplantation of pediatric en bloc kidneys with FK506 immunosuppression. *Transplant Proc* 23:3089–3090, 1991.

207. Harmon WE, Alexander SR, Tejani A, et al.: The effect of donor age on graft survival in pediatric cadaver renal transplant recipients. *Transplantation* 54:232–236, 1992.

208. Rosenthal JT, Miserantino DP, Mendez R, et al.: Extending the criteria for cadaver kidney donors. *Transplant Proc* 22:338–340, 1990.

209. Spees EK, et al.: Successful use of cadaver kidneys from diabetic donors for transplantation. *Transplant Proc* 22:378–379, 1990.

210. Abouna GM, Adnani MS, Kumar MS, et al.: Reversal of diabetic glomerulopathy in human cadaveric kidneys after transplantation into nondiabetic recipients. *Lancet* 1:622–624, 1986.

211. Catelao AM, Grino JM, Gonzalez C, et al.: Long term renal function of kidneys transplanted from non-heart beating donors. *Transplant Proc* 23:2584–2586, 1991.

212. Younger SJ, Arnold RM: Ethical, psychosocial, and public policy implications of procuring organs from non-heart beating donors. *JAMA* 269:2769–2772, 1993.

213. Kootstra G, Wijner R, van Hoof JP, et al.: Twenty percent more kidneys through a non-heart beating program. *Transplant Proc* 23:910–912, 1991.

214. Park MS, Barbetti AA, Geer LI, et al.: HLA epitopes depicted by serology. In: PI Terasaki, ed, *Clinical Transplants 1990*. UCLA Tissue Typing Laboratory, Los Angeles, pp 515, 1991.

215. Uryu N, Maeda M, Ota M, et al.: A simple and rapid method of HLA DrB and DQB typing by digestion of PCR amplified DNA with allele specific restriction endonucleases. *Tissue Antigens* 35:20–31, 1990.

216. Bidwell J: DNA-RFLP analysis and genotyping of HLA-Dr and DQ antigens. *Immunol Today* 9:18–23, 1988.

217. Clay TM, Bidwell JL, Howard MR, et al.: PCR fingerprinting for selection of HLA matched unrelated marrow donors. *Lancet* 337:1049–1052, 1991.

218. UNOS Policy 3.3.1, Richmond, VA. United Network for Organ Sharing, 1990.

219. Terasaki PI, Takemoto S, Mickey MR: A report on 128 six antigen matched cadaver kidney transplants. *Clin Transplant* 3:301–305, 1989.

220. Takemoto S, Terasaki PI, Cecka JM, et al.: The UNOS Scientific Renal Transplant Registry. Survival of nationally shared HLA matched kidney transplants from cadaveric donors. *N Engl J Med* 327:834–839, 1992.

221. Takemoto, Carnahan E, Terasaki PI: Report on 604 six antigen matched transplants. In: PI Terasaki, ed, *Clinical Transplants 1990*. UCLA Tissue Typing Laboratory, Los Angeles, pp 485–495, 1991.

222. Terasaki PI, Cecka JM, Gjertson DW, et al.: A ten year prediction for kidney transplant survival. In: PI Terasaki, ed, *Clinical Transplants 1992*. UCLA Tissue Typing Laboratory, Los Angeles, pp 501, 1993.

223. Gjertson DW, Terasaki PI: The large center variation in half-lives of kidney transplants. *Transplantation* 52:357–361, 1992.

224. Matas AJ, Frey DJ, Gillingham KJ, et al.: The impact of HLA matching on graft survival and on sensitization after a failed transplant. Evidence that failure of poorly matched renal transplants does not result in increased sensitization. *Transplantation* 50:599–605, 1990.

225. Cicciarelli J, Terasaki PI, Mickey R: The effect of zero HLA class I and II mismatching in CSA treated kidney patients. *Transplantation* 43:636–640, 1987.

226. Gilks W, Bradley B, Gore S, et al.: Substantial benefits of tissue matching in renal transplantation. *Transplantation* 43:669–674, 1987.

227. Mytillneos J, Scherer S, Dunckley H, et al.: DNA HLA-Dr typing results of 4000 kidney transplants. *Transplantation* 55:778–782, 1993.

228. Ichikawa Y, Hashimoto M, Nojima M, et al.: The significant effect of HLA-DrB1 matching on long term kidney graft outcome. *Transplantation* 56:1368–1371, 1993.

229. Takemoto S, Terasaki PI, Gjertson DW, et al.: Equitable allocation of HLA compatible kidneys for local pools and for minorities. *N Engl J Med*, in press.

230. Najarian JS, Gillingham KJ, Sutherland DR, et al.: The impact of the quality of initial graft function in cadaver kidney transplantation. *Transplantation* 57:812–815, 1994.

231. Gaston RS, Ayres JD, Dooley LG, et al.: Racial equity in renal transplantation: the disparate impact of HLA based allocation. *JAMA* 270:1352–1356, 1993.

232. Foca N, Reed E, Rohowsky C, et al.: Influence of race on the predictability of MLC identity by HLA-Dr matching. *Transplantation* 35:35–39, 1983.

233. Milford E, Ratner L, Yunis E: Will transplant immunogenetics improve graft survival in blacks? Racial variability in the accuracy of tissue typing for organ donation. *Transplant Proc* 19:30–32, 1987.

234. Lazda VA: The impact of HLA frequency differences in races in the access to optimally HLA matched cadaver renal transplants. *Transplantation* 53:352–357, 1992.

235. Barger B, Shroyer TW, Hudson SL, et al.: The impact of the UNOS mandatory sharing policy on recipients of the black and white races—experience at a single center. *Transplantation* 58:770–774, 1992.

236. Lazda VA: An evaluation of a local variance of the UNOS point system on the distribution of cadaver kidneys to waiting minority recipients. *Transplant Proc* 23:901–902, 1991.

237. Rubin RH: Impact of CMV infection on organ transplant recipients. *Rev Infect Dis* 12:S754–S766, 1990.

238. Chou S: Acquisition of donor strains of CMV by renal transplant recipients. *N Engl J Med* 314:1418–1423, 1986.

239. Grundy JE, Super M, Lui S, et al.: The source of CMV infection in sero positive renal allograft recipients is frequently the donor kidney. *Lancet* 16:132–135, 1988.

240. Hibberd PL, Tolkoff-Rubin NE, Cosimi AB, et al.: Symptomatic CMV disease in the sero positive renal transplant recipient treated with OKT3. *Transplantation* 53:68–72, 1992.

241. Snydman DR, Werner BG, Heinze B, et al.: Use of CMV

immune globulin to prevent CMV disease in renal transplant patients. *N Engl J Med* 317:1049–1054, 1987.

242. Balfour H, Chace BA, Stapleton IT, et al.: A randomized placebo controlled trial of oral acyclovir for the prevention of CMV disease in recipients of renal allografts. *N Engl J Med* 320:1381–1387, 1989.

243. Dunn DL, Gillingham KJ, Kramer MA, et al.: A prospective, randomized study of acyclovir vs ganciclovir plus human immune globulin prophylaxis of CMV infection after solid organ transplantation. *Transplantation* 57:876–884, 1994.

244. Hibberd PL, Tolkoff-Rubin NE, Doran M, et al.: Pre-emptive therapy with ganciclovir during OKT3 administration. *Proc ASTS* 11:125, 1992.

245. Preiksaitis JK, Diaz-Mitoma F, Mirzayans F, et al.: Quantitative oropharyngeal EBV virus shedding in renal and cardiac transplant recipients. *J Infect Dis* 166:986–994, 1992.

246. Denning D, Weiss LM, Flechner SM: Transmission of EBV by a transplanted kidney with activation by OKT3 antibody. *Transplantation* 48:141–144, 1989.

247. Stephanian E, Gruber SA, Dunn DL, et al.: Post-transplant lymphoproliferative disorders. *Transplant Rev* 5:120–129, 1991.

CHAPTER 65

Immunosuppression and Treatment of Rejection

M. ROY FIRST

INTRODUCTION

The introduction in the 1980s of cyclosporine and monoclonal antibodies represented a major therapeutic advance in solid organ transplantation. The United Network for Organ Sharing (UNOS) has recently released the 1- and 2-year graft and patient survival rates for solid organ transplants (1). These survival rates are illustrated in Table 1. Currently, there are a number of promising new immunosuppressive agents on the horizon, and it appears likely that further advances will be made in our ability to control the immune response (2,3). A dynamic interaction exists between basic immunology and clinical transplantation. Advances in immunobiology have resulted in a better understanding of the immunological events involved in the recognition of and response to transplant antigens and have led to a better understanding of the action of various immunosuppressive agents. This chapter reviews the mechanisms involved in the immune response, how currently used immunosuppressive agents act, the possible role for future immunosuppressive drugs, the current approach to clinical immunosuppressive therapy, and the diagnosis and treatment of acute rejection.

THE IMMUNE RESPONSE AND GRAFT REJECTION

The pivotal cells in the rejection process are a small population of T lymphocytes that bear receptors for incompatible major histocompatibility complex (MHC) antigens of the donor graft. These cells initiate a series of cellular interactions within the immune system. The initial step involves the interaction between the graft histocompatibility antigens and the host antigen-presenting cells (APCs). An APC (either a macrophage or a dendritic cell) is capable of taking up antigens and presenting them to lymphocytes in a recognizable form. Class I antigens, HLA-A and HLA-B, are found on the cell membrane of almost all nucleated cells, while Class II antigens, HLA-DR, have a more restricted tissue distribution and are present on B

lymphocytes, monocytes, and dendritic cells (4). T-cell activation and proliferation occur as a result of an encounter between donor-specific T-cell clones and graft antigens. The T-cell antigen recognition complex/T-cell receptor (TCR) includes the CD3 complex and two antigen-binding, clone-specific immunoglobulin-like chains (5). Activation of the T cells results in a cascade of events resulting in graft rejection. Activation of macrophages, dendritic cells, or other accessory cells is required for full T-cell activation (5-7). This cascade is initiated by presentation of incompatible graft antigens by APCs to the host. Class II antigens are responsible for initiation of the immune response and are recognized by T-helper cells bearing the distinctive CD4 marker. The incompatible portion of the Class II molecule is recognized by the TCR. The CD4 protein then binds to a separate region of the HLA Class II, thereby strengthening the attachment of CD4+ T cells to the Class II APCs (5). Cytotoxic T cells bearing the CD8 proteins are activated by recognition of HLA Class I molecules. The TCRs recognizes the incompatible portion of the Class I molecule, while the CD8 protein binds to domains of the molecule, adding strength to the attachment of the antigen-bearing cell. Direct cell–cell contact between T cells and accessory cells and/or stimulation of accessory cells by soluble T-cell products causes accessory cell activation.

Once activated, the T-helper cells release a number of lymphokines, including interleukin (IL)-2, interferon (INF)-γ, and IL-6. Activated CD4+ lymphocytes also release macrophage-stimulating factor, which stimulates production of IL-1 by macrophages (8,9). Formation of IL-2 growth factor receptor and release of IL-2 is of central importance in T-cell activation (5,6). Antigen-activated IL-2-stimulated T cells release B-cell activation factors (IL-4, IL-5, IL-6) that enable antigen-activated B-cells to elaborate antibodies directed against the graft, causing humoral rejection (5,10,11). The interaction of soluble IL-2 and high-affinity cellular IL-2 receptors stimulates proliferation of antigen-activated CD4+ helper T cells and CD8+ cytotoxic T cells (12). IL-2 release also stimulates activation of the cytotoxic capacity of cytotoxic T cells (5,13) and the release of INF-γ (10), which in turn activates the

Suki, WN and Massry SG (eds), Suki and Massry's Therapy of Renal Diseases and Related Disorders, Third Edition. ISBN 978-1-4757-6634-9.
©*1998, Kluwer Academic Publishers, Boston/Dordrecht/London. All rights reserved.*

Table 1. One- and two-year graft and patient survival rates, by organ for transplants between October 1, 1987, and December 31, 1991 (1)

Organ	No.	Graft survival (%)[a]		Patient survival (%)[a]	
		1 year	2 year	1 year	2 year
Kidney (cadaveric)	30,307	78.9 ± 0.2	72.8 ± 0.3	93.0 ± 0.1	90.0 ± 0.2
Kidney (living)	8,185	91.0 ± 0.3	87.4 ± 0.4	97.1 ± 0.2	95.6 ± 0.2
Liver	9,810	66.7 ± 0.5	62.3 ± 0.5	73.9 ± 0.5	69.4 ± 0.5
Pancreas	1,638	72.7 ± 1.1	65.2 ± 1.3	89.2 ± 0.8	84.1 ± 1.0
Heart	7,032	81.0 ± 0.5	76.2 ± 0.5	81.6 ± 0.4	77.0 ± 0.5
Heart–lung	197	55.4 ± 3.2	47.7 ± 3.4	55.4 ± 3.2	48.8 ± 3.4
Lung	550	65.8 ± 1.9	53.1 ± 2.6	67.2 ± 1.9	57.7 ± 2.5

[a] Survival rates computed using Kaplan–Meier method (mean ± standard error).

cytodestructive activities of macrophages. INF-γ also stimulates cells of the transplant, such as tubular and endothelial cells that normally do not express Class II HLA molecules, to express such molecules (5,14,15), and enhances expression of Class I antigens (16), thereby changing the biology of the allograft so that it is more susceptible to rejection (17). Lymphokines also recruit host lymphocytes, macrophages, and polymorphonuclear leukocytes into the graft and stimulate bone marrow to produce more inflammatory cells (17).

T cells perform many activities that coordinate the complex process of allograft rejection. Both delayed-type hypersensitivity (mediated by CD4+ cells) and cytotoxic responses (mediated by CD8+ cells), as well as antibody-mediated rejection, play a role in allograft rejection (18). The T-cell activation sequence in allograft rejection and the site of action of immunosuppressive drugs, described below, are outlined in Figure 1.

ACTION OF CURRENTLY USED IMMUNOSUPPRESSIVE AGENTS

Corticosteroids

Corticosteroids are important agents in preventing rejection. For maximal suppression, corticosteroids need to be present at the initiation of the immune response. Corticosteroids act primarily on IL-1 production from macrophages early in the induction phase of T-cell activation. Steroids inhibit production of tumor necrosis factor- (TNF-) α and eicosanoids by macrophages (19,20) and prevent the formation of appropriate amounts of the nuclear factor of activated T cells (NFAT), which activates the IL-2 gene (21,22). In addition, steroids inhibit T-cell activation indirectly by inhibiting expression of Class II MHC antigens on macrophage cell surfaces (23,24). Because IL-2 expression is facilitated by stimulation of T cells by IL-1 and/or IL-6, corticosteroids indirectly block expression of IL-2 (25,26). Additionally, corticosteroids directly block activation of the IL-2, IL-4, and INF-γ genes in T cells. It appears that the inhibitory effects of corticosteroids on cytokine gene

transcription are produced by the capacity of activated glucocorticoid receptors to directly bind to glucocorticoid response elements present within the regular sequence of many cytokine genes (5). Steroids also inhibit migration of immune cells to the site of inflammation and have nonspecific immunosuppressive and anti-inflammatory effects. In the prevention of rejection, steroids are used in combination with azathioprine and/or cyclosporine.

Azathioprine

Azathioprine is the imidazole derivative of 6-mercaptopurine. It is metabolized to 6-mercaptopurine, which in turn is metabolized to 6-thioinosinic acid, an active metabolite that is incorporated into developing cellular strands of DNA, thereby inhibiting purine nucleotide synthesis and metabolism and altering the synthesis and function of cellular RNA (27,28). This interruption of purine synthesis and salvage pathways markedly reduces mitosis of rapidly dividing cells. As an antimetabolite, azathioprine acts in a crucial step in both B- and T-lymphocyte activation. The drug acts at a relatively distal site in the lymphocyte-activation cascade. Since antigen recognition and stimulation of lymphocytes causes rapid cell division of helper and cytotoxic T lymphocytes, azathioprine will reduce the proliferation of these activated cells. The drug also has some nonspecific anti-inflammatory effects. Azathioprine will affect all rapidly dividing cells, such as lymphocytes, hematopoietic cells, and various endothelial cells. Its main side effects include myelosuppression and gastrointestinal intolerance. It also may cause hepatotoxicity, alopecia, and an increased risk of infection and neoplasia development (28). Azathioprine, together with steroids, had been the mainstay of antirejection immunotherapy for solid organ transplantation prior to the advent of cyclosporine, and remains a key component of triple immunosuppression in combination with steroids and cyclosporine (29).

Cyclophosphamide

Cyclophosphamide has an effect on lymphocyte cellular division and mitosis similar to that of azathioprine. It has been used in solid organ transplantation as a substitute for azathioprine. However, its current use in solid organ transplant immunosuppression is limited; azathioprine is generally preferred due to its better risk–benefit ratio. Cyclophosphamide is an alkylating agent, and its activity is dependent on its ability to disrupt cellular growth and mitosis by interfering with the cross-linking of cellular strands of DNA. Metabolic activation of cyclophosphamide is required for the formation of several key active metabolites (28). This drug does have the ability to decrease antibody production. Due to the similar cellular actions of cyclophosphamide and azathioprine, many of the same adverse

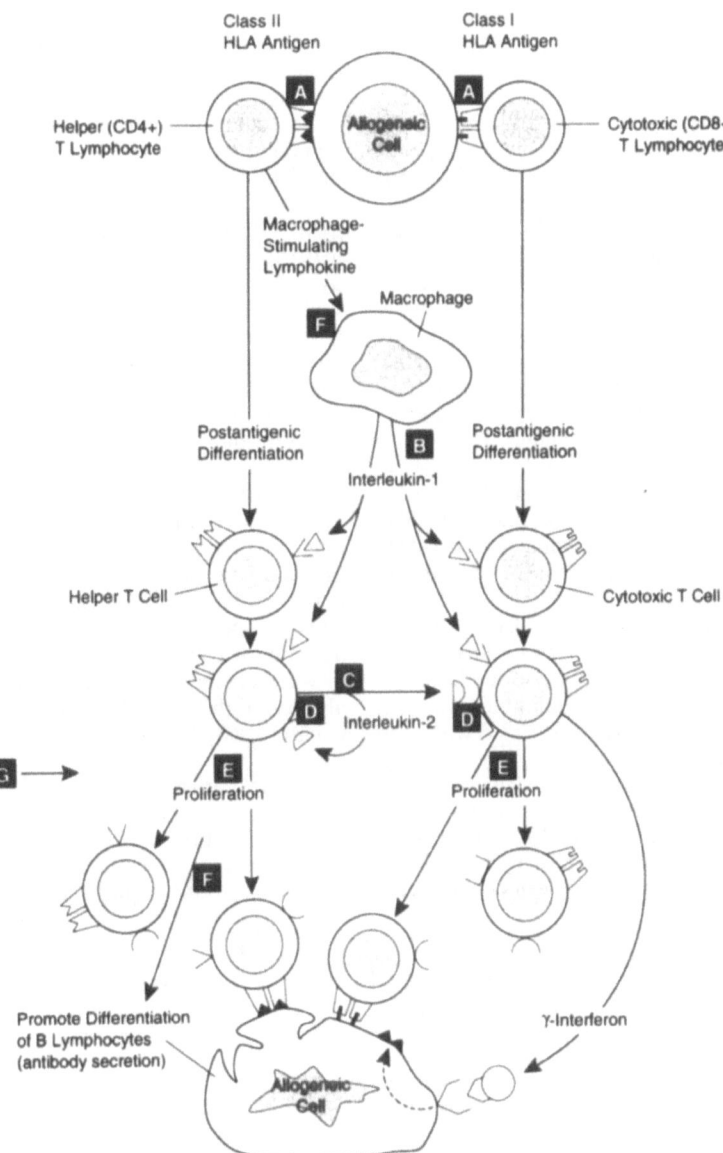

Figure 1. Schematic representation of the immune response leading to allograft recognition and rejection, and sites of action of immunosuppressive drugs. Polyclonal antilymphocyte preparations and OKT3 act at the T-cell receptor site (A). Corticosteroids act primarily on IL-1 production from macrophages early in the induction phase of T-cell activation (B). Cyclosporines and tacrolimus inhibit cytokine, primarily IL-2, synthesis (C). Rapamycin and leflunomide inhibit the action of cytokines (D). Azathioprine, cyclophosphamide, mizoribine, mycophenolate mofetil, and brequinar sodium inhibit DNA and/or RNA synthesis and prevent T-cell proliferation (E). Deoxyspergualin inhibits cell maturation (F). SKF-105685 causes induction of non-specific suppressor cells (G).

effects are noted. Bone marrow suppression appears more commonly with cyclophosphamide, and the development of hemorrhagic cystitis, reported in 2%–40% of cases, can be a particularly troublesome complication (30). Due to the severity of the side effects encountered with this drug, it is rarely used in solid-organ transplant recipients, except in patients with chronic liver disease after transplantation and in instances of toxic reactions to azathioprine.

Cyclosporine A

Cyclosporine A is a small cyclic peptide of fungal origin that has come to play a major role in preventing early allograft rejection episodes and that has resulted in a significant improvement in graft survival rates since its introduction a little more than a decade ago (31). Cyclosporine interferes with the activation phase of T lymphocytes by blocking production of IL-2 from T cells, most likely at the transcription level of IL-2 production (28). It interferes with the antigen-stimulated activation sequence of T cells, thereby blocking T-cell-dependent cellular and humoral mechanisms (5). The drug acts by binding to cytosolic proteins called immunophilins (32,33). Cyclosporine binds to a group of immunophilins called cyclophilins. This binding is critical for the immunosuppressive effect. The active intracellular inhibitor is not the drug alone, but a drug-immunophilin complex (17). The cyclosporine–cyclophilin complex inhibits the action of calcium-activated calcineurin, which is believed to be essential for the activation of DNA-binding proteins (5). The inhibition of IL-2 activity is associated with a decreased response to Class I and II antigens, which are critical for the rejection cascade. It is this selective immunosuppressive activity of cyclosporine that has significantly reduced rejection rates and has improved patient and graft survival associated with solid organ and bone marrow transplants. More recently, cyclosporine A has gained acceptance as a viable treatment for a wide variety of autoimmune disorders, including psoriasis, rheumatoid arthritis, uveitis, and Crohn's disease (34). A major problem with the use of cyclosporine is the difficulty in distinguishing between drug-related nephrotoxicity and acute rejection, since both conditions may present primarily by diminished graft function. Acute rejection episodes in cyclosporine-treated recipients lack the classical signs of fever, graft enlargement, and graft tenderness, features very obvious in the azathioprine-prednisone era. Acute rejection and nephrotoxicity may become manifest despite "therapeutic" drug levels. Hypertension and hyperkalemia may be present in both conditions; moreover, both conditions may coexist. Renal dysfunction is prevalent in nearly all patients treated with cyclosporine (35), with 25%–40% experiencing significant functional impairment (28). With the introduction of cyclosporine, hypertension has become a significant problem in transplant recipients (36–38). Other side effects of cyclosporine therapy include hepatotoxicity, gastrointestinal disturbances, hirsutism, hyperlipidemia, hyperuricemia, glucose intolerance, gingival hyperplasia, hypertrichosis, and neurotoxicity (28,39). A number of well-documented drug interactions with cyclosporine A have been recognized. These interactions may occur as a result of 1) drugs that induce the cytochrome oxidase p-450 enzymes in the liver, thereby accelerating cyclosporine metabolism; 2) drugs that inhibit cytochrome oxidase enzymes, resulting in elevated levels of the parent compound; or 3) drugs that have synergistic nephrotoxicity with cyclosporine A. These interactions, which are illustrated in Table 2, may either reduce or potentiate the therapeutic effect of cyclosporine A, resulting in under-immunosuppression or toxicity, respectively. For these reasons, it is important to monitor clinical and biochemical parameters and cyclosporine blood levels when drugs known to interact with cyclosporine A are either added or discontinued, or when dosages are altered (28). In the long term, it has also been difficult to distinguish chronic cyclosporine nephrotoxicity from chronic rejection.

Polyclonal antilymphocyte agents

Polyclonal antibodies against human lymphoid tissue has been prepared from the serum of a variety of animals immunized with human lymph nodes, thymus, or spleen.

Table 2. Cyclosporine A drug interactions (28)

Decreased concentration	Increased concentration	Synergistic nephrotoxicity
Carbamazepine	Ciprofloxacin	Acyclovir
Isoniazid	Erythromycin	Aminoglycosides
Phenobarbital	Fluconazole	Amphotericin B
Phenytoin	Itraconazole	Furosemide
Rifampicin (rifampin)	Ketoconazole	Ganciclovir
	Metoclopramide	H_2-antagonists
	Methylprednisolone	Melphalan
	Nicardipine	Trimethoprim-sulfamethoxazole
	Verapamil	Nonsteroidal anti-inflammatory drugs
		Vancomycin

Preparations of antibodies used clinically include anti-lymphocyte and antilymphoblast globulin (ALG), antithymocyte globulin (ATG), and antilymphocyte serum (ALS), prepared in horses, rabbits, goats, or sheep. These agents have been used for both induction therapy and reversal of acute rejection episodes (40–42). Polyclonal immune globulins represent a heterogeneous group of antibodies, only a minority of which are specific to T cells. Non-T-cell-specific antibodies account for the greatest binding activity of these preparations. Polyclonal antilymphocyte preparations exert their immunosuppressive effects by complement-mediated lysis and opsonization of lymphocytes and by masking of functioning of important T-cell surface antigens (5,40). Each polyclonal preparation varies in its constituent antibodies. Due to this unpredictable antibody mixture, treatment response and side effects are variable between the different preparations. Allergic reactions to these preparations result in fever and chills. More severe reactions include the development of pruritus, hypotension, acute respiratory distress, and anaphylaxis. Unwanted antibodies can cause thrombocytopenia, granulocytopenia, arthralgia, serum sickness, and immune complex glomerulonephritis (5,28,40). Administration requires 4–6 hours using a central vein catheter. Earlier studies have shown a significant improvement in graft survival in patients receiving a polyclonal antibody for induction together with steroids and azathioprine (40,41). Since the introduction of cyclosporine, the use of these agents has been particularly valuable in patients with acute tubular necrosis who may be more sensitive to the nephrotoxic effects of cyclosporine. In these patients, the institution of cyclosporine therapy can be delayed until good graft function has been obtained. Polyclonal antilymphocyte preparations have also been used successfully in the treatment of steroid-resistant rejection episodes, although monoclonal antibody therapy has tended to supplant polyclonal antilymphocyte preparations for treatment of acute rejection in most instances (43).

Monoclonal antibodies

The development and production of monoclonal antibodies holds promise for a more sophisticated approach to immunosuppressive therapy. Currently, OKT3 is the only monoclonal antibody in widespread use. It was derived by harvesting splenic B cells from mice sensitized with human peripheral T cells and fusing these B cells with myeloma cells. This resulted in an IgG2a monoclonal antibody that reacts with all T cells and approximately 10% of thymocytes (44). OKT3 is a murine monoclonal antibody directed against the epsilon portion of the CD3 receptor on the surface of human T cells (45). The CD3 molecule is closely associated with the TCR, which plays a vital role in T-cell function. OKT3 inhibits the CD3/TCR complex, inactivating lymphocytes. After the first dose of OKT3, lymphocytes are removed from the circulation via opsonization. Following this first dose, lymphocytes return

to the peripheral blood with the CD3 receptor modulated from the surface (46,47). In the initial randomized multicenter study, OKT3 successfully reversed 94% of rejection episodes compared with a 75% reversal in patients treated with steroids (48). Following this initial study, there have been numerous similar experiences reported with OKT3 in reversing primary and steroid-resistant acute renal allograft rejection (40,43,44,47,49–51) as well as acute vascular rejection (52). More recently, OKT3 has been used as an induction therapy. Strategies have varied regarding prophylactic administration of OKT3. It has been used in high-risk patients, such as retransplant recipients or highly sensitized recipients of first grafts (53,54), and in patients with acute tubular necrosis so as to avoid early cyclosporine exposure (55). In a multicenter trial comparing OKT3 induction with triple therapy with cyclosporine, prednisone, and azathioprine, OKT3 prophylaxis significantly delayed the time to first rejection episode, decreased the percentage of patients having rejection, and reduced the number of patients with multiple rejection episodes, and in addition, a greater percentage of rejection episodes in the OKT3 induction group were responsive to steroid therapy (56); however, there was no statistical improvement in short-term graft survival rates. The main side effect with OKT3 is a profound reaction to the first dose (47,48), characterized by pyrexia, chills, tremor, vomiting, and diarrhea. Severe pulmonary edema may develop in patients who are fluid overloaded prior to OKT3 administration (48). This syndrome appears to be related to systemic release of cytokines—TNF, INF, and IL-2 (57–59). OKT3 causes reversible renal dysfunction, also believed to be mediated by high levels of circulating cytokines, thus termed *cytokine nephropathy* (60). The severe first-dose reactions can be minimized by the administration of high-dose methylprednisolone (61), indomethacin (62), pentoxifylline (63), and an anti-TNF monoclonal antibody (64). The development of human antimurine antibody may limit the effectiveness of OKT3, especially if the agent is administered for a second course in the same individual (44,48). The anti-OKT3 response consists of both IgM and IgG antibodies, with approximately 70% of patients exhibiting an IgM response and 50% developing an IgG response (65). The majority of these responses, approximately 60%, are IgG in class and anti-idiotypic in specificity; that is, they react specifically with idiotypic determinants of OKT3 and not with determinants common to other IgG2a antibodies (65,66). Approximately 40% of the antibody responses are anti-isotypic in that they react with determinants common to all IgG2a antibodies (44,65,66). The development of IgG-blocking antibodies, which are anti-idiotypic in specificity, may neutralize the efficacy of OKT3 treatment, while anti-isotypic or IgM anti-idiotypic antibodies have not been shown to neutralize OKT3 immunosuppressive effectiveness (66). The development of anti-OKT3 antibodies can be reduced by the use of high-dose cyclosphosphamide (67), azathioprine (68), and cyclosporine A (68,69). Retreatment with OKT3 has been successful in patients with no antibody formation and low-titer anti-OKT3 antibodies, provided that close monitoring of serum OKT3 levels, circulating CD3 levels, and antibody titers are measured and that appropriate dose adjustments are made (70).

NEW IMMUNOSUPPRESSIVE AGENTS UNDERGOING CLINICAL STUDIES

Over the next few years, we will witness the emergence of many new, potent immunosuppressive agents for use in transplant recipients and in patients with autoimmune diseases. Because each of these agents will display toxic complications at full therapeutic doses, treatment strategies will seek to exploit the synergistic activity of immunosuppressives. This will permit dose reduction and avoidance of toxicity while preserving biological effects and potentiating immunosuppression (2,71–73). New immunosuppressive drugs have been classified according to mechanism of action (73). A modification of this classification is as follows: 1) inhibition of DNA and RNA synthesis (mizoribine, mycophenolate mofetil, brequinar sodium), 2) inhibition of cytokine synthesis (cyclosporines, tacrolimus/FK-506), 3) inhibition of cytokine action (rapamycin, leflunomide), 4) inhibition of cell maturation (deoxyspergualin), and 5) induction of nonspecific suppressor cells (SKF-105685). The sites of action of these drugs are illustrated in Figure 1.

Mizoribine (Bredinin)

Mizoribine (previously termed Bredinin) is a imidazole nucleoside that has been used in Japan for over 10 years. It inhibits inosine monophosphate (IMP) dehydrogenase, an important enzyme in the purine biosynthetic pathway. Inhibition of RNA and DNA synthesis affects both humoral and cell-mediated immune responses (74–76). The immunosuppressive mechanism and potency of mizoribine are similar to those of azathioprine, but mizoribine lacks azathioprine's hepatic toxicity and bone marrow suppression (74–83). Mizoribine has been shown to be synergistic with low-dose cyclosporine in prolonging allograft survival rates in experimental animals (74,78,80). In humans, mizoribine has been effective when used with steroids (77) and with low-dose cyclosporine and prednisolone (79,81–83). In these studies, there was a low graft loss rate beyond the first year, which may be a reflection of mizoribine's ability to prevent chronic graft rejection due to the agent's effect on the B-cell response. However, mizoribine does not appear to be a very potent immunosuppressive agent; in one study, rejection episodes occurred significantly earlier in the mizoribine-treated patients—with more of the rejection being steroid-resistant than in the azathioprine-treated group—and a higher percentage of patients treated with mizoribine were converted to azathioprine due to acute rejection episodes than were converted from

azathioprine to mizoribine (82). Elimination of mizoribine is dependent on renal function, and the dose needs to be adjusted during periods of renal dysfunction (82,84). A major problem encountered with the administration of mizoribine to canine renal allograft recipients is enterotoxicity, which has been associated with renal dysfunction and decreased excretion of the drug, resulting in elevated serum concentrations (84). Elevated serum levels of mizoribine induce angionecrosis of intestinal submucosal arteries, resulting in degeneration, necrosis, and fibrosis of the mucosa (78,84). This side effect has also been described in humans (82). Mizoribine has also been shown to suppress human cytomegalovirus (CMV) replication in vitro (85). Further studies and longer follow-up data will enable clarification of its role as a useful immunosuppressive agent. However, with the development of new drugs that inhibit DNA and RNA synthesis, it does not appear likely that mizoribine will become widely used in the future.

Mycophenolate mofetil (RS-61443)

Mycophenolate mofetil is the ethyl ester of the fungal antibiotic mycophenolic acid. Mycophenolic acid is a potent inhibitor of the enzyme inosine monophosphate dehydrogenase (IMPDH) in the purine biosynthetic pathway, and also inhibits mannose and fucose glycosolation, which is required for activation of human peripheral blood lymphocytes (86–88). Mycophenolic acid is poorly absorbed following oral administration; the use of the prodrug, mycohenolate mofetil, greatly improves the oral bioavailability (86–89). Beta-glucuronidase metabolizes mycohenolate mofetil to mycohenolic acid glucuronide, which is a potent inhibitor of IMP dehydrogenase. Mycophenolic acid glucuronide is secreted into the bile and then converted by intestinal glucuronidase back into active mycophenolic acid; a high concentration is present in the intestine, making this agent a potentially useful drug in future small bowel transplantation (89). This phenomenon may also explain the gastrointestinal toxicity of the drug, which is particularly prominent in dogs. Inhibition of de novo purine synthesis results in powerful inhibition of lymphocyte activation (90–92). Effects of this agent appear to be relatively selective for lymphocytes. In experimental animals, the drug has been shown to prolong skin, heart, kidney, and islet allograft survival and to inhibit development of chronic vascular rejection in rat heart recipients (86,89,93–95). This agent also prolongs heart allograft survival rates in highly sensitized animal recipients when it is combined with cyclosporine (96). Clinical trials with mycohenolate mofetil in human recipients of cadaver renal allograft have shown promising results when used in combination with cyclosporine A and steroids (95,97–99). Present data indicate that the most effective oral dose is between 2000 and 3500 mg/day (98,99). In a single-center study (99), patient and graft survival rates at 2 years were 100% and 95%, respectively, in patients receiving mycophenolate mofetil as part of sequential quadruple immunosuppressive therapy, and no grafts were lost to acute rejection. In another study (100), the addition of mycophenolate mofetil to cyclosporine monotherapy did not influence the occurrence or the severity of acute rejection episodes; however, the dose of mycophenolate mofetil in this study was 200–1000 mg/day. In current Phase III clinical trials, doses of 1500 mg twice daily are being utilized. The drug has also been used as rescue therapy for biopsy-proven rejection refractory to treatment with high-dose steroid, ALG, or OKT3 therapy (99,101). In the larger, multicenter study (101), successful rescue, defined as stabilization or improvement in renal function, was achieved in 52 of 75 patients (69%), with a follow-up time of 8–18 months. Mycophenolate mofetil was instituted within 48 hours of biopsy at a dose of 1000–1500 mg orally twice a day. The success of rescue therapy was related to the quality of renal function at the start of mycophenolate mofetil; patients enrolled with a serum creatinine of 4 mg/dL or less had a rescue rate of 79% compared to 52% in patients with a serum creatinine of more than 4 mg/dL (101). This agent has also been shown to be effective in reversing persistent acute rejection in hepatic allograft recipients resistant to treatment with high-dose steroids and OKT3 (102). This drug appears to show great promise for both induction and maintenance therapy, as well as for rescue of refractory rejection. Additional Phase III clinical studies with this agent are ongoing in Europe and the United States and should be available in the near future. It is anticipated that this drug will receive approval for use in transplant recipients within the next 12 months.

Brequinar sodium

Brequinar sodium is an anticancer agent that inhibits de novo pyrimidine biosynthesis. It noncompetitively inhibits dihydro-orotic acid dehydrogenase, a key enzyme in the synthesis of pyrimidines. This inhibition results in depletion of the nucleotide precursors, uridine and cytidine, which are important in DNA and RNA synthesis (103). Brequinar has been shown to be very effective either alone or in combination with low-dose cyclosporine A in prolongation of heart, liver, and kidney allograft survival in the rat (104–107). In these studies, permanent tolerance developed in approximately 50% of liver recipients and in 90% of kidney recipients after a 30-day course of the drug (105). Brequinar has also been shown to be effective, in combination with cyclosporine, in preventing cardiac allograft rejection in primates (108), and it potentiates the effect of cyclosporine in experimental small bowel transplantation (109). The drug exhibits synergistic activity when used with cyclosporine and rapamycin in rat cardiac allograft recipients (110).

The combination of brequinar with mycophenolate mofetil has resulted in significant prolongation of rat cardiac survival when compared to either agent alone (111). It is possible that the use of these two compounds in combination could result in additive activity due to their individual metabolic effects in inhibiting purine (mycophenolate mofetil) and pyrimidine (brequinar sodium) biosynthesis. Brequinar sodium also inhibits B-cell-mediated immune responses and has been shown to suppress in vivo antibody production (112). In models of accelerated cardiac graft rejection, treatment with brequinar suppresses antidonor IgM and IgG production in the allograft and xenograft recipients, and a close correlation was noted between suppression of antibody production and prolonged graft survival. In addition, brequinar treatment was associated with a reduction in the severity of antibody-mediated vascular lesions in allografts in sensitized recipients (112). Approximately 70% of this drug is cleared by the bile and feces and 30% by the urine. The main side effects are bone marrow suppression and gastrointestinal toxicity. Leukopenia and thrombocytopenia are important side effects with this agent. This agent may become an important addition to the polytherapeutic regimen for the prevention and treatment of human allograft rejection. It is currently in the early stages of clinical studies in renal, hepatic, and cardiac allograft recipients, and one would anticipate that it could be available for use in the next 3–4 years.

Cyclosporines

Cyclosporine A has had a substantial impact on organ transplantation by significantly reducing the rate and severity of rejection episodes (31,39). However, currently available oral formulations of cyclosporine A have markedly variable absorption and disposition, which is of particular concern for a drug that has a narrow therapeutic window (113–115). In addition, renal dysfunction is prevalent in the majority of patients treated with cyclosporine (31,34,35,38,39). These problems have led to the search for formulations with improved bioavailability and to the development of analogues that might be equipotent as immunosuppressive agents but less nephrotoxic.

MICROEMULSION FORMULATION OF CYCLOSPORINE A

Bioavailability following oral administration of cyclosporine A shows marked intrasubject and intersubject variation. The reported bioavailability varied from 10% to 60%, with an overall mean of approximately 29% (116). Poor absorption through the gastrointestinal mucosa is one of the main reasons for the low and variable absolute bioavailability, takes place only in the upper gastrointestinal tract, and requires the presence of bile in the gastrointestinal tract (113). In addition, the poor solubility of the current formulation of cyclosporine A in aqueous fluid of the gastrointestinal tract might be an additional absorption-limiting factor. Recently, a microemulsion formulation of cyclosporine has been introduced for clinical studies. This formulation has been shown to result in improved bioavailability in both normal volunteers (117) and stable renal transplant recipients (118). The new formulation of cyclosporine A immediately forms a transparent microemulsion aqueous fluid, simulating the mixed micellar phase obtained after the digestion of lipid droplets. This fluid allows for release of cyclosporine rapidly in the gastrointestinal tract and uses its entire length for absorption; it allows for the cyclosporine to be kept in solution during dilution by aqueous gastrointestinal fluids, it is able to incorporate a high concentration of cyclosporine in a dissolved and stable state without recrystalization, and its absorption is independent of the presence of bile (119). With the microemulsion formulation of cyclosporine A, bioavailability is increased by 15%–30% and maximum blood cyclosporine concentration by 40%–60%, without change in the trough blood levels (118,120,121). Improved bioavailability has been shown to occur in pediatric (122) and adult (123) liver transplant recipients, diabetics undergoing kidney or kidney and pancreas transplantation (124), cardiac transplant recipients (125), and renal transplant recipients (121,126). In a clinical trial of 300 renal transplant recipients (126), a 1:1 conversion from cyclosporine A to the microemulsion formulation resulted in an increase in the serum creatinine level of 8% and a mean dose decrease of 9%–15%. Currently, the microemulsion formulation of cyclosporine A is undergoing extensive clinical trials in solid organ transplant recipients in Europe and the United States. This formulation of cyclosporine A should be available for clinical use in the next 1–2 years. It is likely that the microemulsion formulation will replace the currently available oral solution and soft gelatin capsules of cyclosporine A. However, the improved bioavailability may result in more acute and chronic toxicity, and close monitoring will be required.

CYCLOSPORINE G (OG37-325)

Cyclosporine G or Nva-2 cyclosporine is a natural analogue of cyclosporine A. It is also a cyclic endecapeptide in which the alpha-aminobutyric acid residue in the second position has been replaced by norvaline. It was developed in an attempt to find a cyclosporine analogue with immunosuppressive activity equivalent to that of cyclosporine A but with less renal toxicity. In vitro and in vivo immunological studies have shown similar immunosuppressive efficacy between cyclosporine A and cyclosporine G (127–129). In renal and heart transplantation in rats, cyclosporine G has been shown to be as effective as cyclosporine A but to cause less nephrotoxicity (127,130). Hepatotoxicity has been reported in experimental animals given cyclosporine G (127,131). In a recent study (132), the toxicity and pharmacokinetics of cyclosporine A and cyclosporine G were compared in an experimental model of chronic cyclosporine-induced nephropathy. In this model, adult male Sprague–Dawley rats given cyclosporine A on a salt-depleted diet developed marked decreases in glomerular filtration rate (GFR) as well as irreversible striped tubulointerstitial injury similar to the histological

lesions seen in human chronic cyclosporine-induced nephrotoxicity. When comparable blood levels of cyclosporine A and cyclosporine G were achieved, cyclosporine A-treated rats had a significantly lower GFR, lower creatinine clearance, and higher serum creatinine level than cyclosporine G-treated animals. Cyclosporine G induced less tubulointerstitial injury than cyclosporine A. Total bilirubin levels were higher in cyclosporine A and cyclosporine G animals than controls, but liver enzymes were not increased with either of the cyclosporines. Liver histology was consistently normal or showed mild fatty changes. Cyclosporine G had a higher clearance than cyclosporine A, lower trough blood levels when given at equivalent doses, smaller area under the curve, higher volume of distribution, and lower renal and hepatic tissue levels. Liver tissue levels were two times higher than renal tissue levels in cyclosporine G-treated animals, a phenomenon not observed with cyclosporine A. These findings were only partially explained by differences in pharmacokinetics and suggest innate differences in tissue uptake and nephrotoxic potential of the two drugs. Differences in drug metabolism and the lower kidney tissue concentration of cyclosporine G may explain the preservation of GFR and the reduced renal cortical and medullary histologic injury with cyclosporine G as compared with cyclosporine A (132). Preliminary results of clinical trials comparing cyclosporine A and cyclosporine G in human transplant recipients have demonstrated similar patient and graft survival rates (133,134). In one study (133), similar nephrotoxicity was seen with both analogues but more hepatotoxicity in cyclosporine G-treated patients. In the other study, less nephrotoxicity but slightly more hepatotoxicity was observed in the cyclosporine G-treated patients (134). In these two studies, patients treated with cyclosporine G had lower serum creatinine levels, higher inulin clearance rates, and lower uric acid levels than the cyclosporine A-treated patients. Cyclosporine G is currently in Phase III clinical studies in Europe and America. It is envisaged that this agent will become available for clinical use in the microemulsion formulation in the next 2–3 years. If the experimental findings are confirmed in the ongoing clinical trials, cyclosporine G may become an important alternative for long-term transplant and nontransplant immunosuppression.

IMM-125

IMM-125 is another cyclosporine analogue. It is the hydroxyethyl derivative of D-serine-8 cyclosporine A. In animal models of autoimmune diseases, IMM-125 was found to be marginally less effective than cyclosporine A (135). It has been shown to cause impairment of kidney and liver function, with histologic changes in these organs. Recently, a European multicenter study with IMM-125 was started. In this study, patients with kidney transplants displaying evidence of cyclosporine A nephrotoxicity are to be switched to treatment with IMM-125. Results of this study are not yet available. However, given the marginally less immunosuppressive efficacy and the potential for hepatotoxicity, this drug does not seem to offer an advance. At the present time, it does not appear that this drug will obtain widespread clinical use.

Tacrolimus (FK-506)

Tacrolimus, previously designated FK-506, was approved for clinical use in liver transplant recipients in the United States by the Food and Drug Administration (FDA) in May 1994. Tacrolimus is a macrolide antibiotic isolated from a soil actinomycete (136). It blocks T-cell activation genes by a mechanism similar to that of cyclosporine A (137–140). It binds to an immunophilin, FK-506 binding protein (FKBP), and prevents signal transduction pathways in T lymphocytes (138,140–143). The drug inhibits alloantigen and mitogen stimulation of T-cell proliferation, as well as the production of IL-2, IL-3, IL-4, INF, and granulocyte-macrophage colony-stimulating factor (137–141). Tacrolimus has an in vitro potency 10–100 times greater than cyclosporine with reference to inhibition of the MLC reaction, generation of cytotoxic T cells, and expression of IL-2 receptors on T cells (137–141). It is also substantially more potent than cyclosporine in suppressing B-cell activation (140,144,145). Tacrolimus has been shown to be highly effective in preventing rejection and suppressing a variety of spontaneous and experimental autoimmune diseases in animals (137,139,140,146–148). Tacrolimus was first used in clinical kidney transplantation at the University of Pittsburgh. The early results revealed patient and graft survival rates similar to those achieved with cyclosporine-based immunosuppression, despite less favorable immunological characteristics in the tacrolimus group (149). The incidence of hypertension and freedom from steroid use were statistically better with tacrolimus, and serum cholesterol and uric acid levels were lower in the tacrolimus-treated patients than in the cyclosporine-treated patients. The other initial clinical experience with tacrolimus in kidney transplant recipients has been reported from Japan (150), where good patients and graft survival rates were obtained but approximately 30% of patients were withdrawn from tacrolimus due to side effects. In a randomized trial of 204 patients utilizing tacrolimus in a double-drug regimen (FK-506/prednisone) versus a triple-drug regimen (FK-506/azathioprine/prednisone), actuarial 1-year patient and graft survival rates for the two-drug and three-drug regimens were 95% and 90% versus 91% and 82%, respectively (151). Rejection rates were less in the three-drug regimen (37%) versus the two-drug regimen (51%). Tacrolimus has also been used at the University of Pittsburgh in an attempt to salvage renal allograft with ongoing rejection failing cyclosporine immunosuppression (152). In 54 patients, all treated for rejection prior to conversion from cyclosporine to tacrolimus, successful conversion (defined as a return to baseline serum creatinine and/or improvement in the

postconversion allograft biopsy) occurred in 70% of cases. Conversion was more successful in patients with acute cellular rejection (76%) than in those with vascular rejection (69%). In another study, conversion from cyclosporine to tacrolimus in renal allograft recipients with chronic rejection was not successful (153). Initial clinical experience, also from the University of Pittsburgh, with tacrolimus in pediatric renal, hepatic, cardiac, lung, islet, small bowel, and combined transplants have resulted in good patient and graft survival rates and the ability to substantial reduce, or withdraw steroids (154). However, the majority of the reports from the University of Pittsburgh have been comparative studies rather than randomized trials. Recently, reports of two large randomized trials comparing tacrolimus and cyclosporine in liver transplant recipients have been published (155,156). In both the U.S. and European studies, patient and graft survival at 1 year was similar; however, significantly less acute rejection, steroid-resistant rejection, and refractory rejection were noted in the tacrolimus-treated patients. On the other hand, tacrolimus was associated with more patients being withdrawn from the studies due to adverse events(155,156). The side effects of tacrolimus are similar to those seen with cyclosporine and include nephrotoxicity, neurotoxicity, gastrointestinal tract complaints, induction of diabetes, infection, and malignancy. Like cyclosporine, tacrolimus demonstrates significant nephrotoxicity. Approximately 5% of tacrolimus-treated patients were withdrawn from the U.S. multicenter liver transplant trial because of nephrotoxicity (157). Like cyclosporine A nephrotoxicity, tacrolimus-induced nephrotoxicity appears to be dose related. The clinical presentation and the morphology of tacrolimus-induced nephrotoxic changes are identical to those of cyclosporine (140,158–160). The incidence of nephrotoxicity appears to be higher in adults than in pediatric transplant recipients. In the U.S. multicenter liver transplant trial, 13% of tacrolimus-treated pediatric patients experienced an increase in serum creatinine, compared with 37% of adult patients (157). Tacrolimus has also been associated with neurotoxicity. Neurological adverse effects associated with posttransplant tacrolimus immunosuppression most commonly developed during the intravenous phase of drug administration and can be categorized as major (aphasia, seizures, confusion, psychosis, encephalopathy, coma) and minor (tremors, headache, sleep disturbances, nightmares, paresthesia) neurotoxicity (161). Tacrolimus therapy has been associated with hyperglycemia after liver, kidney, and heart transplantation (155–157,160). In the U.S. multicenter liver transplant trial, 18% of patients taking tacrolimus and 14% taking cyclosporine A were hyperglycemic (156), while in the main phase of the European study, the frequency of hyperglycemia was 31% in the tacrolimus group versus 20% in the cyclosporine A group (155). In renal allograft recipients randomized to therapy with either of these two drugs, diabetes mellitus developed in 20% treated with tacrolimus and 7% treated with cyclosporine A (162). The incidence of new-onset diabetes mellitus in allograft recipients treated with tacrolimus appears to be much lower among the pediatric than the adult population (157,163). Tacrolimus has been shown to inhibit glucose-induced insulin release at high concentrations (164). The incidence of hypertension appear to be less with tacrolimus-based immunosuppression than with cyclosporine A-based immunosuppression (149). In addition, there appears to be less severe elevations of the serum uric acid level (149), and in liver transplant recipients, FK-506 has been associated with lower triglycerides, cholesterol, and LDL levels at 6 months and 1 year when compared with cyclosporine A (149,165). In the U.S. liver study, the frequency of gastrointestinal symptoms was significantly higher with tacrolimus, which is not surprising considering the macrolide structure of tacrolimus (156). Serious infections and lymphoproliferative disease, related to overall immunosuppression rather than to an individual agent per se, appeared to occur with similar frequency in tacrolimus- and cyclosporine A-treated allograft recipients (140,157). However, a high incidence of lymphoproliferative disease has been reported in pediatric patients receiving tacrolimus (154). Gingival hyperplasia and hirsutism, which commonly occur with cyclosporine therapy, have not been reported with tacrolimus (166). Based on the initial clinical reports, tacrolimus appears to be a promising new agent for use in solid organ transplant recipients. Currently, a number of Phase III multicenter studies are under way in Europe and the United States that compare tacrolimus-based immunosuppression to cyclosporine-based immunosuppression. Tacrolimus has been reported to exhibit pharmacologic antagonism with cyclosporine A, even when both agents are used in low doses (167). However, in a recent study, combination therapy with tacrolimus and cyclosporine at suboptimal doses proved to be effective in prolonging canine lung allografts (168). This agent should become available for use in other transplant recipients in the next 1–2 years.

Sirolimus (rapamycin)

Rapamycin has recently been given the generic name of sirolimus. It is a macrolide antibiotic derived from a soil bacterium and is structurally related to tacrolimus (139,142). Despite the structural similarity to tacrolimus, sirolimus suppresses graft rejection by interfering with cytoplasmic biochemical cascades that transduce signals from cell membranes to the nucleus. Sirolimus also binds to FKBP, but does not inhibit cytokine gene transcription in T cells; rather, it blocks signals transduced from IL-2 receptors to the nucleus (139,142,143,169–174). Binding of sirolimus to its FKBP inhibits p70S6 kinase activity, which is essential for ribosomal phosphorylation and cell cycle progression (142,173). Sirolimus is strongly synergistic with cyclosporine but has an antagonistic response when administered with tacrolimus due to competition for the same FKBP (139,169–171,175). Thus, while both sirolimus and

tacrolimus bind to the FKBP, these agents have highly distinctive mechanisms of action. The drug has been shown to prolong survival rates in a variety of experimental transplant models (139,169,176–178). Sirolimus also inhibits humoral immune responses (174) and has been shown to be effective in reversing ongoing graft rejection in animal models (179,180). This agent has also been effective in delaying and preventing graft vessel disease, frequently encountered in patients with long-surviving grafts (181). Sirolimus mitigates chronic graft vessel disease in rat transplant models (182) and inhibits DNA synthesis in smooth muscle cell cultures more effectively than cyclosporine A, tacrolimus, mycophenolic acid, and deoxyspergualin (183). Therefore, this agent may have a future role in the prevention of chronic allograft rejection and accelerated atheromatous disease in transplant recipients (181). Toxicity studies in rats have shown that sirolimus causes focal myocardial necrosis, increased blood glucose levels, thymic involution, and thrombocytopenia, with little impairment of renal or hepatic function (177,181,184). Vasculitis, which has been observed in dogs, has not been observed in the rat model (139). Sirolimus is in the early phases of clinical experimentation as both an agent for maintenance immunosuppression and for the treatment of acute rejection. The marked synergism between rapamycin and cyclosporine in experimental animals offers an appealing approach for clinical studies. Brequinar sodium has been shown to potentiate the synergistic effect of suboptimal doses of rapamycin and cyclosporine A in prolonging rat cardiac allograft survival (110,185). Sirolimus blocks the immunosuppressive pathway at a different point from other recognized immunosuppressants, and theoretically, a more specific and less toxic effect could be achieved by a combination approach with lower doses of cyclosporine A. It is envisaged that this agent may be available for clinical use in the next 3–5 years.

Leflunomide

Leflunomide is an isoxazol derivative that is well absorbed in man and rapidly converted to its active open-ring form that strongly inhibits T-cell and B-cell proliferation (186–188). Some in vitro studies have shown that the drug inhibits IL-2-induced T-cell proliferation (186,187), while other studies have shown that the drug suppresses IL-2 receptor expression (188). Leflunomide may exert its immunosuppressive effect by inhibiting tyrosine kinase activity, which is involved in the IL-2 signal transduction pathway (186,187). In experimental animals, leflunomide has been shown to prolong survival of skin, kidney, and cardiac transplants (186,188,189). Combining leflunomide with cyclosporine significantly increases survival of allografts in comparison to either agent alone (186,189). In animals with established acute rejection of cardiac allografts, leflunomide was superior to cyclosporine in its ability to reverse such a reaction (186). This agent is in the early stages of development. However, its strong synergism with cyclosporine A raises the possibility that this compound may have application in man for modification of alloresponsiveness.

Deoxyspergualin

15-Deoxyspergualin is an antitumor antibiotic from a soil bacillus. It is another immunosuppressive agent that has been developed and evaluated largely in Japan. It has been shown to have immunosuppressive activity in several animal systems. It decreases the late hypersensitivity responses and inhibits autoimmunity and antibody production (190–195). In vitro studies with this drug have shown that it suppresses macrophage function, blocks IL-1 production, inhibits production of oxygen-derived radicals in monocytes, decreases the expression of Class II antigens on splenic macrophages, decreases cytoxic T-lymphocyte proliferation, induces long-term immunological unresponsiveness, and inhibits antibody production (139,190–195). It has been shown to be effective in prolonging allograft survival rates and reversing allograft rejection in a number of animal transplant models (139,190,192,196,197). The drug exhibits strong synergism with cyclosporine A (190,194) and with FK-506 (198). In clinical studies from Japan, 15-deoxyspergualin has been used as part of induction therapy in living related and cadaveric renal transplant recipients. In these studies, the incidence of rejection in the first month was 30%–50%; however, most of these rejections were reported to be mild and were reversed by steroid therapy (199–201). The drug has also been reported to be effective in reversing acute renal allograft rejection in 80%–90% of cases when combined with methylprednisolone (202–204). This drug is currently undergoing clinical evaluation in Europe and the United States. It has been shown to be effective in the treatment of renal allograft rejection (205,206) and in refractory cases of liver (207) and kidney transplant (208) rejection. The main side effect of 15-deoxyspergualin is bone marrow suppression. Other side effects include perioral numbness and gastrointestinal tract disturbances (200,201). A major drawback with this agent is its very poor bioavailability after oral administration. In clinical studies, 15-deoxyspergualin has been given by intravenous infusion; thus, it appears that the drug's role will be as a short-term agent for induction and/or for the treatment of acute rejection episodes. It will probably be another 3–5 years before it becomes available for clinical use.

SKF-105685

SKF-105685 is an azaspirane with a novel effect on the immune system. Azaspiranes have been shown to effectively ameliorate the manifestations of adjuvant-induced arthritis, experimental allergic encephalitis, and models of murine lupus nephritis in experimental animals (209). Although its exact mechanism of action remains unknown, SKF-105685 has been shown to cause a dose-dependent stimulation of suppressor activity in normal rat splenocytes (210). Studies in rodents and dogs have demonstrated the unique ability of the compound to induce the generation of suppressive cell activity in the spleen, bone marrow, and lymph nodes, which occurs in the absence of myelotoxicity (209–211). These cells lack the surface markers characteristic of mature T cells, B cells, macrophages, or natural killer (NK) cells (211–213) and are resistant to x-irradiation, being similar to the cells generated by total lymphoid irradiation (TLI). When administered for 5–7 days pretransplant, SKF-105685 abrogated the acute rejection response and significantly prolonged graft survival in rats; it was also shown to have a synergistic effect when combined with low-dose cyclosporine A administered posttransplantation (211–213). The agent has also been shown to ameliorate renal allograft rejection in rats (214). In these studies, SKF-105685 resulted in only a modest reduction in the intensity of the interstitial inflammatory cell infiltration. Renal hemodynamics were improved in the azaspirane-treated animals to a level out of proportion to the modest improvement in histopathological changes. SKF-105685 produced dramatic suppression of allograft eicosanoid production (214). These eicosanoids may play an important role in the pathogenesis of allograft rejection. SKF-105685 is in the early phases of development, and more studies are needed to evaluate its therapeutic potential. However, due to its novel mode of action and possible synergy with other immunosuppressive agents, this drug may have a future in the management of human organ transplantation and other immunologically mediated diseases.

MONOCLONAL ANTIBODIES IN EXPERIMENTAL STUDIES

A number of monoclonal antibodies have been used in experimental studies. These are reviewed briefly below.

WT 32

A murine IgG2a monoclonal antibody directed against the epsilon portion of the CD3 determinant, WT 32 results in first-dose reactions and transient increases in serum creatinine levels similar to those seen with OKT3 (215). It has been shown to be effective in reversing acute allograft rejection. It appears to be a safe and reliable monoclonal antibody with results similar to those obtained with OKT3 (47).

BMA 031

BMA 031 is an IgG2b mouse antihuman antibody that has been used to prevent and treat allograft rejection (216–218), as well as graft-versus-host disease (GVHD) following allogeneic bone marrow transplantation (219). High levels of TNF occur 1 hour after the first dose of BMA 031, but increases in levels of other cytokines have not been recorded (216). BMA 031 does not produce first-dose reactions, suggesting that TNF alone is not sufficient to induce this syndrome. In contrast to OKT3, this monoclonal antibody does not modulate the TCR/CD3 complex (220). BMA 031 eliminates more than 90% of CD3+ T cells after the first dose (216). However, by the tenth day of therapy, preoperative levels of CD3-positive cells appear in the circulation (221). BMA 031 induces an intense and very rapid sensitization that neutralizes its therapeutic effect (216,221).

T10B9.1A-31

T10B9.1A-31 is a murine IgM monoclonal antibody directed against the TCR determinant. It is nonmitogenic to human lymphocytes, does not induce significant cytokine production, and therefore does not result in significant first-dose reactions (222–224). In clinical trials, it has been effective as a prophylactic agent and for reversing acute renal allograft rejection (223,224). The main disadvantage of T10B9.1A-31 is its relatively short half-life, necessitating administration every 8 hours.

Anti-interleukin-2 monoclonal antibodies

An ideal immunosuppressive agent would target only those cells involved in the specific response against a graft, leaving intact the remainder of the host immunologic repertoire (47). Since IL-2 receptors are produced only by activated T cells, some B cells, and macrophages, various monoclonal antibodies have been tested that have been directed selectively against cells bearing such receptors. Anti-Tac is a murine IgG2a monoclonal antibody that inhibits binding of IL-2 to the high-affinity receptor and prevents assembly of its two chains (47). In a randomized control trial, this agent, in combination with low-dose azathioprine, cyclosporine, and steroids, was compared to standard doses of these three immunosuppressive agents. A significant reduction in the incidence of early graft rejection was noted in the anti-Tac group, although long-term functional results did not differ (225). Another anti-IL-2-receptor monoclonal antibody, 33B3.1, has been used as an induction agent in primary cadaveric kidney and kidney/pancreas allograft recipients. This antibody was well tolerated and appeared to match the potency of antithymocyte globulin as prophylaxis against acute rejection, with fewer side effects (226,227).

Anti-CD4 monoclonal antibodies

Preliminary trials have been conducted in human allograft recipients using anti-CD4 monoclonal antibodies (228–231). This agent appears to hold promise in preventing acute rejection episodes, but further studies are needed. Currently multicenter studies are under way in the U.S. and Europe using anti-CD4 monoclonal antibodies.

Antilymphocyte function-associated antigen (LFA-1) and anti-intercellular adhesion molecule-1 (ICAM-1/CD54) monoclonal antibodies

LFA-1 is a member of the integrin family of molecules involved in cell–cell interactions. The interaction of LFA-1 with its ligands, ICAM-1 and ICAM-2, is important for the effector cell to bind to the target cell (232,233). Anti-LFA-1 monoclonal antibodies have been effective in preventing graft rejection following bone marrow transplantation (234–236) but were not effective in the treatment of acute cellular rejection in cadaveric renal allograft recipients (237). ICAM-1 is a surface protein that acts as a ligand for LFA-1 (232). It has recently been used for induction therapy following human renal transplantation in high-risk cadaver recipients. Adequate serum levels of the monoclonal antibody were associated with less delayed graft function and rejection (238).

Anti-T12 monoclonal antibodies

Anti-T12 is a mouse IgM monoclonal antibody directed against the T12 antigen, which is present on 65%–75% peripheral blood lymphocytes. It has been used with a moderate degree of success in the treatment of acute renal allograft rejection in humans (239).

EXPERIMENTAL PROTOCOLS AIMED AT INDUCING TOLERANCE

The ultimate goal of transplantation tolerance is induction of a specific unresponsiveness to donor alloantigens, with retention of full reactivity to all other nonself antigens.

Total lymph node irradiation/total lymphoid irradiation (TLI)

TLI has been used by several groups as an immunosuppressive protocol for kidney transplantation (240–244). The irradiation is delivered to the lymph nodes of the neck, the axilla, the mediastinum, and the aortic, iliac, and pelvic lymph nodes. TLI has been used together with low-dose prednisone, low-dose prednisone and cyclosporine, conventional immunosuppression, posttransplant ALG, and cyclosporine (240–244). These protocols resulted in a rejection-free course in almost half the patients. However, TLI is associated with leukopenia and a high incidence of infectious complications. Moreover, a kidney needs to be obtained within a relatively short period of completing the TLI. These difficulties have prevented TLI from gaining wider acceptance as part of the overall immunosuppressive protocol for transplant recipients. It would appear that TLI might result in the induction of acquired tolerance. In cadaveric renal transplant recipients treated with TLI, a short course of ATG, and low doses of steroids, steroids were withdrawn in the majority of patients (243). In an evaluation of three recipients preconditioned with TLI, the proliferative response of peripheral blood lymphocytes of the recipients to the donors or donor type cells was specifically reduced or absent in the MLR reaction; it was also demonstrated that two of these patients had an intact response to the donor's cells in the MLR prior to transplantation (243). Thus, the hyporesponsiveness posttransplantation was not only antigen specific but also acquired.

Donor-specific bone marrow infusion and donor-specific blood transfusion

In experimental animals, a strategy utilizing ALS and donor bone marrow cells has resulted in the creation of tolerance in adult animals (245). Administration of rabbit ATG for 5 days posttransplantation and donor bone marrow infusion on day 12 posttransplant resulted in long-term survival of allogeneic renal allografts in outbred rhesus monkeys (246). The organ graft recipients did not require any maintenance immunosuppressive therapy. Clinical adaptation of the tolerance-inducing protocol of ALG and infusion of bone marrow has been reported in cadaveric renal allografts who were transfused with cryopreserved donor-specific bone marrow cells 7 days after completion of a 10–14 days of ALG (247). The recipients also received cyclosporine, prednisone, and azathioprine. A study group of 57 patients was compared to a group of 54 recipients of the contralateral cadaveric kidneys who were treated with a sequential immunosuppressive regimen of ALG, cyclosporine A, prednisone, and azathioprine. The inclusion of donor-specific bone marrow cells in the treatment regimen resulted in significant improvement in cadaveric renal allograft survival—90% at 12 months in the donor-specific bone marrow infusion group compared with 71% in the control group (247). The infusion of donor-specific bone marrow cells also resulted in a decrease in the responsiveness of the peripheral blood mononuclear cells of the recipients in the MLC reaction. However, renal function and the number of rejection episodes were not different between the two groups of patients. Moreover, some selection bias occurred in favor of the bone marrow infusion group by virtue of the fact that patients were excluded from the bone marrow group if an early rejection episode occurred. Similar studies have been reported in living related donor and cadaveric recipients of kidney transplants using donor-specific blood transfusions (248,249). This approach has resulted in a low rate of graft loss due to rejection.

CURRENT APPROACHES TO CLINICAL IMMUNOSUPPRESSIVE THERAPY

Different approaches have been used by various groups with reference to both induction and maintenance immunosuppressive therapy. Ideally, one would like to be able to craft specific immunosuppressive therapy for each patient

that would provide a balance that would prevent rejection and eliminate the infectious complications of overimmunosuppression. Induction therapy with monoclonal or polyclonal antilymphocyte antibody therapy has been reported to result in improved graft survival, but with a higher rate of infectious complications, particularly those of viral origin (40,41,250). A recent study revealed a markedly reduced incidence of CMV infection with OKT3 induction as compared to ALG induction (251). Data from the UCLA transplant registry suggest that induction with ALG or OKT3 statistically improved graft survival in high-risk groups, especially in recipients of kidneys with delayed graft function and in kidneys from older donors (252). However, no consensus exists as to whether one should employ quadruple immunosuppressive or triple immunosuppressive therapy in induction protocols (253).

Sequential quadruple induction therapy involves the administration of methylprednisolone and azathioprine intraoperatively. This is followed by the daily administration of either a polyclonal or monoclonal antilymphocyte antibody preparation. Cyclosporine A is introduced once good urine output has been established and once the serum creatinine has fallen below a level of 3–5 mg/dL. The cyclosporine A is then overlapped with the antilymphocyte antibody preparation until therapeutic blood levels have been obtained. Thereafter, patients are maintained on triple therapy with cyclosporine A, azathioprine, and prednisone or prednisolone. This approach allows for the administration of adequate immunosuppression while protecting the kidney from the nephrotoxic insults of cyclosporine during the recovery phase from the ischemia time associated with cadaveric transplantation.

Triple drug therapy using cyclosporine A, azathioprine, and steroids can be used as initial immunosuppressive therapy in living related donor recipients and in cadaveric recipients with good early transplant function. In these protocols, cyclosporine is generally started at the time of surgery and is given by intravenous infusion with a rapid conversion to oral therapy. Alternatively, azathioprine and methylprednisolone can be given intraoperatively; the renal function and urine output are then judged within 12 hours of transplantation, and a decision is made as to whether to institute cyclosporine immunosuppression or anti-lymphocyte antibody therapy. This approach would appear to be the most logical one in the attempt to provide adequate induction immunosuppressive therapy while minimizing the problems of over-immunosuppression and the effect of cyclosporine A on an ischemic kidney. The induction and maintenance protocols currently employed in the University of Cincinnati Medical Center renal transplant program are illustrated in Table 3.

Opinions also vary as to the nature of maintenance immunosuppressive therapy. Clearly, long-term immunosuppressive therapy should be tailored to the individual's needs, based on the immune reactivity of the patient and the toxic effects encountered from the different immunosuppressive agents. Long-term steroid therapy is associ-

Table 3. Induction and maintenance immunosuppressive protocols at the University of Cincinnati Medical Center

Situation	Induction	Maintenance
HLA-identical LRD transplant	1. Cyclosporine A 3 mg I.V. by constant infusion started day before transplant and converted to oral cyclosporine A by day 3–4; target level 300–400 ng/mL (TDx). 2. Methylprednisolone 125 mg I.V. intra-operatively; then prednisone 1 mg/kg/day p.o., reduced by 5 mg/day until 20 mg/day. 3. Azathioprine 3 mg/kg I.V. intraoperatively, then 1.5 mg/kg/day oral dosing.	1. If stable after 1 year, slowly taper and then discontinue prednisone. 2. If stable after 2 years, slowly taper and then discontinue cyclosporine A.
HLA-nonidentical LRD transplant	Same as above.	If stable after 1 year, slowly taper and then discontinue prednisone.
First cadaver transplant with PRA <50%	1. Steroids and azathioprine as above. 2. Evaluate urine output during first 6–12 hours. If good urine output and decreasing serum creatinine level, triple therapy (cyclosporine A, steroids, azathioprine). If poor urine output and no fall in serum creatinine (ATN), induction with polyclonal antilymphocyte antibody, and introduction of cyclosporine A when serum creatinine <4 mg/dL.	If stable after 1 year, slowly taper and then discontinue prednisone.
Cadaver transplant with PRA >50%, and/or repeat transplant	1. Steroids and azathioprine as above. 2. Induction with OKT3, and introduction of cyclosporine A when serum creatinine <4 mg/dL.	Maintain long-term triple therapy.
Experimental protocols	1. Donor-specific blood transfusion 24 hours pretransplant in cadaver and HLA-nonidentical LRD transplants. 2. Donor-specific bone marrow infusion 24 hours pretransplant in cadaver transplants. 3. Mycophenolate mofetil. 4. Brequinar sodium. 5. Tacrolimus. 6. Rapamycin.	

ated with a number of well-known side effects. The use of alternate-day steroid therapy has been shown to be as effective as daily therapy in controlling the activity of several autoimmune diseases, with a substantially lower incidence of side effects. Alternate-day steroids result in a reduction in the incidence of hypertension, Cushingoid features, obesity, cataract formation, hyperlipidemia, and avascular necrosis of bone after transplantation (254–257). However, changing to alternate-day steroids in renal transplant recipients may carry a substantial risk of precipitating acute rejection episodes (258). Similar improvements in side effects have been reported in studies in which steroids were discontinued altogether (259,260). However, once again, this approach has been associated with a substantial risk of acute rejection (258,261). A recent Canadian study revealed a high incidence of late allograft dysfunction following steroid withdrawal (262). In our program, we have successfully discontinued steroids in approximately 130 living related and cadaveric kidney transplant recipients; these patients were preselected for discontinuation of steroids on the basis of a relatively benign posttransplant course, as indicated by the presence of good transplant function at 1 year and absence of significant rejection episodes during the first year (263). Steroids were successfully withdrawn in these selected patients, provided that the withdrawal was done slowly and the patients were monitored closely (263).

Several studies have reported that azathioprine can be omitted without subsequent deterioration in renal function (264–267). However, in other studies, azathioprine withdrawal or dose reduction has been associated with reduced graft survival (268–271). In most of these patients, azathioprine had been discontinued due to leukopenia, hepatotoxicity, severe infections, or development of malignancy. These reports all come from the precyclosporine era. Currently, many transplant centers employ cyclosporine A and prednisone without azathioprine for maintenance therapy (272–274), some use cyclosporine monotherapy (274–276), and others employ triple drug therapy (29,277–279).

Cyclosporine A has clearly been shown to improve graft survival rates in all mismatched transplant recipients (31,280–284). However, concern remains regarding the potential chronic and permanent damage to the kidney with long-term cyclosporine administration (31,35,285). For this reason, several authors have advocated limiting cyclosporine administration to the first few months after transplantation, when the risk of graft loss due to rejection is the highest, and converting to conventional immunosuppressive therapy thereafter (286,287). The improved renal function after conversion must, however, be balance against the increased risk of acute rejection episodes, which may result in loss of kidney function. In a recent meta-analysis, cyclosporine withdrawal was associated with an increased rate of acute rejection episodes, but this association did not impact on graft survival (288). However, the follow-up after transplantation in this study averaged only 27 months. In other studies, the development of acute rejection episodes has clearly been shown to have a negative impact on the development of chronic rejection and ultimate graft failure (289–293). The most compelling reasons against withdrawing cyclosporine comes from the large number of patients followed in the Collaborative Transplant Study (294). Withdrawal of cyclosporine after 1 year was associated with an increased graft loss over the subsequent 4 years, so the benefit gained by cyclosporine administration during the first posttransplant year was negated. Discontinuing cyclosporine for economic reasons has been associated with an increased graft loss rate due to rejection (295). In a number of studies on cyclosporine-treated recipients with follow-up of 5 years, stable renal function has been reported (296–299). It would appear that the outcome after discontinuing cyclosporine may be largely dependent on the reason for conversion. In general, there is little evidence to indicate that long-term cyclosporine administration results in progressive deterioration of kidney graft function, and discontinuation of cyclosporine runs a considerable risk of acute rejection and eventual graft loss. However, in individual patients, it is clear that long-term cyclosporine administration is unacceptable due to the development of chronic nephrotoxicity (31,35,285). On the basis of the available data, cyclosporine therapy should be maintained over the long term. Questions remain as to the optimal maintenance dose of cyclosporine. It would appear that doses of less than 4–5 mg/kg/day may be associated with the development of chronic allograft rejection (300).

In conclusion, the ideal approach is to tailor immunosuppressive therapy, both induction and maintenance, according to the individual patient's response to the transplant and his or her tolerance of immunosuppressive drugs. With this approach, it may be possible to maximize immunosuppression without encountering overimmunosuppression.

ACUTE REJECTION

Timing and incidence of acute rejection

Acute renal allograft rejection may occur at any time but is experienced most commonly during the first few months after transplantation. Based upon the analysis of over 40,000 kidney transplants reported to the UNOS Scientific Renal Transplant Registry between October 1987 and August 1992 (291), 24% of recipients of first cadaver grafts experienced one or more rejection episodes during the initial transplant hospitalization and 52% during the first 6

months. At 12 months, only 40% of patients remained rejection free. Patients who experienced any rejection during the first 6 months had a 72% 1-year graft survival rate, compared with 95% for those who remained rejection free (p < 0.001). Recipients of transplants from living donors had a significantly lower incidence of rejection episodes during their initial hospitalization. In these patients, a clear effect of histocompatibility was noted in comparing the incidence of rejection in HLA-identical sibling transplants (8% at discharge, 32% at one year), with that in one-haplotype-disparate transplants (22% at discharge, 52% at 1 year; p < 0.01 at each time point). In other living donors, rejections occurred in 25% at discharge and 56% at 1 year, similar to the figures for cadaver transplants (291). Histocompatibility also influenced the incidence of rejection in first cadaver donor transplants. The incidence of rejection decreased as the recipient age increased; patients under the age of 16 have the highest incidence prior to discharge (28%) and at 1 year (70%) compared with 17% and 47% at the same intervals in patients over 60 years of age. Donor age was also shown to have a significant effect on rejection episodes, with transplants from pediatric and older donors having a higher reported incidence of rejections than those from donors aged 16–30 years, especially after hospital discharge. Prior sensitization significantly increased the incidence and severity of rejections that occurred during the transplant hospitalization, and these were more pronounced in retransplanted patients. The incidence of late rejections (>6 months) was significantly higher among black (20%) than among white (13%) or Hispanic (14%) recipients. The majority of acute rejection episodes occur within 60 days of transplantation. In two large series, from the University of Minnesota (292) and Ohio State University (293), approximately two thirds of acute rejection episodes occurred within this time period.

Diagnosis of acute rejection

Acute rejection is the main cause of allograft dysfunction after renal transplantation. Acute rejection episodes may be manifested clinically by the development of fever, oliguria, weight gain, edema, hypertension, and the presence of an enlarged, tender graft. However, in cyclosporine-treated recipients, the classical features are frequently absent, and the most common presentation of acute rejection may be an asymptomatic rise in the serum creatinine level. An increase in the serum creatinine level of more than 20% is the cardinal feature of acute rejection in patients on cyclosporine. A variety of tests have been devised in an attempt to increase the diagnostic accuracy of acute rejection. Biochemical changes that accompany the increase in serum creatinine level include an increase in the BUN, reduced fractional excretion of sodium (301), and an increase in urinary protein excretion (302).

Nonspecific features of immune activation and graft injury may be present. Evidence of immune activation may be manifested by increased lymphokine secretion. Measurements of soluble cytokines or their receptors, such as IL-1, IL-2, IL-2R, IL-6, IFN-γ, and TNF-α (303–309), and acute phase proteins (310–312) in the body fluids of renal allograft recipients may give some information on the immunological events. In addition, the appearance of lymphocyturia has been reported in relationship to immunological rejection in the graft (313–315).

Fine-needle aspiration biopsy (FNAB) has been used as a non-invasive method for monitoring of renal allograft rejection (316–318). In experienced hands, FNAB has been shown to be a reliable method for diagnosing acute cellular rejection and is most useful during the first postoperative months. It may also help in the differentiation of acute cellular rejection from acute cyclosporine nephrotoxicity. However, it is of limited value in the diagnosis of acute vascular rejection, chronic rejection, chronic cyclosporine nephrotoxicity, and recurrence of original disease (317,318). It must be stressed that FNAB has been proven to be an effective adjunct to the diagnosis only in institutions that are experienced in its use, and this fact has precluded its routine introduction at most transplant centers.

A number of radiologic changes have been described in acute rejection. Duplex sonography has been used to reflect manifestations of the underlying histopathologic process (319). Development of interstitial edema and cellular infiltration may result in an increase in the size of the transplant, which becomes globular in shape. The corticomedullary junction becomes indistinct, and medullary pyramids are larger and more hypoechoic and lose their triangular shape. In more severe cases, the renal cortical echotexture becomes inhomogeneous, with patchy areas of hypoechogenicity, reflecting the underlying cortical edema in areas of increased echogenicity due to infarction and hemorrhage (319,320). Episodes of acute rejection are associated with an increase in the peripheral resistance in graft vasculature due to vasoconstriction, compression of the small vessels by surrounding edema, cellular infiltration, and in severe cases of vascular rejection, vasculitis, and vascular thrombosis. These events may result in a marked increase in the peripheral vascular resistance in the kidney and secondary changes in the Doppler spectral pattern of the transplant vasculature (321). There is a marked increase in the pulsatility of the Doppler waveform with a decrease or absence of forward diastolic flow. Severe cases are associated with dampening of the systolic flow as well as a reversal of flow in diastole. The pulsatility of the waveform results in an increase in the resistive index (RI). However, limitations exist in renal transplant sonograms. If the rejection episode is mild, the renal transplant may appear normal and the flow pattern may not demonstrate any change. Doppler changes associated with acute rejection are not always specific and may occur in severe cases of acute tubular necrosis, cyclosporine toxicity, or hydronephrosis. Nevertheless, sonography remains a useful diagnostic modality for detecting mechanical problems associated with the allograft, such as peritransplant collections (hematomas, abscesses, urinary leaks, lymphoceles), hydronephrosis, renal vein thrombosis, and renal artery thrombosis.

Radionuclides have also been used as an ancillary method for diagnosis of acute allograft rejection (322). These techniques allow for the assessment of renal perfusion and function and are of greatest benefit when sequential scans are performed (322,323). Acute allograft rejection may be characterized by a marked, sudden decrease in both perfusion and function of the transplanted kidney. Differentiation of acute rejection from acute tubular necrosis and cyclosporine toxicity may be extremely difficult unless repetitive isotope nuclear scans are obtained. The diagnosis of acute rejection superimposed on either acute tubular necrosis or cyclosporine toxicity is also difficult without sequential scans.

Magnetic resonance imaging (MRI) and magnetic resonance spectroscopy (MRS) have also been used for evaluating renal allograft dysfunction (324). These techniques are effective in detecting perinephric fluid collections (325). A decrease in the corticomedullary differentiation on MRI has been described in acute rejection. However, MRI has not proven to be sensitive or specific enough in the differentiation of acute rejection from acute tubular necrosis and cyclosporine toxicity. To date, there is little information regarding the value of MRS in human allografts. However, it may be a more sensitive method of differentiating acute rejection from acute tubular necrosis and cyclosporine toxicity.

Percutaneous needle biopsy of the allograft remains the most reliable method for diagnosis of acute rejection and for differentiating it from other causes of transplant dysfunction. Percutaneous biopsy of the renal allograft is a safe and effective method for the diagnosis of allograft dysfunction. At the University of Cincinnati Medical Center, sonographically guided biopsies using an automated gun were performed on an outpatient basis in 105 patients (326). Significant hematuria requiring admission occurred in 2% of cases, and adequate tissue for diagnosis was available in 99% of biopsies. Results of the biopsy were available within 6 hours, permitting a decision to be made as to whether acute rejection was present and giving an indication as to the best management for the patient. If findings indicated acute rejection severe enough to require antilymphocyte antibody therapy, patients were then admitted. If the rejection episode was relatively mild and could be treated with steroids, the patient was discharged and treated as an outpatient. If the findings indicated cyclosporine nephrotoxicity, dose adjustments were made and the patient was followed as an outpatient. Renal biopsy most accurately confirms the diagnosis of rejection, aids in the differential diagnosis of graft dysfunction, and allows for assessment of the likelihood of response to antirejection therapy. For these reasons, in ideal circumstances, allograft biopsy should be done early in all patients

Table 4. Differential diagnosis of acute renal allograft dysfunction

	Early (0–90 days)	Late (>90 days)
Medical	1. Acute rejection	1. Acute rejection
	2. Delayed graft function	2. Cyclosporine nephrotoxicity
	3. Acute cyclosporine nephrotoxicity	3. Chronic rejection
	4. Prerenal/volume contraction	4. Prerenal/volume contraction
	5. Other drug toxicities	5. Other drug toxicities
	6. Infection	6. Infection
	7. Recurrent disease	7. De novo/recurrent disease
Mechanical	1. Lymphocele	1. Renal artery stenosis
	2. Ureteric obstruction	2. Ureteric obstruction
		3. Urine leak
		4. Vascular thrombosis

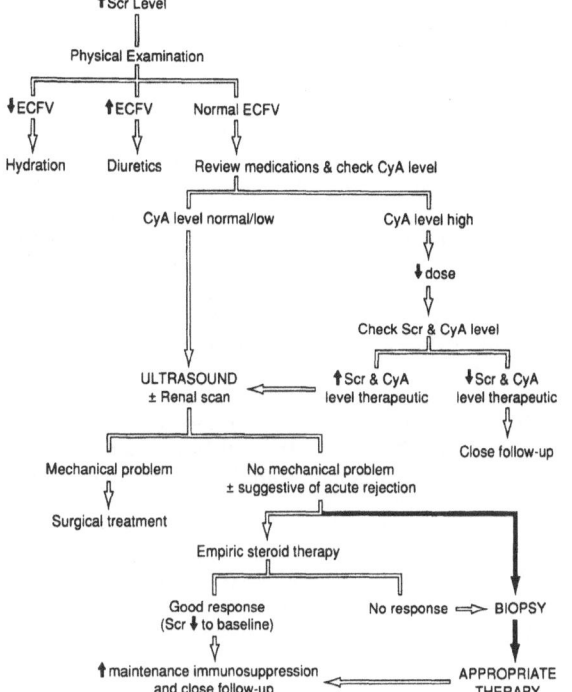

Figure 2. The approach to the renal transplant recipient with an increase in the serum creatinine level. Bold lines indicate the suggested approach to be taken under ideal circumstances.

with allograft dysfunction (increase in serum creatinine >20% from baseline).

Differential diagnosis of acute allograft dysfunction

The differential diagnosis of acute allograft dysfunction can be divided into medical and mechanical problems and into those occurring early (<90 days) and later (>90 days)

after transplantation. Acute rejection is the most common cause of graft dysfunction in both the early and late periods. However, the differential diagnosis differs according to the time frame. Table 4 illustrates the differential diagnosis of acute allograft dysfunction. The medical and mechanical problems encountered in the early and late periods are outlined according to the probability of occurrence.

The approach to the renal transplant recipient with a rise in serum creatinine level is illustrated in Figure 2. In the patient who has a rise in the serum creatinine level of more than 20%, a complete physical examination should be the initial approach. Important features include temperature, weight changes, urine output, presence of peripheral edema, blood pressure, and examination of the renal allograft. The state of the extracellular fluid volume (ECFV) needs to be assessed. If clinical evidence of volume contraction is present, the patient should be given intravenous fluids and then reevaluated. If the ECFV is expanded, diuretics should be administered. In the patient with a clinical normal ECFV, the medications need to be checked carefully in order to assess whether the patient is taking medications correctly or is taking any medications that may cause renal dysfunction or may interfere with cyclosporine metabolism, resulting in either toxic or subtherapeutic levels. Potential cyclosporine drug interactions are indicated in Table 2. If the cyclosporine level is high, the dose should be reduced appropriately and the cyclosporine level and serum creatinine level rechecked. If reducing the dose results in a fall in cyclosporine level to the therapeutic range and a fall in the serum creatinine level, close follow-up is indicated. If the serum creatinine level remains elevated, an ultrasound and possibly a renal scan should be performed. In the patient who has renal dysfunction and a normal or low cyclosporine level, an ultrasound should be the initial approach. If the ultrasound reveals evidence of a mechanical problem (lymphocele, ureteric obstruction, urinary leak), appropriate surgical treatment should be instituted. If no mechanical problem is present, and if the ultrasound and/or renal scan are suggestive of acute rejection, one might either treat the episode by empiric steroid therapy or proceed directly to allograft biopsy. If empiric steroid therapy results in a good response (serum creatinine level returns to baseline), then maintenance immunosuppression should be increased and the patient followed closely. If there is no response to empiric steroid therapy, an allograft biopsy should be performed without delay, and appropriate therapy instituted according to the biopsy findings. However, empiric therapy for suspected rejection might result in overimmunosuppression. Therefore, it is strongly recommended that early allograft biopsy be performed to diagnose the cause of renal dysfunction in patients in whom mechanical factors have been excluded.

Histologic classification of acute rejection

The Banff classification of renal allograft pathology has three distinct diagnostic categories of acute rejection based on histologic severity (327). This classification is based more on the severity of tubulitis and arteritis than the severity of the interstitial infiltrate. Acute rejection is classified as Grades I (mild), II (moderate), and III (severe). There is also a category referred to as *borderline changes*, which is indicated by mild lymphocytic invasion of tubules (tubulitis). In Grade I rejection, there is widespread interstitial infiltrate with moderate tubulitis. In Grade II rejection, there is widespread interstitial infiltrate with severe invasion of tubules and/or mild or moderate intimal arteritis. In Grade III acute rejection, there is a widespread interstitial infiltrate with severe tubulitis and/or severe intimal arteritis and/or transmural arteritis, fibrinoid change, and medial smooth muscle cell necrosis, often with patchy infarction and interstitial hemorrhage.

The introduction of the Banff classification has resulted in a standardized schema for transplant pathology and classification of renal rejection severity. Hopefully, this standardized classification system will be adopted universally and will promote international uniformity in the reporting of renal allograft pathology. This may facilitate the performance of multicenter trials of new therapies in renal transplantation and ultimately may lead to the improvement of the care of renal transplant recipients. The classification has already been adopted for international multicenter trials of many new immunosuppressive agents. However, concerns have been expressed about the treatment recommendations made by the Banff group. This is the case with regard to the recommendation that borderline changes should not be treated; many clinicians and pathologists believe that the presence of tubulitis in the renal biopsy specimen is indicative of invasion of the allograft by activated lymphocytes, and that such changes always warrant treatment (328). At the other end of the spectrum, the Banff group recommendation that severe rejection should often not be treated due to poor outcome is open to dispute (52). These problems aside, this classification remains a most important contribution that hopefully will lead to standardizing both the classification and treatment of acute renal allograft rejection.

Treatment of acute rejection

The principles of management of acute rejection episodes include rapid and accurate diagnosis and prompt administration of antirejection therapy. Ideally, the doses and duration of antirejection therapy should result in reversal of the rejection episode while at the same time not resulting in excessive impairment of host defense mechanisms and consequent opportunistic infections. Currently, corticosteroids and antilymphocyte antibodies represent the main components of antirejection treatment protocols. There is a wide range of different opinions as to the best method of antirejection therapy.

CORTICOSTEROIDS

Increased doses of corticosteroids have been the mainstay of treatment of acute cellular rejection since the early days of transplantation (329). However, the best route and dosage for steroid treatment of renal allograft rejection remains to be determined, and whether steroids should continue to be the agent of first choice for acute rejection is also a subject of increasing controversy (258). Intravenous methylprednisolone has been employed as the treatment of first choice by many transplant units. Doses of methylprednisolone have varied between 250 mg and 1 g daily for 3–4 days. When low-dose and high-dose intravenous methylprednisolone therapies were compared in double-blind randomized studies, there were no significant differences in rejection reversal or graft function (330,331), although in one study patients receiving high doses tended to have greater reductions in serum creatinine levels, while patients receiving low doses tended to have fewer infections (330). These studies suggest that the corticosteroid doses in clinical use in the mid-1970s may have been excessive (258). Following the administration of intravenous methylprednisolone, it is common to increase the dose of oral prednisone therapy and then to taper this fairly rapidly. Oral doses of prednisone or prednisolone ranging from 150 to 600 mg/day and tapered over 1–3 weeks have also been shown to be effective in reversing acute renal allograft rejection (258). Rejection reversal rates of 56%–72% have been reported with oral steroids, compared to 60%–76% with intravenous methylprednisolone (332–334). However, oral steroids were associated with a higher frequency of gastrointestinal bleeding, aseptic necrosis of bone, diabetes, hypertension, fluid retention, and infection (332,333); this higher frequency of adverse effects appears to be related more closely to the duration of therapy than to the total dose administered (331).

POLYCLONAL ANTI-T-CELL ANTIBODIES

Polyclonal anti-T-cell antibodies have been shown to successfully reverse more than 90% of acute rejection episodes (41). In controlled trials, antilymphocyte antibody preparations for first-line treatment of acute rejection have resulted in a more rapid reversal of rejection, fewer repeat rejection episodes, and better long-term graft survival than steroids in living related donor and cadaveric recipients in both azathioprine/steroid-treated and cyclosporine-treated recipients (41,335–338). These agents have also been effective in the treatment of steroid-resistant rejection episodes (339–343). Anti-T-cell antibody is generally administered for 10–14 days, with the dose varying according to the preparation being used. Currently, monoclonal antibody therapy with OKT3 has largely supplanted polyclonal antilymphocyte agents for the treatment of acute rejection episodes.

OKT3

In the original multicenter study (48), OKT3 was shown to be effective in reversing first acute rejection episodes in 94% of cases compared to 75% of patients treated with intravenous methylprednisolone. One-year graft survival was also significantly improved (62% versus 45%). A number of uncontrolled studies have shown OKT3 to be effective in reversing acute rejection episodes when used as first-line therapy or as rescue therapy (45–47,49–52,344–347). OKT3 is administered as a daily intravenous dose of 5 mg for 10–14 days.

A rational approach to the therapy of acute rejection

In deciding upon the approach to the treatment of acute rejection, one must always consider the risk/benefit ratio for doing an early renal biopsy, the value and drawbacks of empiric versus definitive therapy, and the overall effect on the patient of intensifying immunosuppression. The benefits of steroid therapy for acute rejection include the ease of administration; steroids can be administered on an outpatient basis and are an inexpensive treatment modality. On the other hand, potential problems with steroid therapy need to be considered. These include the possibility that if the acute rejection episode is not completely reversed, there is an increased probability of chronic rejection, an increased risk of recurrent rejection episodes, and a number of well-known and serious steroid-induced side effects; in addition, if steroids fail, one would need to intensify immunosuppression further by giving antilymphocyte antibody therapy over and above steroid therapy. The major benefits of antilymphocyte antibody therapy in first-line treatment for rejection are that these antibodies have been shown to be significantly more effective than steroids in reversing the rejection process. However, this needs to be balanced against the fact that they are far more expensive, usually require hospitalization, and carry an increased risk of the development of viral and lymphoproliferative diseases. There are a number of unanswered problems regarding the therapy of acute rejection. Issues that need to be addressed include the following: What constitutes steroid resistance or failure? How long and at what doses should steroids or antilymphocyte preparations be given? What is the best approach to initial therapy? Should prophylactic

antiviral therapy be given together with antilymphocyte agents in order to prevent viral and lymphoproliferative disease? Clearly, additional studies are warranted to determine the agent of choice for first-line treatment of allograft rejection (258).

A number of studies have clearly demonstrated the importance of early diagnosis and effective therapy of acute rejection episodes. In the UCLA Transplant Registry (280), the effect of an acute rejection episode during the initial hospitalization on graft survival at 1 and 3 years was calculated. In patients with no acute rejection episodes, 1- and 3-year graft survival rates were 86% and 72%, respectively. In those with one rejection episode, respective graft survival rates were 68% and 53%, and in patients with more than one rejection episode, the survival rates fell to 57% and 46%, respectively. This analysis illustrates the adverse effect of one or more acute rejection episodes on short-term and medium-term graft survival. The UCLA Transplant Registry (289) has also examined the severity of the initial acute rejection episode, as measured by the degree of rise in the serum creatinine level, on 1-year graft survival rates. In patients with no rejection, the 1-year graft survival rate was 88%. In those who had a mild increase in the serum creatinine (<1.5 mg/dL), 1- year graft survival was 84% (no significant difference from those patients with no acute rejection). In patients with a moderate rise in serum creatinine (1.5–3.5 mg/dL), 1- year graft survival rate fell to 70% ($p < 0.005$ compared to patients with no acute rejection), while in patients with a severe rise in serum creatinine (>3.5 mg/dL), graft survival rate at 1 year was down to 44% ($p < 0.001$ compared to patients with no acute rejection). This is the only study that relates severity of rejection, as measured by the increase in the serum creatinine level, with graft outcome. The adoption of the Banff classification (327) will allow for an assessment of the effect of histologic severity on graft outcome. A study from the State University of New York Health Science Center (290) evaluated the effect of early acute rejection on the incidence of late rejection and transplant outcome. The incidence of late rejection in patients who had experienced an early rejection was 35% compared to 17% in those without an early rejection ($p < 0.001$). Serum creatinine levels at 1 and 5 years were significantly lower in those patients who had not experienced an acute rejection episode (2.4 vs. 1.7 mg/dL and 2.5 vs. 1.7 mg/dL at 1 and 5 years, respectively). Actuarial graft survival (from 100% at 3 months posttransplant) at 1 year was 93% in those patients without an early acute rejection, compared to 85% in those with an acute rejection episode ($p < 0.05$). Corresponding 5-year graft survival rates were 75% and 54%, respectively ($p < 0.001$). In the study from Ohio State University (293), actuarial 8-year graft survival was 83% in patients with no rejection episodes, 69% in those with one rejection episode, and 45% in those with more than one rejection episode. In the study from the University of Minnesota (292), in both related donor and cadaveric recipients, biopsy-proven chronic rejection and graft loss due to chronic rejection was an infrequent occurrence in patients who had not experienced a preceding acute rejection episode. These rates increased significantly in patients with early (≤60 days) acute rejection, and were even more pronounced in patients with a late (>60 days) acute rejection episode. These studies clearly illustrate the adverse effect of acute rejection episodes on short- and long-term graft survival. Future immunosuppressive therapy needs to be aimed at eliminating first-rejection episodes and preventing the onset of a devastating second-rejection episode.

As outlined above, approaches to the treatment of first episodes of acute rejection remain varied. Treatment of rejection should be designed for the individual patient. One needs to consider a number of recipient risk factors, including whether the transplant is the first or a subsequent one, the level of sensitization prior to transplantation, and the severity of the rejection process. At the University of Cincinnati Medical Center, the decision on treatment of acute rejection has been based on histologic severity (52). Mild acute cellular rejection is treated with a 3–4-day course of 250 mg of intravenous methylprednisolone, while moderate and severe acute cellular rejection and acute vascular rejection are treated with a 10–14-day course of OKT3. Using this approach, first-line treatment with OKT3 has resulted in rejection reversal (serum creatinine level returned to baseline) in over 90% of patients, which is clearly superior to the reversal rate with steroid therapy. In patients receiving OKT3, ganciclovir is administered for 21–28 days as prophylaxis against the development of CMV infection and EBV-induced lymphoproliferative disease (348).

CONCLUSION

At the present time, the only approved drugs for the prevention and treatment of acute renal allograft rejection in the United States are steroids, azathioprine, cyclosporine A, OKT3, and antithymocyte globulin. With these drugs, cadaveric 1- year graft survival rates have been around 80%. However, a significant number of grafts are subsequently lost due to the development of chronic rejection. The rapid advances in immunobiology and immunopharmacology over the past 15 years have led to the promise of an exciting future in organ transplantation. The introduction of new immunosuppressive drugs and monoclonal antibodies holds the promise of improving the results even further. However, the shortage of organs remains a major limitation to the widespread application of solid organ transplantations throughout the world. In order to meet this demand, it will be necessary to establish successful xenotransplantation programs. Hopefully, the introduction of new and more potent immunosuppressive agents and the exciting developments in molecular biology, genetic engineering, and tolerance induction will allow such programs to become a practical reality in the not-too-distant future.

REFERENCES

1. *Annual Report of the U. S. Scientific Registry of Transplant Recipients and the Organ Procurement and Transplant Network, Executive Summary.* U.S. Department of Health and Human Services, Library of Congress Catalog Card Number 93-060966, p 22, 1993.
2. First MR: Transplantation in the nineties. *Transplantation* 53:1–11, 1992.
3. First MR: New immunosuppressive drugs. *Am J Kidney Dis* 19:3–9, 1992.
4. Thorsby E: Structure and function of HLA-molecules. *Transplant Proc* 19:29–35, 1987.
5. Strom TB, Tilney NL: Immunobiology and immunopharmacology of graft rejection. In: RW Schrier, CW Gottschalk, eds, *Diseases of the Kidney.* Little, Brown, Boston, pp 2879–2910, 1993.
6. Weiss A, Imboden J, Hardy K, Manger B, Terhorst C, Stobo J: The role of the antigen receptor complex in T-cell activation. *Annu Rev Immunol* 4:593–619, 1986.
7. Williams JM, DeLoria D, Hansen JA, Dinarello CA, Loertscher R, Shapiro HM, Strom TB: The events of primary T cell activation can be staged by use of sepharose bound anti-T3 (64.1) monoclonal antibody and interleukin-1. *J Immunol* 135:2249–2255, 1985.
8. Moore RN, Oppenheim JJ, Farrar JJ, Carter CS, Waheed A, Shadduck RK: Production of LAF (IL-1) by macrophages activated by colony stimulating factors. *J Immunol* 125:1302–1305, 1980.
9. Smith KA, Lachman LB, Oppenheim JJ, Favata MF: The functional relationship of the interleukins. *J Exp Med* 151:1551–1556, 1980.
10. Farrar WL, Johnson HM, Farrar JJ: Regulation of the production of immune interferon and cytotoxic T lymphocytes by interleukin-2. *J Immunol* 126:1120–1125, 1981.
11. Inaba K, Granelli-Piperno G, Steinman RM: Dendritic cells induce T lymphocytes to release B cell-stimulating factors by an interleukin-2-dependent mechanism. *J Exp Med* 158:2040–2057, 1983.
12. Cantrell DA, Smith KA: The interleukin-2 T cell system: a new cell growth model. *Science* 224:1312–1316, 1984.
13. Moscovitch-Lopatin M, Petrillo RJ, Pankewycz O, Hadro E, Bleackley CR, Strom TB, Wieder KJ: Interleukin-2 counteracts the inhibition of cytotoxic T lymphocytes by cholera toxin in vitro and in vivo. *Eur J Immunol* 21:1439–1444, 1991.
14. Kelley VE, Fiers W, Strom TB: Cloned human interferon-gamma, but not interferon-beta or -alpha, induces expression of HLA-DR determinants by fetal monocytes and myeloid leukemia cell lines. *J Immunol* 132:240–245, 1984.
15. Pober JS, Gimbrone MA, Cotran RS, Reiss CS, Burakoff SJ, Fiers W, Ault KA: Ia expression by vascular endothelium is inducible by activated T cells and by human gamma-interferon. *J Exp Med* 157:1339–1353, 1983.
16. Fabre JW, Milton AD, Spencer S, Settaf A, Houssin D: Regulation of alloantigen expression in different tissues. *Transplant Proc* 19:45–49, 1987.
17. Lu CY, Sicher SC, Vazquez MA: Prevention and treatment of renal allograft rejection: new therapeutic approaches and new insights into established therapies. *J Am Soc Nephrol* 4:1239–1256, 1993.
18. Hall BM: Cellular infiltrates in allografts. *Transplant Proc* 19:50–56, 1987.

19. Han J, Thompson B, Beutler B: Dexamethasone and pentoxifylline inhibit endotoxin-induced cachectin/tumor necrosis factor synthesis at separate points in the signaling pathway. *J Exp Med* 172:391–394, 1990.

20. Lee SW, Tsou AP, Chan H, Thomas J, Petrie K, Euglei EM, Allison AC: Glucocorticoids selectively inhibit the transcription of the interleukin-1 beta gene and decrease the stability of interleukin-1 beta gene mRNA. *Proc Natl Acad Sci USA* 85:1204–1208, 1988.

21. Vacca A, Felli MP, Farina AR, Martinotti S, Maroder M, Screpanti I, Meco D, Petrangeli E, Frati L, Golino A: Glucocorticoid receptor-mediated suppression of the interleukin-2 gene expression through impairment of the cooperativity between nuclear factor of activated T cells and AP-1 enhancer elements. *J Exp Med* 175:637–646, 1992.

22. Northrop JP, Crabtree GR, Mattila PS: Negative regulation of interleukin-2 transcription by the glucocorticoid receptor. *J Exp Med* 175:1235–1245, 1992.

23. Zimmer T, Jones PP: Combined effects of tumor necrosis factor-alpha, prostaglandin E2, and corticosterone on induced Ia expression on murine macrophages. *J Immunol* 145:1167–1175, 1991.

24. Politis AD, Sivo J, Driggers PH, Ozato K, Vogel SN: Modulation of interferon consensus sequence binding protein mRNA in murine peritoneal macrophages: induction by INF-γ and down-regulation by INF-α, dexamethasone, and protein kinase inhibitors. *J Immunol* 148:801–807, 1992.

25. Knudsen PJ, Dinarello CA, Strom TB: Glucocorticoids inhibit transcription and post-transcription of interleukin-1. *J Immunol* 139:4129–4134, 1987.

26. Zanker B, Walz G, Wieder KJ, Strom TB: Evidence that glucocorticoids block expression of the human interleukin-6 gene by accessory cells. *Transplantation* 49:183–185, 1990.

27. Elion GB: Biochemistry and pharmacology of purine analogues. *Fed Proc* 26:898–904, 1967.

28. Rossi SJ, Schroeder TJ, Hariharan S, First MR: Prevention and management of the adverse effects associated with immunosuppressive therapy. *Drug Safety* 9:104–131, 1993.

29. First MR, Alexander JW, Wadhwa N, Penn I, Munda R, Fidler JP, Weisskittel P: The use of low dose cyclosporine, azathioprine and prednisone in renal transplantation. *Transplant Proc* 18 (Suppl 1):132–135, 1986.

30. Levine LA, Richie JP: Urological complications of cyclophosphamide. *J Urol* 141:1063–1069, 1989.

31. First MR: Renal allograft survival after 1 and 10 years: Comparison between pre-cyclosporin and cyclosporin data. *Nephrol Dial Transplant* 9:90–97, 1993.

32. Schreiber SL: Chemistry and biology of the immunophilins and their immunosuppressive ligands. *Science* 251:283–287, 1991.

33. Walsh CT, Zydowsky LD, McKeon FD: Cyclosporin A, the cyclophilin class of peptidylprolyl isomerases, and blockade of T cell signal transduction. *J Biol Chem* 267:13115–13118, 1992.

34. Feutren G, Mihatsch MJ: Risk factors for cyclosporine-induced nephropathy in patients with autoimmune disease. *N Engl J Med* 326:1654–1660, 1992.

35. Myers B: Cyclosporine nephrotoxicity. *Kidney Int* 30:964–974, 1986.

36. Curtis J, Luke R, Jones P, Diethelm A: Hypertension in cyclosporine renal transplant recipients is sodium dependent. *Am J Med* 85:134–138, 1988.

37. First MR, Neylan JF, Rocher LL, Tejani A: Hypertension after renal transplantation. *J Am Soc Nephrol* 4 (Suppl 1):S30–S36, 1994.

38. Kahan BD: Cyclosporine nephrotoxicity: pathogenesis, prophylaxis, therapy, and prognosis. *Am J Kidney Dis* 8:323–331, 1986.

39. Kahan BD: Cyclosporine. *N Engl J Med* 321:1725–1738, 1989.

40. Cosimi AB, Delmonico FL: Antilymphocyte antibody therapy. In: JF Burdick, LC Rascusen, K Solez, GM Williams, eds, *Kidney Transplant Rejection: Diagnosis and Treatment*. Marcel Dekker, New York, pp 541–565, 1992.

41. Filo RS, Smith EJ, Leapman SB: Therapy of acute cadaveric renal allograft rejection with adjunctive antithymocyte globulin. *Transplantation* 30:444–449, 1980.

42. Streem SB, Novick AC, Braun WE, Steinmuller D, Greenstreet R: Low-dose maintenance prednisone and antilymphoblast globulin for the treatment of acute rejection. *Transplantation* 35:420–424, 1983.

43. Diflo T, Monaco AP: Clinical immunosuppressive drug therapy. In: AW Thomson, GRD Catto, eds, *Immunology of Renal Transplantation*. Edward Arnold, London, pp 255–263, 1993.

44. O'Connelll PJ, Corpier CL, Steele A, Strom T: Monoclonal antibody therapy. In: AW Thomson, GRD Catto, eds, *Immunology of Renal Transplantation*. Edward Arnold, London, pp 281–302, 1993.

45. Cosimi AB, Colvin RB, Burton RC, Rubin RH, Goldstein G, Kung PC, Hansen WP, Delmonico FL, Russel PS: Use of monoclonal antibodies to T-cell subsets for immunologic monitoring and treatment in recipients of renal allografts. *N Engl J Med* 305:308–314, 1981.

46. Cosimi AB: OKT3: first-dose safety and success. *Nephron* 46:12–18, 1987.

47. Schroeder TJ, First MR: Monoclonal antibodies in organ transplantation. *Am J Kidney Dis* 23:138–147, 1994.

48. Ortho Multicenter Study Group: A randomized clinical trial of OKT3 monoclonal antibody for acute rejection of cadaveric renal transplants. *N Engl J Med* 313:337–342, 1985.

49. Thistlethwaite JR, Gaber AO, Haag BW, Arouson AJ, Broelsch CE, Stuart JK, Stuart FP: OKT3 treatment of steroid-resistant renal allograft rejection. *Transplantation* 43:176–184, 1987.

50. Norman DJ, Shield CF: OKT3: first-line therapy or last option? *Transplant Proc* 18:949–953, 1986.

51. Norman DJ, Barry JM, Bennett WM, Leone M, Henell K, Funnell B, Hubert B: The use of OKT3 in cadaveric renal transplantation that is unresponsive to conventional anti-rejection therapy. *Am J Kidney Dis* 11:90–93, 1988.

52. Schroeder TJ, Weiss MA, Smith RD, Stephens GW, Carey M, First MR: The efficacy of OKT3 in vascular rejection. 51:312–315, 1991.

53. Schroeder TJ, First MR, Mansour ME, Alexander JW, Penn I: Prophylactic use of OKT3 in immunological high risk renal transplant recipients. *Am J Kidney Dis* 14 (Suppl 2):14–18, 1989.

54. Cardella CJ, Blake P, Cattran D, Cole E: Prophylactic OKT3 in renal retransplantation. *Transplant Proc* 21:3373–3374, 1989.

55. Benvensky AJ, Cohen D, Stegall MD, Hardy MA: Improved results using OKT3 as induction immunosuppression in cadaver kidney recipients. *Transplantation* 49:321–327, 1990.

56. Norman DJ, Kahana L, Stuart FP, Thistlethwaite JR, Shield CF, Monaco A, Dehlinger J, Wu SC, Vanhorn A, Haverty

TP: A randomized clinical trial of induction therapy with OKT3 in kidney transplantation. *Transplantation* 55:44–50, 1993.

57. Abramooowicz D, Schandene L, Goldman M, Crusiaux A, Vereestraeten P, De Pauw L, Wybran J, Kinnaert P, Dupont E, Toussaint C: Release of tumor necrosis factor-alpha, interleukin-2 and interferon-gamma in serum after injection of OKT3 monoclonal antibody in kidney transplant recipients. *Trsansplantation* 47:606–608, 1989.

58. Chatenoud L, Reuter A, Legendre C, Gevaert Y, Kreis H, Franchimont P, Bach JF: Systemic reaction to the anti-T-cell monoclonal antibody OKT3 in relation to serum levels of tumor necrosis factor and interferon-gamma. *N Engl J Med* 320:1420–1421, 1989.

59. Suthanthiran M, Fotino M, Giggio RR, Cheigh JS, Stenzel KH: OKT3 associated adverse reactions: mechanistic basis and therapeutic options. *Am J Kidney Dis* 14 (Suppl 2):39–44, 1989.

60. First MR, Schroeder TJ, Hariharan S: The OKT3-induced cytokine release syndrome: renal effects (cytokine nephropathy). *Transplant Proc* 25 (Suppl 1):25–26, 1993.

61. Chatenoud L, Legendre C, Ferran C, Bach J, Kreis H: Corticosteroid inhibition of the OKT3-induced cytokine-release syndrome: dosage and kinetic prerequisites. *Transplantation* 51:334–338, 1991.

62. First MR, Schroeder TJ, Hariharan S, Alexander JW, Weiskittel P: The effect of indomethacin on the febrile response following OKT3 therapy. *Transplantation* 53:91–94, 1992.

63. Alegre M, Gastadello K, Abramoowicz D, Kinnaert P, Vereerstraeten P, De Pauw L, Vandenabeele P, Moser M, Leo O, Goldman M: Evidence that pentoxifylline reduces anti-CD3 monoclonal antibody-induced cytokine release syndrome. *Transplantation* 52:674–679, 1991.

64. Chatenoud L: OKT3-induced cytokine-release syndrome: preventive effect of anti-tumor necrosis factor monoclonal antibody. *Transplant Proc* 25 (Suppl 1):47–51, 1993.

65. Jaffers GJ, Fuller TC, Cosimi AB, Russell PS, Winn HJ, Colvin RB: Monoclonal antibody therapy: anti-idiotypic and non-anti-idiotypic antibodies to OKT3 aristing despite intense immunosuppression. *Transplantation* 41:572–578, 1986.

66. Chatenoud L, Baudrihaye MF, Kreis H, Goldstein G, Bach JF: Restriction of the human in vivo response against the mouse monoclonal antibody OKT3. *J Immunol* 137:830–838, 1986.

67. Nelson PW, Jaffers GJ, Fuller TC, Cosimi AB, Colvin RB: Reduction of immune response to OKT3 monoclonal antibody. *Transplant Proc* 17:644–645, 1985.

68. Schroeder TJ, First MR, Mansour ME, Hurtubise PE, Hariharan S, Ryckman FC, Munda R, Melvin DB, Penn I, Balistreri WF, Alexander JW: Antimurine antibody formation following OKT3 therapy. *Transplantation* 49:48–51, 1990.

69. Hricik DE, Mayes JT, Schulak JA: Inhibition of anti-OKT3 antibody generation by cyclosporine: results of a prospective randomized trial. *Transplantation* 50:237–240, 1990.

70. First MR, Schroeder TJ, Hurtubise PE, Mansour ME, Penn I, Munda R, Balistreri WF, Alexander JW, Melvin DB, Fidler JP, Ryckman FC, Brunson ME: Successful retreatment of allograft rejection with OKT3. *Transplantation* 47:88–91, 1989.

71. Kahan BD: Synergism: how assessed and how achieved. *Clin Transplantation* 5:534–539, 1991.

72. Groth CG, Ohlman S, Gannedahl G, Ericzon BG: New immunosuppressive drugs in transplantation. *Transplant Proc* 25:2681–2683, 1993.

73. Morris RE: Primer on new small molecule immunosuppressants. *Transplant Soc Bull* 1:15–21, 1993.

74. Kamata K, Okubo M, Ishigamori E, Masaki Y, Uchida H, Watanabe K, Kashiwagi N: Immunosuppressive effect of bredinin on cell-mediated and humoral immune reactions in experimental animals. *Transplantaion* 35:144–145, 1983.

75. Turka LA, Dayton J, Sinclair G, Thompson CB, Mitchell BS: Guanine ribonucleotide depletion inhibits T cell activation: mechanism of action of the immunosuppressive drug mizoribine. *J Clin Invest* 87:940–948, 1991.

76. Dayton JS, Turka LA, Thompson CB, Mitchell BS: Comparison of the effects of mizoribine with those of azathioprine, 6-mercaptopurine, and mycophenolic acid on T lymphocyte proliferation and purine ribonucleotide metabolism. *Mol Pharmacol* 41:671–676, 1992.

77. Tajima A, Hata M, Ohta N, Ohtawara Y, Suzuki K, Aso Y: Bredinin treatment in clinical kidney allografting. *Transplantation* 38:116–118, 1984.

78. Gregory CR, Gourley IM, Cain GR, Broaddus TW, Cowgill LD, Willits NH, Patz JD, Ishizaki G: Effects of combination cyclosporine/mizoribine immunosuppression on canine renal allograft recipients. *Transplantation* 45:856–859, 1988.

79. Marumo F, Okubo M, Yokota K, Uchida H, Kumano K, Endo T, Watanabe K, Kashiwagi N: A clinical study of renal transplant patients receiving triple-drug therapy— cyclosporine A, mizoribine, and prednisolone. *Transplant Proc* 20 (Suppl 1):406–409, 1988.

80. Hayashi R, Suzuki S, Shimatani K, Watanabe H, Kenmochi T, Fukuoka T, Niiya S, Amemiya H: Synergistic effect of cyclosporine and mizoribine on graft survival in canine organ transplantation. *Transplant Proc* 22:1676–1678, 1990.

81. Mita K, Akiyama N, Nagao T, Sugimoto H, Inoue S, Osakabe T, Nakayama Y, Yokota K: Advantages of mizoribine over azathioprine combination therapy with cyclosporine for renal transplantation. *Transplant Proc* 22:1679–1681, 1990.

82. Kokado Y, Ishibahi M, Jiang H, Takahara S, Sonoda T: Low-dose ciclosporin, mizoribine and prednisolone in renal transplantation: a new triple-drug therapy. *Clin Transplant* 4:191–197, 1990.

83. Lee HA, Slapak M, Venkatraman G, Mason J, Digard N, Wise M: Mizoribine as an alternative to azathioprine in triple-therapy immunosuppressant regimens in cadaveric renal transplantation. *Transplant Proc* 25:2699–2700, 1993.

84. Gregory CR, Gourley IM, Cain GR, Patz JD, Imondi KA, Martin JA: Mizoribine serum levels associated with enterotoxicity in the dog. *Transplantation* 51:877–881, 1991.

85. Shiraki K, Ishibashi M, Okuno T, Kokado Y, Takahara S, Yamanishi K, Sonoda T, Takahashi M: Effects of cyclosporine, azathioprine, mizoribine, and prednisolone on replication of human cytomegalovirus. *Transplant Proc* 22:1682–1685, 1990.

86. Morris RE, Hoyt EG, Murphy MP: Mycophenolic acid morpholinoedthylester (RS-61443) is a new immunosuppressant that prevents and halts heart allograft rejection by selective inhibition of T- and B-cell purine synthesis. *Transplant Proc* 22:1659–1662, 1990.

87. Allison AC, Almquist SJ, Muller CD, Eugui EM: In vitro immunosuppressive effects of mycophenolic acid and an es-

ter pro-drug, RS-61443. *Transplant Proc* 23 (Suppl 2):10–14, 1991.

88. Eugui EM, Mirkovich A, Allison AC: Lymphocyte-selective antiproliferative and immunosuppressive activity of mycophenolic acid and its morpholinoethyl ester (RS-61443) in rodents. *Transplant Proc* 23 (Suppl 2):15–18, 1991.

89. Platz KP, Eckhoff DE, Hullet DA, Sollinger HW: RS-61443 studies: review and proposal. *Transplant Proc* 23 (Suppl 2): 33–35, 1991.

90. Sollinger HW, Eugui EM, Allison AC: RS-61443: mechanism of action, experimental and early clinical results. *CLin Transplant* 5:523–526, 1991.

91. Eugui EM, Almquist SJ, Muller CD, Allison AC: Lymphocyte-selective cytostatic and immunosuppressive effects of mycophenolic acid in vitro: role of deoxyguanosine nucleotide depletion. *Scand J Immunol* 33:161–173, 1991.

92. Eugui EM, Mirkovich A, Allison AC: Lymphocyte-selective antiproliferative and immunosuppressive effects of mycophenolic acid in mice. *Scand J Immunol* 33:175–183, 1991.

93. Hao L, Lafferty KJ, Allison AC, Eugui EM: RS-61443 allows islet allografting and specific tolerance in mice. *Transplant Proc* 22:876–879, 1990.

94. Morris RE, Wang J, Blum JR, Flavin T, Murphy MP, Almquist SJ, Chu N, Tam YL, Kaloostian M, Allison AC, Eugui EM: Immunosuppressive effects of the morpholinoethyl ester of mycophenolic acid (RS-61443) in rat and nonhuman primate recipients of heart allografts. *Transplant Proc* 23 (Suppl 2):19–25, 1991.

95. Platz KP, Sollinger HW, Hullett DA: RS-61443—A new, potent immunosuppressive agent. *Transplantation* 51:27–31, 1991.

96. Knechtle SJ, Wang J, Beesku M, Burlingham WJ, Sollinger HW, Belzer FO: Effect of RS-61443 in preventing rejection in sensitized recipients. *Surg Forum* 41:380–381, 1990.

97. Sollinger HW, Deierhoi MH, Belzer FO, Diethelm AG, Kauffman RS: RS-61443—A phase I clinical trial and pilot rescue study. *Transplantation* 53:428–432, 1992.

98. Deierhoi MH, Solinger HW, Diethelm AG, Belzer FO, Kauffman RS: One-year follow-up results of a phase I trial of mycophenolate mofetil (RS61443) in cadaveric renal transplantation. *Transplant Proc* 25:693–694, 1993.

99. Deierhoi MH, Kauffman RS, Hudson SL, Barber WH, Curtis JJ, Julian BA, Gaston RS, Laskow DA, Diethelm AG: Experience with mycophenolate mofetil (RS61443) in renal transplantation at a single center. *Ann Surg* 217:476–484, 1993.

100. Salaman JR, Griffin PJA, Johnson RWG, Kohlhaw K, Land W, Moore R, Pichlmayr R, Sells R: Controlled trial of RS-61443 in renal transplant patients receiving cyclosporine monotherapy. *Transplant Proc* 25:695–696, 1993.

101. Sollinger HW, Belzer FO, Deierhoi MH, Diethelm AG, Gonwa TA, Kauffman RS, Klintmalm GB, McDiiarmid SV, Roberts J, Rosenthal JT, Tomlanovich SJ: RS-61443: rescue therapy in refractory kidney transplant rejection. *Transplant Proc* 25:698–699, 1993.

102. Klintmalm GB, Ascher NL, Busuttil RW, Deierhoi M, Gonwa TA, Kauffman R, McDiarmid S, Poplawski S, Sollinger H, Roberts J: Rs-61443 for treatment—resistant human liver rejection. *Transplant Proc* 25:697, 1993.

103. Simon P, Townsend RM, Harris RR, Jones EA, Jaffe BD: Brequinar sodium: inhibition of dihydrorotic acid dehydrogenase, depletion of pyrimidine pools, and consequent inhibition of immune functions in vitro. *Transplant Proc* 25 (Suppl 2):77–80, 1993.

104. Makowka L, Cramer DV: Brequinar sodium: a new immunosuppressive drug for transplantation. *Transplant Sci* 2:50–54, 1992.

105. Cramer DV, Chapman FA, Jaffee BD, Jones EA, Knoop M, Hreha-Eiras G, Makowka L: The effect of a new immunosuppressive drug, brequinar sodium, on heart, liver, and kidney allograft rejection in the rat. *Transplantation* 53:303–308, 1992.

106. Cramer DV, Chapman FA, Makowka L: Prevention of vascularized allograft and xenograft rejection in rodents by brequinar sodium. *Transplant Proc* 25 (Suppl 2):23–28, 1993.

107. Cosenza CA, Cramer DV, Eiras-Hreha G, Cajulis E, Wang HK, Makowka L: Evaluation of the use of brequinar sodium and cyclosporine combination therapy for preventing rat cardiac allograft rejection. *Transplant Proc* 25 (Suppl 2):57–58, 1993.

108. Makowka L, Tixier D, Chaux A, Hill D, O'Neill P, Eiras-Hreha G, Wu GD, Cunneen S, Cajulis E, Zajac I, Jaffee BD, Chapman FA, Cramer DV: Use of brequinar sodium for preventing cardiac allograft rejection in primates. *Transplant Proc* 25 (Suppl 2):48–53, 1993.

109. Collins BH, Areford ML, Fabian MA, Jaffee BD, Bollinger RR: Brequinar sodium potentiates the effects of cyclosporine in experimental small bowel transplantation. *Transplant Proc* 25 (Suppl 2):37–39, 1993.

110. Stepkowski SM, Kahan BD: Synergistic activity of the triple combination: cyclosporine, rapamycin, and brequinar. *Transplant Proc* 25 (Suppl 2):29–31, 1993.

111. Hullett DA, Sollinger HW: Mycopyhenolate mofetil and brequinar sodium: new immunosuppressive agents. *Transplant Proc* 25 (Suppl 2):45–47, 1993.

112. Yasunaga C, Cramer DV, Cosenz CA, Tuso PJ, Chapman FA, Barnett M, Mu GD, Putnam BA, Makowka L: Effect of brequinar sodium on in vivo antibody production. *Transplant Proc* 25 (Suppl 2):40–44, 1993.

113. Ptachinski RJ, Burckart GJ, Venkataramanan R: Cyclosporine concentration determinations for monitoring and pharmacokinetic studies. *J Clin Pharmacol* 26:358–366, 1986.

114. Lindholm A, Welsh M, Rutzky L, Kahan BD: The adverse impact of high cyclosporine clearance rates on the incidence of acute rejection and graft loss. *Transplantation* 55:985–993, 1993.

115. Meyer MM, Munar M, Udeaja J, Bennett W: Efficacy of area under the curve cyclosporine monitoring in renal transplantation. *J Am Soc Nephrol* 4:1306–1315, 1993.

116. Ritschel WA, Adolph S, Ritschel GB, Schroeder T: Improvement of peroral absorption of cyclosporine A by microemulsions. *Methods Find Exp Clin Pharmacol* 12:127–134, 1990.

117. Kovarik JM, Mueller EA, Johnston A, Hitzenberger G, Kutz K: Bioequivalence of soft gelatin capsules and oral solution of a new cyclosporine formulation. *Pharmacotherapy* 13:613–617, 1993.

118. Mueller EA, Kovarik JM, van Brel JB, Lison AE, Kutz K: Pharmacokinetics and tolerability of a microemulsion formulation of cyclosporine in renal allograft recipients—a concentration-controlled comparison with the commercial formulation. *Transplantation* 57:1178–1182, 1994.

119. Vonderscher J, Meinzer A: Rational for the development of Sandimmune Neoral. *Transplant Proc* 26:2925–2927, 1994.

120. Holt DW, Mueller EA, Kovarik JM, van Bull JB, Kutz K: The pharmacokinetics of Sandimmune Neoral: a new oral formulation of cyclosporine. *Transplant Proc* 26:2935–2939, 1994.

121. Kahan BD, Dunn J, Fitts C, Van Buren D, Wombolt D, Pollak R, Carson R, Alexander JW, Chang C, Choc M, Wong R: The Neoral formulation: improved correlation between cyclosporine trough levels and exposure in stable renal transplant recipients. *Transplant Proc* 26:2940–2943, 1994.

122. Superina RA, Strong DK, Acal LA, DeLuca E: Relative bioavailability of Sandimmune and Sandimmune Neoral in pediatric liver recipients. *Transplant Proc* 26:2979–2980, 1994.

123. Trull AK, Tan KKC, Tan L, Alexander GJM, Jamieson NV: Enhanced absorption of new oral cyclosporin microemulsion formulation, Neoral, in liver transplant recipients with external biliary diversion. *Transplant Proc* 26:2977–2978, 1994.

124. Storck M, Mickley V, Grab C, Steinbach G, Abendroth D: Cyclosporine levels in diabetic (Type I) patients undergoing kidney and pancreas transplantation: role of a new galenic formulation. *Transplant Proc* 26:2996–2998, 1994.

125. Fiocchi R, Mamprin F, Gamba A, Glauber M, Catania S, Cattaneo G, Torre L, Bertocchi C, Ruhrmann R, Colombo D, Binetti G, Ferrazzi P: Pharmacokinetic profile of cyclosporin A in long-term heart transplanted patients treated with a new oral formulation. *Transplant Proc* 26:2994–2995, 1994.

126. Neumayer HH, Farber L, Haller P, Kohnen R, Maibucher A, Schuster A, Vollmer J, Waiser J: Conversion from Sandimmun to Sandimmun Neoral in patients with stable renal allografts: results after one month. *Transplant Proc* 26:2944–2988, 1994.

127. Duncan JI, Thomson AW, Simpson JG, Davidson RJL, Whiting PH: A comparative toxicology study of cyclosporine and Nva-2 cyclosporine in Sprague–Dawley rats. *Transplantation* 42:395–399, 1986.

128. McKenna RM, Szturm K, Jeffrey JR, Rush DN: Inhibition of cytokine production by cyclosporine A and G. *Transplantation* 47:343–348, 1989.

129. Hiestand PC, Traber R, Borel JF: Pharmacological studies with norvaline 2–cyclosporine (SD2 OG 37-325) in comparison with cyclosporin (Sandimmun): a summary. *Transplant Proc* 26:2999–3001, 1994.

130. Hagberg RC, Hoyt EG, Billingham ME, Sibley RK, Scarnes VA, Baldwin JC: Comparison of cyclosporin A and G with and without azathioprine regarding immunosuppressive activity, toxicity, and pharmacokinetics in Lewis rats. *J Heart Transplant* 7:359–369, 1988.

131. Masri MA, Naiem M, Pingle S, Daar AS: Cyclosporine A versus cyclosporine G: a comparative study of survival, hepatotoxicity, nephrotoxicity, and splenic atrophy in BALB/c mice. *Transplant Int* 1:13–18, 1988.

132. Burdmann EA, Andoh TF, Rosen S, Lindsley J, Munar MY, Elzinga LW, Bennett WM: Experimental nephrotoxicity, hepatotoxicity and pharmacokinetics of cyclosporin G versus cyclosporin A. *Kidney Int* 45:684–691, 1994.

133. Huser B, Thiel G, Oberholzer M, Beveridge T, Bianchi L, Mihatsch MJ, Landmann J: The efficacy and tolerability of cyclosporine G in human kidney transplant recipients. *Transplantation* 54:65–69, 1992.

134. Henry ML, Tesi RJ, Elkhammas EA, Ferguson RM: A randomized, prospective, double-blinded study of cyclosporine vs. OG37-325 in cadaveric renal transplantation—a preliminary report. *Transplantation* 55:748–752, 1993.

135. Hiestand PC, Graber M, Hurtenbach U, Herrmann P, Cammisuli S, Richardson BP, Eberle MK, Donatsch P, Ryffel B, Borel JF: New cyclosporine derivative SD2IMM125: in vitro and in vivo pharmacologic effects and toxicologic evaluation. *Transplant Proc* 25:691–692, 1993.

136. Kino T, Hatanaka H, Miyata S, Inamura N, Nishiyama M, Yajima T, Goto T, Okuhara M, Kohsaka M, Aoki H: FK506, a novel immunosuppressant isolated from a streptomyces. Immunosuppressive effect of FK506 in vitro. *J Antibiot* 40:1256–1260, 1987.

137. Thompson AW: FK-506: profile of an important new immunosuppressant. *Transplant Rev* 4:1–13, 1990.

138. Johansson A, Moller E: Evidence that the immunosuppressive effects of FK-506 and cyclosporine are identical. *Transplantation* 50:1001–1007, 1990.

139. Wood RP, Katz SM, Kahan BD: New immunosuppressive agents. *Transplant Sci* 1:34–46, 1991.

140. Peters DH, Fittow A, Plosker GL, Faulds D: Tacrolimus: a review of its pharmacology and therapeutic potential in hepatic and renal transplantation. *Drugs* 46:746–794, 1993.

141. Bierer BE, Schreiber SL, Burakoff SJ: Mechanisms of immunosuppression by FK506. Preservation of T cell transmembrane signal transduction. *Transplantation* 49:1168–1170, 1990.

142. Bierer BE, Somers PK, Wandless TJ, Burakoff SJ, Schreiber SL: Probing immunosuppressant action with a nonnatural ligand *Science* 250:556–559, 1990.

143. Van Duyne GD, Standaert RF, Karplus PA, Schreiber SL, Clardy J: Atomic structure of FKBP-FK506, an immunophilinimmunosuppressant complex. *Science* 252:839–842, 1991.

144. Suzuki N, Sakane T, Tsunematsu T: Effects of a novel immunosuppressive agent, FK506, on human B cell activation. *Clin Exp Immunol* 79:240–245, 1990

145. Lagodzinski Z, Gorski A, Stepien-Sonpniewska B, Wasik M: Effect of FK506 on B-cell responses. *Transplant Proc* 23:942–943, 1991.

146. Ochiai T, Nakajima K, Nagata M, Suzuki T, Asano T, Uematsu T, Goto T, Hori S, Kenmochi T, Nakagoori T, Isono K: Effect of a new immunosuppressive agent, FK506, on heterotopic cardiac allotransplantation in the rat. *Transplant Proc* 19:1284–1286, 1987.

147. Murase N, Kim D, Todo S, Cramer DV, Fung JJ, Starzl TE: Suppression of allograft rejection with FK506. *Transplantation* 50:186–189, 1990.

148. Hildebrandt A, Meiser B, Human P, Reichenspurner H, Rose A, Odell J, Reichart B: FK506: short- and long-term treatment after cardiac transplantation in nonhuman primates. *Transplant Proc* 23:509–510, 1991.

149. Starzl TE, Fung J, Jordan M, Tzakis A, McCauley J, Johnston J, Iwaki Y, Jain A, Alessiani M, Todo S: Kidney transplantation under FK506. *JAMA* 264:63–67, 1990.

150. Japanese FK506 Study Group: Japanese study of FK506 in kidney transplantation: results of an early phase II study. *Transplant Proc* 23:3071–3074, 1991.

151. Fung JJ, Shapiro R, Armitage J, Starzl TE: Influence of FK506 in clinical transplantation. In: AW Thomson, TE Starzl, eds, *Immunosuppressive Drugs: Developments in Anti-Rejection Therapy*. Edward Arnold, London, pp 121–128, 1994.

152. Jordan ML, Shapiro R, Vivas CA, Scantleburg VP, Darras FS, Carrieri G, McCauley J, Demetris AJ, Randhawa P, Jensen C, Hakala TR, Fung JJ, Starzl TE: FK506 salvage of renal allografts with ongoing rejection failing cyclosporine immunosuppression. *Transplant Proc* 25:638–640, 1993.

153. Jordan ML, Shapiro R, Jensen CWP, Scantleburg V, Fung J, Tzakis A, McCauley J, Jain A, Demetris AJ, Randhawa P, Simmons RL, Hakala TR, Starzl TE: FK506 conversion of renal allografts failing cyclosporine immunosuppression. *Transplant Proc* 23:3078–3081, 1991.

154. Tzakis AG, Reyes J, Todo S, Nour B, Shapiro R, Jordan M, McCauley J, Armitage J, Fung JJ, Starzl TE: Two-year experience with FK506 in pediatric patients. *Transplant Proc* 25:619–621, 1993.

155. European FK506 Multicenter Liver Group: Randomized trial comparing tacrolimus (FK506) and cyclosporin in prevention of liver allograft rejection. *Lancet* 344:423–428, 1994.

156. The U.S. Multicenter FK506 Liver Study Group: A comparison of tacrolimus (FK506) and cyclosporine for immunosuppression in liver transplantation. *N Engl J Med* 331:1110–1115, 1994.

157. Klintmalm G: A review of FK506: a new immunosuppressant agent for the prevention and rescue of graft rejection. *Transplant Rev* 8:53–63, 1994.

158. McCauley J: The nephrotoxicity of FK506 as compared with cyclosporine. *Curr Opin Nephrol Hypertens* 2:662–669, 1993.

159. Demetris AJ, Banner B, Fung J, Shapiro R, Jordan M, Starzl TE: Histopathology of human renal allograft rejection under FK506: a comparison with cyclosporine. *Transplant Proc* 23:944–946, 1991.

160. Japanese FK506 Study Group: Japanese study of FK506 on kidney transplantation: results of a late phase II study. *Transplant Proc* 25:649–654, 1993.

161. Eidelman BH, Abu-Elmagd K, Wilson J, Fung JJ, Alessiani M, Jain S, Takaya S, Todo SN, Tzakis A, Van Thiel D, Shannon W, Starzl TE: Neurologic complications of FK506. *Transplant Proc* 23:3175–3178, 1991.

162. Scantleburg V, Shapiro R, Fung J, Tzakis A, McCauley J, Jordan M, Jensen C, Hakala T, Simmons R, Starzl TE: New onset diabetes in FK-506 vs cyclosporine-treated kidney transplant recipients. *Transplant Proc* 23:3169–3170, 1991.

163. Carroll PB, Rilo H, Reyes J, Alejandro R, Zeng Y, Ricordi C, Tzakis A, Shapiro R, Starzl TE: FK-506-associated diabetes mellitus in the pediatric transplant population is a rare complication. *Transplant Proc* 23:3171–3172, 1991.

164. Carroll PB, Boschero AC, Li M-Y, Tzakis AG, Starzl TE, Atwater L: Effect of the immunosuppressant FK506 on glucose-induced insulin secretion from adult rat islets of Langerhans. *Transplantation* 51:275–278, 1991.

165. Jindal RM, Popescu I, Emre S, Schwartz ME, Boccagni P, Meneses P, Mor E, Sheiner P, Miller CM: Serum lipid changes in liver transplant recipients in a prospective trial of cyclosporine versus FK506. *Transplantation* 57:1395–1397, 1994.

166. Fung JJ, Alessiani M, Abu-Elmagd K, Todo S, Shapiro R, Tzakis A, Van Thiel D, Armitage J, Jain A, McCauley J, Selby R, Starzl TE: Adverse effects associated with the use of FK506. *Transplant Proc* 23:3105–3108, 1991.

167. Vathsala A, Goto S, Yoshimura N, Stepkowski S, Chou T-C, Kahan BD: The immunosuppressive antagonism of low doses of FK506 and cyclosporine. *Transplantation* 52:121–128, 1991.

168. Fukuse T, Hirai T, Yokomise H, Hasegawa S, Hirata T, Muro K, Inui K, Hitomi S, Wada H: Combined therapy with FK-506 and cyclosporine for canine lung allotransplantation: immunosuppressive effects and blood trough levels. *J Heart Lung Transplant* 12:941–947, 1993.

169. Kahan BD, Chang JY, Sehgal SN: Preclinical evaluation of a new potent immunosuppressive agent, rapamycin. *Transplantation* 52:185–191, 1991.

170. Dumont FJ, Staruch MJ, Koprak SL, Melino MR, Sigal NH: Distinct mechanism of suppression of murine T cell activation by the related macrolides FK-506 and rapamycin. *J Immunol* 144:251–258, 1990.

171. Kahan BD, Gibbons S, Tejpal N, Chou TC, Stepkowski S: Synergistic effect of the rapamycin/cyclosporine combination: median effect analysis of in vitro performances by human T lymphocytes in PHA, CD3 and MLR proliferative and cytotoxicity assays. *Transplant Proc* 23:1090–1091, 1991.

172. Chang JY, Sengal SN, Bansbach CC: FK506 and rapaymcin: novel pharmacological probes of the immune response. *Trends Pharmacol Sci* 12:218–223, 1991.

173. Morris RE: Rapamycins: antifungal, antitumor, antiproliferative and immunosuppressive macrolides. *Transplant Rev* 6:39–87, 1992.

174. Daloze P, Chen H, Luo H, Xu D, Wu J: Rapaymcin's longterm effect on humoral and cellular immune responses in the rat. *Transplant Proc* 25:721–722, 1993.

175. Kimball PM, Kerman RH, Kahan BD: Production of synergistic but nonidentical mechanisms of immunosuppression by rapamycin and cyclosporine. *Transplantation* 51:486–490, 1991.

176. Morris RE, Wu J, Shorthouse R: A study of the contrasting effects of cyclosporine, FK 506, and rapamycin on the suppression of allograft rejection. *Transplant Proc* 22:1638–1641, 1990.

177. Collier DSJ, Calne R, Thiru S, Lim S, Pollard SG, Barron P, Dacosta M, White RJ: Rapamycin in experimental renal allografts in dogs and pigs. *Transplant Proc* 22:1674–1675, 1990.

178. Stepkowski SM, Chen H, Daloze P, Kahan BD: Prolongation by rapamycin of heart, kidney, pancreas, and small bowel allograft survival in rats. *Transplant Proc* 23:507–508, 1991.

179. Chen HF, Wu JP, Lu HY, Daloze PM: Reversal of ongoing rejection of allografts by rapamycin. *Transplant Proc* 23:2241–2242, 1991.

180. Wang M, Stepkowski SM, Ferraresso M, Kahan BD: Rapamycin rescue therapy delays rejection of major (MHC) plus minor (non-MHC) histoincompatible heart allografts in rats. *Transplantation* 54:704–709, 1992.

181. Boyle MJ, Kahan BD: Immunosuppressive role of rapamycin in allograft rejection. In: AW Thomson, TE Starzl, eds, *Immunosuppressive Drugs: Developments in Anti-Rejection Therapy*. Edward Arnold, London, pp 129–140, 1994.

182. Meiser BM, Billingham ME, Morris RE: Effects of cycl0sporine, FK506 and rapamycin on graft vessel disease. *Lancet* 338:1297–1298, 1991.

183. Gregory CR, Pratt RE, Huie P, Shorthouse R, Dzau VJ, Billingham ME, Morris RE: Effect of treatment with cyclosporine, FK506, rapamycin, mycophenolic acid or deoxyspergualin on vascular muscle proliferation in vitro and in vivo. *Transplant Proc* 25:770–771, 1993.

184. Whiting PH, Woo J, Adam BJ, Hasan NU, Davidson RJ, Thomson AW: Toxicity of rapamycin—a comparative and

combination study with cyclosporine at immunotherapeutic doses in the rat. *Transplantation* 52:203–208, 1991.

185. Kahan BD, Tejpal N, Gibbons-Stubbers S, Tu Y, Wang M, Stepkowski S, Chou TC: The synergistic interactions in vitro and in vivo of brequinar sodium with cyclosporine or rapamycin alone and in triple combination. *Transplantation* 55:894–900, 1993.

186. Williams JW, Xiao F, Foster PF, Chong A, Sharma S, Bartlett R, Sankarg HN: Immunosuppressive effects of leflunomide in a cardiac allograft model. *Transplant Proc* 25:745–746, 1993.

187. Chong AS-F, Finnegan A, Jiang XL, Gebel H, Sankarg HN, Foster P, Williams JW: Leflunomide, a novel immunosuppressive agent: the mechanism of inhibition of T cell proliferation. *Transplantation* 55:1361–1366, 1993.

188. Kuchle CCA, Thoenes GH, Langer KH, Schorlemmer HU, Bartlett RR: Prevention of kidney and skin allograft rejection in rats by leflunomide, a new immunosuppressive agent. *Transplant Proc* 23:1083–1086, 1991.

189. Schorlemmer HU, Seiler FR, Bartlett RR: Prolongation of allogeneic transplanted skin grafts and induction of tolerance by leflunomide, a new immunosuppressive isoxazol derivative. *Transplant Proc* 25:763–767, 1993.

190. Reichenspurner H, Hildebrandt A, Human PA, Boehm DH, Rose AG, Odell JA, Reichart B, Schorlemmer HU: 15-deoxyspergualin for induction of graft nonreactivity after cardiac and renal allotransplantation in primates. *Transplantation* 50:181–185, 1990.

191. Waaga AM, Jlrichs K, Krzymanski M, Treumer J, Hansmann ML, Rommel T, Muller-Ruchholtz W: The immunosuppressive agent 15-deoxyspergualin induces tolerance and modulates MHC-antigen expression and interleukin-1 production in the early phase of rat allograft responses. *Transplant Proc* 22:1613–1614, 1990.

192. Valdivia LA, Monden M, Gotoh M, Nakano Y, Tono T, Mori T: Evidence that deoxyspergualin prevents sensitization and first-set cardiac xenograft rejectoion in rats by suppression of antibody formation. *Transplantation* 50:132–136, 1990.

193. Tepper MA, Petty B, Bursuker I, Pasternak RD, Cleaveland J, Spitalny GL, Schacter B: Inhibition of antibody production by the immunosuppressive agent, 15-deoxyspergualin. *Transplant Proc* 23:328–331, 1991.

194. Yuh DD, Morris RE: 15-deoxyspergualin is a more potent and effective immunosuppressant than cyclosporine but does not effectively suppress lymphoproliferation in vivo. *Transplant Proc* 23:535–539, 1991.

195. Gannedahl G, Karlsson-Parra A, Totterman TH, Tufveson G: 15-deoxyspergualin inhibits antibody production in mouse to rat heart transplantation. *Transplant Proc* 25:778–780, 1993.

196. Schorlemmer HU, Dickneite G, Seiler FR: Treatment of acute rejection epsiodes and induction of tolerance in rat skin allotransplantation by 15-deoxyspergualin. *Transplant Proc* 22:1626–1630, 1990.

197. Nemoto K, Hayashi M, Ito J, Saguwara Y, Mae T, Fujil H, ABE F, Takeuchi T: Deoxyspergualin in lethal murine graft-versus-host disease. *Transplantation* 51:712–715, 1991.

198. Yabuuchi H, Nakajima Y, Segawa M, Kanehiro H, Murao Y, Hisanaga M, Yoshimura A, Wada T, Nakagawa K, Nakano H: Prominent prolongation of islet xenograft survival in combination therapy with FK 506 and 15-deoxyspergualin. *Transplant Proc* 23:859–861, 1991.

199. Okazaki H, Sato T, Jimbo M, Senga S, Amada N, Oguma S: Prophylatic use of deoxyspergualin in living related renal transplantation. *Transplant Proc* 23:1094–1095, 1991.

200. Koyama I, Amemiya H, Taguchi Y, Wanatage T, Nagashima N, Suzuki S, Omoto R: Prophylatic use of deoxyspergualin in a quadruple immunosuppressive protocol in renal transplantation. *Transplant Proc* 23:1096–1098, 1991.

201. Okazaki H, Sato T, Amada N: Further study of deoxyspergualin prophylaxis in living related renal transplantation. *Transplant Proc* 25:772–773, 1993.

202. Takahashi K, Ota K, Tanabe K, Oba S, Teraoka S, Toma H, Agishi T, Kawaguchi H, Ito K: Effect of a novel immunosuppressive agent, deoxyspergualin, on rejection in kidney transplant recipients. *Transplant Proc* 22:1606–1612, 1990.

203. Amemiya H, Dohi K, Otsubo O, Endo T, Nagano S, Ishibashi M, Hirano T, Sato K, Kurita T, Fukao K: Markedly enhanced therapeutic effect of deoxyspergualin on acute rejection when combined with methylprednisolone in kidney recipients. *Transplant Proc* 23:1087–1089, 1991.

204. Amemiya H, Taguchi Y, Fukao K, Isono K, Omato R, Ota K, Kosaki M, Takagi H, Oka T, Sonoda T, Orita K, Dohi K: Establishment of rejection therapy with deoxyspergualin by multicentral controlled clinical studies in renal recipients. *Transplant Proc* 25:730–733, 1993.

205. Borg AJ, Ohlman S: 15-deoxyspergualin treatment of graft rejection in man: effect on mononuclear cells. *Transplant Int* 5:219–225, 1992.

206. Ohlman S, Zilg H, Schindel F, Lindholm A: Pharmacokinetics of 15-deoxyspergualin studied in renal transplant patients receiving the drug during graft rejection. *Transplant Int* 7:5–10, 1994.

207. Groth CG, Ohlman S, Ericzon BG, Barkholt L, Reinholt FP: Deoxyspergualin for liver graft rejection. *Lancet* 336:626, 1990.

208. Matas AJ, Gores PK, Kelley SL, Bielefield-Skrokov M, Kinaszezuk M, Gruessner RWG, Najarian JS: Pilot evaluation of 15-deoxyspergualin for refractory acute renal transplant rejection. *Clin Transplant* 8:116–119, 1994.

209. Badger AM, DiMartino MJ, Talmadge JE, Picker DH, Schwartz DA, Dorman JW, Mirabelli CK, Hanna N: Inhibition of animal models of autoimmune disease and the induction of non-specific suppressor cells by SK&F 105685 and related azaspiranes. *Int J Immunopharmacol* 11:839–846, 1989.

210. Badger AM, King AG, Talmadge JE, Schwartz DA, Picker DH, Mirabelli CK, Hanna N: Induction of non-specific suppressor cells in normal Lewis rats by a novel azaspirane SK&F 105685. *J Autoimmunol* 3:485–500, 1990.

211. Badger AM, Albrightson-Winslow CR, Kupiec-Weglinski JW: SK&F 105685: a novel immunosuppressive compound with efficacy in animal models of autoimmunity and transplantation. *Transplant Proc* 23:194–195, 1991.

212. Schmidbauer G, Hancock WW, Badger AM, Kupiec-Weglinski JW: Induction of nonspecific x-irradition-resistant suppressor cell activity in vivo and prolongation of vascularized allograft survival by SK&F 105685, a novel immunomodulatory azaspirane. *Transplantation* 55:1236–1243, 1993.

213. Schmidbauer G, Hancock WW, Badger AM, Kupiec-Weglinski JW: SK&F treatment induces suppressor cell activity and modulates cell adhesion properties in rat recipients of cardiac allografts. *Transplant Proc* 25:758–760, 1993.

214. Fan P-Y, Albrightson CR, Howell DN, Best C, Badger AM, Coffman TM: The azaspirane SKF 105685 ameliorates renal

allograft rejection in rats. *J Am Soc Nephrol* 3:1680–1685, 1993.

215. Tax WJM, van de Heijden HMW, Willems HW, Hoitsma AJ, Berden JHM, Capel PJA, Koene RAP: Immunosuppression with monoclonal anti-T3 antibody (WT32) in renal transplantation. *Transplant Proc* 19:1905–1907, 1987.

216. Chatenoud L, Ferran C, Legendre C, Kurile R, Kreis H, Bach JF: Immunological follow-up of renal allograft recipients treated with BMA 031 (anti-TCR) monoclonal antibody. *Transplant Proc* 22:1787–1788, 1990.

217. Dendorfer U, Hillebrand G, Kasper C, Smely S, Weschka M, Hammer C, Racenberg J, Gurland HJ, Land W: Effective prevention of interstitial rejection crises in immunological high risk patients following renal transplantaton: use of high doses of the new monoclonal antibody BMA 031. *Transplant Proc* 22:1789–1790, 1990.

218. Pfeffer PF, Ohlman S, Jakobsen A, Fauchald P, Leivestad T, Tyden G, Flatmark A: A Scandinavian two-center study of BMA031 in steroid-resistant rejection of renal grafts. *Transplantation* 56:304–307, 1993.

219. Schlitt HJ, Kurrle R, Wonigiet K: T cell activation by monoclonal antibody directed to different epitopes on the human T cell receptor/CD3 complex: evidence for two different modes of activation. *Eur J Immunol* 19:1649–1655, 1989.

220. Kurrle R, Kanzy EJ, Racenberg J, Lang W, Seiler FR: BMA 031—a TCR-specific monoclonal antibody for clinical application. *Transplant Proc* 21:1017–1019, 1989.

221. Smely S, Weschka M, Hillebrand G, Dendorfer U, Krombach F, Kurrle R, Land W, Hammer C: Prophylactic use of the new monoclonal antibody BMA 031 in clinical kidney transplantation. *Transplant Proc* 22:1785–1786, 1990.

222. Waid TH, Lucas BA, Amlot P, Janossy G, Yacoub M, Cammisuli S, Jezek D, Rhoades J, Brown S, Thompson JS: T10B9.1A-31 anti-T-cell monoclonal antibody: preclinical studies and clinical treatment of solid organ allograft rejection. *Am J Kidney Dis* 14 (Suppl 2):61–70, 1989.

223. Waid TH, Lucas BA, Thompson JS, Brown SA, Munch L, Prebeck RJ, Jezek D: Treatment of acute cellular rejection with T10B9.1A-31 or OKT3 in renal allograft recipients. *Transplantation* 53:80–86, 1992.

224. Waid TH, Lucas BA, Thompson JS, Brown S, Moore D, Amlot P, Janossy G: Treatment of acute cellular kidney allograft rejection with T10B9.1A-31 anti-T-cell monoclonal antibody. *Transplant Proc* 21:1778–1784, 1989.

225. Kirkman RL, Shapiro ME, Carpenter CB, Milford EL, Ramos EL, Tilney NL, Waldmann TA, Zimmerman CE, Strom TB: Early experience with anti-Tac in clinical renal transplantation. *Transplant Proc* 21:1766–1768, 1989.

226. Cantarovich D, LeMauff B, Hourmant M, Giral M, Denis M, Jacques Y, Soulillou JP: Anti-IL2 receptor monoclonal antibody (33B3.1) in prophylaxis of early kidney rejection in humans: a randomized trial versus rabbit antithymocyte globulin. *Transplant Proc* 21:1769–1771, 1989.

227. Cantarovich D, LeMauff B, Hourmant M, Dantal J, Baatard R, Denis M, Jacques Y, Karam G, Paineau J, Soulillou JP: Prevention of acute rejection episodes with an anti-interleukin 2 receptor monoclonal antibody: results after combined pancreas and kidney transplantation. *Transplantation* 57:198–203, 1994.

228. Norman DJ, Bennett WM, Cobanoglu A, Hershberger R, Hosenpud JD, Meyer MM, Misiti J, Ott G, Ratkovec R, Shihab F, Vitow C, Barry JM: Use of OKT4A (a murine monoclonal anti-CD4 antibody) in human organ transplanta-

tion: initial clinical experience. *Transplant Proc* 25:802–803, 1993.

229. Morel P, Vincent C, Cordier G, Panaye G, Carosella E, Revillard JP: Anti-CD4 monoclonal antibody administration in renal transplanted patients. *Clin Immunol Immunopathol* 56:311–322, 1990.

230. Reinke P, Volk HD, Miller H, Neuhaus K, Fietze E, Herberger J, Herberger D, Baehr RV, Emmrich F: Anti-CD4 therapy of acute rejection in long-term renal allograft recipients. *Lancet* 338:702–703, 1991.

231. Meiser BM, Reiter C, Ebel M, Uberfuhr P, Wenke K, Reichenspurner H, Rieber E, Riethmuller G, Reichart B: A new chimeric monoclonal CD4 antibody for prevention of rejection after heart transplantation. *Transplant Proc* 24:1734, 1992.

232. Marlin SD, Springer TA: Purified intercellular adhesion molecule-1 (ICAM-1) is a ligand for lymphocyte function associated antigen (LFA1). *Cell* 51:813–819, 1987.

233. Stauton DE, Dustin MI, Springer TA: Functional cloning of ICAM-2, a cell adhesion ligand for LFA1 homologous to ICAM-1. *Nature* 339:61–64, 1989.

234. Dijken PJV, Ghayur T, Mauch P, Down J, Burakoff SJ, Ferrara JLM: Evidence that anti-LFA1 in vivo improves engraftment and survival after allogeneic bone marrow transplantation. *Transplantation* 49:882–886, 1990.

235. Fischer A, Griscelli C, Blanche S, Deist FL, Veber F, Lopez M, Delaage M, Olive D, Mawas C, Janossy G: Prevention of graft failure by anti-LFA1 monoclonal antibody in HLA matched bone marrow transplantation. *Lancet* 2:1058–1061, 1986.

236. Maraninchi D, Mawas C, Reiffers J, Gaspard MH, Laurent G, Stoppa A, Hirn M, Delaage M: Anti-LFA1 monoclonal antibody and bone marrow graft rejection in adults. *Lancet* 2:579–580, 1988.

237. LeMauff B, Hourrmant M, Rougier JP, Hirn M, Dantal J, Baatard R, Cantarovich D, Jacques Y, Soulillou JP: Effect of anti-LFA1 (CD11a) monoclonal antibodies in acute rejection in human kidney transplantation. *Transplantation* 52:291–296, 1991.

238. Haug CE, Colvin RB, Delmonico FL, Auchincloss H, Tolkoff-Rubin N, Preffer FI, Rothlein R, Norris S, Scharschmidt L, Cosimi AB: A phase I trial of immunosuppression with anti-ICAM-1 (CD54) mAB in renal allograft recipients. *Transplantation* 55:766–772, 1993.

239. Milford EL, Carpenter CB, Kirkman RL, Tilney NL, Mazoujian G, Strom TB, Lazarus JM, Schlossman SF, Guttmann RD, Lowry R, Rocher L, Campbell DA, Salomon DR, Pfaff WW: Anti-T12 monoclonal antibody therapy of acute renal allograft rejection. *Transplant Proc* 19:1910, 1987.

240. Levin B, Hoppe RT, Collins G, Miller E, Waer M, Bieber G, Girinsky T, Strober S: Treatment of cadaveric renal transplant recipients with total lymphoid irradiation, antithymocyte globulin, and low-dose prednisone. *Lancet* 2:1321–1325, 1985.

241. Vanrenterghem Y, Waer M, Roels L, Michielsen P: A controlled trial comparing pretransplant total lymophoid irradiation versus posttransplant cyclosporine in type I diabetic cadaveric kidney graft recipients: short-term results. *Transplant Proc* 19:1542–1543, 1987.

242. Myburgh JA, Meyers AM, Botha JR, Thompson PD, Smith JA, Browde S, Lakier R: Wide field low-dose total lymphoid irradiation in clinical kidney transplantation. *Transplant Proc* 19:1974–1977, 1987.

243. Strober S, Dhillon M, Schubert M, Holm B, Engleman E, Benike C, Hoppe R, Sibley R, Myburgh JA, Collins G: Acquired immune tolerance to cadaveric renal transplants. *N Engl J Med* 321:28–33, 1989.

244. Molajoni ER, Bachetoni A, Anti P, Poli L, Caricato M, Pretagostini R, Vetere A, Bertoco P, Alfani D, Cortesini R: Eight-year actuarial graft and patient survival of kidney transplants in highly immunized recipients pretreated with total lymphoid irradiation: a single-center experience. *Transplant Proc* 25:776–777, 1993.

245. Monaco AP, Wood ML: Studies of heterologous antilymphocyte serum in mice. Optimal cellular antigen for induction of immunologic tolerance with antilymphocyte serum. *Transplant Proc* 2:489–496, 1970.

246. Thomas JM, Carver FM, Foil MB, Pryor WH, Larkin EW, Hall WR, Haisch CE, Thomas JM: Renal allograft tolerance induced with ATG and donor bone marrow in outbred rhesus monkeys. *Transplantation* 36:104–106, 1983.

247. Barber WH, Mankin JA, Laskow DA, Deierhoi MH, Julian BA, Curtis JJ, Diethelm AG: Long-term results of a controlled prospective study with transfusion of donor-specific bone marrow in 57 cadaveric renal allograft recipients. *Transplantation* 51:70–75, 1991.

248. Salvatierra O, Vincenti F, Amend W, Potter D, Iwaki Y, Opelz G, Terasaki P, Duca R, Cochrum K, Hanes D, Stoney RJ, Feduska NJ: Deliberate donor-specific blood transfusions prior to living related renal transplantation: a new approach. *Ann Surg* 192:543–552, 1980.

249. Alexander JW, First MR, Davies CB, Campbell P, Babcock GF: Donor-specific transfusion-induced tolerance in animals and man: a therapeutic strategy. *Transplant Sci* 3:72–75, 1993.

250. Rubin RJ, Cosimi AB, Hirsch MS, Herrin JT: Effects of antithymocyte globulin on cytomegalovirus infection in renal transplant recipients. *Transplantation* 31:143–145, 1981.

251. Hanto DW, Jendrisak MD, So SKS, McCullough CS, Rush TM, Michalski SM, Phelam D, Mohanakumar T: Induction immunosuppression with antilymphocyte globulin or OKT3 in cadaver kidney transplantation: results of a single institution prospective randomized trial. *Transplantation* 57:377–384, 1994.

252. Cecka JM, Gjertson D, Terasaki PI: Do prophylactic antilymphocyte globulins (ALG and OKT3) improve renal transplant survival in recipient and donor high risk groups? *Transplant Proc* 25:548–549, 1993.

253. Pfaff WW, Patton PR, Howard RJ, Brunson ME, Ramos EL, Fennell RS, Peterson JC, Scornik JC: Immunosuppression without prophylaxtic antilymphocyte preparations. In: P Terasaki, J Cecka, eds, *Clinical Transplants 1992*. UCLA Tissue Typing Laboratory, Los Angeles, pp 237–248, 1993.

254. Curtis JJ, Galla JH, Kotchen TA, Lucas B, McRoberts JW, Luke RG: Prevalence of hypertension in a renal transplant population on alternate-day steroid therapy. *Clin Nephrol* 5:123–127, 1976.

255. Diethelm AG, Sterling WA, Hartley MW, Morgan JM: Alternate-day prednisone therapy in recipients of renal allografts. *Arch Surg* 111:867–870, 1976.

256. Dumler F, Levin NW, Szego G, Vulpetti AT, Preuss LE: Longterm alternate day steroid therapy in renal transplantation. *Transplantation* 34:78–82, 1982.

257. Curtis JJ, Galla JH, Woodford SY, Lucas BA, Luke RG: Effect of alternate-day prednisone on plasma lipids in renal transplant recipients. *Kidney Int* 22:42–47, 1982.

258. Hricik DE, Almawi WY, Strom TB: Trends in the use of glucocorticoids in renal transplantation. *Transplantation* 57:979–989, 1994.

259. Kupin W, Venkat KK, Oh HK, Dienst S: Complete replacement of methylprednisolone by azathioprine in cyclosporine-treated primary cadaveric renal transplant recipients. *Transplantation* 45:53–55, 1988.

260. Hricik DE, Whalen CC, Lautman J, Bartucci MR, Moir EJ, Mayes JT, Schulak JA: Withdrawal of steroids after renal transplantation—clinical predictors of outcome. *Transplantation* 53:41–45, 1992.

261. Hricik DE, O'Toole M, Schulak JA, Herson J: Steroid-free, cyclosporine-based immunosuppression after renal transplantation: a meta-analysis of controlled trials. *J Am Soc Nephrol* 4:1300–1305, 1993.

262. Sinclair NRStC: Low-dose steroid therapy in cyclosporine-treated renal transplant recipients with well-functioning grafts. *Can Med Assoc J* 147:613–614, 1992.

263. Hariharan S, Schroeder TJ, Weiskittel P, Alexander JW, First MR: Prednisone withdrawal in HLA identical and one haplotype-matched live-related donor and cadaver renal transplant recipients. *Kidney Int* 44 (Suppl 43):30–35, 1993.

264. Sheriff MHR, Yayha T, Lee HA: Is azathioprine necessary in renal transplantation? *Lancet* 1:118–120, 1978.

265. Schmidt P, Kapsa H, Zazgornik J, Pils P, Balcke P: Renal graft acceptance without azathioprine. *Lancet* 2:314, 1978.

266. Dandavino R, Trunet P, Descamps B, Kreis H: Prolonged withdrawal of azathioprine in kidney transplantation. *Transplant Proc* 10:655–657, 1978.

267. Ozaki A, Iwasaki Y, Miyajima T: Withdrawal of azathioprine after renal transplantation. *Transplant Proc* 12:513–514, 1980.

268. Haesslein HC, Pierce JC, Lee HM, Hume DM: Leukopenia and azathioprine management of renal homotransplantation. *Surgery* 71:598–604, 1972.

269. Woods JE, de Weerd JH, Johnson WJ, Anderson CF: Splenectomy in renal transplantation—influence on azathioprine sensitivity. *JAMA* 218:1430–1431, 1972.

270. Toussaint C, Kinnaert P, Vereerstraeten P, Dupont E, Van Geertruyen J: Azathioprine is necessary in kidney transplantation. *Transplantation* 27:145–146, 1979.

271. Parfrey PS, Hutchinson TA, Lowry RP, Knaack J, Guttmann RD: The role of azathioprine reduction in late renal allograft failure. *Transplantation* 39:147–151, 1985.

272. Starzl TE, Weil III R, Iwatsuki S, Klintmalm G, Schroter GPJ, Koep LJ, Iwaki Y, Terasaki PI, Porter KA: The use of cyclosporin and prednisone in cadaver kidney transplantation. *Surg Gynecol Obstet* 151:17–26, 1980.

273. Kahan BD, Mickey R, Flechner SM, Lorber MI, Wideman CA, Kerman RH, Terasaki P, Van Buren CT: Risk factors for cadaveric donor allograft survival in cyclosporine-prednisone-treated recipients. *Transplant Proc* 19:1835–1838, 1987.

274. MacDonald AS, Daloze P, Dandavino R, Jindal S, Bear L, Dossetor JB, Klassen J, Stiller CR, Lockwood B, Reeve CE, and the Canadian Transplant Group: A randomized study of cyclosporine with and without prednisone in renal allograft recipients. *Transplant Proc* 19:1865–1872, 1987.

275. European Multicentre Trial Group: Cyclosporin in cadaveric renal transplantation: one-year followup of a multicentre trial. *Lancet* 2:986–989, 1983.

276. Merion RM, White DJG, Thiru S, Evans DB, Calne RY: Cyclosporine: five years' experience in cadaver renal transplantation. *N Engl J Med* 310:148–154, 1984.

277. Simmons RL, Canafax DM, Strand M, Ascher NL, Payne WD, Sutherland DER, Najarian JS: Management and prevention of cyclosporine nephrotoxicity after renal transplantation: use of low doses of cyclosporine, azathioprine and prednisone. *Transplant Proc* 17 (Suppl 1):266–275, 1985.

278. Fries D, Hiesse C, Charpentier B, Rieu P, Neyrat N, Cantarovich M, Ouziala, Bellamy J, Benoit G: Triple combination of low-dose cyclosporine, azathioprine and steroids in first cadaver donor renal allografts. *Transplant Proc* 19:1911–1914, 1987.

279. Henry ML, Sommer BG, Ferguson RM: Triple drug therapy: an alternative regimen in renal transplantation. *Transplant Proc* 19:1920–1921, 1987.

280. Terasaki PI, Cecka JM, Lim E, Takemoto S, Cho Y, Gjertson D, Ogura K, Koyama H, Mitsuishi Y, Yuge J, Cohn M: Overview. In: P Terasaki, ed, *Clinical Transplants 1991.* UCLA Tissue Typing Laboratory, Los Angeles, pp 409–430, 1992.

281. Ihorogood J, van Houwelingen JC, van Rood JJ, Zantvoort FA, Scheuder GMT, Persijn GG: Factors contributing to longterm kidney graft survival in Eurotransplant. *Transplantation* 54:152–158, 1992.

282. Opelz G: Collaborative Transplant Study: 10-year report. *Transplant Proc* 24:2342–2355, 1992.

283. European multicenter trial of cyclosporine in renal transplantation: 10-year follow-up. *Transplant Proc* 25:527–529, 1993.

284. Opelz G: Superior long-term kidney graft survival in patients on maintenance immunosuppression with cyclosporine and azathioprine. *Transplant Proc* 25:1289–1290, 1993.

285. Myers BD, Newton L, Oyer P: The case against the indefinite use of cyclosporine. *Transplant Proc* 23:41–42, 1991.

286. Hoitsma AJ, Van Lier HJJ, Wetzels JFM, Berden JHM, Koene RAP: Cyclosporin treatment with conversion after three months versus conventional immunosuppression in renal allograft recipients. *Lancet* 1:584–586, 1987.

287. Morris PJ, Allen RD, Thompson JF, Chapman JR, Ting A, Dunnill MS, Wood RFM: Cyclosporin conversion versus conventional immunosuppression: long-term followup and histological evaluation. *Lancet* 1:586–591, 1987.

288. Kasiske BL, Heim-Duthoy K, Ma JZ: Elective cyclosporine withdrawal after renal transplantation: a meta-analysis. *JAMA* 269:395–400, 1993.

289. Cecka JM, Terasaki PI: Early rejection episodes. In: P Terasaki, ed, *Clinical Transplants 1989.* UCLA Tissue Typing Laboratory, Los Angeles, pp 425–434, 1990.

290. Sumrani N, Delaney V, Daskalakis P, Hong JH, Cacciarelli TV, Sommer BG: The detrimental effect of early rejection on long-term renal allograft outcome. *Transplant Proc* 24:1750–1752, 1992.

291. Koyama H, Cecka JM: Rejection episodes. In: PI Terasaki, JM Cecka, eds, *Clinical Transplants 1992.* UCLA Tissue Typing Laboratory, Los Angeles, pp 391–403, 1993.

292. Basadonna GP, Matas AJ, Gillingham KJ, Payne WD, Dunn DL, Sutherland DER, Gores PF, Gruessner RWG, Najarian JS: Early versus late acute renal allograft rejection: impact on chronic rejection. *Transplantation* 55:993–995, 1993.

293. Tesi RJ, Henry ML, Eldhammas EA, Ferguson RM: Predictors of long-term primary cadaveric renal transplant survival. *Clin Transplant* 7:345–352, 1993.

294. Stiller CR, Opelz G: Should cyclosporine be continued indefinitely? *Transplant Proc* 23:36–40, 1991.

295. Sanders CE, Curtis JJ, Julian BA, Gaston RS, Jones PA, Laskow DA, Deierhoi MH, Barber WH, Phil D, Diethelm AG: Tapering or discontinuing cyclosporine for financial reasons—A single-center experience. *Am J Kidney Dis* 21:9–15, 1993.

296. Thiel G, Mihatsch M, Landmann J, Hermle M, Brunner FP, Harder F: Is cyclosporin-A induced nephrotoxicity in recipients of renal allograft progressive? *Transplant Proc* 17 (Suppl 1):169–178, 1985.

297. Tilney NL, Milford EL, Carpenter CB, Lazarus JM, Strom TB, Kirkman RL: Long-term results of cyclosporine treatment in renal transplantation. *Transplant Proc* 18:179–185, 1986.

298. Snider J, Francis DMA, Kincaid-Smith P, Walker RG: Long-term graft survival and renal function in cyclosporin-treated renal allograft recipients: lack of evidence of nephrotoxicity. *Clin Transplant* 7:25–27, 1993.

299. Lewis R, Podbielski J, Sprayberry S, Munsell M, Katz S, Rubin M, Kimball P, Van Buren CT, Kerman R, Kahan B: Stability of renal allograft glomerular filtration rate associated with long-term use of cyclosporine A. *Transplantation* 55:1014–1017, 1993.

300. Almond PS, Matas A, Gillingham K, Dunn DL, Payne WD, Gores P, Gruessner R, Najarian JS: Risk factors for chronic rejection in renal allograft recipients. *Transplantation* 55:752–757, 1993.

301. Hong CD, Kapoor BS, First MR, Pollak VE, Alexander JW: Fractional excretion of sodium after renal transplantation. *Kidney Int* 16:167–178, 1979.

302. Sethi K, First MR, Pesce AJ, Fidler JP, Pollak VE: Proteinuria following renal transplantation. *Nephron* 18:49–59, 1977.

303. Woloszczuk W, Troppmair J, Leiter E: Relationshop of interferon-gamma and neopterin levels during stimulation with alloantigens in vivo and in vitro. *Transplantation* 41:716–719, 1986.

304. Maury CPJ, Teppo AM: Serum immunoreactive interleukin 1 in renal transplant recipients. *Transplantation* 45:143–147, 1988.

305. McKenna RM, Rush DN, Bakkestad-Legare P, Jeffrey JR: Interleukin 2, interferon, and lymphotoxin in renal transplant recipients. *Transplantation* 45:76–81, 1988.

306. van Oers MHJ, van der Heyden AA, Aaren LA: Interleukin 6 in serum and urine of renal transplant recipients. *Clin Exp Immunol* 71:314–319, 1988.

307. Colvin RB, Preffer FI, Fuller TC, Brown MC, Ip SH, Kung PC, Cosimi AB: A critical analysis of serum and urine interleukin-2 receptor assays in renal allograft recipients. *Transplantation* 48:800–805, 1989.

308. McLaughlin PJ, Aikawa A, Davies HM: Evaluation of sequential plasma and urinary tumor necrosis factor alpha levels in renal allograft recipients. *Transplantation* 51:1225–1229, 1991.

309. Schroeder TJ, Helling T, McKenna RM, Rush D, Jeffrey JR, Brewer B, Martin LA, Traylor D, Fisher RA, First MR, Muth KL: A multicenter study to evaluate a novel assay for quantitation of a soluble interleukin 2 receptor in renal transplant recipients. *Transplantation* 53:34–40, 1992.

310. Maury CPJ, Teppo AM, Eklund B, Ahonen J: Serum amyloid A protein: a sensitive indicator of renal allograft rejection in humans. *Transplantation* 36:501–504, 1983.

311. Edwards LC, Helderman JH, Hamm LL, Ludwin D, Gailiunas P, Hull AR: Noninvasive monitoring of renal

transplant function by analysis of beta2-microglobulin. *Kidney Int* 23:767–770, 1983.

312. Cohen DJ, Benvenisty AI, Meyer E, Hardy MA: Serum C-reactive protein concentrations in cyclosporine-treated renal allograft recipients. *Transplantation* 45:919–922, 1988.

313. Schumann GB, Burleson RL: Importance of urine cytology in renal transplantation. *Transplantation* 23:186–188, 1977.

314. Fidler JP, Dajani F, First MR, Munda R, Alexander JW: Value of urine cytology in renal transplantation. *Transplantation* 26:133–135, 1978.

315. Dooper IMM, Bogman MJT, Hoitsma AJ, Maas CN, Vooijs PG, Koene RAP: Immunocytology of urinary sediments as a method of differentiating acute rejection from other causes of declining renal graft function. *Transplantation* 52:266–271, 1991.

316. von Willebrand E: Fine-needle aspiration cytology of human renal allografts. *Clin Immunol Immunopathol* 17:309–322, 1980.

317. Hayry P, von Willebrand E: Monitoring of human renal allograft rejection with fine-needle aspiration cytology. *Scand J Immunol* 13:87–97, 1981.

318. Belitsky P, Campbell J, Gupta R: Serial biopsy controlled evaluation of fine needle aspiration in renal allograft rejection. *Lab Invest* 53:580–585, 1985.

319. Sheth S: Evaluation of acute renal transplant rejection with duplex sonography. In: JF Burdick, LC Racusen, K Solez, GM Williams, eds, *Kidney Transplant Rejection: Diagnosis and Treatment*. Marcel Dekker, New York, pp 459–470, 1992.

320. Rigsby CM, Taylor KW, Weltin GG, Garnes PB, Bia M, Princethol RA, Kashgarian M, Flye WM: Renal allografts in acute rejection: evaluation using duplex sonography. *Radiology* 158:375–378, 1986.

321. Rifkin MD, Needleman L, Pasto ME, Kurtz AB, Foy PM, McGlynn E, Canino C, Baltarowich OH, Pennell RB, Goldberg BB: Evaluation of renal transplant rejection by Doppler examination. Value of the resistive index. *Am J Radiol* 148:759–762, 1987.

322. Camargo EE, Sostre S: Radionuclides in the evaluation of kidney transplant rejection. In: JF Burdick, LC Racusen, K Solez, GM Williams, eds, *Kidney Transplant Rejection: Diagnosis and Treatment*. Marcel Dekker, New York, pp 471–485, 1992.

323. Dubovsky EV, Russel CD: Radionuclide evaluation of renal transplants. *Semin Nucl Med* 18:181–198, 1988.

324. Tempany CMC, Yang A: Magnetic resonance imaging and magnetic resonance spectroscopy. In: JF Burdick, LC Racusen, K Solez, GM Williams, eds, *Kidney Transplant Rejection: Diagnosis and Treatment*. Marcel Dekker, New York, pp 487–502, 1992.

325. Geisinger MA, Risius B, Jordan ML, Zelch M, Novick AC, George CR: Magnetic resonance imaging of renal transplants. *Am J Radiol* 143:1229–1234, 1984.

326. Mahoney MC, Racadio JM, Merhar GL, First MR: Safety and efficacy of kidney transplant biopsy: Tru-cut needle vs sonographically guided biopty gun. *Am J Roentgen* 160:325–326, 1993.

327. Solez K, Axelsen RA, Benediktsson H, Burdick JF, Cohen AH, Colvin RB, Croker BP, Droz D, Dunnill MS, Halloran PF, Hayry P, Jennette JC, Keown PA, Marcussen N, Mihatsch MJ, Morozumi K, Racusen LC, Ramos EL, Rosen S, Sachs DH, Salomon DR, Sanfilippo F, Verani R, von Willebrand E, Yamaguchi Y: International standardization of criteria for the histologic diagnosis of renal allograft rejection: the Banff working classifications of kidney transplant pathology. *Kidney Int* 44:411–422, 1993.

328. Rush D, Jeffrey J, Gough J: Protocol biopsies in stable renal transplant patients under triple immunosuppression: results at 6 months. *Transplant Proc* 26:2576, 1994.

329. Goodwin WE, Kaufman JJ, Mims MM, Turner RD, Glassock R, Goldman R, Maxwell MM: Human renal transplantation: clinical experience with six cases of renal homotransplantion. *J Urol* 89:13–24, 1963.

330. Kauffman HM, Stromstad SA, Sampson D, Stawicki AT: Randomized steroid therapy of human kidney transplant rejection. *Transplant Proc* 11:36–38, 1979.

331. Park GD, Bartucci M, Smith MC: High- versus low-dose methylprednisolone for acute rejection episodes in renal transplantation. *Nephron* 36:80–83, 1984.

332. Mussche MM, Ringoir SMG, Lameire NH: High intravenous doses of methylprednisolone for acute cadaveric renal allograft rejection. *Nephron* 16:287–291, 1976.

333. Gray D, Shepherd H, Daar A, Oliver DO, Morris PJ: Oral versus intravenous high-dose steroid treatment of renal allograft rejection. *Lancet* 1:117–118, 1978.

334. Orta-Sibu N, Chantler C, Bewick M, Haycock G: Comparison of high-dose intravenous methylprednisolone with low-dose oral prednisolone in acute renal allograft rejection in children. *Br Med J* 285:258–260, 1982.

335. Shield CF, Cosimi AB, Tolkoff-Rubin N, Rubin RH, Herrin J, Russel PS: Use of antilymphocyte globulin for reversal of acute rejection. *Transplantation* 28:461–464, 1979.

336. Nowygrod R, Appel G, Hardy MA: Use of ATG for reversal of acute allograft rejection. *Transplant Proc* 13:469–472, 1981.

337. Hoitsma AJ, Reekers P, Kreftenberg JG, van Lier HJJ, Capel PJA, Koene RAP: Treatment of acute rejection of cadaveric renal allografts with rabbit antithymocyte globulin. *Transplantation* 33:12–16, 1982.

338. Broyer M, Niaudet P, Bijaoui, Gagnadoux MF: Treatment of acute rejection crisis by antilymphocyte globulins: a randomized prospective study in pediatric kidney transplant recipients. *Transplant Proc* 19:1886–1888, 1987.

339. Hardy MA, Nowygrod R, Erlberg A, Appel G: Use of ATG in treatment of steroid-resistant rejection. *Transplantation* 29:162–164, 1980.

340. Light JA, Alijani MR, Biggers JA, Oddenino K, Reinmuth B: Antilymphocyte globulin (ALG) reverses irreversible allograft rejection. *Transplant Proc* 13:475–481, 1981.

341. Griffin PJA, Williams GT, Salaman JR: Antilymphocyte globulin for the treatment of steroid non-responsive acute renal allograft rejection. *Clin Nephrol* 21:115–117, 1984.

342. Matas AJ, Tellis VA, Quinn T, Glichlick D, Soberman R, Weiss R, Karwa G, Veith FJ: ALG treatment of steroid-resistant rejection in patients receiving cyclosporine. *Transplantation* 41:579–583, 1986.

343. Veremis SA, Maddux MS, Pollak R, Kline SS, Mozes MF: Alternative antirejection treatment with steroids or antilymphoblast globulin in renal transplant patients receiving cyclosporine. *Transplant Proc* 19:1893–1895, 1987.

344. Deierhoi MH, Barber WH, Curtis JJ, Julian BA, Luke RB, Hudson S, Barger BO, Diethelm AG: Treatment of acute rejection by monoclonals. A comparison of OKT3 monoclonal antibody and corticosteroids in the treatment of acute renal allograft rejection. *Am J Kidney Dis* 11:86–89, 1988.

345. Tesi RJ, Elkhammas EA, Henry ML, Ferguson RM: OKT3 for primary therapy of the first rejection episode in kidney transplants. *Transplantation* 55:1023–1029, 1993.

346. Cosimi AB, Burton RC, Colvin RB, Goldstein G, Delmonico FL, LaQuaglia MP, Tolkoff-Rubin N, Rubin RH, Herrin JT, Russell PS: Treatment of acute renal allograft rejection with OKT3 monoclonal antibody. *Transplantation* 32:535–539, 1981.

347. Alamartine E, Bellakoul R, Berthoux F: Randomized prospective study comparing OKT3 and antithymocyte globulins for treatment of the first acute cellular rejection of kidney allografts. *Transplant Proc* 26:273–274, 1994.

348. Anderson P, Schroeder TJ, Hariharan S, First MR: Incidence of post-transplant lymphoproliferative disease in OKT3 treated renal transplant recipients. *Clin Transplant* 7:582–585, 1993.

CHAPTER 65

Immunosuppression and Treatment of Rejection

M. ROY FIRST

INTRODUCTION

The introduction in the 1980s of cyclosporine and mono-clonal antibodies represented a major therapeutic advance in solid organ transplantation. The United Network for Organ Sharing (UNOS) has recently released the 1- and 2-year graft and patient survival rates for solid organ transplants (1). These survival rates are illustrated in Table 1. Currently, there are a number of promising new immunosuppressive agents on the horizon, and it appears likely that further advances will be made in our ability to control the immune response (2,3). A dynamic interaction exists between basic immunology and clinical transplantation. Advances in immunobiology have resulted in a better understanding of the immunological events involved in the recognition of and response to transplant antigens and have led to a better understanding of the action of various immunosuppressive agents. This chapter reviews the mechanisms involved in the immune response, how currently used immunosuppressive agents act, the possible role for future immunosuppressive drugs, the current approach to clinical immunosuppressive therapy, and the diagnosis and treatment of acute rejection.

THE IMMUNE RESPONSE AND GRAFT REJECTION

The pivotal cells in the rejection process are a small population of T lymphocytes that bear receptors for incompatible major histocompatibility complex (MHC) antigens of the donor graft. These cells initiate a series of cellular interactions within the immune system. The initial step involves the interaction between the graft histocompatibility antigens and the host antigen-presenting cells (APCs). An APC (either a macrophage or a dendritic cell) is capable of taking up antigens and presenting them to lymphocytes in a recognizable form. Class I antigens, HLA-A and HLA-B, are found on the cell membrane of almost all nucleated cells, while Class II antigens, HLA-DR, have a more restricted tissue distribution and are present on B

lymphocytes, monocytes, and dendritic cells (4). T-cell activation and proliferation occur as a result of an encounter between donor-specific T-cell clones and graft antigens. The T-cell antigen recognition complex/T-cell receptor (TCR) includes the CD3 complex and two antigen-binding, clone-specific immunoglobulin-like chains (5). Activation of the T cells results in a cascade of events resulting in graft rejection. Activation of macrophages, dendritic cells, or other accessory cells is required for full T-cell activation (5-7). This cascade is initiated by presentation of incompatible graft antigens by APCs to the host. Class II antigens are responsible for initiation of the immune response and are recognized by T-helper cells bearing the distinctive CD4 marker. The incompatible portion of the Class II molecule is recognized by the TCR. The CD4 protein then binds to a separate region of the HLA Class II, thereby strengthening the attachment of CD4+ T cells to the Class II APCs (5). Cytotoxic T cells bearing the CD8 proteins are activated by recognition of HLA Class I molecules. The TCRs recognizes the incompatible portion of the Class I molecule, while the CD8 protein binds to domains of the molecule, adding strength to the attachment of the antigen-bearing cell. Direct cell–cell contact between T cells and accessory cells and/or stimulation of accessory cells by soluble T-cell products causes accessory cell activation.

Once activated, the T-helper cells release a number of lymphokines, including interleukin (IL)-2, interferon (INF)-γ, and IL-6. Activated CD4+ lymphocytes also release macrophage-stimulating factor, which stimulates production of IL-1 by macrophages (8,9). Formation of IL-2 growth factor receptor and release of IL-2 is of central importance in T-cell activation (5,6). Antigen-activated IL-2-stimulated T cells release B-cell activation factors (IL-4, IL-5, IL-6) that enable antigen-activated B-cells to elaborate antibodies directed against the graft, causing humoral rejection (5,10,11). The interaction of soluble IL-2 and high-affinity cellular IL-2 receptors stimulates proliferation of antigen-activated CD4+ helper T cells and CD8+ cytotoxic T cells (12). IL-2 release also stimulates activation of the cytotoxic capacity of cytotoxic T cells (5,13) and the release of INF-γ (10), which in turn activates the

Suki, WN and Massry SG (eds), Suki and Massry's Therapy of Renal Diseases and Related Disorders, Third Edition. ISBN 978-1-4757-6634-9.
©1998, Kluwer Academic Publishers, Boston/Dordrecht/London. All rights reserved.

cyclosporine. Some of the recipients demonstrate an incomplete distal renal tubular acidosis (RTA), most probably due to an isolated secretory defect in the distal nephron. No association was found between occurrence of distal RTA and rejection or late graft function. The incomplete distal RTA was also found by Aguilera et al. in patients with idiopathic uveitis treated with cyclosporine A (6).

Our own study (7), which was performed in the 1980s in renal living related and cadaver graft recipients treated with steroids and azathioprine, documented the occurrence of complete and incomplete distal tubular acidosis only in cadaver graft recipients with warm ischemia time longer than 15 minutes and in those patients whose acute rejection episodes were treated with oral prednisolone. The defect was not found in the living related kidney recipients nor in those cadaver recipients treated with I.V. methylprednisolone. The defect did not require any treatment and disappeared spontaneously with time. The acetazolamide loading test revealed occurrence of proximal tubular dysfunction in the same recipients.

METABOLIC BONE DISEASE

Successful kidney transplantation is almost always associated with several abnormalities in the locomotor system. Metabolic bone disease can be caused by 1) an incomplete resolution of pretransplant uremic derangement and/or 2) posttransplant immunosuppressive therapy, and 3) actual renal function. Preexisting accumulation of β_2-microglobulin and disorders associated with diabetes mellitus Type I often fail to improve and lead to skeletal defects despite excellent allograft function. In the diabetic, combined renal–pancreas transplant population, osteoarticular destruction has been observed (8). Most likely, this outcome is due to periarticular and intramedullar fat necrosis associated with pancreatitis.

Osteomalacia associated with aluminium overload may resolve after transplantation. Symptoms of aluminium-related bone disease disappear over a wide range of plasma creatinine levels (9); therefore, in most cases, no specific treatment is required. However, bone histomorphometric examination, performed before and 1 year after successful renal transplantation in 20 patients described by Bertolome and coworkers, showed good recovery of bone resorption (well correlated with serum, parathyroid hormone (PTH) concentration) but slow removal of aluminum deposits and small improvement in bone formation indices (10). Aluminium disappearance from bone surfaces seems to be independent of graft function. In 167 successful renal transplant recipients examined for locomotor complications by Agarwal and Owen, tendonitis of the supraspinatus and calcaneal tendons was found in 12 patients (7.8%) with pretransplant hyperphosphatemia and posttransplant hypercalcemia, and spontaneous tendon ruptures were observed in four patients (2.4%) (11).

Sustained, severe hyperparathyroidism may accelerate bone loss, contribute to the risk of osteonecrosis (partly attributed to posttransplant steroid therapy), and cause hypercalcemia and hypophosphatemia. Hypercalcemia can be defined as a total serum calcium concentration above 11 mg/dL in the presence of normal albumin and globulin concentrations or serum ionized calcium above 6 mg/dL. The incidence of hypercalcemia in renal transplant recipients ranges from 10% to 50% and can be detected as early as the first day after surgery. Posttransplant hypercalcemia has been classified by Partiff (12) as early severe, transient, and persistent (lasting longer than 1 year). In about 10% of cases, early hypercalcemia occurs due to the sustained secretion of parathyroid hormone by the hyperplastic gland. Early, transient, and persistent hypercalcemia may all also be caused by phosphorus depletion due to posttransplant phosphaturia, use of phosphorus-binding antacid, or rapid tapering of the steroid dose. Last but not least, another cause of transient hypercalcemia is posttransplant treatment with prolonged half-life metabolites of vitamin D and the normalization of vitamin D metabolism.

Lack of resolution of hypercalcemia after normalization of vitamin D metabolism in the presence of a well-functioning kidney suggests that the process of involution of the parathyroid gland is slow. This is the reason for the slow resolution of bone changes in osteitis fibrosa.

The posttransplant occurrence of hypocalcemia in patients who underwent pretransplant parathyroidectomy should alert the physician to the possibility of malignancies in immunocompromised graft recipients or ectopic PTH production. Hypercalcemia is the effect of an osteolytic destruction mediated by many humoral factors such as interleukin-1, TGF-α, TGF-β, prostaglandins, procathepsin D, $1,25(OH)_2$ vitamin D_3, or ectopic production of PTH-related protein.

The resolution of radiologic changes in hyperparathyroidism can be observed as early as 3 months after transplantation but may persist for more than 1 year. If the signs and symptoms of hyperparathyroidism do not resolve despite good kidney function, parathyroidectomy should be considered. The indications for this procedure include prolonged elevation of PTH concentration and alkaline phosphatase activity, increasing signs of hyperparathyroidism in x-ray examination, metastatic calcification, pruritus, osteonecrosis, and proximal myopathy. Those last two can also be induced or aggravated by steroid therapy. One should remember that high alkaline phosphatase activity as well as proximal myopathy can be observed in patients presenting with osteomalacia. Severe early hypercalcemia may require urgent subtotal parathyroidectomy. Parathyroidectomy is also indicated when allograft recipients develop calculi and/or nephrocalcinosis. Surgery may be the required mode of treatment if data indicate that hypercalcemia is contributing to hypertension.

In phosphate-depleted recipients, phosphorus supplementation should be prescribed cautiously.

Long-term glucocorticoid treatment directly inhibits bone formation due to a decreased calcium absorption from the gastrointestinal tract and an increased calcium excretion with urine (13). Glucocorticoids decrease osteocalcine, osteopontin, and fibronectin synthesis and inhibit integrin expression on osteoblasts, impairing their attachment to the bone. The decreased concentration of circulating osteocalcin is dose related. It can be used as a measure of PTH-mediated effects on bone turnover. It has been postulated that glucocorticoids increase cyclic-AMP response to PTH (14). The response of bone cells and bone organ culture is biphasic with respect to time and dose (15).

There is evidence that the most rapid bone loss occurs within the first few months of therapy, with only age-associated loss thereafter (16,17). Calcium malabsorption seems to occur only with higher doses of prednisolone (15–20 mg daily) (18), while a dose of 8–10 mg/day has no such effect. Treatment with low doses (below 10 mg of prednisone per day) influences bone loss to a minimal or even an undetectable degree. In the majority of patients, with exception of the very few who did not experience rejection episodes during the first year after transplantation, there is no possibility to discontinue the steroid treatment. Therefore, the low-dose steroid protocol should be used, with high intravenous pulses of methylprednisolone rather than oral prednisone to combat rejection (18).

The currently used immunosuppressive protocols, in contrast to the previous ones, are based on cyclosporine A combined with prednisone rather than on azathioprine in combination with prednisone. All three drugs are frequently used together. There is some evidence that cyclosporine A—the most widely used posttransplant immunomodulatory agent acting mainly on T cells—also has a direct effect on bone and cartilage cells (17). Cyclosporine A apparently inhibits in vitro bone resorption induced by interleukin-1, $1,25(OH)_2D_3$, PTH, and PGE_2. The deleterious effect of cyclosporine A on bone can be alleviated by concomitant administration of PGE_2 (19). In vivo, it protects against bone and cartilage loss in adjuvant arthritis. Cyclosporin A causes high-turnover osteopenia in rats. In contrast to patients on an azathioprine–prednisone protocol, those on cyclosporine A–prednisone therapy frequently demonstrate an isolated rise in bone-derived serum alkaline phosphatase activity without overt symptoms of bone disease. Despite this rise in alkaline phosphatase activity, the radiological lesions improved, while bone mass remained stable (20).

An avascular necrosis of the femoral head is the most debilitating skeletal complication. It is related partly to pretransplant metabolic bone disease but mostly to posttransplant immunosuppressive therapy with glucocorticoids and cyclosporin A. The relationship between osteonecrosis and immunosuppressive therapy, especially cyclosporine administration, was recently studied in 224 transplant patients. The incidence of aseptic necrosis of the femoral head in patients receiving prednisone plus azathioprine was found to be 9.3%, while the incidence was 18% in patients given cyclosporine A plus prednisone. The complication was not observed in patients treated with the triple drug regimen (21). Patients on double drug therapy received higher doses of cyclosporine A in comparison with those on the triple drug regimen. Avascular necrosis of the hip presenting severe pain occurs 1–3 years following kidney transplantation. Several years ago, the incidence of osteonecrosis reached 15% and then fell dramatically to about 2% after the introduction of low-dose steroid therapy (22). Patients with preexisting or sustained hyperparathyroidism, as well as those receiving high doses of steroids due to uncontrolled rejection episodes, are at higher risk of developing bone necrosis. The posttransplant weight gain and iron overload due to multiple pretransplant blood transfusions are another risk factor for the development of osteonecrosis. Iron overload causes marrow fibrosis and osteopenia, which would make the femoral head more vulnerable to osteonecrosis. No treatment for bone aseptic necrosis has been described. Prosthetic total hip replacement has been used with excellent results in more severe states of the disease.

Osteoporosis prevention is based on concomitant administration of calcium, vitamin D or its active metabolites, and fluoride. However, careful adjustment of doses to kidney function, serum calcium, and PTH levels is necessary. Hormonal replacement therapy in perimenopausal and postmenopausal female kidney recipients is also used in the prevention of posttransplant osteoporosis. (According to Lukert and coworkers, bone density measured in the lumbar spine with DXA (23) in postmenopausal or amenorrheic women on estrogen replacement therapy increased significantly within 1 year in comparison to the age-matched controls.) Dose–response effects of estrogen on bones have been demonstrated. The necessary daily dose is 0.625 mg of conjugated estrogens (Premarin®), 15 μg of ethinyloestradiol, 1–2 mg of micronized estradiol or estradiol valerate (Progynova®), and 25–50 μg of transdermal estradiol (Estraderm®) (23). The possibility of estrogen-induced increased risk of malignancies in immunosuppressed females must be considered.

Treatment with sodium fluoride could be considered as a preventive or a therapeutic procedure, depending on whether the agent was prescribed at the onset of therapy or later on; however, sodium fluoride should be withdrawn when the patient's plasma creatinine level rises above 2 mg/dL. In double-blind controlled trials, an approximately 8% increase in bone mass per year can be observed with this treatment in 60%–70% of osteoporotic patients. However, in 30%–40% of patients, sodium fluoride has no effect on the increase of bone mass. One should remember that the incidence of bone fissures affecting bones of the lower limbs is significantly increased when doses of elemental fluoride are greater than 25 mg/day or in the case of an unrecognized renal insufficiency (24). Our unpublished data have proven the usefulness of this treatment.

Calcitonin inhibits osteoclast-mediated bone resorption, although this agent is not used for prevention but for treatment of corticosteroid-induced osteoporosis. It has an additional analgesic effect (25).

The efficacy of biphosphonates has been established in the treatment of states characterized by increased bone resorption. Intermittent administration of biphosphonates, which is expected to decrease bone resorption and to provide a drug-free period in which bone formation may proceed at a normal rate, leading to a positive calcium balance, was able to increase trabecular bone density for a period of up to 3 years. There are some indications that continuously given pamidronate can prevent glucocorticoid-induced bone loss. There is no information about the effects of biphosphonates on nonvertebral fractures. New biphosphonates are of great value for the management of hypercalcemia in pregnancy (26).

The importance of osteoporosis prevention in renal transplant recipients was strongly supported by an elegant study by Kwan (27), who demonstrated that bone mineral density (BMD) of the lumbar spine had fallen progressively at 3 months with no evidence of recovery at 6 months. We have studied 51 transplant recipients during the first year after kidney transplantation who were treated with a triple drug immunosuppressive regimen consisting of low-dose prednisone, cyclosporine A, and azathioprine. Twenty-three patients additionally received 25-hydroxy-vitamin D_3 in a daily dose of 40 µg and 3 g of calcium carbonate. During the first year after transplantation, patients without preventive treatment showed a decrease in BMD of 6% in the lumbar spine and of 3%–6% in different regions of the proximal femur. The number of new deformities of vertebral bodies was closely correlated with the decrease in BMD of the lumbar spine. Treatment with 25-hydroxy-vitamin D_3 and calcium reduced the decrease in BMD in all evaluated regions to less than 1% and prevented new vertebral crush fractures (28).

It is well established that physical activity may inhibit bone loss and perhaps even increase bone mass. Therefore, it is generally recommended that osteoporotic subjects should take regular physical exercise, e.g., brisk walking, social dancing, and group aerobics. Swimming is less effective. Regardless of its effectiveness, physical activity after kidney transplantation improves general physical performance and feelings of well-being.

PHOSPHATE METABOLISM

Hypophosphatemia develops in 20%–45% of renal allograft recipients with good function of the transplanted kidney. Hypophosphatemia can be divided into three categories: very early (12–24 hours posttransplantation), early, and late. In all three categories, an inappropriate phosphaturia due to 1) sustained hyperparathyroidism or 2) a renal phosphate wasting syndrome, independent of the PTH level and occurring in the absence of other proximal tubule dysfunction, seems to be the major pathogenic factors of hypophosphtemia.

The correlation between low maximal tubular phosphorus reabsorption corrected for glomerular filtration rate and serum PTH level is well documented (29). Although this correlation might play a major role in posttransplant hypophosphatemia, other studies suggest an important role for a selective phosphate leak that could be attributed to the presence of only one kidney (30). Pabico found a low tubular phosphate reabsorption corrected for GFR in healthy kidney donors (31), but according to others, transplant recipients demonstrate lower values of maximal phosphate reabsorption than donors, despite comparable kidney function (30,31). It could be explained by a relative calcitriol deficiency in the transplanted patients (32). Intestinal malabsorption (partly due to the use of phosphate-binding antacid and steroids, which inhibit renal phosphorus transport, but also secondary to inadequate vitamin D levels), tubular dysfunction caused by chronic rejection, and an inadequate phosphorus intake are other factors that might play a role in establishing the posttransplant phosphorus level. Intravascular volume expansion and osmotic diuresis play a major role in the pathogenesis of phosphaturia and the subsequent hypophosphatemia of the "very early" category.

Hypophosphatemia is observed mainly during the first year after transplantation but also for a longer period in 20%–25% of patients. The disorder is usually asymptomatic. Severe and prolonged hypophosphatemia can lead to osteomalacia and fractures, as well as changes in the central nervous system. Oral phosphate supplementation can be dangerous due to its stimulation of PTH, but in severe hypophosphatemia it may be prescribed. Some patients may benefit from careful administration of vitamin D or its metabolites. Monitoring of serum and urine calcium levels as well as kidney function is necessary in these cases.

MAGNESIUM METABOLISM

Despite a well-functioning allograft, successful renal transplantation is often accompanied by hypomagnesemia. In the immediate posttransplant period, this outcome is due to increased urinary losses of magnesium.

Excretion of 20%–30% of the filtered magnesium load and profound hypomagnesemia can be caused by an increased extracellular fluid volume, administration of large amounts of diuretics, and a polyuric phase of acute tubular necrosis. "Late" hypomagnesemia might be induced by long-term diuretic therapy and hypercalcemia. Hypomagnesemia should alert the physician to consider the possibility of concomitant malignancies and hyperaldosteronism. However, a posttransplant immunosuppressive regimen with glucocorticoids and cyclosporine A is the major cause of this disorder.

According to Markell et al. (32), renal transplant recipients treated with prednisolone and cyclosporine A exhibit marked deficits of ionized magnesium concentrations, with a smaller deficit in total magnesium as compared to controls. Values for ionized and total calcium did not differ. Ionized magnesium concentration was related to cyclosporine through level total and cholesterol but not to serum creatinine level, time after transplantation, or dose of cyclosporine. The ratio of ionized calcium to ionized magnesium was elevated in transplant recipients. It appears from this study that the deficit in ionized magnesium is common in the late posttransplant period in cyclosporine-treated recipients and that the ionized magnesium concentration may serve as a more sensitive parameter than the measurement of the total magnesium level. Moreover, the ionized magnesium level correlates well with the cyclosporin level. This fact is of clinical importance during I.V. treatment with cyclosporine, since hypomagnesemia predisposes to seizures.

Nozne et al. (33), in an elegant study performed on rats treated with cyclosporine (5–15 mg/kg/day), has proven that intracellular migration of magnesium plays as important a role in the pathogenesis of cyclosporine-induced hypomagnesemia as the impaired renal conservation of magnesium.

Hypermagnesemia may occur in those transplant recipients, who are treated with drugs containing magnesium without dose correction for GFR.

AMYLOIDOSIS

Dialysis amyloidosis after renal transplantation

β_2-microglobulin, a plasma protein with almost exclusively renal metabolism, was identified as the major factor in dialysis amyloidosis. The progression of amyloid arthropathy in patients undergoing hemodialysis is evident. No treatment for dialysis arthropathy has yet been described. A switch to high-flux dialysis or hemofiltration has not been convincingly successful, despite decreasing β_2-microglobulin concentrations. Some authors suggest that renal transplantation should be a treatment method of choice for dialysis arthropathy (34,35). After transplantation, an immediate improvement in symptoms was observed. The radiological picture of amyloid bone deposits remained unaltered for up to 4 years, but transplantation prevented the growth of cysts and improved the clinical status of the patients (35).

Kidney transplant amyloidosis in familial mediterranean fever (FMF)

FMF is an autosomal recessive disease, expressed clinically by acute febrile attacks and the insidious development of AA amyloidosis. Persistent proteinuria in an FMF patient is almost invariably a sign of amyloidosis (32).

Amyloid kidney disease progresses from proteinuria through nephrosis to uremia and finally to end-stage kidney disease. Therefore, in these patients, kidney transplantation is the only alternative to dialysis.

The literature data suggest that appropriate doses of colchicine may prevent, retard, or reverse the development of amyloidosis in kidneys transplanted to FMF patients.

Livneh et al. (36) conclude, that the development of amyloidosis in FMF kidney graft recipients is inevitable at colchicine doses lower than 1 mg/day, unpredictable at 1 mg/day, and usually preventable with 1.5 mg/day or more.

Recurrent amyloidosis in a renal allograft

Recurrent amyloidosis is a rare but well-documented event in renal transplant recipients. Recurrent AA amyloid deposition in renal allografts has been shown in 15% of patients transplanted for rheumatologic diseases and in 14% transplanted for chronic infection. Recurrence rates, based on clinically indicated biopsies, may reach 26% of patients who survive beyond 12 months after transplantation.

Graft loss from recurrent amyloidosis was observed in 5% of patients with renal amyloidosis accompanying rheumatologic diseases (37). An improved or stabilized renal function and decreased proteinuria were shown following steroid, chlorambucil, or cyclophosphamide therapy. Treatment was directed towards control of the underlying disease, which was responsible for amyloid formation.

HYPERURICEMIA AND GOUT IN RENAL ALLOGRAFT RECIPIENTS

Cyclosporin-induced hyperuricemia has been recognized as a common metabolic consequence of therapy, occurring in 30%–80% of renal allograft recipients (38). Hyperuricemia is more frequent in cyclosporin- than in azathioprine-treated patients (39). Independent of nephrotoxicity, this complication occurs in 30%–80% of patients treated with cyclosporin but in up to 30% of patients treated with azathioprine (40).

Renal transplant recipients treated with CsA have impaired tubular urate handling that occurs within the first 3 months after transplantation (41). In cyclosporin nephrotoxicity, urate retention is primarily mediated by an increased tubular reabsorption and therefore an impaired tubular secretion of urate.

Several factors play a role in the cyclosporin-associated decrease of urate clearance, so the cause of hyperuricemia is probably multifactorial (40,41). The chronic renal insufficiency is associated with a subsequent decline in urate secretion due to loss of effective renal mass.

The use of diuretics in cyclosporin-treated patients increased the tendency to retain urate. Literature data suggest that avoiding diuretic therapy for cyclosporin-related hypertension could decrease the hyperuricemia (38,41,42). Therefore, treatment of these patients with furosemide must be restricted as much as possible (41).

Although transplant-related immunosuppressive medications, including prednisone, azathioprine, and cyclosporin, probably suppress clinical evidence of inflammation and modulate the degree of synovitis, they do not slow the rate of tissue uric acid deposition and the risk of chronic tophaceous gout (38).

The combination of allopurinol (quite effective in decreasing serum acid levels via the inhibition of xanthine oxidase) with azathioprine (also metabolized on this pathway) may result in leukopenia. Allopurinol in low doses may be cautiously added to azathioprine after a 50%–75% reduction of the azathioprine dose (38).

MYOPATHY AFTER RENAL TRANSPLANTATION

Variable degrees of myopathy symptoms are observed in approximately 10% of renal transplant recipients; the legs are the most affected area. In most cases, this outcome is due to glucocorticoid treatment, but some recipients develop proximal weakness ascribed to severe hypophosphatemia or treatment with cyclosporin (43). Diffuse pain and increased serum concentrations of muscle enzymes due to rhabdomyolysis were observed in patients treated with lovastatin and cyclosporin simultaneously. The risk of rhabdomyolysis appeared to be increased in patients simultaneously treated with gemfibrozil, nicotinic acid, and erythromycin (44).

METABOLIC STATUS OF THE MYOCARDIUM FOLLOWING RENAL TRANSPLANTATION

Congestive cardiac failure is observed in about 40% of patients on chronic dialysis. In many cases, myocardial dysfunction is caused by uremic cardiomyopathy, but cardiac failure and myocardial dysfunction in dialysis patients may be caused by multiple factors. Accumulation of toxic substances (such as urea nitrogen), acidosis, hyperkalemia and hyperparathyroidism, deficiency of essential metabolites, hypocalcemia, B1 hypovitaminosis, and deficiency of carnitine and selenium become significant during the uremic state. These myocardial-depressive factors are rapidly corrected after successful transplantation, which clinically results in marked improvement of myocardial function. Abouna et al. suggest that renal transplantation should be the treatment of choice in all dialysis patients with compromised cardiac function and no coronary or valvular disease, since both uremia and the myocardial dysfunction may be successfully reversed (45).

HYPERLIPIDEMIA IN RENAL TRANSPLANT RECIPIENTS

The incidence of hyperlipidemia in patients after renal transplantation ranges from 16% to 73%, depending on the time when serum lipids are examined (46). In different studies, this incidence ranged from 22% to 53% (47). Two years after transplantation, hyperlipidemia was detected in 51% and after 10 years in 25% of patients (48).

Atherosclerosis is an important clinical manifestation of hyperlipidemia (49). In renal transplant recipients, atherosclerotic vascular disease is a major cause of morbidity and mortality. The risk of myocardial infarction has been estimated to be 25 times greater than in normal age- and sex-matched population (50).

The European Dialysis and Transplant Association registry shows that cardiovascular disease accounts for approximately 32% of all deaths in kidney graft recipients (46). The histological features of glomerulosclerosis are similar to those observed in atherosclerosis, and lesions characteristic for the latter can also be observed in vessel walls during chronic rejection of the kidney graft (51). It was reported that glomerular hypercellularity and expansion of the mesangial matrix might be present within weeks after initiating a high cholesterol intake (52). There are receptors for low-density lipoprotein (LDL) and oxidized LDL on mesangial cells, which thereby can accumulate lipid material. LDL cholesterol may be the cause of monocyte adherence to vascular endothelial cells, and this adherence can also occur in a glomerulus (53).

There is evidence indicating that lipids might cause progressive glomerular injury. In several animal species, lipogenic diets lead to focal glomerulosclerosis. A decrease in serum lipids and cholesterol is associated with a diminution of structural and functional renal injury. Many mechanisms have been suggested by which hyperlipidaemia might accelerate glomerular damage. Thus, high cholesterol diets might lead to significant de novo glomerular injury and worsen the existing renal disease (52). Therefore, the role of lipids in the pathogenesis of chronic rejection and progressive graft failure attracts increasing interest (49).

The mechanism of development of an abnormal lipid metabolism after renal transplantation has not yet been clarified. These abnormalities might be caused by several factors. Immunosuppression, obesity, high blood glucose levels, proteinuria, and concomitant treatment with diuretics or β-blockers were related to lipid abnormalities after renal transplantation (46). Although there was no clear relationship with the type of applied immunosuppressive regimen (49), the development of hyperlipidemia was associated with CsA and steroid treatment (47).

Lipoprotein (a) (Lp(a)), a variant of LDL that is both atherogenic and thrombogenic, has recently gained the attention of researchers (54). In the transplant patient population, Lp(a) concentrations were normal; however, an impaired graft function was associated with raised lipid–lipoprotein levels, including TC, LDL, and Lp(a) (49), similarly to atherosclerosis. Unlike LDL, Lp(a) is not affected by age, sex, or diet. There is increasing evidence that elevated Lp(a) concentration is an independent risk factor for coronary heart disease, and that this increased risk is potentiated by the elevated LDLs. In patients with an Lp(a) concentration greater than 30 mg/dL, the relative risk for myocardial infarction is estimated to be 1.75 (55). Cyclosporin might cause an increase in plasma Lp(a) concentration (50), although in the cyclosporin group there is no relationship between steroid dose and Lp(a) levels.

Cyclosporin is known to be highly lipophilic; up to 50% of the drug is transported in plasma, mainly due to binding to lipoproteins. Binding of cyclosporin to LDL and possibly to Lp(a) could lead to an impaired clearance of lipoproteins, thereby resulting in their elevated plasma concentrations (50). Alternatively, cyclosporin may interfere with Lp(a) metabolism via a hepatic mechanism or a nephrotoxic effect.

A low-cholesterol diet, which is necessary to maintain normal cholesterol levels, alone does not change lipid profiles in a significant way (47), and many patients are not able to keep the restricted diet for a long time.

Lovastatin

Lovastatin can be especially effective in the treatment of hyperlipidemia in the nephrotic syndrome. Renal breakdown of mevalonic acid in the nephrotic syndrome is decreased, resulting in an increased substrate delivery for cholesterol synthesis to the liver (56). Lovastatin, which is an HMG-CoA reductase inhibitor, blocks the formation of mevalonic acid and cholesterol synthesis. A decrease in intracellular cholesterol leads to enhancement of LDL-receptor expression on liver cells and peripheral tissues (57). As a consequence, LDL clearance is increased (53).

Although 10 mg/day of lovastatin induced a 12% decrease in total and LDL cholesterol, an additional 15% decrease was observed when the dose was increased to 20 mg/day. The treatment, which is supposed to cause a decrease in lipid concentrations, was composed of 20 mg lovastatin per day in all patients who received simultaneous immunosuppression with cyclosporin and prednisolone (58). After 6 months of lovastatin treatment, Lp(a) levels showed a 30%–40% decrease. The total cholesterol level was decreased by about 30%, LDL cholesterol and triglycerides were decreased by about 35%, and high-density lipoprotein (HDL) cholesterol was increased by 10% (58).

Rises in hepatic transaminases have been reported to occur in 1%–3% of lovastatin-treated patients. Lovastatin therapy has been occasionally associated with cholestatic jaundice (46).

Kosiske (59) reported an increase in the leukocyte count of renal transplant patients treated with azathioprine and lovastatin. Other adverse effects of lovastatin previously reported in a general population include gastrointestinal disorders, headaches, rash, pruritus, hepatic toxicity, and cataracts (60). None of these symptoms was clinically evident after lovastatin treatment (46,60).

Both lovastatin and CsA appear to be catabolized by the P450IIIA cytochrome system in liver. The serum CsA levels do not increase significantly after introduction of the lovastatin treatment, and the mean levels remain within the therapeutic range. The major concern in using lovastatin for the treatment of renal transplant patients is the potential occurrence of muscle damage during the concurrent therapy. However, lovastatin in doses of 20 mg/day or lower seems not to induce rhabdomyolysis (58,60).

Provastatin

Part of the provastatin molecule has a structure similar to a molecule of HMG-CoA. Since provastatin competes with HMG-CoA for HMG-CoA reductase, it does not completely block cholesterol synthesis. Provastatin is water soluble and therefore seldom enters cells other than hepatocytes, in contrast to lovastatin, which is lipophilic and enters nonhepatic cells. This might be the cause of provastatin's insignificant inhibition of cholesterol synthesis by muscle cells and almost no association with rhabdomyolysis (47).

Gemfibrozil

Gemfibrozil, a fibric acid derivative, reduces hypertriglyceridemia and hypercholesterolemia while increasing HDL levels. Gemfibrozil significantly decreases the total-cholesterol:HDL ratio and triglycerides, with significant trends towards lowering total cholesterol by 15% and increasing HDL by 19%. In combination with a low-carbohydrate diet, gemfibrozil markedly improves lipoprotein levels in hyperlipidemic renal transplant patients, with no induction of any evident toxicity (61).

Cholestyramine

Cholestyramine, a nonabsorbable resin that binds cholesterol in an intestinal lumen, affects bile-dependent intestinal absorption of cyclosporin in an adverse and unpredictable manner (61).

Nicotenic acid

Nicotinic acid causes aggravation of hyperglycemia and increased plasma uric acid levels in diabetic patients. Therefore, nicotinic acid is relatively contraindicated due to the contribution of cyclosporin to the elevation of uric acid levels, especially in the transplanted diabetic patient population (61).

IMPACT OF OBESITY ON RENAL TRANSPLANTATION

Obesity was identified as an independent risk factor for successful renal transplantation. During the initial hospital period, the mortality rate was increased in the obese population. Obese patients had a worse survival rate and a higher incidence of serious complications following renal transplantation as compared to nonobese controls. This outcome was due to a combination of adverse factors, including cardiac, pulmonary, endocrinologic, and surgical ones. In transplant recipients, the effects of immunosuppressive agents may add to morbid factors (62). More wound complications and an increased demand for insulin therapy occurred in obese patients in comparison to control patients (63). Interestingly, obese patients with functioning allografts had similar short- and long-term graft function as compared to controls. The decreased allograft survival rates in the obese group were directly related to the decreased patient survival, since no increase in immunologic loss of allografts was observed (62).

Since obesity appears to be an independent risk factor in patients undergoing transplantation, these patients should make every attempt to lose weight before renal transplantation (62,63).

It is worth mentioning that obesity significantly impacts CsA deposition, since CsA is lipophilic. Therefore, according to Flechner et al. (64), CsA should be given to obese patients based on their IBW (Ideal Body Weight) in order to achieve a comparable drug concentration in the early transplant period. Dosing according to the ABW (Actual Body Weight) resulted in elevated serum cyclosporin levels during the first posttransplant week.

POSTTRANSPLANT DIABETES MELLITUS IN RENAL TRANSPLANT RECIPIENTS

Posttransplant diabetes mellitus frequently develops in older patients with pretransplant postprandial hyperglycemia (65).

Besadonna et al. (66) reviewed their experience of 1275 renal transplants in diabetic patients as compared to 1561 nondiabetic transplant recipients. They concluded that graft loss did not occur more often in the diabetic than in the nondiabetic population. The risk of developing posttransplant diabetes mellitus appeared to be greatest in the first 4 months after transplantation (65).

It was previously documented (67) that both insulin resistance and insulin deficiency were necessary for the development of diabetes in kidney transplant patients.

Steroids

Steroids are a well-recognized cause of posttransplant hyperglycemia (68). The tissue content of glycogen, which is synthesized at high and low blood glucose levels, is increased even in a fasting individual.

Several mechanisms have been suggested to explain steroid-induced insulin resistance: decreased numbers and affinity of insulin receptors; an impaired suppression of hepatic glucose production by insulin; an impaired peripheral glucose uptake; and activation of the glucose/fatty acid cycle (67).

Hricik (69) reported that discontinuation of insulin or oral hypoglycemic agents after complete withdrawal of prednisone in patients maintained on prednisone, azathioprine, and steroids was possible within 4 months after discontinuation of steroids in 7 of 8 patients with posttransplant diabetes mellitus.

Cyclosporin

Diabetes mellitus recognized as a complication of renal transplantation traditionally was attributed to the steroid therapy (70). Nevertheless, several investigators have described a higher incidence of posttransplant diabetes mellitus in patients receiving CsA in comparison to historical controls who received azathioprine and prednisone (69). A retrospective review revealed that posttransplant diabetes developed in 12.9% of previously nondiabetic kidney transplant recipients maintained on prednisone, azathioprine, and CsA, in comparison to 9.6% of patients maintained on azathioprine and prednisone.

Cyclosporin has been shown to inhibit insulin secretion in rats (71); however, there are no data from human studies. It is generally believed that cyclosporin exerts a direct toxic effect on pancreatic cells, since this outcome has been demonstrated in animal studies (65).

It was reported (69) that insulin therapy could be withdrawn within 3 months in 6 of 8 patients who had been converted from CsA to azathioprine, despite continued treatment with prednisone. Based on current knowledge, the beneficial effects of CsA for renal transplant survival outweigh significantly the possible risk of induction of diabetes mellitus (66).

Patients on immunosuppression converted from CsA to azathioprine require careful monitoring in order to avoid rejection episodes.

Extrarenal complications

Extrarenal, secondary complications in diabetic patients continue to be a problem. Diabetic neuropathy proceeds slowly after successful renal transplantation (72). Similarly, in successfully transplanted diabetics who have been nonuremic for at least 10 years, retinopathy proceeds in all patients, although visual activity remains stable in two thirds of the recipients (67).

Patients with posttransplant diabetes mellitus had higher mean hemoglobin levels than controls and a higher incidence of avascular bone necrosis (65).

Diabetic nephropathy

De novo occurrence of diabetic nephropathy in renal allografts was not frequently reported. It should be considered in diabetic transplant patients with proteinuria, nephrotic syndrome, or impairment of graft function. Hypertension and suboptimal diabetes control might cause an acceleration in the development of glomerular lesions (73).

POSTTRANSPLANT ERYTHROCYTOSIS

ERYTHROCYTOSIS DEVELOPED BETWEEN 6 WEEKS AND 30 MONTHS AFTER TRANSPLANTATION

Posttransplant erythrocytosis is a relatively common condition in cyclosporin-treated patients, affecting 3%–16% of all transplants. It is frequently mild and can be spontaneously reversed over a 1–3 years period. The etiology of posttransplant erythrocytosis remains unclear (74).

Various causes have been suggested for increased red cell production, including graft artery stenosis, hydronephrosis, graft rejection, and cyclosporin toxicity. In the majority of cases, excessive production of erythropoietin (Epo) was shown and the hormone was produced by native kidneys (74–78).

Posttransplant erythrocytosis is associated with an increased incidence of thromboembolic episodes and hypertension. Thromboembolic events occur in 20% of patients suffering from posttransplant erythrocytosis (79). Nonetheless, due to recognized serious sequelae, phlebotomy was recommended when hematocrit was greater than 51%. Alternative treatment approaches have included bilateral native nephrectomies. More recently, the usefulness of adenosine antagonist theophylline in reducing serum erythropoietin levels and hematocrit in renal transplant recipients was demonstrated (80). Theophylline is generally well tolerated, but in some patients may cause headaches, nervousness, insomnia, and an increase in blood pressure.

Enalapril is also effective and safe in reducing erythropoietin and hematocrit levels in renal transplant recipients (80).

Angiotensin-converting enzyme (ACE) inhibitors were recently described in a number of clinical settings as reducing the circulating erythropoietin levels (80).

There is a general agreement that enalapril and other ACE inhibitors should be used with great caution in kidney transplant recipients.

Before administration of ACE inhibitors, renal artery stenosis should be excluded (using Doppler ultrasound ex-amination), the endogenous renin–angiotensin system should be inhibited by withdrawing diuretics for a day, and intravascular fluid volume should be expanded with physiologic saline. After such protective measures, no significant reduction in creatinine clearance was observed.

ACE inhibitors offer the additional advantages of slowing down the progression of renal insufficiency and reducing proteinuria and hyperlipidemia associated with proteinuria (80–82).

STEROID SUPPLEMENTATION IN RENAL TRANSPLANT RECIPIENTS

Brombert et al. (83) reported that adrenal function suppression was not common in renal allograft recipients receiving baseline prednisone immunosuppression (5–10 mg/day) and that the demands of physiologic stress were met by a combination of endogenous adrenal function and exogenous baseline immunosuppressive doses of glucocorticoids.

A prospective study on the demand for increased doses of glucocorticoids during periods of stress (sepsis, metabolic abnormalities, and surgery) was set up for 40 renal allograft recipients admitted to the hospital with a significant physiologic stress. They received only their baseline prednisone immunosuppression and no supraphysiologic or stress doses of glucocorticoids. The clinical course of these patients revealed no evidence of adrenal insufficiency. Perhaps allograft recipients, who receive additional immunosuppressants such as cyclosporin and azathioprine, have better control of cytokine production (proinflammatory lymphokines and monokines, e.g., IL-1, TNF, IL-6) than patients receiving steroids alone. These drugs may mimic certain steroid effects and reduce stress-related requirements for steroids (83).

It should be mentioned, that patients with other types of diseases, that are treated chronically with corticosteroids (e.g., asthma or SLE) may have qualitatively different physiologic demands and responses.

ADVERSE EFFECTS OF DRUGS USED FOR IMMUNOSUPPRESSION IN KIDNEY ALLOGRAFT RECIPIENTS (Table 1)

Cyclosporin (Sandimmune)(CsA)

Unlike other cytotoxic immunosuppressants, CsA does not cause myelosuppression. Nowadays, tremor, gingival hyperplasia, and hirsutism are definitely less common, probably due to appropriate dosing regimens. Nephrotoxicity, the major toxic effect of CsA, is pronounced during two periods: 1) the first weeks after transplantation, especially when acute tubular necrosis is present, and 2) when kidney graft function is impaired, with creatinine level higher than 3 mg% (250–300 mmol/L).

Table 1. Immunosuppressive agents—clinical toxicity

	Steroid	Cyclosporin	Azathioprine
Electrolyte disturbances			
(Na/K)	+		
(Ca)	+		
Hypertension	+	+	
Hyperglycemia (diabetes mellitus)	+	+	
Peptic ulcer	+		
Osteoporosis	+		
Myopathy	+		
Subcapsular cataract	+		
Arrest of growth	+		
Nephrotoxicity		+	
Myelosuppression			+
Hepatotoxicity		+	+
Hyperuricemia		+	
Hyperlipidemia	+	+ (?)	
Increased susceptibility to infections	+	+	+
Increased incidence of malignancies	+	+	+

Cyclosporin-induced renal dysfunction has been proposed to be of three types: an acute (reversible) decrease in renal blood flow, associated with the decrease in glome··· lar filtration; an acute thrombotic microangiopathy (partially reversible); and chronic (irreversible) renal damage (84).

Glucocorticoids

The anti-inflammatory properties of glucocorticoids are related to their inhibitory impact on production of prostaglandins in different cells (85). In addition to pituitary–adrenal suppression, the principal complications resulting from prolonged glucocorticoid therapy are fluid and electrolyte disturbances, hypertension, hyperglycemia, peptic ulcers, osteoporosis, myopathy, behavioral disturbances, posterior subcapsular cataracts, arrest of growth, Cushing's habitus (central obesity, striae), and increased susceptibility to infections (86).

In patients given high doses of steroids (15 mg/kg), urinary PGE2 was significantly reduced. It was previously documented that glomerular filtration in patients with renal disease depended on intact renal cyclooxygenase. High steroid boluses might theoretically be harmful for patients with renal dysfunction. A transient increment of the creatinine level is actually observed relatively often in the early phase of steroid pulse therapy introduced for kidney graft rejection treatment (85).

Azathioprine

Azathioprine (imuran) toxicity is mainly manifested in the blood and gastrointestinal system (84). Leukopenia, thrombocytopenia, and slight anemia are the symptoms of toxicity affecting blood cells. Nausea and vomiting, especially in the morning, are the gastrointestinal effects, which do not stop the treatment. Liver dysfunction is the most severe complication and is especially dangerous when HBV or HCV infection coexist. We would strongly advise against the use of azathioprine in patients with postviral hepatitis. Occasionally, hepatic venoocclusive disease could be observed. Allopurinol should be avoided during the administration of imuran or the imuran dose should be reduced by 75%, since allopurinol reduces the oxidation of active mercaptopurine to inactive metabolites.

METABOLIC SIDE EFFECTS OF OKT3

Most transplant centers consider antilymphocyte antibodies to be an important element of their immunosuppressive regimens. Clinical trials have shown the effectiveness of antilymphocyte antibodies in reversing steroid-resistant rejections. There is no controversy about their use in this situation (87).

The best-described side effect of OKT3 is the cytokine release syndrome (CRS) caused by cytokines released from T cells and monocytes. TNF seems to play a particularly pivotal role (88). This clinical syndrome is composed of high fever, chills, headaches, diarrhea, and vomiting that can be observed immediately after injecting the first dose of OKT3 (88). A capillary leak syndrome induced by the released cytokines in the presence of volume overload can lead to pulmonary edema. Hemodynamic changes include depressed systemic vascular resistance, hypotension, tachycardia, and probably direct myocardial depression.

During OKT3 therapy, cytokine encephalopathy can be observed. The symptoms may include hallucinations, seizures, and coma, but in general these are benign and self-limited (90). Coagulation and fibrinolysis after the first dose of OKT3 are activated in two phases. The initial phase seems to be associated with complement activation and the later phase with the release of cytokines (91). Preinjection of steroids, indomethacin, and antihistamines reduces the severity of CRS (88,90). It was recently shown that pretreatment with pentoxyphylline (20 mg/kg I.V.) reduced the TNF release after the first injection of OKT3 (92). Upon subsequent doses of OKT3, the severity of CRS was definitely less expressed.

GROWTH RATES IN CHILDREN TREATED WITH GROWTH HORMONE AFTER RENAL TRANSPLANTATION

Transplanted children often display spontaneous growth acceleration, and one third of them end up as small adults. Janssen et al. documented that human growth hormone (rhGH) treatment in 1 U/kg/wk doses for 1–3 years improved the growth of children after transplantation and on dialysis. rhGH treatment did not change the renal graft function deterioration rate (93). However, treatment with growth hormone might affect renal function in these children by any of several mechanisms—direct effects, glomerular hyperfiltration, differential growth, or immunologic processes (94).

Van Dop et al. used growth hormone at a dose of 0.3–0.35 mg/kg/wk (1 mg was approximately 2 U). The authors concluded that transplanted children with poor growth after kidney transplantation responded to treatment with an accelerated linear growth, without concomitant accelerated skeletal maturation (94).

The decrease in creatinine clearance that occurred among these patients demonstrates that every child with renal allograft subjected to treatment with growth hormone should be closely monitored for its adverse effects. However, the increase in predicted adult stature and potential adult height that result from treatment with growth hormone may outweigh the risks.

RENAL TRANSPLANTATION IN ELDERLY PATIENTS

The increasing age of the population accepted for chronic dialysis has increased the demand for transplantation (95). From the ethical point of view, age cannot be the sole criterion in allocating any type of medical therapy (96). Patients of age 60 years or more constitute about half the patients accepted for dialysis. In order to achieve optimal results for kidney transplantation in older patients, patient survival rate after transplantation should be equal to or greater than survival on dialysis. Low-risk patients (free of diabetes and heart disease) do very well after kidney transplantation, with a $3^{1}/_{2}$-year survival probability of 91%. In comparison, mortality rates for dialysis patients of age 60 and older were estimated to be as high as 20% per year (1-year survival rate: about 80%). Cardiac arrest was the major cause of early graft loss (96). The benefits for elderly patients who underwent renal transplantation were smaller than for younger patients. For example, muscular strength did not improve as in the younger patients (95).

RENAL FUNCTION AFTER PREGNANCY IN RENAL TRANSPLANT RECIPIENTS

Female kidney-transplanted patients generally tolerate pregnancy well, and in individual cases, good graft function continues throughout the pregnancy (97). However, pregnancy seems to bring an increased risk of long-term reduced renal function and shorter graft survival. The increase in serum creatinine concentration, registered during the pregnancy period at 3 months and at 1 year after delivery, was higher than in matched control patients without pregnancy at corresponding periods after transplantation (98).

Pregnancy is associated with approximately a 9% risk of allograft rejection and a 5% risk of a permanent impairment of renal function. Pregnant women on azathioprine and steroids have an increased uric acid clearance. Hyperuricemia can be also induced by cyclosporin. Thus, hyperuricemia in pregnant women taking cyclosporin does not necessarily signify preeclampsia (especially in the absence of hypertension, proteinuria, and edema) but may reflect cyclosporin nephrotoxicity (97).

Although 80% of neonates born to mothers with transplanted kidneys were below the mean gestational age, the weight and length at birth were within normal ranges, and no severe intrauterine growth retardation was documented. There was no higher risk of other developmental disturbances (97). However, the risk of nonfatal neonatal complications (primarily metabolic and infectious) was 4%–5%, and additionally 4% for intrauterine deaths and 4% for neonatal deaths (99).

REFERENCES

1. Gutshe HU, Delz E, Lüneburg E, et al.: Effect of cyclosporine on the proximal tubular function of the rat kidney (abstract). *Kidney Int* 637, 1984.
2. Dieperink H, Starklint H, Leyssac PP: Nephrotoxicity of cyclosporine—an animal model of nephrotoxic effect of cyclosporine on overall renal and tubular function in conscious rats. In: BD Kahad, ed, *Cyclosporine.* Grune and Stratton, New York, p 520, 1984.
3. Battle DC, Gutterman C, Tarka J, Prasad R: Effect of short term cyclosporine A administration on urinary acidification. *Clin Nephrol* 25 (Suppl):162–169, 1986.
4. Adu D, Michael J, Turney J, Master P: Hypercalcemia in cyclosporine treated renal allograft recipients. *Lancet* 2:370–371, 1983.

5. Heering P, Grabensee B: Influence of cyclosporin A on renal tubular function after kidney transplantation. *Nephron* 59:66–70, 1991.

6. Aguilera S, Deray, Desjobert H, et al.: Effects of cyclosporine on tubular acidification function in patients with idiopatic uveitis. *Am J Nephrol* 12:425–430, 1992.

7. Gradowska L: Wydzielanie jonu wodorowego przez przes-zczepioną nerkę. *Pol Arch Med Wewn* 61(5):373, 1979.

8. Derfus BA, Carrera GF, Komorowski RM, Ryan LM: Severe arthropathy and osteopathy following combined renal pancreas transplantation. *Transplantation* 53:678–681, 1992.

9. Nordal KP, Dahl E, Halse J, Aksnes L, Thomassen Y, Flatmark A: Aluminium metabolism and bone histology after kidney transplantation, a one year follow-up study. *J Clin Endocrinol Metab* 74(5):1140–1145, 1992.

10. Bertolone G, Anchiami M, Bonuci E, et al.: Dynamics of bone aluminium over one year of functioning renal graft. *Nephron* 64(4):540–546, 1993.

11. Agarwal S, Owen R: Tendinitis and tendon ruptures in succesful renal transplant recipients. *Clin Orthop* 252:270–275, 1990.

12. Partiff AM: Hypercalcemia hyperparathyroidism following renal transplantation: diferential diagnosis management and implications for cell population control in the parathyroid gland. *Miner Electrolyte Metab* 8:92–112, 1982.

13. Reid IR: Pathogenesis and treatment of steroid osteoporosis. *Clin Endocrinol* 30:83–103, 1989.

14. Rude RK, Gruber HE, Oldham SB: Cortisone-induced osteoporosis, effect on bone adenylate cyclase. *Miner Electrolyte Metab* 19(2):71–77, 1993.

15. Gallagher JA, Beresford JN, Mac Donald BR, Russell RG: Hormone target cell interactions in human bone. In: Christiansen et al., eds, *Osteoporosis*. Glostrup Hospital pp 431–439, 1984.

16. Cascio VLO, Bonucci V, Imbimbo E, et al.: Bone loss after glucocorticoid therapy. *Calcif Tissue Int* 36:435–438, 1984.

17. Russel RG, Graveley R, Skjodt H: The effects of cyclosporine A on bone end cartilage.*Br J Rheumatol* 32 (Suppl 1):42–46, 1993.

18. Bosch SA, Raymakers JA, Huber-Bruning O: Acute changes in calcium and bone metabolism during methylprenisolone pulse therapy in rheumatoid arthritis. *Br J Rheumatol* 27:215–219, 1988.

19. Katz JA, Jee WS, Jaffe II, et al.: Prostaglandin E_2 alleviates cyclosporine A induced bone loss in rats. *J Bone Miner Res* 7(10):191–200, 1992.

20. Briner VA, Landmann J, Brunner FP, Thiel G: Cyclosporin A induced transient rise in plasma alkaline phosphatase in kidney transplant patients. *Transplant Int* 6(2):99–107, 1993.

21. Russel RG, Graveley R, Coxon F, Skjodt H, Del-Poco E, Elford P, Mackenzie A: Cyclosporine A mode of action and effects on bone and joint tissues. *Scand J Rheumatol Suppl* 95:8–9, 1992.

22. Sato K, Satoni S, Oguma S, Ohkohchi N, Ozaki H: Relationship between aseptic necrosis of femoral head bone and immunosuppressive therapy, especially CsA administration. *Nippon Geka Gakkai Zasshi* 94(8):832–839, 1993.

23. Lukert BP, Johnson BE, Robinson RG: Estrogen and progesterone replacement therapy reduces glucocorticoid-induced bone loss. *J Bone Miner Res* 7(9):1063–1069, 1992.

24. Kunz D: Treatment of common osteoporosis with fluoride: current trends. *Rev Rhum Mal Osteoartic* 59:39–45, 1992.

25. Olbricht T, Benkert G: Glucocorticoid-induced osteoporosis,

pathogenesis, prevention and treatment with special regard to rheumatic disease. *J Intern Med* 234(3):237–244, 1993.

26. Papapoulos SE, Landsan JO, Bijvoet OL, et al.: The use of biphosphonates in the treatment of osteoporosis. *Bone* 13 (Suppl 1):s41–s49, 1992.

27. Kwan JT, Almond MK, Ewans K, Cunningham J: Changes in total body mineral content and regional bone mineral density in renal patients following renal transplantation. *Miner Electrolyte Metab* 18:166–168, 1992.

28. Tałałaj M, Gradowska L, Durlik M, et al.: Prevention of glucocorticoid-induced osteoporosis with 25-hydroxyvitamin D in kidney transplant patients. Abstracts, XXX Congress of EDTAP, 6, 1993.

29. Rosenbaum RW, Hruska KA, Kokor A, Anderson C, Slatopolsky E: Decreased phosphate reabsorption after renal transplantation: evidence for a mechanism independent of calcium and parathyroid hormone. *Kidney Int* 19:568–578, 1981.

30. Graf H, Kovarik J, Stummvoll HK, Wolf A, Pinggerra WF: Handling of phosphate by the transplanted kidney. *Proc Eur Dial Transplant Assoc* 16:624–628, 1979.

31. Pabico RC, McKenna BA, Freeman RB: Renal function before and after unilateral nephrectomy in renal donors. *Kidney Int* 8:166–175, 1975.

32. Markell NS, Altura BT, Barbour RL, Altura BK: Ionized and total magnesium levels in cyclosporine-treated renal transplant recipients; relationship with cholesterol and cyclosporine level. *Clin Sci (Colch)* 85(3):315–318, 1993.

33. Nozue T, Kobayashi A, Sako A, et al.: Evidence that cyclosporine causes both intracellular migration and inappropiate urinary excretion of magnesium in rats. *Transplantation* 55(2):346–349, 1993.

34. Stethi P, Brown EA, Maini RN, Gower PE: Renal transplantation for dialysis arthropathy. *Lancet* ii:448–449, 1988.

35. Campistol JM, Ponz E, Munoz-Gomez J, Oppenheimer F, Ricard MJ, Vilardell J, Andreu J: Renal transplantation for dialysis amyloidosis. *Transplant Proc* 24:118–119, 1992.

36. Livneh A, Zemer D, Siegal B, Leor A, Sohar E, Pras M: Colchicine prevents kidney transplant amyloidosis in Familial Mediterranean Fever. *Nephron* 60:418–422, 1992.

37. Harrison KL, Alpers ChE, Daris CL: De novo amyloidosis in a renal allograft: a case report and review of the literature. *Am J Kidney Dis* 22:468–476, 1993.

38. Burack DA, Gryffith BP, Thompson ME, Kahl LE: Hyperuricemia and gout among heart transplant recipients receiving cyclosporine. *Am J Med* 42:141–145, 1992.

39. Delaney V, Sumrani N, Daskelakis P, Hong JH, Sommer BG: Hyperuricemia and gout in renal allograft recipients. *Transplant Proc* 24:1773–1774, 1992.

40. Lin HY, Rocher LL, Mc Quillan MA, Schaltz S, Pallella TD, Fox IH: Cyclosporine-induced hyperuricemia and gout. *N Engl J Med* 321:287–292, 1989.

41. Noordzij TC, Leunissen KML, Ven Hooff JP: Renal handling of urate and the incidence of gout arthritis during cyclosporine and duvetic ure. *Transplantation* 52:64–66, 1991.

42. Marcen R, Gallego N, Gamez C, Orofino L, Ortuno J: Hyperuricemia after kidney transplantation in patients treated with cyclosporine. *Am J Med* 93:354–355, 1992.

43. Julian BA, Guarles LD, Niemann KMW: Musculoskeletol complications after renal transplantation: pathogenesis and treatment. *Am J Kidney Dis* 19:99–120, 1992.

44. Marais GE, Larson KK: Rhabdomyolysis and acute renal failure induced by combination lovastatin and gemfibrozil therapy. *Ann Intern Med* 112:228–230, 1990.

45. Abouna GM, Kumar MSA, Silva OSG, Samhan M, Cheriyan G, At Abdulla I., White AG: Reversal of myocardial dysfunction following renal transplantation. *Transplant Proc* 25:1034–1035, 1993.
46. Castelao AM, Grino JM, Anders E, Gliverent S, Seron D, Castineiras MJ, Roca M, Galceran JM, Gonzalez MT, Alisina J: HMGCoA reductase inhibitors lovastatin and simvastatin in the treatment of hypercholesterolemia after renal transplantation. *Transplant Proc* 25:1043–1046, 1993.
47. Yoshimura N, Oka T, Okamato M, Ohmori Y: The effect of Pravastatin on hyperlipidemia in renal transplant recipients. *Transplantation* 53:94–99, 1992.
48. Nicholas ML, Alexandre GPJ: The evolution of hyperlipidemia late after renal transplantation. *Proc Eur Dial Transplant Assoc* 16:339, 1979.
49. Moore R, Thomas D, Morgan E, Wheeler D, Griffin P, Salaman J, Rees A: Abnormal lipid and lipoprotein profiles following renal transplantation. *Transplant Proc* 25:1060–1061, 1993.
50. Webb AT, Plant M, Reaveley DA, O'Donnell M, Luck VA, O'Connor B, Seed M, Brown EA: Lipid and lipoprotein (a) concentration in transplant patients.
51. Diamond JR: In: WF Keane, JH Stein, eds, *Contemporary Issues in Nephrology*. Vol *24: Lipids and Renal Disease*. Churchill Livingstone, New York, 109–1, 1990.
52. Schmitz PG, Kasiske BL, O'Donnel MP, Keane WF: Lipids and progressive renal injury. *Semin Nephrol* 9:354–369, 1989.
53. Appel G: Lipid abnormalites in renal disease. *Kidney Int* 39:169–183, 1991.
54. Scott J: Lipoprotein (a): trombogenesis linked to atherogenesis at last. *Nature* 341:22–23, 1989.
55. Kostner GM, Avogaro P, Cazzolato G, Marth E, Bittolobon G, Quinci GB: Lipoprotein Lp (a) and the risk for myocardial infarction. *Atherosclerosis* 38:51–61, 1991.
56. Hopper J, Ryan P, Lee JC, Rosenman W: Lipoid nephrosis in 31 adult patients. *Medicine (Baltimore)* 49:321–341, 1970.
57. Curry RC, Roberts WC: Status of the coronary arteries in the nephrotic syndrome. *Am J Med* 63:183–192, 1977.
58. Traindl O, Reaoling S, Frauz M, Watschinger B, Klauser R, Pidlich H, Widhelm K, Pohonka E, Kovorik J: Treatment of hyperlipidemic kidney graft recipients with Lovastatin: effect on LDL-cholesterol and lipoprotein (a). *Nephron* 62:394–398, 1992.
59. Kasiske BL, Tortorice KL, Heim-Dilthoy KL, Goryance JM, Rao V: Lovastatin treatment of hypercholesterolemia in renal transplant recipients. *Transplantation* 49:95, 1990.
60. Chueng AK, De Vault GA, Gregory MC: A perspective study on treatment of hypercholesterolemia with Lovastatin in renal transplant patients receiving cyclosporine. *J Am Soc Nephrol* 3:1884–1891, 1993.
61. Knigkt RJ, Vathsala A, Schoeuberg L, Comel S, Weinberg RB, Goldstein RA, Lewis RM, Van Buren CT, Kohen BD: Treatment of hyperlipidemia in renal transplant patients with gemfibrozil and dietary modification. *Transplantation* 53:224–225, 1991.
62. Gill IS, Hodge EE, Novick AC, Steinmuller DR, Garred D: Impact of obesity on renal transplantation. *Transplant Proc* 25:1047–1048, 1993.
63. Holley JL, Shapiro R, Lopatin WB, Tzakis AG, Hakela TR, Starz TE: Obesity as a risk factor following cadaver renal transplantation. *Transplantation* 49:387–389, 1990.
64. Flechner SM, Kolbeiusson ME, Tam J, Lum B: The impact of body weight on cyclosporine pharmacokinetics in renal transplant recipients. *Transplantation* 47:806–810, 1989.
65. Rao M, Jacob CK, Shastry JCM: Post-renal transplant diabetes mellitus—retrospective study. *Nephrol Dial Transplant* 7:1039–1042, 1992.
66. Basadonna G, Matas AJ, Nojarian JS: Kidney transplantation in diabetic patient: The University of Minnesota experience. *Kidney Int* 42:S-193–S-196, 1992.
67. Ekstrand AV, Eriksson JG, Gronhagen-Riska C, Ahonen PJ, Groop LC: Insulin resistance and insulin deficiency in the pathogenesis of posttransplantation diabetes in man. *Transplantation* 53:563–569, 1992.
68. Feinstein EI, Wanner Ch, Bohler J, Horl WH: Endocrine and metabolic disorders following kidney transplantation. *Am J Nephrol* 12:363–368, 1992.
69. Hricik DE, Bartucci MR, Moir EJ, Mayes JT, Schulak JA: Effects of steroid withdrawal on posttransplant diabetes mellitus in cyclosporine-treated renal transplant recipients. *Transplantation* 51:374–377, 1991.
70. Ruiz JO, Simmons RL, Callender CO, Kjellstrand CM, Buselmeier TJ, Nojerien JS: Steroid-induced diabetes in renal transplant patients: pathogenetic factors and prognosis *Surgery* 73:759, 1973.
71. Seemayer TA, Murphy GF, Marliss EB: Glucose tolerance in the rat. *Diabetes* 34:1309, 1985.
72. Najarian JS, Kaufmant DB, Fryd DS, Mc Hugh L, Mauer SM, Remsay RC, Kennedy WR, Navarro X., Goetz FC, Sutherland DER: Long-term survival following kidney transplantation in 100 Type I diabetic patients. *Transplantation* 47:106–113, 1989.
73. Kelly JJ, Walker RG, Kinceid-Smith P: De novo diabetic nodular glomerulosclerosis in renal allograft. *Transplantation* 53:688–689, 1992.
74. Innes A, Pol CR, Deunis MJ, Ryan JJ, Morgan AG, Burolen RR: Posttransplant erythrocytosis and immunosuppression with cyclosporin: a case control study. *Nephrol Dial Transplant* 6:588–591, 1991.
75. Wolff M, Jelkmann W: Erythropoiesis and erythropoietin levels in renal transplant recipients. *Klin Wochensch* 69:53–58, 1991.
76. Hammond D, Winnick S: Paraneoplastic erythrocytosis and ectopic erythropoietins. *Ann N Y Acad Sci* 230:219–227, 1974.
77. Rell K, Koziak K, Jarzyło I, Lao M, Gaciong Z: Correction of posttransplant erythrocytosis with enalapril. *Transplant Int*, in press.
78. Sauron C, Bertoux P, Bertoux F, Alamartine E, Diob N, Broyet C, Hecini J: New insights and treatment in posttransplant polycythemia (erythrocytosis) of renal recipients. *Transplant Proc* 25:1032–1033, 1993.
79. Gaston RS, Julian BA, Barker CV, Diethelm AG, Curtis JJ: Enalapril: safe and effective therapy for posttransplant erythrocytosis. *Transplant Proc* 25:1029–1031, 1993.
80. Conlon P, Fawell J, Donohoe J, Carmody M, Walsche JJ: The beneficial effect of enalapril on erythrocytosis after renal transplantation. *Transplantation* 56:217–219, 1993.
81. Brunner HR: ACE inhibitors in renal disease. *Kidney Int* 42:463–479, 1992.
82. Hermans MP, Brichard SM, Colin I, Borgies P, Ketelslegers JM, Lambert AE: Long-term reduction of microalbuminuria after 3 years of angiotensin-converting enzyme inhibitors by Perindopril in hypertensive insulin-treated diabetic patients. *Am J Med* 92 (Suppl 4B):102S–107S, 1992.
83. Bromberg JS, Alfrey EJ, Barker CF, Chavin KD, Dafoe DC, Holland T, Noji A, Perloff LJ, Zellers LA, Grossman RA: Adrenal suppression and steroid supplementation in renal

transplant recipients. *Transplantation* 51:385–390, 1991.

84. Handschumacher RE: Immunosuppressive agents. In: AG Goodman, TW Rall, AS Nies, P Toylor, eds, *The pharmacological Basis of Therapeutics*. Pergamon Press, New York, p 14–1276, 1991.

85. Rota S, Rembaldi A, Gaspari F, Noris M, Daina E, Benigni A, Aerna A, Donadelli R, Remuzzi G, Garattini S: Methyl-prednisolone dosage effects on peripheral lymphocyte subpopulations and eicosanoid synthesis. *Kidney Int* 42:981–990, 1992.

86. Haynes RC: Adrenocorticotropic hormone: adrenocortical steroids and their synthetic analogs: inhibitors of the synthesis and actions of adrenocortical hormones. In: AG Goodman, TW Rall, SA Nies, P Taylor, eds, *The Pharmacological Basis of Therapeutics*. Pergamon Press, New York, p 14–1276, 1991.

87. Norman DJ: Antilymphocyte antibodies in the treatment of allograft rejection: targets, mechanisms of action, monitoring and efficacy. *Semin Nephrol* 12:315–324, 1992.

88. Leimenstoll G, Zabel P, Schroeder P, Schlaak M, Niedermayer W: Suppression of OKT-3-induced Tumor Necrosis Factor Alfa formation by Pentoxifylline in renal transplant recipients. *Transplant Proc* 25:561–563, 1993.

89. Kreis H: Antilymphocyte globulin in kidney transplantation. *Kidney Int* 42:S-188–S-192, 1992.

90. Shihab F, Barry JM, Bennet WM, Mayer MM, Norman DJ: Cytokine-related encephalopathy induced by OKT-3: incidence and predisposing factors. *Transplant Proc* 25:564–565, 1993.

91. Berge RJM, Reasveld MHM, van Diepen FNJ, Hack CE: Activation of coagulation and fibrinolysis during treatment with OKT-3. *Transplant Proc* 25:566–567, 1993.

92. Alegre ML, Gasteldello K, Abramowicz D, Kiunaert P, Vereestreeten P, De Pauw L, Vandenebelle P, Moser M, Leo O, Goldmen M: Evidence that pentoxifylline reduces anti-CD3 monoclonal antibody induced cytokine release syndrome. *Transplantation* 52:674–679, 1991.

93. Janssen F, Van Damme-Lombaerts R, Van Dyck M, Hall M, Proesmans W, Goos G, Kinnaert P: Effects of recombinant human growth hormone on graft function in renal transplanted children and adoltescents: three-year experience of a Belgian study group. *Transplant Proc* 25:1049–1050, 1993.

94. Van Dap C, Jobs KL, Donohoue PA, Bock GH, Fivush BA, Hormau WE: Accelerated growth rates in children treated with hormone after renal transplantation. *J Pediatr* 120:244–250, 1992.

95. Neberg G, Nilsson B, Hallste G, Haljamac V, Norden G, Blohme I: Renal transplantation in elderly patients: survival and complications. *Transplant Proc* 25:1062–1063, 1993.

96. Schulak JA, Mayes JT, Jonston KH, Hricik DE: Kidney transplantation in patients aged sixty years and older. *Surgery* 108:7–733, 1990.

97. Salmela KT, Kyllonen LEJ, Holmberg Ch, Gronhagen-Riska C: Impaired renal function after pregnancy in renal transplant recipients. *Transplantation* 56:1372–1375, 1993.

98. Bumgardner GL, Matas AJ: Transplantation and pregnancy. *Transplantation Rev* 6:139–162, 1992.

CHAPTER 67

Transplantation in Inherited, Systemic, and Metabolic Diseases

ELEANOR D. LEDERER

INTRODUCTION

The population of end-stage renal disease patients continues to grow for a variety of reasons. Advances in renal replacement therapies have resulted in relaxed criteria for patient acceptance into renal failure programs. Improved medical management of nonrenal diseases such as diabetes and atherosclerosis has added to the end-stage renal disease population by allowing the emergence of progressive renal failure. Finally, more elderly patients are being added to dialysis programs as a consequence of the aging of the general population. The challenges posed by the variety of medical problems in this growing, diverse population have been met by innovative approaches to renal replacement therapy. The purpose of this chapter is to describe the experience of renal transplantation in several systemic, metabolic, and inherited conditions. Consonant with the theme of this book, the chapter will emphasize selection criteria, unique treatment techniques, and specialized follow-up considerations.

METABOLIC DISEASES

Diabetes

Diabetes mellitus is responsible for ESRD in 25%–30% of patients presenting for renal replacement therapy. The optimal therapy for these patients, long considered high-risk candidates for transplantation, continues to be controversial. The widespread use of cyclosporine has yielded short-term results in these patients that are comparable to those in nondiabetics in some centers (1–16). With the exception of a few reports, diabetics do not appear to have an increased incidence of early death from infections, graft thrombosis, or acute rejection. Despite promising early results, however, long-term patient survival is inferior in diabetics, resulting in inferior long-term graft survival statistics. In fact, if death with a functioning renal transplant is not considered a graft loss, the long-term graft survival results for diabetic and nondiabetic patients are similar (5).

This finding suggests that diabetics are not high-risk candidates from an immunologic standpoint.

Selection of diabetic candidates who would be likely to enjoy the optimal benefit from renal transplantation thus depends on an evaluation of nonimmunologic risk factors. Because the excessive mortality in these patients is primarily a result of aggressive cardiovascular disease (17–19), attention to pretransplant cardiovascular status and risk factors is of utmost importance. Lemmers et al. (20) tracked the occurrence of peripheral vascular disease, coronary artery disease, and cerebrovascular disease during the course of 123 renal allografts in 101 patients over 6 years. Four-year patient survival was 65%. Of the 30 patient deaths, 57% were secondary to vascular disease. Six-year living related graft survival was 61%, and cadaveric graft survival was 28%. Nineteen of 64 graft losses were secondary to death with a functioning allograft. Of the 41 patients who had evidence of vascular disease prior to transplantation, 32 (nearly 80%) had another vascular event posttransplant. On the other hand, of the 60 patients who had no evidence of vascular disease prior to transplant, 26 (about 44%) had a vascular event posttransplant. In all, 12 patients sustained cerebrovascular events; 14 patients had a coronary artery event, 11 of which were fatal; and 25 patients underwent amputation. Peripheral vascular disease occurred most commonly pretransplantation and posttransplantation. Pretransplant coronary artery disease was predictive of a post-transplant coronary event. Using echocardiographic evaluation of transplant candidates, Weinrauch and colleagues noted that the 3-year patient survival for those with known coronary artery disease, an increased left ventricular end-diastolic diameter, and decreased circumferential shortening velocity was 42%, compared to 82% in patients with a normal left ventricular end-diastolic diameter (21). Thus, both coronary artery disease and left ventricular dysfunction are risk factors for increased mortality. Due to the high incidence of silent myocardial ischemia in diabetics, reliance on symptoms to identify those with preoperative coronary risk factors is inadequate. The optimal screening algorithm for evaluation of cardiac risk, however, is not yet known. Some cen-

Suki, WN and Massry SG (eds), Suki and Massry's Therapy of Renal Diseases and Related Disorders, Third Edition. ISBN 978-1-4757-6634-9.
©1998, Kluwer Academic Publishers, Boston/Dordrecht/London. All rights reserved.

ters simply refer all patients for cardiac catheterization. However, due to the expense and potential morbidity of catheterization, others have attempted to stratify patients into low- or high-risk candidates, forgoing catheterization in the low-risk group. Manskie et al. compared historical and EKG findings with cardiac catheterization in 141 diabetics with far-advanced renal insufficiency and no chest pain or history of myocardial infarction (22). Of those patients over age 45, 14 of 16 had significant coronary artery disease. In those less than age 45, a smoking history of less than five pack years, fewer than 25 years of diabetes, and no ST changes on EKG were highly predictive of an absence of coronary artery disease. These investigators suggested that all patients over age 45 and those less than 45 with one of the risk factors undergo catheterization. Other investigators have attempted to use echocardiogram and stress thallium to identify patients at high risk for coronary artery disease (23–28). The center-to-center variability in experience makes it difficult to recommend the use of any one modality for all centers. Nonetheless, noninvasive techniques have clearly proved to be useful. Thus, the presence of a specific expertise may help a center formulate its own individualized screening algorithm. If significant coronary artery disease is identified, there is now evidence that surgical intervention can successfully decrease the incidence of future cardiac events (29).

Another diabetic complication that may have an impact on results of renal transplantation is neuropathy, particularly bladder dysfunction and gastroparesis. Several studies now show that diabetics and other patients with bladder dysfunction or urinary diversion can be successfully transplanted (30). In most patients, the degree of bladder dysfunction is slight enough that no specific intervention is required. However, other patients have been managed quite successfully with intermittent catheterization (31). Gastroparesis poses the potential risk of poor immunosuppressive drug absorption (32). While depressed cyclosporine absorption has been documented in some patients, this problem has not emerged as a major impediment to renal transplantation of diabetics.

Management of diabetic transplant recipients is similar immunologically to that of nondiabetics. Autonomic neuropathy, however, does confer a higher anesthetic risk, as amply documented by reports of sudden death in diabetics undergoing renal transplantation, even diabetics with normal coronaries (33,34). Supplemental oxygen, extended postoperative cardiac monitoring, and attention to fluid and electrolyte status are strategies that have been suggested to avert such complications. Perioperative diabetic control is most flexibly managed with an initial insulin infusion, followed by frequent subcutaneous injections of short-acting insulin (35). Long-term complications that require special attention in the diabetic include progressive microangiopathy resulting in neuropathy, retinopathy, and recurrent nephropathy; progressive atherosclerotic disease; an increased incidence of posttransplant

erythrocytosis; an increased incidence of hyperlipidemia; and an increased incidence of clinically significant bone disease (36–48). Diabetic glomerulopathy recurs pathologically in normal kidneys transplanted into diabetics within 2 years but can be ameliorated by intensive metabolic control and avoided by simultaneous pancreas transplantation (49–52). Kidney transplantation ameliorates motor but not sensory uremic peripheral neuropathy; however, with standard diabetes control, diabetic neuropathy continues to progress after transplantation. Macrovascular disease has been discussed. Preoperative vascular evaluation and correction of coronary artery disease and postoperative attention to cardiac risk factors, including hyperlipidemia and hypertension, are suggested to improve the high incidence of vascular mortality. Hypercholesterolemia can be treated with HMG-CoA-reductase inhibitors if liver functions and creatine kinase are monitored. Hypertension is a significant risk factor for posttransplant mortality in this population. The calcium channel blockers have the potential advantage of ameliorating cyclosporine-induced renal vasoconstriction. Whether ACE inhibition will be useful in preventing recurrent diabetic nephropathy is unknown; however, these agents may be useful in the treatment of erythrocytosis in the hypertensive diabetic transplant patient.

In summary, diabetic patients with end-stage renal disease presenting for consideration for renal transplantation should be counseled as follows. Immunologically, they are not at a higher than normal risk. Preoperative cardiovascular evaluation is important to identify patients who are at high risk for posttransplant vascular morbidity and mortality. Diabetic patients without significant vascular disease who undergo transplantation tend to survive longer than those who remain on dialysis. On the other hand, in the presence of significant vascular disease, transplantation confers no survival benefit. In either case, due to the high incidence of cardiovascular mortality in diabetics, risk factor reduction will be a major postoperative priority. The microangiopathic complications of diabetes progress, although intensive diabetic control or pancreas transplantation may slow this process. Clearly, risk factor reduction and metabolic control are successful only with substantial patient input.

Obesity

Over 25% of American adults are overweight. Although difficult to dissect from associated risk factors, obesity appears to be an independent risk factor for insulin resistance, hyperlipidemia, certain cancers, sleep apnea, and mortality from coronary artery disease (53). For the potential transplant recipient, obesity confers a greater surgical risk (54,55) and the potential for accelerated allograft failure secondary to hyperfiltration (56). Weight gain after transplantation is not correlated with pretransplant obesity (57). In a study comparing obese (body mass index greater than 30) and nonobese individuals undergoing renal transplantation, Holley and coworkers (55) found that obese individuals had an increased incidence of early graft dysfunction, wound complications, reintubations, intensive care unit admissions, and the development of diabetes. Mortality was higher, and 1-year graft survival was decreased (66% compared to 84% in nonobese patients). To determine the potential impact of instituting a weight-restriction policy on access to our transplant list, we determined the body mass index of all referrals for 1 year and deferred activation in individuals with a body mass index greater than 32. Approximately 10% of our patient referrals exceeded the target weight. Of these, half achieved their weight loss goals and were activated on the transplant list within 6 months. From these results, we predict that adherence to this policy would exclude about 5% of all referrals. Whether pretransplant weight loss will reduce the occurrence of the above complications has not been tested. These patients should therefore be counseled concerning their risks. With the paucity of data concerning this condition and the difficulty in treating it, no universal policy recommendations can be made.

PARAPROTEINEMIAS

Amyloidosis

Amyloidosis is a systemic illness characterized by the deposition of a characteristic protein in various organs, including the kidney. Primary (AL) amyloid protein is a light chain protein, whereas secondary (AA) amyloid protein is a non-light chain protein. Twenty-five to fifty percent of individuals with amyloid develop renal insufficiency (58). The few series documenting experience with transplantation in patients with amyloid generally include a mixture of both types, the majority being of the AA variety. Many, but not all, reports suggest a low rejection rate but a high early mortality rate in these recipients, resulting in somewhat inferior short-term results (58–65). However, if graft losses associated with patient death are excluded, graft survival is equivalent to that in other diseases. Pathologic recurrence of amyloid has been shown to be as high as 40%, but loss of transplant function secondary to recurrent disease is uncommon. Interestingly, significant gastrointestinal intolerance of cyclosporine has been described in some reports (66). Although most investigators advise screening potential recipients for amyloid involvement of other organs, especially the heart, no guidelines are offered to indicate what degree of involvement should exclude the candidate. Given reasonable cardiac and liver function, these candidates should be accepted. In consideration of the known early mortality and low rejection rate, overimmunosuppression should be avoided. If tolerated, colchicine 1.5 g/day should be added to the posttransplant

regimen, since a few series suggest that this drug will prevent recurrence of disease (67–68).

Monoclonal gammopathies

This group of illnesses includes multiple myeloma, monoclonal gammopathy of unknown significance, and idiopathic light chain deposition disease. Monoclonal gammopathy of unknown significance very rarely causes renal failure. On the other hand, renal failure is a relatively common complication of both light chain deposition disease and multiple myeloma. Acute renal failure can occur in the setting of severe hypercalcemia or hyperuricemia, volume depletion, pyelonephritis, or nephrotoxins, and is oftentimes reversible. However, the process of light chain deposition in the renal interstitium with resulting inflammation and fibrosis leads to progressive, irreversible renal failure in both myeloma and light chain deposition disease (69). The experience with transplantation in either of these illnesses is quite limited. Recent isolated case reports of renal transplantation for idiopathic light chain deposition disease have yielded varying results. In one, there was no recurrence up to 44 months (70), while in another, there was recurrence with loss of the allograft after $2 \frac{1}{2}$ years (71). Previous case reports attest to a high rate of recurrence, 6 of 9 individual cases and 3 of 4 in a small series (72–80). The mortality in one series of nine patients was about 50% at 9 years. While renal failure secondary to myeloma is a common occurrence, the transplantation experience is small secondary to accelerated mortality and an understandable reluctance to transplant an individual with a known malignancy (58,81,82). The clinical course of multiple myeloma varies from a rapidly fatal one to a relatively prolonged smoldering course, and there is no evidence that immunosuppression accelerates the course of this illness.

There are no established criteria for transplantation of patients with either multiple myeloma or light chain deposition disease. For multiple myeloma, important prognostic factors in determining long-term survival are relative rapidity of disease progression and the response to chemotherapy. In the author's opinion, it is reasonable to consider a patient with multiple myeloma for renal transplantation if, after remission, the course on dialysis for 1 year has been stable without evidence of recurrent disease. On the other hand, patients with light chain deposition disease are generally not treated as for multiple myeloma and therefore continue to excrete light chains of proven nephrotoxicity. Due to our limited understanding of the mechanism of light chain toxicity and our limited ability to ameliorate the toxicity, our ability to prevent recurrence of disease is also limited. Again, the rapidity of the development of renal failure may have some prognostic significance in predicting rapidity of recurrence. Anecdotal reports suggest that maintenance of a large urine volume, alkalinization of the urine, and even plasmapheresis can be considered for patients with either idiopathic light chain deposition disease or multiple myeloma who demonstrate persistent or recurrent light chain proteinuria.

CONNECTIVE TISSUE DISEASES

Systemic lupus erythematosus

Renal failure remains a major cause of morbidity and mortality in patients with systemic lupus erythematosus (SLE). Of the many ways that SLE can affect the kidney, membranous nephropathy, chronic sclerosing glomerulonephritis, and diffuse proliferative glomerulonephritis are the pathologic lesions most likely to lead to renal failure. Generally, patients with renal lupus suffer multiple extrarenal manifestations as well; however, once they reach end-stage renal disease, most of the clinical and serologic manifestations of the disease disappear (83).

Initial predictions that this disease would invariably recur in transplanted kidneys, with resulting destruction of the allograft, have not been realized. There are reported cases of recurrence, clinically and pathologically; however, they are uncommon (84,85). In 12 documented case reports, recurrent lupus has occurred in patients who were transplanted. Some of these patients were transplanted while they were serologically active, and some developed hypocomplementemia after transplant. However, as a screen, lupus serology and complement level are not always useful to predict who will or will not experience a recurrence. The major cause of allograft failure is chronic rejection. Several recently reported series attest to the success of renal transplantation in this population (86–95). Goss et al. (86) demonstrated excellent patient and graft survival of 92.8% and 62.5%, respectively, at 43.7 months mean follow-up. Another series reported by the Dutch Working Party on Systemic Lupus Erythematosus showed 1- and 5-year patient survival of 87% and graft survival of 68% and 54%, respectively (88). Rivera (90) and Cheigh (91) also reported results in their lupus transplant recipients that were comparable to nonlupus patients. On the other hand, Nyberg et al. (89) did not report as favorable an experience; however, they noted that patients treated with cyclosporine fared much better than those treated with azathioprine. Interestingly, despite the immunologic nature of this disease, few investigators have reported a higher incidence of acute rejection in these patients.

The following recommendations can be made concerning transplantation of individuals with systemic lupus erythematosus. It is probably advisable to transplant these patients during clinical and serologic inactivity. In particular, the serum complement level appears to have some predictive value. However, this recommendation is tempered by the knowledge that the ability of lupus serology to predict recurrence is unproven. A waiting period of a year on dialysis is also advisable for two reasons. First, the clinical activity of the disease can be monitored and allowed to abate. Second, some patients who develop renal failure

requiring dialysis regain enough kidney function to come off dialysis. This phenomenon occurs more frequently in patients who have experienced an explosive course culminating in renal failure. Thus, the waiting time on dialysis would ensure that the patient truly has end-stage renal disease. Because these patients come to transplantation with a background of immunosuppression, they may demonstrate manifestations of long-term side effects of steroids and/or cytotoxic agents. These patients should be given cyclosporine and should be considered for steroid-sparing regimens. Follow-up of these patients should not differ significantly from other patients. There is no evidence that routine monitoring of lupus serology is helpful. These patients tend to suffer from aseptic necrosis and pancreatitis with a higher frequency than nonlupus patients (96).

Antiphospholipid syndrome

First described by Conley and Hartman (97), the antiphospholipid syndrome (APS) is increasingly recognized as a cause of renal failure. The syndrome may present alone, in which case the major renal finding is that of a thrombotic microangiopathy (98,99), or in conjunction with an autoimmune syndrome, most commonly SLE. When nephropathy complicates lupus-associated APS, the renal pathology generally is similar to that seen with SLE alone (100). Both primary and secondary APS, are characterized by recurrent thromboses, hemorrhage, thrombocytopenia, recurrent spontaneous abortions, and neuropsychiatric disorders. The experience in transplantation of these individuals has only very recently been described. Radhakrishnan and colleagues reported eight cases of transplantation in individuals with SLE and positive anti-cardiolipin antibodies (101). Compared to SLE patients without antibodies, the APS patients did not differ in age, sex, duration of disease, number of rejections, or renal function after 1 year. On the other hand, the APS patients had a greater number of thrombotic events, including thrombotic microangiopathy on a graft biopsy, systemic embolization from valvular heart disease, and pulmonary embolus. Pretransplant thrombotic events were predictive of posttransplant events. Other reports attest to the high incidence of thrombotic or hemorrhagic events after transplantation, as well as the high incidence of graft dysfunction secondary to microangiopathy, presumably recurrent disease (102–104). In one case, severe thrombocytopenia with central nervous system thrombosis responded to intravenous immunoglobulin (105).

The following recommendations can be made concerning renal transplantation in patients with primary APS or APS complicating SLE. All patients with a history of recurrent thrombotic events and patients with SLE should be screened for APS. Transplantation during clinical remission is also recommended. Because many of these patients consistently demonstrate antibody even in the absence of clinical disease, serologic remission is not necessary. However, serial measurement of titers of antibody in individual patients may allow the transplant team to monitor disease activity and anticipate clinical relapse. For patients with known thrombotic events, anticoagulation with heparin followed by coumadin at the time of transplantation may be advisable; however, no studies have been performed to support this approach. For acute clinical flares, treatment with immunoglobulin may be helpful.

Vasculitides

Vasculitides, inflammatory diseases of the arterial tree, are an uncommon but well-recognized cause of renal failure. Recent advances in early diagnosis and therapy have uncovered significant differences in the clinical manifestations and response to treatment. The discovery of antineutrophil cytoplasmic antibodies (ANCAs) has resulted in the ability to diagnose some of these diseases on the basis of the clinical picture without invasive procedures to obtain tissue, has allowed better classification of these diseases, and has offered a noninvasive method for following some of these patients. Like SLE, vasculitides are felt to have an autoimmune pathogenetic basis. Unlike lupus, where disease recurrence in the transplanted kidney is uncommon and a rare cause of graft loss, these diseases recur in the transplanted kidney with a predictably high incidence and may cause loss of the allograft.

WEGENER'S GRANULOMATOSIS

Antineutrophil cytoplasmic antibodies have proven to be of perhaps the most usefulness in the diagnosis and clinical monitoring of Wegener's granulomatosis, a particular form of vasculitis (106,107). Classically, the disease involves the upper and lower airways with a granulomatous necrotizing arteritis of the medium- to small-sized arterioles and a segmental nectrotizing glomerulonephritis. Refinement of aggressive therapeutic modalities has converted this disease from one with a uniformly fatal prognosis to one where prolonged survival is the rule. Over 90% of the patients achieve at least a partial remission with therapy. Nonetheless, 10-year mortality is still in the range of 20% (108).

Renal manifestations occur in up to 80% of cases with renal failure, complicating about 10% overall. Numerous case reports of transplantation for Wegener's granulomatosis can be found in the literature. Initial reports, where azathioprine and prednisone alone were used, demonstrated a high rate of recurrence, leading to graft loss in many cases (109,110). Interestingly, the use of cyclosporine has not made a significant difference in the rate of recurrence, but the addition of cyclophosphamide to the regimen has been shown to induce remissions in recurrent cases (111,112).

From the case reports and the few series available (113,114), the following recommendations can be made concerning transplantation of patients with Wegener's granulomatosis. Clinical disease quiescence is mandatory.

However, serologic manifestations do not disappear in all patients, and many patients with positive ANCA titers have been transplanted without experiencing immediate disease activation in the transplanted kidney. Because patients who have undergone transplantation after years on dialysis have experienced recurrence of disease, no firm and fast recommendations can be made concerning a waiting period. Current recommendations for treatment of the disease suggest a 2-year period of treatment with cyclophes-pherncide to ensure remission. Whether or not to monitor ANCA levels is controversial. Because in some patients disease activity correlates to ANCA titer, because an increase in ANCA titer has been demonstrated to presage disease recurrence, and because treatment of a rising ANCA titer has been shown to decrease recurrence rate, the author recommends periodic ANCA measurement in patients in whom disease activity and ANCA titer have previously correlated (107). Moreover, due to the demonstrated efficacy of cyclophosphamide in this disease, the author recommends addition of cyclophosphamide to the long-term immunosuppressive regimen. In programs that use triple immunosuppression, cyclophosphamide can replace azathioprine. Whether cyclophosphamide should be added to cyclosporine or replace it in dual therapy immunosuppression has not been tested; however, our recommendation would be to add cyclophosphamide. Another acceptable option would be to maintain usual cyclosporine immunosuppression, to monitor ANCA levels, and to add cyclophosphamide for evidence of disease recurrence. Because the rate of disease recurrence is so high (up to 50%), clinical and/or serologic monitoring for disease recurrence is critical in these patients.

HENOCH–SCHÖNLEIN PURPURA

Hecnoch–Schönlein disease, a small vessel vasculitis, is characterized by necrotizing glomerulonephritis, purpura, arthritis, and gastrointestinal vasculitis (melena, abdominal pain). The disease tends to occur more frequently in children than adults, but more frequently leads to renal failure in adults (115). In this disorder, the ANCA is not as helpful for diagnostic or therapeutic purposes. Thus, the diagnosis is generally made on clinical grounds with the demonstration of the mesangial IgA deposition in the face of typical clinical findings. The literature documents 74 transplants in 67 patients with the disease, spanning nearly 30 years of renal transplantation. Thus, these patients have been treated with a multitude of immunosuppressive regimens. A recent report on a series of 14 transplants in 10 patients, with a review of the subject, documented an incidence of clinical recurrence of disease in up to one third of patients, with loss of the allograft attributable to recurrent disease in 10% (116). The authors noted that recurrences occurred despite transplantation after prolonged clinical quiescence and despite aggressive triple drug immunosuppression. Recurrences leading to graft failure were associated with a rapid initial course of disease and were more likely to occur in adults. Thus, the author recommends that transplantation is best suited to individuals with a relatively indolent course of their disease. No recommendations can be made concerning length of time on dialysis prior to transplantation or alterations in immunosuppressive regimen.

OTHER VASCULITIDES

Transplantation for renal failure secondary to polyarteritis nodosa is scarcely reported. Of eight reported patients in 1980 (117), four had functioning transplants 1–4 years after transplantation without evidence of disease recurrence, as demonstrated on renal biopsy. Since these data predate the use of cyclosporine, it is not possible to make any predictions concerning the success of this modality with the use of cyclosporine. No contraindications to transplantation short of active clinical disease are apparent.

Transplantation for renal failure secondary to Goodpasture's syndrome is equally scarce. Similar to Wegener's granulomatosis and Henoch–Schonlein purpura, recurrent disease appears to be relatively common, even years after transplantation and even when the transplantation occurs during a period of clinical quiescence (118–120). Patient and graft survival have been reportedly inferior for patients with Goodpasture's syndrome compared to patients with idiopathic nephrotic syndrome or IgA nephropathy, two diseases with excellent survival statistics (121). Most investigators recommend transplantation during clinical and serologic quiescence. Successful transplantation has occurred in the face of a positive antiglomerular basement membrane antibody titer. However, most reports of recurrent nephritis have occurred in individuals who were transplanted with persistently positive serology. Whether serial monitoring of the anti-GBM titer is advisable is not known. However, due to the incidence of late recurrence, unexplained renal dysfunction should prompt a search for disease activity.

INHERITED DISORDERS

Polycystic kidney disease

The recent discovery of the gene locus for the mutation responsible for polycystic kidney disease (PKD) will undoubtedly revolutionize the ability to diagnose and treat this common renal disease (122). For the present, however, PKD continues to be responsible for renal failure in up to 5% of those entering end-stage renal disease programs (123). Besides control of hypertension, no therapies have made a substantial difference in the relentless progression toward renal failure for afflicted individuals. These patients usually reach end-stage renal disease in their late 30s to 50s. Despite a wide array of extrarenal manifestations, patients with end-stage renal disease secondary to PKD come to renal replacement therapy with few medical problems other than hypertension.

Early series demonstrated that patients with PKD who underwent renal transplantation enjoyed a high success rate. The recent experience with transplantation in the cyclosporine era continues to document the success of this technique in these individuals (124–129). Three large, recently published series show 1- and 5-year patient survival rates of 93%–95% and 81%–90%, respectively (127–129). One- and five-year graft survival rates are 83% and around 70%, respectively. These results compare very favorably with the results in patients with primary glomerulopathies. Florijn and coworkers have suggested that these individuals suffer a higher rate of cardiovascular morbidity and mortality with long-term follow-up; however, while quite obvious for azathioprine-treated individuals, this trend was not as apparent in cyclosporine-treated patients (130). In general, PKD patients tend to be older, and cardiovascular abnormalities have been well described in these patients. Nonetheless, the results of renal transplantation in patients with PKD speak for themselves, and the authors recommend renal transplantation.

Evaluation of PKD transplant candidates should center around screening for the renal and extrarenal manifestations of the disease, which may cause future complications. Due to the known cardiac and cardiovascular complications (131), echocardiography and peripheral vascular noninvasive evaluation are suggested. Cerebral aneurysms occur, but only in a small minority (132). Therefore, screening for this potentially lethal complication should be reserved for either those with suggestive symptoms or those with a known family history of cerebral aneurysms. Although diverticuli at an early age have been reported, unless the patient has a history suggestive of lower gastrointestinal bleeding or prior diverticulitis, routine screening is not recommended (133). In general, the other extrarenal manifestations of the disease such as liver cysts are generally clinically unimportant and do not warrant preoperative evaluation. One issue that frequently arises is the question of pretransplant nephrectomy (134,135). Since the procedure has a defined mortality and confers no survival benefit when performed on a routine basis, the authors feel that bilateral nephrectomy should be reserved for specific indications—infection, uncontrollable hypertension, or massive replacement of the abdominal cavity that would preclude transplantation.

The follow-up of these patients should also be tailored toward early diagnosis and prevention of known complications. Due to the high incidence of cardiovascular disease, control of hypertension, hypercholesterolemia, and other modifiable risk factors is an important adjunct therapy. Unexplained abdominal pain or fever should prompt consideration of diverticulitis. If pretransplant valvular heart disease is discovered, endocarditis precautions should be instituted.

As for other renal diseases, graft survival from a living related donor is superior, and with careful screening of potential donors, this option is acceptable. In the future, screening of donors will likely be performed routinely using genetic techniques. For the present, it is recommended that all potential donors undergo evaluation for the presence of hypertension, renal cysts, or inability to achieve maximal urinary concentration. Ultrasound is acceptable for donors over age 30. CT may be required for younger donors.

Alport's syndrome

Alport's syndrome encompasses a group of hereditary diseases characterized by progressive renal failure variably associated with hematuria, sensorineural deafness, retinal, and ocular lens changes (136). Most cases are inherited in an X-linked dominant pattern, but other families demonstrate an autosomal-recessive pattern. The disease is a result of several mutations in the gene that encodes the $\alpha 5$ chain of Type IV collagen, leading to distinctive changes in the glomerular basement membrane (137). The transplantation experience reported during the precyclosporine era documented excellent results in Alport's patients, comparable to other groups of patients. In 1975 the ASC/NIH Renal Transplant Registry reported a 2-year graft survival of 53% and a 2-year patient survival of 71% (138). Milliner et al. reported a nearly 80% 6-year graft survival in 1987 (139). A more recent series reported in 1991, encompassing patients undergoing renal transplantation from 1968 to 1988, confirmed the previous excellent results with respective patient and graft survivals at 5 years of 96% and 75% and at 10 years of 77% and 42% (140). In all these studies, the major cause of graft loss was rejection. In 1987, Milliner reported that three allografts studied pathologically demonstrated linear anti-GBM staining and one kidney also demonstrated 75% crescents, suggesting the development of de novo crescentic glomerulonephritis of the Goodpasture's variety. The recent discovery that the glomerular basement membrane (GBM) of patients with Alport's syndrome lacks the Goodpasture's antigens offers a pathophysiologic basis for these phenomena. It has been postulated that the Goodpasture's antigen present in the transplanted kidney is recognized as a foreign antigen by Alport's patients, leading to the development of an antibody response. Although there are now several published examples of anti-GBM nephritis occurring posttransplantation, the full-blown entity resulting in clinically significant disease is surprisingly rare (141–143). However, the finding of linear immunofluorescence is quite common. Thus, positive anti-GBM immunofluorescence is not necessarily indicative of active disease and does not constitute a rationale for treatment in the absence of clinical findings.

The following recommendations concerning transplantation can be made. Living related and cadaveric renal transplantation are very reasonable options. The graft and patient survival are excellent. No changes need be made in either evaluation of potential recipients or selection of immunosuppressive therapy. Deterioration of kidney function is most likely to be caused by rejection, as for other kidney transplant recipients; however, the possibility of anti-GBM nephritis needs to be kept in mind and investigated if clinically indicated. Screening of potential living related donors at the present time is done on clinical grounds; however, in the future, genetic techniques will likely be used. The evaluation should exclude individuals with microscopic hematuria, proteinuria, sensorineural deafness, or hypertension. In the author's opinion, asymptomatic female carriers should not be chosen, since the long-term effects of nephrectomy in this clinical situation are not known.

Sickle cell disease

Several renal pathologies accompany heterozygous or homozygous hemoglobin S disease, though the renal and the extrarenal manifestations are predictably more severe in the homozygous state (144). End-stage renal disease complicates only about 4% of the total affected population; however, the prognosis for these individuals is dismal, with a reported survival of 4 years on dialysis (145). The high mortality in these patients is a result of progressive extrarenal organ dysfunction, such as liver failure and cardiomyopathy. Efforts to ameliorate the anemia with high-dose erythropoietin have failed, necessitating frequent transfusions (146,147).

The clinical experience with renal transplantation for sickle cell nephropathy is scattered and contradictory. In one of the few published series, Chatterjee reported in 1987 a 1-year graft survival of 82% for living related transplants and 62% for cadaveric renal transplants (148). These results were reasonably comparable to non-sickle-cell patients; however, they were somewhat offset by a relatively high 1-year mortality of 12%. A more recent, smaller series from Johns Hopkins University (149) and several case reports present both dramatic successes and spectacular failures in transplanting these individuals (150–152). Several problems unique to the sickle cell patient emerge from a review of this literature. The frequency of painful sickle cell crises and even multiorgan failure crises increases after successful renal transplantation, necessitating repeated transfusions. Rejection episodes can be complicated by the development of intrarenal sickling, thus exacerbating renal dysfunction and complicating therapy. Moreover, OKT3 has been implicated in triggering painful crises, presumably secondary to cytokine release. Recurrent disease as manifested by hyposthenuria and frank sickle cell nephropathy have been reported.

The author recommends consideration of renal transplantation for patients suffering from sickle cell disease, recognizing the paucity of data. Evaluation of potential recipients should exclude individuals with advanced liver or cardiac disease. Some investigators recommend against living related donation; however, living related transplantation has been successfully accomplished and in the opinion of the author should not be summarily dismissed as an option (153). Living related donation has the potential of presenting the recipient with a transplant having little ischemic damage and a close immunologic match, thus minimizing the chances of initial transplant dysfunction and later rejection. Moreover, the recipient condition can be optimized as well. Should a living related donor not be available, cadaveric donation is also acceptable; however, in the opinion of the author, the use of kidneys with a long ischemic time should be avoided. Due to the reported occurrence of painful crises, the author recommends pretransplant transfusion to a greater than 50% hemoglobin A. These patients should maintain a well-hydrated and well-oxygenated state with supplemental fluid and supplemental oxygen. Some authors have recommended the early use of low-dose dopamine as well to maintain excellent renal perfusion. OKT3 should be avoided. For long-term immunosuppression, hydroxyurea may be substituted for azathioprine to enhance production of hemoglobin F and to reduce the occurrence of painful crises and transfusion requirements.

Primary hyperoxaluria

The deficiency of the hepatic peroxisomal enzyme alanine:glyoxylate aminotransferase (AGT) results in excessive accumulation of oxalate in multiple organ systems (154). Deposition in the kidney leads to renal failure. Treatment of individuals with end-stage renal disease secondary to primary hyperoxaluria has been an exercise in frustration. Those patients who remain on hemodialysis suffer continued deposition of oxalate, leading to arthropathy, peripheral neuropathy, retinopathy, osteodystrophy, vasculopathy, and cardiomyopathy (155). Renal transplantation performed using conventional techniques has generally resulted in rapid failure of the organ, presumably secondary to accelerated deposition of oxalate in the transplanted kidney (156). The success or failure of the allograft does not seem to correlate with residual AGT activity as demonstrated by liver biopsy (157). A prolonged period on dialysis prior to dialysis, however, may be a poor prognostic factor.

In response to these dismal results, three strategies have evolved to deal with the unique challenges of this disease—renal transplantation with aggressive recipient conditioning, combined liver and kidney transplantation, and isolated liver transplantation prior to the development of renal failure. Scheinman et al. published a series of 11 patients who had undergone an aggressive conditioning protocol prior to transplantation (158). Ten of the transplants were from living related donors, one factor that may have influenced their results. The conditioning protocol consisted of aggressive pretransplant dialysis to reduce the oxalate load, high-dose pyridoxine, neutral phosphate magnesium, and aggressive posttransplant diuresis. Of eight patients who received a transplant within a year of the onset of end-stage renal disease, seven had functioning transplants after a mean of 31 months of follow-up. The two patients who received transplants after 3 years or more

on dialysis lost their transplants, as did the recipient of the cadaveric transplant. Long-term follow-up of these patients has demonstrated that even in the face of reasonable initial kidney function, continued oxalate deposition results in progressive cardiomyopathy, vasculopathy, and bone disease. Moreover, 3-year graft survival in one large series was only about 20%. More recently, several groups have performed combined kidney and liver transplantation in order to replace the failed organ and to prevent recurrence of disease by providing a source for AGT. While theoretically appealing, the results have been mixed (159–173). Case reports have shown that successful double transplant results in regression of bone disease and cardiomyopathy and prevention of disease recurrence. On the other hand, the procedure is associated with substantial morbidity and mortality. Watts et al., reporting on nine patients who underwent combined transplantation, had only four long-term survivors (166). Recommendations from a workshop on combined liver–kidney transplantation were recently published in *Nephrology, Dialysis and Transplantation*. Drawing on results of 22 combined transplants, the participants found that 1-year graft survival was better in combined transplants and that prolonged dialysis period prior to transplantation was associated with extensive systemic deposition of oxalate. The oxalate burden resulted in prolonged hyperoxaluria, potentially damaging the kidney. The authors recommended that the diagnosis of primary hyperoxaluria be confirmed by liver biopsy and planned at a GFR of 25 mL/min. In a few rare instances, preemptive liver transplantation has been performed. Clearly, the diagnosis has to be confirmed by measurement of AGT activity, and the transplant needs to be performed at a GFR of 60 mL/min or greater.

There is no consensus on the best form of transplantation for end-stage renal disease secondary to primary hyperoxaluria. The most conservative approach is simple renal transplantation. In the opinion of the authors, this approach is quite acceptable, especially if a living related donor is available. The transplant should be planned before dialysis is necessary to minimize the oxalate burden. The recipient should receive high-dose pyridoxine (500 mg/ 1.73 m^2/day, neutral phosphate (2 g elemental phosphate/ 1.73 m^2/day), magnesium (5–10 mEq/1.73 m^2/day), and aggressive pretransplant dialysis. After transplantation, forced diuresis with a noncalciuric diuretic such as a thiazide should be maintained to allow excretion of the oxalate load. If renal transplantation fails or if extrarenal disease is present, then combined organ transplantation should be contemplated. The role of preemptive liver transplantation is still undefined.

Hereditary cystinosis

Nephropathic cystinosis, an autosomal-dominant disorder, is a lysosomal storage disease characterized by lysosomal accumulation of cystine and development of renal failure in early childhood (174). Children affected with this disorder also suffer from extrarenal organ involvement, including myopathy, mental retardation, hypothyroidism, and visual impairment. A recently published report from the National Institutes of Health demonstrates that aggressive early cystine depletion therapy with cysteamine is effective in preventing renal failure (175). Less than adequate treatment, defined as treatment beginning beyond the age of 2 years, resulted in postponement but not prevention of end-stage renal disease. This finding raises the possibility that routine early diagnosis and intervention may abolish nephropathic cystinosis as a cause of end-stage renal disease.

Despite the rarity of the disorder, several series have been published documenting the immediate and long-term results of transplantation (176–178). In both the azathioprine and cyclosporine eras, patient and graft survival are comparable to that of noncystinosis patients. Superior catch-up growth, however, is seen in cyclosporine-treated patients (178). Biopsies of transplanted kidneys have documented the presence of cystine crystals in cells that are infiltrating the graft. However, recurrent cystinosis leading to graft failure has not been reported. Transplantation of the kidney alone does not supply enough of the deficient enzyme to prevent other systemic complications of the disease, since long-term follow-up of transplanted patients reveal persistence of extrarenal organ involvement (179–182). Visual impairment is seen in about 25%. Thyroid replacement is required in almost all recipients. When looked for, myopathy has been documented in up to 25% of patients. Hormonal evaluation of male patients has revealed a picture of hypergonadotropic hypogonadism with permanently retarded sexual development.

The very respectable results documented over the last 25–30 years support a strong recommendation for renal transplantation in end-stage renal disease secondary to nephropathic cystinosis. The recipients should be treated with cyclosporine to enhance growth and development. Otherwise, no specific recommendations for immunosuppressive therapy are warranted. With the success of cysteamine in preventing end-stage renal disease, the authors recommend cysteamine supplementation (50–60 mg/kg/day in four divided doses) after transplantation of these individuals in the hope that the extrarenal manifestations may be ameliorated. Living related transplantation is encouraged. Donation from an asymptomatic carrier is acceptable (176).

Fabry's disease

Fabry's disease, angiokeratoma corporis diffusum, is an X-linked recessive disorder of α-galactosidase deficiency. This uncommon cause of end-stage renal disease is characterized by the widespread systemic deposition of ceramide trihexoside, resulting in the clinical picture of burning paresthesias, anhidrosis, erythematous skin lesions, and renal failure in the third to fourth decade of life (183). The

published transplantation experience for this disorder is meager. Initial case reports by Philippart (184) and Desnick (185) documented the presence of detectable levels of the missing enzyme in the serum of the recipients, raising the hope that the transplanted kidney would provide sufficient enzyme to prevent recurrence in the allograft and ameliorate progressive injury. These hopes were dashed by later reports of death secondary to progressive cardiac involvement and by small series that demonstrated inferior patient survival at 1 and 5 years of 57% and 26%, respectively, compared to 92% and 78% in a control group (186–188). Moreover, surviving patients suffered early cardiovascular, infectious, and intestinal complications. In light of these findings, the author offers the following recommendations. Renal transplantation is feasible but may be associated with a slightly higher mortality. Pathologic but not clinical recurrence of disease in the allograft has been documented (189). Progression of extrarenal disease is expected, but the degree of disability produced is highly variable. These patients should be screened for significant extrarenal disease and transplantation should be discouraged, particularly if significant cardiac involvement is found (190). Potential living donors should be screened for carrier status. Symptomatic males can be excluded outright from consideration. Asymptomatic males and females can be screened by measurement of serum α-galactosidase activity. Affected males and heterozygous females should be excluded as donors.

Miscellaneous

Transplantation has been carried out in a small number of other inherited diseases, and these are listed here for interest. Mesangial proliferative glomerulonephritis with a predominant IgA deposition is seen in 64% and 94% of renal biopsies performed in Navajo and Zuni Indians, respectively, suggesting a genetic predisposition in these populations. The few reports of transplantation suggest acceptable results for both living related and cadaveric grafts. Recurrence pathologically but not clinically has been reported (191). Due to the occurrence of occult disease in asymptomatic individuals, potential donors may require biopsy before clearance.

The results of serial renal biopsies in a renal transplant recipient who had lecithin cholesterol acyltransferase deficiency were recently reported (192). No evidence of disease was seen at 1 month posttransplant. Pathologic findings of advanced disease were described for a biopsy performed 3.5 years later; however, the patient had a serum creatinine of 2.0 mg/dL.

Concerns about infectious and oncologic sequelae of immunosuppression notwithstanding, a patient with Wiskott–Aldrich syndrome who underwent successful renal transplantation was also recently described (193). The immunosuppressive protocol was adjusted to avoid antilymphocyte preparations and to reduce the total chronic immunosuppressive burden.

Finally, renal transplantation has also recently been described in a patient with Liddle's syndrome (pseudoaldosteronism) complicated by renal failure (194). The characteristic hypokalemia seen with this disease, caused by mutations in the beta subunit of the epithelial sodium channel, disappeared following transplantation, as would be expected from the pathogenesis of the disease.

REFERENCES

1. Ekberg H, Persson NH, Kallen R, Persson MO: Reduced patient survival in diabetic recipients of renal transplants. *Transplant Proc* 26:1759–1760, 1994.
2. Cheigh JS, Riggio RR, Stenzel KH, Green R, Tapia L, Schechter N, Suthamthiran M, Stubenbord WT, Rubin AL, Riehle RA: Kidney transplantation in insulin dependent diabetic patients: improved survival rehabilitation. *Transplant Proc* 21:2016–2017, 1989.
3. Lewis RM, Janney RP, Golden DL, Kerr ND, Van Buren CT, Kerman RH, Kahan BD: Stability of renal allograft function associated with long-term cyclosporine immunosuppressive therapy—five year follow-up. *Transplantation* 47:266–272, 1989.
4. Matas AJ, Gillingham KJ, Sutherland DER: Half-life and risk factors for kidney transplant outcome—importance of death with function. *Transplantation* 55:757–761, 1993.
5. Hirschl MM, Heinz G, Sunder-Plassman G, Derfler K: Renal replacement therapy in Type 2 diabetic patients: 10 years' experience. *Am J Kidney Dis* 20:564–568, 1992.
6. Thorogood J, van Houwelingen JC, van Rood JJ, Zantvoort FA, Schreuder GM, Persijn GG: Factors contributing to long-term kidney graft survival in Eurotransplant. *Transplantation* 54:152–158, 1992.
7. McMillan MA, Briggs JD, Junor BJ: Outcome of renal replacement treatment in patients with diabetes mellitus. *Br Med J* 301:540–544, 1990.
8. Burke G, Esquenazi V, Charagozloo H, Roth D, Strauss J, Kyriakides S, Milgrom M, Ranjan D, Contreras N, Rosen A: Long-term results of kidney transplantation at the University of Miami. *Clin Transplant* 215–228, 1989.
9. Frohnert PP, Sterioff S: Twenty-five years of renal transplantation at Mayo Clinic. *Clin Transplant* 3:267–274, 1989.
10. Najarian JS, Kaufman DB, Fryd DS, McHugh L, Mauer SM, Ramsay RC, Kennedy WR, Navarro X, Goetz FC, Sutherland DE: Long-term survival following kidney transplantation in 100 type I diabetic patients. *Transplantation* 47:106–113, 1989.
11. Lindholm A, Ohlman S, Alberchtsen D, Tufveson G, Persson H, Persson NH: The impact of acute rejection episodes on long-term graft function and outcome in 1347 primary renal transplants treated by 3 cyclosporine regimens. *Transplantation* 56:307–315, 1993.
12. Rischen Vos J, van der woude FJ, Tegzess AM, Zwinderman AH, Gooszen HC, van den Akker PJ, van Es LA: Increased morbidity and mortality in patients with diabetes mellitus after kidney transplantation as compared with non-diabetic patients. *Nephrol Dial Transplant* 7:433–437, 1992.
13. Yoon YS, Bang BK, Jin DC, Ahn SJ, Yoon JY, Park YH, Koh YB: Factors influencing long-term outcome of living-donor kidney transplantation in the cyclosporine era. *Clin Transplant* 6:257–266, 1992.
14. Reissell E, Lindgren L, Tikkanen I, Ahonen J: Renal transplantations from the same kidney donor: outcome of diabetic and nondiabetic patients. *Scand J Urol Nephrol* 26:403–408, 1992.
15. Laskow DA, Diethelm AG, Hudson SL, Deierhoi MH, Barber WH, Barger BO, Gaston RS, Julian BA, Curtis JJ: Analysis of 22 years experience in living-related transplantation at the University of Alabama in Birmingham. *Clin Transplant* 5:179–191, 1991.
16. Manivel C, Kyriakides P, Payne WD, Dunn DL: Renal transplant function after ten years of cyclosporine. *Transplantation* 53:316–323, 1992.
17. Hirschl MM, Derfler K, Heinz G, Sunder-Plassmann G, Waldhausl W: Long-term follow-up of renal transplantation in type 1 and type 2 diabetic patients. *Clin Invest* 70:917–921, 1992.
18. Hirschl MM, Heinz G, Sunder-Plassmann G, Derfler K: Renal replacement therapy in type 2 diabetic patients: 10 years' experience. *Am J Kidney Dis* 20:564–548, 1992.
19. Grenfell A, Bewick M, Snowden S, Watkins PJ, Parsons V: Renal replacement for diabetic patients: experience at King's College Hospital 1980–1989. *Q J Med* 85:861–874, 1992.
20. Lemmers MJ, Barry JM: Major role for arterial disease in morbidity and mortality after kidney transplantation in diabetic recipients. *Diabetes Care* 14:295–301, 1991.
21. Weinrauch LA, D'Elia JA, Monaco AP, Gleason RE, Welty F, Nishan PC, Nesto RW: Preoperative evaluation for diabetic renal transplantation: impact of clinical, laboratory, and echocardiographic parameters on patient and allograft survival. *Am J Med* 93:19–28, 1992.
22. Manske CL, Thomas W, Wang Y, Wilson RF: Screening diabetic transplant candidates for coronary artery disease: identification of a low risk subgroup. *Kidney Int* 44:617–621, 1993.
23. Trochu JN, Cantarovich D, Renaudeau J, Patra O, du Roscoat P, Helias J: Assessment of coronary artery disease by thallium scan in type 1 diabetic uremic patients awaiting combined pancrease and renal transplantation. *Angiology* 42:302–307, 1991.
24. Cottier D, Pfisterer M, Muller-Brand J, Thiel G, Burkart F: Cardiac evaluation of candidates for kidney transplantation: value of exercise radionuclide angiocardiography. *Eur Heart J* 11:832–838, 1990.
25. Camp AD, Garvin PJ, Hoff J, Marsh J, Byers SI, Chaitman RR: Prognostic value of intravenous dipyridamole thallium imaging in patients with diabetes mellitus considered for renal transplantation. *Am J Cardiol* 65:1459–1633, 1990.
26. Brown KA, Rimmer J, Haisch C: Noninvasive cardiac risk stratification of diabetic and nondiabetic uremic renal allograft candidates using dipyridamole-thallium-201 imaging and radionuclide ventriculography. *Am J Cardiol* 64:1017–1021, 1989.
27. Morrow CE, Schwartz JS, Sutherland DER, Simmons RL, Ferguson RM, Kjellstrand CM, Najarian JS: Predictive value of thallium stress testing for coronary and cardiovascular events in uremic diabetic patients before renal transplantation. *Am J Surg* 146:3331–3335, 1983.
28. Philipson JD, Carpenter BJ, Itzkoff J, Hakala TR, Rosenthal JT, Taylor RJ, Puschett JB: Evaluation of cardiovascular risk for renal transplantation in diabetic patients. *Am J Med* 81:630–634, 1986.
29. Manske CL, Wang Y, Rector T, Wilson RF, White CW:

Coronary revascularization in insulin-dependent diabetic patients with chronic renal failure. *Lancet* 340:998–1002, 1992.

30. Gill IS, Hayes JM, Hodge EE, Novick AC: Clean intermittent catheterization and urinary diversion in the management of renal transplant recipients with lower urinary tract dysfunction. *J Urol* 148:1397–1400, 1992.

31. Friedman EA, Cohen C, Lowder G, Laungani GB, Butt KMH: Cystopathy does not preclude successful kidney transplantation in diabetics. *Kidney Int* 29:429, 1986.

32. Munda R, Schroeder TJ, Pedersen SA, Clardy CW, Wadhwa NK, Myre SA, Stephens GW, Pesce AJ, Alexander JW, First MR: Cyclosporine pharmacokinetics in pancreas transplant recipients. *Transplant Proc* 20:487–490, 1988.

33. Thomas AN, Pollard BJ: Renal transplantation and diabetic autonomic neuropathy. *Can J Anaesth* 36:590–592, 1989.

34. Reissell E, Yli Hankala A, Orko R, Lindgren L: Sudden cardiorespiratory arrest after renal transplantation in a patient with diabetic autonomic neuropathy and prolonged QT interval. *Acta Anaesthesiol Scand* 38:406–408, 1994.

35. Gavin LA: Management of diabetes mellitus during surgery. *West J Med* 151:525–529, 1989.

36. Braun WF: Long-term complications of renal transplantation (clinical conference). *Kidney Int* 37:1363–1378, 1990.

37. Pirsch JD, D'Alessandro AM, Sollinger HW, Knechtle SJ, Reed A, Kalayoglu M, Belzer FO: Hyperlipidemia and transplantation: etiologic factors and therapy. *J Am Soc Nephrol* 2:S238–S242, 1992.

38. Ong CS, Pollock CA, Caterson RJ, Mahony JF, Waugh DA, Ibels LS: Hyperlipidemia in renal transplant recipients: natural history and response to treatment. *Medicine (Baltimore)* 73:215–223, 1994.

39. Nisbeth U, Lindh E, Ljunghall S, Backman U, Fellstrom B: Fracture frequency after kidney transplantation. *Transplant Proc* 26:1764, 1994.

40. Hasslacher C, Borgholte G, Ritz E, Wahl P: Impact of hypertension on prognosis in IDDM. *Diabete Metab* 15:338–342, 1989.

41. Vathsala A, Weinberg RS, Schoenberg L, Grevel J, Goldstein RA, Van Buren CT, Lewis RM, Kahan BD: Lipid abnormalities in cyclosporine–prednisone-treated renal transplant recipients. *Transplantation* 48:37–43, 1989.

42. Muller-Felber W, Landgraf R, Scheuer R, Wagner S, Reimers CD, Nusser J, Abendroth D, Illner WD, Land W: Diabetic neuropathy 3 years after successful pancreas and kidney transplantation. *Diabetes* 42:1482–1486, 1993.

43. Julian BA, Quarles LD, Niemann KM: Musculoskeletal complications after renal transplantation: pathogenesis and treatment. *Am J Kidney Dis* 19:99–120, 1992.

44. Sumrani NB, Daskalakis P, Miles AM, Sarkar S, Markell MS, Hong JH, Friedman EA, Sommer BG: Erythrocytosis after renal transplantation. A prospective analysis. *ASAIO J* 39:51–55, 1993.

45. Landgraf R, Nusser J, Muller W, Landgraf-Leurs MM, Thurau S, Ulbig M, Kampik A, Lachenmayr B, Hillebrand G, Schleibner S: Fate of late complications in type I diabetic patients after successful pancrease kidney transplantation. *Diabetes* 38 (Suppl 1):33–37, 1989.

46. Larsen JL, Larson CE, Hirst K, Miller SA, Ozaki CF, Taylor RJ, Stratta RJ: Lipid status after combined pancreas–kidney transplantation and kidney transplantation alone in type I diabetes mellitus. *Transplantation* 54:992–926, 1992.

47. Ekstrand A, Groop L, Pettersson E, Gronhagen-Riska C, Laatikainen L, Matikainen E, Seppalainen AM, Laasonen E,

Summanen P, Ollus A: Metabolic control and progression of complications in insulin-dependent diabetic patients after kidney transplantation. *J Intern Med* 232:253–261, 1992.

48. Laatikainen L, Summanen P, Ekstrand A, Groop L: Ophthalmological follow-up of diabetic patients after kidney transplantation. *Ger J Ophthalmol* 2:24–27, 1993.

49. Mauer SM, Goetz FC, McHugh LE, Sutherland DE, Barbosa J, Najarian JS, Steffes MW: Long-term study of normal kidneys transplanted into patients with type I diabetes. *Diabetes* 38:516–512, 1989.

50. Osterby R, Nyberg G, Hedman L, Karlberg I, Persson H, Svalander C: Kidney transplantation in type 1 (insulin-dependent) diabetic patients. Early glomerulopathy. *Diabetologia* 34:668–674, 1991.

51. Barbosa J, Steffes MW, Sutherland DE, Connett JE, Rao KV, Mauer SM: Effect of glycemic control on early diabetic renal lesions. A 5 year randomized controlled clinical trial of insulin-dependent diabetic kidney transplant recipients. *JAMA* 272:600–606, 1994.

52. Cheung AT, Cox KL, Ahlfors CE, Bry WI: Reversal of microangiopathy in long-term diabetic patients after successful simultaneous pancrease–kidney transplants. *Transplant Proc* 25:1310–1333, 1993.

53. Pi-Sunyer FX: Medical hazards of obesity. *Ann Intern Med* 119:655–660, 1993.

54. Pirsch JD, Armbrust MJ, Knechtle SJ, D'Alesandro AM, Sollinger HW, Heisey DM, Belzer FO: Obesity as a risk factor following renal transplantation. *Transplantation* 59:631–647, 1995.

55. Holley JL, Shapiro R, Lopatin WB, Tzakis AG, Hakala TR, Starzl TE: Obesity as a risk factor following cadaveric renal transplantation. *Transplantation* 49:387–389, 1990.

56. Terasaki PI, Koyama H, Cecka JM, Gjertson DW: The hyperfiltration hypothesis in human renal transplantation. *Transplantation* 57:1450–1454, 1994.

57. Johnson CP, Gallagher-Lepak S, Zhu Y-R, Porth C, Kelber S, Roza AM, Adams MB: Factors influencing weight gain after renal transplantation. *Transplantation* 56:822–827, 1993.

58. Brown JH, Doherty CC: Renal replacement therapy in multiple myeloma and systemic amyloidosis. *Postgrad Med J* 69:672–678, 1993.

59. Kilicturgay S, Haberal M: Transplantation for renal amyloidosis. *Ren Fail* 15:629–633, 1993.

60. Isoniemi H, Eklund B, Hockerstedt K, Salmela K, Ahonen J: Renal transplantation in amyloidosis. *Transplant Proc* 21:2039–2040, 1989.

61. Heering P, Kutkuhn B, Frenzel H, Linke RP, Grabensee B: Renal transplantation in amyloid nephropathy. *Int Urol Nephrol* 21:339–347, 1989.

62. Brown JH, Maxwell AP, Bruce T, Murphy RG, Doherty CC: Renal replacement therapy in multiple myeloma and systemic amyloidosis. *Ir J Med Sci* 162:213–217, 1993.

63. Kilicturgay S, Tokyay R, Arslan G, Rilgin N, Haberal M: The results of transplantation of patients with amyloid nephropathy. *Transplant Proc* 24:1788–1789, 1992.

64. Shmueli D, Lustig S, Nakache R, Yussim A, Bar-Nathan N, Shaharahani F, Shapira Z: Renal transplantation in patients with amyloidosis due to familial Mediterranean fever. *Transplant Proc* 24:1783–1784, 1992.

65. Hartmann A, Holdaas H, Fauchald P, Nordal KP, Berg KJ, Talseth T, Leivestad T, Brekke TB, Flatmark A: Fifteen years' experience with renal transplantation in systemic amyloidosis. *Transplant Int* 5:15–18, 1992.

66. Cohen SL, Boner G, Shmueli D, Yusim A, Rosenfeld J, Shapira Z: Cyclosporin: poorly tolerated in familial Mediterranean fever. *Nephrol Dial Transplant* 4:201–204, 1989.

67. Zemer D, Livneh A, Pras M, Schar F: Familial Mediterranean fever in the colchicine era: the fate of one family. *Am J Med Genet* 45:340–344, 1993.

68. Livneh A, Zemer D, Siegal R, Laor A, Sohar F, Pras M: Colchicine prevents kidney transplant amyloidosis in familial Mediterranean fever. *Nephron* 60:418–422, 1992.

69. Johnson WJ, Kyle RA, Pineda AA, O'Brien PC, Holley KE: Treatment of renal failure associated with multiple myeloma. *Arch Intern Med* 150:863–869, 1990.

70. David-Neto E, Ianhez LE, Chocair PR, Saldanha LB, Sabbaga E, Arap S: Renal transplantation in systemic light chain deposition (SLCD): a 44 month follow-up without recurrence. *Transplant Proc* 21:2128–2129, 1989.

71. Alpers CE, Marchioro TL, Johnson RJ: Monoclonal immunoglobulin deposition disease in a renal allograft: probable recurrent disease in a patient without myeloma. *Am J Kidney Dis* 13:418–423, 1989.

72. Cosio FT, Pence TV, Shapiro FL, Kjellstrand: Severe renal failure in multiple myeloma. *Clin Nephrol* 15:206–210, 1981.

73. Walker F, Bear RA: Renal transplantation in light chain multiple myeloma. *Am J Nephrol* 3:34–37, 1983.

74. Gerlag PGG, Koene RAP, Berden JHM: Renal transplantation in light chain nephropathy: case report and review of the literature. *Clin Nephrol* 25:101–104, 1986.

75. Spence RK, Hill GS, Goldwein MI, Grossman RA, Barker CF, Perloff LJ: Renal transplantation for end-stage myeloma kidney. *Arch Surg* 114:950–952, 1979.

76. Humphrey RL, Wright JR, Zachary JB, Sterioff S, DeFronzo RA: Renal transplantation in multiple myeloma. *Ann Intern Med* 83:651–653, 1975.

77. De Lima JJG, Kourilsky O, Meyrier A, Morel-Maroger L, Sraer JD: Kidney transplantation in multiple myeloma. *Transplantation* 31:223–224, 1981.

78. Medical Staff Conference: The kidney in multiple myeloma. *West J Med* 129:41–59, 1978.

79. Briefel GR, Spees EK, Humphrey RL, Hill GS, Saral R, Zachary JB: Renal transplantation in a patient with multiple myeloma and light chain nephropathy. *Surgery* 93:579, 1983.

80. Penn I: Kidney transplantation following treatment of tumors. *Transplant Proc* 18:16–20, 1986.

81. Ingo N, Palmer AB, Severn A, Trafford JA, Mufti GH, Taube D, Parsons V: Chronic dialysis in patients with multiple myeloma and renal failure: a worthwhile treatment. *Q J Med* 73:903–910, 1989.

82. Iggo N, Parsons V: Renal disease in multiple myeloma: current perspectives. *Nephron* 56:229–233, 1990.

83. Coplon NS, Diskin CJ, Petersen J, Swenson RS: The long-term clinical course of systemic lupus erythematosus in end-stage renal disease. *N Engl J Med* 308:186–190, 1983.

84. Ward LA, Jelveh Z, Feinfeld DA: Recurrent membranous lupus nephritis after renal transplantation: a case report and review of the literature. *Am J Kidney Dis* 23:326–329, 1994.

85. Nyberg G, Blohme I, Persson H, Glausson M, Svalandar C: Recurrence of SLE in transplanted kidneys: a follow-up transplant biopsy. *Nephrol Dial Transplant* 7:1116–1123, 1992.

86. Goss JA, Cole BR, Jandrisak MD, McCullough CS, So SK, Windus DW, Hanto DW: Renal transplantation for systemic lupus erythematosus and recurrent lupus nephritis. A single-center experience and a review of the literature. *Transplantation* 52:805–810, 1991.

87. Krishnan G, Tharker I, Angstadt JD, Canelli JP: Multicenter analysis of renal allograft survival in lupus patients. *Transplant Proc* 23:1755–1756, 1991.

88. Nossant HC, Swaak TJ, Berden JH: Systemic lupus erythematosus after renal transplantation: patient and graft survival and disease activity. The Dutch Working Party on Systemic Lupus Erythematosus. *Ann Intern Med* 114:183–188, 1991.

89. Nyberg G, Karlberg I, Svalandar C, Hedman I, Blohme I: Renal transplantation in patients with systemic lupus erythematosus: increased risk of early graft loss. *Scand J Urol Nephrol* 24:307–313, 1990.

90. Rivera M, Marcen R, Pascual J, Naya MT, Orofino I, Ortuno J: Kidney transplantation in systemic lupus erythematosus nephritis: a one-center experience. *Nephron* 56:148–151, 1990.

91. Cheigh JS, Kim H, Stenzel KH, Tapia I, Sullivan JF, Stubenbord W, Riggin RR, Rubin AI: Systemic lupus erythematosus in patients with end-stage renal disease: long-term follow-up on the prognosis of patients and the evolution of lupus activity. *Am J Kidney Dis* 16:189–185, 1990.

92. Bitker MO, Barrou B, Qurhama S, Mouquet C, Chartier-Kastler E, Luciani J, Chatelain C: Renal transplantation in patients with systemic lupus erythematosus. *Transplant Proc* 25:2172–2173, 1993.

93. Cheigh JS, Stenzel KH: End-stage renal disease in systemic lupus erythematosus. *Am J Kidney Dis* 21:2–8, 1993.

94. Bumgardner GL, Mauer SM, Ascher NL, Payne WD, Dunn DL, Fryd DS, Sutherland DE, Simmons RL, Najarian JS: Long-term outcome of renal transplantation in patients with systemic lupus erythematosus. *Transplant Proc* 21:2031–2032, 1989.

95. Sokunhi D, Wadhwa NK, Waltzer WD, Rapaport FT: Renal transplantation in patients with end-stage renal disease secondary to systemic lupus erythematosus. *Transplant Proc* 25:3328–3333, 1993.

96. Padilla R, Pollak VF, Peace A, Kent KS, Gilinsky NH, Daddens JA: Pancreatitis in patients with end-stage renal disease. *Medicine (Baltimore)* 73:8–20, 1994.

97. Conley CL, Hartman RC: A hemorrhagic disorder caused by circulating anticoagulant in patients with disseminated lupus erythematosus. *J Clin Invest* 31:621–622, 1952.

98. Amigo MC, Garcia-Torres R, Robles M, Bochicchio T, Reyes PA: Renal involvement in primary antiphospholipid syndrome. *J Rheumatol* 19:1181–1185, 1992.

99. Farrugia E, Tores VE, Gastineau D, Michet CJ, Holley KE: Lupus anticoagulant in systemic lupus erythematosus: a clinical and renal pathological study. *Am J Kidney Dis* 20:463–471,1992.

100. Hughson MD, Nadasdy T, McCarty GA, Sholer C, Min KW, Silva F: Renal thrombotic microangiopathy in patients with systemic lupus erythematosus and the antiphospholipid syndrome. *Am J Kidney Dis* 20:150–158, 1992.

101. Radhakrishnan J, Williams GS, Appel BG, Cohen DJ: Renal transplantation in anticardiolipin antibody-positive lupus erythematosus patients. *Am J Kidney Dis* 23:286–289, 1994.

102. Sitter T, Spannagl M, Schiffl H: Anticardiolipin antibodies and lupus anticoagulant in patients treated with different methods of renal replacement therapy in comparison to patients with systemic lupus erythematosus. *Ann Hematol* 65:79–82, 1992.

103. Pasquali S, Banfi G, Zucchelli A, Moroni, Ponticelli C, Zucchelli P: Lupus membranous nephropathy: long-term outcome. *Clin Nephrol* 39:175–182, 1993.

104. Marcen R, Pascual J, Quereda C, Pardo A, Mampaso F, Orofino L, Teruel JL, Ortuno J: Lupus anticoagulant and thrombosis of kidney allograft vessels. *Transplant Proc* 22:1396–1398, 1990.

105. Sturfelt G, Mousa F, Jonsson H, Nived O, Thysell H, Wollheim F: Recurrent cerebral infarction and the antiphospholipid syndrome: effect of intravenous gammaglobulin in a patient with systemic lupus erythematosus. *Ann Rheum Dis* 49:939–941, 1990.

106. Kallenberg CGM, Brouwer E, Weening JJ, Tervaert JWC: Anti-neutrophil cytoplasmic antibodies: current diagnostic and pathophysiological potential. *Kidney Int* 46:1–15, 1994.

107. Jennette JC, Falk RJ: Antineutrophil cytoplasmic autoantibodies and associated diseases: a review. *Am J Kidney Dis* 15:517–529, 1990.

108. Hoffman GS, Kerr GS, Leavitt RY, Hallahan CW, Lebovics RS, Travis WD, Rottem M, Fauci AS: Wegener granulomatosus: an analysis of 158 patients. *Ann Intern Med* 116:488–998, 1992.

109. Steinman TI, Jaffe BF, Monaco AP, Wolff SM, Fauci AS: Recurrence of Wegener's granulomatosis after kidney transplantation. Successful reinduction of remission with cyclophosphamide. *Am J Med* 68:458–460, 1980.

110. Curtis JJ, Diethelm AG, Herrera GA, Crowell WT, Whelchel JD: Recurrence of Wegener's granulomatosis in a cadaver renal allograft. *Transplantation* 36:452–454, 1983.

111. Rosenstein ED, Ribot S, Ventresca E, Kramer N: Recurrence of Wegener's granulomatosis following renal transplantation. *Br J Rheumatol* 33:869–871, 1994.

112. Boubenider SA, Akhtar M, Alfurayh O, Algazlan S, Taibah K, Qunibi W: Late recurrence of Wegener's granulomatosis presenting as tracheal stenosis in a renal transplant patient. *Clin Transplant* 8:5–9, 1994.

113. Rich LM, Piering WF: Ureteral stenosis due to recurrent Wegener's granulomatosis after kidney transplantation. *J Am Soc Nephrol* 4:1516–1521, 1994.

114. Kuross S, Davis T, Kjellstrand CM: Wegener's granulomatosis with severe renal failure: clinical course and results of dialysis and transplantation. *Clin Nephrol* 16:172–180, 1981.

115. Weiss JH, Bhathma DB, Curtis JJ, Lucas BA, Luke RG: A possible relationship between Henoch–Schonlein syndrome and IgA nephropathy. *Nephron* 22:582, 1978.

116. Mueldes Q, Pirson Y, Cosyns J-P, Squifflet J-P, van Ypersele de Strihou C: Course of Henoch–Schonlein nephritis after renal transplantation: report on ten patients and review of the literature. *Transplantation* 58:1179–1186, 1994.

117. Montalbert C, Carvallo A, Broumand B, Noble D, Anstine LA, Currier CB: Successful renal transplantation in polyarteritis nodosa. *Clin Nephrol* 14:206–209, 1980.

118. Wilson CB, Dixon FJ: AntiGBM antibody induced glomerulonephritis. *Kidney Int* 3:74–89, 1973.

119. Beleil OM, Coburn JW, Shinaberger JH, Glassrock RJ: Recurrent glomerulonephritis due to anti-glomerular basement membrane antibodies in two successive allografts. *Clin Nephrol* 1:377–380, 1973.

120. Almkuist RD, Buckalew VM, Hirszel P, Maher JF, James PM, Wilson CB: Recurrence of antiglomerular basement membrane antibody mediated glomerulonephritis in an isograft. *Clin Immunol Immunopathol* 18:54, 1981.

121. Lim EC, Terasaki PI: Outcome of kidney transplantation in different diseases. *Clin Transplant* 4:461–469, 1990.

122. Harris PC, Ward CJ, Peral B, Hughes J: Polycystic kidney disease 1: identification and analysis of the primary defect. *J Am Soc Nephrol* 6(4):1125–1133, 1995.

123. Parfrey PS: Hereditary renal diseases. *Curr Opin Nephrol Hypertens* 2:192–200, 1993.

124. Lim EC, Terasaki PI: Outcome of renal transplantation in different primary diseases. *Clin Transplant* 5:293–303, 1991.

125. Delaney V, Sumrani N, Butt KM, Hong JH: The impact of cyclosporin in patients with adult polycystic kidney disease following transplantation. *Nephron* 59:537–542, 1991.

126. Fitzpatrick PM, Torres VE, Charboneau JW, Offord KP, Holley KE, Zincke H: Long-term outcome of renal transplantation in autosomal dominant polycystic kidney disease. *Am J Kidney Dis* 15:536–543, 1990.

127. Jacobs C, Selwood NH: Renal replacement therapy for end-stage renal failure in France: current status and evolutive trends over the last decade. *Am J Kidney Dis* 25:188–195, 1995.

128. Fenton S, Desmeules M, Copleston P, Arbus G, Froment D, Jeffrey J, Kjellstrand C: Renal replacement therapy in Canada: a report from the Canadian Organ Replacement Register. *Am J Kidney Dis* 25:134–150, 1995.

129. Disney APS: Demography and survival of patients receiving treatment for chronic renal failure in Australia and New Zealand: report on dialysis and renal transplantation treatment from the Australia and New Zealand Dialysis and Transplant Registry. *Am J Kidney Dis* 25:165–175, 1995.

130. Florijn KW, Chang PC, van der Woude FJ, van Bockel JH, van Saase JLCM: Long-term cardiovascular morbidity and mortality in autosomal dominant polycystic kidney disease patients after renal transplantation. *Transplantation* 57:73–81, 1994.

131. Timio M, Monarca C, Pede S, Gentili S. Verdura C, Lolli S: The spectrum of cardiovascular abnormalities in autosomal dominant polycystic kidney disease: a 10 year follow-up in a five-generation kindred. *Clin Nephrol* 37:245–250, 1992.

132. Levey AS, Pauker SG, Kassirer JP: Occult intracranial aneurysms in polycystic kidney disease. *N Engl J Med* 308:986–990, 1983.

133. Abramson SJ, Berdon WE, Laffey K, Ruzal-Shapiro C, Nash M, Baer J: Colonic diverticulitis in young patients with chronic renal failure and transplantation. *Pediatr Radiol* 21:352–354, 1991.

134. Rayner BL, Cassidy MJ, Jacobsen JE, Pascoe MD, Pontin AR, van Zyl Smit R: Is preliminary binephrectomy necessary in patients with autosomal dominant polycystic kidney disease undergoing renal transplantation? *Clin Nephrol* 34:122–124, 1990.

135. Warholm C, Rekola S, Roll M: Fatal outcome of bilateral nephrectomy in a patient with polycystic kidney disease. *Scand J Urol Nephrol* 26:201–203, 1992.

136. Kashtan CE, Michael AF: Hereditary nephritis. *Semin Nephrol* 9:135–146, 1989.

137. Knebelmann B, Antignac C, Gubler M-C, Grunfeld J-P: A molecular approach to inherited kidney disorders. *Kidney Int* 44:1205–1216, 1993.

138. Advisory Committee to the Renal Transplant Registry: Renal transplantation in congenital and metabolic diseases—a report from the ASC/NIH Renal Transplant Registry. *JAMA* 232:148–153, 1975.

139. Milliner DS, Pierdes AM, Holley KE: Renal transplantation in Alport's syndrome. Anti-glomerular basement membrane glomerulonephritis in the allograft. *Mayo Clin Proc* 57:35–43, 1987.

140. Peten E, Pirson Y, Cosyns JP, Squifflet JP, Alexandre GP, Noel LH, Grunfeld JP, van Ypersele de Strihou C: Outcome of thirty patients with Alport's syndrome after renal transplantation. *Transplantation* 52:823–826, 1991.

141. Diaz JI, Valenzuela R, Gephardt G, Novick A, Tubbs RR: Anti-glomerular and anti-tubular basement membrane nephritis in a renal allograft recipient with Alport's syndrome. *Arch Pathol Lab Med* 118:728–731, 1994.

142. Berardinelli L, Pozzoli E, Raiteri M, Canal R, Tonello G, Tarantino A, Vegeto A: Renal transplantation in Alport's syndrome. Personal experience in twelve patients. *Contrib Nephrol* 80:131–134, 1990.

143. Goldman M, Depierreux M, De Pauw L, Vereerstraeten P, Kinnaert P, Noel LH, Grunfeld JP, Toussaint C: Failure of two subsequent renal grafts by anti-GBM glomerulonephritis in Alport's syndrome: case report and review of the literature. *Transplant Int* 3:82–85, 1990.

144. Allon M: Renal abnormalities in sickle cell disease. *Arch Intern Med* 150:501–510, 1990.

145. Powars D, Elliott-Mills D, Chan L: Chronic renal failure in sickle cell disease: risk factors, clinical course, and mortality. *Ann Intern Med* 115:614–622, 1991.

146. Tomson CR, Edmunds ME, Chambers K, Bricknell S, Feehally J, Walls J: Effect of recombinant human erythropoietin on erythropoiesis in homozygous sickle cell anemia and renal failure. *Nephrol Dial Transplant* 7:817–821, 1992.

147. Powe NR, Griffiths RI, Greer JW, Watson AJ, Anderson GF, de Lissovoy G, Herbert RJ, Eggers PW, Milam RA, Whelton PK: Early dosing practices and effectiveness of recombinant human erythropoietin. *Kidney Int* 43:1125–1133, 1993.

148. Chatterjee SN: National study in natural history of renal allografts in sickle cell disease or trait: a second report. *Transplant Proc* 19:33–35, 1987.

149. Montgomery R, Zibari G, Hill GS, Ratner LE: Renal transplantation in patients with sickle cell nephropathy. *Transplantation* 58:618–642, 1994.

150. Tomson CR: End stage renal disease in sickle cell disease: future directions. *Postgrad Med J* 68:775–778, 1992.

151. Spector D, Zachary JB, Sterioff S, Millan J: Painful crisis following renal transplantation in sickle cell anemia. *Am J Med* 64:835–839, 1978.

152. Miner DJ, Jorkasky DK, Perloff LJ, Grossman RA, Tomaszewski JE: Recurrent sickle cell nephropathy in a transplanted kidney. *Am J Kidney Dis* 10:306–313, 1987.

153. Brennan DC, Lippmann BJ, Shenoy S, Lowell JA, Howard TK, Flye MW: Living unrelated renal transplantation for sickle cell nephropathy. *Transplantation* 59:794–795, 1995.

154. Williams HE, Smith LH: Primary hyperoxaluria. In: JB Stanbury, JB Wyngaarden, DS Fredrickson, eds, *The Metabolic Basis of Inherited Disease*. McGraw Hill, New York, pp 182–204, 1978.

155. Milliner DS, Eickholt JT, Bergstralh EJ, Wilson DM, Smith LH: Results of long-term treatment with orthophosphate and pyridoxine in patients with primary hyperoxaluria. *N Engl J Med* 331:1553–1558, 1994.

156. Cameron JS: Recurrent disease in renal allografts. *Kidney Int Suppl* 43:S91–S94, 1993.

157. Katz A, Freese D, Danpura CJ, Scheinman JI, Mauer SM: Success of kidney transplantation in oxalosis is unrelated to residual hepatic enzyme activity. *Kidney Int* 42:1408–1411, 1992.

158. Scheinman JI, Namarian JS, Mauer SM: Successful strategies for renal transplantation in primary oxalosis. *Kidney Int* 25:804–811, 1984.

159. Watts RWE, Roles K, Morgan SH: Successful treatment of primary hyperoxaluria type 1 by combined hepatic and renal transplantation. *Lancet* 2:474–475, 1987.

160. Lloveras JJ, Durand D, Dopre C, Rischman P, Fourtanier G, Ton-That H, Suc JM: Combined liver kidney transplantation in primary hyperoxaluria type I. Prevention of the recidive of calcium oxalate deposits in the renal graft. *Clin Nephrol* 38:128–131, 1992.

161. Rodby RA, Tyszka TS, Williams JW: Reversal of cardiac dysfunction secondary to type 1 primary hyperoxaluria after combined liver–kidney transplantation. *Am J Med* 90:498–504, 1991.

162. Toussaint C, De Pauw L, Vienne A, Sevenois PA, Quintin J, Gelin M, Pasteels JL: Radiological and histological improvement of oxalate osteopathy after combined liver–kidney transplantation in praimary hyperoxaluria type 1. *Am J Kidney Dis* 21:54–63, 1993.

163. Scheinman JI: Primary hyperoxaluria: therapeutic strategies for the 90's. *Kidney Int* 40:389–399, 1991.

164. Lloveras JJ, Dupre-Goudable C, Rey JP, Sporer P, Durand D, Ton-That H, Suc JM: The European experience of liver–kidney transplantation for primary hyperoxaluria type I. Prevention of recurrent intrarenal oxalate deposits. *Presse Med* 20:2016–2018, 1991.

165. Watts RW, Danpure CJ, De Pauw L, Toussaint C: Combined liver–kidney and isolated liver transplantations for primary hyperoxaluria type 1: the European experience. The European study Group on Transplantation in Hyperoxaluria Type 1. *Nephrol Dial Transplant* 6:502–511, 1991.

166. Watts RW, Morgan Sh, Danpure CJ, Purkiss P, Calne RY, Rolles K, Baker LR, Mansell MA, Smith LH, Merion RM: Combined hepatic and renal transplantation in primary hyperoxaluria type I. Clinical report of nine cases. *Am J Med* 90:179–188, 1991.

167. Broyer M, Brunner FP, Brynger H, Dykes SR, Ehrich JH, Fassbinder W, Geerlings W, Rizzoni G, Selwood NH, Tufveson G: Kidney transplantation in primary oxalosis: data from the EDTA Registry. *Nephrol Dial Transplant* 5:332–336, 1990.

168. Ruder H, Otto G, Schutgens RB, Querfeld U, Wanders RJ, Herzog KH, Wolfel P, Pomer S, Scharer K, Rose GA: Excessive urinary oxalate excretion after combined renal and hepatic transplantation for correction of hyperoxaluria type 1. *Eur J Pediatr* 150:56–58, 1990.

169. dePauw L, Gelin M, Danpure CJ, Vereerstreeten P, Adler M, Abramowicz D, Toussaint C: Combined liver–kidney transplantation in primary hyperoxaluria type 1. *Transplantation* 50:886–887, 1990.

170. Janssen F, Hall M, Schurmans T, De Pauw L, Hooghe L, Gelin M, Goyens P, Kinnaert P: Combined liver and kidney transplantation in primary hyperoxaluria type 1 in children. *Transplant Proc* 26:110–111, 1994.

171. Shaked A, Thompson M, Wilkinson AH, Nuesse B, el Khoury GF, Rosenthal JT, Danovich GM, Busuttil RW: The role of combined liver/kidney transplantation in end-stage hepato-renal disease. *Am Surg* 59:606–609, 1993.

172. Fauchald P, Flatmark A, Jellum E, Sodal G, Jorstad S: Com-

bined hepatic and renal transplantation in primary hyperoxaluria type 1 (PH1): long-term results. *Transplant Proc* 26:1799–1800, 1994.

173. Cochat P, Scharer K: Should liver transplantation be performed before advanced renal insufficiency in primary hyperoxaluria type 1? *Pediatr Nephrol* 7:326–327, 1993.

174. Theodoropoulos DS, Krasnewich D, Kaiser Kupfer MI, Gahl WA: Classic nephropathic cystinosis as an adult disease. *JAMA* 270:2200–2204, 1993.

175. Markello TC, Bernardini IM, Gahl WA: Improved renal function in children with cystinosis treated with cysteamine. *N Engl J Med* 328:1157–1162, 1993.

176. Almond PS, Matas AJ, Nakleh RE, Morel P, Troppmann C, Najarian JS, Chavers B: Renal transplantation for infantile cystinosis: long-term follow-up. *J Pediatr Surg* 28:232–238, 1993.

177. Ehrich JH, Brodehl J, Byrd DI, Hossfeld S, Hoyer PF, Leipert KP, Offner G, Wolff G: Renal transplantation in 22 children with nephropathic cystinosis. *Pediatr Nephrol* 5:708–714, 1991.

178. Offner G, Hoyer PF, Ehrich JH, Pichlmayr R, Brodehl J: Paediatric aspects of renal transplantation: experience of a single centre. *Eur J Pediatr* 151:S16–S22, 1992.

179. Charnas LR, Luciano CA, Dalakas M, Gilliatt RW, Bernardini I, Ishak K, Cwik VA, Fraker D, Brushart TA, Gahl WA: Distal vacuolar myopathy in nephropathic cystinosis. *Ann Neurol* 35:181–188, 1994.

180. Chik CL, Friedman A, Merriam GR, Gahl WA: Pituitary-testicular function in nephropathic cystinosis. *Ann Intern Med* 119:568–578, 1993.

181. Winkler L, Offner G, Krull F, Brodehl J: Growth and pubertal development in nephropathic cystinosis. *Eur J Pediatr* 152:244–249, 1993.

182. Almond PS, Morel P, Troppmann C, Matas, Najarian JS, Chavers B: Progression of infantile cystinosis after renal transplantation. *Transplant Proc* 23:1386, 1991.

183. Desnick RJ, Sweeley CC: Fabry's disease: galactosidase deficiency. In: JB Stanbury, JB Wyngaarden, DS Fredickson, JL Goldstein, MS Brown, eds, *The Metabolic Basis of Inher-*

ited Disease, 5th ed. McGraw Hill, New York, pp 906–944, 1983.

184. Philippart M: Fabry disease: kidney transplantation on an enzyme replacement therapy. *Birth Defects* 9(2):81–87, 1973.

185. Desnick RJ, Allen KY, Simmons RL, Woods JE, Anderson CF, Najarian JS, Krivit W: Fabry disease: correction of the enzymatic deficiency by renal transplantation. *Birth Defects* 9(2):88–96, 1973.

186. Ramos EL: Recurrent diseases in the renal allograft. *J Am Soc Nephrol* 2:109–121, 1991.

187. Maizel SE, Simmons RL, Kjellstrand C, Fryd DS: Ten year experience in renal transplantation in Fabry's disease. *Transplant Proc* 13:57–59, 1981.

188. Donati D, Novario R, Gastaldi L: Natural history and therapy of uremia secondary to Fabry's disease: an European experience. *Nephron* 46:353–360, 1983.

189. Mosnier JF, Degott C, Bedorssian J, MOlas G, Degos F, Pruna A, Potet F: Recurrence of Fabry's disease in a renal allograft eleven years after successful renal transplantation. *Transplantation* 51:759–762, 1991.

190. Schweitzer EJ, Drachenberg CB, Bartlett ST: Living kidney donor and recipient evaluation in Fabry's disease. *Transplantation* 54:924–927, 1992.

191. Hoy WE, Megill DM: End-stage renal disease in southwestern Native Americans, with special focus on the Zuni and Navajo Indians. *Tranplant Proc* 21:3906–3908, 1989.

192. Horina JH, Wirnsberger G, Horn S, Roob JM, Ratschek M, Holzer H, Pogglitsch H, Krejs GJ: Long-term follow-up of a patient with lecithin cholesterol acyltransferase deficiency syndrome after kidney transplantation. *Transplantation* 56:233–236, 1993.

193. Webb MC, Andrews PA, Koffman CG, Cameron JS: Renal transplantation in Wiskott–Aldrich syndrome. *Transplantation* 56:1585, 1993.

194. Noblins M, Kleinknecht D, Dommergues JP, Nazaret C, Garay RP, Jullien M, Guillot M, Fries D, Charpentier B: Liddle syndrome (or pseudo-hyperaldosteronism). Long-term development and erythrocyte potassium flow study in 4 cases. *Arch Fr Pediatr* 49:685–691, 1992.

CHAPTER 68

Complications of Renal Transplantation

PETER J. MORRIS

INTRODUCTION

Although complications following renal transplantation are now fewer than in the earlier years of transplantation, they are nevertheless still responsible for appreciable morbidity and even mortality in the transplant recipient. Such complications are diverse in nature, ranging from technical problems related to the surgery to more widespread effects related to immunosuppression and/or poor renal function.

TECHNICAL

Vascular

Transplant renal artery thrombosis as a primary event is, fortunately, a relatively rare complication in experienced units, for it will almost certainly result in loss of the transplanted kidney, even if recognized early with immediate exploration. It may be recognized during the operation after revascularization of the kidney due to an intimal flap caused by damage to the artery during removal of the kidney from the donor. However, it is generally due to technical error producing twisting or kinking of the renal artery when the kidney is placed in its extraperitoneal pouch. It should be suspected in any patient who suddenly becomes anuric within 48 hours of surgery, and, although rapid confirmation of arterial occlusion may be obtained by duplex ultrasound examination or isotope renography, the problem is of such urgency that it may be more appropriate to return the patient immediately to the operating room for exploration. If the blood supply cannot be reconstituted within 90 minutes, warm ischemia will almost certainly cause irreversible damage to the graft. In the later weeks after transplantation, renal artery thrombosis may occur as a secondary event after arteriolar thrombosis in an acutely rejecting kidney.

However, in contrast, thrombosis of the renal vein has become a relatively common vascular complication after transplantation in the cyclosporine era. Certainly, in the precyclosporine era, it occurred as a result of kinking or twisting of the vein (1), compression of the vein by a swollen kidney due to rejection or acute tubular necrosis (2). However, following the first report of six cases of renal vein thrombosis in 79 patients receiving cyclosporine (3), there have been a number of other reports confirming this much higher incidence of renal vein thrombosis in most centers (4,5), and it is of interest to note that in reports of randomized trials of new immunosuppressive agents, one consistently sees a significant number of renal vein thromboses recorded. In one report from a large center (6), a low incidence of renal vein thrombosis was noted, but it may be relevant that in that center sequential immunosuppressive therapy is practiced, with the introduction of cyclosporine when renal function is established. Cyclosporine has been associated with a number of risk factors that could be responsible for an increased tendency for thrombosis. These include reduction in renal blood flow (7), increased production of thromboxane and decreased production of prostacyclin (8–10), and enhanced platelet aggregation (11), together with a sustained enhancement of in vitro hemostasis and reduced thrombolysis in the early postoperative period (12). Venous thrombosis may also be more common in diabetes (13), which is certainly our experience in Oxford.

Classically, the patient with a functioning kidney who develops renal vein thrombosis complains of sudden pain over the transplanted kidney and becomes virtually anuric, while on examination a large tender kidney is found. The diagnosis can be confirmed by immediate duplex scanning of the kidney. Although immediate surgery can sometimes allow evacuation of the clot in the vein, this is unusual. However, the patient should always be explored, since often the kidney will be ruptured with considerable perigraft hemorrhage (14). Late renal vein thrombosis usually secondary to iliac vein thrombosis on the side of the graft may occur, but does not necessarily result in loss of the kidney. Hematuria and proteinuria are common, but the kidney will not necessarily be swollen due to the perigraft fibrosis that exists around a long-surviving kidney.

Prevention of acute renal vein thrombosis is obviously the desirable option, but apart from care taken to avoid the predisposing technical factors such as kinking or twisting of the vein, the only other approach is prophylactic anticoagulation. However, if a major defect induced by cyclosporine is a platelet defect, then heparin prophylaxis is not likely to be helpful (and indeed will lead to a significant incidence of postoperative hemorrhage). Aspirin prophylaxis, e.g., 75 mg/day, may be of value, and this is our practice. Certainly since introducing prophylactic aspirin for 1 month from the time of transplantation in our patients some years ago (all of whom receive triple therapy as immunosuppressive therapy), there has been a dramatic decrease in the incidence of renal vein thrombosis in Oxford. But of course this represents no more than anecdotal experience and needs to be tested in a large prospective randomized trial.

Renal artery stenosis occurs with a frequency ranging from 1.5% to 7%, but it should be noted that when routine angiography is carried out in patients with hypertension after transplantation, a much higher incidence is found (15–18). When it occurs in the early months after transplantation, it often affects the anastomotic site itself and is due to a technical defect. More often it presents from 3 months to 2 years after transplantation with poorly controlled hypertension and deterioration in graft function, the latter often precipitated by the use of angiotensin-converting enzyme (ACE) inhibitors (19,20). Such stenoses typically lie distal to the site of anastomosis (Figure 1), and although they occur quite frequently, they are often not of functional significance. While the lesion may be demonstrated angiographically, it may be difficult to establish that it is the cause of hypertension and/or renal dysfunction, since both these factors may be due to vascular changes associated with chronic rejection. A renal biopsy may be helpful if it excludes chronic rejection, and renal-vein renin studies may be of value in determining the functional significance of a radiologic stenosis. ACE inhibitors may also be used as a diagnostic test, but this test should be performed in hospital (21).

The treatment of a proven functional renal artery stenosis should be angioplasty in the first instance in most cases, especially for the common lesion distal to the anastomosis. The success rate reported in the literature is extremely variable, with initial success rates ranging from 58% to 76% and a low to high recurrence rate (15–17,22). Surgical reconstruction, although associated with a high success rate in experienced hands, is often a very difficult technical procedure and should be restricted to the management of lesions with failed angioplasty or recurrent stenoses after angioplasty (16,23).

Secondary hemorrhage is an uncommon but life-threatening complication after transplantation and is due to infection at the anastomosis. The source of sepsis may be contamination from the graft itself, but in any event the infection is usually introduced at the time of operation. It is fortunate that prophylactic antibiotics have reduced the incidence of this problem, since it inevitably requires graft nephrectomy and occasionally also the ligation of the external iliac artery if this has been used for renal revascularization. Surprisingly, such a ligation does not always require the insertion of a vascular graft, but if arterial reconstruction is deemed necessary, it should always be delayed if possible due to the associated infection.

Urologic

The two principal urologic complications after transplantation are ureteric obstruction and urine leakage (24–26). When obstruction occurs early in the posttransplant period, it is generally due to technical reasons at the site of implantation of the ureter into the bladder or twisting of the ureter. Oliguria or anuria in the immediate posttransplant period should make one suspect such problems. The diagnosis is confirmed by ultrasonography in the first instance (25,26), followed by antegrade pyelography to define the exact site of obstruction. Early surgical revision is required. Ureteric obstruction by hematoma after a percutaneous needle biopsy is occasionally encountered, but this outcome usually resolves spontaneously over a few days without active intervention. At times remote from the transplant operation, ureteric obstruction is often due to ureteric stricture formation, which is presumed to reflect ischemic damage to the ureter. Again, ultrasonography and an antegrade pyelogram or an intravenous urogram will confirm the diagnosis, which should always be considered when a gradual deterioration in renal function is seen, especially without evidence of significant chronic rejection. Ureteric strictures may be treated by balloon catheter dilatation and insertion of a double J stent, although formal surgical reconstruction is often necessary (26).

Urine leakage usually occurs from the lower end of the ureter due to ischemia of this structure, perhaps as a result of skeletonization of the ureter at donor nephrectomy (26). Leakage from the cystotomy made at the time of ureteric implantation is relatively uncommon nowadays. Urine leakage is often not evident until at least 1 week after transplantation, and often several weeks pass before the diagnosis becomes obvious. Oliguria is noted in association with fever, local tenderness, and swelling. Ultrasonography followed by antegrade pyelography or intravenous urography allows a definitive diagnosis (27). Surgery should be undertaken as soon as possible, since a delay will undoubtedly result in infection, making the inevitable surgery more difficult and hazardous.

There has been a marked reduction in the incidence of urologic complications, both obstruction and leakage, in recent years in the Oxford Transplant Unit (28). While the surgical techniques have remained constant, the immunosuppression protocols have changed significantly. From 1975 to 1979, when high-dose steroids (initially 100 mg prednisolone/day) were used, the rate of urologic complications was 15%. In later years, although a variety of protocols have been used, the steroid dose has been significantly lower (initially 20 mg/day), and primary urologic complications now affect only about 2% of transplants, with an

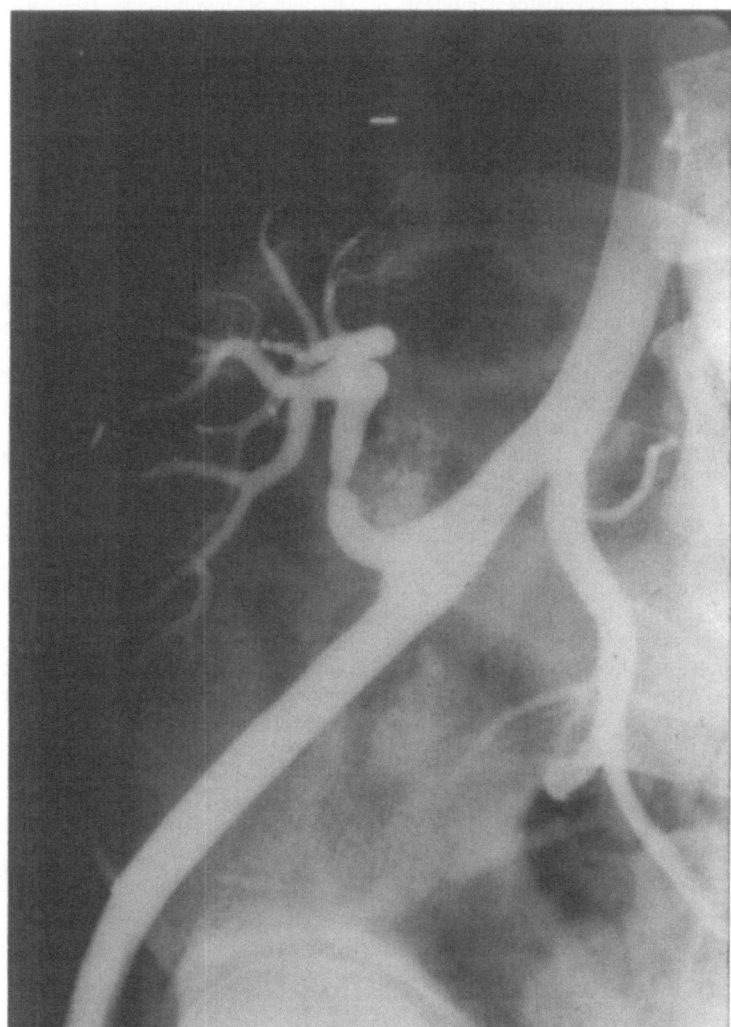

Figure 1. Angiogram showing transplant renal artery stenosis distal to the site of arterial anastomosis (renal artery end-to-side to external iliac artery).

overall complication rate remaining constant at around 4.5%.

Urological complications can be avoided to some extent by careful attention to the removal of the donor kidney and its implantation (26). Management of complications has been revolutionized by the development of minimally invasive techniques such as antegrade and retrograde insertion of stents and balloon dilatation of stenoses, all of which have reduced the need for operative intervention. However, it is important not to persist too long with these less invasive techniques if early correction of the defect is not achieved.

Other urologic complications such as vesicoureteric reflux in the transplanted kidney associated with repeated infection may require reimplantation of the donor ureter with an antireflux procedure, while in an increasingly elderly male population with a renal transplant, bladder outflow obstruction requiring transurethral resection of the prostate is seen with increasing frequency.

Lymphatic

While lymph drainage in the first few days after transplantation is often evident if a suction drain has been inserted, this drainage is rarely a problem. The major complication associated with the lymphatics is lymphocele formation, which usually occurs in the first 3 months after transplantation and presents as a large cystic mass in the vicinity of the kidney. A lymphocele always arises from the host lymphatics and is caused by a failure to ligate those lymphatics that were divided during exposure of the iliac vessels (29). Presenting features are due to the pressure of the lymphocele on the surrounding structures. Pressure on the ureter may reduce renal function, pressure on the iliac vein may cause swelling of the leg, and strangury and diarrhea may occur due to pressure on the bladder and rectum, respectively (Figure 2). Ultrasonography allows definitive diagnosis, and the initial management is aspiration under ultrasonographic control. After two or three aspirations, the lymphocele often does not recur, but if continuing problems are met then fenestration into the peritoneal cavity is performed, and this may be achieved with laparoscopic techniques as well as by open surgery (22).

Wound

Prevention of contamination during donor nephrectomy, careful aseptic technique during transplantation, and the use of prophylactic antibiotics should ensure that the incidence of wound infection after the transplant operation is no more than 3%. This complication is serious, since deep sepsis may involve the vascular anastomoses and cause

secondary hemorrhage (see Vascular section above). When wound infection occurs, adequate drainage must be provided immediately, and appropriate antibiotic therapy should be introduced.

INFECTION

Incidence

Although the last decade has seen a decrease in the incidence of serious infections after transplantation, this complication remains a significant hazard for the transplant recipient, especially in the early months after surgery (30). The fall in incidence is primarily due to a general reduction in immunosuppressive therapy and, in particular, to modern low-dose steroid regimens. The reduction in morbidity and mortality from infection is also in some part due to fewer rejection episodes requiring additional high-dose steroid therapy immunosuppressive treatment in the cyclosporine era. A greater awareness of the hazard of infection and more aggressive diagnosis and treatment have also made a significant contribution. While postoperative bacterial chest infection and bacteriuria are not uncommon in transplant recipients, these rarely pose significant problems, unlike infections due to a variety of pathogens that may be encountered rather late in the posttransplant period.

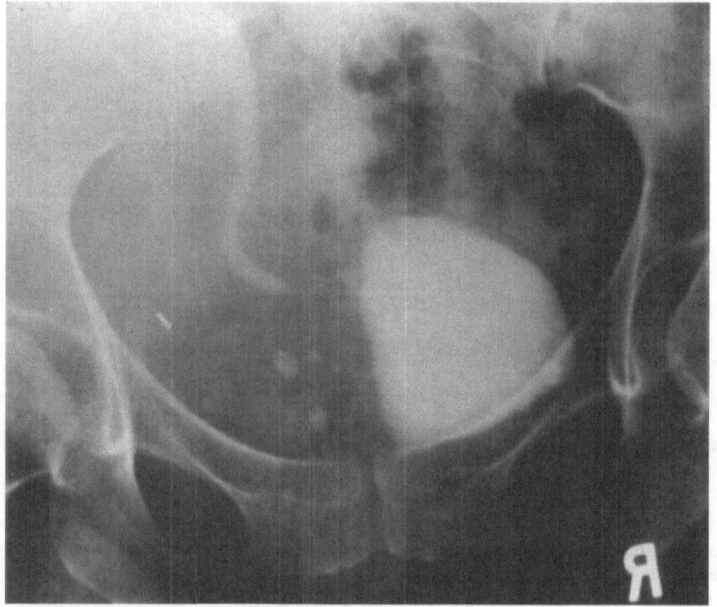

Figure 2. Urogram showing bladder filling defect due to posttransplantation lymphocele.

After transplantation, the most common presentation of an infection is fever. Although this may have a relatively trivial origin, such as gastroenteritis or influenza, thorough investigation is always required and, depending on the clinical features, may involve chest radiography; ultrasonography of the transplant wound area; cultures from the mouth and access sites; cultures of sputum, urine, blood, and stool; viral antibody titers; and even lumbar puncture. If the diagnosis remains elusive, the possibility of cytomegalovirus (CMV) infection, in particular, or tuberculosis or fungal infection should be excluded by intensive investigation. Antibiotics should be withheld until an organism is identified if this is feasible, but on occasion empirical therapy is justified, especially in the neutropenic patient.

Pulmonary infection

Pulmonary infection is a major cause of morbidity and mortality after renal transplantation. The diagnosis of fever in association with a pulmonary infiltrate on a chest radiography may be difficult to ascertain, and it is first necessary to exclude pulmonary edema, infarction, or hemorrhage as a cause of the radiologic appearance. It is worthy of note that in the first few weeks after transplantation, chest infections are usually due to those bacteria commonly encountered as pulmonary pathogens after any form of surgery. Opportunistic infections, on the other hand, such as those due to CMV, pneumocystis, legionella, nocardia, and fungi, occur after the first postoperative month, and such organisms are encountered especially in the first year after transplantation (30,31), with a declining incidence in later years, especially in those with good renal function on minimal immunosuppression. Pneumococcal pneumonia, however, may occur at any time and may run an aggressive course, leading to death, unless diagnosed and treated early.

The radiologic appearance may assist diagnosis. Rapidly progressive changes tend to be associated with bacterial infections, whereas a less rapid progression may indicate a viral or fungal causation. Consolidation is more commonly a feature of bacterial infection, whereas interstitial shadowing is compatible with viral or pneumocystis infection. Nodular infiltrates are associated with infection due to streptococcus, nocardia, tuberculosis, or fungi. While radiography is of undoubted importance in the management of the transplant patient with pulmonary infection, definitive diagnosis can only be made after identification of the responsible pathogen, and an aggressive approach to the acquisition of suitable specimens for bacteriologic study is needed. Although it is generally wise to withhold antibiotics until the pathogen has been identified, the condition of individual patients may make this approach unrealistic. Empirical treatment of suspected bacterial pneumonia must cover staphylococci, pneumococci, hemophilus, legionella, and gram-negative organisms, and a satisfactory antibiotic choice is flucloxacillin

plus erythromycin in conjunction with an aminoglycoside. Suspected pneumocystis infection will often respond to high-dose cotrimoxazole, and in practice all four of the above drugs tend to be administered. If a definitive diagnosis is not reached or if empirical antibiotic treatment is started without a response within 24 hours, bronchoscopy with bronchial alveolar lavage or open-lung biopsy is indicated (30).

CYTOMEGALOVIRUS PNEUMONIA

CMV pneumonia does not occur in the first month after transplantation. A fever associated with changes on a chest radiograph, occurring between 1 and 4 months after transplantation in a patient who was seronegative at the time of operation and who received a kidney from a seropositive donor, should be regarded as due to CMV infection when all other causes of fever and pulmonary infiltrate have been excluded. A leukopenia may develop in association with this infection, requiring a reduction in immunosuppression. Azathioprine, in particular, if being used with cyclosporine, may have to be discontinued. Therapy for a CMV pneumonitis is ganciclovir, which has replaced the use of hyperimmune globulin. CMV is discussed further in the section on viral infections (below).

PNEUMOCYSTIS CARINII PNEUMONIA

Pneumocystis carinii pneumonia was once relatively common in transplant recipients who presented with a fever, often associated with some dyspnea, but with few other physical signs. Radiography shows diffuse pulmonary shadowing with a linear distribution (Figure 3). High-dose cotrimoxazole is the treatment of choice. This infection may now be occurring more frequently with the use of cyclosporin, but this increased incidence probably reflects a much higher diagnosis rate with the use of bronchoscopy and bronchial lavage. Prophylactic cotrimoxazole has been used for some years now in Oxford and elsewhere during the first 6 months after transplantation, and this agent has virtually eliminated this form of pneumonia from transplant units as a primary infection.

PULMONARY TUBERCULOSIS

While the incidence of tuberculosis varies according to the region, it is undoubtedly more common in transplant recipients than in the general population. Symptoms are often nonspecific, and the site of infection may be outside of the lungs. Established cases are treated with rifampicin and isoniazid, but both drugs are metabolized in the liver, and rifampicin, in particular, is a potent inducer of hepatic enzymes. Such enzyme induction renders cyclosporin an unwise choice for immunosuppression, and this drug is better replaced by azathioprine if rifampicin is the chosen treatment.

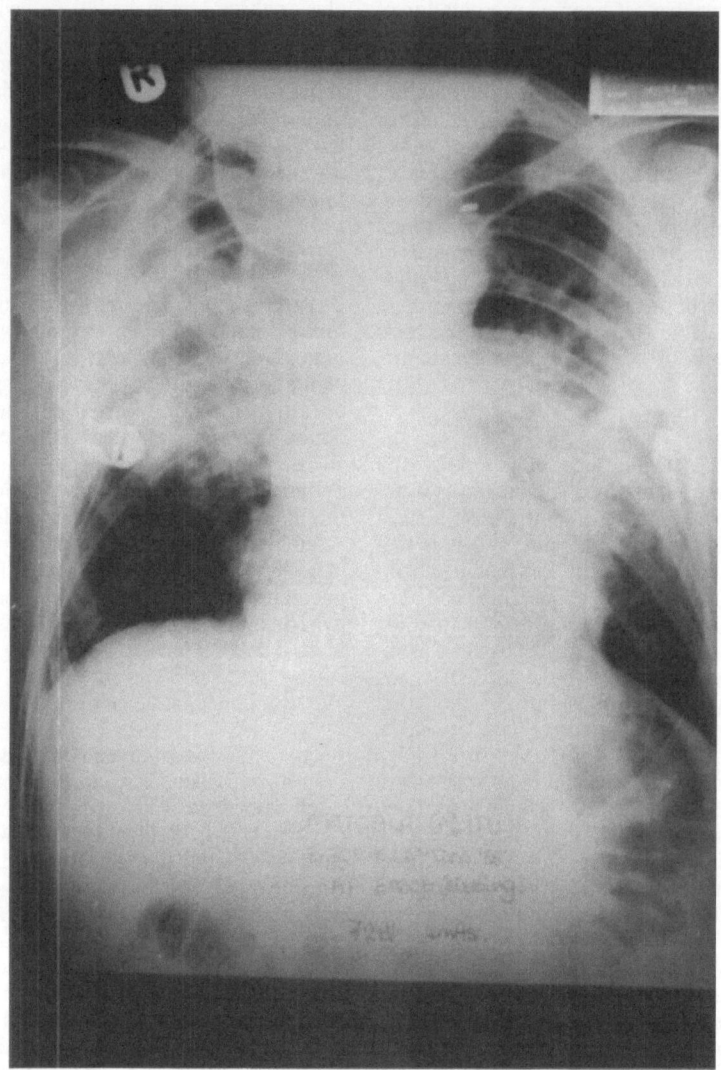

Fgure 3. Pulmonary shadowing on a chest radiograph due to *Pneumocystis carinii* pneumonia in a transplant recipient.

LEGIONELLA PNEUMONIA

The recent increase in the incidence of legionella pneumonia is probably due to an increasing awareness and identification of the organism, which proliferates in stagnant water and is often spread via air conditioning systems and showers (32). In the early stages, the chest radiograph shows irregular, nodular shadows, which may progress rapidly to lobar or diffuse consolidation. Identification of legionella usually requires direct immunofluorescent staining, and the organism may be cultured from sputum or biopsy samples on specialized media. The drug of choice is high-dose erythromycin.

Urinary tract infection

A bacteriuria nearly always occurs in the first few weeks after transplantation due to the presence of an indwelling catheter for some days after the operation. Such a bacteriuria generally clears on removal of the catheter, especially in the presence of a good urine output. If it does not clear within a few days of catheter removal, or if a frank urinary tract infection is evident, active treatment with an appropriate antibiotic is warranted, since the continuing presence of bacteria in the urinary tract is a potential cause of septicemia in the immunosuppressed patient.

Wound infection

Wound infection is a serious complication that has been discussed earlier. In cases of deep infection, diagnosis may be aided by ultrasonography or computerized tomography, but treatment should be prompt and consists of adequate drainage and appropriate antibiotic therapy.

Septicemia

Septicemia is not uncommon and is usually due to gram-negative organisms from the urinary tract. *Staphylococcus, Listeria,* and *Candida* may also cause septicemia. While the results of blood cultures are being awaited, broad-spectrum antibiotic treatment should be started, and an aggressive search for the focus of infection should be made. The treatment of such a focus depends on its nature and site.

Viral infections

CYTOMEGALOVIRUS (CMV)

CMV infection is the most important of the viral infections encountered in transplant recipients and takes two forms (30,31,33). The first is a primary infection and gives rise to more concern than the second, which is a secondary or reactivated infection. Primary infection occurs in patients who are seronegative at the time of transplantation and who receive a kidney from a seropositive donor (34) (Table 1). Transmission of infection with the kidney is far more common than transmission by blood transfusion (33), which has never been noted in the Oxford Transplant Unit.

Primary CMV infection often presents as a fever in the second or third month after transplantation, although it will occur much earlier in patients treated with antilymphocyte reagents such as OKT3 or ALG. It may be

associated with neutropenia. Atypical lymphocytes may be seen on the blood film. Leukopenia will require a reduction in immunosuppression, especially if azathioprine has been used, and this drug in particular may need to be discontinued, putting the kidney at some risk of rejection. Primary CMV infection may cause pneumonia and, less commonly, hepatitis, arthralgia, splenomegaly, myalgia, and gastrointestinal ulceration. Renal function may deteriorate during the early stages of infection, and a glomerulopathy may occur (35). The infection is self-limiting within a period of 3 weeks, but great care is required to exclude other causes of fever in these patients until the diagnosis is firmly established. Early diagnosis is now possible using a variety of techniques to detect CMV antigen before the appearance of CMV- specific IgM antibodies. The polymerase chain reaction may be used to detect CMV in early cultures (36), but the direct detection of CMV antigen in peripheral blood leukocytes is proving to be extremely reliable in Oxford not only for early diagnosis but also for surveillance after ATG or OKT3 therapy (37,38).

Treatment of CMV infection may be expectant if the infection is a reactivation, but the tendency is to treat a primary infection with ganciclovir in that established infection, especially pneumonitis, is more resistant to treatment (30,39,40). An alternative drug, foscarnet, which is active against all the herpes group viruses, including CMV, may also be used in these infections, but it is nephrotoxic (41).

Primary infection can be prevented by avoiding transplantation of a kidney from a seropositive donor into a seronegative recipient (Table 1), and this should be considered among the selection criteria for the donor and recipient. Vaccination against CMV has been evaluated in seronegative recipients, and although the incidence of infection was not decreased, the severity of the infection was reduced (42,43). High-titered CMV immunoglobulin has been used prophylactically with success (44), and high-dose acyclovir, although of no value in treating the disease, has been claimed to decrease the incidence of primary CMV infection (45). Prophylactic ganciclovir in patients at high risk of CMV infection, i.e., seronegative patients given ATG or OKT3, is of value (46), but must be given for at least 4 weeks.

HERPES SIMPLEX VIRUS (HSV)

Latent HSV infection may commonly be reactivated in immunosuppressed patients, especially in the early weeks after transplantation or in association with later complications. Local lesions are painted with 35% idoxuridine in dimethylsulphoxide or treated with acyclovir cream. If the local infection is severe, however, or if systemic infection has occurred, acyclovir chemotherapy should be started immediately, since widespread infection may occasionally cause death (30). The results of treatment with acyclovir for HSV infection are generally good provided treatment is started early, and side effects are minimal.

Table 1. Incidence of cytomegalovirus infection in 306 consecutive cadaver renal transplant recipients in Oxford with respect to CMV antibody status of donor and recipient (34)

	Recipient CMV+		Recipient CMV−	
	Donor CMV+	Donor CMV−	Donor CMV+	Donor CMV−
No. patients	84	98	60	64
No. infected	52 (62%)	52 (53%)	38 (63%)	0
	Reactivation		Primary infection	

VARICELLA ZOSTER

Varicella zoster is again a frequently encountered problem occurring at any stage after transplantation in up to 3% of patients (34), and acyclovir is the treatment of choice. Patients who are seronegative for varicella antibody should avoid contact with children with chicken pox. Prophylactic hyperimmune globulin should be given after accidental contact, since chicken pox, although rare, can be an extremely virulent infection in a transplant recipient.

EPSTEIN–BARR VIRUS (EBV)

EBV is an occasional cause of a glandular fever-like illness in immunosuppressed patients. Although such an illness is not itself a major problem, patients taking cyclosporin may be especially prone to EBV infection due to suppression of the generation of T-cytotoxic cells against EBV-infected B lymphocytes, which in turn may cause an acute lymphoproliferative disorder or even a polyclonal lymphoma (see Primary Cancer section below).

HEPATITIS B VIRUS

Transplantation in patients who are carriers of the hepatitis B antigen is a relatively common problem in many countries. Graft survival in hepatitis B antigen carriers is rather better than in noncarriers, reflecting some innate immune defect in addition to the effect of immunosuppressive drugs. There is great concern in carrier patients, however, about the progression of liver disease, which may accompany immunosuppression, even leading to liver failure (47–49). In these patients who are positive for HBeAg/HBV DNA, there is a particularly high risk of death from liver failure, and these patients possibly should not be transplanted (50). If transplantation is chosen, then a case can be made for selecting only those patients who have a normal liver biopsy. In countries where hepatitis B is relatively common within the renal failure population, all new patients who are hepatitisB antibody negative should be vaccinated. All staff in renal units should be vaccinated against the hepatitisB virus.

HEPATITIS C VIRUS (HCV)

HCV is responsible for most non-A, non-B hepatitis (51). In renal units, the prevalence of HCV infection ranges from 2% to 30%, depending on the part of the world. HCV can be transmitted by organ transplantation (52), so kidneys from donors who have antibody for HCV should not be used in countries where the prevalence of HCV is low. Interferon-gamma has been used to treat HCV-positive patients with liver dysfunction, and improvement has been noted (53). However, prolonged therapy is required, and there is a risk of inducing rejection of a renal allograft in a transplant patient.

HUMAN IMMUNODEFICIENCY VIRUS I (HIV I)

HIV can be transmitted with an organ allograft from an HIV-positive donor (54). Renal transplantation in HIV-positive patients has a bad outcome; 63% of patients in one series died within 5 years, since the disease displayed a more rapid progress in these immunosuppressed patients (55). The only treatment available is zidovudine, together with prophylaxis against *Pneumocystis carinii*.

OTHER VIRAL INFECTIONS

Many viruses commonly cause infections in the transplant patient. Fortunately, most of these are a nuisance rather than a potential threat to life. They include parainfluenza, influenza A, influenza B, polyoma, and papilloma viruses.

Bacterial infections

Bacterial infections are common after transplantation, and many have already been described in this section. Some rather less common bacteria also have to be remembered that may affect the transplant recipient even many years after the operation.

LISTERIA MONOCYTOGENES

Listeria monocytogenes may cause infection at any time after transplantation but usually after increased or excessive immunosuppression. This infection is the single most common cause of meningoencephalitis in transplant recipients, and as soon as cerebrospinal fluid and blood cultures have been obtained, any patient with this condition should be given ampicillin as the drug of choice (30).

CLOSTRIDIUM DIFFICILE

Pseudomembranous colitis (PMC) is due to infection of the colon by *Clostridium difficile* and, although it typically occurs in patients who have been exposed to broad-spectrum antibiotics, it may pose special problems in units where the organism has become endemic. Such a situation is likely in any unit with a large continuous ambulatory peritoneal dialysis program with its inevitable antibiotic-treated recurrent peritonitis. The drug of choice in PMC is oral vancomycin, but *Clostridium difficile* is highly infectious, and appropriate steps must be taken to avoid spread within the transplant unit (56).

NOCARDIA

Nocardia usually causes a respiratory illness with unproductive cough and malaise associated with a fever. Chest radiographs show a nodular pulmonary infiltrate. Spread to the brain, skin, and joints may result in local abscess formation. Sulphonamide is the drug of choice and must be given for at least 2 months. Some have suggested that treatment continue for 1 year.

Although not very common, possible infection with mycobacterium should be considered if an unusual infective process is encountered, especially in transplant recipients with a past history of active tuberculosis. In transplant patients, extrapulmonary tuberculosis occurs just as often as pulmonary tuberculosis. If there is a past history of tuberculosis and doubt exists about the adequacy of previous treatment, prophylactic antituberculous chemotherapy should be given for the first 12 months after transplantation.

Fungal infection

While not particularly common in the transplant recipient, the possibility of fungal infection should be considered when fever and pneumonia occur in the presence of increased or excessive immunosuppression.

CANDIDA

Candida is the most common fungal infection after transplantation and is often associated with debility from other complications, including other infections. Its most severe local manifestation is esophageal candidiasis, which should respond to local nystatin, but the rare septicemia will require treatment with fluconazole.

ASPERGILLUS

Aspergillus may cause pneumonia and may disseminate to many sites, including the brain, skin, kidney, and alimentary tract. It is treated with amphotericin B and occasionally with the addition of 5-flucytosine.

COCCIDIOIDES

Coccidioides is rare in Europe but common in certain parts of North America. Lesions occur in the lungs, liver, brain, and spleen, and may be due to primary infection or reactivation of latent infection. Again, amphotericin B is the treatment of choice.

CRYPTOCOCCUS

Cryptococcus is a rare cause of pneumonitis and meningitis in immunosuppressed patients. Amphotericin B is again the treatment of choice, together with 5-flucytosine.

HISTOPLASMA

Histoplasma may be a primary infection or the result of reactivation of a latent infection. Fever, skin lesions, and pneumonitis are seen, and again amphotericin B is the treatment of choice.

Protozoal and helminthic infection

Pneumocystis carinii is by far the most common of the protozoal and helmimthic organisms encountered in the transplant patient. However, infections due to *Giardia, Schistosoma, Toxoplasma, Leishmania,* and *Strongyloides* may be encountered. Many of these organisms have marked geographic limits, and knowledge of these is helpful in diagnosis (30).

CARDIOVASCULAR COMPLICATIONS

Cardiovascular disease is a major cause of death in the general population and is even more pronounced in transplant recipients. No less than a quarter of deaths after renal transplantation in North America and Europe are due to cardiovascular complications (57). Much of the risk is associated with the underlying cause of renal failure, and patients whose renal impairment is due to hypertensive disease or diabetes mellitus fare particularly badly in this respect. Correction of risk factors, such as hypertension, obesity, and hyperlipidemia, is of major importance in the transplant patient, and although no direct evidence exists that smoking is a risk factor in the transplant population, its role in the normal population is well established, and it would seem unlikely that it does not similarly have a deleterious effect after transplantation. Strenuous efforts should be made to persuade potential transplant recipients to stop smoking. The tendency to transplant increasing numbers of elderly and diabetic patients, combined with the longer graft survival that can now be achieved, will ensure that cardiovascular complications will become even more prominent in the future. The emphasis should be on prevention by correction of risk factors.

Hypertension

Although uremia itself may be associated with hypertension, elevated blood pressure also remains a major problem in those with functioning allografts. Despite improvements in renal function after operation, there must be new causes for hypertension, a problem that affects well over half of recipients of kidneys between 6 months and 3 years after surgery (58). Hypertension is also recognized as the most common complication in long-term survivors after transplantation, affecting about half of these patients (59). The causes of such hypertension may include rejection, the influence of disease in the native kidneys, transplant renal artery stenosis, and immunosuppressive drugs, in particular cyclosporine.

Hypertension is more common in recipients of cadaver grafts than in recipients of kidneys from living related donors, which suggests that rejection is a significant factor in the high incidence of hypertension after transplantation. Chronic rejection, in particular, has a direct relationship with hypertension, and acute rejection too is often accompanied by elevation of blood pressure. This outcome may involve the renin–angiotensin system in the allograft, but reports are conflicting (60–62).

Some patients have poorly controlled hypertension attributable to disease of the native kidneys and may benefit from bilateral nephrectomy (63). This operation is a major one, however, and if the kidneys are small, an alternative approach is bilateral renal embolization, a minor procedure with little morbidity that has been used with some success in the Oxford Transplant Unit (64).

The problem of transplant renal artery stenosis has been discussed earlier. When other causes of hypertension have been excluded, percutaneous transluminal angioplasty is a useful initial approach, for while the results in Oxford have not been particularly good, the technique has never resulted in graft loss, and other units have reported good results. Reconstructive surgery can then be reserved for those in whom angioplasty fails.

Steroid immunosuppressive therapy contributes to hypertension, although modern low-dose steroid protocols are less hazardous in this respect. It is now apparent that the incidence of hypertension in patients treated with cyclosporine, with or without steroids, is probably greater than that seen in patients treated with prednisolone and azathioprine (65,66).

Hyperlipidemia

Hypercholesterolemia is common after renal transplantation, and there is an association between serum cholesterol at the time of transplantation and subsequent cardiovascular disease (67).

Both ischemic heart disease and cerebrovascular disease are more common in hyperlipidemic renal transplant patients (68). Serum lipoprotein (a), an independent risk factor for cardiac disease, is also elevated in renal transplant patients (69). In addition to dietary advice, transplant patients with significant elevation of cholesterol should be treated. The HMG coenzyme A reductive inhibitors are effective (70) and although there was concern about interactions with cyclosporine being associated with rhabdomyolysis (71), these concerns have not been borne out with further experience.

Deep venous thrombosis

Deep venous thrombosis has occurred in 8% of transplant recipients in Oxford, the incidence increasing with age (72). Although it has been suggested that thromboembolic events in general occur with increased frequency in patients receiving cyclosporine (73), others have not found such an association (74). Deep venous thrombosis exhibits two peaks in incidence, the first at the expected time about 1 week after the transplant operation and the second,

larger peak at about 4 months. It is noteworthy that a functioning allograft will largely correct the anemia and hemostatic defect associated with chronic renal failure by 4 months. The 4-month peak in incidence, and indeed all thrombosis distant to the time of the transplant operation itself, is usually associated with some complication requiring prolonged bed rest or further surgery. Thus, prophylaxis for thrombosis should be mandatory in patients with such complications. Our policy has been to investigate any significant leg swelling by venography and more recently by duplex scanning, or, if pulmonary symptoms suggest embolism, to carry out a ventilation/perfusion isotope scan of the lungs, whether or not such symptoms are accompanied by lower limb swelling. Treatment is immediate anticoagulation with heparin followed by oral warfarin for at least 4 months, since pulmonary embolism is responsible for about 4% of deaths in transplant recipients.

CANCER

Primary cancer

The incidence of cancer in transplant patients ranges from 1.6% in Europe to 24% in Australia (75,76). Much of the difference is accounted for by the very high incidence of skin cancers in Australia. Transplant recipients also have a significantly increased risk of developing malignant lymphoma, but even if lymphoma and skin cancer are excluded, the transplant population still has a greater incidence of nearly all forms of cancer compared with the normal population. Increased susceptibility to neoplasia is due to several factors alone or in combination, which include depression of immune surveillance, increased susceptibility to oncogenic virus infection, chronic antigenic stimulation in the presence of immunosuppression, and a direct neoplastic action of immunosuppressive agents themselves.

Skin cancer is the most common cancer encountered in transplant recipients, even in areas not known for a high incidence of such neoplasia in the general population. Squamous cell carcinoma is the most common type, and it may be very aggressive in the immunosuppressed patient, leading to death from metastatic disease. Bowen's disease, malignant melanoma, and basal cell carcinoma are also not infrequent in transplant recipients. Patients who develop skin cancers continued to do so even after treatment of specific lesions. In some cases, immunosuppression has to be discontinued and the kidney abandoned in order to save life. When immunosuppression is withdrawn, new skin cancers do not occur. Due to the high incidence of this disease in warm climates, a serious attempt must be made at prevention. Transplant recipients should be advised on suitable clothing while in the sun, and barrier creams should be used. Retinoids have a place in the management of patients with multiple and recurrent skin cancers, but prolonged therapy is difficult due to side effects (77).

Malignant (non-Hodgkin) lymphomas occur 50–100 times more frequently in the transplant population than in the general population and account for nearly one third of all cancers in transplant recipients (75,76). Nowadays these lymphomas are often described as lymphoproliferative disease, of which two types are recognized and for which differing treatments are appropriate (78). The first type is due to infection by the Epstein–Barr virus and presents as an infectious mononucleosis-like illness within 1 year of transplantation. The fever and general lymphadenopathy often progress rapidly to a fatal conclusion, although withdrawal of immunosuppression will lead to regression in some patients. More recently, treatment with acyclovir without discontinuing immunosuppressive therapy has met with some success. The second type of lymphoproliferative disease presents as a local solid tumor, often confined to the central nervous system. This disease responds to conventional therapy for non-Hodgkin's lymphoma, but it is often more aggressive than that seen in the general population, with short remissions and an eventually fatal outcome. In this type of disease, neither discontinuing immunosuppression nor acyclovir appear to have any beneficial effect. The clinician should be aware that these two types of disease tend to merge, both in their presentation and in their histologic cytogenetic classification, which shows a spectrum ranging from polymorphic diffuse B-cell hyperplasia through a polymorphic B-cell lymphoma to a monomorphic B-cell lymphoma.

The behavior, and thus the treatment, of other cancers varies according to the cell type and site. Usually the treatment is not significantly different from that of the disease when it occurs in the general population. It is appropriate for the transplant recipient to adopt those prophylactic measures available to the general population, and in particular the increased incidence of cervical cancer in female transplant patients suggests that an annual cervical smear is a wise precaution.

Transferred cancer

Cancer has occasionally been transferred accidentally in the transplanted kidney from a cadaver donor with undetected neoplasia (75). If metastatic disease is present in the allograft, it will soon appear in the recipient. Rapid spread tends to occur in the immunosuppressed patient, and treatment is withdrawal of immunosuppression and graft nephrectomy followed by a return to dialysis. This approach will occasionally lead to the regression of disease.

GASTROINTESTINAL COMPLICATIONS

Perforation or hemorrhage from a peptic ulcer is associated with a high mortality in the transplant patient. Patients with indigestion are endoscoped and placed on histamine-receptor blockers (cimetidine or ranitidine) if evidence of ulceration or gastritis is found. Surgery is re-

stricted to failed medical treatment or recurrent ulceration, but this is rare. All patients with a past history of peptic ulcer disease without evidence of active ulceration at the time of transplantation receive prophylactic ranitidine during the first few months after transplantation. If perforation or hemorrhage occur, these complications are treated promptly and aggressively by surgery.

Diverticular disease is no more common in transplant recipients than in the general population, but the problems of hemorrhage or sepsis, should they occur, pose an especially grave risk to the transplant recipient. Should a complication of diverticulosis occur after transplantation, it must be treated aggressively, and abscess formation or sepsis is an indication for early surgery.

The problems of gastrointestinal infection have been discussed previously. Pseudomembranous colitis may occur especially in units where *Clostridium difficile* is endemic (30). A necrotizing enterocolitis is also seen occasionally, which may result in gangrene of the colon and even the small bowel. When gangrene occurs it is uniformly fatal and, although the cause is unknown, may be associated with CMV infection. Solitary ulcers may also occur in the bowel, notably in the cecum. These may bleed or perforate and require urgent surgery. Here to, CMV infection is often the cause.

BONE COMPLICATIONS

Most bone complications after transplantation are due to steroid therapy. Avascular necrosis may affect many joints, including the wrists, elbows, knees, ankles, and shoulders, but it is most commonly seen in the hips, where it tends to occur bilaterally. This complication tends to occur between 1 and 3 years after transplantation, and pain is the common presenting feature. Although the incidence of avascular necrosis has been as high as 15% in transplant recipients, with modern low-dose steroid immunosuppressive regimens this incidence has dropped dramatically (79). Eventually, patients with avascular necrosis will require surgery. Replacement of the hip joint is well tolerated in transplant recipients and should be considered early to improve rehabilitation. Osteoporosis is the other principal steroid-related bone complication, although with low-dose steroid protocols this too has declined in incidence. Nevertheless, even low doses of steroid are likely to produce a significant degree of osteoporosis in postmenopausal women. Hormone replacement therapy should be given to most postmenopausal women with a renal transplant.

GROWTH IN CHILDREN

Retardation of growth in children with end-stage renal failure is well known, and although the rate of growth generally improves after successful transplantation, catch-up growth is less common and some reduction in eventual stature is likely. Growth rate is related both to the age of the child and to renal function, but it is the use of steroids in immunosuppressive regimens that causes most retardation after successful transplantation. While the use of alternate-day steroids improves the situation to some extent, a limitation of potential stature is still probable (80). When cyclosporine is used as the main immunosuppressive agent, on the other hand, especially if used without steroids, a normal growth rate is possible, and even catch-up growth may be seen (81,82).

CATARACTS

Posterior lenticular cataracts occur in up to 10% of transplant recipients, and this outcome was a more common complication associated with high-dose steroid therapy. While most cataracts remain small and cause little disability, some are large and require ophthalmic surgery to the lens (83).

SPECIFIC COMPLICATIONS OF DRUG THERAPY

Many complications of drug therapy have already been mentioned, especially in the case of steroid therapy. It would be inappropriate, however, to end this chapter without listing several important complications that are related to specific drugs. Azathioprine may cause bone marrow depression, hepatic dysfunction, and hair loss. Cyclosporine may cause nephrotoxicity, hepatic dysfunction, gingival hypertrophy, hypertrichosis, neurasthesia, and fluid retention. The more severe of these complications, when they occur, may require a reduction in the dosage or even withdrawal of the appropriate drug. Detailed descriptions of these specific drug complications are provided elsewhere in this volume.

REFERENCES

1. D'Apuzzo V, Bretscher D, Oetliker O, Nachbur B: Renal vein thrombosis in kidney allografts. *Lancet* 2:975–976, 1973.
2. Sorensen BL, Hald T, Nissen HM: Silent iliac compression syndrome as a cause of renal vein thrombosis after transplantation. *Scand J Urol Nephrol* 6 (Suppl 15):75–77, 1972.
3. Merion RM, Calne RY: Allograft renal vein thrombosis. *Transplant Proc* 17:1746–1750, 1985.
4. Jones RM, Murie JA, Ting A, Dunnill MS, Morris PJ: Renal vascular thrombosis of cadaveric renal allografts in patients receiving cyclosporin, azathioprine and prednisolone triple therapy. *Clin Transplant* 2:122–126, 1988.
5. Akyol AM, Briggs JD, Junor BJR, et al.: Renal vein thrombosis after cadaveric renal transplantation. Presented to the Association of Surgeons of Great Britain and Ireland, Oxford, 1991.
6. Gruber SA, Chavers B, Payne WD, et al.: Allograft renal vascular thrombosis: lack of increase with cyclosporine immunosuppression. *Transplantation* 47:475–478, 1989.
7. McKenzie N, Deviveni R, Vezina W, Keown P, Stiller C: The effect of cyclosporin on organ blood flow. *Transplant Proc* 17:1973–1975, 1985.
8. Petric R, Freeman D, Wallace C, McDonald J, Stiller C, Keown P: Effect of cyclosporine on urinary prostanoid excretion, renal blood flow and glomerulotubular function. *Transplantation* 45:883–889, 1988.
9. Brown Z, Neild GH: Cyclosporine inhibits prostacyclin production by cultured human endothelial cells. *Transplant Proc* 19:1178–1180, 1987.
10. Neild GH, Rocchi G, Imberti L, et al.: Effect of cyclosporin A on prostacyclin synthesis by vascular tissue. *Thromb Res* 32:373–379, 1983.
11. Vanrenterghem Y, Roels L, Lerut T, et al.: Thromboembolic complications and haemostatic changes in cyclosporin-treated cadaveric kidney allograft recipients. *Lancet* 1:999–1002, 1985.
12. Baker LR, Tucker B, Kovacs IB: Enhanced in vitro hemostasis and reduced thrombolysis in cyclosporine-treated renal transplant recipients. *Transplantation* 49:905–909, 1990.
13. Bergentz SE, Bergqvisst D, Bornmyr S, Brunkwall J, Husberg B: Venous thrombosis and cyclosporin. *Lancet* 2:101–102, 1985.
14. Richardson AJ, Higgins RM, Jaskowski AJ, et al.: Spontaneous rupture of renal allografts: the importance of renal vein thrombosis in the cyclosporin era. *Br J Surg* 77:558–560, 1990.
15. Roberts JP, Ascher NL, Fry DS, et al.: Transplant renal artery stenosis. *Transplantation* 48:580–583, 1989.
16. Benoit G, Hiesse C, Icard P, et al.: Treatment of renal artery stenosis after renal transplantation. *Transplant Proc* 19:3600–3601, 1987.
17. Greenstein SM, Verstandig A, McLean GK, et al.: Percutaneous transluminal angioplasty, the procedure of choice in the hypertensive renal allograft recipient with renal artery stenosis. *Transplantation* 43:29–32, 1987.
18. Morris PJ, Yadav R, Kincaid-Smith P, Anderson J, Hare WSC, Johnson N, Johnson W, Marshall VC: Renal artery stenosis in renal transplantation. *Med J Aust* 1:1255–1257, 1971.
19. Curtis JJ, Luke RG, Whelchel JD, Diethelm AG, Jones P, Dustan HP: Inhibition of angiotensin-converting enzyme in renal-transplant recipients with hypertension. *N Engl J Med* 308:377–381, 1983.
20. Tilney NL, Rocha A, Strom TB, Kirkman RL: Renal artery stenosis in transplant patients. *Ann Surg* 199:454–460, 1984.
21. Hricik DE: Antihypertensive and renal effects of enalapril in post-transplant hypertension. *Clin Nephrol* 27:250–259, 1987.
22. Gray DW: Vascular and lymphatic complications after renal transplantation. In: PJ Morris, ed, *Kidney Transplantation: Principles and Practice*, 4th ed. WB Saunders, Philadelphia, pp 314–329, 1994.
23. Morris PJ: Renovascular hypertension: the indications for and results of surgery. In: P Bell, C Jamieson, CV Ruckley, eds, *Surgical Management of Vascular Disease*. WB Saunders, philadelphia, pp 739–750, 1992.
24. Mundy AR, Podesta ML, Bewick M, Rudje CJ, Ellis FG: The urological complications of 1000 renal transplants. *Br J Urol* 53:397–402, 1981.
25. Loughlin KR, Tilney NL, Richie JP: Urological complications in 718 renal transplant patients. *Surgery* 95:297–302, 1984.
26. Cranston D: Urological complications after renal transplantation. In: PJ Morris, ed, *Kidney Transplantation: Principles and Practice*, 4th ed. WB Saunders, Philadelphia, pp 330–338, 1994.

27. Petrek J, Tilney NL, Smith EH, Williams JS, Vineyard GC: Ultrasound in renal transplantation. *Ann Surg* 185:441–447, 1975.

28. Jaskowski A, Jones RM, Murie JA, Morris PJ: Urological complications in 600 consecutive renal transplants. *Br J Surg* 74:922–925, 1987.

29. Griffiths AB, Fletcher EW, Morris PJ: Lymphocele after renal transplantation. *Aust NZ J Surg* 49:626–628, 1979.

30. Cohen J, Hopkin J, Kurtz J: Infectious complications after renal transsplantation. In: PJ Morris, ed, *Kidney Transplantation: Principles and Practice*, 4th ed. WB Saunders, Philadelphia, pp 364–389, 1994.

31. Rubin RH, Wolfson JS, Cosimi AB, Tolkoff-Rubin NE: Infections in the renal transplant recipient. *Am J Med* 70; 405–411, 1981.

32. Tobin JO'H, Beare J, Dunnill MS, Fisher-Hoch S, French M, Mitchell RG, Morris PJ, Meurs MF: Legionnaire's disease in a transplant unit: isolation of the causative agent from shower baths. *Lancet* 2:118–121, 1980.

33. Rubin RH: The problem of cytomegalovirus infection in transplantation. In: PJ, Morris, NL Tilney, eds, *Progress in Transplantation II*. Churchill Livingstone, Edinburgh, pp 89–114, 1984.

34. Warrell MJ, Chinn I, Morris PJ, Tobin JO: The effects of viral infection on renal transplants and their recipients. *Q J Med* 49:219–231, 1980.

35. Richardson WP, Colvin RB, Cheeseman H, Tolkoff-Rubin NE, Herrin JT, Cosimi AB, Collins AB, Hirsch MS, McCluskey RT, Russell PS, Rubin RH: Glomerulopathy associated with cytomegalovirus uremia in renal allografts. *N Engl J Med* 305:57–63, 1981.

36. Einsele H, Steidle M, Vallbracht A, et al.: Early occurrence of CMV infection after BMT as demonstrated by PCR technique. *Blood* 77:1104–1110, 1991.

37. van der Bij W, Schirm J, Torensma R, et al.: Comparison of viremia and antienemia for detection of cytomegalovirus in blood. *J Clin Microbiol* 26:2531–2535, 1988.

38. van der Bij W, Torensma R, van Son WJ, et al.: Rapid immunodiagnosis of active cytomegalovirus infection by monoclonal antibody staining of blood leucocytes. *J Med Virol* 25:179–188, 1988.

39. Collaborative DHPG Treatment Study Group: Treatment of serious cytomegalovirus infections with 9-(1.3-dihydroxy-2-propoxymethyl) guanine in patients with AIDS and other immunodeficiences. *N Engl J Med* 314:801–805, 1986.

40. Reed EC, Bowden RA, Dandliker PS, et al.: Treatment of cytomegalovirus pneumonia with ganciclovir and intravenous cytomegalovirus immunoglobulin in patients with bone marrow transplants. *Ann Intern Med* 109:783–788, 1988.

41. Deray G, Martinez F, Katlama C, et al.: Foscarnet nephrotoxicity: mechanism, incidence and prevention. *Am J Nephrol* 9:316–321, 1989.

42. Plotkin SA, Starr SE, Friedman HM, et al.: Effect of Town live virus vaccine on cytomegalovirus disease after renal transplant. A controlled trial. *Ann Intern Med* 114:525–531, 1991.

43. Plotkin SA, Higgins R, Kurtz JB, Morris PJ, Campbell DA, Shope TC, Spector SA: Dankner WM Multicenter trial of Towne strain attenuated virus vaccine in seronegative renal transplant recipients. *Transplantation* 58:1176–1178, 1994.

44. Snydman DR, Werner GB, Tilney NC, et al.: Final analysis of primary cytomegalovirus disease prevention in renal transplant recipients with a cytomegalovirus-immune globulin: comparison of the randomized and open-label trials. *Transplant Proc* 23:1357–1360, 1991.

45. Balfour HH, Chace BA, Stapleton MD, et al.: A randomized placebo-controlled trial of oral acyclovir for the prevention of cytomegalovirus disease in recipients of renal allografts. *N Engl J Med* 320:1381–1387, 1989.

46. Merigan TC, Renlund DG, Keay S, et al.: A controlled trial of gangiclovir to prevent cytomegalovirus disease after heart transplantation. *N Engl J Med* 326:1182–1186, 1992.

47. Pirison Y, Alexandre GP, van Ypersele de Strihou C: Long-term effects of HBs antigenemia on patient survival after renal transplantation. *N Engl J Med* 296:194–196, 1977.

48. Parfrey PS, Forbes RDC, Hutchinson TA, Beaudoin JG,Dauphine WD, Hollomby DJ, Guttmann RD: The clinical and pathological cause of hepatitis B liver disease in renal transplant recipients. *Transplantation* 37:461–466, 1984.

49. La Quaglia MP, Tolkoff-Rubin NE, Dienstag JL, Cosimi AB, Herrin JT, Kelly M, Rubbin RH: Impact of hepatitis on renal transplantation. *Transplantation* 32:504–507, 1981.

50. Fairley CK, Mijch A, Gust ID, et al.: The increased risk of fatal liver disease in renal transplant patients who are hepatitis Be antigen and/or HBY DNA positive. *Transplantation* 52:497–500, 1991.

51. Alter HJ, Purcell RH, Shih JW, et al.: Detection of antibody to hepatitis C virus in prospectively followed transfusion recipients with acute and chronic non-A, non-B hepatitis. *N Engl J Med* 321:1494–1500, 1989.

52. Pereira BJG, Milford EL, Kirkman RL, Levey AS: Transmission of hepatitis C by organ transplantation. *N Engl J Med* 325:454–460, 1991.

53. Davis Gl, Balart LA, Schiff ER, et al.: Treatment of chronic hepatitis C with r recombinant interferon alpha. A multi center randomized, controlled trial. *N Engl J Med* 321:1501–1506, 1989.

54. L'Age-Stehr J, Schwarz A, Offermann G, et al.: HTLV-III in renal transplant recipients. *Lancet* 2:1361–1362, 1985.

55. Lang P, Niaudert P, and the Groupe Cooperatif de Transplantation d'Ile de France. HIV infection in renal transplant patients. In: JL Touraine et al. eds, *Transplantation and Clinical Immunology*, vol 23. Excerpta Medica, Amsterdam, pp 221–••, 1991.

56. Ritchie DB, Jennings LC, Lynn KL, Bailey RR, Cook HB: Clostridium difficile-associated colitis: cross-infection in predisposed patients with renal failure. *NZ Med J* 95:265–266, 1982.

57. Raine AEG: Cardiovascular complications after renal transplantation. In: PJ Morris, ed, *Kidney Transplantation: Principles and Practice*, 4th ed. WB Saunders, Philadelphia, pp 339–355, 1994.

58. Raine AEG: Cardiovascular complications after renal transplantation. In: PJ Morris, ed, *Kidney Transplantation: Principles and Practice*, 3rd ed. WB Saunders, Philadelphia, pp 575–601, 1988.

59. Kirkman RL, Strom TB, Weir MR, Tilney NL: Late mortality and morbidity in recipients of long-term renal allografts. *Transplantation* 34:347–351, 1982.

60. Bennett WM, McDonald WJ, Lawson RK, Potter GA: Post-transplant hypertension: Studies of cortical blood flow and the renal pressor system. *Kidney Int* 6:99–108, 1974.

61. Dustan HP: Inhibition of angiotensin converting enzyme in renal transplant recipients with hypertension. *N Engl J Med* 308:377–381, 1983.

62. Linas SL, Miller PD, McDonald KM, Stables DP, Katz F, Weil R, Schrier RW: Role of the renin–angiotensin system in post-transplantation hypertension in patients with multiple kidneys. *N Engl J Med* 298:1440–1444, 1978.

63. Curtis JJ, Luke RG, Diethelm AG, Whelchel JD, Jones P: Benefits of removal of native kidneys in hypertension after renal transplantation. *Lancet* 2:729–745, 1985.

64. Taylor HM, Benjamin IS, Morris PJ: Control of hypertension after renal transplantation by embolisation of host kidneys. *Lancet* 2:424–427, 1984.

65. Bennett WM, Porter GA: Cyclosporine-associated hypertension. *Am J Med* 85:131–133, 1988.

66. Schachter M: Cyclosporine A and hypertension. *J Hypertens* 6:511–516, 1988.

67. Kasiske BL: Risk factors for accelerated atherosclerosis in renal transplant recipients. *Am J Med* 84:985–992, 1988.

68. Vathsala, A, Weinberg RB, Schoenberg L, et al.: Lipid abnormalities in cyclosporine–prednisolone-treated renal transplant recipients. *Transplantation* 48:37–43, 1989.

69. Webb AT, Plant M, Reaveley DA, et al.: Lipid and lipoprotein (a) concentrations in renal transplant patients. *Nephrol Dial Transplant* 7:636–641, 1992.

70. Grundy SM: HMG-CoA reductase inhibitors for treatment of hypercholesterolemia. *N Engl J Med* 319:24–33, 1988.

71. Kasiske BL, Tortorice KL, Heim-Duthoy KL, et al.: Lovastatin treatment of hypercholesterolemia in renal transplant recipients. *Transplantation* 49:95–100, 1990.

72. Allen RD, Michie CA, Murie JA, Morris PJ: Deep venous thrombosis after renal transplantation. *Surg Gynecol Obstet* 164:137–142, 1987.

73. Vanrenterghem Y, Roels L, Lerut T, Gruwez J, Michielsen P, Gresele P, Deckmyn H, Colucci M, Arnout J, Vermylen J: Thromboembolic complications and haemostatic changes in cyclosporin-treated cadaveric kidney allograft recipients. *Lan-cet* 1:999–1002, 1985.

74. Allen RD, Michie CA, Morris PJ, Chapman JR: Venous thrombosis and cyclosporin. *Lancet* 2:1004, 1985.

75. Sheil AGR: Cancer in dialysis and transplant patients. In: PJ Morris, ed, *Kidney Transplantation: Principles and Practice*, 4th ed. WB Saunders, Philadelphia, pp 390–400, 1994.

76. Penn I: The changing pattern of post-transplant malignancies. *Transplant proc* 23:1101–1103, 1991.

77. Venning VA: Non-malignant skin lesions in renal transplant patients. In: PJ Morris, ed, *Kidney Transplantation: Principles and Practice*, 4th ed. WB Saunders, Philadelphia, pp 401–411, 1994.

78. Hanto DW, Simmons RL: Lymphoproliferative disease in immunosuppressed patients. In: PJ Morris, NL Tilney, eds, *Progress in Transplantation*, vol 1. Churchill Livingstone, New York, pp 186–208, 1994.

79. Walker RG, D'Apice AJ: Non-specific immunosuppression: azathioprine and steroids. In: PJ Morris, ed, *Kidney Transplantation: Principles and Practice*, 4th ed. WB Saunders, Philadelphia, pp 202–214, 1994.

80. Fine R, Ettenger R: Renal transplantation in children. In: PJ Morris, ed, *Kidney Transplantation: Principles and Practice*, 4th ed. WB Saunders, Philadelphia, pp 412–459, 1994.

81. Klare B, Walter JV, Hahn H, Emmrich P, Land W: Cyclosporin in renal transplantation in children. *Lancet* 2:692, 1984.

82. Fletcher SM, Conley SB, van Buren CT, Rose G, Kerman R, Kahan BD: Impact of cyclosporin on renal function and growth in pediatric renal transplant recipients. *Transplant Proc* 17:1284–1288, 1985.

83. Shun-Shin GA, Ratcliffe P, Brou AJ, Brown NP, Sparrow JM: The lens after renal transplantation. *Br J Opthalmol* 74:261–271, 1990.

CHAPTER 69

Essential Hypertension

MICHAEL A. WEBER

THE HISTORY OF HYPERTENSION

Hypertension is a common condition and is estimated to exist in over 50 million Americans (1). It is probably the most commonly treated chronic condition dealt with by primary care physicians. This observation represents a marked change from the days when only severe hypertension was considered worthy of treatment, and reflects a growing appreciation of the cardiovascular risks associated with even modest elevations of blood pressure.

It was over 150 years ago that high blood pressure was observed to be a consequence of glomerulonephritis. Several decades passed, however, before the reverse was also noted—namely, that hypertension could be a primary condition and that renal disease might be one of its outcomes. Because effective antihypertensive therapy was not yet available, the natural history of this condition—regardless of whether it began as hypertension or intrinsic renal disease—often culminated in end-stage renal failure. Routine measurement of blood pressure was not yet considered a necessary part of the physical examination, and hypertension generally went undiagnosed or unacknowledged. For many patients, the first known manifestation of their hypertension was the clinical picture of end-stage renal disease or other major events such as myocardial infarction, heart failure, or stroke. This period of the early history of hypertension, in which the kidney—either primarily or secondarily—appeared to be pivotal could be labeled the *renal era* of hypertension.

Clinical awareness

Despite excellent work by physiologists, pathologists, and especially clinical pioneers in the discipline of nephrology, the widespread awareness of hypertension has been created largely by statisticians and epidemiologists. Actuarial data generated by the life insurance industry, together with findings published from such epidemiologic sources as the Framingham Study, have shown that the relationship between blood pressure and the probability of cardiovascular events is a continuum. Accordingly, even small increases in blood pressure potentially carry a risk. Of course, the fact that high blood pressure may be associated with adverse cardiovascular outcomes does not, of itself, justify the use of blood-pressure-lowering therapy. The term *essential* hypertension actually implies that high blood pressure could be an appropriate response to an ongoing vascular pathology and might in fact be necessary to ensure adequate perfusion of vital organs. Accordingly, until recently physicians were appropriately cautious in undertaking the treatment of asymptomatic hypertension.

The chief breakthrough in the history of hypertension came from major clinical trials published for the first time in the 1970s and the 1980s, demonstrating significant reductions in such events as strokes and heart failure in patients treated for mild to moderate hypertension (2–4). Another major factor in providing incentives for the treatment of hypertension was the availability in more recent decades of innovative antihypertensive drugs, including beta blockers, angiotensin-converting enzyme (ACE) inhibitors, and calcium antagonists that effectively decrease blood pressure without causing unacceptable adverse effect. This period in the history of hypertension, in which this condition became popularized and understood as a result of major epidemiologic studies and clinical trials, could be termed the *epidemiologic era.*

The role of vascular biology

Our understanding of hypertension has continued to advance, however, and there has been perceptible progress even since to beginning of the 1990s. Two key factors have worked to challenge clinicians and investigators working in this area. First, it has become apparent that although stroke and some other cardiovascular complications have been reduced effectively by treatment, hypertensive patients still experience an unacceptably high incidence of ischemic heart disease. Part of the explanation for this disappointing outcome has been the realization that high blood pressure rarely exists alone but more typically is part of a syndrome of cardiovascular risk factors. These con-

Suki, WN and Massry SG (eds), Suki and Massry's Therapy of Renal Diseases and Related Disorders, Third Edition. ISBN 978-1-4757-6634-9.
©*1998, Kluwer Academic Publishers, Boston/Dordrecht/London. All rights reserved.*

comitant metabolic, cardiac, vascular, and renal changes are discussed in more detail below.

The second principal factor has been the growth of the disciplines of molecular and cellular biology, which are being applied increasingly to the study of vascular disease. It has become possible to study the mechanisms by which proliferative and degenerative changes occur in the vascular wall and to speculate how these pathologic changes could be exaggerated in hypertensive patients and could lead to premature coronary disease. It is becoming clear that these broader clinical and tissue characteristics of hypertension appear to be part of an inherited system of abnormalities that predispose to cardiovascular disease. Thus, the history of hypertension now appears to have moved into a new *vascular era* in which this condition serves as a paradigm that helps illustrate the fuller spectrum of cardiovascular diseases.

DIAGNOSIS OF HYPERTENSION

Over the years, there has been a steady reduction in the level of blood pressure at which a clinical diagnosis has been made. A vivid example of the data that have propelled these changes is shown in Figure 1. These findings are derived from the long-term follow-up of young and middle-aged men who were originally enrolled in the Multiple Risk Factor Intervention Trial (MRFIT) (5). A review of the relationship between diastolic blood pressure and the risk of a major cardiovascular event, as shown in Figure 1, suggests that the risk starts to accelerate as diastolic blood pressures enter the low 90s. This finding appears to confirm (see below) the recommendation that hypertension should be diagnosed when diastolic blood pressures fall into this range.

The importance of metabolic blood pressure

The data on systolic blood pressure clearly are more compelling. Cardiovascular risk appears to start increasing quite steeply with systolic blood pressures still in the 130s. Moreover, when compared with diastolic blood pressure, the risk associated with systolic hypertension appear to rise more steeply. Physicians generally have depended primarily on diastolic blood pressure values to guide the diagnosis of hypertension, and they might be surprised at the danger associated with relatively modest increases in systolic blood pressure. But actuarial data from life insurance sources appear to confirm this concept. As shown in Table 1, there are meaningful reductions in life expectancy in young to middle-aged men with relatively modest increases in systolic blood pressure.

This heightened awareness of the importance of systolic blood pressure has resulted in recent changes to diagnostic recommendations provided in the Fifth Report of the Joint National Committee on the Detection, Evaluation ad Treatment of High Blood Pressure (JNC V) (1). These recommendations are shown in detail in Table 2. As with its previous reports, the JNC continues to regard diastolic blood pressure of under 85 mmHg as being normal and has characterized the range of 85–89 mmHg as "high normal." No specific treatment is suggested for this latter range, although physicians are advised that such patients should be followed on a regular basis to determine whether or not they might fall into either the normal range or, alternatively, be shown to be hypertensive. When diastolic criteria are used, hypertension exists when the blood pressure values are 90 mmHg or higher. These measurements, obtained in the seated position, should be performed in duplicate and repeated on at least two further occasions to confirm the diagnosis.

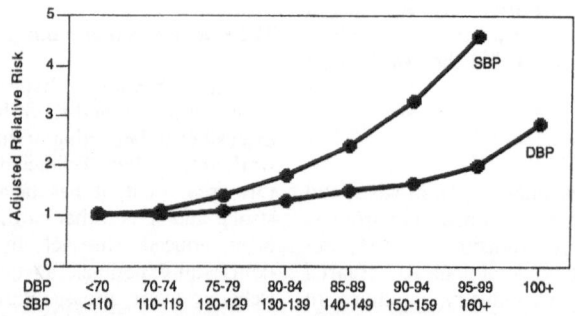

Adjusted Relative Risk of CV Mortality in Men Screened for MRFIT

Adapted from National High Blood Pressure Education Program Working Group. Arch Intern Med 153:186,1993

Figure 1. A comparison of the relative risks of cardiovascular (CV) mortality as a function of systolic (SBP) and diastolic blood pressure (DBP) in men screened for the Multiple Risk Factor Intervention Trial (MRFIT).

Table 1. Reduced life expectancy in men (years)

Systolic blood pressure	Age		
	35	45	55
130 mmHg	4	3	1
140 mmHg	9	6	4
150 mmHg	16	12	6

Report of Statistical Bureau, Metropolitan Life Insurance Co. (Based on experience of 26 life insurance companies.)

Table 2. Classification of blood pressure for adults aged 18 years and older[a]

Category	Systolic, mmHg	Diastolic, mmHg
Normal[b]	<130	<85
High normal	130–139	85–89
Hypertension[c]		
Stage 1 (mild)	140–159	90–99
Stage 2 (moderate)	160–179	100–109
Stage 3 (severe)	180–209	110–119
Stage 4 (very severe)	≥210	≥120

[a] Not taking antihypertensive drugs and not acutely ill. When systolic and diastolic pressures fall into different categories, the higher category should be selected to classify the individual's blood pressure status. For instance, 160/92 mmHg should be classified as Stage 2, and 180/120 mmHg should be classified as Stage 4. Isolated systolic hypertension is defined as a systolic blood pressure of 140 mmHg or more and a diastolic blood pressure of less than 90 mmHg and staged appropriately (e.g., 170/85 mmHg is defined as Stage 2 isolated systolic hypertension).

In addition to classifying stages of hypertension on the basis of average blood pressure levels, the clinician should specify presence or absence of target-organ disease and additional risk factors. For example, a patient with diabetes and a blood pressure of 142/94 mmHg plus left ventricular hypertrophy should be classified as having "Stage 1 hypertension with target-organ disease (left ventricular hypertrophy)" and with another major risk factor (diabetes)." This specificity is important for risk classification and management.

[b] Optimal blood pressure with respect to cardiovascular risk is less than 120 mmHg systolic and less than 80 mmHg diastolic. However, unusually low readings should be evaluated for clinical significance.

[c] Based on the average of two or more readings taken at each of two or more visits after an initial screening.

The systolic recommendations, as shown in Table 2, represent important new changes. Values in the range of 130–139 mmHg are now classed as "high normal," and true hypertension begins at 140 mmHg. Reference to Figure 1 confirms that systolic values in the 140s carry equally as much risk as diastolic values in the 90s and thus confirms the validity and importance of the JNC V diagnostic recommendations. It should also be noted that the systolic

Table 3. Independent predictors of carotid stenosis (Normotensive and hypertensive patients, *N* = 366)

Systolic BP ≥ 160 mmHg	7.5	<0.001
Diastolic BP < 75 mmHg	3.7	0.001

From Sutton-Tyrrell et al.: *Stroke* 24:355, 1993, with permission.

recommendations apply to all adults over the age of 18; these recommendations are not limited just to elderly patients of all ages or to any other age group. The JNC report further argues that hypertension should be diagnosed for either a high systolic or a high diastolic value; it is not necessary that both readings be in the hypertensive range. Except in young people, it is relatively uncommon for patients to have high diastolic but normal systolic values. Thus, it is quite likely that many patients will be diagnosed with hypertension primarily on the basis of increases in their systolic values.

More about blood pressure

It has long been appreciated by clinicians that systolic and diastolic blood pressures have different patterns with aging. Whereas systolic blood pressure tends to rise steadily throughout life, the diastolic pressure plateaus during young adulthood and middle age and actually starts to fall in later life. The physiologic explanation for these disparate patterns is complex, but it appears to be related primarily to progressive stiffening of the large and small vessels of the arterial circulation. The new concept of *vascular overload* recently has been described in detail (6). In essence, the three factors that contribute to overload are the systolic blood pressure, reflected waves (simply expressed, the rapid return of the pulse wave from more distal to more central parts of the arterial circulation), and reduced compliance (conceptually equivalent to increased arterial stiffness).

All three of these factors become especially important with aging. Reduced compliance actually is best predicted by the presence of an increased pulse pressure—that is, a relatively high systolic and a relatively low diastolic blood pressure. One clinical example of this is shown in Table 3 (7). In this observation of patients aged 65 or older, the presence of carotid disease (which is a useful noninvasive surrogate for coronary disease) was related separately to systolic and diastolic blood pressures. Not surprisingly, as shown in Table 3, high systolic pressures (≤160 mmHg) were strongly predictive of the presence of disease. But of great interest, patients with low diastolic values (*less than* 75 mmHg) were more likely than individuals with higher diastolic pressures to have evidence for significant carotid disease. Thus, especially in older individuals, the relationship between blood pressure and cardiovascular disease appears to be more complex than was previously though.

HYPERTENSION IN THE ELDERLY

The successful completion of major clinical trials of the treatment of hypertension in the elderly in the early 1990s has given strong support to the importance of diagnosing and treating this condition. It has long been known that hypertension, especially the increases in systolic blood pressure, is highly prevalent in older individuals. Increases in systolic blood pressure appear to occur as part of the aging process, and it is no surprise that hypertension can potentially be diagnosed in a large proportion of older individuals. Moreover, this process, which was once widely considered to be a normal part of aging, is associated with marked increases in the risks of major cardiovascular events (8). The differing contributions of systolic and diastolic blood pressures as predictors of risk were discussed earlier.

Because hypertension apparently is so common in elderly patients, it has been difficult to persuade physicians that the condition is worthy of treatment. There has been concern that if the elevated systolic blood pressure of the elderly is a reflection of progressive vascular changes, then antihypertensive treatment could in theory neutralize an appropriate compensatory mechanism required to sustain perfusion of critical circulation, thereby increasing rather than decreasing the risk of ischemic events. This concern has been highlighted by the alleged phenomenon of the J-shaped curve, a claim that excessive reduction of diastolic blood pressure—especially in older hypertensive individuals with underlying ischemic coronary disease—can actually precipitate fatal cardiovascular events (9).

These concerns have all been rebutted powerfully by the results of three pivotal clinical trials recently completed in elderly hypertensives. The Systolic Hypertension in the Elderly Program (SHEP) in the United States (10), the Medical Research Council (MRC) Trial in the Elderly performed in Britain (11), and the Swedish Trial in Old Patients (STOP) Hypertension Trial in Scandinavia (12) have all convincingly shown the benefit of treating elderly patients who have isolated or predominant systolic hypertension. These trials all produced highly significant reductions in strokes and in other critical cardiovascular events such as heart failure; there were also decreases in the incidence of cardiac and coronary events, although these findings were less convincing. Importantly, there were no upper age limits for these benefits; patients well into their 80s appeared to benefit just as much as younger patients and thus should be diagnosed and managed in a similar fashion.

The choice of drugs

The principal drugs used in these clinical trials were diuretics and beta blockers. It should be remembered that the time required to complete these studies, including the planning phase, patient recruitment, the multi-year clinical observations, and the time required to collect, analyze, and publish the data, adds up to a substantial period. Thus, at the time when these studies were originally conceived, the investigators responsible for their planning still regarded diuretics and beta blockers as appropriate contemporary drugs. Unfortunately, information concerning the prognostic effects of such newer agents as ACE inhibitors, alpha blockers, and calcium antagonists in this population is not yet available.

Despite the positive results in the studies in the elderly, it is important not to extrapolate these findings into recommendations for the treatment of younger individuals in whom different pathophysiologic mechanisms might be relevant (see below). Moreover, the highly selective fashion in which patients were chosen for the clinical trials in the elderly, especially SHEP (10), together with other questions and issues that arose during the conduct of these studies (10–12) should serve to emphasize that care must be taken in interpreting the roles of specific drug classes. Now that the benefits of antihypertensive treatment in the elderly have been established, physicians should individualize the selection of drugs for their patients based on the full picture of physical findings, concomitant conditions, and laboratory findings both before and during the administration of treatment.

THE SYNDROME CONCEPT

Hypertension rarely exists as high blood pressure alone. In general, it appears to comprise a syndrome of cardiovascular and metabolic abnormalities, some of which are listed in Table 4. Many of these features are independent risk factors, which helps explain why hypertension is so commonly associated with coronary disease and other atherosclerotic outcomes. A further key feature of this syndrome is that many of its components appear to be inherited. Although familial clusterings of findings can be explained by environmental as well as by genetic causes, the consistency with which these abnormalities are found in the offspring of hypertensive parents suggests a true inheritance, especially since these findings have been reported in adult offspring who have spent many years away from their parental homes. Although it seems most convenient to refer to these findings as the Hypertension Syndrome (13), the condition has also been referred to as Syndrome X (14) or the Deadly Quartet (15).

Table 4. Features of hypertension

---

1. High blood pressure: relationship between blood pressure fluctuations and cardiovascular events
2. Lipid abnormalities: amplified coronary risk in hypertension
3. Underlying insulin resistance and glucose intolerance
4. Trucal obesity
5. Early changes in renal functional reserve
6. Changes in left ventricular structure and function
7. Reduced compliance of arterial circulation

Blood pressure and the hypertension syndrome

The relationships between blood pressure and cardiovascular outcomes have already been discussed. The development of ambulatory blood pressure monitoring techniques, however, has further helped characterize possible relationships between blood pressure and outcomes. It has been shown that there is a clear circadian pattern (see Figure 2) of blood pressure throughout the 24-hour period; pressures tend to be high during the daytime hours, but then fall steadily during the evening to their lowest values during sleep. Blood pressure then rises sharply during the early morning hours. It is during this morning period that there appears to be an increased incidence of stroke and coronary ischemic events (16,17), perhaps influenced by the rapidly changing hemodynamic measurements. Neurohumoral factors are also activated in the morning, further adding to the challenge of finding antihypertensive therapy that is effective during this critical time period.

Lipid factors

Lipid abnormalities are closely associated with high blood pressure. Interestingly, the normotensive offspring of hypertensive parents can be shown to have significantly higher plasma total cholesterol values than carefully matched individuals who do not have a positive family history (18). Not surprisingly, therefore, epidemiologic surveys have shown a close link between cholesterol and blood pressure values in the general community (19), helping to explain why lipid abnormalities are so common in

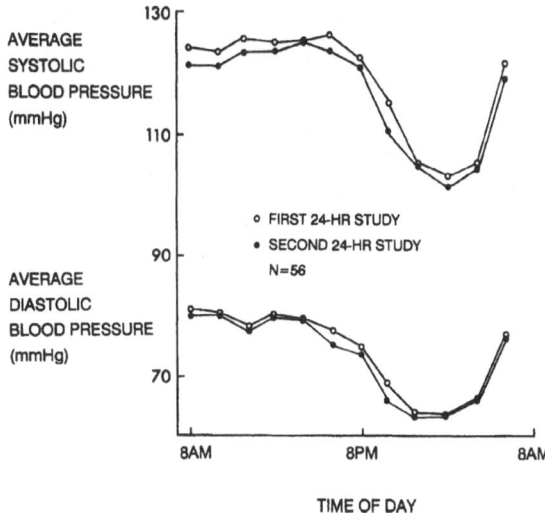

Figure 2. Whole-day blood pressure profiles, measured 2 weeks apart by ambulatory monitoring, in 56 normal volunteers undergoing their routine daily activities.

hypertension. Indeed, it has been suggested that 40% of hypertensive patients have unequivocal lipid abnormalities, whereas an additional 40% have borderline changes in their lipid profiles (1).

The concurrent presence of high blood pressure and high cholesterol measurements is of clinical importance, for there is an exaggerated risk of coronary events when these two risk factors occur together. This finding has therapeutic implications as well. For example, it has been demonstrated that effective reduction of coronary events during antihypertensive therapy requires a reduction both in blood pressure and in concomitant cholesterol abnormalities; treating just one or the other of these problems is less effective (20). The reason for the common concurrence of these two problems has not yet been fully elaborated. Possible explanations include a single common underlying etiology, such as increased sympathetic activity; it is also possible that LDL cholesterol itself might produce direct effects on arterial tissue that could increase vascular tone.

Glucose and insulin metabolism

Glucose intolerance frequently coexists with hypertension, especially in overweight persons. A major community survey has shown that hypertensive individuals are twice as likely as normotensives to have evidence for glucose intolerance (21). Interestingly, glucose intolerance is even more common in treated hypertensives, presumably reflecting the adverse effects of such commonly used agents as diuretics on insulin sensitivity (21).

Insulin resistance appears to be an intrinsic property of hypertension. Figure 3 shows the effects on plasma glucose and plasma insulin concentrations in carefully matched groups of normal volunteers and untreated hypertensives subjected to standard glucose tolerance testing (22). The hypertensives, who in this study were relatively lean, has a similar glucose profile to that in the normal volunteers, but it is quite clear that their plasma insulin concentrations throughout the period of hyperglycemia were approximately twice as high as in the normals. Thus, even though they are not necessarily clinically diabetic, hypertensives as a group appear to require more insulin than normals to clear glucose from the plasma.

This strong evidence for insulin resistance has been confirmed by other investigators (23,24). Even in young men with borderline hypertension, plasma insulin concentrations appear to be significantly higher than in normal controls, and it has also been shown that their insulin-mediated glucose uptake correlates inversely with systolic blood pressure (24). This trait might be inherited; as shown in Figure 4, normotensive young adults with a positive family history of hypertension have significantly higher fasting plasma insulin concentrations and insulin; glucose ratios (an index of insulin resistance) than their matched counterparts without a positive family history (18).

These increases in plasma insulin concentrations are not

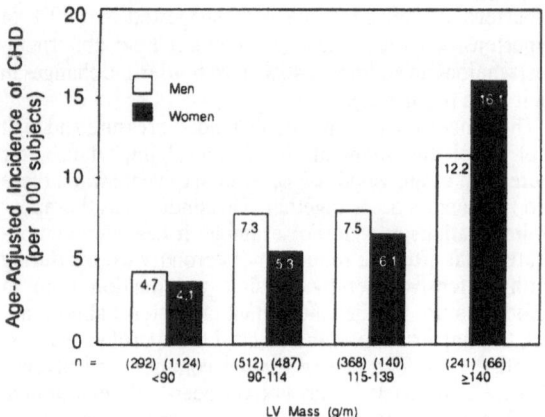

Figure 3. Mean (+SEM) plasma glucose concentrations before and after the 75 oral glucose challenge in the four experimental groups.

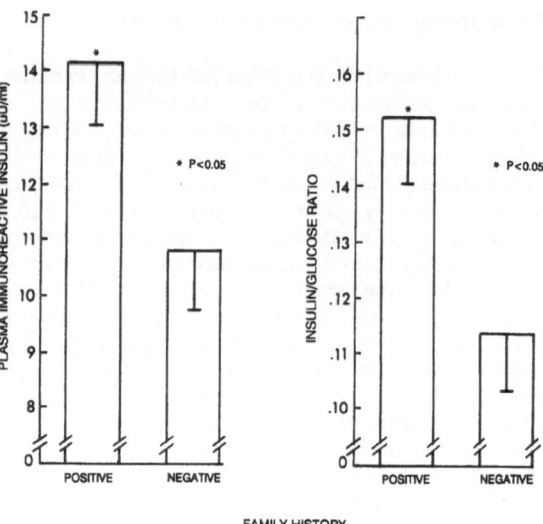

FAMILY HISTORY

Figure 4. Plasma immunoreactive insulin concentrations and the insulin-glucose ratio in subjects with and without a family history of hypertension. Plotted values are means + SEM.

benign. For example, there is preliminary evidence to indicate that hyperinsulinemia might actually contribute to the elevated blood pressure of hypertension: it decreases renal sodium excretion, induces hypertrophy of vascular smooth muscle, and stimulated the sympathetic nervous system, all of which are potential contributors to increased blood pressure (25). Insulin also produces adverse effects on the lipid profile. Hyperinsulinemia has been shown to be associated with increased triglyceride and decreased high-density lipoprotein (HDL) cholesterol plasma concentrations (26). This constellation of findings helps explain why disorders of glucose and insulin metabolism are though to be a major factor in accelerating the process of atherosclerosis (25,27). Indeed, this characteristic of hypertension might be one of the reasons for the high incidence of coronary events in these patients, a possibility that emphasizes the importance of treating hypertension as a full syndrome rather than simply as a problem of high blood pressure.

The heart in hypertension

Structural changes of the heart associated with hypertension have been viewed traditionally as a compensatory response to sustained high blood pressure. A changing perspective, based largely on studies using echocardiographic assessment of left ventricular wall thickness, now envisages left ventricular hypertrophy (LVH) as an independent risk factor for cardiovascular disease.

The presence of echocardiographic LVH portends serious cardiovascular consequences. As shown in Figure 5, both men and women experience substantial (3–4-fold) increases in coronary heart disease in the presence of LVH (28,29). The presence of LVH also is associated with increased cardiovascular mortality. Importantly, the influence of left ventricular mass on risk remains even after

statistical adjustments for other factors such as age, diastolic blood pressure, cigarette smoking, diabetes mellitus, antihypertensive treatment, and lipid abnormalities. Indeed, it has been claimed that echocardiographic LV mass is a better predictor of cardiovascular morbidity and mortality than blood pressure, cholesterol levels, or gender (30).

As with the other findings described as part of the hypertension syndrome, it appears that LVH also may be an inherited characteristic. When university students in their early 20s were divided into two groups on the basis of the presence or absence of a family history of hypertension, those with a positive family history had significantly greater echocardiographic measurements of septal and posterior wall thickness as well as left ventricular muscle mass index (31). Since there was no difference in blood pressure between these two groups of young people, it seems probable that some other inherited factor was responsible for the increased left ventricular wall thickness in the group with a positive family history.

Functional changes in the left ventricle also may appear early. Doppler echocardiography, which characterizes LV diastolic function by calculating the ratio of late to early LV diastolic filling, has also shown that young people with a family history of hypertension have changes in their diastolic function (32). Although the clinical importance—if any—of these early changes in diastolic function has not yet been established, this finding again highlights the familial tendency of the cardiovascular characteristics of hypertension.

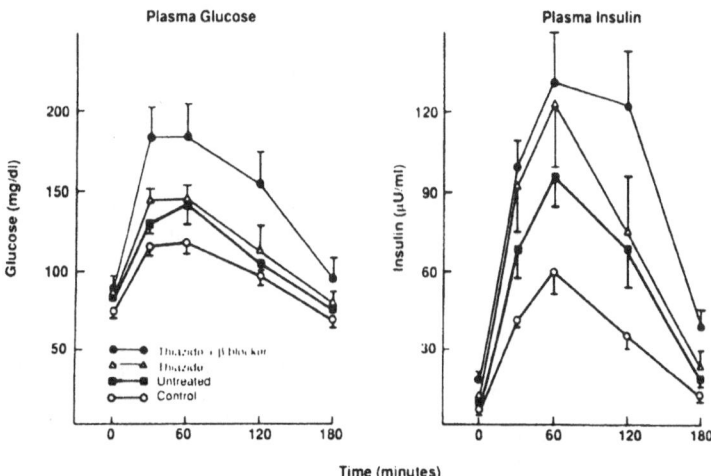

Figure 5. Left ventricular (LV) mass and age-adjusted, 4-year incidence of coronary heart disease (CHD) per 100 subjects in the Framingham Heart Study (corrected for height). Adapted from Levy D, et al.: *N Engl J Med* 322:1516, 1990.

Arterial changes

Changes similar to those occurring in the heart can also be demonstrated in the peripheral arterial circulation. Evidence for stiffening of both the large and small arteries—measured as reduced arterial compliance—occurs early in hypertension and can also be shown to be affected by the presence of a positive family history of hypertension (33). These arterial changes can be independent of blood pressure itself, and may be related to increased activity of the sympathetic nervous system and the renin–angiotensin system (34). The effector hormones of these systems, norepinephrine and angiotensin II, both have been shown to stimulate the growth of cardiac myocytes, and it is likely that a similar mechanism affects tissues of the peripheral arterial circulation. It is noteworthy that increased activity of both the sympathetic and the renin systems is a further characteristic of the offspring of hypertensive parents (18).

Hypertension and the kidney

As discussed earlier, there is a strong relationship between hypertension and kidney disease; renal pathology can cause hypertension, as well as result from it. Although detailed discussion of these renal changes is beyond the scope of this chapter, it is of interest to briefly consider the early changes in renal function that are part of the hypertension syndrome. An early renal characteristic of hypertension, similar to that observed in patients with juvenile diabetes, is a tendency to glomerular hypertension that apparently results, at least in part, from excessive vasoconstriction of the efferent arteriole. This change in glomeru-

lar hydraulic pressure produces an increased filtration fraction, resulting in increased glomerular filtration rate and a tendency to proteinuria. A study of normotensive young adults has indicated that those with a positive family history for hypertension already display evidence for increased glomerular filtration and a tendency to proteinuria, despite their own normal blood pressures (18).

Observations in young schoolchildren have extended this observation. Investigators tested the ability of children with one hyperensive parent to increase their endogenous creatinine clearance (a measure of glomerular filtration rate) in response to an oral protein load. This increase can be used as a measure of the renal functional reserve. A substantial number of these young children with a hypertensive parent were found to lack the ability to increase their creatinine clearance in response to the protein challenge (35).

Other studies have compared renal blood flow and glomerular filtration rate (based on clearance of PAH and inulin) in a large group of children and young adults classified according to the presence of absence of a family history of hypertension (36). Individuals with two hypertensive parents had significantly lower renal blood flow and higher renal vascular resistance and filtration fraction than the children of normotensive parents. Individuals with just one hypertensive parent were intermediate between the other two groups. It appears reasonable to assume that these inherited characteristics might be predictive of later renal disease, especially since glomerular hyperfiltration will probably lead to premature glomerulosclerosis. Nevertheless, in the absence of longitudinal observations in these individuals, we cannot be certain that these early functional changes will result in established renal disease.

EVALUATION OF HYPERTENSIVE PATIENTS

Blood pressure

Although the blood pressure criteria described earlier should usually be used to diagnose hypertension clinically, there is growing interest in the problem of white-coat hypertension. Studies with automated ambulatory blood pressure monitoring have shown that between 20% and 30% of patients with hypertension diagnosed in the office or clinic appear to have predominantly normal blood pressures at other times (37). The cause of this discrepancy is not clear, but white-coat hypertension can persist during multiple office visits (38). Patients with this condition have not yet been well characterized clinically, and we cannot be certain that they are truly normal. However, since their ambulatory blood pressures do not usually respond to antihypertensive therapy, it may be helpful to identify these individuals. The recent JNC V report (1) has recognized that 24-hour ambulatory blood pressure monitoring can be helpful in evaluating patients in whom white-coat hypertension is suspected. In general, this technique probably is not required in patients with an established susceptibility for cardiovascular events, including those with evidence for target organ involvement, concomitant risk factors, or a strong family history of cardiovascular disease.

Secondary hypertension

Underlying causes of hypertension are not common in adults, and there is little justification for extensive diagnostic studies on a routine basis. Renal disease is probably the most common cause of secondary hypertension and can readily be diagnosed by routine blood and urine studies. Abnormalities in potassium, which might be indicative of adrenocortical factors, are also easily found. Clues to the presence of underlying causes include hypertension of sudden onset. A poor blood pressure response to normally effective forms of treatment, or a loss of control in patients already established on treatment, especially if the effects of potentially conflicting drugs or poor patient compliance have been ruled out, is a further indicator of secondary hypertension.

Target organ damage

Evaluation of target organs affected by hypertension is critical. Evidence for changes in organs such as the kidneys, the heart, or the optic fundi provides an incentive for aggressive antihypertensive therapy and can provide a baseline for judging long-term responses. Moreover, findings such as renal dysfunction, proteinuria, or left ventricular hypertrophy can guide the selection of specific antihypertensive agents.

Cardiovascular risk assessment

Because high blood pressure is commonly associated with other cardiovascular risk factors such as lipid abnormalities, changes in glucose tolerance, and left ventricular hypertrophy, it is important to devise treatment strategies that address each of the risk factors in individual patients. It is improbable that patients will be adequately protected from coronary events if concomitant metabolic and cardiovascular risk factors are ignored. Information about the overall risk profile can guide the selection of antihypertensive therapy as well as suggest other forms of drug therapy or life-style modification.

Pretreatment baseline

Yet a further reason to perform pretreatment assessment is to provide a baseline against which possible drug-induced changes can be measured. Several of the commonly used antihypertensive agents produced effects on lipid metabolism, insulin sensitivity, electrolytes, and renal function; it is important to quantify potential adverse metabolic effects during long-term therapy.

Strategy for the routine workup

The overall clinical assessment of hypertensive patients can be accomplished conveniently and inexpensively. Indeed, a routine clinical chemistry profile, which includes lipid and glucose measurements obtained following an overnight fast, can provide useful information on risk factors, target organ involvement, and even some forms of secondary hypertension. Complete blood count, urinalysis, and electrocardiography (ECG) are further simple tests that can strengthen the evaluation. A careful 24-hour urine collection for creatinine, protein, and sodium is another inexpensive test that provides a valuable measure of renal function prior to therapy. Elevated plasma creatinine and reduced creatinine clearance indicate that renal dysfunction is present. Elevated plasma calcium and reduced plasma phosphorus concentrations raise the suspicion that primary hyperparathyroidism may be the cause of hypertension. Persistent hypokalemia points toward primary aldosteronism as the underlying cause of hypertension. Although the ECG is a useful screening test for ischemic heart disease and LVH, it lacks the sensitivity of echocardiography for measuring more subtle—and prognostically important—changes in the structure and function of the LV wall. Although potentially of great value, echocardiography is not yet recommended as part of the routine evaluation of every hypertensive patient.

ISSUES IN TREATMENT

Life-style changes

Hypertension most commonly is treated with antihypertensive drugs, but there remains a place for nonpharmacologic strategies. Although life-style modifications have never been tested in controlled clinical trials to determine whether they affect cardiovascular prognosis, they can favorably influence several risk factors. Weight loss, for example, is associated with improvement in the lipid profile, increased insulin sensitivity, and reduced sympathetic drive. Reduction of alcohol intake to one or two drinks daily is a further approach towards reducing blood pressure. Although results have been inconsistent, standard programs of aerobic exercise similarly are associated with a downward trend in blood pressure. Cessation of cigarette smoking removes a powerful cardiovascular risk factor. Moreover, since blood pressure is increased during the act of smoking and for a period of several minutes after each cigarette, it is likely that cessation of smoking in heavy smokers could have meaningful cumulative benefits on blood pressure as well. It is noteworthy that the Fifth Report of the JNC in 1993 has strongly advocated these lifestyle strategies as an important cornerstone of treatment and has additionally speculated that the application of these strategies in the community at large might have primary prevention effects on hypertension and cardiovascular disease.

Special groups

Because hypertension is so clinically diverse, there is a natural tendency to consider patients in different groups. These include the elderly; women; black patients; patients with diabetes mellitus; and patients with renal insufficiency.

As discussed previously, systolic hypertension in the elderly is an excellent target for antihypertensive therapy; there is a strong probability of protection against stroke and other cardiovascular events, and there appears to be no upper age limit to these benefits. Hypertension in women is relatively uncommon until the postmenopausal age groups. At that stage, hypertension becomes as common in women as in men, and the associated cardiovascular risk also approaches that observed in men. Interactions between antihypertensive drugs and postmenopausal hormone replacement therapy are not well understood, although there is evidence that estrogen replacement might reduce the incidence of hypertension and the likelihood of cardiovascular events.

Hypertension has always been common within the black community, and it carries a heavy toll of cerebrovascular and renal complications. Socioeconomic factors have played a part in the relatively poor response of black patients to antihypertensive therapy, but even when treatment is readily available there has been a tendency for certain complications—especially renal insufficiency—to progress. This finding may be explained partly by the widespread belief that hypertension in black patients responds well to diuretic therapy. Although this probably is true as far as blood pressure is concerned, diuretics may not be optimal for renal protection in this highly susceptible group. Although ACE inhibitors have not been specifically studied in black patients for this indication, their ability to preserve renal blood flow and decrease glomerular hyperfiltration might offer a further measure of protection against deteriorating renal function and glomerulosclerosis.

Diabetic patients with hypertension offer a special challenge because good prognosis depends on excellent control of both glucose metabolism and blood pressure. Renal protection, as in black patients, is a primary goal of antihypertensive therapy; the ACE inhibitors and calcium channel blockers might, in addition, offer protection against the accelerated atherosclerotic process that is characteristic of diabetes. These newer agents do not produce the adverse metabolic effects often attributed to diuretics and beta blockers; nevertheless, in patients with diabetes and renal insufficiency, diuretics are often necessary for adequate control of blood pressure.

Renal insufficiency

The special issues involved in managing hypertension in patients with renal insufficiency and other hypertension subgroups are dealt with elsewhere in this volume. Hypertension remains and important cause of end-stage renal disease in the United States. There is strong evidence that effective and aggressive management of hypertension slows the rate of decline of renal function in patients with renal insufficiency. Beyond this general observation, it has been noted that ACE inhibitors confer yet further benefits. Inhibition of the renin–angiotensin system within the kidney appears to reduce glomerular hypertension as well as protect glomerular basement membrane and mesangial structures. As a consequence, the renal functional reserve appears to be maintained, and typically there is a reduction in proteinuria (39). Care must be taken to avoid hyperkalemia when using these drugs, and an unexpected, large decrease in glomerular filtration rate could be an indication of unsuspected underlying bilateral renal artery disease. Some of the calcium channel blockers, including verapamil and diltiazem, may also have renal protective effects; there appear to be some differences among the dihydropyridine agents in their renal effects, and it is not yet possible to make firm recommendations regarding their use in hypertensive patients with renal disease.

SELECTING ANTIHYPERTENSIVE AGENTS

Controversy

Most physicians now believe that any of the currently available antihypertensive drugs, especially the ACE inhibitors, calcium channel blockers, alpha-adrenergic blockers, beta-adreneric blockers, and diuretics can be suitable for starting and maintaining antihypertensive therapy. Because hypertensive patients have differing underlying mechanisms for their high blood pressure, and also have differing concomitant risk factors and other diseases, this broad selection of drugs enables physicians to individualize treatment.

It was surprising, therefore, that the recent JNC V report

regressed to an earlier recommendation and suggested that diuretics and beta blockers be generally preferred as first-step treatment (1). Two rationales have been offered: first, that diuretics and beta blockers are the only drugs shown to produce significant reductions in stroke and other cardiovascular endpoints in controlled clinical trials; and second, that these older drugs are cheaper. These arguments are, at best, highly tenuous. Although it is true that these older drugs have been effective in preventing stroke and cardiovascular events, the most convincing evidence has been in elderly patients with isolated or predominant systolic hypertension. Studies using diuretics and beta blockers in younger patients selected for diastolic hypertension has been far less convincing, especially where coronary disease—which is the major cause of illness and death in hypertension—is concerned.

Thus, the JNC's extrapolation to the broad spectrum of hypertension seems unjustified. Moreover, it ignores indirect but progressively more convincing evidence from several sources that newer drug classes have beneficial effects on the heart, the kidneys, and the vasculature. Because long-term prospective studies of cardiovascular outcomes with these newer agents will not be completed for several years, it is appropriate that thoughtful physicians, confronting the full picture of cardiovascular risk in their hypertensive patients, will choose from among the full array of available agents. Moreover, even the JNC V report acknowledges that for patients with such major concomitant risk factors as lipid and glucose abnormalities—who might actually be a majority of hypertensives—individualized care should not necessarily begin with diuretics or beta blockers.

The rationale for treating hypertension

The objective of treating essential hypertension is to protect patients from major cardiovascular and renal events. It appears that almost any form of antihypertensive therapy can be effective in reducing the incidence of stroke and heart failure, suggesting that these are predominantly hemodynamic problems that can be addressed by a meaningful reduction in blood pressure. But it is clear that the reduction in coronary events in hypertensive patients during treatment has been disappointing (40), and it is evident that a fresh look must be given to this important problem.

Coronary disease in hypertension

Prevention of coronary disease remains the principal and largely unresolved therapeutic problem of hypertension. The connection between hypertension and coronary disease obviously is somewhat indirect, especially when it is realized that the coronary vessels comprise a low pressure circulation that is perfused only during diastole. Thus, while high levels of blood pressure can increase LV wall stress, which in turn can affect coronary reserve and produce ischemia, the development of coronary pathology clearly goes beyond high blood pressure alone. Rather, it is an issue of the multiple components that lead to atherosclerosis and alterations in coronary function.

The coronary hypothesis in hypertension

Three chief components contribute to vascular disease, which includes the coronary vessels. First are the proliferative–hypertrophic changes mediated by the neuroendocrine and paracrine abnormalities that characterize hypertension; second are the commonly recognized risk factors, such as chronic hypertension and the other metabolic and cardiovascular abnormalities that exaggerate and accelerate the underlying pathologic changes; and third are the effects of acute hemodynamic changes, specifically sharp fluctuations in blood pressure and heart rate that can destabilize the vascular lesions.

Hypertension can be regarded as an inherited condition in which fundamental abnormalities predispose to atherosclerosis. These factors could be excessive activity of the sympathetic and the renin–angiotensin systems, and in addition could include abnormalities of local tissue paracrine factors such as endothelin—which has powerful constrictor and growth-promoting properties—and nitric oxide, deficiencies of which could allow pathologic changes to advance more readily. The components of the hypertension syndrome, including all the endocrine, metabolic and cardiovascular abnormalities described earlier, clearly have the potential to contribute to these pathologic changes.

Relevance of age

Obviously, the proliferative and risk factor components are most important in young and middle-aged individuals, since they set up the pathologic changes that will eventually lead to clinical problems. In elderly people, however, especially those with isolated or predominant systolic hypertension, it is reasonable to assume that this form of vascular pathology is already far advanced. It seems probable that high blood pressure and tachycardia, especially acute hemodynamic changes or fluctuations, can provide the precipitating factors that convert an underlying pathologic lesion into a clinical event. Thus, in older individuals it is the hemodynamic factor that is the chief problem. Not surprisingly, therefore, the treatment of hypertension in the elderly—as exemplified by the SHEP, MRC, and STOP trials described earlier (10–12)—can be effective in preventing major cardiovascular events in these patients. It is likely that any antihypertensive drug that can lower blood pressure, and especially reduce blood pressure variability, will be effective in this setting.

Hemodynamic issues

Hemodynamic variability appears just as important as high blood pressure itself in leading to ischemic events (41). In this context, it is especially interesting that a subanalysis of

Table 5. Principal properties of major drug classes

	Diuretics	Beta blockers	Calcium channel blockers	ACE inhibitors	Alpha blockers
Hemodynamic	+	+	+	+	+
Metabolic	−	−	0	0	+
Antiproliferative	0	0 (?)	+	+	+

+, beneficial; −, adverse; 0, neutral.
Definitions:
Hemodynamic: effects on blood pressure (perhaps including ability to reduce its variability);
Metabolic: including effects on lipid and glucose metabolism;
Antiproliferative: human or experimental evidence of ability to inhibit adverse vascular wall proliferative changes.

the STOP trial (42) showed that patients receiving drug therapy, but whose on-treatment blood pressures were identical to those observed in a matched subgroup of placebo-treated patients, nevertheless had significantly fewer events. The only plausible explanation for this beneficial action of the drugs is that, even though they failed to produce chronic antihypertensive effects, they modified or buffered excessive hemodynamic variability.

It is also of note that the MRC trial in the elderly (11) reported that diuretics but not beta blockers appeared to protect against coronary events; it is easy to conjecture that beta blockers, despite their apparent antihypertensive efficacy, tend to "unmask" vasoconstrictor alpha receptors in arterial tissue through their blockade of beta receptors, thereby creating a situation of heightened hemodynamic variability. The mechanism by which those effects promote coronary events is not clear, but it could be speculated that surges of hemodynamic activity, either through associated neuroendocrine stimulation or perhaps by increasing LV wall stress, can acutely decrease coronary flow and additionally increase the likelihood of thrombotic activity.

The available drug classes

Based on this reasoning, the treatment of hypertension might differ in older patients as compared with younger individuals. In older patients, probably any antihypertensive agent that can reduce blood pressure and diminish variability will be effective in reducing events. On the other hand, the effective long-term protection of younger individuals seems to require that the proliferative and risk-factor aspects of hypertension be equally well addressed. Table 5 summarizes the effects of the five most commonly used drug groups on the hemodynamic, concomitant risk factor, and proliferative aspects hypertension.

It is obvious that all antihypertensive drugs currently available significantly reduce blood pressure. But as shown in Table 5, there appear to be important differences among the drug classes in their effects on concomitant risk factors and on proliferative changes. These differences might be important in selecting antihypertensive agents, especially for younger and middle-aged patients in whom prevention of atherosclerosis is a primary goal.

Final comment

The coronary hypothesis in hypertension still awaits further refinement and the application of appropriate clinical and basic science studies to test its validity. Nevertheless, it is already clear that hypertension is a condition linked to intrinsic abnormalities of vascular biology as well as to high blood pressure and other commonly recognized cardiovascular risk factors. The evaluation and treatment of hypertensive patients must take this full picture into account.

REFERENCES

1. Joint National Committee on Detection, Evaluation, and Treatment of High Blood Pressure: The Fifth Report of the Joint National Committee on Detection, Evaluation, and Treatment of High Blood Pressure (JNC V). *Arch Intern Med* 153:154–183, 1993.
2. Veterans Administration Cooperative Study Group on Antihypertensive Agents: Effects of treatment on morbidity in hypertension. II. Results in patients with diastolic blood pressure averaging 90 through 114 mmHg. *JAMA* 213:1143–1151, 1970.
3. Medical Research Council Working Party: MRC trial of treatment of mild hypertension: principal results. *Br Med J* 291:97–104, 1985.
4. Report by the Management Committee: The Australian Therapeutic Trial in Mild Hypertension. *Lancet* 1:1261–1267, 1980.
5. Stamler J, Stamler R, Neaton JD: Blood pressure and diastolic, and cardiovascular risks. U.S. Population Data. *Arch Intern Med* 153:598–615, 1993.

6. Franklin SF, Weber MA: Measuring hypertensive cardiovascular risk: the vascular overload concept. *Am Heart J*, in press.

7. Sutton-Tyrrell K et al.: *Stroke* 24:355, 1993.

8. Probstfield JL, Furberg CD: Systolic hypertension in the elderly: controlled or uncontrolled. In. ED Frohlich, ed, *Preventive Aspects of Coronary Heart Disease*. FA Davis Philadelphia, pp 65–84, 1990.

9. Hansson L: What are we really achieving with long-term drug therapy. *Am J Hypertens* 1:414–420, 1988.

10. Prevention of stroke by antihypertensive drug treatment in older persons with isolated systolic hypertension: final results of the Systolic Hypertension in the Elderly Program (SHEP). *JAMA* 265:3255–3264, 1991.

11. MRC Working Party: Medical Research Council Trial of Treatment of Hypertension in Older Adults: principal results. *Br Med J* 304:405–412, 1992.

12. Dahlof B, Lundholm L, Hansson L, et al.: Morbidity and mortality in the Swedish Trial in Old Patients with Hypertension (STOP-Hypertension). *Lancet* 338:1281–1285, 1991.

13. Alderman MH, Madhavan S, Ooi WL, et al.: Association of the renin–sodium profile with the risk of myocardial infarction in patients with hypertension. *N Engl J Med* 324:1098–1104, 1991.

14. Reaven GM: Role of insulin resistance in human disease (1988 Banting Lecture). *Diabetes* 37:1595–1607, 1989.

15. Kaplan NM: The deadly quartet: upper body obesity, glucose intolerance, hypertriglyceridemia, and hypertension. *Arch Intern Med* 139:1514–1520, 1989.

16. Agnoli A, Manfredi M, Mossuto L, Piccinelli A: Rapport entre les rythmes hemeronyctaux de la tension arterielle et sa pathogenie de l'insuffisance vasculaire cerebrale. *Rev Neurol* 131:597–606, 1975.

17. Meyers A, Dewar HA: Circumstances attending 100 sudden deaths from coronary artery disease with coroners' necropsies. *Br Heart J* 37:1133–1143, 1975.

18. Neutel JM, Smith DHG, Graettinger WF, Weber MA: Heredity and hypertension. Impact on metabolic characteristics. *Am Heart J* 124:435–440, 1992.

19. Hjerman I, Helgeland A, Holme I: *J Epidemiol Community Health* 32:117–124, 1978.

20. Sammelsson O, Wilmhelmsen L, Anderson OK, Pennert K, Berglund G: Cardiovascular morbidity in relation to change in blood pressure and serum cholesterol levels in treated hypertension. *JAMA* 285:1768–1776, 1987.

21. Modan M, Halkin H, Lusky A, Segal P, Fuchs Z, Chetrit A: Hyperinsulinemia is characterized by jointly disturbed plasma VLDL, LDL, and HDL levels, *Arteriosclerosis* 8:227–236, 1988.

22. Swislocki ALM, Hoffman BB, Reaven GM: Insulin resistance, glucose intolerance and hyperinsulinemia in patients with hypertension. *Am J Hypertens* 2:419–423, 1989.

23. Ferrannini E, Buzzigoli G, Bonadonna R, et al.: Insulin resistance in essential hypertension. *N Engl J Med* 320:702–706, 1989.

24. Falkner B, Hulman S, Tannenbaum J, Kushner H: Insulin resistance and blood pressure in young black men. *Hypertension* 15:705–711, 1990.

25. Reaven GM: Insulin resistance, hyperinsulinemia, and hypertriglyceridemia in the etiology and clinical course of hypertension. *Am J Med* 90 (Suppl 2A):7S–12S, 1991.

26. Zavaroni I, Bonora E, Pagliara M, et al.: Risk factors for coronary artery disease in health persons with hyperinsulinemia and normal glucose tolerance. *N Engl J Med* 320: 702–706, 1989.

27. Stamler R, Stamler J, Schoenberger JA, et al.: Relationship of glucose tolerance to prevalence of ECG abnormalities and to 5-year mortality from cardiovascular disease: findings of the Chicago Heart Association Detection Project in Industry. *J Chronic Dis* 32:817–828, 1979.

28. Levy D, Garrison RJ, Savage DD, Kannel WB, Castelli WP: Left ventricular mass and incidence of coronary heart disease in an elderly cohort: the Framingham Heart Study. *Ann Intern Med* 110:101–107, 1989.

29. Levy D, Garrison RJ, Savage DD, Kannel WB, Castelli WP: Prognostic implications of echocardiographically determined left ventricular mass in the Framingham Heart Study. *N Engl J Med* 322:1561–1566, 1990.

30. Koren MJ, Devereux RB, Casale PN, Savage DD, Laragh JH: Relation of left ventricular mass and geometry to morbidity and mortality in uncomplicated essential hypertension. *Ann Intern Med* 114:345–352, 1991.

31. Celentano A, Galderisi M, Garofalo M, et al.: Blood pressure and cardiac morphology in young children of hypertensive subjects. *J Hypertens* 6 (Suppl 4):S107–S109, 1988.

32. Graettinger WF, Neutel JM, Smith DHG, Weber MA: Left ventricular diastolic filling alterations in normotensive young adults with a family history of systemic hypertension. *Am J Cardiol* 68:51–56, 1991.

33. Weber MA, Smith DHG, Neutel JM, Graettinger WF: Arterial properties of early hypertension. *J Hum Hypertens* 5:417–423, 1991.

34. Neutel JM, Smith DHG, Graettinger WF, Weber MA: Dependency of arterial compliance on circulating neuroendocrine and metabolic factors in normal subjects. *Am J Cardiol* 69:1340–1344, 1992.

35. Grunfeld B, Perelstein E, Simsolo R, Gimenez M, Romero JC: Renal function reserve and microalbuminuria in offspring of hypertensive parents. *Hypertension* 15:257–261, 1990.

36. Van Hooft IMS, Grobbee DE, Derkx FHM, de Leeuw PW, Schalekamp MADH, Hofman A: Renal hemodynamics and the renin–angiotensin–aldosterone system in normotensive subjects with hypertensive and normotensive parents. *N Engl J Med* 324:1305–1311, 1991.

37. Drayer JIM, Weber MA, Nakamura DK: Automated ambulatory blood pressure monitoring: a study in age-matched normotensive and hypertensive men. *Am Heart J* 109:1334–1338, 1985.

38. Weber MA, Cheung DG, Graettinger WF, Lipson JL: Characterization of antihypertensive therapy by whole-day BP monitoring. *JAMA* 259(22):3281–3285, 1988.

39. Lewis EJ, Hunsicker LG, Bain RP, et al.: The effect of angiotensin-converting-enzyme inhibition on diabetic nephropathy. *N Engl J Med* 329:1456–1462, 1993.

40. MacMahon S, Peto R, Cutler J, Collin R, Sorlie P, Neaton J, Abbott R, Godwin J, Dyer A, Stamler J: Blood pressure, stroke and coronary heart disease. Part I: prolonged differences in blood pressure: prospective observational studies corrected for the regression dilution bias. *Lancet* 335:765–774, 1990.

41. Deedwania PC, Nelson JR: Pathophysiology of silent myocardial ischemia during daily life. *Circulation* 82:1296–1304, 1990.

42. Ekbom T, Dahlof B, Hansson L, Lindholm L, Oden A, Schersten B, Wester PO: The stroke preventive effect in elderly hypertensives cannot fully be explained by the reduction in office blood pressure—Insights from the Swedish Trial in Old Patients with Hypertension (STOP-Hypertension). *Blood Pressure* 1:168–172, 1992.

CHAPTER 70

Renal and Renovascular Hypertension

GEORGES MOURAD, JEAN-MICHEL HALIMI, JEAN RIBSTEIN & ALBERT MIMRAN

INTRODUCTION

Renal parenchymal disease and renovascular abnormalities are the most common causes of secondary hypertension. In clinical practice, a search for renal disease (i.e., proteinuria, abnormal urinary sediment, increased serum creatinine) should be undertaken in the presence of any newly diagnosed hypertension; however, only selected patients should be screened for renovascular disease. In recent years, the challenge in the management of patients with renal parenchymal disease has focused on the influence of strict control of hypertension on the rate of deterioration of renal function with time. In several experimental models, the use of antihypertensive agents has proved efficient in preventing the decline in renal function as well as the extent of glomerulosclerosis; interestingly, all antihypertensive medications were not equally effective in this regard. A number of questions remain unsettled in humans: Can adequate control of blood pressure slow down renal deterioration? Which drug should be used? What is the optimal level of arterial pressure? Although ischemic renovascular disease has recently emerged as an important cause of renal failure, the potential of revascularization to improve or preserve renal function is still a matter of debate.

RENAL PARENCHYMAL DISEASES AND DIALYSIS

Hypertension may be present in patients with normal serum creatinine, but its prevalence strikingly increases with the progression of the decline in renal function. Whether the development and maintenance of hypertension results from the progression of renal lesions or is the main reason for functional deterioration is often difficult to establish. Nevertheless, it is universally accepted that optimal control of hypertension is crucial in the management of these patients.

Treatment of hypertension in acute renal disease

Hypertension associated with acute renal disease is usually volume mediated (as suggested by the usual favorable response to volume depletion) and subsides with resolution of the underlying process. Hypertension occurs in approximately 40% of patients with acute renal failure (1); however, its prevalence is higher in vascular and glomerular diseases (73%) than in tubular necrosis (15%). In the latter group, hypertension mainly results from the rapid reduction in glomerular filtration rate and consequently salt and water retention, whereas in the acute nephritic syndrome, hypertension may be present in the absence of a marked decline in glomerular filtration rate. Surprisingly, in rapidly progressive glomerulonephritis, blood pressure is normal or slightly elevated, even in patients with severe renal failure and fluid retention.

Induction of abundant diuresis by high-dose, intravenous diuretics (i.e., furosemide 500–1000 mg/day) or rapid ultrafiltration is usually associated with the return of blood pressure to normal. In addition to the removal of excess fluid, dialysis may be transiently indicated to relieve severe uremic symptoms. When antihypertensive drugs are needed, calcium antagonists (CAs) or other vasodilators are the most useful agents. Since in the acute phase of renal failure plasma renin activity is normal or depressed, beta blockers and angiotensin-converting enzyme (ACE) inhibitors are not expected to be of great value except in patients in whom activation of the renin–angiotensin system is achieved by vigorous volume depletion.

Rationale for treating hypertension in chronic renal parenchymal disease

As shown in Table 1, the prevalence of hypertension varies according to the nature of the renal lesions and significantly increases with the degree of renal failure (from 20% of patients with near normal renal function (2) to 85%–90% in end-stage renal failure), age, male sex, and genetic

Suki, WN and Massry SG (eds), Suki and Massry's Therapy of Renal Diseases and Related Disorders, Third Edition. ISBN 978-1-4757-6634-9.

Table 1. Prevalence of hypertension in renal parenchymal diseases

Renal pathology	% hypertensive
Glomerular diseases	50
Membranoproliferative GN	85
Focal and segmental glomerulosclerosis	65
Membranous GN	51
IgA nephropathy	43
Minimal change disease	34
Polycystic kidney disease	50–75
Pyelonephritis and analgesic nephropathy	20–30
Vascular diseases (vasculitis, HUS, . . .)	70

Table 2. Mechanisms of hypertension in renal parenchymal disease

Extracellular fluid volume expansion
   Positive correlation between blood pressure and blood volume or exchangeable sodium; favorable effect of diuretics and sodium restriction in nondialysis patients, and ultrafiltration in dialysis patients

Activation of "pressor" systems
   Renin–angiotensin system (? intrarenal > systemic)
   Increased sympathetic nervous system activity
   Antidiuretic hormone
   Endothelin

Deficiency of "depressor" systems
   Kinins?
   Vasodilator prostaglandins
   Atrial natriuretic peptide
   Nitric oxide (through accumulation of the endogenous arginine analogue antagonist ADMA)
   Medullary neutral lipid

predisposition to hypertension. Other reported factors include geographic variations—20%–30% in patients with chronic pyelonephritis and analgesic nephropathy in Europe and North America versus 50% in Australia.

The mechanisms of the development and maintenance of hypertension in patients with chronic renal parenchymal disease are summarized in Table 2.

Although no specific data are available, it is likely that adequate control of blood pressure is associated with a decrease in cardiovascular mortality and morbidity in patients with renal parenchymal diseases, as is the case in patients with essential hypertension. In addition, a beneficial effect of blood pressure control on the progression of renal failure has been unequivocally demonstrated in patients with malignant hypertension (3) and in those with clinical diabetic nephropathy, in whom antihypertensive treatment was shown to reduce the slope of the reciprocal of plasma creatinine versus time (4,5); treatment also prevented the progression from incipient to clinical nephropathy (6). Whether this finding holds true in nondiabetic renal disease is subject to debate. Three important issues are open to discussion:

1. Does blood pressure control retard the progression of renal deterioration? When the progression of renal failure was retrospectively evaluated in 86 patients with various causes of renal failure on maintenance dialysis, it was observed that patients with diastolic blood pressure of 90 mmHg or less had a slower decline in their predialysis renal function than those with diastolic blood pressure of more than 90 mmHg (7). In a prospective study conducted in 17 patients, it was demonstrated that additional reduction of diastolic pressure from 93 to 90 mmHg was associated with a significant change in the slope of the decline in renal function in most patients (8). In contrast, other studies have suggested that for a similar degree of blood pressure control, the initial nature and severity of the disease are primary determinants of the rate of progression of renal failure (9).

2. Is there any particular benefit associated with the use of specific antihypertensive agents? Animal studies demonstrated a strong beneficial effect of ACE inhibitors when compared to other antihypertensive agents in

the progression of the renal lesions observed in streptozotocin-induced diabetes and subtotal nephrectomy (10); however, the clinical evidence to support this proposition is rather scarce. In short-term studies assessing the effect of ACE inhibitors in patients with chronic renal failure of various etiologies and nephrotic-range proteinuria, it was demonstrated that arterial pressure control by ACE inhibitors resulted in a decrease in proteinuria, whereas the use of atenolol or CAs such as nifedipine or nitrendipine did not reduce proteinuria despite a similar effect on arterial pressure. The filtration fraction only fell in response to ACE inhibitors, whereas it remained unchanged with the other treatments, thus suggesting that the antiproteinuric effect of ACE inhibitors may be a result of preferential postglomerular dilation and possibly a decrease in intraglomerular capillary pressure (11). The long-term effect of ACE inhibitors was assessed in 30 patients with a progressive decline in renal function during a 12–24-month period during which hypertension was controlled by propranolol, hydralazine, and furosemide; the switch to captopril was associated with similar control of blood pressure and a complete arrest of the progression of renal failure as assessed by the reciprocal of serum creatinine and isotopic evaluation of glomerular filtration rate for the remaining 33 months of follow-up (12). No difference in the rate of progression of renal failure was observed when nifedipine and captopril were compared prospectively in parallel groups during a follow-up period of 3 years (13). It is important to emphasize that the effect of antihypertensive treatment on the progression of renal disease was shown to be related to the extent of the decrease in proteinuria within a follow-up period of 24 months, whatever the class of medication used (14). Actually, ACE inhibitors seem to be more effective than beta blockers in reducing proteinuria (15).

3. Finally, what is the optimal level of blood pressure that should be achieved? Although interesting studies provided evidence that antihypertensive treatment associated with a small diastolic blood pressure decline (from 78 to 73 mmHg) resulted in significant prevention of the progression from incipient to clinical nephropathy in normotensive patients with insulin-dependent diabetes mellitus (6), no study addressed this issue in patients with nondiabetic renal disease. It is reasonable to assume that all efforts should be undertaken in order to achieve a final diastolic blood pressure of 85 mmHg or less, at least in patients without evidence of atheromatous disease. To date, no argument for the superiority of any class of antihypertensive agent has been provided.

Practical aspects of treatment before dialysis (Table 3)

REDUCTION IN DIETARY SODIUM AND DIURETIC THERAPY

As a general rule, restriction of sodium to 80–100 mmol/day and water to 1000–1500 mL/day should be the first step of management. With this approach, blood pressure is usually lowered in most patients with renal parenchymal disease. If sodium restriction is insufficient or not accepted, diuretics may be added. The efficacy of thiazide diuretics is limited in chronic renal failure (CRF), and these drugs are generally considered to be ineffective when glomerular filtration rate is lower than 30 mL/min; however, a synergistic effect with loop diuretics may be observed. Loop-acting diuretics promote sodium and water excretion even in advanced renal failure, and large doses (500–1000 mg/day) may be used without major side effects. Potassium-sparing agents given alone are contraindicated in CRF due to the high risk of hyperkalemia, especially in patients with a glomerular filtration rate less than 50 mL/min, hyporeninemic hypoaldosteronism such as diabetics, interstitial nephritis, and polycystic kidney disease, as well as subjects chronically treated by ACE inhibitors.

Worsening of renal function may be observed during diuretic treatment; body weight, orthostatic and clinostatic blood pressure, and renal function should be carefully assessed in order to achieve optimal "dry weight." Interestingly, it was observed in a retrospective study that long-term use of diuretics was associated with a worse evolution of renal function than other antihypertensive agents (16).

If blood pressure is not controlled, hypotensive drugs are indicated.

HYPOTENSIVE DRUGS

Drugs used in chronic renal failure are essentially the same as those used in patients with normal renal function; however, dose reduction may be required with the use of drugs

Table 3. Antihypertensive drugs in renal parenchymal disease

Class	Products	Dosage (mg/day)		Common side effects in CRF
		Initial	Maximum	
Diuretics	Hydrochlorothiazide	25	100	Prerenal acute renal failure
	Furosemide	40	500–1000	Hypokalemia, metabolic alkalosis, hyponatremia
				Hyperuricemia and gout
β-blockers	Propranolol	40	480	Orthostatic hypotension and bradycardia
	Pindolol	10	60	Decrease in renal blood flow
	Atenolol	25	100	
α- and β-blockers	Labetalol	200	1000	
α-blockers	Prazosin	1	20	Orthostatic hypotension
	Terazosin	1	20	Salt retention
Central agents	Clonidine	0.2	1	Salt retention (associated with diuretics)
	Methyldopa	500	1500	Hypotension
ACE inhibitors	Captopril	25	100	Hyperkalemia
	Enalapril	5	20	Acute renal failure, particularly in patients with renal ischemia (hypovolemic patients, diuretics, cardiac failure)
				Acute renal failure in patients with bilateral RAS or RAS in a single kidney
Calcium antagonists	Nifedipine	20	100	Flush
	Diltiazem	60	360	Peripheral edema
	Nicardipine	20	100	
Vasodilators	Minoxidil	5	20	Salt retention (should be associated with diuretics)
	Hydralazine	50	150	Tachycardia

with pharmacokinetic characteristics dependent on glomerular filtration rate. Usually, hypotension is the first symptom of overdose.

In clinical practice, except for ACE inhibitors, no consistent reduction of daily dosage is required. It is well demonstrated that ACE inhibitor treatment is associated with drug accumulation in CRF. The maximal recommended dose of these agents is 50% of the usual dose given to patients with normal renal function. In addition, doses of less than 20% of the usual dose should be given initially to patients already on diuretic therapy in order to avoid a drastic fall in arterial pressure. Finally, since atheromatous renovascular disease may often be present in older patients with progressive renal deterioration, serum creatinine should be measured within 1 week following initiation of treatment.

Whatever the means used to control blood pressure, initiation of treatment and effective lowering of blood pressure usually result in a decrease in renal perfusion and worsening of renal failure. In the majority of cases, the initial deterioration is only transient, and the rate of progression of renal failure is decreased in the long term.

OTHER RECOMMENDATIONS.

In addition to hypertension, patients with CRF usually have other risk factors of cardiovascular disease: hyperlipidemia, obesity, alcohol, diabetes, and smoking. Meticulous attention must be given to the elimination or treatment of these factors in order to improve blood pressure control and decrease cardiovascular mortality.

Treatment of hypertension in dialysis patients

As early as 1969, it was shown that in 35 of 40 hypertensive patients with end-stage renal disease, blood pressure became normal when dry weight was obtained by dialysis; in the five patients in whom blood pressure remained elevated despite fluid removal, plasma renin activity was 10 times higher than in the volume-responsive group (17). These observations led to the individualization of the so-called *volume-dependent* and *renin-dependent* types of hypertension. As recently shown by Charra et al. (18), gentle dialysis treatment for 8 hours three times per week provides a perfect control of arterial pressure in almost all patients (98% of 445), without any need of antihypertensive drugs; this study suggests that persistence of hypertension in dialysis patients indicates nonoptimal fluid removal rather than activation of the pressor compounds. Some practical measures may be helpful in providing adequate fluid removal while alleviating hypotension: 1) low-rate ultrafiltration over a period of time higher than the usual 3–4 hours of dialysis; 2) the use of a dialysate with a sodium concentration of 138–142 mmol/L or more, and newer dialysis membranes allowing unlimited ultrafiltration; and 3) dietary sodium and water restriction in anuric patients in order to limit the interdialytic weight gain.

In those patients in whom ultrafiltration and maintenance of an appropriate dry weight do not adequately control hypertension, antihypertensive medications are indicated. Most drugs increase vascular instability and may cause frequent and profound hypotensive episodes during dialysis. Thus, dosage and schedule must be arranged in order to decrease the action of these drugs during dialysis sessions. In our experience, the tolerance to CAs and low-dose ACE inhibitors is usually good, whereas central agents and peripheral α_1-adrenergic antagonists often cause drastic arterial pressure decrements during dialysis. Centrally acting drugs such as clonidine and related compounds may be responsible for rebound hypertension resulting from the rapid removal of the medications by dialysis.

The availability of new drugs and dialysis techniques and the inconvenience of anemia, increased transfusion requirements, loss of residual renal function, and permanent hypotension associated with the anephric state have made the use of binephrectomy no longer necessary for the treatment of hypertension.

Hypertension and recombinant human erythropoietin (rhEpo)

In early trials, 35%–45% of dialysis patients receiving rhEpo became hypertensive within 3 months following initiation of treatment, more frequently when hematocrit was rapidly corrected (≥1.5%/week) (19). A few cases of malignant hypertension with seizures were reported. rhEpo-induced hypertension was attributed to an increase in total peripheral resistance, due to the suppression of anemia-associated vasodilation and a rise in blood viscosity, proportional to the increment in hematocrit. However, volume expansion and a direct vasoconstrictive effect of rhEpo may play an important role.

Prevention of rhEpo-associated hypertension may be obtained by administration of small doses of rhEpo, the use of the subcutaneous route, the monitoring of hematocrit every 2 weeks, and reduction of rhEpo doses according to hematocrit. The target level of hematocrit should be 35% or less in normotensive and 30% or less in previously hypertensive patients. rhEpo must be transiently withdrawn when hematocrit increases abruptly (≥5% after 3–4 weeks of treatment). In patients with rhEpo-associated hypertension and neurological symptoms, a phlebotomy may be performed (-300 mL of blood). Dialysis-induced ultrafiltration (with or without hemodilution), vasodilators, and beta blockers may be indicated.

ACCELERATED HYPERTENSION

The terms *malignant hypertension* and *accelerated hypertension* currently refer to the same clinical condition, characterized by a diastolic arterial pressure above 130 mmHg, retinal hemorrhages, and exudates with or without papilledema and progressive renal impairment. Renal failure results from rapid glomerular ischemia due to fibrinoid necrosis and proliferative endarteritis of interlobular arteries and downstream arterioles. A renal underlying disease was detected in approximately 50% of patients in earlier series and 80% in more recent ones (3), including renal artery stenosis (up to 41% of such patients) (20), glomerulonephritis, IgA nephropathy, and the antiphospholipid syndrome. Factors predisposing to malignant hypertension include discontinuation of drug treatment and smoking (21). Although formal epidemiological surveys have not been conducted, malignant hypertension has probably become a rare disease in westernized countries (3) due to the wide availability and efficacy of antihypertensive treatments, whereas its prevalence is still significant in less developed areas (22).

Since high blood pressure per se is the major determinant of visceral complications, treatment should aim to reduce blood pressure by all means available. Parenteral vasodilating agents such as sodium nitroprusside, diazoxide (given as a small loading dose and subsequent maintenance doses), and more recently nicardipine are most useful (Table 4). However, the use of any powerful drug is hampered by the risk of an abrupt fall in arterial pressure with attendant neurological complications, including blindness. Thus, except for patients with dissecting aneurysm of the aorta and acute left ventricular failure, immediate lowering of arterial pressure should be avoided; in the presence of hypertensive encephalopathy, the decrease in arterial pressure should be progressive (20%–25% reduction of mean arterial pressure over 3–6 hours) and carefully monitored (target pressure no lower than 180/100 mmHg within the first 48 hours except in truly recent diseases, such as acute glomerulonephritis in a child).

Several oral medications (including diuretics, beta blockers, or other sympatholytic drugs, often given in combination) also proved capable of halting the course of malignant hypertension (22). It was claimed that some drugs might have salutary renal effects in addition to the lowering of arterial pressure (23). Since the renin–angiotensin

Table 4. Selected medications used in the treatment of acute hypertension

Drug	Administration	Action		Dosage			Comments
		Onset	Duration	Initial	Maximal	Units	
Vasodilators[a]							
Sodium nitroprusside	I.V. infusion	<1 min	2–3 min	0.25	10	µg/kg/min	Most hypertensive emergencies, when fine titration desirable. May worsen intracranial hypertension. Risk of toxicity beyond 48 hr, higher in hepatic and renal failure
Nicardipine	I.V. infusion	1–5 min	3–6 hr	5	15	mg/hr	Most hypertensive emergencies. Local reaction of peripheral veins beyond 48 hr
Adrenergic inhibitors[b]							
α Phentolamine mesylate	I.V. bolus I.V. infusion	1 min	5 min	5 1	20 20	mg µg/min	Catecholamine excess
α + β Labetalol	I.V. bolus I.V. infusion	5–10 min	3–6 hr	1 1	3 5	mg/kg µg/kg/min	Most hypertensive emergencies, except acute heart failure
β Esmolol	I.V. bolus then infusion	1 min	30 min	500 50	200	µg/kg/min "	Aortic dissection, postoperative
Central Clonidine	I.M.	1 hr	4–8 hr	0.15	0.9	mg/dose	
Angiotensin-converting enzyme inhibitors							
Enalapril	I.V. bolus	2–4 hr	8–12 hr	1.25	5	mg/6 hr	Acute left ventricular failure
Captopril	Oral	30 min	6 hr	12.5	50	mg	Monitor renal function in the presence of sodium depletion and atherosclerosis
Diuretics[c]							
Furosemide	I.V. oral	10 min 1 hr	3–6 hr 12–18 hr	20	250–500 (in renal failure)	mg	Mild vasodilating effect prior to diuresis

[a] Other agents include glyceryl trinitrate and hydralazine; nifedipine 10–20 mg qid may also be used orally, but titration is not precise.
[b] Other agents include trimetaphan camsylate, urapidil, ganfacine, methyldopa.
[c] Other agents include bumetanide.

system is highly activated, it was claimed that ACE inhibitors may be more efficient than previously available agents. However, the use of ACE inhibitors (often associated with diuretics) may be complicated by a consistent and sometimes dramatic deterioration of renal function resulting from impaired renal autoregulation due to diseased small renal vessels. Nevertheless, several reports suggest that inhibition of the renin–angiotensin system may provide a mean of reversing the process of malignant nephrosclerosis, which may lead to interruption of dialysis in some patients (24).

UNILATERAL PARENCHYMAL RENAL DISEASE

More than four decades ago, Smith (25) reviewed 47 selected cases in which ablation of a unilateral small kidney resulted in cure of hypertension; the primary renal disease included arterial occlusion, pyelonephritis, hypoplasia, radiation sclerosis, tumor, compressive cyst, and hydronephrosis. Subsequent larger series indicated that the success rate was only one in four patients operated upon, and renal artery stenosis emerged as the only common cause of "surgically curable" hypertension.

Hydronephrosis

An increase in arterial pressure may accompany the pain of renal colic. In selected patients with short-term hydronephrosis and hypertension, successful restoration of urine flow was followed by a reduction in arterial pressure, and activation of the renin–angiotensin system was documented in several such cases (26). Most patients with long-standing hydronephrosis are normotensive. Hypertension was actually noted in 20 of 101 consecutive patients with unilateral hydronephrosis and in 23 of 101 age- and sex-matched control subjects; higher age and smaller estimated kidney volume were noted in hypertensive as compared to normotensive cases. Surgical treatment (14 nephrectomies, 12 ureteroplasties) resulted in sustained cure of hypertension in 15 patients; the renal-vein renin ratio was 1.5 or greater in most cured patients (27). In another study, hypertension was present in only 10 of 101 adults presenting with unilateral ureteropelvic junction obstruction and persisted in eight of them postoperatively (28). Of note, in experimental unilateral ureteral occlusion, hypertension tends to resolve with time even though renal injury often progresses (29). Taken together, these data suggest that hydronephrosis rarely cause permanent hypertension and that the surgical decision should be based on urological considerations.

Chronic atrophic pyelonephritis and segmental hypoplasia

Atrophic pyelonephritis is a form of renal scarring, frequently associated with vesicoureteral reflux and recurrent urinary infections. In two adult series, hypertension was present in 10 of 45 (30) and 12 of 29 patients (31); arterial pressure declined in only one third of patients in whom a unilateral pyelonephritic kidney was removed. The finding of extensive parietal thickening and luminal narrowing in the interlobar and arcuate arteries suggested that ischemia was the cause of both parenchymal loss and hypertension (30). However, peripheral renin activity and the renal vein-renin ratio were usually within normal limits (31). In addition, increased arterial pressure was associated with no measurable change in plasma renin activity in a dog model of vesicoureteral reflux combined with ascending infection (29). In fact, the pathogenesis of renal atrophy is obscure, probably multifactorial, and the role of chronic pyelonephritis as a cause of hypertension has probably been overestimated. A number of adult patients may present with essential hypertension coincidental to chronic interstitial nephritis; in addition, hypertensive subjects may be more vulnerable to urinary infection than the general population (32).

The spectrum of renal dysplasia encompasses several heterogeneous malformations characterized by abnormal parenchymal development commonly associated with urinary tract obstruction but not hypertension. No convincing data support the role of global hypoplasia as a cause of hypertension, in contrast with segmental hypoplasia, first identified by Ask-Upmark. In an autopsy study of 11,058 adults, 31 cases of aglomerular segmental hypoplasia (half of them hypertensive) were found among 144 subjects with a small unilateral kidney; in addition, unilateral nephrectomy improved or cured hypertension in 12 of 21 patients followed up for more than 1 year, whereas partial nephrectomy constantly failed to alter arterial pressure (33).

It is often suspected that failure of the removal of a unilateral small kidney to improve hypertension results from coexistent renal damage in the remaining kidney. Although this is often the case, it is noteworthy that in eight patients presenting with hypertension and a unilateral small kidney (secondary to unilateral agenesis or dysplasia and reflux), a significant fibrodysplasic stenosis was present on the artery supplying the contralateral kidney; revascularization led to normalization of arterial pressure in all cases (34).

Renal trauma, extracorporeal shock wave lithotripsy, and radiation nephritis

Perinephric hemorrhage following blunt trauma often goes unnoticed (35) and may result in hypertension after intervals varying from a few days to several years. The hematoma plays the same role as cellophane wrapped around one or both kidneys in experimental models of hypertension (the *Page kidney*). In humans as well as animals, elevated peripheral renin activity and the efficacy of blockade of the renin system argue for an angiotensinogenic mechanism (36). Hypertension developing early after injury may resolve spontaneously over the ensuing months (37) and should be treated conservatively. Although partial nephrectomy was advocated in some cases of persistant hypertension (38), removal of the whole kidney is the method of choice; cure or improvement of hypertension was documented in 15 of 17 such patients (35), whereas percutaneous drainage often failed, especially when a fibrous capsule was present (39). Other mechanisms may lead to hypertension after trauma, including arteriovenous fistulae secondary to penetrating wounds and renal artery occlusion following road traffic accidents.

Extracorporeal shock wave lithotripsy is thought to create renal ischemic changes and/or perirenal hematoma with alterations in arterial pressure and transient proteinuria (40). The clinical relevance of such observations warrants further investigation, since in the largest series to date (731 patients), the rise in diastolic arterial pressure averaged 0.8 mmHg and the incidence of de novo hypertension 2.4%, as compared to a decrease of 0.9 mmHg in 171 controls treated by ureteroscopy or spontaneous stone passage (41).

Hypertension is almost constant when renal irradiation results in renal vascular damage (42). Progression to the accelerated stage may occur in approximately 50% of cases with early hypertension and 30% of those with later onset (more than 18 months). Although a cure of hypertension by nephrectomy was reported in two cases of unilateral radiation nephropathy (43), medical management is preferred, especially when a long time interval elapsed between irradiation and the occurrence of hypertension and when the renal insult is bilateral. Inhibitors of the renin–angiotensin system are expected to be efficient. In fact, in a rat model of unilateral renal irradiation in which hypertension precedes renal failure by several weeks, enalapril reduced glomerular sclerosis more markedly than hydrochlorothiazide (44).

RENOVASCULAR DISEASE

Renovascular disease represents only 1%–5% of all causes of hypertension; however, it is increasingly recognized as an important cause of renal failure (45). The exact prevalence of renovascular disease in the general population is unknown; in necropsy studies, significant renal artery stenosis was found in 25% of subjects over 40 (46), whereas in angiographic studies, renal artery stenosis was documented in 15% (including 4% bilateral) of 1235 patients undergoing cardiac catheterization (47) and approximately 30% of those with peripheral vascular disease (48). Of note, almost half the patients with more than 50% narrowing of one or both renal arteries were normotensive, and four fifths had normal serum creatinine (47).

Renovascular disease as a cause of hypertension and renal failure

Clinical clues relevant for the diagnosis of renovascular disease include accelerated/malignant hypertension (up to

a prevalence of 41% among white patients) (20); unilateral small kidney; onset of hypertension in patients under 20 or over 50; refractory hypertension despite three or more classes of antihypertensive medications and features of ischemic nephropathy, such as progressive azotemia in an elderly patient or in a patient with refractory hypertension on medical treatment; and renal failure following administration of antihypertensive agents and especially ACE inhibitors, particularly when combined with diuretics (45). Of note, acute reversible renal deterioration following ACE inhibitors was associated with renovascular disease in 17 of 28 patients (49) and was often, but not always (50), related to a fall in arterial pressure. Other presentations include severe hypertension, sometimes associated with nephrotic range proteinuria in the setting of unilateral renal artery thrombosis (51), and recurrent episodes of pulmonary edema associated with hypertension and renal failure in bilateral renovascular disease (52).

Renal failure is of major concern in all patients with atheromatous renovascular disease; in contrast to fibromuscular dysplasia, atheromatous renovascular disease was shown to progress in 44% of patients within a mean follow-up period of 52 months, and total occlusion occurred in 39% of those with 75%–99% initial stenosis within a mean follow-up period of 13 months (53). Of interest, there is no close correlation between anatomical progression, control of arterial pressure, and deterioration of renal function (53). In addition, cholesterol embolism may be an important contributive factor to progression of atherosclerotic renovascular disease to end-stage renal disease. According to Mailloux et al. (54), patients with renovascular disease represent 16% of all patients entering dialysis programs and have the worst 5-year survival rate on dialysis in comparison to patients with other causes of ESRD.

Screening for renovascular disease is justified in patients with high clinical suspicion of renovascular hypertension or ischemic nephropathy. In contrast to the significant value of screening tests in the setting of unilateral renovascular disease and normal renal function (sensitivity and specificity of up to 80%–85% for duplex ultrasound and renal scintigraphy), most tests proved to be unreliable when renal function was altered and/or bilateral renal artery stenosis was present (55). The place of spiraled computerized to mography (CT) scan and magnetic resonance imaging as major diagnostic tools remains to be determined. The decision for angiography—which remains the "gold standard" diagnostic test—rests mainly on clinical grounds and must be carefully weighed against risks of contrast nephropathy, particularly in diabetes mellitus, renal failure, hypercalcemia, or myeloma. Whether nonionic iodinated compounds or CO_2 will reduce the incidence of contrast nephropathy remains to determined. Of interest, in bilateral renovascular disease, renal scintigraphy is useful not only as a diagnostic tool but also when revascularization is chosen, the side contributing most to the renal impairment being treated first.

Medical treatment versus revascularization

Revascularization, the logical treatment of renovascular disease, resulted in the cure of hypertension in 60% of patients with fibromuscular dysplasia and 15%–20% of those with atheromatous lesions (56). The renal-vein renin ratio and arterial pressure response to long-term (2–3 months) ACE inhibitors appeared to be the most useful predictors of the arterial pressure response to intervention (57,58). In addition, revascularization is associated with fewer cardiovascular events than medical treatment; in a prospective study conducted three decades ago in patients with renovascular disease and severe hypertension, death (mostly from myocardial infarction and stroke) occurred in 30% of those who underwent surgery and in 70% of those treated medically within a 7- to 14-year follow-up period (59). Finally, revascularization may better preserve renal function than medical treatment in the absence of irreversible parenchymal damage. In the study of Dean et al. (60), conducted in 41 patients with renovascular disease who were randomly selected for nonoperative management and repeated angiographic studies, five progressed to complete occlusion within 6–102 months after the initial evaluation, and 17 were converted to the surgical treatment group due to progressive degradation of renal function and/or loss of renal size, despite satisfactory arterial pressure control. Medical treatment is still indicated when intervention is not possible due to anatomical constraints or poor clinical status.

Whether antihypertensive agents differ with regard to renovascular disease remains controversial. In a double-blind, prospective study comparing enalapril combined with hydrochlorothiazide and standard triple therapy (hydrochlorothiazide, timolol, hydralazine), arterial pressure was controlled in 96% of patients on the enalapril-based treatment and 82% of patients on triple-drug regimen. However, serum creatinine rose by more than 0.3 mg/dL in 10 of 49 patients treated with enalapril and in 1 of 39 in the other group; most patients who developed an acute reversible renal deterioration during ACE inhibition had a severe stenosis (80%–90% or more) or bilateral renovascular disease (61). Recently, CAs (alone or associated with beta-adrenergic blockers) were shown to allow adequate control of arterial pressure without significant alteration in renal function (62). In a retrospective study conducted in 78 patients who were submitted to serial angiography, 11 of 14 patients in whom occlusion developed and 31 of 64 patients without occlusion were on ACE inhibitor therapy; no consistent difference in arterial pressure was noted between the patients who did and those who did not develop complete occlusion (63). However, renal artery occlusion was reported in some patients treated with non-ACE inhibitor medications in whom arterial pressure was abruptly lowered, suggesting that the risk of renal artery occlusion associated with ACE inhibitors (or any other antihypertensive medications) may result from a marked and/or prolonged decrease in arterial pressure (64). It is noteworthy that in two-kidney, one-clip hypertensive rats, irreversible cessation of renal function and atrophy of the clipped kidney resulted from ACE inhibitors but not from comparative treatment (65).

Angioplasty versus surgical revascularization

In nonazotemic patients, the choice between percutaneous transluminal angioplasty (PTA) and surgery is based on anatomical considerations; ostial lesions are preferentially treated by surgery, whereas nonostial lesions could benefit from either PTA or surgery.

In azotemic patients with unilateral renovascular disease, revascularization was associated with improved renal function in 30% of cases, whether it was done by PTA (66–68) or surgery (69–71). In bilateral or single-kidney stenosis, surgery was followed by improvement in renal function in 30%–60% of azotemic patients (52,69,70,72–74); however, lower figures were obtained with PTA (67,68,75). In such patients, the mortality rate (6%–30%) was usually comparable for surgery and PTA. Failure to improve renal function following revascularization was associated with a 25%–40% short-term progression to end-stage renal failure after PTA (76) as compared to 10%–20% after surgery (52,72,74) (Table 5).

Predictors of renal functional response to revascularization

The various parameters proposed to predict functional response to revascularization, including total and split renal function, renal-vein renin determinations, and angiographic and histologic findings, are of poor predictive value (69,77). Extreme azotemia was considered as an indicator of poor prognosis; however, it was shown that some patients with advanced renal failure could benefit from surgery (70,71), even in cases of renal artery occlusion (70). Kidney size of less than 8 cm and proteinuria are of pejorative value, since they usually indicate diffuse parenchymal damage and may preclude retrieval of renal function following intervention.

We prospectively assessed the predictive value of several parameters in 26 patients with atheromatous renovascular disease (9 unilateral, 11 bilateral, 6 solitary kidney) and basal serum creatinine higher than 1.2 mg/dL. Glomerular filtration rate (^{99m}Tc-DTPA clearance) was measured prior to and within an average of 17 months following revascularization. Degradation of glomerular filtration rate by more than 15% occurred in only 1 of 14 patients with no proteinuria prior to revascularization, whereas improvement of glomerular filtration rate was observed in only 1 of 12 proteinuric patients. Interestingly, a striking inverse correlation was observed between basal urinary albumin excretion and the change in glomerular filtration rate resulting from revascularization.

In the treatment of renovascular disease, interest has recently focused on preventing the degradation of the pro-

Table 5. Renal function outcome following revascularization in patients with atheromatous renovascular disease

	n	Follow-up (months)	Outcome[a] Improved (%)	Deteriorated (included HD) (%)	Dialysis (%)	Death (%)	Serum creatinine Before (μmol/L)	After (μmol/L)	Creatinine clearance Before (mL/min)	After (mL/min)
Surgery										
Unilateral disease										
Hansen 1992 (69)	16	24	31	13	—	—	—	—	15.7	16
Novick 1983 (70)	16	24	75	0	0	0	198	148	—	—
Dean 1991 (80)	12	1	33	9	—	—	—	—	25.9	29.1
Bilateral disease										
Hansen 1992 (69)	54	24	54	16	—	—	—	—	15.3	21.5
Novick 1983 (70)	16	24	56	0	0	0	211	148	—	—
Dean 1985 (71)	11	1	100	0	0	0	451	248	—	—
Dean 1991 (80)	41	1	66	12	—	—	—	—	21.4	33.8
Solitary kidney										
McCready 1987 (72)	17	33	79[b]	21	12	24	327	195	—	—
Novick 1983 (70)	14	24	50	21	0	7	243	213	—	—
Askari 1982 (73)	30	72	60	20	0	5	202	165	—	—
Flatmark 1980 (74)	9	27	22	11	11	22	267	167	—	—
PTA										
Unilateral disease										
Madias 1981 (78)	13	7	31	0	0	0	125	116	—	—
Mahler 1982 (81)	8	24	13	0	0	0	150	142	—	—
Bilateral disease										
Tykarski 1993 (66)	13	—	62	0	0	0	456	260	—	—
Canzanello 1988 (68)	18	16	61[b]	39	—	—	186	212	—	—
Flechner 1982 (82)	8	6	50	38	0	0	294	279	—	—
Solitary kidney										
Martinez-Amenos 1991 (67)	10	22	21	—	0	0	275	246	—	—
Canzanello 1988 (68)	19	21	42[b]	58	—	—	398	434	—	—
Madias 1982 (75)	10	6	44	33	1	0	344	351	—	—
Weinberger 1986 (76)	9	17	11	40	30	78	410	499	—	—

[a] Improved and deteriorated are defined as a change in serum creatinine of <20% and <20%, respectively.
[b] Improved or stable.
Serum creatinine was higher than 12 mg/Dl in all patients. HD, hemodialysis.

gression of the renal function, rather than on the control of hypertension. Medical treatment should be proposed only in those patients with overall poor medical condition and in the absence of high-grade (>90%) stenosis. PTA should be preferred in patients with nonstial unilateral renovascular disease, since this procedure is repeatable and cost-effective, except when aortic reconstruction is indicated. In the absence of renal functional impairment, PTA and surgery are probably equally effective in lowering arterial pressure. When unilateral renovascular disease is associated with renal failure, likely nephrosclerosis of the contralateral kidney probably precludes improvement of renal function, despite revascularization. In azotemic patients with bilateral or single-kidney stenosis, surgery may provide better results than PTA for preservation of renal function. However, it would be unwise to make formal recommendations in the absence of a randomized trial. The experience of the operator (radiologist or surgeon) is probably a prominent factor. Large studies are needed to evaluate the efficacy of new techniques such as atherectomy or stenting in renovascular disease.

RENIN-SECRETING TUMORS

The diagnosis of renin-secreting tumors is based on the presence of severe hypertension associated with hyperreninemia and ultimately normalization of arterial pressure following removal of the tumor and with high levels of renin or prorenin in the tumor tissue (79). The term *primary reninism* was first proposed in order to discriminate between secondary reninism resulting from renal artery stenosis or thrombosis and compression of the renal pedicle by renal or extra-renal tumors. Both renal and extrarenal (mostly malignant) renin-secreting tumors exist. Among renal tumors are rare cases of clear cell carcinoma, nephroblastoma (Wilms' tumor, always found in childhood), and benign juxtaglomerular cell tumors. To date, 41 cases of these benign tumors have been reported in rather young subjects (70% in patients younger than 30 years), usually presenting with severe hypertension that may be in the accelerated phase (17% of patients) associated with hypokalemia (61% of cases). Proteinuria is observed in 55% of patients, rarely within the nephrotic range. Renal function is always normal. In such patients, pharmacological blockade of the renin–angiotensin system results in sometimes drastic decrements in arterial pressure. Since the demonstration of high renin dependence of hypertension may be suggestive of unilateral renovascular disease, attempts are usually made to eliminate this etiology. In fact, the absence of renovascular cause is highly suggestive of the existence of a renin-secreting tumor. Renal arteriography is positive in approximately half of patients (demonstration of a radiolucent zone) when the size of the tumor is higher than 15 mm in diameter. The best diagnostic tool is presently computerized tomography, which was positive in 11 of 12 patients. Unequivocal diagnosis is achieved by the demonstration of lateralization of renin secretion by renal-vein catheterization. Juxtaglomerular cell tumors are smaller than 16 mm in 40% of cases, and the maximum size is 50 mm. Following nephrectomy and preferably tumorectomy, which was recently performed in most patients, arterial pressure returns to normal limits within days after the operation.

REFERENCES

1. Bonomini V, Campieri C, Scolari MP, Vangelista A: Hypertension in acute renal failure. *Contrib Nephrol* 54:152–157, 1987.
2. Johnston PA, Davison AM: Hypertension in adults with idiopathic glomerulonephritis and normal serum creatinine. A report from the MRC glomerulonephritis registry. *Nephrol Dial Transplant* 8:20–24, 1993.
3. Kincaid-Smith P: Malignant hypertension. *J Hypertens* 9:893–899, 1991.
4. Mogensen CE: Long-term antihypertensive treatment inhibiting progression of diabetic nephropathy. *Br Med J* 285:685–686, 1982.
5. Parving HH, Smidt UM, Andersen AR, Sveendsen PAA: Early aggressive antihypertensive treatment reduces rate of decline in kidney function in diabetic nephropathy. *Lancet* 1:1175–1178, 1983.
6. Mathiesen ER, Hommel E, Giese J, Parving HH: Efficacy of captopril in postponing nephropathy in normotensive insulin-dependent diabetic patients with microalbuminuria. *Br Med J* 303:81–86, 1991.
7. Brazy PC, Stead WW, Fitzwilliam JF: Progression of renal insufficiency: role of blood pressure. *Kidney Int* 35:670–674, 1989.
8. Bergström J, Alvestrand A, Bucht H, Gutierez A: Progression of chronic renal failure in man is retarded with more frequent clinical follow-ups and better blood pressure control. *Clin Nephrol* 25:1–6, 1986.
9. Alberti O, Locatelli F, Graziani G, and the Northern Italian Cooperative Study Group: Hypertension and chronic renal insufficiency: the experience of Northern Italian Cooperative Study Group. *Am J Kidney Dis* 21 (Suppl 2):124–130, 1993.
10. Anderson S, Rennke HG, Brenner BM: Therapeutic advantage of converting enzyme inhibitors in arresting progressive renal disease associated with systemic hypertension in the rat. *J Clin Invest* 77:1993–2000, 1986.
11. Smith WGJ, Dharmasena AD, El Nahas AM, Thomas DM,

Coles GA: Short-term effect of captopril on renal haemodynamics in chronic renal failure. *Nephrol Dial Transplant* 4:696–700, 1989.
12. Rodicio JL, Alcazar JM, Ruilope LM: Influence of converting enzyme inhibition on glomerular filtration rate and proteinuria. *Kidney Int* 38:590–594, 1990.
13. Zucchelli P, Zuccala A, Borghi M, Fusaroli M, Sasdelli M, Stallone C, Sanna G, Gaggi R: Long-term comparison between captopril and nifedipine in the progression of renal insufficiency. *Kidney Int* 42:452–458, 1992.
14. Aperloo AJ, DeZeeuw D, DeJong PE: Short-term antiproteinuric response to antihypertensive treatment predicts long-term GFR decline in patients with non-diabetic renal disease. *Kidney Int* 45 (Suppl 45):S174–S178, 1994.
15. Hannedouche T, Landais P, Goldfarb B, El-Esper N, Fournier A, Godin M, Durand D, Chanard J, Mignon F, Suc JM, Grünfeld JP: Blood pressure control in non diabetic chronic renal failure: a prospective controlled study comparing ACE inhibition versus conventional antihypertensive therapy. *Br Med J* 309:833–837, 1994.
16. Brazy PC, Fitzwilliam JF: Progressive renal disease: role of race and antihypertensive medications. *Kidney Int* 37:1113–1119, 1990.
17. Vertes V, Cangiano JL, Berman LB, Gould A: Hypertension in end-stage renal disease. *N Engl J Med* 280:978–981, 1969.
18. Charra B, Calemard E, Ruffet M, Chazot C, Terrat JC, Vanel T, Laurent G: Survival as an index of adequacy of dialysis. *Kidney Int* 41:1286–1291, 1992.
19. Esbach JW, Aquiling T: The long-term effect of recombinant human erythropoïetin on the cardiovascular system. *Clin Nephrol* 38:S98–S103, 1992.
20. Davis BA, Crook JE, Vestal RE, Oates JA: Prevalence of renovascular hypertension in patients with grade III or IV hypertension retinopathy. *N Engl J Med* 301:1273–1276, 1979.
21. Isles C, Brown JJ, Cumming AMM: Excess smoking in malignant-phase hypertension. *Br Med J* 1:579–581, 1979.
22. Ramos O: Malignant hypertension: the Brazilian experience. *Kidney Int* 25:209–217, 1984.
23. Elliott WJ, Weber RR, Nelson KS, Oliner CM, Fumo MT, Gretler DD, McCray GR, Murphy MB: Renal and hemodynamic effects of intravenous fenoldopam versus nitroprusside in severe hypertension. *Circulation* 81:970–977, 1990.
24. Mourad G, Mimran A, Mion C: Recovery of renal function in patients with accelerated malignant nephrosclerosis on maintenance dialysis with management of blood pressure by captopril. *Nephron* 41:166–169, 1985.
25. Smith HW: Hypertension and urologic disease. *Am J Med* 4:724–743, 1947.
26. Belman BA, Kropp KA, Simon NM: Renal pressor hypertension secondary to unilateral hydronephrosis. *N Engl J Med* 278:1133–1136, 1968.
27. Wanner C, Lüscher TF, Schollmeyer P, Vetter W: Unilateral hydronephrosis and hypertension: cause or coincidence? *Nephron* 45:236–241, 1987.
28. Clark WR, Malek RS: Ureteropelvic junction obstruction. Observations on the classic type in adults. *J Urol* 138:276–279, 1987.
29. Vaughan ED, Sosa RE: Hypertension and hydronephrosis. In: JH Laragh, BM Brenner, eds, *Hypertension: Pathophysiology, Diagnosis, and Management*. Raven Press, New York, pp 1601–1607, 1990.
30. Kincaid-Smith P: Vascular obstruction in chronic pyelonephritic kidneys. *Lancet* 2:1263–1268, 1955.

31. Bailey RR, McCrae CU, Maling TMJ, Tisch G, Little PJ: Renal vein renin concentration in the hypertension of unilateral reflux nephropathy. *J Urol* 120:21–23, 1978.

32. Shapiro AP, Sapira JD, Scheib ET: Development of bacteriuria in hypertensive population. A 7-year follow-up study. *Ann Intern Med* 74:861–868, 1971.

33. Batzenschlager A, Weill-Bousson M, Guerbaoui M: Hypoplasie segmentaire aglomérulaire du rein. Complication hypertensive et résultats de la chirurgie. *Sem Hop Paris* 50:609–613, 1974.

34. de Jong PE, van Bockel JH, de Zeeuw D: Unilateral renal parenchymal disease with contralateral renal artery stenosis of the fibrodysplasia type. *Ann Intern Med* 110:437–445, 1989.

35. Sufrin G: The Page kidney: a correctable form of arterial hypertension. *J Urol* 113:450–454, 1975.

36. McCune TR, Stone WJ, Breyer JA: Page kidney: case report and review of the literature. *Am J Kidney Dis* 18:593–599, 1991.

37. Elias AN, Anderson GH, Dalakos TG, Streeten DHP: Renin angiotensin involvement in transient hypertension after renal injury. *J Urol* 119:561–562, 1978.

38. Stockigt JR, Sacharias N, Wood AS, Dugdale LM: Segmental renin sampling and partial nephrectomy in renal hypertension. *Arch Intern Med* 136:1297–1298, 1976.

39. Sterns RH, Rabinowitz R, Segal AJ, Spitzer RM: "Page kidney". Hypertension caused by chronic subcapsular hematoma. *Arch Intern Med* 145:169–171, 1985.

40. Knapp PM, Kulb TB, Lingeman JE: Extracorporeal shock wave lithotripsy induced perirenal hematoma. *J Urol* 139:700–703, 1988.

41. Lingeman JE, Woods JR, Toth PD: Blood pressure changes following extracorporeal shock wave lithotripsy and other forms of treatment for nephrolithisasis. *JAMA* 263:1789–1794, 1990.

42. Madrazo A, Schwartz G, Churg J: Radiation nephritis. A review. *J Urol* 114:822–827, 1975.

43. Luston RW: Radiation nephritis: a long-term study of 54 patients. *Lancet* 2:1221–1225, 1961.

44. Juncos LI, Carrasco Dueñas S, Cornejo JC, Broglia CA, Cejas H: Long-term enalapril and hydrocholorothiazide in radiation nephritis. *Nephron* 64:249–255, 1993.

45. Jacobson HR: Ischemic renal disease: an overlooked clinical entity? *Kidney Int* 34:729–743, 1988.

46. Holley KE, Hunt JC, Brown AL, Kincaid OW, Sheps SG: Renal artery stenosis. *Am J Med* 37:14–22, 1964.

47. Harding MB, Smith LR, Himmelstein SI, Harrison K, Phillips HR, Schwab SJ, Hermiller JB, Davidson CJ, Bashore M: Renal artery stenosis: prevalence and associated risk factors in patients undergoing routine cardiac catheterization. *J Am Soc Nephrol* 2:1608–1616, 1992.

48. Olin JW, Melia M, Young JR, et al.: Prevalence of atherosclerotic renal artery stenosis in patients with atherosclerosis elsewhere. *Am J Med* 188:46–51, 1990.

49. Mimran A, Ribstein J, Du Cailar G: Converting enzyme inhibitors and renal function in essential and renovascular hypertension. *Am J Hypertens* 4:7s–14s, 1991.

50. Hricik D, Browning PJ, Kopelman R, Goorno WE, Madias NE, Dzau VJ: Captopril-induced functional renal insufficiency in patients with bilateral renal-artery stenoses or renal-artery stenosis in a solitary kidney. *N Engl J Med* 308:373–376, 1983.

51. Zimbler MS, Pickering TG, Sos TA, Laragh JH: Proteinuria in renovascular hypertension and the effects of renal angioplasty. *Am J Cardiol* 59:406–408, 1987.

52. Messina LM, Zelenock GB, Yao KA, Stanley JC: Renal revascularization for recurrent pulmonary edema in patients with poorly controlled hypertension and renal insufficiency: a distinct subgroup of patients with atherosclerotic renal artery occlusive disease. *J Vasc Surg* 15:73–82, 1992.

53. Schreiber MJ, Pohl MA, Novick AC: The natural history of atherosclerotic and fibrous renal artery disease. *Urol Clin North Am* 11:383–392, 1984.

54. Mailloux LU, Bellucci AG, Mossey RT, Napolitano B, Moore T, Wilkes BM, Bluestone PA: *Am J Med* 84:855–862, 1988.

55. Mann SJ, Pickering TG: Detection of renovascular hypertension. State of the Art: 1992. *Ann Intern Med* 117:845–853, 1992.

56. Libertino JA, Beckman CF: Surgery and percutaneous angioplasty in the management of renovascular hypertension. *Urol Clin North Am* 21:235–243, 1994.

57. Atkinson AB, Brown JJ, Cumming AMM, Fraser R, Lever AF, Leckie BJ, Morton JJ, Robertson JIS: Captopril in renovascular hypertension: long-term use in predicting surgical outcome. *Br Med J* 284:689–693, 1982.

58. Pickering TG, Sos TA, Vaughan ED, et al.: Predictive value and changes of renin secretion in hypertensive patients with unilateral renovascular disease undergoing successful renal angioplasty. *Am J Med* 76:398–404, 1984.

59. Hunt JC, Sheps SG, Harrisson EG, et al.: Renal and renovascular hypertension: a reasoned approach to diagnosis and management. *Arch Intern Med* 133:988–999, 1974.

60. Dean RH, Kieffer RW, Smith BL, Oates JA, Nadeau JHJ, Hollifield JW, DuPont WD: Renovascular hypertension: anatomic and renal function changes during drug therapy. *Arch Surg* 116:1408–1415, 1981.

61. Franklin SS, Smith RD: A comparison of enalapril plus hydrochlorothiazide with standard triple therapy in renovascular hypertension. *Nephron* 44 (Suppl 1):73–82, 1986.

62. Ribstein J, Mourad G, Mimran A: Contrasting effects of captopril and nifedipine on renal function in renovascular hypertension. *Am J Hypertens* 1:239–244, 1988.

63. Postma CT, Hoefnagels WHL, Barentsz JO, DeBoo T, Thien T: Occlusion of unilateral stenosed renal arteries—relation to medical treatment. *J Hum Hypertens* 3:185–190, 1989.

64. Shaw AB, Gopalka SK: Renal artery thrombosis caused by antihypertensive treatment. *Br Med J* 285:1617, 1982.

65. Michel JB, Dussaule JC, Choudat L, Auzan C, Nochy D, Corvol P, Menard J: Effects of antihypertensive treatment in one-clip, two kidney hypertension in rats. *Kidney Int* 29:1011–1020, 1986.

66. Tykarski A, Edwards R, Dominiczak AF, Reid JL: Percutaneous transluminal renal angioplasty in the management of hypertension and renal failure in patients with renal artery stenosis. *J Hum Hypertens* 7:491–496, 1993.

67. Martinez-Amenos A, Rama H, Sarrias X, Galceran J, Alsina J, Montanya X: Percutaneous transluminal angioplasty in the treatment of renovascular hypertension. *J Hum Hypertens* 5:97–100, 1991.

68. Canzanello VJ, Millan VG, Spiegel JE, Ponce SP, Kopelman RI, Madias NE: Percutaneous transluminal renal angioplasty in management of atherosclerotic renovascular hypertension: results in 100 patients. *Hypertension* 13:163–172, 1989.

69. Hansen KJ, Starr SM, Sands RE, Burkart JM, Plonk GW, Dean RH: Contemporary management of renovascular disease. *J Vasc Surg* 16:319–331, 1992.

70. Novick AC, Ziegelbaum M, Vidt DG, Gifford RW, Pohl MA,

Goormastic M: Trends in surgical revascularization for renal artery disease. *JAMA* 257:498–501, 1987.

71. Dean RH, Englund R, Dupont WD, Meacham PW, Plummer WD, Pierce R, Ezell C: Retrieval of renal function by revascularization. *Ann Surg* 202:367–375, 1985.

72 McCready RA, Daugherty ME, Nightbert EJ, Hyde GL, Freedman AM, Ernst CB: Renal revascularization in patients with a single functioning ischemic kidney. *J Vasc Surg* 6:185–190, 1987.

73. Askari A, Novick AC, Stewart BH, Straffon RA: Surgical treatment of renovascular disease in the solitary kidney: results in 43 cases. *J Urol* 127:20–23, 1982.

74. Flatmark A, Jervell J, Sodal G: Surgical correction of renovascular hypertension in patients with one kidney. *Scand J Urol Nephrol* 14:81–83, 1980.

75. Madias NE, Kwon OJ, Millan VG: Percutaneous transluminal renal angioplasty. A potentially effective treatment for preservation of renal function. *Arch Intern Med* 142:693–697, 1982.

76. Weinberger MH, Grim CE, Luft FC, Yune HY: Percutaneous transluminal angioplasty in complicated renal vascular hypertension. *Nephron* 44 (Suppl 1):51–53, 1986.

77. Pickering TG, Sos TA, Saddekni S, Rozenblit G, James GD, Orenstein A, Helseth G, Laragh JH: Renal angioplasty in patients with azotemia and renovascular hypertension. *J Hypertens* 4: (Suppl):S667–S669, 1986.

78. Madias NE, Ball JT, Millan VG: Percutaneous transluminal renal angioplasty in the treatment of unilateral atherosclerotic renovascular hypertension. *Am J Med* 70:1078–1084, 1981.

79. Mimran A: Renin-secreting tumors. In: JD Swales, *Textbook of Hypertension*. Blackwell Scientific Publications, Oxford, pp 858–864, 1993.

80. Dean RH, Tribble RW, Hansen KJ, O'Neil E, Craven TE, Redding JF: Evolution of renal insufficiency in ischemic nephropathy. *Ann Surg* 213:446–456, 1991.

81. Mahler F, Probst P, Haertel M, Weidman P, Krneta A: Lasting improvement of renovascular hypertension by transluminal dilatation of atherosclerotic and nonatherosclerotic renal artery stenoses. *Circulation* 65:611–617, 1982.

82. Flechner S, Novick AC, Vidt D, Buonocore E, Meaney T: The use of percutaneous transluminal angioplasty of renal artery stenosis in patients with generalized atherosclerosis. *J Urol* 127:1072–1075, 1982.

CHAPTER 71

Posttransplant Hypertension

DAVID A. LASKOW & JOHN J. CURTIS

INTRODUCTION

The main cause of death in the general population is cardiovascular disease, for which hypertension is a significant risk factor. It is not surprising, therefore, to find that the principal cause of mortality in renal failure patients is cardiovascular disease and that cardiovascular deaths occur at a much earlier age than in the general population (1,2).

Similarly, postrenal transplant hypertension is a risk factor for early atherosclerotic disease, which Brunner et al. have demonstrated is a frequent cause of late morbidity and mortality after renal transplantation (3). Multiple studies have confirmed that post-transplant hypertension is associated not only with an increased mortality but also with de-creased graft survival (4–6). It is unclear whether posttransplant hypertension in itself causes this shift in graft survival or, as suggested by Cheigh, is merely a reflection of allograft dysfunction (7). Overall, posttransplant hypertension occurs in the majority of renal allograft recipients, negatively affecting both patient survival and graft function.

Posttransplant hypertension differs from the essential hypertension that is seen in the general population. In contrast to essential hypertension, factors such as age, gender, race, and family history have little association with posttransplant hypertension. Posttransplant hypertension is multifactorial; many of the contributing factors are correctable or can be ameliorated with adjustments in drug therapy. Although there may be factors such as central nervous system or genetic predisposition that do not imply a primary role of the kidney, it is convenient to focus on factors *intrinsic* or *extrinsic* to the allograft, since this approach can help identify reversible causes of posttransplant hypertension (Figure 1).

INTRINSIC CAUSES OF HYPERTENSION

Chronic rejection

Early in the transplant experience, prior to the use of cyclosporine, chronic rejection was recognized as the lead-

ing cause of posttransplant hypertension (8,9). The histology of chronic rejection is nonspecific and resembles that of nephrosclerosis and chronic cyclosporine (CsA) nephropathy. Chronic rejection is mostly a vascular phenomenon, as reflected by narrowing of the small renal arteries, interstitial fibrosis, and evidence of glomerular ischemia. Chronic rejection is usually recognized by a slow gradual drop in glomerular filtration rate (GFR), mild proteinuria, and the development of chronic hypertension over months and years. Initially, there is an early decrease in renal blood flow despite relative maintenance of GFR in chronic rejection (9). The decrease in renal blood flow is eventually accompanied by a decrease in GFR and an overall increase in renal vascular resistance. In addition, the decrease in renal blood flow results in ischemia which leads to the activation of the renin–angiotensin axis. Since the pathophysiology of chronic rejection is poorly understood, it is not surprising that currently there is no specific treatment (10). The hypertension associated with chronic rejection is often progressive, as is the loss of renal function, and eventually may require several antihypertensive agents. The hemodynamic changes resulting in the hypertension seen in chronic rejection may coexist or be exacerbated by the use of cyclosporine. Patients with chronic rejection may respond favorably with a decrease in blood pressure in reaction to a downward adjustment in their CsA dose (11).

Acute rejection

Hypertension is also closely associated with acute rejection, and indeed new-onset hypertension may be an early marker for such an event (12). The changes in renal hemodynamics seen with acute rejection—decrease in effective renal plasma flow (ERPF), decreased GFR, increased renal vascular resistance (RVR), and an activation of the renin–angiotensin system—are similar to those seen with chronic rejection (13,14). The importance of the renin–angiotensin system in acute and chronic rejection is implied by the attenuation of the hemodymanic changes with converting enzyme inhibitors. In contrast to chronic rejection,

Suki, WN and Massry SG (eds), Suki and Massry's Therapy of Renal Diseases and Related Disorders, Third Edition. ISBN 978-1-4757-6634-9.
©*1998, Kluwer Academic Publishers, Boston/Dordrecht/London. All rights reserved.*

Intrinsic causes of hypertension
  Chronic rejection
  Acute rejection
  Recurrent disease
Extrinsic causes of hypertension
  Native kidneys
  Renal artery stenosis
  Drugs
    Corticosteroids
    Cyclosporine
    FK-506

Figure 1. The common causes of hypertension after renal transplantation can be divided into two groups: those due to intrinsic allograft damage and those due to extrinsic causes.

the hypertension associated with acute rejection is reversible, as are the changes in the renal hemodynamics. Clearly, not only angiotensin but also a whole host of vasoactive substances released during an episode of acute rejection may contribute to the changes in renal hemodynamics. The effect of these vasoactive components of rejection— nitric oxide, prostaglandins, and endothelin—are diminished with successful treatment of acute rejection. It is somewhat ironic that high-dose steroids, which would exacerbate hypertension from other causes, are the drug of choice in treating first-time episodes of acute rejection and its accompanying hypertension.

Recurrent disease

Recurrence of the primary renal pathology in the allograft varies according to the original disease. While most idiopathic forms of glomerulonephritis and the glomerulonephritis associated with systemic disease have been reported to recur occasionally, focal glomerulosclerosis recurs frequently and is often associated with heavy proteinuria and severe hypertension (15). In patients who originally lost their renal function to hematuria uremic syndrome (HUS), it is impossible to distinguish between recurrent disease and de novo HUS associated with cyclosporine. Clinically, de novo and recurrent HUS are both associated with severe hypertension and microangiopathic hemolytic anemia. In the majority of recipients with recurrent disease, the diagnosis is suspected when hypertension and proteinuria are greater than that seen with chronic rejection and may be confirmed with renal biopsy. The hypertension associated with recurrent disease often worsens with progressive loss in renal function.

EXTRINSIC CAUSES OF HYPERTENSION

Native kidney hypertension

Pretransplant hypertension is a common problem in the end-stage renal failure patient; however, the majority of

hypertension seen in the dialysis population is not renin dependent. In fact, it has been estimated that only 10%– 20% of hypertension seen in dialysis is renin mediated (16,17). The incidence of native kidney renin-dependent hypertension posttransplant is difficult to determine. Prior to the use of cyclosporine, Van Ypersele suggested that 25% of posttransplant hypertension might be related to the patients' native kidneys (4). The role of native kidneys in posttransplant hypertension is dramatically demonstrated by the phenomenon of 'curing' the hypertension with bilateral native nephrectomy years after transplantation (18). In addition, the prevalence of hypertension is significantly higher in patients with native kidneys left in situ as opposed to patients who underwent bilateral nephrectomy prior to transplantation (18). Graft survival was also significantly increased in those patients who underwent bilateral native nephrectomy (19). Subsequent to bilateral native nephrectomy in renal allograft recipients, Curtis et al. demonstrated that despite the resultant lowering of mean arterial pressure (MAP) and cardiac output, there was an increase in renal blood flow (18). These results suggested that the diseased native kidneys caused a marked increase in renal vascular resistance in the allograft, which maintained GRF through a rise in filtration fraction. They noted that identical changes in the renal blood flow and MAP occurred after the administration of captopril in these patients prior to bilateral nephrectomy. The response to captopril and the finding of elevated plasma renin activity suggest that the renin–angiotensin system in the native kidney plays a major role in this form of hypertension. Prior to the use of cyclosporine, investigators found that in hypertensive patients a response to angiotensin-converting enzyme (ACE) inhibitors indicates native kidney disease that would respond to bilateral native nephrectomy (18,20,21). Coffman et al. (22), in a rat model of transplant hypertension, have been able to reproduce this exact phenomenon. Unfortunately, cyclosporine vasoconstriction of the afferent arterioles and the resultant decrease in renal blood flow and increase in renal vascular resistance form the overriding pathology, even in the face of concomitant native kidney disease. It is therefore not surprising to find that the use of ACE inhibitors is ineffective in identifying native-kidney-induced hypertension in patients receiving cyclosporine (23). Although native-kidney-induced hypertension behaves as if it is mediated by the renin–angiotensin system, renal-vein renin levels do not appear to be a reliable indication of patients whose hypertension will respond to bilateral native nephrectomy (24). Thus, in the postcyclosporine era, the incidence and diagnosis of native-kidney-induced hypertension is indeterminate.

Although the renin–angiotensin system is believed to be responsible for native-kidney-induced hypertension, Converse et al. have suggested that native diseased kidneys can result in increased sympathetic nerve activity (25). It is possible that there is more than one mechanism by which the native kidney induces hypertension. It is extremely interesting that ACE-inhibitor therapy is effective in treating native-kidney-induced hypertension and also in treating posttransplant erythrocytosis, which may be similarly related to native kidney disease (26).

The decision to schedule bilateral nephrectomy has become more relevant since the availability of erythropoietin has negated a major reason for reluctance to perform this surgery (27). Indeed, pretransplant and posttransplant bilateral native nephrectomy appears to have regained some popularity. Although embolization of the native kidneys remains an option, we have been daunted by its associated morbidity and continue to recommend a surgical approach.

Renal artery stenosis

Renal artery stenosis, an extrinsic form of posttransplant hypertension, deserves special consideration since it is often correctable with invasive procedures. The diagnosis of renal artery stenosis is suspected in recipients with poorly controlled blood pressure despite maximum medical therapy, and often may be associated with worsening renal function (28). Unfortunately, worsening hypertension and renal function are also associated with chronic rejection, acute rejection, chronic cyclosporine nephrotoxicity, recurrence of the original disease, and de novo glomerulonephritis. The physical examination of patients with renal artery stenosis offers little additional help in substantiating the diagnosis. Bruits, originally thought to be present in 100% of cases with renal artery stenosis, may be completely absent (29). In addition, bruits when present may be secondary to native atherosclerotic disease.

The diagnosis of renal artery stenosis has been reported to be as low as 1.5% and as high as 23% (29–31). The difference in reported incidences can be explained by several facts. First, reports often do not differentiate between anatomically narrowed renal arteries and functionally significant stenosis (32). In addition, determination of the functional significance of stenosis can vary by tests and center. Each center may have its own criteria for obtaining arteriograms; therefore, centers using arteriograms as a screening test report a much higher incidence of renal artery stenosis (32). Finally, the overall outcome may be influenced by factors unique to each center; the use of pediatric donors less than age 4 is not universally accepted, the percent of living related donors varies by center, and surgical techniques vary at each center (31,33). These factors, as well as differences in determining functionality of the stenosis, are responsible for the large discrepancies in the reported incidence of renal artery stenosis.

A test dose of ACE inhibitors may be useful as a diagnostic tool to identify clinically significant renal artery stenosis (34,35). Patients with renal artery stenosis are dependent on vasoconstriction of the efferent arterioles to maintain an effective GFR. Therefore, administration of an ACE inhibitor in the presence of renal artery stenosis results in an immediate and marked fall in GFR (34). Prior to the use of cyclosporine, challenge with an ACE inhibitor was an excellent way of identifying patients with renal artery stenosis. Unfortunately, in patients receiving cyclosporine, a potent vasoconstrictor of afferent arteri-

oles, GFR also depends on efferent vasoconstriction (36–38). Similar renal hemodynamic conditions exist when there is intrarenal small vessel disease, as seen in chronic rejection (39). A decrease in GFR in response to an ACE inhibitor is not unique for renal artery stenosis, but it identifies those patients whose renal function is dependent on postglomerular constriction. Although a lack of deterioration of renal function after administration of an ACE inhibitor strongly argues against the diagnosis of renal artery stenosis, a definitive diagnosis remains dependent on angiographic imaging.

Duplex color flow Doppler and ultrasound scans may be effective in identifying patients with renal artery stenosis. At this time, the predicted value of color duplex scanning is 56% (40). Therefore, arteriographic confirmation is still required.

The cause for renal artery stenosis may vary and can be due to technical factors associated with the anastomosis, acute angles or "kinking" of a long donor renal artery, atherosclerotic lesions, cyclosporine toxicity, or immunologic factors (31,33,41,42). Technical factors associated with renal artery stenosis can be diminished by using an aortic patch whenever possible during cadaveric transplantation. In addition, kinking of the artery may be reduced by leaving as much perivascular tissue surrounding the vessels as possible. It is also important when harvesting the right kidney to leave a segment of the vena cava that would allow for lengthening of this vessel, minimizing the discrepancy in length between the right renal vein and right renal artery.

Use of kidneys from donors less than 4 years old has been shown to be an important risk factor for developing renal artery stenosis (33). In view of all the technical reasons for developing renal artery stenosis, one would expect to see a higher incidence in the living related population. Contrary to intuition, however, there is a greater incidence of renal artery stenosis in cadaveric kidneys as compared to live donor allografts (29,31). Consistent with this finding is the report that the incidence of renal artery stenosis has a direct relationship to the frequency of acute rejection (42). There is speculation that vascular manifestations of acute rejection may result in renal artery stenosis. This notion is supported in a separate report demonstrating that 36% of the patients with renal artery stenosis who went on to lose their grafts had chronic rejection (43). In addition, cyclosporine has been associated with narrowing of major renal arteries (44).

The physiologic status of a patient with posttransplant hypertension secondary to renal artery stenosis is best reflected in the experimental one- kidney Goldblatt model, in which one kidney is clipped and the other removed. In this model, there is early stimulation of the renin–angiotensin system with volume expansion and sodium retention, which in turn suppresses the renin–angiotensin system. The overall result is the hypertensive patient with low to normal renin levels, as described by Kornerup (45). In the outpatient setting, renin levels are not as clinically useful as diuretic treatment and can convert a volume-dependent form of hypertension into renin-dependent hypertension (46). Useful information is only obtained under standardized conditions and diet.

The early experience with percutaneous transluminal angioplasty (PTA) for the treatment of renal artery stenosis was very encouraging (47,48). However, with more experience and long-term follow-up, a more defined role for PTA has been described. Immediate angiographic improvement in the stenosis has been reported to be as high as 90% (49). However, there is a large discrepancy in the reported complications and recurrence rate postdilatation (30,31,50). Roberts et al. reported poor results in 80% of the patients undergoing PTA of their stenosis; PTA resulted in graft loss of 16% in their patients (31). Even in centers with successful PTA programs, reported incidences of 10% graft loss have been noted (50). The difference in reported rates of successful dilatation may be secondary to patient selection. Those strictures located at the anastomosis or caused by kinking are associated with a lower success rate and an increased incidence of complications as compared to postanastomotic stenosis. In addition, the difference may be explained by the definition of "success." All patients that have successful dilatation of their stenosis do not enjoy a corresponding decrease in blood pressure or improvement in renal function. In summary, surgical intervention is often difficult and requires an experienced surgical team. Surgical intervention may enjoy a lower incidence of recurrence: 15% with surgical intervention versus 40% with PTA intervention (30). In view of the post-PTA course and ease of the procedure, it is still preferred as the initial approach for most stenotic lesions. Renal artery stenosis secondary to kinking may be the exception, and surgery should be the first choice of treatment.

Drug effects

The immunosuppressive drugs used in transplantation have long been recognized as important extrinsic factors associated with posttransplant hypertension. In the 1970s, steroids were thought to be an important factor in causing posttransplant hypertension. In the 1980s, the role of steroids and their relationship to hypertension were overshadowed when cyclosporine was added to the immunosuppressive armamentarium. In the 1990s, the addition of FK-506 has only served to widen the differential diagnosis of posttransplant hypertension.

Although the mechanism by which synthetic glucocorticoids may cause hypertension is unknown, this linkage of causality has been assumed ever since Popoutzer's landmark paper in 1973 (51). Prior to the cyclosporine era, it was believed that steroids were a major contributing factor to posttransplant hypertension (52). Whitworth has been able to demonstrate an increase in blood pressure in humans after administration of glucocorticoids in low doses (52). The patients all had an increase in urinary sodium excretion, suggesting that the increase in blood pressure

was not associated with any mineralocorticoid effects. Other investigators have not been able to demonstrate any relationship between prednisone and hypertension (53–56). Indeed, Hall et al. demonstrated a decrease in mean arterial pressure in dogs, which they felt was caused by chronic renal vasodilation, increased excretion of sodium, and volume depletion (57).

Most recently, Suzuki, reporting on an individual with Cushing's syndrome, demonstrated that cortisol was a determining factor in the patient's hypertension (58). He effectively argued against the importance of mineralocorticoid effects and the reninangiotensin system and speculated that cortisol may enhance vascular reactivity. Unfortunately, it is difficult to find a corresponding model of renal transplant chronic therapy with small doses of prednisone to confirm Popovtzer's proposal. Most clinical studies in the renal transplant population have demonstrated a benefit from both dose reduction and dose spacing of steroids (59,60). The improvement in blood pressure after steroid withdrawal has been modest, implying conversely that steroids are seldom responsible for severe hypertension.

Cyclosporine became widely available in 1983 and quickly gained wide acceptance in the transplant community. The magnitude of cyclosporine-associated hypertension and nephrotoxicity was not recognized until after its worldwide distribution and usage. Cyclosporine not only increased the incidence of posttransplant hypertension but also was unique in its pathophysiology.

In the precyclosporine era, most forms of posttransplant hypertension were mediated by the renin–angiotensin system (13,34,61,62). Approximately 50% of all patients exhibited mild to moderate hypertension (4,46,63). The administration of cyclosporine has resulted in a new, iatrogenic form of posttransplant hypertension. Similar to essential hypertension, cyclosporine-induced hypertension appears to be associated with sodium retention and increased vascular resistance that is responsive to salt restriction (64). In addition, like long-term essential hypertension-induced nephrosclerosis, the renal histology in patients receiving cyclosporine initially appears normal, but with time demonstrates renal scarring and vascular narrowing (15,65). Unlike hypertension precyclosporine, renin levels are often normal or low in patients with cyclosporine-induced hypertension (66–68). Clearly, the diagnosis and management of posttransplant hypertension has been complicated by the introduction of cyclosporine.

The mechanism of cyclosporine-induced hypertension remains poorly understood but is related to cyclosporine-induced alterations in renal hemodynamics, as is cyclosporine-associated nephrotoxicity. It has been graphically demonstrated that cyclosporine is a potent vasoconstrictor of the afferent arterioles in both animal and human models (69–72). There is a consensus that cyclosporine increases both mean arterial pressure and renal vascular resistance and decreases renal blood flow and glomerular filtration rate (68,72). Alteration in the above parameters can be induced acutely with the administration of cyclosporine. The rapidity and reversibility of these changes highlight cyclosporine's effect on the renal vasculature (73,74).

Early on, studies in rats and mice stated that cyclosporine was a potent stimulator of the renin–angiotensin system (75–78). The vasoconstriction of the afferent arterioles and decreased GFR were the result of this stimulation. These findings were not supported by Bantle et al., who demonstrated decreased renin activity in cyclosporine recipients with posttransplant hypertension (66). Staner et al., like Bantle, et al., were unable to demonstrate elevated renin levels in patients undergoing cyclosporine therapy; these patients had little response to ACE inhibition therapy (67). It has been suggested that the differences between these animal and human results are due to the chronic nature of cyclosporine administration in humans (66). It has been postulated that with the initial use of cyclosporine, the renin–angiotensin system is stimulated, but with long-term volume expansion, it is suppressed. Unfortunately, this argument could not be supported by clinical studies. In humans, the renin–angiotensin system does not appear to be stimulated by cyclosporine administered for short- or long-term therapy (21,79–83). The conflict between animal and human studies remains unclear but cannot be attributed to the length of cyclosporine use. The animal studies may not reflect the clinical use of cyclosporine in humans, since the animals were given large doses that often led to nausea, vomiting, and volume depletion.

Other possible mediators responsible for the vasoconstriction of the afferent arterioles and resultant renal hemodynamic changes have been proposed. Coffman et al. suggest that thromboxane and/or inhibition of the vasodilatory prostaglandins might be responsible for these changes (84). Thromboxane A_2 (TxA_2), a potent vasoconstrictor released from renal endothelial cells, is believed to be stimulated by cyclosporine (84). Data from animal and human studies again do not provide a clear answer (82,83,85–88). Gladue et al. were able to prevent and reverse cyclosporine nephrotoxicity in rats and humans with the administration of damzegrel, a specific inhibitor of thromboxane synthetase (89). Conversely, Weir et al. administered CGS12970, another thromboxane synthetase inhibitor, to renal transplant recipients and noted a decrease in GFR (90). Other clinical trials designed to test inhibition of the vasoconstrictive effects of thromboxane have been unsuccessful (91). Mason et al. concluded that neither the renin–angiotensin system nor prostaglandins are the major mediators of the vasoconstriction associated with cyclosporine (92).

Most recently, endothelin and nitric oxide have been implicated in cyclosporine-induced nephrotoxicity (91–93). Endothelin-induced vasoconstriction of the afferent arterioles appears to be secondary to calcium-dependent contraction of the vascular smooth muscle. Endothelin release from the renal vascular endothelial cells is stimulated by cyclosporine administration (94). The afferent arterioles are particularly sensitive to endothelin-induced vasoconstriction, since this area is rich in endothelin receptors. Bunchman et al. demonstrated that both calcium channel blockers and antiendothelin antibodies inhibit the effect of endothelin on isolated afferent arterioles (95). Cyclosporine not only increases plasma endothelin levels but also inhibits the production of nitric oxide, an endothelial-dependent vasodilator (95–97). Clinically, it has been recognized that calcium channel blockers are an effective agent in treating cyclosporine-induced hypertension and nephrotoxicity (98,99). Animal and human studies have demonstrated that endothelin-induced vasoconstriction is attenuated by calcium channel blockers, thus substantiating the clinical use of these agents (92,94,97).

Overall, cyclosporine-induced nephrotoxicity and associated hypertension probably result from an interplay between cyclosporine activation of various vasoconstrictors and the inhibition of various vasodilators. Nonrenal mechanisms may also play a role in cyclosporine-induced hypertension and nephrotoxicity. There are both animal and human studies that implicate the nervous system as a possible nonrenal cause for these adverse effects (100–102). Moss et al. have demonstrated increases in nerve activity in the rat gentifemoral nerve with the infusion of cyclosporine (101). This increase in nerve activity was associated with increased sodium retention by the kidneys, which is a hallmark of cyclosporine-induced hypertension (64). This observation was further supported by Murray et al., who demonstrated that the renal hemodynamic changes associated with cyclosporine administration could be ameliorated by the administration of an alpha-1 antagonist or actual deenervation of the kidney (70). The increase in sympathetic activity associated with cyclosporine administration has also been reported in the cardiac transplant population, whose kidneys have never been deenervated (103). This Finding may explain why cardiac recipients have the highest incidence of posttransplant hypertension. The overall incidence of cyclosporine-induced hypertension is a result of the interplay between a myriad of intrarenal and extrarenal factors. Fortunately, the hypertension associated with cyclosporine is usually modest in nature and is decreased with dose reduction or withdrawal unless fixed histologic changes associated with renal impairment occur.

FK-506 is a new immunosuppressive agent that was granted FDA approval in 1994 for its use in liver transplantation (104). The clinical use of FK-506 will increase with this approval, as will the list of potential factors in transplant hypertension. Similar to the intracellular mechanism of cyclosporine, FK506 binds to an immunophilin, FK506 binding protein (FKBP) (105,106). The FK-FKBP complex binds to and inhibits the action of calcineurin, which is believed to be necessary for the translocation of cytosolic nuclear factors of Tcell activation (NF-AT) (107–111). NF-AT appear to be responsible for the expression of IL-2 by antigen stimulated cells. The translocation of NF-AT appears to be dependent on calcinurin mediated dephosphorylation (111). Consistent with, and perhaps because of, the similarities in the mode of action between cyclosporine and FK506 is the finding that both agents are associated with nephrotoxicity and hypertension. Lyson et al. have demonstrated increased sympathetic activity and arterial pressure in rats receiving either cyclosporine or FK506 (112). They postulate that calcineurin, a cellular target of both the FK506-and the CSA-immunophilin complexes, plays a pivotal role in mediating both immunosuppression and alteration in sympathetic activity of both these agents. The renal hemodynamic changes after administration of FK-506 are the same as with cyclosporine: decrease in renal blood flow, decrease in GRF, and increase in renal vascular resistance. Curtis et al. have also demonstrated that, as with cyclosporine, patients receiving FK-506 have an increased sodium absorption and are slightly volume-expanded (113). The nephrotoxicity has been attributed to alteration in prostaglandin metabolism and increased endothelin secretion (114,115). Rats receiving FK506 demonstrated an increase in thromboxane B_2 excretion, indirectly demonstrating an increased production of thromboxane A_2 (116). In addition, FK506 has been demonstrated to stimulate increased production of the endothelin from cultured renal tubular cells (115). Clinical trials comparing FK506 and cyclosporine in heart, liver and kidney transplantation suggest that there is a lower incidence of post-transplant hypertension in those patients receiving FK506 (117,118,119). If the mode of action, mechanism of nephrotoxicity, and changes in renal hemodynamics are similar, how can one explain the reported differences in the incidence of posttransplant hypertension? During clinical trials, patients receiving FK-506 uniformly received fewer steroids than those patients receiving cyclosporine (120,121). In addition, in the renal transplant population, the reported incidence of acute rejection is less in patients on FK-506 therapy; one can postulate that there is a lower incidence of chronic rejection and hence subsequent hypertension (122,123). Overall, the exact incidence of posttransplant hypertension due to FK-506 and its mechanism need to be more fully explored.

THERAPY

In general, the causes of postrenal transplant hypertension are multifactorial. The majority of the renal allograft recipients undergo steroid, cyclosporine, and/or FK-506 immunosuppressive therapy with intact native kidneys. There is invariably some alteration in blood flow at the surgical anastomosis. Over time, allografts suffer some form of immunologic damage, which also alters renal blood flow. While it is often difficult to identify a single predominant factor responsible for posttransplant hypertension, it is important to entertain and address all the above possibilities in a single individual when planning management. In the case of hypertensive patients with normal renal func-

tion, chronic rejection and recurrent disease are unlikely to be causative factors in elevated blood pressure. Therefore, one can assume that cyclosporine is a major contributing factor. Since hypertension associated with cyclosporine is believed to be related to its renal vasoconstriction effects, two classes of potent renal vasodilatation have been employed: ACE inhibitors and calcium antagonists. These two classes of drugs are considered to be *renoprotective* in that they maintain or increase renal blood flow despite decreasing systemic hypertension. In theory, calcium channel blockers should be the ideal antihypertension agent for cyclosporine-induced hypertension. They appear to mitigate many of the untoward side effects of cyclosporine, since they have a preferential vasodilating effect on the afferent arteriole, increase renal blood flow, and can cause a natriuresis. Unfortunately, there are very few randomized prospective trials that compare these two classes of drug in the treatment of cyclosporine-induced hypertension. Mourand et al. have demonstrated that there is no difference in blood pressure control over a 3-year period in those patients treated with ACE inhibitor therapy as compared to calcium channel blocker therapy (126). Curtis et al. have also demonstrated almost identical decreases in blood pressure with short-term administration (48 hours) of either calcium channel blockers or ACE inhibitors (98). However, while these drugs appeared to be similar in their ability to decrease blood pressure, calcium channel blockers were more effective in reducing renal vascular resistance. Other investigators have reported similar effects of calcium channel blockers on renal blood flow and blood pressure in short-term human trials (99,125). Feehally noted in a retrospective study that hypertensive patients on cyclosporine who were treated with nifedipine had good blood pressure control, less nephrotoxicity and fewer rejection episodes (126). The decrease in rejection episodes is notable, and it is conceivable that calcium channel blockers may add to the immunosuppressive effects of cyclosporine (127). It is important to note that not all calcium channel blockers interact with cyclosporine in the same fashion. In general, the dihydropyridine agents do not appear to interfere significantly with the metabolism of cyclosporine, whereas the nondihydropyridine derivates may increase cyclosporine blood levels by 40%–50% (128,129).

Some investigations have taken advantage of this interaction to markedly decrease the cyclosporine dose while maintaining cyclosporine blood levels, thereby decreasing the patient's cost. Others believe this approach unduly complicates the patient's immunosuppressive management and use only the dihydropyridine calcium channel blockers. Some clinicians continue to support the use of ACE inhibitors based on their effectiveness at controlling blood pressure. However, in cyclosporine-treated recipients, ACE inhibitors need to be used cautiously, since their use has been associated with reversible renal failure, hyperkalemia, and anemia.

In addition to the use of calcium channel blockers, we

recommend the concomitant use of diuretic therapy in most patients on cyclosporine, based on the evidence that patients receiving cyclosporine are slightly volume expanded and have increased sodium retention. Diuretics need to be used judiciously, since cyclosporine-treated patients are prone to marked increases in their BUN and creatinine with volume depletion (130). Despite the concern that diuretic therapy may exacerbate the problem of hyperuremia, hyperlipidemia, and erythrocytosis, we continue to recommend a sodium-restricted diet and furosemide therapy for hypertensive patients receiving cyclosporine (131–133).

Lastly, cyclosporine dose may be cautiously reduced in an effort to help control blood pressure. Unfortunately, cyclosporine may have a continued effect on blood pressure even at lower doses. Discontinuation of cyclosporine for hypertension is not practical, since this approach is associated with an increased incidence of acute rejection (134,135).

If, in this group of patients with good renal function, blood pressure remains poorly controlled despite three-drug therapy, hypertension mediated through the renin-angiotension system secondary to renal artery stenosis or native kidney disease should be considered. A positive captopril test, although not conclusive, would suggest renal artery stenosis. As discussed previously, the particular method for correcting the stenosis would depend on its location and length of time from transplant. If the workup for renal artery stenosis is negative, then native kidney disease must be considered. Unfortunately, most immunosuppression protocols employ cyclosporine, which has the effect of ACE inhibitors on native kidneys and the concomitant increase in blood flow in the transplanted allograft. Despite the difficulties in identifying patients who would derive maximal benefit from bilateral native nephrectomies, we continue to recommend this procedure in those patients with excellent renal function (serum creatinine < 2.0) and urinary protein less than 500 mg who at 1 year continue to require more than three antihypertensive medications and in whom renal artery stenosis has been excluded.

REFERENCES

1. US Renal Data System: *USRDS 1990 Annual Data Report.* National Institutes of Health, National Institute of Diabetes and Digestive and Kidney Disease, Bethesda, MD, August 1990.
2. Fabrega AJ, Lopez-Boado M, Gonzalez S: Problems in the long-term renal allograft recipient. *Crit Care Clin* 6:979–1005, 1990.
3. Brunner FP, Broyer M, Brynger H, Challah S, Fassbinder W, Oules R, Rizzoni G, Selwood NH, Wing AJ: Combined report on regular dialysis and transplantation in Europe XV, 1984. In: AM Davison, PJ Guillov, eds, *Proceedings of the European Dialysis and Transplant Association.* Bailliere Tindal, London, pp 5–79, 1985.
4. Van Ypersele de Strihou C, Vereerstraeten P, Wauthier M, Toussaint C, Pirson Y, De Plaen JF, Vanherweghem JL, Dautrebande J, Kinnaert P, van Geertruyden J, Dupont E, Alexandre GP: Prevalence, etiology and treatment of late post-transplant hypertension. *Adv Nephrol Necker Hosp* 12:41–60, 1983.
5. Luke RG, Curtis JJ, Jones P, Whelchel JD, Diethelm AG: Mechanisms of posttransplant hypertension. *Am J Kidney Dis* 5:A79–A84, 1985.
6. Cheigh JS: Hypertension in kidney transplant recipients. In: JS Cheigh, eds, *Hypertension in Kidney Disease.* Martinus Nijhoff, Boston, pp 115–146, 1986.
7. Cheigh JS, Wang J, Fine P, et al.: Hypertension and decreased graft survival in long-term kidney transplant recipients (abstract). American Society of Nephrology, Washington, DC, 1984.
8. Knight RJ, Kerman RH, Welsh M, Golden D, Schoenberg L, Van Buren CT, Lewis RM, Kahan BD: Chronic rejection in primary renal allograft recipients under cyclosporine-prednisone immunosuppressive therapy. *Transplantation* 51(2):355–359, 1991.
9. Dubovsky EV, Curtis JJ, Luke RG, Jones P, Edwards SM, Keller F, Whelchel JD, Diethelm AG: Captopril as a predictor of curable hypertension in renal transplant recipients. *Contrib Nephrol* 56:117–123, 1987.
10. Paul LC, Fellstrom B: Chronic vascular rejection of the heart and the kidney—have rational treatment options emerged? (review). *Transplantation* 53(6):1169–1179, 1992.
11. Gaston RS: Hypertension in the renal transplant recipient. In: Shaul, Massry, Glassock,eds, *Massry and Glassock's Textbook of Nephrology.* 3rd ed. Williams and Wilkins, Baltimore, 1995.
12. Curtis JJ: Distinguishing the causes of post-transplantation hypertension. *Pediatr Nephrol* 5:108–111, 1991.
13. Gunnells JC Jr, Stickel DL, Robinson RR: Episodic hypertension associated with positive renin assays after renal transplantation. *N Engl J Med* 274:543–547, 1966.
14. Curtis JJ: Hypertension: a common problem for kidney transplant patients. *Kidney* 18(2):5, 1985.
15. Remuzzi G, Bertani T: Renal vascular and thrombotic effects of cyclosporine (review). *Am J Kidney Dis* 13(4):261–272, 1989.
16. Brunner HR, Laragh JH, Baer L, Newton MA, Goodwin FT, Krakoff LR, Bard RH, Buhler FR: Essential hypertension: renin and aldosterone, heart attack and stroke. *N Engl J Med* 286:441–449, 1972.
17. Vertes V, Cangiano JL, Berman LB, Gould A: Hypertension in end-stage renal disease. *N Engl J Med* 280:978–981, 1969.
18. Curtis JJ, Luke RG, Diethelm AG, Whelchel JD, Jones P: Benefits of removal of native kidneys in hypertension after renal transplantation. *Lancet* 2(8458):739–742, 1985.
19. The 13th report of the human renal transplant registry. *Transplant Proc* 9(1):9–26, 1977.
20. Haber E: The renin–angiotensin system and hypertension (review). *Kidney Int* 15(4):427–444, 1979.
21. Mimran A, Mourad G, Ribstein J: The renin–angiotensin system and renal function in kidney transplantation. *Kidney Int Suppl* 30:S114–S117, 1990.
22. Coffman TM, Himmelstein S, Best C, Klotman PE: Post-transplant hypertension in the rat: effects of captopril and native nephrectomy. *Kidney Int* 36:35–40, 1989.
23. Curtis JJ: Cyclosporine and hypertension. *Clin Transplant* 4:337–340, 1990.

24. Curtis JJ, Lucas BA, Kotchen TA, Luke RG: Surgical therapy for persistent hypertension after renal transplantation. *Transplantation* 31(2):125–128, 1981.

25. Converse RL, Jacobsen TN, Toto RD, Jost CM, Cosentino F, Fouad-Tarazi F, Victor RG: Sympathetic overactivity in patients with chronic renal failure. *N Engl J Med* 327(27):1912–1918, 1992.

26. Gaston RS, Julian BA, Diethelm AG, Curtis JJ: Effects of enalapril on erythrocytosis after renal transplantation. *Ann Intern Med* 115:954–955, 1991.

27. Ettenger RB, Mark J, Grimm P: The impact of recombined human erythropoietin therapy on renal transplantation. *Am J Kidney Dis* 18(4 Suppl 1):57–61, 1991.

28. Tilney NL, Rocha A, Strom TB, Kirkman RL: Renal artery stenosis in transplant patients. *Ann Surg* 199:454–460, 1984.

29. Lacombe M: Arterial stenosis complicating renal allotransplantation in man: a study of 38 cases. *Ann Surg* 181:283–288, 1975.

30. Benoit G, Moukarzel M, Hiesse C, Verdelli G, Charpentier B, Fries D: Transplant renal artery stenosis: experience and comparative results between surgery and angioplasty. *Transplant Int* 3:137–140, 1990.

31. Roberts JP, Ascher NL, Fryd DS, Hunter DW, Dunn DL, Payne WD, Sutherland DE, Castaneda-Zuniga W, Najarian JS: Transplant renal artery stenosis. *Transplantation* 48(4):580–583, 1989.

32. Morris PJ, Yadav RV, Kincaid-Smith P, Anderton J, Hare WS, Johnson N, Johnson W, Marshall VC: Renal artery stenosis in renal transplantation. *Med J Aust* 1:1255–1257, 1971.

33. Trompeter RS, Bewick M, Haycock GB, Chantler C: Renal transplantation in very young children. *Lancet* 1(8321):373–375, 1983.

34. Curtis JJ, Luke RG, Whelchel JD, Diethelm AG, Jones P, Dustan HP: Inhibition of angiotensin-converting enzyme in renal-transplant recipients with hypertension. *N Engl J Med* 308:377–381, 1983.

35. Hricik DE: Antihypertensive and renal effects of enalapril in post-transplant hypertension. *Clin Nephrol* 27:250–259, 1987.

36. Myers BD, Sibley R, Newton L, et al.: The long-term course of cyclosporine-associated chronic nephropathy. *Kidney Int* 33(2):590–600, 1988.

37. Ahmad T, Coulthard MG, Eastham EJ: Reversible renal failure due to the use of captopril in a renal allograft recipient treated with cyclosporine. *Nephrol Dial Transplant* 4:311–312, 1989.

38. Murray BM, Venuto RC, Kohli R, Cunningham EE: Enalapril-associated acute renal failure in renal transplants: possible role of cyclosporine. *Am J Kidney Dis* 16(1):66–69, 1990.

39. Davin JC, Mahieu PR: Captopril-associated renal failure with endarteritis but not renal artery stenosis in transplant recipient. *Lancet* 1(8432):820, 1985.

40. Erley CM, Duda SH, Wakat JP, Sokler M, Reuland P, Muller-Schauenburg W, Schareck W, Lauchart W, Risler T: Noninvasive procedures for diagnosis of renovascular hypertension in renal transplant recipients—a prospective analysis. *Transplantation* 54:863–867, 1992.

41. Munda R, Alexander JW, Miller S, First MR, Fidler JP: Renal allograft artery stenosis. *Am J Surg* 134:400–403, 1977.

42. Macia M, Paez A, Tornero F, De Oleo P, Hidalgo L, Barrientos A: Post-transplant renal artery stenosis: a possible immunological phenomenon. *J Urol* 145:251–252, 1991.

43. McMullin ND, Reidy FJ, Koffman CG, Rigden SP, Haycock G, Chantler C, Bewick M: The management of renal transplant artery stenosis in children by percutaneous transluminal angioplasty. *Transplantation* 53(3):559–563, 1992.

44. Sawaya B, Provenzano R, Kupin WL, Venkat KK: Cyclosporine-induced renal macroangiopathy. *Am J Kidney Dis* 12(6):534–537, 1988.

45. Kornerup HJ, Pedersen EB, Fjeldborg O: Kidney transplant artery stenosis. Interrelationship between blood pressure, kidney function, renin-aldosterone system and body sodium content. *Proc Eur Dial Transplant Assoc* 14:377–385, 1977.

46. Pollini J, Guttman RD, Beaudoin JG, Morehouse DD, Klassen J, Knaack J: Late hypertension following renal allotransplantation. *Clin Nephrol* 11:202–212, 1979.

47. Sniderman RW, Sprayregen S, Sos TA, Saddekni S, Hilton S, Mollenkopf F, Soberman R, Cheigh JS, Tapia L, Stubenbord W Jr, Tellis V, Veith FJ: Percutaneous transluminal dilation in renal transplant arterial stenosis. *Transplantation* 30:440–444, 1980.

48. Lohr JW, MacDougall ML, Chonko AM, Diederich DA, Grantham JJ, Savin VJ, Wiegmann TB: Percutaneous transluminal angioplasty in transplant renal artery stenosis: experience and review of the literature. *Am J Kidney Dis* 7(5):363–367, 1986.

49. Thomas CP, Riad H, Johnson BF, Cumberland DC: Percutaneous transluminal angioplasty in transplant renal arterial stenoses: a long-term follow-up. *Transplant Int* 5:129–132, 1992.

50. Greenstein SM, Verstandig A, McLean GK, Dafoe DC, Burke DR, Meranze SG, Naji A, Grossman RA, Perloff LJ, Barker CF: Percutaneous transluminal angioplasty, the procedure of choice in the hypertensive renal allograft recipient with renal artery stenosis. *Transplantation* 43:29–32, 1987.

51. Popovtzer MM, Pinnggera W, Katz FH, Corman JL, Roninette J, Lanois B, Haglrimson CG, Starzel TE: Variations in arterial blood pressure after kidney transplantation. Relation to renal function, plasma renin activity, and the dose of prednisone. *Circulation* 47:1297–1305, 1973.

52. Whitworth JA, Gordon D, Andrews J, Scoggins BA: The hypertensive effect of synthetic glucocorticoids in man: role of sodium and volume. *J Hypertens* 7(7):537–549, 1989.

53. Sampson D, Albert DJ: Alternate-day therapy with methylprednisolone after renal transplantation. *J Urol* 109(3):345–348, 1973.

54. Jackson SH, Beevers DG, Myers K: Does long-term low-dose corticosteroid therapy cause hypertension? *Clin Sci (Colch)* 61 (Suppl 7):381s–383s, 1981.

55. McHugh MI, Tanboga H, Marcen R, Liano F, Robson V, Wilkinson R: Hypertension following renal transplantation: the role of the host's kidney. *Q J Med* 49(196):395–403, 1980.

56. Cohen SL: Hypertension in renal transplant recipients: role of bilateral nephrectomy. *Br Med J* 3(871):78–81, 1973.

57. Hall JE, Morse CL, Smith MJ, Young DB, Guyton AC: Control of arterial pressure and renal function during glucocorticoid excess in dogs. *Hypertension* 2(2):139–148, 1980.

58. Suzuki H, Shibata H, Murakami M, Nakamoto H, Kondo K, Saruta T: Case report: hypertension in Cushing's syndrome. *Am J Med Sci* 303:329–332, 1992.

59. Curtis JJ, Galla JH, Kotchen TA, Lucas B, McRoberts JW, Luke RG: Prevalence of hypertension in a renal transplant population on alternate-day steroid therapy. *Clin Nephrol* 5(3):123–127, 1976.

60. Siegel RR, Luke RG, Hellebusch AA: Reduction of toxicity of corticosteroid therapy after renal transplantation. *Am J Med* 53(2):159–169, 1972.

61. McDonald JC, Bethea MC, Lindsey ES, Gonzalez FM, Garbus SB: Hypertension and renin activity in human renal transplantation. *Ann Surg* 179:580–586, 1974.

62. Curtis JJ, Luke RG, Jones P, Diethelm AG, Whelchel JD: Hypertension after successful renal transplantation. *Am J Med* 79:193–200, 1985.

63. Wauthier M, Vereerstraeten P, Pirson Y, Toussaint C, Alexandre GP, Kinnaert P, Van Geertruyden H, van Ypersele de Strihou C: Prevalence and causes of hypertension late after renal transplantation. *Proc Eur Dial Transplant Assoc* 19:566–571, 1983.

64. Curtis JJ, Luke RG, Jones P, Diethelm AG: Hypertension in cyclosporine-treated renal transplant recipients is sodium dependent. *Am J Med* 85:134–138, 1988.

65. Mihatsch MJ, Thiel G, Ryffel B: Histopathology of cyclosporine nephrotoxicity. *Transplant Proc* 20 (3 Suppl 3):759–771, 1988.

66. Bantle JP, Boudreau RJ, Ferris TF: Suppression of plasma renin activity by cyclosporine. *Am J Med* 83:59–64, 1987.

67. Stanek B, Kovarik J, Rasoul-Rockenschaub S, Silberbauer K: Renin–angiotensin–aldosterone system and vasopressin in cyclosporine-treated renal allograft recipients. *Clin Nephrol* 28:186–189, 1987.

68. Bellet M, Cabrol C, Sassano P, Leger P, Corvol P, Menard J: Systemic hypertension after cadaveric transplantation: effect of cyclosporine on the renin–angiotensin–aldosterone system. *Am J Cardiol* 56:927–931, 1985.

69. English J, Evan A, Houghton DC, Bennett WM: Cyclosporine-induced acute renal dysfunction in the rat. Evidence of arteriolar vasoconstriction with preservation of tubular function. *Transplantation* 44:135–141, 1987.

70. Murray BM, Paller MS, Ferris TF: Effect of cyclosporine administration on renal hemodynamics in conscious rats. *Kidney Int* 28:767–774, 1985.

71. Youngelman DF, Kahng KU, Rosen BD, Dresner LS, Wait RB: Effects of chronic cyclosporine administration on renal blood flow and intrarenal blood flow distribution. *Transplantation* 51(2):503–509, 1991.

72. Curtis JJ, Luke RG, Dubovsky E, Diethelm AG, Whelchel JD, Jones P: Cyclosporine in therapeutic doses increases renal allograft vascular resistance. *Lancet* 2(8505):477–479, 1986.

73. Cunningham C, Gavin MP, Whitney PH, Burke MD, Macintyre F, Thomson AW, Simpson JG: Serum cyclosporin levels, hepatic drug metabolism and renal tubulotoxicity. *Biochem Pharmacol* 33(18):2857–2861, 1984.

74. Paller MS, Murray BM: Renal dysfunction in animal models of cyclosporine toxicity. *Transplant Proc* 17(4) (Suppl 1):155–159, 1985.

75. Baxter CR, Duggin GG, Hall BM, Horvath JS, Tiller DJ: Stimulation of renin release from rat renal cortical slices by cyclosporin A. *Res Commun Chem Pathol Pharmacol* 43(3):417–423, 1984.

76. Perico N, Benigni A, Bosco E, Rossini M, Orisio S, Ghilardi F, Piccinelli A, Remuzzi G: Acute cyclosporine A nephrotoxicity in rats: which role for the renin–angiotensin system and glomerular prostaglandins? *Clin Nephrol* 25 (Suppl 1):S83–S88, 1986.

77. Nahman NS Jr, Cosio FG, Mahan JD, Henry ML, Ferguson RM: Cyclosporine nephrotoxicity in spontaneously hypertensive rats. *Transplantation* 45:768–772, 1988.

78. Duggin GG, Baxter C, Hall BM, Horvath JS, Tiller DJ: Influence of cyclosporine A (CSA) on intrarenal control of GFR. *Clin Nephrol* 25 (Suppl 1):S43–S45, 1986.

79. Klassen DK, Solez K, Burdick JF: Effects of cyclosporine on human renal allograft renin and prostaglandin production. *Transplantation* 47:1072–1075, 1989.

80. Sturrock NDC, Lang CC, Struther AD: The renin angiotensin axis is suppressed after initiation of cyclosporine in man (abstract). In: HE Eliahous, A Lasna, Y Bar-khayim, eds, *XIIth International Congress of Nephrology*, Jerusalem, Israel, p 542, June 1993.

81. Curtis JJ: Hypertension and kidney transplantation. *Curr Opin Nephrol Hypertensi* 1:100–105, 1992.

82. Nieszporek T, Grzeszczak W, Kokot F, Zukovska-Szczechowska E, Wiecek A, Kusmierski S, Szkodny A: Does the kind of immunosuppressive therapy influence plasma renin activity, aldosterone and vasopressin in patients with a kidney transplant? *Int Urol Nephrol* 21:233–240, 1989.

83. Zukowska-Szczechowska E, Kokot F, Grzeszczak W, Wocial B: Plasma levels of adrenaline and noradrenaline, plasma renin activity and arterial blood pressure in patients after kidney transplantation. (Polish). *Pol Arch Med Wewn* 86(4):254–262, 1991.

84 Coffman TM, Carr DR, Yarger WE, Klotman PE: Evidence that renal prostaglandin and thromboxane production is stimulated in chronic cyclosporine nephrotoxicity. *Transplantation* 43:282–285, 1987.

85. Deray G, Le Hoang P, Cacoub P, et al.: Effects of cyclosporine on plasma renin activity, catecholamines and prostaglandins in patients with idiopathic uveitis. *Am J Nephrol* 8:298–304, 1988.

86. Tresham JJ, Whitworth JA, Scoggins BA, Bennett WM: Cyclosporine-induced hypertension in sheep. The role of thromboxanes. *Transplantation* 49(1):144–148, 1990.

87. Wilkie ME, Beer JC, Newman D, Raftery MJ, Marsh FP: Evidence that the risks of misoprostol outweight its benefits in stable cyclosporine-treated renal allograft recipients. *Transplantation* 54(3):565–567, 1992.

88. Boers M, Bensen WG, Ludwin D, Goldsmith CH, Tugwell P: Cyclosporine nephrotoxicity in rheumatoid arthritis: no effect of short term misoprostol treatment. *J Rheumatol* 19:534–537, 1992.

89. Gladue RP, Newborg MF: The protective effects of the thromboxane synthetase inhibitor Dazmegrel on nephrotoxicity in cyclosporine-treated rats. *Transplantation* 52(5):837–841, 1991.

90. Weir MR, Klassen DK, Burdick JF: A pilot study to assess the ability of an orally available selective thromboxane synthase inhibitor to improve renal function in cyclosporine-treated renal transplant recipients. *J Am Soc Nephrol* 2:1285–1290, 1992.

91. Adams MB: Enisoprost in renal transplantation. The Enisoprost Renal Transplant Study Group. *Transplantation* 53:338–345, 1992.

92 Mason J: The pathophysiology of Sandimmune (cyclosporine) in man and animals. *Pediatr Nephrol* 4:686–704, 1990.

93. Kon V, Sugiura M, Inagami T, Harvie BR, Ichikawa I, Hoover RL: Role of endothelin in cyclosporine-induced glomerular dysfunction. *Kidney Int* 37:1487–1491, 1990.

94. Awazu M, Sugiura M, Inagami T, Ichikawa I, Kon V: Cyclosporine promotes glomerular endothelin binding in vivo. *J Am Soc Nephrol* 1:1253–1258, 1991.

95. Bunchman TE, Brookshire CA: Cyclosporine-induced synthesis of endothelin by cultured human endothelial cells. *J Clin Invest* 88(1):310–314, 1991.

96. Perico N, Ruggenenti P, Gaspar F, Mosconi L, Benigni A, Amuchastegui CS, Gasparini F, Remuzzi G: Daily renal hypoperfusion induced by cyclosporine in patients with renal transplantation. *Transplantation* 54(1):56–60, 1992.

97. Diederich D, Yang Z, Luscher TF: Chronic cyclosporine therapy impairs endothelium-dependent relaxation in the renal artery of the rat. *J Am Soc Nephrol* 2(8):1291–1297, 1992.

98. Curtis JJ, Laskow DA, Jones BA, Gaston RS, Luke RG: Captopril-induced fall in glomerular filtration rate in cyclosporine-treated hypertensive patients. *J Am Soc Nephrol* 3:1570–1574, 1993.

99. Copur MS, Tasdemir I, Turgan C, Yasavul U, Caglar S: Effects of nitrendipine on blood pressure and blood ciclosporine A level in patients with posttransplant hypertension. *Nephron* 52:227–230, 1989.

100. Berg KJ, Holdaas H, Endresen L, Fauchald P, Hartmann A, Pran T, Solbu D: Effect of isradipine on renal function in cyclosporine-treated renal transplant patients. *Nephrol Dial Transplant* 6:725–730, 1991.

101. Moss NG, Powell SL, Falk RJ: Intravenous cyclosporine activates afferent and efferent renal nerves and causes sodium retention in innervated kidneys in rats. *Proc Natl Acad Sci USA* 82:8222–8226, 1985.

102. Lyson T, McMullan DM, Ermel LD, Morgan BJ, Victor RG: Mechanism of cyclosporine-induced sympathetic activation and acute hypertension in rats. *Hypertension* 23(5):667–675, 1994.

103. Scherrer U, Vissing SF, Morgan BJ, Rollins JA, Tindall RS, Ring S, Hanson P, Mohanty PK, Victor RG: Cyclosporine-induced sympathetic activation and hypertension after heart transplantation. *N Engl J Med* 323(11):693–699, 1990.

104. Kino T, Hatanaka H, Miyata S, et al.: FK-506, a novel immunosuppressant isolated from a Streptomyces. II. Immunosuppressive effect of FK-506 in vitro. *J Antibiot (Tokyo)* 40:1256–1265, 1987.

105. Harding MW, Galat A, Uehling DE, Schreiber SL: A receptor for the immunosuppressant FK506 is a *cis-trans* peptidyl-prolyl isomerase. *Nature* 341(6244):758–760, 1989.

106. Siekierka JJ, Hung SH, Poe M, Lin CS, Sigal NH: A cytosolic binding protein for the immunosuppressant FK506 has peptidyl-prolyl isomerase activity but is distinct from cyclophilin. *Nature* 341(6244):755–757, 1989.

107. Clipstone NA, Crabtree GR: Identification of calcineurin as a key signalling enzyme in T-lymphocyte activation. *Nature* 357(6380):695–697, 1992.

108. O'Keefe SJ, Tamura J, Kincaid RL, Tocci MJ, O'Neill EA: FK506- and CsA-sensitive activation of the interleukin-2 promoter by calcineruin. *Nature* 357 (6380):692–694, 1992.

109. Liu J, Albers MW, Wandless TJ, Luan S, Alberg DG, Belshaw PJ, Cohen P, MacKintosh C, Klee CB, Schreiber SL: Inhibition of T cell signaling by immunophilin–ligand complexes correlates with loss of calcineurin phosphatase activity. *Biochemistry* 31:3896–3901, 1992.

110. DeFranco AL: Signal transduction. Immunosuppressants at work. *Nature* 352(6338):754–755, 1991.

111. McCaffrey PG, Perrino BA, Soderling TR, Rao A: NF-ATp, a T lymphocyte DNA-binding protein that is a target for calcineurin and immunosuppressive drugs. *J Biol Chem* 268:3747–3752, 1993.

112. Lyson T, Ermel LD, Belshaw PJ, Alberg DG, Schreiber SL, Victor RG: Cyclosporine- and FK506-induced sympathetic activation correlates with calcineurin-mediated inhibition of T-cell signaling. *Circ Res* 73(3):596–602, 1993.

113. Curtis JJ, Laskow DA, Jones PA: Sodium sensitivity of blood pressure: FK506 compared to CSA treated renal transplant recipients (Abstract). American Society of Transplant Physicians, 13th Annual Meeting, p 90, 1994.

114. Yamada K, Sugisaki Y, Akimoto M, Yamanaka N: FK 506-induced juxtaglomerular apparatus hyperplasia and tubular damage in rat kidney—morphologic and biologic analysis. *Transplant Proc* 24:1396–1398, 1992.

115. Moutabarrik A, Ishibashi M, Fukunaga M, et al.: FK506-induced kidney tubular cell injury. *Transplantation* 54:1041–1047, 1992.

116. Benigni A, Chiabrando C, Piccinelli A, Perico N, Gavinelli M, Furci L, Patino O, Abbate M, Bertani T, Remuzzi G: Increased urinary excretion of thromboxane B$_2$ and 2,3-dinor-TxB2 in cyclosporine A nephrotoxicity. *Kidney Int* 34:164–174, 1988.

117. Shapiro R, Jordan M, Fung J, McCauley J, Johnston J, Iwaki Y, Tzakis A, Hakala T, Todo S, Starzl TE: Kidney transplantation under FK 506 immunosuppression. *Transplant Proc* 23 (1 Pt 1):920–923, 1991.

118. Fung J, Abu-Elmagd K, Jain A, et al.: A randomized trial of primary liver transplantation under immunosuppression with FK 506 vs cyclosporine. *Transplant Proc* 23(6):2977–2983, 1991.

119. Armitage JM, Kormos RL, Fung J, et al.: Preliminary experience with FK506 in thoracic transplantation. *Transplantation* 52(1):164–167, 1991.

120. Demetris AJ, Fung JJ, Todo S, McCauley J, Jain A, Takaya S, Alessiani M, Abu-Elmagd K, Van Thiel DH, Starzl TE: Conversion of liver allograft recipients from cyclosporine to FK506 immunosuppressive therapy—a clinicopathologic study in 96 patients. *Transplantation* 53:1056–1062, 1992.

121. Tzakis AG, Fung JJ, Todo S, Reyes J, Green M, Starzl TE: Use of FK 506 in pediatric patients. *Transplant Proc* 23 (1, Pt 2):924–927, 1991.

122. Klintmalm GB, Goldstein R, Gonwa T, et al.: Use of FK506 for the prevention of recurrent allograft rejection after successful conversion from cyclosporine for refractory rejection. US Multicenter FK 506 Liver Study Group. *Transplant Proc* 25 (1, Pt 1):635–637, 1993.

123. Laskow DA, Vincenti F, Neylan J, Mendez R, Matas A: Phase II FK506 multicenter concentration control study: one-year follow-up. *Transplant Proc*, in press.

124. Mourad G, Ribstein J, Mimran A: Converting-enzyme inhibitor versus calcium antagonist in cyclosporine-treated renal transplants. *Kidney Int* 43(2): 419–425, 1993.

125. Sorensen SS, Skovbon H, Eiskjaer H, Thomsen K, Pedersen EB: Effect of felodipine on renal haemodynamics and tubular sodium handling in cyclosporine-treated renal transplant recipients. *Nephrol Dial Transplant* 7:69–78, 1992.

126. Feehally J, Walls J, Mistry N, Horsburgh T, Taylor J, Veitch PS, Bell PR: Does nifedipine ameliorate cyclosporine A nephrotoxicity? *Br Med J (Clin Res Ed)* 295 (6593):310, 1987.

127. Corteza Q, Shen S, Revie D, Chretien P: Effect of calcium channel blockers on in vivo cellular immunity in mice. *Transplantation* 47(2):339–342, 1989.

128. Howard RL, Shapiro JI, Babcock S, Chan L: The effect of calcium channel blockers on the cyclosporine dose requirement in renal transplant recipients. *Ren Fail* 12(2):89–92, 1990.

129. Endresen L, Bergan S, Holdaas H, Pran T, Sinding-Larsen B, Berg KJ: Lack of effect of the calcium antagonist isradipine on cyclosporine pharmacokinetics in renal transplant patients. *Ther Drug Monit* 13(6):490–495, 1991.

130. Laskow DA, Curtis JJ, Luke RG, Julian BA, Jones P, Deierhoi MH, Barber WH, Diethelm AG: Cyclosporine-induced changes in glomerular filtration rate and urea excretion. *Am J Med* 88(5):497–502, 1990.

131. Curtis JJ: Hypertension and kidney transplantation. *Am J Kidney Dis* 7(3):181–196, 1986.

132. Tiller DJ, Hall BM, Horvarth JS, Duggin GG, Thompson JF, Sheil AG: Gout and hyperuricaemia in patients on cyclosporin and diuretics (letter). *Lancet* 1(8426):453, 1985.

133. Pollak R, Maddux MS, Cohan J, Jacobsson PK, Mozes MF: Erythrocythemia following renal transplantation: influence of diuretic therapy. *Clin Nephrol* 29(3):119–123, 1988.

134. Sanders CE, Curtis JJ, Julian BA, Gaston RS, Jones PA, Laskow DA, Deierhoi MH, Barber WH, Diethelm AG: Tapering or discontinuing cyclosporine for financial reasons—a single-center experience. *Am J Kidney Dis* 21(1):9–15, 1993.

135. Flechner SM, Lorber M, Van Buren C, Kerman R, Kahan BD: The case against conversion to azathioprine in cyclosporine-treated renal recipients. *Transplant Proc* 17(4) (Suppl 1):276–281, 1985.

CHAPTER 72

The Catheter

GRANNUM R. SANT & EDWIN M. MEARES, JR.

INTRODUCTION

Urinary catheters are widely used to manage urinary tract obstruction and incontinence, facilitate surgical repair of the genitourinary tract, provide access to the upper urinary tract (kidneys and ureters), and monitor urine output. Indwelling urethral catheters are an important cause of hospital-acquired (nosocomial) infection. In his landmark editorial, "The Case Against the Catheter," Beeson (1), emphasized the morbidity of catheterization and stressed that "the decision to use this instrument should be made with the knowledge that it involves the risk of producing a serious disease which is often difficult to treat." This editorial initially led to widespread and unfounded fears of catheterization. A redefinition of the indications for catheterization and a flurry of research aimed at reducing the catheter-associated morbidity then followed.

The pathogenesis of catheter-related urinary tract infection (UTI) is now better understood, and alternative methods of urinary drainage and bladder management have replaced the indwelling urethral catheter. The benefits of catheterization in the management of various conditions outweigh its potential complications. To minimize morbidity and mortality, urethral catheters must be used judiciously and removed at the earliest opportunity. Alternative drainage methods include intermittent catheterization, external "condom" catheter drainage, percutaneous nephrostomy tubes, suprapubic cystostomy, and ureteral stents (2–4). The widespread use of these alternative drainage techniques is associated with a variety of infectious and noninfectious complications. There should always be strict indications for catheterization of the urinary tract, techniques for catheter insertion must be safe and aseptic, and every effort should be made to prevent infection during the period of drainage. Importantly, the patient must be left with a sterile urinary tract after catheter removal.

TYPES OF URINARY CATHETERS

Urinary catheters are of various shapes and sizes (Table 1). Catheter diameter is measured on the French (F) scale; this can be converted to millimeters by dividing by three. The three-way Foley catheter, which has a third lumen for continuous or intermittent bladder irrigation, is used to prevent clot retention (e.g., post-TURP) or to administer drugs (e.g., alum, prostaglandins, etc.) in order to control cyclophosphamide- or radiation-induced hemorrhage. Indwelling catheters are made of soft latex rubber, silicone, or silastic and feature a balloon (Foley) or phalanges (Malecot and de Pezzer) to prevent dislodgement. Catheters that are used to bypass urethral strictures or bladder neck contractures are fashioned from woven silk, gum elastic, or plastic and have a distal curvature (coude) to facilitate passage. Small plastic, polyethylene, or glass catheters are suitable for intermittent catheterization. The hydrophilic coating of some newer catheters reduce catheter irritation and trauma and increase patient comfort.

Percutaneous suprapubic cystostomy catheters are usually polyethylene or silastic (8–14F in diameter). When a suprapubic catheter is inserted during an open surgical procedure, a large Foley, Malecot, or de Pezzer catheter is used to drain blood and urine.

Most ureteral catheters (3–8F in diameter) are made of soft polyethylene or silicone. Self-retaining catheters, fashioned to remain for prolonged periods within the ureter, have terminal "pigtails" or J-hooks (double J stent) (3,5).

Percutaneous nephrostomy catheters are seldom larger than 14F in diameter and usually made of polyethylene. They are anchored by suture attachment to the skin. Some also have a terminal "pigtail" that coils within the collecting system. During surgical procedures, large Foley, Malecot, or de Pezzer catheters are used for nephrostomy drainage; alternatively, soft polyethylene tubes may be used to minimize trauma to the renal pelvis and kidney.

COMMON INDICATIONS FOR URINARY CATHETERIZATION

Urinary retention

Common causes of acute urinary retention—sudden inability to void—include benign prostatic hyperplasia (BPH), bladder neck contracture, neuropathic bladder dysfunc-

Suki, WN and Massry SG (eds), Suki and Massry's Therapy of Renal Diseases and Related Disorders, Third Edition. ISBN 978-1-4757-6634-9.
©1998, Kluwer Academic Publishers, Boston/Dordrecht/London. All rights reserved.

Table 1. Common types of urinary catheters

Urethral
  Simple (straight)
  Retention (Foley balloon)
  Coude tip (curved tip)
  Three-way (Foley balloon)
Suprapubic
  Mushroom (dePezzer)
  Winged tip (Malecot)
  Percutaneous (Stamey, Cystocath)
Nephrostomy
  Open insertion (dePezzer, Malecot, Foley)
  Percutaneous insertion (angiocatheters, polyethylene tubes)
Ureteral stents
  External (standard ureteral catheters)
  Internal (double-J catheters)
External condom type

tion, trauma, gross hematuria with obstructing clots, and acute prostatitis. Temporary postoperative retention can occur following inguinal, perirectal, or pelvic surgical, procedures.

Acute bladder overdistention requires prompt relief. An initial attempt to pass a well-lubricated Foley catheter (size 18–22 F) should be made. Smaller catheters (12–14 F) lack "body" and frequently coil at the external urethral sphincter or bladder neck in men. Inability to insert a standard Foley catheter should be followed by an attempt to pass a coude-tip catheter. The curved tip facilitates passage through the external sphincter and over the median prostatic lobe. If these attempts are unsuccessful, a urologist trained in the use of filiforms and followers should be consulted. Alternatively, the bladder can be drained suprapubically by needle aspiration or a small cystostomy tube inserted using local anesthesia. Percutaneous drainage minimizes urethral trauma, avoids dissemination of urethral bacteria into the bloodstream, and allows radiographic/endoscopic evaluation of the lower urinary tract. An inexperienced person should never attempt to insert a catheter using a metal catheter guide, lest severe urethral or prostatic trauma results.

In acute urinary retention due to progressive prostatism and benign prostatic hyperplasia, the catheter should remain indwelling until definitive surgery is performed. This decompresses the overdistended bladder detrusor and promotes earlier postoperative return of effective voiding. Postoperative retention is usually managed by intermittent or short-term (i.e., a few days) urethral catheterization. Restoration of normal voiding can be enhanced by administration of alpha-1-adrenergic blockers, e.g., prazosin (1 mg orally twice daily) or terazosin (2–5 mg daily). These drugs relax the smooth muscle of the bladder neck and prostate and reduce the dynamic component of bladder outlet obstruction (6). Intermittent catheterization is recommended for the initial management of retention in acute spinal cord injury during the phase of spinal shock (7).

Techniques of intermittent catheterization are discussed below.

Urinary incontinence

Incontinence results from urethral incompetence ("stress"), uninhibited detrusor contractions ("urge"), urinary fistulas ("total"), or urinary retention ("overflow"). In the evaluation of incontinence, catheterization measures postvoid residual (PVR) urine volume, introduces radiographic contrast for delineation of fistulas, and helps to study detrusor-sphincter function by means of cystometrography (CMG) and voiding cystourethrography (VCUG).

Stress incontinence is a major problem in women, especially in the postmenopausal age groups. The etiology is multifactorial, and many women with urinary incontinence experience significant lowering of their quality of life. Surgical cure of female stress incontinence is achieved by resuspension of the bladder neck into the true pelvis and restoration of urethral competence. Complete sphincteric dysfunction (e.g., neuropathic, postsurgical, radiation injury) produces severe incontinence (Type III) that is difficult to correct surgically. Intractable incontinence can result in decubitus ulcers, cellulitis, and bacteremia and morbidity exceeding that normally produced by an indwelling catheter. In women, alternative methods of management include indwelling catheters, surgical closure of the bladder neck plus suprapubic cystostomy, creation of a vesicostomy, or proximal urinary diversion, e.g., ileal conduit. The most common cause of incontinence in men follows radical prostatectomy for prostate cancer. Management options include penile clamps, condom catheters, collagen injections and artificial sphincters. Penile clamps (e.g., Cunningham clamps) are poorly tolerated and can cause urethral fistulas or diverticula, whereas condom catheters can cause urethral obstruction, penile skin abrasions, and urinary tract infection (8). Complications of condom catheter drainage are discussed later.

Uninhibited bladder contractions (detrusor instability) causing mild incontinence can be treated with oral anticholinergic drugs, e.g., propantheline, oxybutinin (Ditropan®), Urispas®, Levsinex®, etc. In severe incontinence due to uninhibited bladder contractions, intermittent catheterization plus large doses of oral anticholinergics are needed for continence and effective bladder drainage. If bladder paralysis is not achieved or if drug side effects become intolerable, supravesical urinary diversion may be required.

Demyelinating diseases of the central nervous system, e.g., multiple sclerosis and traumatic injuries involving the cervical or thoracic spinal cord, present special management problems. Patients may be incontinent and may incompletely empty their bladders due to bladder–external sphincter dyssynergia (9). Hydroureteronephrosis develops due to high intravesical pressures produced by the simultaneous occurrence of uninhibited detrusor and external urethral sphincter contractions. Effective therapy of dyssynergia in men usually requires external sphincterotomy, which results in low intravesical pressure and total incontinence. Bladder drainage is then achieved using an external condom catheter.

Urinary fistulas

Fistulas occur in the upper or lower urinary tract. The most common fistulas encountered in clinical practice are vesicovaginal or ureterovaginal fistulas complicating gynecologic pelvic surgery and vesicoenteric fistulas occurring as a result of colonic diverticular disease or cancer. The diagnosis is usualy suspected clinically (e.g., infections, constant vaginal urine leakage) and is confirmed radiologically. Computerized tomography (CT) scanning is recommended for visualization of vesicoenteric fistulas. Introduction of radiographic contrast, e.g., retrograde ureteropyelography, cystography, and urethrography, confirms the site and size of urinary fistulas.

If recognized early, urinary fistulas (e.g., vesicovaginal, vesicointestinal) may close spontaneously following temporary urinary diversion above the level of the fistula. Initial treatment of renal pelvic or ureteral fistulas consists of percutaneous or open nephrostomy drainage or a double-J ureteral catheter to divert urine. Vesical fistulas are managed by indwelling catheters or suprapubic cystotomy drainage. Spontaneous closure of chronic or large vesical fistulas is unusual, and these fistulas usually require surgical repair, chronic indwelling catheter drainage, or permanent proximal urinary diversion, e.g., ileal conduit.

Hydroureteronephrosis

Obstruction of the urinary collecting system proximal to a pelviureteric, ureteric, or subvesical obstruction can be managed by placement of a catheter proximal to or through the obstruction. Surgical correction of the obstructing lesion is then performed as the patient's condition and disease state permit. Percutaneous drainage of the obstructed renal pelvis was introduced by Goodwin (10). Percutaneous nephrostomy tubes are also used to define obstructive lesions by antegrade pyelography, to obtain urine for culture, to assess renal function and creatinine clearances, and to define the hydrodynamic significance (e.g., Whitaker test) of obstruction (11,12). Percutaneous drainage is occasionally used for long-term palliative management.

Ureteral stents (e.g., Stamey stent), which are used for temporary urinary diversion, exit the urethra and are anchored to indwelling catheters to prevent migration (upward or downward) or dislodgement. Ascending renal infection is an obvious disadvantage of this form of catheterization. Internal double-J ureteral catheters are designed to prevent migration and are widely used for temporary relief of upper-tract obstruction and as an adjunct to ureteroscopy and extracorporeal shock wave lithotripsy (ESWL) (13,14). Percutaneous nephrostomy drainage and internal ureteral stents are excellent methods to manage symptomatic renal obstruction due to stones in pregnant women. They allow delay in definitive surgical correction until after delivery (15).

Trauma and hematuria

Urethral catheterization is used in multiple-trauma patients to monitor urinary output, especially if they are in shock and are hemodynamically unstable. When a male patient suffers a pelvic fracture, the integrity of the urethra must be assessed before urethral catheterization is attempted. Once a normal urethra is visualized by means of retrograde urethrography, a Foley balloon catheter can be passed transurethrally and a cystogram done to assess bladder integrity. If the urethrogram shows significant urethral disruption, the bladder should be preferentially drained by a percutaneous suprapubic catheter or by a suprapubic tube placed at open cystostomy.

A large Foley catheter (22 F or 24 F) is used for patients with gross hematuria. The large lumen permits clot irrigation and passage of new clots. The catheter allows egress of urine, monitoring of the hemorrhage, collapse of the bladder wall with concomitant contraction of bleeding vessels, and tamponade of prostatic or urethral bleeding.

Urinary infection

Voided urine specimens in women are frequently contaminated by periurethral bacterial flora; frequently, collection of a urine sample by "in-and-out" or "straight" catheterization is necessary for accurate diagnosis of UTI. Suprapubic needle bladder aspiration remains the least morbid and most accurate method of obtaining a urine sample for culture (16). The site of an infection (upper versus lower tract) can be localized by passage of ureteral catheters into the renal pelvis and procurement of differential renal and bladder cultures (17). Percutaneous aspiration of the renal pelvis for culture may prove necessary when ureteral catheterization is difficult or impossible, e.g., after ureteroneocystostomy or ileal loop urinary diversion.

An obstructed, infected urinary tract requires prompt drainage by ureteral catheters, stents, or nephrostomy tubes (percutaneous or open). Intermittent urethral catheterization is an excellent adjunct in the therapy of cystitis associated with chronic retention or indwelling catheters (4,18).

Miscellaneous

Urethral catheterization is required for instillation of radiographic contrast for cystourethrography, etc.; intravesical pharmacotherapy for bladder carcinoma (e.g., Thiotepa®, BCG) and interstitial cystitis (e.g., dimethyl sulfoxide (DMSO), etc.); and dissolution of struvite calculi. Ureteral and nephrostomy catheters are used to deliver these agents to the renal pelvis and ureter in selected patients (19).

The widespread use of percutaneous and extracorporeal shock wave lithotripsy has led to increased use of ureteral catheters and percutaneous nephrostomy tubes (20). These applications are dealt with later in this chapter.

INDWELLING URETHRAL CATHETERS

Incidence of infection

Of patients hospitalized in the U.S.A., 5% develop hospital-acquired or nosocomial infections, 40% of which arise from the urinary tract (21,22). Catheterization and instrumentation account for 80% of hospital-acquired UTIs. Between 15% and 20% of all hospitalized patients undergo catheterization, and 1%–3% develop bacteremia, with a mortality rate of about 10% (21). Severe catheter-associated infections occur in patients with catheters left in situ for prolonged periods (23). The National Nosocomial Infections Study (NNIS) (22) and the Study of the Efficiency of Nosocomial Infection Control (SENIC Project) (24). indicate that urethral catheterization frequently precedes the development of hospital-acquired UTIs.

The rate of infection with in-and-out catheterization in hospitalized women is about 6%, compared to less than 1% in outpatients (21,25). Single in-and-out catheterization is used to relieve temporary obstruction, to obtain urine from patients unable to provide a clean-catch specimen, to measure postvoid residual urine volumes, and to allow radiographic or urodynamic study of the lower urinary tract. The risk of infection with single catheterization is increased in the elderly, the debilitated, the immunosuppressed, the diabetic, the pregnant woman prior to delivery or postpartum, and patients with significant postvoid residuals (26). Women catheterized during labor are 2–5 times more susceptible to infection compared to their noncatheterized counterparts (27).

The incidence of infection associated with indwelling urethral catheters in hospitalized patients has diminished during the past 30 years, mainly as a result of closed systems of urinary drainage (28). About 95% of patients develop significant bacteriuria within 96 hours of open urinary catheter drainage (29,30). Most catheters are left indwelling for short periods of time—a mean of 2 days and a median of 4. The incidence of bacteriuria with Foley catheters averages 5% per day, and bacteriuria is universally present in all catheterized patients after 3–4 weeks, despite the use of closed drainage systems. The SENIC Project documented a linear relationship between the duration of closed drainage and the incidence of UTI (24).

Diagnosis

Kass defined UTI as more than 100,000 bacteria per milliliter of urine (29). Many still use this criterion to define catheter-related UTI; however, others accept lower colony counts (10,000/mL or 1000/mL) as significant levels of bacteriuria in catheterized or symptomatic patients (32,33).

Urine samples for culture are best obtained from catheterized patients by needle aspiration of the catheter. The catheter is cleansed with alcohol or idophor solution at its junction with the collecting tube. It is then punctured with a 21-gauge (or smaller) needle connected to a syringe and urine aspirated (34). The accuracy of this technique was confirmed by Bergqvist et al. (35), who found that cultures taken from the distal end of the catheter agreed with those obtained by catheter puncture and percutaneous bladder aspiration. Interruption of the "closed" drainage system to obtain a urine sample should not be done due to the risk of contamination.

Pathogenesis of catheter-associated UTI's

Urethral catheterization can innoculate the bladder with bacteria from the perineum, the urethral meatus, or the urethra (26,34). Thorough cleansing temporarily eradicates resident bacteria from the perineum and periurethral areas. The distal third of the male urethra is sometimes colonized by coliforms or *Pseudomonas*; the female urethra, however, is frequently colonized by pathogenic bacteria from the vagina and introitus (36–38). During catheterization, these urethral bacteria can be displaced into the bladder and cause infection (Table 2). About 1% of healthy, nonhospitalized patients subjected to a single catheterization develop bacteriuria (21,39). The rate of infection is higher in patients prone to urethral and meatal bacterial colonization, i.e., female, elderly, bedridden, and debilitated patients (26,34). Fecal perineal contamination in incontinent patients also increases the risk of catheter-associated UTIs (23).

Other sources of catheter contamination include inadequate sterilization of instruments, catheters, antiseptic solutions, and even the hands of personnel (40,41). There is a correlation between the professional training of the person who inserts the catheter and the incidence of bacteriuria. Women catheterized by licensed practical nurses develop about twice the incidence of bacteriuria during the first 48 hours after catheterization as those catheterized by registered nurses or physicians (42).

Table 2. Catheter-associated UTIs

40% of all nosocomial infections
Significant causes
   Periurethral bacterial migration
   Catheter surface bacterial biofilm
   Altered bladder defenses (GAGs, etc.)
Less significant causes
   Retrograde spread from distal urethra
   Drainage bag contamination
   Break in closed drainage system

The incidence of urethral bacterial colonization exceeds the rate of infection following in-and-out catheterization, and this finding suggests that intrinsic defense mechanisms exist in the bladder. If the bladder empties completely and the bladder defense mechanisms are intact, UTIs seldom occur (43). A bacterial antiadherence mechanism resides in the mucopolysaccharide glycosaminoglycan (GAG) layer of the bladder mucosa. A GAG deficiency may make the bladder more susceptible to infection. Indwelling catheters may adversely affect the GAG protective layer with increased bacterial adherence, colonization, and infection (44).

The major pathway of infection in patients with indwelling catheters is the extraluminal migration of bacteria in the periurethral space (Table 2) (38,42,45). About 70% of catheter-associated nosocomial urinary tract infections are preceded by colonization of the urinary meatus (38,46). Pericatheter colonization is enhanced by the accumulation of urethral secretions that are normally cleared by normal voiding.

Bacteria can also enter the catheter drainage bag or tubing and ascend within the catheter lumen against the direction of urine flow (47). Infection by this route generally occurs within 12–24 hours after the drainage bag becomes infected (30,31). Sites of entry of bacteria into a collecting system include the junctions between catheter and drainage tube, drainage tube and collecting bag, and the drainage spigot of the collecting bag (Figure 1) (42,47,48,49). Elimination of the open junction between the drainage tube and collecting bag markedly reduces infection associated with an indwelling urethral catheter (50). Interruption of the junction between the catheter and drainage tube for irrigation or drug instillation increases the rate of bacteriuria (42,51).

Geographical grouping of high-risk catheterized patients, e.g., the immunosuppressed, the debilitated, those receiving antimicrobics, and those in intensive care units, may lead to bacteriuria caused by multidrug-resistant organisms owing to passive carriage on the hands of attendants (41). Indeed, epidemics of nosocomial, catheter-associated bacteriuria have been traced to the transfer of pathogens on the contaminated hands of hospital staff attendants from one drainage-bag spigot to another. To prevent this iatrogenic form of infection, medical staff must wash their hands carefully between attending each patient.

Bacterial isolates in catheter-associated UTIs are usually those organisms found in the gastrointestinal tract of the host. Strains of *Escherichia coli*, species of *Klebsiella* and *Enterobacter*, and enterococci constitute about 50% of isolates found in patients who have not received antibiotics (52). *Staphylococcus epidermidis*, non-Group-D streptococci, and yeast account for one third of the isolates, especially in patients receiving antibiotics (23,52). Organisms such as *Pseudomonas* and *Serratia* cause infections late during hospitalization, particularly in patients receiving broad-spectrum antibiotics, bladder irrigations,

antineoplastic agents, or immunosuppressive drugs (51–53).

Urinary catheters and stents present a potentially colonizable surface for bacteria. Colonization may be asymptomatic or may cause bacteremia and clinical UTIs. Sessile bacteria trapped and growing in an exopolysaccharide glycocalyx biofilm differ from free-growing planktonic bacteria, i.e., they are relatively protected from antibiotics, antibodies, phagocytic cells, etc. (54). Successful treatment of biofilm-related UTIs requires either 1) removal of the catheter or 2) very high antibiotic levels, usually more than 20 times the MIC (Minimum Inhibitory Concentration) for planktonic bacteria (55). Antibiotic efficacy against biofilm bacteria can be enhanced by electric field stimulation.

Risk factors for bacteriuria in catheterized patients (Table 3) include duration of catheterization, inadequate care of the drainage bag and closed drainage system, female gender, diseases such as diabetes mellitus or renal failure, and systemic immunosuppression. Many nursing home patients have indwelling catheters for urinary incontinence (particularly females) or prostatic obstruction. Some bacteria (e.g., *Providencia stuartii* and *S. epidermidis*) readily adhere to catheter surfaces and are frequent causes of catheter-associated bacteriuria. Urease-producing bacteria such as the *Proteus* species hydrolyze urea to ammonia, increase urinary pH, and predispose to the formation of struvite and apatite stones.

Complications

Closed urinary catheter drainage and other preventive measures reduce the rate of catheter-related UTI. However, infected patients experience significant morbidity. At least 70% of symptomatic nosocomial bacteriuria are catheter related (21,24). While most patients experience cystitis, others develop prostatitis, epididymitis, or pyelonephritis. A special risk exists if infection occurs with urea-splitting bacteria, such as the *Proteus* species—namely, the rapid formation of infected struvite and apatite stones.

Bacteremia is a significant threat to patients with indwelling catheters. Patients with catheters are 5–8 times more susceptible to bacteremia than noncatheterized pa-

Table 3. Risk factors for nosocomial UTIs

Female sex
Prolonged catheterization
Age
Debilitating disease
Immunosuppression
Granulocytopenia
Malnutrition
Alcoholism
Prolonged hospitalization

tients (24). The risk of bacteremia increases with the duration of catheterization and reaches 10% by 37 days (24). Sixty-five percent of bacteremias in the SENIC Project occurred in patients with urinary catheters, and the mortality rate was about 10% (21,53). Acute bacterial prostatitis, prostatic abscess, and epididymitis may complicate indwelling catheter drainage in men.

Noninfectious complications of chronic urethral catheterization include bladder calculi, contracted noncompliant bladders, vesicoureteral reflux, urethral incompetence, urethral stricture, urethral fistula, and bladder carcinoma. The incidence of bladder carcinoma is higher in catheterized patients as a result of chronic irritation and squamous metaplasia of the epithelium. The highest risk of bladder cancer is in patients managed with indwelling Foley catheters for more than 10 years (56). Chronic catheter use also causes polypoid cystitis and nephrogenic adenoma. The latter is a nonmalignant metaplastic transformation of the bladder epithelium (57). Polypoid cystitis is a benign reactive lesion (58).

Proper fixation of an indwelling catheter to the lower abdomen or upper thigh reduces the risk of urethral stricture. Strictures may occur in patients having open heart surgery, probably as a result of mucosal ischemia (59). Catheter encrustation is common on catheters left in situ for more than 7–10 days. Calcium, magnesium, phosphorus, and urea nitrogen make up about 40% of the dry weight of encrusted material. Encrustation can be retarded by bladder irrigation with 10% hemiacidrin solution (Renacidin®) or the oral administration of acetohydroxamic acid (Lithostat®). Both agents prevent precipitation of struvite and apatite salts and thereby impede the formation of bladder calculi (60). Nonlatex catheters, e.g., silicone, may cause less urethritis, catheter encrustation, and stone formation compared to latex catheters (60).

The Foley balloon may on occasion not deflate, which makes catheter removal impossible (61). The balloon can be ruptured by injection of mineral oil or ether. Care must then be taken to ensure that balloon fragments do not remain in the bladder, since these may predispose to infection and stone formation. The usual reason the balloon fails to deflate is mechanical collapse of the catheter material in the channel leading to the balloon. This collapse can be overcome by insertion of a fine catheter stylet, such as one from a CVP manometer, to clear the channel (62). The balloons of all catheters should be tested, i.e., inflated and deflated exvivo before they are inserted into the urinary tract. After prostatic surgery, a 30-mL balloon catheter is used to prevent slippage of the balloon into the prostatic fossa; however, this large balloon may cause troublesome postoperative bladder spasms.

In quadriplegics, bladder distension from obstruction to catheter drainage can lead to autonomic dysreflexia. This outcome typically occurs in patients with high spinal cord injury (above T7) and is manifested by hypertension, severe headache, sweating and piloerection above the level of the lesion, facial flushing, and bradycardia (63). Auto-nomic dysreflexia can be life-threatening and requires prompt treatment. Dysreflexia is caused by the uninhibited sympathetic discharge triggered by the bladder distension, and bradycardia results from reflex baroreceptor activation in the carotid sinus and aortic arch. Treatment consists of prompt decompression of the bladder and the use of an alpha-sympatholytic agent, e.g., phentolamine, prazosin, etc. (63,64). Chronic, mild dysreflexia may be treated pharmacologically with oral agents, e.g., prazosin 1 mg orally twice daily. Occasionally, devastating complications may occur as a consequence of urinary tract catheterization, e.g., bladder gangrene and perforation (65,66).

PREVENTION AND MANAGEMENT OF CATHETER-ASSOCIATED BACTERIURIA

Indications for catheterization

Catheterization of the urinary tract should be limited to situations where the benefits outweigh the potential risks and complications. The best prophylaxis against catheter-related bacteriuria is avoidance of catheterization. When catheterization is required, in-and-out or intermittent catheterization is preferable to indwelling catheterization—either Foley or suprapubic.

Aseptic catheterization

Catheter insertion should be performed under aseptic conditions by trained personnel after thorough cleansing of the meatus and perineum with an antiseptic solution. Antiseptic solutions should be tested periodically to rule out bacterial contamination. The use of aseptic technique in the handling of the collecting apparatus, especially when the catheter–drainage tubing junction is assembled or when this seal is broken for irrigation, is important.

Closed urinary drainage system

Closed drainage systems reduce the frequency of catheter-associated bacteriuria. In 1928, Dukes (67) first described the potential benefits of such a system. However, four decades passed before closed drainage became popular after studies showed that closed systems reduce the rate of catheter-associated infection from 80% to 15%–30% (42,68). The incidence of bacteriuria rises sharply, however, whenever the integrity of the closed system is breached. The drainage bag should remain below the level of the patient and never be inverted; the drainage spigot must not be contaminated (69). The points of bacterial entry into the urinary drainage system are illustrated in Figure 1: 1) the urethral meatus and around the catheter; 2) the junction between the catheter and collection tubing; 3) the connection of the drainage tubing to the collection bag and reflux from the bag to the tubing; and 4) the mouth of the bag drainage spigot.

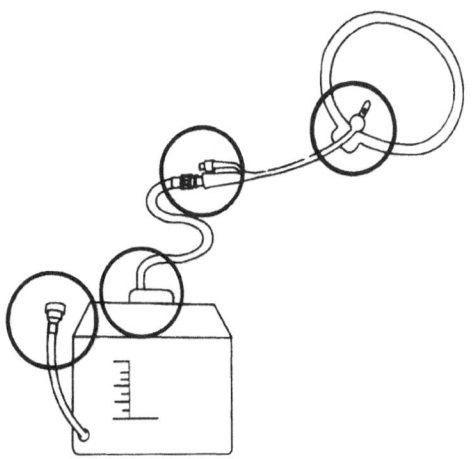

Figure 1. Potential sites of bacterial contamination in catheter drainage system.

Prophylaxis of extraluminal bacterial migration

Extraluminal pericatheter migration of bacteria is the main cause of catheter-associated bacteriuria (38,46). Trials of daily cleansing regimens show that neither once-daily cleansing with green soap and water nor twice-daily applications of povidone-iodine solution and ointment is more beneficial than no meatal care in preventing bacteriuria (70). The antiseptic benefits of meatal care in women may be negated by the adverse effect of urethral manipulation, which may enhance entry of bacteria into the bladder, whether or not the woman is catheterized (71). On the other hand, crusting occurs frequently at the catheter–meatal interface in men, and cleansing is a welcome comfort measure.

Conventional urethral catheters are made of latex. No significant differences in the rate of bacteriuria have been noted between latex, sialastic, polyvinylchloride, or hydropolymer-coated indwelling catheters (72,73). Moreover, antibiotic-impregnated catheters do not reduce infection rates, probably because the antibacterial activity is short-lived (74). Hydrophylic coating of latex catheters reduces catheter encrustation and precipitation of magnesium ammonium phosphate. However, it is unclear whether this effect potentiates antibiotic therapy of established catheter-related bacteriuria (75).

Antibacterial therapy—prophylaxis and cure

If catheters are left in situ long enough, bacteria gain access to the bladder, drainage tubing, and drainage receptacle, despite all efforts at prevention. Antibacterial therapy can be directed at prophylaxis or cure of established infection.

Bladder irrigation with antimicrobial solutions (e.g., 0.25% acetic acid, neomycin-polymyxin solution) tempo-rarily lower the incidence of catheter-associated UTI. Irrigation can be intermittent or continuous via a three-way Foley catheter. However, continuous bladder irrigation is expensive, requires extra nursing time, and can cause discomfort and gross hematuria (76). Superinfection with resistant bacteria or yeast may develop after extended periods of irrigation. The addition of bacitracin to neomycin/polymyxin reduces the chance of superinfection with gram-positive cocci (77). Currently, bladder irrigations are of limited use in the management of indwelling catheters.

Antiseptic solutions placed in drainage bags of closed urinary drainage systems inhibit ascending bladder infections (30,31,48). Oxycyanide, formalin, chlorhexidine, hydrogen peroxide (3%), and povidone-iodine have been recommended as drainage bag additives to reduce catheter-associated bacteriuria (48,78). Overall, it appears that periodic instillation of disinfectants into drainage bags is ineffective in reducing, the rate of bacteriuria (79,80).

Systemic antibiotics and urinary antiseptics have been disappointing when used to prevent UTIs in patients with indwelling catheters. The rate of infection is seldom reduced, and antibiotic-resistant organisms may emerge (32,76,81). The use of antimicrobics combined with strict closed urinary drainage of short duration can keep the urinary tract sterile or delay the onset of infection (82–84). The system should be cultured at least weekly and contaminated systems replaced promptly.

Prior to catheter removal, a urine culture should be obtained and appropriate antibacterial therapy instituted to ensure a sterile urinary tract after removal. If the urine is sterile at the time of catheter removal, antibacterial therapy usually is not necessary. An exception is the high-risk patient who suffers from debilitating disease (76,85).

Catheter care teams

Catheter care teams can minimize catheter-associated bacteriuria and its sequelae (84,86). Undoubtedly, the education of personnel regarding the importance of handwashing, the use of aseptic technique in catheter handling and care of the drainage bag, the avoidance of unnecessary disruption of a closed drainage system, and the wisdom of physical separation of catheterized patients, as well as their urine measuring equipment, will reduce the rate of infection (41,49). Some, however, argue that availability of a catheter care team may increase the tendency of physicians to manage their patients with catheterization.

GUIDELINES FOR CATHETER MANAGEMENT

1. Strict indications for catheterization must exist.
2. Intermittent catheterization is preferred to indwelling catheterization.
3. Closed drainage system is recommended.

4. Aseptic insertion of urethral catheters is mandatory. The catheter should be secured to minimize movement.
5. Irrigation of the catheter is kept to a minimum; however, aseptic technique must be used when irrigation is required.
6. Prophylactic, systemic antibiotics are not routinely indicated. Symptomatic infections require therapy based on urine culture and sensitivity testing.
7. Asymptomatic bacteriuria should not be treated until just before the catheter is removed. Exceptions include infections caused by urease-producing bacteria.
8. Catheterized patients with bacteriuria should be isolated from catheterized patients who are noninfected to minimize cross-contamination.
9. Prior to removal of the catheter, patients with positive urine cultures should be started on pathogen-specific antimicrobial therapy.
10. At the time of insertion or removal of the catheter, patients with bacteriuria (especially due to enterococcus) who have heart murmurs, valvular heart disease, or prosthetic devices should receive prophylactic antimicrobial therapy to prevent bacterial endocarditis or infection of the prosthesis.
11. Members of the hospital staff must be educated regarding all aspects of this system: urinary drainage, catheterization, and asepsis.

INTERMITTENT CATHETERIZATION

Intermittent catheterization is the method of choice for bladder drainage in acute spinal cord injury patients. Sterile intermittent catheterization was introduced by Guttmann to control urinary infection, rehabilitate the bladders, and render patients catheter free (87).

Intermittent catheterization requires trained personnel or a well-motivated patient with manual dexterity. Intermittent catheterization may not be practical in quadriplegics who are unable to self-catheterize. The usual catheterization regime requires q 6 hours catheterization. The volumes drained and the state of continence between catheterizations are monitored, and every effort is made to limit the volumes to 400–600 mL (4,7). Larger volumes require more frequent catheterization. Incontinence should be evaluated urodynamically to pinpoint its cause, e.g., hyperreflexia, bladder neck incompetence, and select appropriate pharmacologic therapy. Anticholinergics paralyze the detrusor muscle, and alphasympathomimetics (e.g., ephedrine, phenyl propanolamine) increase urethral and bladder neck competence.

The advantages of intermittent catheterization over indwelling Foley catheters include less bacteriuria and infection, increased patient comfort, and less interference with the patient's social and sexual life. Intermittent catheterization is frequently utilized in patients with spinal cord injury, in patients with neurogenic bladder dysfunc-tion, and for short-term management of urinary retention (18,88,89).

Sterile versus clean intermittent catheterization

Sterile intermittent catheterization was initially used in spinal-cord-injury patients because urethral or suprapubic drainage carries a high risk of infection, sepsis, and renal failure. Its effectiveness in paraplegics and quadriplegics quickly became apparent (87). Bacteriuria (continuous or intermittent) occurs in about 50% of patients on intermittent catheterization, but its significance is not fully known. Some clinicians recommend oral proplylaxis with nitrofurantoin or vitamin C plus methenamine mandelate or bladder instillations with neomycin–polymyxin solution to reduce bacteriuria (7,90,91). Asymptomatic bacteriuria is, however, usually left untreated in patients who regularly empty their bladders by intermittent catheterization (92). Symptomatic patients should be cultured and treated with appropriate antimicrobics. Urethritis and epididymoorchitis may occur early in the course of intermittent catheterization; therefore, oral antibiotics may be prescribed for patients during the first few weeks of the program (93).

Bladder infection occurs secondary to decreased bladder resistance and vascularity resulting from bladder overdistension (18). Prevention of overdistension by frequent catheterization allows the natural bladder defenses to overcome any bacteria introduced into the bladder during "clean" catheterization. Clean intermittent catheterization is widely used in adults and children to manage urinary retention, detrusor areflexia, and bladder dysfunction. Clean catheterization more often leads to asymptomatic bacteriuria than does sterile intermittent catheterization; however, each is a safe and effective method of bladder drainage that allows preservation of the patient's self-esteem, avoids the use of external collecting devices, and minimizes the occurrence of significant infection and urosepsis. Sterile intermittent catheterization is recommended for hospitalized patients to avoid the risk of nosocomial UTIs, whereas nonhospitalized patients are adequately managed with clean catheterization.

Careful instruction in the technique of clean self-intermittent catheterization is required. Motivation and a good understanding of the external genitalia and urethral anatomy are prerequisites. The catheter size (8–16 F) varies with the age of the patient; rubber, plastic, glass, or metal catheters are used. In clean intermittent catheterization, soap and water are used to cleanse the catheter and external genitalia. Only water-soluble lubricants, e.g., K-Y jelly, are recommended. The catheter is boiled in hot water for about 5 minutes daily and stored in a clean, dry container between catheterizations.

Besides bacteriuria and incontinence, other complications of intermittent catheterization occur (93). Mechanical problems secondary to adductor spasms, obesity, hypospadiac external urethral openings, and edema can make catheter insertion difficult. Whole catheters or tips of catheters can be "lost" inside the bladder. Bladder calculi, usually calcium phosphate, can result from the introduction of oil-based lubricants or pubic hair into the bladder. These stones may be asymptomatic or cause recurrent infection, bladder spasms, or sudden interruption of urinary drainage. They can be managed by endoscopic removal or lithotripsy.

NEPHROSTOMY TUBES

Nonsurgical catheter placement within the renal pelvis (*percutaneous nephrostomy*) was first used by Goodwin to drain a hydronephrotic renal pelvis (10). It is now used to treat hydronephrosis, in endourological manipulations, for postoperative urinary drainage, for percutaneous stone dissolution, to determine of renal function, and to assess the degree of upper-tract obstruction (the Whitaker pressure-perfusion test) (2,11,12).

Large-diameter (18–22 F) Malecot or de Pezzer catheters can be placed in the renal pelvis during surgery (e.g., pyelolithotomy, anatrophic nephrolithotomy) to allow urinary drainage and permit postoperative access for radiograhic study or chemolysis of residual stone fragments (19). Smaller tubes (8–14 F) can be inserted percutaneously using local anesthesia and an angiographic guide wire controlled by fluoroscopy, ultrasound, or computerized tomography (2). The nephrostomy tract can be dilated using fascial or balloon dilators (24–32 F) to allow access to the renal pelvis for endourological manipulation, e.g., stone removal or ultrasonic lithotripsy (94,95). The nephrostomy tube is left in situ for 24–72 hours to monitor bleeding, to prevent urinary extravasation, and to provide urinary drainage.

Percutaneous nephrostomy tube placement and percutaneous stone removal (*percutaneous nephrolithotomy*) can be complicated by bleeding (95). This bleeding, mainly venous, is generally controlled by the tamponade effect of the rigid nephroscope sheath used for stone manipulation. Postmanipulation, a large nephrostomy tube is left in the renal pelvis for drainage and a parenteral diuretic reduces clot formation (96,97).

Significant arterial bleeding occurs in less than 1% of patients following percutaneous stone removal with hemorrhage from a segmental branch of the renal artery, a pseudoaneurysm, or an arteriovenous fistula (96,98). Acute hemorrhage is manifested by gross hematuria or bleeding through or around the nephrostomy tube, either continuously or intermittently. Blood transfusions are given as needed, and an effort is made to control the bleeding using a Foley balloon or angiographic balloon for tamponade of the nephrostomy tract. Persistent bleeding is managed by renal angiography and selective embolization of the bleeding vessel. If angiographic embolization is unsuccessful, surgical exploration, often resulting in partial or total nephrectomy, is necessary.

Other complications of percutaneous endourology include urine extravasation and sepsis. Renal pelvic tears can lead to extravasation of fluid into the retroperitoneal space. Absorption of this fluid leads to fluid overload, hyponatremia, and hyperammonemia if glycine is used as an irrigant. Strict monitoring of fluid ingress and egress during percutaneous surgery is necessary (97). Prophylactic antibiotics are routinely administered to reduce the chance of urosepsis.

Mechanical problems occur with nephrostomy tubes (99). The tube may become dislodged or blocked by sediment or clots. Dislodgement is prevented by anchoring the tube to the skin with a nonabsorbable silk or nylon suture. Self-retaining nephrostomy tubes (e.g., Cope, Foley, Circle) reduce the chance of migration or dislodgement. If a tube is dislodged completely, the tract can usually be renegotiated using a guide wire and a new tube inserted under fluoroscopic control. Tube blockage is prevented by intermittent, gentle irrigations with normal saline, the use of a large diameter tube, and frequent tube changes. A high fluid intake with a brisk diuresis is also helpful (99). Skin care at the catheter entry site consists of cleansing with antiseptics and sterile dressing changes.

Percutaneous chemolysis is a useful adjunct for dissolving struvite renal calculi. Chemolysis is generally used for residual fragments after open renal stone surgery, extracorporeal shock wave lithotripsy, or percutaneous lithotripsy. A 10% hemiacidrin solution (Renacidin®) is useful for dissolving triple phosphate calculi, whereas alkalinating agents (e.g., bicarbonate, Tham-E) dissolve uric acid and cystine calculi (19). Sepsis is a potential complication of percutaneous irrigation, especially when infected struvite calculi are present. Marked elevations in renal pelvic pressure (>30 cm H_2O) should be avoided by the use of a three-way irrigation system incorporating a manometer. This prevents backflow of urine and fluid into the vascular system and reduces the risk of bacteremia. Hemiacidrin solution contains magnesium, and excessive absorption can lead to hypermagnesemia with resultant neuromuscular paralysis. Serum magnesium levels should be monitored daily. Urine cultures are obtained frequently, and appropriate pathogen-specific antimicrobial drugs are administered during irrigation (19).

Nephrostomy tubes can cause bacteriuria. The responsible organisms are commonly gram-positive skin bacteria (staphylococci and streptococci) that enter through or alongside the nephrostomy tube (100). Appropriate antimicrobial agents are used to treat symptomatic infections and at the time of tube removal.

URETERAL STENTS

Ureteroscopic procedures, percutaneous endourology, and extracorporeal shock wave lithotripsy (ESWL) have led to widespread use of ureteral stents (101,102). Stents are used to prevent obstruction by stone fragments (*steinstrasse*) following ESWL lithotripsy, to push ureteral stones back into the renal pelvis and thus allow ESWL treatment, and to stent the ureter following ureteroscopic manipulation and ureteral dilatation. Stents also relieve obstructive uropathy (e.g., metastatic retroperitoneal disease, benign retroperitoneal fibrosis), manage ureteral fistulas, and prevent leaks after ureteral surgery. The use of stents to bypass obstructions and for temporary or palliative drainage has reduced the need for open surgery in many urologic conditions (102).

Ureteral stents are external or internal. The distal ends of external ureteral stents traverse the urethra and are usually fixed externally to an indwelling catheter using silk ligatures. Stent migration (upward or downward) potential, the threat of ascending upper-tract infection, and patient discomfort make external stents unsuitable for long-term use.

Internal or indwelling ureteral stents have the advantage of not requiring a Foley catheter for external fixation. The double-J ureteral catheter is the most widely used internal stent. J configurations at the upper and lower ends prevent migration. Stents are made from polymers, including polyethylene, polyurethane, silicone, and C-flex (a copolymer of silicone) (103). Silicone stents are the most widely used due to their biocompatibility, pliability and flexibility. However, stents made of polyurethane, C-flex, or Urosoft are used to bypass obstructions and to overcome the flexibility of silicone stents. The softness of silicone ensures patient comfort, although ureteral placement over a guide wire may prove difficult.

Endoscopic, retrograde insertion via the cystoscope or the ureteroscope is the most common technique of stent placement. Stents are usually inserted over a guide wire under fluoroscopic control. Attention to stent position, size (usually 3–8 F in diameter), and length (20–30 cm) is important. Improper stent selection can lead to traumatic bleeding from the renal pelvis or bladder, trigonal irritation, and poor urinary drainage. Stents can also be inserted in an antegrade fashion via a percutaneous approach or by open surgery (102).

Ureteral stents can cause vesicoureteral reflux, microscopic hematuria, pyuria, encrustation, and irritative bladder symptoms (Table 4) (103). Urosepsis is uncommon, unless the stent becomes occluded. Bladder irritation (frequency, urgency, pain) generally indicates that the stent is too long, with its distal end resting on the trigone or bladder neck. If these symptoms persist, the stent should be replaced with a shorter one. Pyuria is common in patients with indwelling stents and represents a reaction to the stent's foreign material. Infection occurs in less than 10% of patients with indwelling stents (104). Urine cultures should be obtained at least monthly in patients with indwelling stents; appropriate antibiotics should be prescribed as indicated. Encrustation of ureteral stents occurs commonly, especially in patients with bacteriuria or urolithiasis. Catheter encrustation can lead to struvite stone formation, which may necessitate treatment with

Table 4. Complications of double-J ureteral stents

Encrustation
Migration
   Upward
   Downward
Stent "fracture"
Infection
   <10%
Reflux
Pain/discomfort
Miscellaneous
   Pyuria
   Hematuria
   Nondrainage

percutaneous renal pelvic irrigation or open surgical removal (105). Encrustation can be retarded by promoting adequate hydration and an acidic urine. Long-term antimicrobial suppression, frequent abdominal x-ray studies, and short periods of internal stenting are recommended to reduce the occurrence of catheter encrustation and stone formation (106). The common stent complications are listed in Table 4.

Upward stent migration can cause obstruction, sepsis, or stone formation. Displaced stents generally can be retrieved from below by using the ureteroscope or from above by a percutaneous approach. Nondisplaced internal stents usually are removed or replaced via the cystoscope. Internal stents can be removed without cystoscopy if, during placement, a nonabsorbable suture is tied to the bladder end of the stent, exteriorized through the urethra, and taped to the penis or abdomen. A gentle tug on the suture usually suffices to remove the stent (107). Breakage can occur due to stent damage at the time of insertion or overzealous use of force during endoscopic removal (108). Stents used for long-term drainage must be changed frequently, especially in elderly, debilitated patients who tend to forget about their stents, become dehydrated, and thus promote catheter encrustation and stone formation. Patients with ureteral stents must be monitored carefully and evaluated promptly if fever, flank pain, gross hematuria, azotemia, or infection develop.

EXTERNAL CONDOM CATHETER DRAINAGE

Condom catheters are external collecting devices used in incontinent men with central nervous system disease (e.g., cerebrovascular accidents), postprostatectomy incontinence, and detrusor hyperreflexia, e.g., quadriplegia or multiple sclerosis (109). Condom drainage is not suitable for women.

Various types of condom catheters are commercially available. They can also be constructed makeshift by using a condom or a finger cot. The condom part of the catheter is fixed to the penile shaft using tincture of benzoin, tape, and a surgical adhesive to provide a skin bond. Patients with short penile shafts have difficulty in keeping the condom on the penis, but this problem can be corrected by insertion of a penile prosthesis to provide increased length and rigidity.

Incontinent patients managed with condom catheters have a high rate of bacteriuria, particularly with *Proteus* and *Pseudomonas* species (110,111). Bacteria from the penis, perineum, and scrotum colonize the condom part of the collecting device, and this bacterial reservoir leads to ascending bacterial infection. Urine cultures are unreliable with the condom in place; instead, the condom device should be removed, the penis cleaned, and a midstream or catheterized specimen obtained.

Poorly fitted condom devices can cause penile skin maceration, skin breakdown, skin necrosis, urethrocutaneous fistulas, and obstruction to urinary flow. These problems can be avoided by careful application of the catheter, prevention of kinking of the tubings, and frequent patient monitoring. The latter is particularly important in patients with neuropathic bladders who have absent or reduced penile sensation, since skin breakdown and pressure necrosis may go undetected due to lack of pain sensation (112).

SUPRAPUBIC CATHETERS

Because indwelling urethral catheters have many problems, suprapubic catheters are good alternatives (113). They are well tolerated, require less nursing care than indwelling urethral catheters, avoid ascending pericatheter urethral infection, and generally prevent prostatitis and epididymitis.

Suprapubic catheters are inserted percutaneously or during open surgical procedures. Percutaneous suprapubic catheters (e.g., Stamey suprapubic catheter, sialistic Cystocath) are inserted at the bedside using local anesthesia. The patient should have a full bladder before the tube is inserted; otherwise, the bowel may be damaged. If the bladder is not palpable, a spinal needle (#20) should be inserted percutaneously into the bladder, urine aspirated, and the bladder distended with sterile saline. Patients who have undergone previous lower abdominal or pelvic surgery may have bowel or peritoneum attached to the bladder, which often makes them better candidates for open suprapubic cystostomy than for percutaneous cystostomy.

Percutaneous suprapubic catheters are used in various situations (114,115). They are preferred to indwelling urethral catheters in men who develop acute urinary retention associated with acute bacterial prostatitis. The suprapubic tube is also used following anti-incontinence surgery (e.g., Stamey urethropexy, Burch colposuspension) to minimize infection and to monitor residual urine during postoperative voiding trials.

The suprapubic catheter is well tolerated, and its short-term use produces few complications. Bladder irritability can develop if the catheter tip abuts the bladder trigone.

This is managed by adjustment of catheter position or use of oral anticholinergics, e.g., oxybutynin chloride, propantheline bromide, etc. Bacteriuria may occur via spread of skin bacteria alongside the tube into the bladder; however, bacteriuria rates are less with suprapubic tubes than with indwelling urethral catheters. The long-term use of suprapubic tubes, especially in the debilitated and elderly patient, results in a chronic foreign body reaction, with the risk of chronic cystitis, bladder contracture, bladder stones, and possible malignant transformation of the bladder epithelium.

REFERENCES

1. Beeson PB: Editorial: the case against the catheter. *Am J Med* 24:1–3, 1958.
2. Fowler JE Jr, Meares EM Jr, Goldin RA: Percutaneous nephrostomy: Techniques, indications and results. *Urology* 6:428–434, 1975.
3. Finney RP: Experience with new double J ureteral catheter stents. *J Urol* 120:678–681, 1978.
4. Perkash I: Intermittent catheterization: the urologist's point of view. *J Urol* 111:356–360, 1974.
5. Gibbons RP, Correa RJ Jr, Cummings KB, Mason JT: Experience with indwelling ureteral stent catheter. *J Urol* 115:22–26, 1976.
6. Leventhal A, Pfau A: Pharmacologic management of post-operative overdistention of the bladder. *Surg Gynecol Obstet* 146:347–348, 1978.
7. Anderson RU: Non-sterile intermittent catheterization with antibiotic prophylaxis in the acute spinal cord injured male patient. *J Urol* 124:392–394, 1980.
8. Hirsh DD, Fainstein V, Musher DM: Do condom catheter collecting systems cause urinary tract infection? *JAMA* 242:340–341, 1979.
9. Fam BA, Rossier AB, Blunt K, Gabilondo FB, Sarkarati M, Sethi J, Yalla SV: Experience in the urologic management of 120 early spinal cord injury patients. *J Urol* 119:485–487, 1978.
10. Goodwin WE, Casey WC, Woolf W: Percutaneous trocar (needle) nephrostomy in hydronephrosis. *JAMA* 157:891–894, 1955.
11. Pfister RC, Newhouse JH: Interventional percutaneous pyeloureteral techniques. II. Percutaneous nephrostomy and other procedures. *Radiol Clin North Am* 17:351–362, 1979.
12. Whitaker RH: Methods of assessing obstruction in dilated ureters. *Br J Urol* 45:15–23, 1973.
13. Huffman JL, Bagley DH, Lyon ES: Extending cystoscopic techniques into the ureter and renal pelvis—experience with ureteroscopy and pyeloscopy. *JAMA* 250:2002–2005, 1983.
14. Campbell RJ, Griffith DP: Exchange ureteral stent insertion using pullout suture after extracorporeal shock wave lithotripsy. *Urology* 29:653–655, 1987.
15. Cass AS, Smith CS, Gleich P: Management of urinary calculi in pregnancy. *Urology* 28:370–372, 1986.
16. Stamey TA, Pfau A: Urinary infections: a selective review and some observations. *Calif Med* 113:16–35, 1970.
17. Fairley KF, Bond AG, Brown RB, Habersberger P: Simple test to determine the site of urinary tract infection. *Lancet* 2:427–428, 1967.
18. Lapides J, Diokno AC, Gould FR, Lowe BS: Further observations of self-catheterization. *J Urol* 116:169–171, 1976.

19. Sant GR, Blaivas JG, Meares EM Jr: Hemiacidrin irrigation in the management of struvite calculi: longterm results. *J Urol* 1048–1050, 1983.

20. Dretler SP: Management of "steinstrasse." *Endourology* 1:1–2, 1986.

21. Meares EM Jr: Nosocomial urinary tract infections. *Infect Surg* 5:278–280, 1986.

22. Allen JR, Hightower AW, Martin SM, Dixon RE: Secular trends in nosocomial infections: 1970–1979. *Am J Med* 70:389–392, 1981.

23. Sant GR: Urinary tract infections in the elderly. *Sem in Urol* 5:126–153, 1987.

24. Haley RW, Hooton TM, Culver DH, Stanley RC, Emori TG, Hardison CD, Quade D, Shachtman RH, Schaberg DR, Shah BV, Schatz GD: Nosocomial infections in U.S. hospitals, 1975–1976. Estimated frequency by selected characteristics of patients. *Am J Med* 70:947–959, 1981.

25. Marple CD: The frequency and character of urinary tract infections in an unselected group of women. *Ann Intern Med* 14:2220–2239, 1941.

26. Turck M, Goffe B, Peterdorf RG: The urethral catheter and urinary tract infection. *J Urol* 88:834–837, 1962.

27. Brumfitt W, Davies BI, Rosser E: Urethral catheter as a cause of urinary-tract infection in pregnancy and puerperium. *Lancet* 2:1059–1062, 1961.

28. Finkelberg R, Kunin CM: Clinical evaluation of closed urinary drainage systems. *JAMA* 207:1657–1662, 1969.

29. Kass EH: Asymptomatic infections of the urinary tract. *Trans Assoc Am Physicians* 69:56–63, 1956.

30. Kunin CM, McCormack RC: Prevention of catheter-induced urinary tract infections by sterile closed drainage. *N Eng J Med* 274:1155–1161, 1966.

31. Martin CM, Bookrajian EN: Bacteriuria prevention after indwelling urinary catheterization. A controlled study. *Arch Intern Med* 110:703–711, 1962.

32. Warren JW, Platt R, Thomas RJ, Rosner B, Kass EH: Antibiotic irrigation and catheter-associated urinary tract infections. *N Engl J Med* 299:570–573, 1978.

33. Stark R, Maki D: Bacteriuria in the catheterized patient. What quantitative level of bacteriuria is relevant. *N Eng J Med* 311:560–564, 1984.

34. Turck M, Stamm W: Nosocomial infection of the urinary tract. *Am J Med* 70:651–654, 1981.

35. Bergqvist D, Bronnestam R, Hedelin H, Stahl A: The relevance of urinary sampling methods in patients with indwelling foley catheters. *Br J Urol* 52:92–95, 1980.

36. Helmholtz HF: Determination of the bacterial content of the urethra. A new method, with results of a study of 82 men. *J Urol* 64:158–162, 1950.

37. Cox CE: The urethra and its relationship to urinary tract infection: the flora of the normal female urethra. *South Med J* 59:621–626, 1966.

38. Garibaldi RA, Burke JP, Britt MR, Miller WA, Smith CB: Meatal colonization and catheter-associated bacteriuria. *N Engl J Med* 303:316–318, 1980.

39. Guze LB, Beeson PB: Observations on the reliability and safety of bladder catheterization for bacteriologic study of the urine. *N Eng J Med* 255:474–475, 1956.

40. Hardy PG, Ederer GM, Matsen JM: Contamination of commercially packaged urinary catheter kits with pseudomonad EO-l. *N Engl J Med* 282:33–35, 1970.

41. Maki DG, Hennekens CH, Bennett JV: Prevention of catheter-associated urinary tract infection. An additional measure. *JAMA* 221:1270–1271, 1972.

42. Garibaldi RA, Burke JP, Dickman ML, Smith CB: Factors predisposing to bacteriuria during indwelling urethral catheterization. *N Engl J Med* 291:215–219, 1974.

43. Cox CE, Hinman F Jr: Experiments with induced bacteriuria, vesical emptying and bacterial growth on the mechanism of bladder defense to infection. *J Urol* 86:739–748, 1961.

44. Daifuku R, Stamm WE: Bacterial adherence to bladder urothelial cells in catheter-associated urinary tract infection. *N Eng J Med* 314:1208–1213, 1986.

45. Kass EH, Schneiderman LJ: Entry of bacteria into the urinary tract of patients with inlying catheters. *N Engl J Med* 256:556–557, 1957.

46. Bultitude MI, Eykyn S: The relationship between the urethral flora and urinary infection in the catheterized male. *Br J Urol* 45:678–683, 1975.

47. Weyrauch HM, Bassett BJ: Ascending infection in an artificial urinary tract. *Stanford Med Bull* 9:25–29, 1951.

48. Maizels M, Schaeffer AJ: Decreased incidence of bacteriuria associated with periodic instillations of hydrogen peroxide into the urethral catheter drainage bag. *J Urol* 123:841–845, 1980.

49. Rutala WA, Kennedy VA, Loflin HB, Sarrubbi FA: Serratia marcescens nosocomial infections of the urinary tract associated with urine measuring containers and urinometers. *Am J Med* 70:659–663, 1981.

50. Gillespie WA, Lennon GG, Linton KB, Slade N: Prevention of catheter infection of urine in female patients. *Br Med J* 2:12–16, 1962.

51. Schaberg DR, Weinstein RA, Stamm WE: Epidemics of nosocomial urinary tract infection caused by multiple resistant gram-negative bacilli: Epidemiology and control. *J Infect Dis* 133:363–366, 1976.

52. McCormack RC: Nosocomial urinary tract infections. In: EW Hook, GL Mandell, JM Gwaltney Jr, MA Sande, eds, *Current Concepts of Infectious Diseases*. New York, John Wiley & Sons, pp 233–240, 1977.

53. Krieger JN, Kaiser DI, Wenzel RP: Nosocomial urinary tract infections. Secular trends, treatment and economics in a university hospital. *J Urol* 130:102–106, 1983.

54. Costerton JW, Cheny KJ, Greesey GG, et al.: Bacterial biofilms in nature and disease. *Ann Rev Microbiol* 41:435, 1987.

55. Nickel J: Bacterial biofilms in urological infectious diseases. *Dial Pediatr Urol* 14:7, 1991.

56. Locke JR, Hill DE, Walzer Y: Incidence of squamous cell carcinoma in patients with long-term catheter drainage. *J Urol* 133:1034–1035, 1985.

57. Ritchey ML, Novicki DE, Schultenover SJ: Nephrogenic adenoma of bladder: a report of 8 cases. *J Urol* 131:537–539, 1984.

58. Ekelund P, Johansson S: Polypoid cystitis: a catheter-associated lesion of the human bladder. *Acta Pathol Microb Scand* 87A:179, 1979.

59. Elhilali MM, Hassouna M, Abdel-Hakim A, Teijeira J: Urethral stricture following cardiovascular surgery: role of urethral ischemia. *J Urol* 135:275–277, 1986.

60. Burns JR, Gauthier JF: Prevention of urinary catheter encrustations by acetohydroxamic acid. *J Urol* 132:455–456, 1984.

61. Kelly TWJ, Griffiths GL: Balloon problems with Foley catheters. *Lancet* 2:1310, 1983.

62. Kleeman FJ: Technique for removal of Foley catheter when

balloon does not deflate. *Urology* 21:416, 1983.

63. McGuire EJ, Wagner FM, Weiss RM: Treatment of autonomic dysreflexia with phenoxybenzamine. *J Urol* 115:53, 1976.

64. Texter JH Jr, Reece RW, Hranowsky N: Pentolinium in the management of autonomic hyperreflexia. *J Urol* 116:350–351, 1976.

65. Busse K, Altwein JE: Catheter-induced bladder gangrene. *J Urol* 112:461–462, 1974.

66. Freed JS, Krespi Y: Urologic catheter—unusual complication. *N Y State J Med* 79:1892–1893, 1979.

67. Dukes C: Urinary infections after excision of the rectum: their cause and prevention. *Proc R Soc Med* 22:259–270, 1928.

68. Miller A, Linton KB, Gillispie WA, Slade N, Mitchell JP: Catheter drainage and infection in acute retention of urine. *Lancet* 1:310–312, 1960.

69. Buddington WT, Graves RC: Management of catheter drainage. *J Urol* 62:387–393, 1949.

70. Burke JP, Garibaldi RA, Britt MR, Jacobson JA, Conti M, Alling DW: Prevention of catheter-associated urinary tract infections. Efficacy of daily meatal care regimen. *Am J Med* 70:655–658, 1981.

71. Bran JL, Levison ME, Kaye D: Entrance of bacteria into the female urinary bladder. *N Engl J Med* 286:626–629, 1972.

72. Tidd MJ, Gow JG, Pennington JH, Shelton J, Scott MR: Comparison of hydrophilic polymer-coated latex, untreated latex and PVC indwelling balloon catheters in the prevention of urinary infection. *Br J Urol* 48:285–291, 1976.

73. Monson T, Kunin CM: Evaluation of a polymer-coated indwelling catheter in prevention of infection. *J Urol* 111:220–222, 1974.

74. Butler HK, Kunin CM: Evaluation of polymyxin catheter lubricant and impregnanted catheters. *J Urol* 100:560–566, 1968.

75. Miller JM: The effect of hydron on latex urinary catheters. *J Urol* 113:530, 1975.

76. Andriole VT: Hospital acquired urinary infections and the indwelling catheter. *Urol Clin North Am* 451–469, 1975.

77. Fincke BG, Friedland G: Prevention and management of infection in the catheterized patient. *Urol Clin North Am* 3:313–321, 1976.

78. Webb JK, Blandy JP: Closed urinary drainage into plastic bags containing antiseptic. *Br J Urol* 40:585–588, 1968.

79. Thompson RL, Haley CE, Searcy MA, Guenthner SM, Kaiser DL, Groschel DHM, Gillenwater JY, Wenzel RP: Catheter-associated bacteriuria: failure to reduce attack rates using periodic instillations of a disinfectant into urinary drainage systems. *JAMA* 251:747–751, 1984.

80. Kunin CM: The drainage bag additive saga. *Infect Control* 6:261–262, 1985.

81. Brocklehurst JC, Brocklehurst S: The management of indwelling catheters. *Br J Urol* 50:102–105, 1978.

82. Britt MR, Garibaldi RA, Miller WA, Hebertson RM, Burke JP: Antimicrobial prophylaxis for catheter-associated bacteriuria. *Antimicrob Agents Chemother* 11:240–243, 1977.

83. Turck M, Petersdorf RG: The role of antibiotics in the prevention of urinary tract infections. *J Chronic Dis* 15:683–689, 1962.

84. Shapito SR, Santamarina A, Harrison JH: Catheter-associated urinary tract infections: incidence and a new approach to prevention. *J Urol* 112:659–663, 1974.

85. Chodak GW, Plaut ME: Systemic antibiotics for prophylaxis in urologic surgery: a critical review. *J Urol* 121:695–699, 1979.

86. Stamm WE: Guidelines for prevention of catheter-associated urinary tract infections. *Ann Intern Med* 82:386–390, 1975.

87. Guttmann L: Initial treatment of traumatic paraplegia. *Proc Royal Soc Med* 47:1103, 1954.

88. Firlit CF, Canning JR, Lloyd FA, Cross RR, Brewer RJ Jr: Experience with intermittent catheterization in chronic spinal cord injury patients. *J Urol* 114:234–236, 1975.

89. Kyker J, Gregory JG, Shah J, Schoenberg HW: Comparison of intermittent catheterization and supravesical diversion in children with meningomyelocele. *J Urol* 118:90–91, 1977.

90. Anderson RU: Prophylaxis of bacteriuria during intermittent catheterization of the acute neurogenic bladder. *J Urol* 123:364–366, 1980.

91. Orikasa S, Koyanagi T, Motomura M, Kudo T, Tozashi M, Tsuju I: Experience with non-sterile, intermittent self-catheterization. *J Urol* 115:141–143, 1976.

92. Hinman F Jr: Intermittent catheterization and vesical defenses. *J Urol* 117:57–60, 1977.

93. Klauber GT, Sant GR: Complications of intermittent catheterization. *Urol Clin North Am* 10:557–562, 1983.

94. White EC, Smith AD: Percutaneous stone extraction from 200 patients. *J Urol* 132:437–438, 1984.

95. Segura JW: Endourology. *J Urol* 132:1079–1084, 1984.

96. Segura JW: Percutaneous endourology: vascular complications. *World J Urol* 3:24–26, 1985.

97. Rudy DC, Woodside JR, Borden TA, Ball WS: Adult respiratory distress syndrome complicating percutaneous nephrolithotomy. *Urology* 23:376–377, 1984.

98. Kalash SS, Young JD Jr: Serious complications associated with percutaneous nephrolithotomy. *Urology* 29:290–293, 1987.

99. Roven SJ, Rosen RJ: Percutaneous nephrostomy and maintenance of nephrostomy drainage. *Urology* 23 (Special Issue, Part 1):25–28, 1984.

100. Sant GR, Hawes R, Meares EM Jr: "Bacteriuria" in patients with nephrostomy tubes—implications for antibiotic use in endourology. *J Urol* 135 (Suppl):255A, 1986.

101. El-Kappany H, Gaballah MA, Ghoneim MA: Rigid ureteroscopy for the treatment of ureteric calculi. Experience in 120 cases. *Br J Urol* 58:491–503, 1986.

102. Smith AD: Percutaneous ureteral surgery and stenting. *Urology* 23:37–42, 1984.

103. Culkin DJ, Zitman R, Bundruck WS, et al.: Anatomic, functional and pathologic changes from internal ureteral stent placement. *Urology* 40:385–390, 1992.

104. Dedominicis DFC, Dalforno S, Iori R, et al.: The incidence of post-operative urinary tract infection in patients with ureteric stents. *Br J Urol* 65:10–12, 1990.

105. Spirnak JP, Resnick MI: Stone formation as a complication of indwelling ureteral stents: a report of 5 cases. *J Urol* 134:349–351, 1985.

106. Schulze KA, Wettlaufer JN, Oldani G: Encrustation and stone formation: complication of indwelling ureteral stents. *Urology* 25:616–619, 1985.

107. Siegel A, Altadonna V, Ellis D, Hulbert W, Elder J, Duckett J: Simplified method of indwelling ureteral stent removal. *Urology* 28:429, 1986.

108. Sasagawa I, Nakada T, Akiya T, Umeda K, Sakamoto M, Katayama T: Use of indwelling double-curved ureteral stents and problems after stenting. *Eur Urol* 13:176–179, 1987.

109. Nanninga JB, Rosen J: Problems associated with the use of

external urinary collectors in the male paraplegic. *Paraplegia* 13:56–58, 1975.

110. Johnson ET: The condom catheter: urinary tract infection and other complications. *South Med J* 76:579–582, 1983.

111. Fierer J, Ekstrom M: An outbreak of Providencia stuartii urinary tract infections—Patients with condom catheters are a reservoir of the bacteria. *JAMA* 245:1553–1555, 1981.

112. Steinhardt G, McRoberts W: Total distal penile necrosis caused by condom catheter. *JAMA* 244:11–12, 1980.

113. Bruschchini H, Tanagho EA: Cystostomy drainage: Its efficacy in preventing residual urine and infection. *J Urol* 118:391–393, 1977.

114. Hodgkinson CP, Hodari AA: Trocar suprapubic cystostomy for post-operative bladder drainage in the female. *Gynecology* 96:773–783, 1966.

115. Peatfield RC, Burt AA, Smith PH: Suprapubic catheterization after spinal cord injury: a follow-up report. *Paraplegia* 21:220–226, 1983.

CHAPTER 73

Nonsurgical Management of Vesicourethral Dysfunction

J. KEITH LIGHT

INTRODUCTION

The conservative or nonsurgical treatment of voiding dysfunction has improved significantly, due predominantly to an improved understanding of the basic neurophysiologic mechanisms regulating the function of the bladder, prostate, and urethra. An example is the recent surge in nonsurgical treatment of benign prostatic hyperplasia. Due to the expected increase in the aging population, together with the current cost of traditional surgery, it is expected that knowledge regarding the medical treatment of benign prostatic hyperplasia will rapidly advance over the next few years. As such, this chapter has been expanded to include current knowledge regarding medical treatment of this condition.

A basic understanding of the anatomy and physiology of the lower urinary tract is important when applying the principles of pharmacologic manipulation.

APPLIED NEUROPHYSIOLOGY

The lower urinary tract is innervated by both the autonomic and somatic nervous systems. The function of urine storage and expulsion is controlled by a complex set of reflex mechanisms involving both the central and peripheral circuits.

Autonomic nervous system

Both the parasympathetic and sympathetic components of the autonomic nervous system play a role in the lower urinary tract.

PARASYMPATHETIC NERVOUS SYSTEM

The parasympathetic nervous system via the pelvic nerve originates in the intermediolateral nuclei of the sacral spinal segments S2–S4. Both human and animal experiments suggest that S3 is the main segment affecting detrusor function [1,2]. Stimulation of the pelvic nerve results in a sus-

tained detrusor contraction. Acetylcholine is the main neurotransmitter. Cholinergic receptor sites are found throughout the bladder and posterior urethra, being most common in the bladder body. Most are muscarinic in nature, i.e., atropine characteristically exhibits a complete blocking action at these sites. In most animals species, part of the bladder contraction elicited by electrical stimulation of the pelvic nerve is resistant to atropine. The finding of this atropine resistance in both experimental animals and humans led researchers to believe that acetylcholine was not the sole transmitter, and therefore the search for additional transmitters ensued [3,4]. The concept of nonadrenergic, noncholinergic transmitters and nerves arose, and led to the discovery that several other chemicals were indeed present in the lower urinary tract. These include vasoactive intestinal polypeptide, substance P, enkephalins, and the presence of p nerves—purinergic according to Burnstock and peptidergic according to Baumgarten [5,6]. Adenosine triphosphate was proposed as the nonadrenergic, noncholinergic neurotransmitter. Current opinion, however, holds that the noncholinergic excitatory component in the normal human bladder is very small [7]. Available data, however, do not exclude the possibility that the atropine resistance component of bladder contraction may be important in abnormal detrusor behavior, e.g., instability. This may explain why anticholinergic drugs fail to inhibit involuntary detrusor contractions in some patients. The precise role that the other chemicals play in influencing the function of the lower urinary tract remains to be clarified. These neuropeptides, however, have been demonstrated in nerves in the bladder wall and may act by modulating the effect of the autonomic nervous system on the intrinsic ganglia within the bladder wall.

SYMPATHETIC NERVOUS SYSTEM

The superior hypogastric plexus (presacral nerve) is thought in humans to arise from the intermediolateral cell nuclei of T10–L2. The fibers cross the pelvic brim and continue as the inferior hypogastric plexus to reach the bladder. Sympathetic fibers join with parasympathetic

Suki, WN and Massry SG (eds), Suki and Massry's Therapy of Renal Diseases and Related Disorders, Third Edition. ISBN 978-1-4757-6634-9.
©*1998, Kluwer Academic Publishers, Boston/Dordrecht/London. All rights reserved.*

fibers at this level to form the pelvic plexus. The pelvic plexus, which lies immediately adjacent to the bladder wall, thus receives both sympathetic and parasympathetic fibers, allowing modulation of one system by the other (8). Postganglionic fibers then spread out to supply the entire lower urinary tract. The neurotransmitter is norepinephrine, and consequently, adrenergic receptors are found throughout the bladder, posterior urethra, prostate, and seminal vesicles. Important sex differences occur in the distribution of these adrenergic nerves. They appear to be present in the male bladder neck, but morphologic studies have failed to demonstrate a significant number of catecholamine-containing nerve fibers in the female bladder neck and urethra. Pharmacologic studies, however, have demonstrated sympathetic-induced responses of smooth muscle in the female urethra. The adrenergic receptors are divided into alpha and beta, depending on whether stimulation results in contraction or relaxation, respectively, of the smooth muscle. Alpha receptors are further subdivided into alpha$_1$ and alpha$_2$. The term alpha$_1$ refers to the postjunctional aplha receptor that mediates smooth muscle contraction. *Alpha$_2$* includes a group of presynaptic receptors that are responsible for a negative feedback mechanism inhibiting release of norepinephrine in response to postganglionic neural stimulation. The alpha$_1$ receptor type is thought to predominate in humans.

Although beta receptors are also present in the bladder, estimates of the density very from investigator to investigator. The functional importance of these receptors in the human remains to be settled. Certainly, from the clinical viewpoint, beta blockade in humans does not result in significant changes.

Alpha receptors predominate in the bladder base and urethra, while beta receptors, although sparse, predominate in the bladder body. The sympathetic nervous system thus has the potential to enhance urine storage by relaxing the bladder body through stimulation of beta receptor, by contracting the bladder outlet through stimulation of alpha receptors, and by inhibition of nerve transmission along the pelvic nerve at the level of the pelvic ganglia. The precise role that the sympathetic nervous system plays in regulating bladder function in the normal person is, however, unclear at present. Once again, it may be in the abnormal situation that the sympathetic nervous system becomes important. Significant morphologic and histochemical changes have been described in bladder strips obtained from patients with damage to the parasympathetic nervous system, i.e., decentralized bladders. Phenylephedrine, an alpha-receptor stimulant, resulted in contraction of these bladder muscle strips, whereas there was little effect on normal bladder muscle (9). Similarly, in bladder outflow obstruction, noradrenaline caused contraction of muscle instead of the expected relaxation (10). These studies suggest that there may be an increased alpha-adrenoceptor activity in response to denervation or obstruction.

Calcium has an important role in the excitation–contraction coupling of smooth muscle. The dependence of bladder muscle contractility on the inflow of exogenous calcium or the release of endogenous calcium and the ability to interfere with this process is an additional potential for the mediation of bladder relaxation.

Somatic nervous system

The pudendal nerve arises from the anterior horn cells of the sacral segments S2–S4. This is the motor nerve to the pelvic floor muscles, including the periurethral muscle and striated muscle component of the distal sphincteric mechanism. Whether the somatic fibers reach the sphincter muscle directly through the pudendal nerve or as vegetative fibers running with the pelvic nerves is still in dispute (11,12).

APPLIED ANATOMY

Bladder

The bladder consists of intertwining bundles of smooth muscle. Discrete layers of smooth muscle are absent. Each muscle cell is in close apposition to the adjacent cells, except at certain junctional regions. This is termed a *region of close approach*, where intercellular distances of 10–20 nm occur, and it is through these junctional regions that the spread of an electrical stimulus from cell to cell is thought to occur.

The bladder neck smooth muscle differs histologically and pharmacologically from the detrusor proper. In males, the smooth muscle forms a complete circular collar, perhaps justifying the term *proximal internal urethral sphincter* (13). This collar arrangement is absent in the female (13). As mentioned previously, the male bladder neck has a rich noradrenergic but sparse cholinergic nerve supply. The female bladder, in contrast, has relatively few noradrenergic nerves.

Urethra

The part of the male urethra contributing to continence extends from the bladder neck to and including the membranous urethra. Extension of the smooth muscle from the bladder neck occurs down to the membranous urethra. At this level, a layer of circularly orientated striated muscle fibers is found, termed the *striated component* of the distal urethral sphincter (13). The fibers differ, however, from those of the classic periurethral striated muscle, since they are smaller, are predominantly slow twitch, and are devoid of a muscle spindle (13). These characteristics allow for the sustained contraction that is so necessary for sphincteric function. The distal sphincteric mechanism is therefore composed of both smooth and striated muscle. The classic periurethral muscle plays no part in continence and is responsible for the volitional interruption of the urinary stream.

TREATMENT OF VOIDING DYSFUNCTION

There are a multitude of reasons why voiding does not occur in the smooth coordinated fashion that it is supposed to. A simplified functional approach divides these reasons into two main categories: failure of storage and failure to empty. Frequently, these two problems coexist. It should be remembered that a normal voiding cycle depends on the presence of a stable bladder and a competent sphincteric mechanism. Urodynamic evaluation is often essential in determining which of the two problems occurs so that rational treatment can be planned.

Failure of bladder storage

Any illness resulting in uninhibited detrusor contractions may cause urinary incontinence. Examples are multiple sclerosis, suprasacral spinal cord injuries, and stroke. Therapy is therefore aimed predominantly at controlling or ablating the detrusor contraction. A decrease in outlet resistance from any cause will likewise lead to urinary incontinence.

INHIBITION OF BLADDER CONTRACTILITY

Anticholinergic agents

Since the main excitatory neurotransmitter for detrusor muscle contractility is acetylcholine, atropine and its cogeners will depress uninhibited contractions of any etiology. Atropine sulfate itself, however, is rarely used, although the tablet form is available.

Propantheline (Pro-Banthine®). Propantheline is a quaternary ammonium compound that is thought to competitively inhibit cholinergic transmission in the detrusor muscle and pelvic ganglia (14). In patients with detrusor hyperreflexia, the volume to the first contraction will generally increase and the force of the contraction will decrease, thus increasing the functional bladder capacity, with a proportionate decrease in symptoms. Only the tablet form is now available in the United States. The usual adult dose is 15–30 mg every 4–6 hours per 24 hours. As with all the antimuscarinic agents, troublesome side effects may occur that can interfere with patient compliance. These include inhibition of salivary secretion (dry mouth), blockade of the iris sphincter muscle (pupillary dilatation) and ciliary muscle (blurred vision), tachycardia, drowsiness, and constipation. The last of these may require laxatives in patients with a neuropathic etiology for the voiding dysfunction. Antimuscarinic agents are contraindicated in patients with glaucoma and should be used with caution if significant outflow obstruction is present, since urinary retention may result.

Methantheline (Banthine®). Methantheline is also a quaternary ammonium compound and has a higher ratio of ganglionic blocking to antimuscarinic activity than propantheline. At the clinical level, however, there does not appear to be any significant difference between the two drugs. Methantheline has similar effects on the lower urinary tract. The usual dose is 50–100 mg every 4–6 hours per 24 hours. The side effects and contraindications are similar to propantheline.

Emepronium (Ceteprin®). Emepronium is a synthetic C_{10} quaternary ammonium base with anticholinergic properties. It has enjoyed more popularity and success in Europe than in the United States. The drug is currently unavailable in the United States. The standard adult dose is 100–200 mg every 6 hours. Esophageal erosions have been reported if insufficient fluids are taken with each administration of the drug.

Antispasmodics

Agents that fall into the category of antispasmodics are thought to act directly on the smooth muscle at a site distal to the cholinergic receptor mechanism. The agents also possess some antimuscarinic and local anesthetic properties. There are still some questions as to whether, in fact, the clinical effect is not simply due to their atropinelike effect. Due to the experimental evidence suggesting a different mode of action, however, these agents may be used in conjunction with true anticholinergic agents.

Oxybutynin (Ditropan®). Oxybutynin is a tertiary amine with anticholinergic and musculotropic relaxant activity. The clinical effect is to suppress detrusor contractility. The recommended adult dose is 5 mg 3–4 times per 24 hours. The side effects are similar to propantheline. Hyperthermia may occur secondary to interference with sudomotor responses, and peduncular hallucinosis has been reported.

Flavoxate hydrochloride (Urispas®). Although reported to exhibit a direct inhibitory reaction on smooth muscle in addition to anticholinergic properties, flavoxate hydrochloride appears clinically to be of limited value if used in situations where other agents have failed to control detrusor contractility (15). The adult dose is 100–300 mg 3–4 times per 24 hours. The reported side effects are rare.

Alpha-adrenergic antagonists. The basis for using alpha-adrenergic antagonists is the change in alpha-receptor density that occurs following outflow obstruction and damage to the nerve supply. The detrusor instability that is often present coincident with benign prostatic hypertrophy may improve following administration of these agents (10). With neurologic lesions above the conus medullaris resulting in detrusor hyperreflexia, however, these agents are of little clinical benefit in controlling detrusor contractility. Alpha-adrenergic antagonists have, however, been reported to improve the tonus limb, where decreased compliance has been observed on cystometrogram (16). This finding occurs most commonly in patients with meningomyelocele. Experimental studies in primates with decentralized bladders indicated a separate response to alpha-adrenergic blockade and anticholinergic agents (16). There is thus experimental evidence to try a combination of alpha-antagonists and anticholinergics in patients with this type of bladder. Acquired neurologic lesions (e.g., cauda equina lesions), however, rarely show decreased compliance on cystometry.

Prazosin (Minipress®) (see also under Benign Prostatic Hyperplasia). Prazosin is now widely used in the United States following withdrawal of phenoxybenzamine due to possible mutagenic effects. This drug is thought to act by blocking the postsynaptic alpha-adrenoceptors, i.e., alpha$_1$-receptors. The usual adult dose is 3–6 mg daily in divided doses. Higher doses, which are commonly used to control hypertension, are rarely required to achieve an effect on the bladder. Side effects include dizziness and syncope due to postural hypotension.

Calcium antagonists

The rationale for the use of calcium antagonists has already been described. Both the initial experimental and clinical reports, however, have been disappointing (17,18). Consequently, monotherapy with calcium antagonists was expanded to include the addition of an anticholinergic drug. Success has been encouraging using this combination, at least in the experimental animal (19). Terodiline, which has both anticholinergic and calcium channel blocking effects, has been used with success in humans (20). The precise role that this class of drugs will play in controlling detrusor contractility remains to be clarified.

INCREASING OUTFLOW RESISTANCE

The human urethra contains both cholinergic and adrenergic innervation with both muscarinic and adrenergic receptors. It has been clearly shown that adrenoceptor-stimulating and -blocking drugs are far more important in regulating intraurethral pressure than cholinergic drugs. The predominant adrenoreceptor in humans is the alpha$_1$ subtype.

Alpha-adrenergic agonist

Ephedrine. This drug acts by releasing peripheral noradrenaline but also stimulates beta receptors. The oral adult dose is 25–50 mg, four times per 24 hours. Tachyphylaxis may develop. Pseudoephedrine (Sudafed®) has similar indications. The adult dose is 30–60 mg, four times per 24 hours.

The side effects include anxiety, insomnia, headache, and palpitations. The drug should be used with caution in patients with hypertension, hyperthyroidism, and cardiovascular disease. Urinary retention may be precipitated in the presence of outflow obstruction.

Phenylpropanolamine hydrochloride. This drug has the same properties as ephedrine while causing less central stimulation. The average adult dose is 50 mg, three times per 24 hours. The side effects are the same as ephedrine.

Imipramine and the lower urinary tract

Imipramine hydrochloride, a tricyclic antidepressant, exerts at least three pharmacologic effects on the lower urinary tract, facilitating urinary storage (21). The first is a central and peripheral anticholinergic action at some sites, the second is to block the active reuptake of norepinephrine by the presynaptic nerve, and third is a strong direct inhibitory effect on the bladder smooth muscle. The net clinical result is decreased bladder contractility and an increase in outflow resistance (21). This drug is also used commonly in nocturnal enuresis. In elderly patients, therapy is commenced with a single nighttime dose of 25 mg and is gradually increased until side effects appear or the dose reaches 150 mg (21). The usual adult dose is 25 mg, four times a day, for detrusor instability. The side effects include weakness, fatigue, tremor, mania, sedation, and postural hypotension. The drug is contraindicated when used in conjunction with monoamine oxidase inhibitors, as coma and seizures can be precipitated.

Failure of bladder emptying

Inadequate bladder emptying with large postvoid residuals may be secondary to abnormal detrusor contractility, such as contractions of short duration or poor force, or to an increase in outlet resistance. Therapy is therefore aimed at improving the detrusor contraction or decreasing the outlet resistance.

INCREASING INTRAVESICAL PRESSURE

Acetylcholine, the primary neurotransmitter in humans, cannot be used therapeutically due to actions at the central and ganglionic level and due to rapid hydrolysis by acetylcholinesterase.

Parasympathomimetic drugs

Bethanechol chloride (Urecholine®). This drug is cholinesterase resistant and causes in vivo contraction of bladder muscle. The clinical effectiveness in improving bladder emptying in the majority of patients with both neuropathic and non-neuropathic disease, however, has been disappointing (22,23).

Bethanechol chloride does produce an increase in tension in the bladder muscle but fails to stimulate or facilitate a coordinated sustained detrusor contraction. The drug may be given subcutaneously in doses of 5 mg for postoperative urinary retention and repeated every 6 hours. The usual oral adult dose is 25-100 mg, four times per 24 hours. The side effects include nausea, vomiting, diarrhea, intestinal cramps, sweating, and salivation. Contraindications to the use of this drug are asthma, peptic ulcer, bowel obstruction, cardiac arrhythmia, and bladder outflow obstruction.

DECREASING OUTFLOW RESISTANCE.

The sphincteric mechanism in males, both proximal and distal, and the prostate contain an abundance of adrenergic nerves with alpha adrenoceptors (24,25). The most common cause for organic obstruction in males is benign prostatic hypertrophy. Obstruction from an enlarged prostate may be secondary to either a mechanical effect or a functional effect. The former is produced by the physical presence of the tissue itself, while the latter is mediated through stimulation of the abundant alpha adrenoreceptors, resulting in increased tone of the prostatic smooth muscle. Although the mechanical component may gradually increase, fluctuation of symptoms does not occur. The functional or dynamic component, however, can vary quite rapidly according to the degree of sympathetic stimulation. Not infrequently, a patient with relatively mild prostatic obstruction will develop sudden acute urinary retention due to associated factors such as chilling, nervous tension, or bladder overdistension. This outcome is often transient, and the use of an alpha-blocking agent may abort or relieve the retention. Alpha blockers are also useful in cases with bladder neck obstruction or *dyskinesia*. This condition usually occurs in young males who complain of poor voiding. Urodynamic assessment reveals poor opening of the bladder neck associated with a normal detrusor contraction and relaxation of the striated periurethral muscle. Prazosin (Minipress®) has been found to be effective in reducing the obstructive symptoms of benign prostatic hypertrophy (26).

There is no class of pharmacologic agents that will selectively relax the striated muscle of the pelvic floor. The condition of detrusor-sphincter dyssynergia, where reflex contraction of the pelvic floor muscles occurs simultaneously with a bladder contraction, occurs exclusively in neuropathic voiding dysfunction and results in variable degrees of incomplete bladder emptying. Although skeletal muscle relaxants used to treat muscle spasticity have been tried, the clinical effectiveness of these agents is lacking.

BENIGN PROSTATIC HYPERPLASIA (BPH)

The prostate is the most common organ affected by disease in males above the age of 60 years. The single most common pathological process implicated is benign prostatic hyperplasia (BPH), which is characterized by a gradual increase in both glandular and fibromuscular tissue of the prostate. Enlargement of the prostate gland in males over the age of 60 years assumes importance with two pathological conditions: the first is benign enlargement resulting in bladder outflow obstruction, while the second is prostatic carcinoma. Both may present with identical symptoms of bladder outflow obstruction. For the purposes of this chapter, only benign prostatic hyperplasia will be considered.

The traditional treatment for symptomatic BPH has been transurethral resection of the prostate (TURP). The overall cost of a TURP in the U.S.A. is about $12,000. More than 400,000 TURP were performed in 1988 in the U.S.A. for a total estimated cost of $4.5 billion. The high medical cost of such treatment has naturally focused attention on whether all these surgical procedures are indeed necessary, since health insurance data suggest a surprising fourfold variation in the prostatectomy rate for age-adjusted populations in adjacent regions in the U.S.A. (27). As a result, attempts have been made to clarify and simplify the approach to lower urinary tract symptoms in the male. This has led to the increasing use of symptom scoring systems whereby the patient answers questions with various points being applied to each question. The attempt is to assess the significance of the symptoms and how this affects the patient's quality of life. Traditionally, the symptoms from BPH have been divided into two categories: obstructive symptoms consisting of hesitancy, poor stream, intermittency and a sense of incomplete bladder emptying, and irritative symptoms consisting of diurnal and nocturnal frequency and urgency with urge incontinence. It should be emphasized at this point, however, that several other pathological entities may closely mimic these symptoms and be totally unrelated to coincidental BPH. These pathological conditions include detrusor instability, impaired detrusor contractility, or a combination of both entities. Objective measurements, using a flow rate, have recently been recommended as the only necessary test. This test alone, however, will not distinguish among obstruction, impaired contractility, and overactivity (bladder instability). The current therapeutic trend, therefore, is purely a symptomatic one, tending to neglect the underlying pathophysiology. Complex urodynamic evaluation in the form of pressure–flow studies are required to accurately distinguish the various pathological processes that may mimic bladder outflow obstruction secondary to BPH. It has been estimated that approximately 70% of 70-year-old males develop BPH, but only approximately 40% suffer symptoms of bladder outflow obstruction as a result. It is also important to remember that the size of the prostate gland is totally unrelated to the presence or absence of bladder outflow obstruction.

Histologically, BPH is characterized by a variable increase in both the glandular and stromal components, the latter including the smooth muscle of the prostatic capsule. Bladder outflow obstruction therefore may be purely mechanical from enlargement of the glandular tissue or active due to contraction of the smooth muscle component, predominantly that of the prostatic capsule.

The prostate requires the presence of adequate levels of circulating testosterone in order to develop and grow (28,29). Of the circulating testosterone, 98% is bound, predominately to human serum albumin and sex-hormone-binding globulin. As a consequence, only 2% of free testosterone is available to enter the prostatic cells by simple diffusion. Intracellular testosterone is then converted to the active component, dihydrotestosterone (DHT), by an enzyme called 5-alpha-reductase. The DHT then binds to the nuclear androgen receptors, resulting in a complex but orderly series of changes that gives rise to synthesis and cell replication. A drug that blocks the action of this enzyme, thus preventing formation of the active hormone DHT, could prevent an increase in prostatic size and even reduce the size of existing glandular tissue.

Since the discovery in the 1970s of alpha-adrenergic receptors within the smooth muscle elements of prostatic adenomas, the prostatic capsule, and the bladder neck, the use of a nonhormonal pharmacological agent capable of reducing bladder outflow obstruction caused by BPH became possible (24). Recent molecular biological studies have shown that the alpha-1 receptor (postjunctional) may be further subdivided into alpha-1a, alpha-1b, and alpha-1c subtypes (30). The alpha-1c subtype may be the receptor mediating smooth muscle contraction in the prostate, thus raising the possibility of developing a selective alpha-1c antagonist and thereby avoiding the adverse effects commonly associated with alpha-1 blockers (31).

Medical treatment of BPH

5-ALPHA-REDUCTASE INHIBITORS

Finasteride (Proscar®)

Finasteride is a neutral 4-azasteroid that appears to act as a pure 5-alpha-reductase inhibitor without detectable androgen-blocking properties. The usual dose is 5 mg/day, which must be continued for a minimum of 4–6 months before any apparent benefit may be discerned (32). It is not possible at present, using the minimum invasive studies of symptom score and flow rate, to distinguish between responders and nonresponders. Theoretically, those patients with predominantly glandular (mechanical) rather than stromal (fibromuscular) hyperplasia would be expected to respond better to this form of therapy.

The drug appears to be well tolerated in all reported studies, with the only adverse effects being impotence, reduced libido, and ejaculatory disturbances. These, however, occur in less than 4% of treated patients and are generally reversible on stopping the medication.

Finasteride was approved in 1992 by the FDA for the treatment of BPH and currently is the only 5-alpha-reductase inhibitor thus recommended.

It is important to realize that finasteride decreases the prostatic specific antigen (PSA) values by as much as 46%. Any PSA value, therefore, that fails to drop appropriately following the commencement of finasteride should raise the suspicion of concomitant prostatic carcinoma.

ALPHA-ADRENOCEPTER BLOCKERS

Terazosin (Hytrin®)

There are several alpha-adrenocepter blocking agents on the market that may be used in the treatment of BPH. However, the only one approved by the U.S. Food and Drug Administration (FDA) for treatment of benign prostatic hyperplasia is terazosin (Hytrin).

Terazosin causes rapid relaxation of smooth muscle tone in the bladder neck, prostate capsule, and prostatic urethra, relieving the symptoms of active obstruction. It has no effect on the size of the prostate gland and unlike finasteride does not alter the concentration of PSA. Terazosin is rapidly and almost completely absorbed from the gastrointestinal tract, reaching peak serum concentration 1–2 hours after an oral dose. The drug is metabolized in the liver, and the metabolites are excreted mainly in the bile but also partly in the urine. The elimination half-life of terazosin is approximately 12 hours. Terazosin, unlike other alpha blockers, is specific for the alpha-1 receptor.

Titration of dose is necessary, commencing with 1 mg to be taken at night to avoid the initial hypotensive effect. Therefter, a titrated and stepwise increase in dosage to 2 mg, 5 mg and then 10 mg, once daily has been found most effective in producing a clinical response. The optimum dose of terazosin varies from individual to individual. The average daily dose if tolerated, is 10 mg. There is no evidence that this drug reduces the complications of BPH or the need for future surgery. Side effects include asthenia, postural hypotension, dizziness, somnolence, nasal congestion and impotence.

OTHER ALPHA-ADRENOCEPTOR BLOCKERS

Several other agents in this category are available and have been used in the treatment of BPH. All have potentially the same side effects as already listed above. These agents include prazosin, thymoxamine, indoramin, and doxazosin.

Prazosin (Minipress®)

Prazosin was the first alpha-1-specific adrenoblocker to be intensively studied. Again, because the first-dose phenomenon leads to postural hypotension, it is recommended that the initial dose commence at 0.5 mg twice daily, gradually increasing to 2 mg, twice daily over several weeks (33).

Doxazosin (Cardura®)

Doxazosin, an alpha-1-specific blocker, was originally developed as a treatment for hypertension. It is structurally similar to prazosin but has a more gradual onset of action and a longer half-life.

The initial daily dose should start at 2 mg, increasing to a daily dose of 4–8 mg. No further improvement is noted with a daily dose exceeding 12 mg (34).

INTERMITTENT CATHETERIZATION

Sterile intermittent catheterization was introduced in 1954 in the treatment of patients with spinal cord injury. The clean or nonsterile technique was described in 1972 (35). Since then, this technique has gained wide acceptance by virtue of its simplicity and effectiveness. To be truly effective, it must ensure social continence between catheterizations. This requires a bladder of adequate functional capacity that is capable of storing urine at low pressures, which is often not the case with neuropathic bladders; pharmacology may be necessary to achieve this outcome.

In addition, it is preferable to have the patients catheterize themselves, which for various reasons may not be possible. Intermittent catheterization as a definitive means of bladder drainage is usually performed every 4–6 hours. Care is taken to limit the volume drained to 300–500 cc per catheterization. This may necessitate limiting fluid intake or adjusting the catheterization interval. Bacteriuria is common in this population group but does not appear to have any long-term deleterious effects (36).

Intermittent catheterization may be used to ensure bladder drainage in voiding dysfunction of diverse etiology.

REFERENCES

1. Brindley GS, Polkey CE, Rushton DN: Sacral anterior root stimulators for bladder control in paraplegic and quadriplegic patients. *J Neurol Neurosurg Psychiatry* 45:952, 1983.
2. Juenemann KP, Lue TF, Schmidt RA, Tanagho EA: The clinical significance of sacral and pudendal nerve anatomy. *J Urol* 139:74–80, 1988.
3. Ambache N, Zar MA: Noncholinergic transmission by postganglionic motor neurons in the mammalian bladder. *J Physiol (Lond)* 210:761, 1970.
4. Cowan WD, Daniel EE: Human female bladder and its noncholinergic contractile function. *Can J Physiol Pharmacol* 61:1236, 1983.
5. Burnstock G: Purinergic nerves. *Pharmacol Rev* 24:509, 1972.
6. Baumgarten JG, Holstein AF, Owman CH: Auerbach's plexus of mammals and man: electron microscopic identification of three different types of neuronal processes in mesenteric ganglia of the large intestine from rhesus monkey, guinea-pigs and man. *Z Zellforschung Mikroskop Anat* 106:376, 1970.
7. Sjogren C, Andersson K-E, Husted S, Mattiasson A, Moller-Madsen B: Atropine resistance of transmurally stimulated isolated human bladder muscle. *J Urol* 128:1368, 1982.
8. DeGroat WC, Booth AM, Kriev J: Interaction between sacral parasympathetic and lumbar sympathetic inputs to pelvic ganglia. In: CM Brooks, K Koizani, A Sato, eds, *Integrative Functions of the Autonomic Nervous System.* University of Tokyo Press, Tokyo, pp 234–247, 19.
9. Sundin T, Dahlstrom A, Norlen L, Svedmyr N: The sympa-

10. Perlberg S, Caine M: Adrenergic response of bladder muscle in prostatic obstruction. *Urology* 20:524–527, 1982.
11. Vodusek DB, Light JK: The motor nerve supply of the external urethral sphincter muscles: An electrophysiologic study. *Neurourol Urodynam* 2:193–200, 1983.
12. Gosling JA: The structure of the bladder and urethra in relation to function. *Urol Clin North Am* 6:31–38, 1979.
13. Gosling JA, Dixon JS, Critchley HOD, Thompson SA: A comparative study of the human external sphincter and periurethral levator ani muscles. *Br J Urol* 53:35–41, 1981.
14. Benson GS, Sarshik SA, Raezer D, Wein AJ: Bladder muscle contractility. Comparative effects of and mechanisms of actions of atropine, propantheline, flavoxate, and imipramine. *Urology* 9:31–35, 1977.
15. Briggs RS, Castleden CM, Asher MJ: The effect of flavoxate on uninhibited detrusor contractions and urinary incontinence in the elderly. *J Urol* 123:665–666, 1980.
16. McGuire EJ, Savastano JA: Effect of alpha-adrenergic blockade and anticholinergic agents on the decentralized primate bladder. *Neurourol Urodynam* 4:139–142, 1985.
17. Forman A, Andersson K-E, Hendriksson L, Rud T, Ulmsten U: Effect of nifedipine on the smooth muscle of the human urinary tract. *Acta Pharmacol Toxicol* 43:111–118, 1978.
18. Leval KU, Lutzeyer W: Spontaneous phasic activity of the detrusor: a cause of uninhibited contractions in unstable bladder. *Urologia Int* 35:182–187, 1980.
19. Andersson K-E, Fovaeus M, Morgan E, McLorie G: Comparative effects of five different calcium channel blockers on the atropine-resistant contraction in electrically stimulated rabbit urinary bladder. *Neurourol Urodynam* 5:579–586, 1986.
20. Peters D, et al.: Terodiline in the treatment of urinary frequency and motor urge incontinence. A controlled multicentre trial. *Scand J Urol Nephrol (Suppl)* 87:21–33, 1984.
21. Castleden CM, George CF, Renwick AG, Asher MJ: Imipramine—a possible alternative to current therapy for urinary incontinence in the elderly. *J Urol* 125:318–320, 1981.
22. Wein A, Malloy TR, Shofer F, Raezer DM: The effects of bethanechol chloride on urodynamic parameters in normal women and in women with significant residual urine volumes. *J Urol* 124:397–399, 1980.
23. Light JK, Scott FB: Bethanechol chloride and the traumatic cord bladder. *J Urol* 128:85–87, 1982.
24. Caine M, Raz S, Zeigler M: Adrenergic and cholinergic receptors in the human prostate, prostatic capsule and bladder neck. *Br J Urol* 47:193–202, 1975.
25. Ek A, Alm P, Andersson K-E, Person CG: Adrenergic and cholinergic nerves of the human urethra and urinary bladder. A histochemical study. *Acta Physiol Scand* 99:345–352, 1977.
26. Hedlund H, Andersson K-E, Ek A: Effects of prazosin in patients with benign prostatic obstruction. *J Urol* 130:275–278, 1983.
27. McConnell JD, Barry MJ, Bruskev RC, et al.: *Benign Prostatic Hyperplasia: Diagnosis and Treatment.* HCPR Publication No. 94-0582. Agency for Health Care Policy and Research, Public Health Service, U.S. Department of Health and Human Services, Rockville, MD, February 1994.
28. Isaccs JT, Coffey DT: Changes in DHT metabolism associated with the development of canine benign prostatic hyperplasia.

Endocrinology 108:445–453, 1981.

29. Coffey DS: The endocrine control of normal and abnormal growth of the prostate. In: *Urologic Endocrinology* WB Saunders, Philadelphia, pp 170–193, 1986.

30. Ruffolo PR, Nichols AJ, Stadel JM, Hieble JP: Structure and function of alpha-adrenoreceptors. *Pharmacological Rev* 43:475–505, 1991.

31. Lepor H, Tang R, Shapiro E: The alpha-adrenoceptor subtype mediating the tension in human prostatic smooth muscle. *Prostate* 22:301–308, 1993.

32. Gormley GJ, Stoner E, Bruskevitz RC, and the Finasteride Study Group: The effect of finasteride in men with benign prostatic hyperplasia. *N Engl J Med* 327:1185–1191, 1992.

33. Chapple CR, Stott M, Abrahms PH, Christmas TJ, Milroy EJG: A twelve week placebo-controlled study of prazosin in the treatment of prostatic obstruction due to benign prostatic hyperplasia. *Br J Urol* 70:285–294, 1992.

34. Fawzy A, Sullivan J, Cook M, Gonzalez F: A multicentre sixteen week double blind, placebo-controlled dose response study using doxazosin for the treatment of BPH in patients with mild to moderate hypertension. *J Urol* 149:323A, 1993.

35. Lapides JM, Diokno AC, Silber SJ, Lowe BS: Clean intermittent self-catheterization in the treatment of urinary tract disease. *J Urol* 107:458–461, 1972.

36. Kass EJ, Koff SA, Diokno AC, Lapides J: The significance of bacilluria in children on long-term intermittent catheterization. *J Urol* 126:223–225, 1981.

INDEX

A

AAMI. *See* Association for
  Advancement of Medical
  Instrumentation
Accelerated hypertension, 1198–200,
  1199t. *See also* Hypertension
ACE. *See* Angiotensin converting
  enzyme
Acetazolamide
  duration of action, 38
  onset, 38
  site of action, 36
Acid-base disorders
  metabolic, 332–33
  mixed, 307–18
  clinical manifestations, 311
  diagnosis, 311–16, 312t, *313*
  therapy, 316–17
Acidosis
  lactic, 211–31
  Bifidobacterium, 227
  classification, 212–14, 213t
  diagnosis, *214*, 214–15
  disorders associated with
  catecholamine excess, 225–26
  congenital defects, lactic acid
    metabolism, 226
  D-lactic acid, excessive production
    of, 227
  diabetes, 222–23
  liver disease, 223
  malignancy, 222
  nutritional causes of, 226
  obstructive pulmonary disease, 223
  seizures, 225
  toxins, acidosis due to, 223–25
  Eubacterium, 227
  Lactobacillus, 227
  pathophysiology of, 211–12, *212*, 212t
  phosphofructokinase, inhibition of,
    211

physiology of, 211–12, *212*, 212t
  therapy, *214*, 215–22
  bicarbonate therapy, *212*, 218–20
  calcium administration, 220
  carbicarb, 220t, 220–21
  dialysis, 222
  dichloroacetate, 221, *221*
  improve tissue oxygen delivery, 216–
    18
  magnesium balance, 124
  metabolic
  added acids, 253–55, 254t
  ethylene glycol poisoning, 270
  from gastrointestinal tract, 271–72
  glue-sniffing, *254*, 271
  hyperkalemia, renal tubular acidosis
    with, 272–73
  ketoacidosis, 266t, 266–67
  L-lactic acidosis, 267–69, 268t
  management, 262–66
  NaHCO₃, use of, 262–65
  methanol poisoning, 269–70
  NaHCO₃, loss of, *255*, 255–56
  patient assessment, 256–62
  basis of disorder, determination of,
    256–57
  renal response to, 260–62
  threat to life, 257–60, 258t
  potassium status, management of,
    266, 266t
  renal acidosis, 254t, 272–73
  salicylate intoxication, 270–71
  specific causes of, 266–73
  subgroups of, 253–56, 254t
  respiratory, 294–301
  acute, treatment of, 298–99
  chronic, treatment of, 297t, 299–
    301
  clinical manifestations, 295–96
  diagnosis, 297–98
  etiology, 295, 296–97t

factors influencing development of,
  294–95
  hypercapnia, 295
  plasma electrolyte composition, 295
Acute glomerulonephritis, 387–93, 584
  captopril, 389
  clinical features, 387–88, 388t
  diazoxide, 390
  edema and, 48
  furosemide, 389, 390
  hydralazine, 389
  nifedipine, 389, 390
  nitroprusside, 390
  poststreptococcal glomerulonephritis,
    prevention of, 392
  prognosis, 391–92, 392t, 398
  renal disease, specific therapy, 391–
    92, 392t
  treatment, 388–91
  anemia, 391
  fluid and electrolyte imbalances, 390–
    91
  hospitalization, 388
  hypertension, 388–90, 389t
  hypertensive encephalopathy, 389–
    90t, 390
Acute pericardial tamponade,
  pericarditis, 822
Acute peritoneal dialysis, 915–21
  access, 916–17
  complications, 918t, 918–21
  contraindications, 905–6
  indications, 905–6
  schedules, 917–18
  solutions, 917, 917t
  technique, 917–18
Acute rejection, 1121–26
Acute renal failure, 359–86
  complications, 375–76
  bleeding, 375–76
  cardiopulmonary complications, 375

infections, 375
diagnosis, 361–63
chart review, 361
medical history, 361–62
physical examination, 361–62
urinalysis, 362
urinary indices, 362–63, 363t
urine output pattern, 360t, 362
edama and, 47
etiology of, 359–61
hypernatremia, 12
intrarenal, 360t, 360–61
outcome, 376–78
recovery, 377–78
survival, factors influencing, 376–77
pathogenesis, 363–69
drug-induced, 366–69
heme-pigment-associated, 365
ischemic acute renal failure, 363–65
pathophysiology, 363–69
postrenal acute renal failure, 360, 360t
prerenal acute renal failure, 359, 360t
prevention, 369–71
mannitol, 370–71
overview, 369t, 369–70
sickle cell hemoglobinopathy, 667
treatment, 371–74
conservative management, 371–73
nutrition, 374
renal replacement therapies, 373–74
Acyclovir, for AIDS, 622
Addison's disease, potassium and, 70
ADM. *See* Antidiuretic hormone
ADPKD. *See* Autosomal-dominant polycystic kidney disease
Adrenal failure, in thermally injured, 353
Adrenogenital syndromes, metabolic alkalosis, 202, 203
Aerobacter, kidney stones and, 185
African-Americans, autosomal dominant polycystic kidney disease and, 649
After transplant, metabolic status of myocardium following, 1144
AGN. *See* Acute glomerulonephritis
AIDS
acyclovir, 622
amphotericin B, 622
focal segmental glomerular sclerosis, 417
foscarnet, 622
hypocalcemia, 104
pentamidine, 622
rifampin, 622

sulfadiazine, 622
trimethroprim-sulfamethoxazole, 622
Akdomet, for hypertension in pregnancy, 578
AL amyloidosis, 529–31
clinical features, 530
treatment, 530–31
Albuminuria/blood pressure elevation, glomerular filtration rate and, diabetic renal disease, 607–8
Alcoholism
chronic, end-stage liver disease, 12
magnesium balance, 126
Aldosterone
excess, renal acid excretion, 196–97
potassium balance and, *54*, 55
Alimentary tract, with renal failure, 778
Alkalosis, respiratory, 301–4
clinical manifestations, 303
diagnosis, 303–4
etiology, 302t, 302–3
plasma electrolyte composition, 301–2
treatment, 304
Allopurinol, hyperuricosuria, 170t, 177
Alport's syndrome, transplant, 1159
Alternagel, treatment of hyperphosphatemia, 158
Alu, treatment of hyperphosphatemia, 158
Aluminum, removal of, in renal failure, 885
Aluminum salts, treatment of hyperphosphatemia, 158
Alzheimer's disease
hypomagnesemia and, 129
magnesium balance, 130
Ambulatory peritoneal dialysis, with pregnancy, 591
Amiloride
duration of action, 38
for hypertension, 492
onset, 38
for renal tubular acidosis, 288–89
site of action of, 36
Aminoaciduria, 671–72
Aminoglycoside antibiotics, magnesium balance, 122–23
Amlodipine for hypertension, 493
Ammonium, renal acid excretion, 195
Ammonium acid urate, kidney stones and, 167
Amphogel, treatment of hyperphosphatemia, 158
Amphotericin B
for AIDS, 622

nephrogenic diabetes insipidus and, 26
Amyloidosis, after transplant, 1143
dialysis amyloidosis, 1143
in familial mediterranean fever, 1143
recurrent, renal allograft, 1143
Amyotrophic lateral sclerosis, hypomagnesemia and, 129
Analgesic abuse, focal segmental glomerular sclerosis, 417
Analgesic nephrotoxicity, 735–37
clinical presentation of AN, 735
epidemiology of AN, 735–37, 736t
Androgens
for murine lupus nephritis, 463
for renal failure, 885–86
Anemia, with acute glomerulonephritis, 391
Anesthetics
polyuria, 23
vasopressin levels, 23
Angiographic dye
nephrogenic diabetes insipidus and, 26
polyuria, 26
Angiotensin-converting enzyme inhibitors
nephrotoxicity from, 738
potassium, effect, 69–70
Anhydrase, carbonic, bicarbonate reclamation, *190*, 192–93
Aniline dye, bladder carcinoma and, 705
ANP. *See* Atrial natriuretic peptide
Anti-T12 monoclonal antibodies, 1118
Antibiotic-induced nephrotoxicity, 725–28
acyclovir nephropathy, 728
aminoglycoside antibiotic nephrotoxicity, 725–26
amphotericin B nephropathy, 727–28
carbapenum nephropathy, 727
cephalosporin nephropathy, 726–27
foscarnet, 728
penicillin nephropathy, 726
pentamidine nephropathy, 728
rifampin nephropathy, 727
sulfonamide nephropathy, 727
tetracycline nephropathy, 727
vancomycin nephropathy, 727
Antibiotic selection, for peritonitis, 984–85
gram-negative organisms, 985
gram-positive organisms, 984–85
yeast, gram stain, 985

Anticoagulants, for hypertension in pregnancy, 580
Anticonvulsants, hypocalcemia and, 104
Antidiuretic hormone, fluid and electrolyte disorders and, surgical patient, 336, 336t
Antihymocyte globulin, for murine lupus nephritis, 463
Antihypertensive treatments, diabetic renal disease, 611
  diabetic nephropathy, 612t, 612–13
  intervention trials, normoalbuminuria, 611
  microalbuminuria, 611–12
  proteinuria, 612t, 612–13
Antimicrobials, neuropsychiatric complications, 869
Antineutrophil cytoplasmic antibodies, vasculitic disease, 479
Antioxidants, thrombotic microangiopathy, 521
Antiphospholipid syndrome, transplant, 1156–57
Antiplatelet agents, thrombotic microangiopathy, 520
Antithrombotic treatment, thrombotic microangiopathy, 520–21
Antituberculous drugs, toxicity, renal failure and, 455, 456t
Antiukaliuretic agents
  duration of action, 38
  onset, 38
Aqitation, hypomagnesemia and, 129
ARF. *See* Acute renal failure
Arginine vasopressin, 2
  polyuria, 21
ARPKD. *See* Autosomal-recessive polycystic kidney disease
Arrhythmias, refractory, hypomagnesemia and, 129
Arteriography, genitourinary tuberculosis, 452
Ascites, edema and, 46–47
Ascorbic acid, uremia, 795
Aspergillus species, therapy, end-stage renal disease, endocarditis, 833
Aspirin, low-dose, for hypertension in pregnancy, 581–82
Association for Advancement of Medical Instrumentation, dialysis water treatment, standards, 1021–26, 1022t
Asthma, magnesium balance, 135
Atenolol
  dosage, side effects, 1197

for hypertension, 492
Atheroembolic renal disease, 770
  renal insufficiency and, 770
Atherosclerosis, with systemic lupus erythematosus, 462, 462t
Atrial natriuretic peptide
  polyuria, 23
  vasopressin-mediated water permeability and, 23
Autonomic nervous system dysfunction
  in uremia, 861
  in uremiahemolytic-uremic syndrome, 868
Autosomal dominant polycystic kidney disease, 639–50
  African-Americans, 649
  cardiovascular system, 645–46
  in childhood, 649–50
  counseling, 648–49
  fluid and electrolyte management, 640–41
  gastrointestinal abnormalities, 646–48, *648*
  genetic counseling, 648–49
  hematuria, 642–43
  hypertension, 645
  infection, 643–45, 644t
  lifestyle, 641
  nephrolithiasis, 646, *647*
  pain, 641–42
  physical activity, 641
  pregnancy, 649
  prognosis, 650
  proteinuria, 645
  renal replacement therapy, 650
Autosomal recessive polycystic kidney disease, 650–52
  management, 651–52
AVP. *See* Arginine vasopressin
Azathioprine, 1108
  adverse effects, 1148

B
B$_6$. *See* Pyridoxine
B$_{12}$. *See* Cyanocobalamin
Bacterial endocarditis
  glomerulonephritis in
    clinical features, 397–98
    diffuse glomerulonephritis, 397–98
    focal glomerulonephritis, 397
    epidemiology, 395–96
    glomerular ultrastructure, 397
    immunopathology, 397
    pathologic features, 396
    Staphylococcus aureus, 395–400

therapy, 398
    Staphylococcus aureus, glomerulonephritis in, 395–400
Bacterial infections, transplant, 1176–77
Bacteriuria
  asymptomatic, 439
  catheters and, 1224–25
Barbiturates
  central diabetes insipidus and, 24
  polyuria, 24
  vasopressin levels, 23
Barium intoxication, 60
Bartter's syndrome, 63–64, 679–80
  magnesium, 124
  with metabolic alkalosis, 203
  mineralocorticoid excess, 203–4
Basagel, treatment of hyperphosphatemia, 158
Beans
  magnesium concentration in, 116
  phosphorus content, 843
Bed rest, for hypertension in pregnancy, 578
Benazepril for hypertension, 493
Benign prostatic hyperplasia, 1237–39
  medical treatment, 1238–39
Beta, adrenergic inhibitors for chronic hypertension in pregnancy, 577
Beta-2-microglobulin amyloidosis, 848–49
Beta adrenergic catecholamines, potassium balance and, 53
Beta-adrenoceptor blocking agents
  alpha, combined, for hypertension in pregnancy, 579
  for hypertension in pregnancy, 579
Beverages, phosphorus content, 843
Bezafibrate, nephrotic syndrome, 414
Bicarbonate loads, metabolic alkalosis, 204
Bicarbonate reclamation, 189–94, *190*, 191t
  arterial pCO$_2$, acidity and, 192
  chloride deficiency, 191
  extracellular volume, 190
  glomerular filtration rate, 190–91
  glucose loading, 191t, 194
  phosphate depletion, 193
Bicarbonate regeneration, 189
Bicarbonate therapy, for lactic acidosis, *212*, 218–20
Bifidobacterium, lactic acidosis, 227
Bile salt, diuretic, natriuretic effect of, *551*, 551–52
Bisphosphonates, hypocalcemia and, 104

Bladder, anatomy, 1234
Bladder carcinoma, 704–12
    aniline dye, 705
    continent urinary diversion, *709–10*,
        710–11
    cyclophosphamide, 705
    diagnosis, 706–7
    genetics, 705
    metastatic, treatment, 708–10
    molecular markers, *711*, 711–12
    pathology, 705–6, 706t
    risk factors, 705
    staging, 706–7
    tobacco smoking, 705
    treatment, 707–8
    bladder-sparing, 708
Bladder emptying, failure of, 1236–37
Bladder storage, failure of, 1235–36
Bleeding, with acute renal failure, 375–
    76
Blood loss, iatrogenic, in renal failure,
    883–85, *884*
Blood pressure. *See also* Hypertension
    ambulatory blood pressure
        recordings, 611
    blood pressure elevation, insulin and,
        609
    continuous ambulatory peritoneal
        dialysis, 941–42
    diabetic renal disease, 606, 606t, 608–
        11
    examination evidence of
        dehydration, 323
    hyperfusion, 609
    large vessel disease, 609
    mechanisms of, 609–11, 610t
    relation to kidney function, 608–9
    sickle cell hemoglobinopathy, 666
    sodium, retention of, 609
    systemic, diabetic renal disease, 605
Blood transfusion
    exchange, for poisoning, 753–54,
        754t
    policy, in hypertensive emergencies,
        584
Body water compartments
    electrolyte composition, 319–20
    fluid and electrolyte abnormalities,
        319, *320*
Bone, hypophosphatemia, effect on,
    153
Bone complications, after transplant,
    1179
Bone resorption, inhibition, calcium,
    97–98
BPH. *See* Benign prostatic hyperplasia
Brain, adaptation

    to altered plasma tonicity, 2
    to hypernatremia, 11–12
    to hyponatremia, 1
Breast cancer, hypercalcemia and, 88
Bredinin, 1112
Brequinar sodium, 1113
    rejection, 1113
Buffer composition, hemodialysis fluid,
    1047
Bumetanide
    for hypertension, 492
    site of action of, 36
Bumetanide test, for renal tubular
    acidosis, 288
Burn shock, fluid and electrolyte
    disorders, 351–54, *352*
    vasoconstrictor shock, 352
    young adults, 352–53, *352–53*
Burns with dermal losses, magnesium
    balance, 126

C
Cabbage, magnesium concentration in,
    116
Cadaver donors, transplantation, 1093–
    94
Cadmium, nephrotoxicity, 737–38
Calcitonin
    hypercalcemia and, 96, 97
    hypocalcemia and, 104
Calcitrol deficiency, osteitis fibrosa,
    844, *844*
Calcium
    electrolyte abnormalities, surgical
        patient, perioperative period, 344–
        45
    homeostasis, 85–87, *86*
    hypercalcemia, 87, 87t, 88t, 88–98
    causes, 88–95
    clinical features, 88, 88t
    diagnostic evaluation, 88t, 95–96
    malignancies associated with, 88
    treatment, 96t, 97–98
    hypocalcemia, 87, 87t, 98–107, 99t
    biochemical findings, 101
    causes, 99, 100–105
    clinical features, 99t, 99–100
    diagnostic evaluation, 101t, 105
    treatment, 105–7
    kidney stones and, 167
    magnesium, chemical differentiation,
        115
    metabolism disorders, 85–114
    physiologic functions, 86
Calcium acetate, treatment of
    hyperphosphatemia, 158

Calcium administration, for lactic
    acidosis, 220
Calcium carbonate, treatment of
    hyperphosphatemia, 158
Calcium channel blockers, for
    hypertension in pregnancy, 579
Calcium citrate, treatment of
    hyperphosphatemia, 158
Calcium disorder, 858
Calcium homeostasis, 85–87, *86*
Calcium salts, treatment of
    hyperphosphatemia, 158
Calcium stone, 169t, 169–84
Calcium supplementation, osteitis
    fibrosa, 845
Cancer
    after transplant, 1178–79
    urinary tract, 695–722
    bladder carcinoma, 704–12
    aniline dye, 705
    continent urinary diversion, *709–10*,
        710–11
    cyclophosphamide, 705
    diagnosis, 706–7
    genetics, 705
    metastatic, treatment, 708–10
    molecular markers, *711*, 711–12
    pathology, 705–6, 706t
    risk factors, 705
    staging, 706–7
    tobacco smoking, 705
    treatment, 707–8
    bladder-sparing, 708
    hypernephroma, usage of term, 695
    malignant tumors of kidney, 695–701
    diagnosis, *696–97*, 699–700, 699–700t
    metastases, 701
    pathology, 696–99
    staging, *696–97*, 699–700, 699–700t
    treatment, *698*, 700t, 700–701
    prostate cancer, 712–17
    diagnosis, 714–15
    early, 712–14, 713t, *714*
    pathology, 712
    staging, 714–15
    treatment, *715–16*, 715–17
    renal pelvis, neoplasms of, *701*,
        702–2
    ureter, neoplasms of, *701*, 702–2
Cancer-associated hemolytic uremic
    syndrome, 517–18
Cancer therapy, gastrointestinal
    potassium loss, 61
Candida, vulvovaginitis secondary to,
    437
CAPD. *See* Continuous ambulatory
    peritoneal dialysis

Capillary refill, examination evidence of dehydration, 323
Captopril
  acute glomerulonephritis, 389
  dosage, side effects, 1197
  for hypertension, 493, 496
Carbamazepine
  central diabetes insipidus and, 24
  vasopressin levels, 23
Carbicarb, for lactic acidosis, 220t, 220–21
Carbonic anhydrase
  bicarbonate reclamation, *190*, 192–93
  inhibitors, onset and duration of action, 38
Cardiac arrhythmias
  dialysis, 828–29
  magnesium, 134
  uremia, dialysis, 828–29
Cardiac dysfunction, renal insufficiency and, 773
Cardiac glycosides, magnesium balance, 123–24
Cardiac muscle, hypophosphatemia, 152–53
Cardiac patients, magnesium, 128
Cardiomyopathy, uremic, 822–27, *823*
  etiology, 823–24
  incidence, 822–23
  left ventricular morphology, 824, *825*
  management, 824–27, 826t
Cardiopulmonary bypass, magnesium balance, 125
Cardiopulmonary complications, with acute renal failure, 375
Cardiovascular complications
  transplant, 1177–78
  uremia, 817–39
Cardiovascular disturbances, with renal failure, 777–78
Cardiovascular system
  autosomal dominant polycystic kidney disease and, 645–46
  hypophosphatemia, consequences of, 151
Carpal tunnel syndrome, dialysis and, 863
Cast nephropathy, multiple myeloma, plasma cell dyscrasias, 532–34, *533*, 533t
Cataracts, after transplant, 1180
Catecholamines
  beta adrenergic, potassium balance and, 53
  excess, lactic acidosis, 225–26
  magnesium balance, 125
Catheters, 1219–32

bacteriuria, 1224–25
external condom catheter drainage, 1228–29
indications for, 1219–22
indwelling urethral catheters, 1222–24
intermittent catheterization, 1226–27
management, 1225–26
nephrostomy tubes, 1227
peritoneal, 953–79
  break-in, 966–68
  care of, 966–68
  exit, 966–68
  immediate intraperitoneal segment care, 966
  long-term results, 974–76
  National CAPD Registry survey, 974–75
  swan-neck catheters, 975
  United States Renal Data System Report, 975–76
  peritoneal dialysis, 966
  removal, 973–74
  functioning catheter, with complication, 973–74
  malfunction, 973
  nonfunctioning catheter, 974
  rigid catheters, 953–55
  complications, 954t, 954–55
  insertion, 953–54
  preinsertion, patient assessment, 953
  soft catheters, 955t, 955–58
  complications, 968–73
  early, 968–69
  late, 969–73
  implantation of, 958–66
  catheter preparation, 959
  flange, anchoring, 962
  implantation method, 959–66
  patient preparation, 958–59
  straight, coiled Tenckhoff catheters, 956, *956*
  swan-neck catheters, *956*, 956t, 956–58
suprapubic catheters, 1229
types of, 1219, 1220t
ureteral stents, 1227–28, 1228t
urinary tract infection, 438–39
CCPD. *See* Continuous cyclic peritoneal dialysis
Cell content, solutes, steady state, 1
Cell volume
  determination of, 1
  regulation of, 1, 2t
Central diabetes insipidus, 24t, 24–25
  causes of, 24
  polyuria, 24t, 24–25, 30

Central nervous system depression
  as cause of acute respiratory acidosis, 296
  as cause of chronic respiratory acidosis, 297
Central pontine myelinolysis, 8
Cerebral demyelinating lesions, hyponatremia, 10
Cerebral edema, with diabetic ketoacidosis, 244, 244t
Cerebral salt-wasting syndrome, 9
Cheese, phosphorus content, 843
Chemical contaminants, dialysis water treatment, 1015
Chemotherapeutic agent nephrotoxicity, 729–31
  cisplatin, 729–30
  methotrexate, 730
  nitrosoureas, 730
Chemotherapy
  genitourinary tuberculosis, 452–54, 453t
  for multiple myeloma with plasma cell dyscrasias, 534–35, 535t
Child, autosomal dominant polycystic kidney disease and, 649–50
Children
  fluid and electrolyte abnormalities, 319–34
  body water compartments, 319, *320*
  electrolyte composition, 319–20
  electrolyte, mineral disturbances, 327–32
  hypercalcemia, 330–31, 331t
  hyperkalemia, 329, 329t
  hypernatremia, 324t, 328–29
  hypocalcemia, 330
  hypokalemia, 328t, 329
  hyponatremia, *327*, 327t, 327–28
  magnesium balance disorders, 331–32, 331–32t
  hydration, disorders of, 320–27
  maintenance fluid and electrolyte requirements, 320–22, 321–22t
  overhydration, 326t, 326–27
  maturation of kidney, anatomic, functional, 320
  metabolic acid-base disorders, 332–33
  metabolic acidosis, 332, 332t
  metabolic alkalosis, 332–33, 333t
  hypernatremia in, 12
  thermally injured, fluid and electrolyte disorders, 353
Chlamydia, 437
Chloride-losing diarrhea
  congenital, 204
  with metabolic alkalosis, 203

Chloride shunt syndrome, 680
Chlorothiazide, site of action of, 36
Chlorthalidone
  for hypertension, 492
  onset and duration of action, 38
Chronic peritoneal dialysis, 921–29
  access, 921
  complications, 925t, 925–29
  continuous cyclic, 922t, 923–24
  delivery systems, 921–22
  intermittent, 922t, 922–23
  nocturnal, 922t, 924
  tidal, 924–25
Chronic renal failure
  edema, 47–48
  nutritional status in, 783–85, 784t
  pre dialysis stage, nutrition, 785–86
  with sickle cell hemoglobinopathy,
    667–69
Churg-Strauss vasculitis, 868
Cigarette smoking. *See* Tobacco
    Smoking
Circulating levels of vasopressin, effect
    upon, 23
Cirrhosis, edema and, 46–47
Cisplatin, magnesium balance, 123
Clofibrate
  nephrotic syndrome, 414
  vasopressin levels, 23
Clonidine
  for chronic hypertension in
    pregnancy, 577
  dosage, side effects, 1197
  for hypertension, 492, 496
CMV. *See* Cytomegalovirus
Cocaine, renal complications, 619
Cocoa, magnesium concentration in,
    116
Coffee, phosphorus content, 843
Cola, phosphorus content, 843
Colchicine, nephrogenic diabetes
    insipidus and, 26
Colic, kidney stones and, 168
Collagen-vascular diseases, 868
Collecting duct, loop of Henle, diuretic
    action, 36, 40
Coma, hypomagnesemia and, 129
ConA-induced factors, for murine
    lupus nephritis, 463
Condom catheter drainage, external,
    1228–29
Confusion, hypomagnesemia and, 129
Congestive heart failure
  edema and, 42–45
  therapy, 45
  pulmonary edema, 44–45, 45t
  severe, edema and, 43–44

Connective tissue diseases, transplant,
    1156–58
Continuous ambulatory peritoneal
    dialysis, 935–51, 981
  complications, 944–47
  catheter-related, 944, 944t
  from intra-abdominal pressure, 944–
    45
  membrane failure, 945–46
  metabolic, 946–47
  peritonitis, 944, 944t
  edema, 44
  individualized dialysis, 937–44
  acid-base balance, 942
  adequacy, 937, 937–40
  blood pressure, 941–42
  dietary requirements, 943t, 943–44
  hyperkalemia, 942
  mineral metabolism, 937, 942–43
  sodium balance, 941–42
  nutrition, 790–92
  causes of malnutrition, 791
  malnutrition
  outcome of, 790–91
  prevalence, 790–91
  prevention, protein energy
    malnutrition, 791t, 791–92
  patient selection, 935–36
  advantages of, 935–36, 936t
  contraindications, 936, 936t
  indications, 936, 936t
  patient training, 937
  peritoneal access, 936
  peritonitis, 981
Continuous arteriovenous
    hemofiltration, 1050
Continuous cyclic peritoneal dialysis,
    922t, 923–24
Contraceptive pill, genitourinary
    tuberculosis, 455
Contrast medium
  nephrotoxicity, 728–29
  management, 729
  prevention, 729
  risk factors, 728–29
  renal insufficiency and, 770
Copper, uremia, 795
Coronary heart disease
  end-stage renal disease, infective
    endocarditis in, 830–34
  Aspergillus species, therapy, 833
  clinical presentation, 830–31t, 830–32
  etiology, 830
  fungi candida species, therapy, 833
  management, 832–33t, 832–34
  Pseudomonas aeruginosa, therapy,
    833

Staphylococcus aureus, therapy, 833
Staphylococcus epidermidis, therapy,
    833
Streptococcus, therapy, 833
  hypotension, hemodynamic stability
    and, 829–30, 830t
  in uremia, dialysis, 827–28
  cardiac arrhythmias, 828–29
  ischemic heart disease, 828, 829t
Corticosteroids, 1108
  for murine lupus nephritis, 463
Counseling
  autosomal dominant polycystic
    kidney disease, 648–49
  inherited renal disease, 690–93
  natural history, 690–91
  prenatal diagnosis, 692t, 692–93
  presymptomatic testing, 691–92
  risks, of pregnancy, 691
CPM. *See* Central pontine myelinolysis
Cream cheese, phosphorus content, 843
Cream of wheat, phosphorus content,
    843
Creatinine clearance, progression of
    renal disease and, 757
Cregs, donor selection, 1097
Crescentic glomerulonephritis
  corticosteroids for, 483
  cyclophosphamide for, 483
CRF. *See* Chronic renal failure
Cyanocobalamin, uremia, 795
Cyclophosphamide, 1108–10
  bladder carcinoma and, 705
Cycloserine, detecting hypersensitivity
    to antituberculous drugs, 455
Cyclosporine, 1113–15
  adverse effects, 1147–48
  hemolytic uremic syndrome, 518
  magnesium balance, 123
  for murine lupus nephritis, 463
  nephtrotoxicity, 731t, 731–34
  potassium and, 70
  rejection, 1113–15
Cyclosporine A, 1110, 1110t
Cystic disease, 639–62
  acquired renal cystic disease, 654–55
  management, 654–55, 655t
  autosomal dominant polycystic
    kidney disease, 639–50
  African-Americans, 649
  cardiovascular system, 645–46
  in childhood, 649–50
  counseling, 648–49
  fluid and electrolyte management,
    640–41
  gastrointestinal abnormalities, 646–
    48, 648

genetic counseling, 648–49
hematuria, 642–43
hypertension, 645
infection, 643–45, 644t
lifestyle, 641
nephrolithiasis, 646, *647*
pain, 641–42
physical activity, 641
pregnancy, 649
prognosis, 650
proteinuria, 645
renal replacement therapy, 650
autosomal recessive polycystic
    kidney disease, 650–52
management, 651–52
cystic diseases of renal medulla, 652–
    54
familial juvenile nephronopthisis,
    652–53
medullary cystic disease, 652–53
medullary sponge kidney, 653–54
simple cysts, 655–56
Cystinosis, hereditary, transplant,
    1160–61
Cystinuria, 184–85
Cystitis, acute, 435–38
Cytomegalovirus
magnesium balance, 124
transplantation and, 1098
Cytotoxic drugs
for murine lupus nephritis, 463
for vasculitic disease, complications
    of, 484

D
Deep venous thrombosis, after
    transplant, 1178
Dehydration, fluid and electrolyte
    balance, 322–24t, 322–26
Dehydration tests, interpretation, 28
Delirium, hypomagnesemia and, 129
Demeclocycline
hyponatremia, 8
nephrogenic diabetes insipidus and,
    26
Deoxyspergualin, 1117
rejection, 1117
Deoxyspergualin for murine lupus
    nephritis, 463
Depression, hypomagnesemia and,
    129
Desmopressin, polyuria, 30–31
Diabetes
insulin, role of, 234
with lactic acidosis, 222–23
magnesium balance, 130

origin of term, 233
in Papyrus Ebers, 233
transplant, 1153–54
Diabetes insipidus, hypernatremia, 12
Diabetes mellitus
after transplant, 1146–47
magnesium balance, 126
potassium loss and, 64
Diabetic ketoacidosis, 234–44, *235*
cerebral edema, 244, 244t
clinical manifestations, 235–36, 236t
complications of therapy, 244, 244t
diagnosis, 235–36, 236t
metabolic acidosis, 236–39
phosphorus, 243–44
potassium, 241–43
sodium, 240–41
Diabetic renal disease, 605–17
after transplant, 1147
albuminuria/blood pressure
    elevation, glomerular filtration rate
    and, 607–8
antihypertensive treatments, 611
diabetic nephropathy, 612t, 612–13
intervention trials,
    normoalbuminuria, 611
microalbuminuria, 611–12
proteinuria, 612t, 612–13
blood pressure elevation, 608–11
ambulatory blood pressure
    recordings, 611
blood pressure elevation, insulin and,
    609
hyperfusion, 609
large vessel disease, 609
mechanisms of, 609–11, 610t
relation to kidney function, 608–9
sodium, retention of, 609
diet, protein-reduced, 613
microalbuminuria, 613
normoalbuminuria, 613
proteinuria, 613
glycemic control, 611
intermediary endpoints, final
    endpoints, correlation of, 607–8
intraglomerular pressure, 605
pregnancy, 584, 587
risk factors, 605–7
blood pressure elevation, 606, 606t
glycemia, degree of, 605–6
protein intake, 606
systemic blood pressure in, 605
Dialysates
buffer, 1012–13
calcium, 1010t, 1013–14
composition, 1010t, 1010–14
glucose, 1010–11

potassium, 1014
sodium, 1011–12
Dialysis
cardiovascular complications, 817–
    39
chronic, pregnant patients
    undergoing, 590–91
drugs, 1071–74, 1072–74t
hemofiltration, 1043–64
for lactic acidosis, 222
magnesium metabolism in, 136
neurological complications, 861–64
carpal tunnel syndrome, 863
dialysis disequilibrium syndrome,
    861–62
dialytic encephalopathy, 862–63
intracranial hemorrhage, 863–64
peritoneal, 915–33
acute peritoneal dialysis, 915–21
access, 916–17
complications, 918t, 918–21
contraindications, 905–6
indications, 905–6
schedules, 917–18
solutions, 917, 917t
technique, 917–18
ambulatory, with pregnancy, 591
chronic peritoneal dialysis, 921–29
access, 921
complications, 925t, 925–29
continuous cyclic, 922t, 923–24
delivery systems, 921–22
intermittent, 922t, 922–23
nocturnal, 922t, 924
tidal, 924–25
for poisoning, 750–51t, 751–54
potassium imbalances, 72–73, *73*
ultrafiltration, 1043–64
Dialysis access, 989–1003
peritoneal dialysis, 1001–3
complications, 1002–3
operative technique, 1001–2, *1002*
permanent, 991–1001
temporary, 989–91
Dialysis disequilibrium syndrome, 861–
    62
Dialysis water treatment, 1015t, 1015–
    21
Association for Advancement of
    Medical Instrumentation,
    standards, 1021–26, 1022t
hazards associated with, 1015, 1016t
microbiology, 1018, 1018t
pathogenesis, pyrogenic reactions,
    1020–21, 1020–21t, *1021*
pyrogenic reactions, during dialysis,
    1018–19, 1019t

purification, components of, 1016–18,
    1017
Dialytic encephalopathy, 862–63
Dialyzers, 1005–10
    biocompatibility, 1008t, 1008–10
    characteristics of, 1005–7, 1006t
    types of, 1007t, 1007–8
Diarrhea
    gastrointestinal potassium loss, 61
    losses of fluid and electrolytes, 325
Diazoxide
    acute glomerulonephritis, 390
    for hypertensive emergency, 496
    for severe hypertension in
        pregnancy, 581
Dicarboxylic, 672
    aminoaciduria, 671
Dichloroacetate, for lactic acidosis, 221,
    221
Diet
    for hypertension in pregnancy, 578
    kidney stones and, 174t, 178
    protein, risk factor, renal disease,
        762–64
    protein-reduced, diabetic renal
        disease, 613
    microalbuminuria, 613
    normoalbuminuria, 613
    proteinuria, 613
    renal insufficiency and, 768
    requirements, continuous
        ambulatory peritoneal dialysis,
        943t, 943–44
    sources, potassium, 73
Digestive system, hypophosphatemia,
    effect on, 153
Digoxin, hyperkalemia, 68
Diltiazem
    dosage, side effects, 1197
    for hypertension, 493
Distal renal tube
    acidosis, 277–83, *278*, 278t
    classic, 278–80
    hyperkalemic types of, 280–83
    incomplete, 280
    pseudohypoaldosteronism, 283
    dysfunction
    multiple myeloma with plasma cell
        dyscrasias, 532
    proximal, combined, with multiple
        myeloma with plasma cell
        dyscrasias, 532
Diuresis, forced, for poisoning, 749–51
Diuretics
    conditions for efficacy, 41
    duration of action, 38
    for hypercalcemia, 96

for hypertension in pregnancy, 579–
    80
hyponatremia, 6
    with metabolic alkalosis, 203
    mineralocorticoid excess, 203
    neuropsychiatric complications, 869
    onset of, 38
    potassium loss and, 59t, 61–62
    potassium sparing, 69
    proximally active, *36*, 36t, 39
    resistance to, 41t, 41–42, *42*
    side effects, *36*, 40–41
DKA. *See* Diabetic ketoacidosis
DNA testing, inherited renal disease,
    688–90
Donor selection, for transplantation,
    1079–105
    cadaver donors, 1093–94
    HLA antigens, 1096–98
    living related donors, 1089–92, *1090*
    living unrelated donors, 1092t, 1092–
        93
    pretransplant evaluation of potential
        living donor, 1092t, 1093
Dosing
    adjustment, 1065–75
    regimens, *1070*, 1070–71
Doxazocin for hypertension, 492
Drug abuse. *See under* specific
    substance
Drugs. *See also under* specific drug
    active metabolites, 1074–75, 1075t
    acute renal failure, induced by, 366–
        69
    antituberculous, renal failure and,
        455, 456t
    beta-adrenergic blocking,
        hyperkalemia, 68
    cytotoxic
        for murine lupus nephritis, 463
        vasculitic disease, complications of,
            484
    dialysis, 1065–78, 1072–74t
    vs. diet, hyperuricosuria, 177
    dosing
        adjustment, 1065–75
        regimens, *1070*, 1070–71
    elimination techniques
        dialysis, 753
        criteria for, 754, 754t
        techniques, 750–51t, 751–52
        diuresis, forced, 749–51
        exchange blood transfusion, 753–54,
            754t
        hemoperfusion, 753
        criteria for, 754, 754t
        plasmapheresis, 753–54, 754t

sorbent hemoperfusion, 752–53, 752–
    53t
    half-life, 1069–70
    hyperkalemia induced by, 68
    immunosuppression
        adverse effects, 1147–48, 1148t
        toxic nephropathy from, 731–34
        intoxication, 747–56. *See also*
            Poisoning
    isoniazid, detecting hypersensitivity
        to antituberculous, 455
    lipid-lowering, nephrotic syndrome
        and, 414
    loading dose, 1065–68, 1066t
    magnesium, renal handling of, 121–
        24, 122t
    maintenance dose, 1068–69
    nonsteroidal anti-inflammatory
        potassium, effect, 70
        toxic nephropathy, 734t, 734–35
    renal insufficiency, 769–70
        dosing recommendations, 1066t,
            1075–78, 1076–77t
    renal losses of, diuretics, 121–22
    rifampicin, detecting hypersensitivity
        to antituberculous, 455
    in uremia, 1065–78
Dye, aniline, bladder carcinoma and,
    705

E
E. coli
    peritonitis, 985
    urinary tract infection, 436
ECF. *See* Extracellular fluid
Eclampsia
    edema and, 49
    magnesium sulphate to prevent, 583
    usage of term, 49
Ectopic hyperparathyroidism,
    hypercalcemia and, 89
Edema, 35–52
    acute glomerulonephritis, 48
    acute renal failure, 47
    ascites, 46–47
    cerebral, with diabetic ketoacidosis,
        244, 244t
    chronic renal failure, 47–48
    cirrhosis, 46–47
    congestive heart failure, 42–45
        pulmonary edema, 44–45, 45t
        severe, 43–44
        therapy, 45
    continuous ambulatory peritoneal
        dialysis, 44
    diuretic, *36*, 37–42, 38t

duration of action, 38
efficacy, conditions for, 41
on loop of Henle, *36*, 38t, 39
collecting duct, *36*, 40
early distal loop
metolazone, 40
thiazides, *36*, 36t, 38t, 40
early distal tubule, 40
late distal loop, potassium-sparing agents, *36*, 40
late distal tubule, *36*, 40
onset of, 38
proximally active, *36*, 36t, 39
resistance, 41t, 41–42, *42*
side effects, *36*, 40–41
eclampsia, 49
usage of term, 49
hepatorenal syndrome, 46–47
idiopathic, 48–49
nephron, diuretic agent site of action, 36
nephrotic syndrome, 45–46
with nephrotic syndrome, 45–46, 413
preeclampsia, 49
premenstrual syndrome, 49
sodium, dietary restriction, 36–37, 37t
therapy, 35–36
Effective osmoles, defined, 22
Egg, phosphorus content, 843
Eicosapentanoic acid, for murine lupus nephritis, 463
Electrical burns, fluid and electrolyte disorders, 354
Electrolytes
abnormalities
magnesium depletion, 130–31
surgical patient, perioperative period, 339–47
and hydrogen ion, with renal failure, 778
mineral disturbances, 327–32
hypercalcemia, 330–31, 331t
hyperkalemia, 329, 329t
hypernatremia, 324t, 328–29
hypocalcemia, 330
hypokalemia, 328t, 329
hyponatremia, *327*, 327t, 327–28
urinary, renal tubular acidosis, 284, *286–87*
Embolization, renal
large-vessel, 500–501
small-vessel, 501–2
Emotional disturbances, release of vasopressin, 23
Enalapril
dosage, side effects, 1197
for hypertension, 493, 496

Encephalopathy
dialytic, 862–63
hyponatremic, *6*, 6–8, 7t
differential diagnosis, 7t, 7–8
uremic, 855–57
clinical features, 855
electrophysiological findings, 855–56
maintenance dialysis, 856
morphology, 856
pathophysiology, 856
treatment, 856–57
End-stage renal disease. *See also* Transplantation
patient options in, 1081
pericarditis, therapy, 821
Endocarditis
bacterial
glomerulonephritis in
clinical features, 397–98
diffuse glomerulonephritis, 397–98
focal glomerulonephritis, 397
epidemiology, 395–96
glomerular ultrastructure, 397
immunopathology, 397
pathologic features, 396
Staphylococcus aureus, 395–400
therapy, 398
Staphylococcus aureus, glomerulonephritis in, 395–400
end-stage renal disease, 830–34
Aspergillus species, therapy, 833
clinical presentation, 830–31t, 830–32
etiology, 830
management, 832–33t, 832–34
Endocrine disorders
hypercalcemia and, 93–94
renal insufficiency and, 772
Endoscopy, genitourinary tuberculosis, 452
Endothelial cell dysfunction, thrombotic microangiopathy, 514–15
Endothelin, vasopressin-mediated water permeability and, 23
Environmental toxicants, nephrotoxicity, 740
Epidermal growth factor, vasopressin-mediated water permeability and, 23
Epidural anesthesia, in labor, 584
Epstein-Barr vizoster virus, transplantation and, 1098
Erythrocytosis, after transplant, 1147
Erythropoiesis, inhibition of, in renal failure, 876
Erythropoietin deficiency, in renal failure, 876

Erythropoietin supplementation, in renal failure, 878–83, *879*
Escherichia coli, urinary tract infection, 435
ESRD. *See* End-stage renal disease
Essential hypertension
antihypertensive agents, 1191–93
diagnosis, *1184*, 1184–85
in elderly, 1186
history of, 1183–84
magnesium, 133
metabolic blood pressure, 1184–85, 1185t
patient evaluation, 1190
syndrome concept, 1186t, 1186–89
treatment, 1190–91
Estrogen, brain adaptation, 3
Ethacrynic acid
for hypertension, 492
onset and duration of action, 38
site of action of, 36
Ethambutol
detecting hypersensitivity to antituberculous drugs, 455
genitourinary tuberculosis chemotherapy, *453*, 453–54, 454t
with renal insufficiency, 456
Ethylene glycol poisoning, metabolic acidosis from, 270
Etidronate for hypercalcemia, 96
Eubacterium, lactic acidosis, 227
Exchange blood transfusion, for poisoning, 753–54, 754t
Experimental protocols, rejection, 1118–19
donor-specific blood transfusion, 1119
donor-specific bone marrow infusion, 1119
total lymph node irradiation, 1118–19
total lymphoid irradiation, 1118–19
External condom catheter drainage, 1228–29
Extracellular fluid, osmolality of, 1–19
Extracorporeal hemodialysis therapy, 1051–58
biocompatibility, 1054t, 1054–57, *1055*
coagulation, 1057–58
reuse, hemodialyzers, 1053–54
single-needle dialysis, 1051
toxic substances, leaching of, 1058
uremic toxin removal, 1051–53, 1052t
Extrarenal complications, after transplant, 1146–47

Extremities, myoclonic jerking of, with hypernatremia, 13

F

Fabry's disease, transplant, 1161
Factitious hyperkalemia, 66
Familial hyperkalemic periodic paralysis, 69
Familial hypocalciuric hypercalcemia, 92–93
Familial juvenile nephronopthisis, 652–53
Fanconi syndrome, 677–79, 678t
  multiple myeloma with plasma cell dyscrasias, 532
Felodipine for hypertension, 493
Fetal morbidity, mortality, with systemic lupus erythematosus, 462–63
FHH. *See* Familial hypocalciuric hypercalcemia
Fish, magnesium concentration in, 116
FK-506, rejection, 1115–16
Fleet's phosphasoda, for hypophosphatemia, 154
Fluid and electrolyte disorders
  with acute glomerulonephritis, 390–91
  autosomal dominant polycystic kidney disease, 640–41
  in children, 319–34
  body water compartments, 319, *320*
  electrolyte composition, 319–20
  electrolyte, mineral disturbances, 327–32
  hypercalcemia, 330–31, 331t
  hyperkalemia, 329, 329t
  hypernatremia, 324t, 328–29
  hypocalcemia, 330
  hypokalemia, 328t, 329
  hyponatremia, *327*, 327t, 327–28
  magnesium balance disorders, 331–32, 331–32t
  hydration, disorders of, 320–27
  dehydration, 322–24t, 322–26
  maintenance fluid and electrolyte requirements, 320–22, 321–22t
  overhydration, 326t, 326–27
  maturation of kidney, anatomic, functional, 320
  metabolic acid-base disorders, 332–33
  metabolic acidosis, 332, 332t
  metabolic alkalosis, 332–33, 333t
  renal insufficiency and, 771
  surgical patient, 335–50
  antidiuretic hormone, 336, 336t

consequences of surgery, 335–36
mineralocorticoid activity, 335–36
renal function, 335
intraoperative fluid management, 337–38, 338t
plasma and protein replacement, 338
perioperative period, electrolyte abnormalities in, 339–47
calcium, 344–45
hypercalcemia, 345, 345t
magnesium, 345–46, 346t
phosphorus, 346–47
potassium, 341–44
sodium, 339–41
postoperative period, fluid management in, 339, *339*
volume disorders, 336–37
volume depletion, 336–37, 336–37t
volume overload, 337
in thermally injured, 351–57
burn shock, 351–54, *352*
adrenal failure, 353
concomitant injury, 353
elderly patients, 353
middle-aged adults, 352–53, *352–53*
pediatric patients, 353
vasoconstrictor shock, 352
young adults, 352–53, *352–53*
later postburn period, 354
electrical burns, 354
preexisting diseases, 354
postresuscitation period, immediate, 354–56, *355*
Fluid therapy, intravenous, postoperative, 5
Fluoride, hypocalcemia and, 104
Folate supplementation, in renal failure, 886
Food intake, decreased, with hypernatremia, 13
Foscarnet
  for AIDS, 622
  hypocalcemia and, 104
  magnesium balance, 124
Fosinopril for hypertension, 493
Fructose intolerance, hereditary, 678
Fruit, phosphorus content, 843
Functional maturation of kidney, fluid and electrolyte balance, 320
Fungal infection, transplant, 1177
Fungi candida species, therapy, infective endocarditis, end-stage renal disease, 833
Furosemide
  acute glomerulonephritis, 389, 390
  dosage, side effects, 1197

for hypertension, 492
hypotonic states, 8
nephrogenic diabetes insipidus and, 26
onset and duration of action, 38
site of action of, 36
test, for renal tubular acidosis, 288

G

Gallium nitrate
  hypercalcemia and, 96, 98
  hypocalcemia and, 104
Gastric alkalosis, 198t, 201–2, 201–2t
  pathogenesis of, 201
Gastric drainage, potassium loss and, 62
Gastric juice, losses of fluid and electrolytes, 325
Gastroenteritis, hypernatremia, 12
Gastrointestinal abnormalities, autosomal dominant polycystic kidney disease, 646–48, *648*
Gastrointestinal complications
  after transplant, 1179
  renal insufficiency and, 773
Gastrointestinal potassium losses, 61, 61t
Gastrointestinal system, hypophosphatemia, consequences of, 151
Gemfibrozil, nephrotic syndrome, 414
General anesthesia, 778–80
  central diabetes insipidus and, 24
Genetic counseling
  autosomal dominant polycystic kidney disease, 648–49
  inherited renal disease, 690–93
  natural history, 690–91
  prenatal diagnosis, 692t, 692–93
  presymptomatic testing, 691–92
  risks, of pregnancy, 691
Genetic diagnosis, inherited renal disease, 685–90
  biochemical tests, 687
  clinical diagnosis, 685–87, 686t
  DNA testing, 688–90
  radiological diagnosis, 687–88, 687–88t
  renal pathology, 688
Genitourinary tuberculosis, 451–58
  algorithm for, 457
  chemotherapy, 452–54, 453t
  ethambutol, *453*, 453–54, 454t
  isoniazid, 452–53
  pyrazinamide, 453
  rifampicin, 452

steroids, 454
streptomycin, 453
HIV, 455–56
investigations, 451–52
arteriography, 452
endoscopy, 452
intravenous urogram, 451–52
percutaneous nephrostomy, 452
radiography, 451
retrograde pyelography, 452
management, 452
pyrazinamide, 454
rifampicin, 454
streptomycin, 454
surgery, 456–58
diseased tissue, removal of, 456
follow-up, *457*, 458
reconstructive surgery, 456–58
toxicity, 454–55
antituberculous drugs, renal failure, 455, 456t
contraceptive pill, 455
hepatotoxicity, 455
hypersensitivity, 454–55
rifampicin, 455
Gentamycin, nephrogenic diabetes insipidus and, 26
GH. *See* Growth hormone
Gitelman's syndrome, 679
magnesium balance, 124
Glomerular disease, 623–31
Glomerular filtration rate, nephrotoxicity and, 723
Glomerular sclerosis, focal segmental, 417–19, *418*
Glomerulonephritis, 387–93
in bacterial endocarditis
clinical features, 397–98
diffuse glomerulonephritis, 397–98
focal glomerulonephritis, 397
epidemiology, 395–96
glomerular ultrastructure, 397
immunopathology, 397
pathologic features, 396
Staphylococcus aureus, 395–400
therapy, 398
captopril, 389
chronic, in pregnancy, 585
clinical features, 387–88, 388t
diazoxide, 390
furosemide, 389, 390
hydralazine, 389
lupus, therapy, 465–71
membranoproliferative, *421*, 421–22
nifedipine, 389, 390
nitroprusside, 390
poststreptococcal

immunoglobulin A nephropathy, distinguished, 431
prevention of, 392
pregnancy, 584
renal complications, 584
prognosis, 391–92, 392t
treatment, 388–91
anemia, 391
fluid and electrolyte imbalances, 390–91
hospitalization, 388
hypertension, 388–90, 389t
hypertensive encephalopathy, 389–90t, 390
Glomerulopathies, 630–31
Glomerulosclerosis, 623–30
Glucocorticoids
for hypercalcemia, 96
thrombotic microangiopathy, 520
Glucopenia, release of vasopressin, 23
Glucose loading, bicarbonate reclamation, 191t, 194
Glue-sniffing, metabolic acidosis from, *254*, 271
Glyburide, nephrogenic diabetes insipidus and, 26
Glycemia, diabetic renal disease, 605–6
Glycemic control, diabetic renal disease, 611
Glycinuria, 672
Glycocorticoids, adverse effects, 1148
Glycogen storage disease, untyped, 679
Glycosuria, 672
GM-CSF. *See* Granulocyte-macrophage colony stimulating factor
Gold nephropathy, 739–40
Goodpasture's syndrome, 401–11
clinical features, 403–5, *404*
epidemiology, 401–3
outcome, 407–9, 408t
pathogenesis, 403
pathology, *405–6*, 405–7
treatment, 407–9, 408t
Graft rejection, 1107–8, *1109*. *See also* Transplantation
Gram-negative microorganisms, peritonitis, 985–86
Gram-positive microorganisms, peritonitis, 985
Granulocyte-macrophage colony stimulating factor, magnesium balance, 123
Granulomatous disease, hypercalcemia and, 93
Growth hormone after transplant, 1149
Guanabenz for hypertension, 492
Guanfacine for hypertension, 492

H
Half-life, drugs, 1069–70
Hartnup disease, 671
HCO$_3$. *See* Bicarbonate
HCV. *See* Hepatitis C virus
HDL, 767–75, 803–5
Head and neck cancer, hypercalcemia and, 88
Heart failure, congestive, 42–45
Heavy metals, nephrotoxicity, 740
Helminthic infection, transplant, 1177
Hemangiopericytoma, with metabolic alkalosis, 203
Hematologic disorders
cancer, hypercalcemia and, 88
renal failure, 772–73, 773t, 875–92
clinical features, 875
leukocyte function, 886–87
management, 878, 878t
aluminum, removal of, 885
androgen therapy, 885–86
erythropoietin supplementation, 878–83, *879*
folate supplementation, 886
hyperparathyroidism, correction of, 885
iatrogenic blood loss, iron supplementation, 883–85, *884*
inhibitors, removal of, 885
r-HuEPO, 881
toxins, removal of, 885
transfusion, 878
transplant, 886
pathogenesis
clinical features, 875–77
erythropoietin deficiency, 876
hemolysis, 875–76
inhibition of erythropoiesis, 876
secondary mechanisms, 876–77
polycythemia, 886
thrombocyte, 886–87
function, 887
thrombotic complications, 887
white blood cells, 886–87
Hematopoietic system, hypophosphatemia
consequences of, 151
effect on, 151–52, *152*
Hematuria
autosomal dominant polycystic kidney disease, 642–43
immunoglobulin A nephropathy and, 429–34
clinical course, 430–31
clinical features, 430
differential diagnosis, 431
epidemiology, 429

pathology, 429–30
pathophysiology, 431–32
prognosis, 430–31
treatment, 432–33
antigen entry, prevention of, 432,
432t
immune response, abnormal,
manipulation of, 432–33, 433t
sickle cell hemoglobinopathy, 666
Heme-pigment-associated acute renal
failure, 365
Hemodialysis
buffer composition, 1047
continuous arteriovenous
hemofiltration, 1050
dialysis fluid, 1046
composition, 1046–47
dialyzers, 1005–10
extracorporeal therapy, 1051–58
biocompatibility, 1054t, 1054–57,
1055
cannula/catheter dialysis, 1051
catheter dialysis, 1051
coagulation, 1057–58
reuse, hemodialyzers, 1053–54
single-needle dialysis, 1051
toxic substances, leaching of, 1058
uremic toxin removal, 1051–53,
1052t
hemodiafiltration, 0149, 1049
hemofiltration, 1048, 1048–49
hemoperfusion, 1051
long-term access techniques, 1044
modality, 1058–59
plasma separation, 1050t, 1050–51
sequential ultrafiltration and, 1047
starting, 1058
temporary access techniques, 1043,
1044
Hemoglobinopathy, sickle cell, 663–70
acute renal failure, 667
blood pressure, 666
chronic renal failure, 667–69
hematuria, 666
renal function abnormalities, 663–
66
acid-base homeostasis, renal
acidification and, 665
potassium, renal handling of, 665
renal concentrating defect, 665
renal hemodynamics, 663–65
renal papillary necrosis, 666–67
sickle cell nephropathy, 667–69
outcome, 668
treatment, 668–69
urinary tract infection, 667
Hemolysis, in renal failure, 875–76

Hemolytic uremic syndrome
cancer-associated, 517–18
cyclosporine-associated, 518
epidemic, 516
hereditary, hemolytic uremic
syndrome, 518
postpartum, 517
pregnancy-associated, 517
sporadic, 516–17
thrombotic thrombocytopenic
purpura, 518
acute, 518
chronic, 518
relapsing, 518
Hemolytic-uremic syndrome, 868
Hemoperfusion, hemodialysis, 1051
Hemorrhage, intracranial, dialysis and,
863–64
Henoch-Schonlein nephritis, 484–85
prognostic considerations, 485
renal involvement, 484–85
therapeutic approaches, 485
Heparin
potassium and, 70
thrombotic microangiopathy, 521
Hepatic failure, 12
hypernatremia, 12
Hepatitis, 893–914
anti-HCV diagnostic tests, 895
clinical presentation, 894–95
diagnostic testing for, 894–95
dialysis, 904–6
epidemiology, 894–95
hepatitis B virus, 904–8
syndromes, 906–7
vaccination, 905
hepatitis C virus, 893–904
biology of, 893, 894
infection in ESRD patient, 895–903
in nephrology, 903
transplant, 907–8
Hepatitis B virus, 904–8
syndromes, 906–7
vaccination, 905
Hepatitis C virus, 893–904
biology of, 893, 894
Hepatorenal syndrome, edema and, 46–
47
Heroin, use of
focal segmental glomerular sclerosis,
417
renal complications, 619–20
High-density lipoprotein. See HDL
Hippel-Lindau disease, 868
Histidinuria, 672
HIV, 620t, 620–21
genitourinary tuberculosis, 455–56

HLA antigens, transplantation, 1096–98
HONKS. See Hyperosmolar nonketotic
syndrome
Hormone, brain adaptation, 1
androgens, 3
brain damage, with hypoxic, 4
estrogen, 3
hyponatremia, 2–3
hypoxia, effects of, 3–4
physical factors, effects of, 3
progesterone, and androgens, 3
respiratory insufficiency, 3
vasopressin, 2–3
cerebral effects of, 3
Host defense mechanisms, peritonitis,
981–82, 982
Human immunodeficiency virus. See
HIV
Humoral factors, peritonitis, 982
"Hungry bone" syndrome, magnesium
balance, 125
HUS. See Hemolytic uremic syndrome
Hydralazine
acute glomerulonephritis, 389
dosage, side effects, 1197
for hypertension, 492, 496
in pregnancy, 579, 581
methyldopa with, for hypertension in
pregnancy, 579
Hydration, disorders of, 320–27
dehydration, 322–24t, 322–26
fluid and electrolyte requirements,
320–22, 321–22t
overhydration, 326t, 326–27
Hydrochlorothiazide
dosage, side effects, 1197
for hypertension, 492
onset and duration of action, 38
Hydrogen, renal secretion of, 189–98
bicarbonate reclamation, 189–94, 190,
191t
arterial pCO_2, acidity and, 192
carbonic anhydrase, 190, 192–93
chloride deficiency, 191
extracellular volume, 190
glomerular filtration rate, 190–91
glucose loading, 191t, 194
hypercalcemia, 193
parathyroid hormone, 193
phosphate depletion, 193
potassium, 191–92, 192
bicarbonate regeneration, 189
renal acid excretion, 194–98
ammonium excretion, 195
distal acidification, 195–98
aldosterone excess, 196–97
buffer content, 191t, 197–98, 198t

decreased arterial pH, 197
distal sodium delivery, *194*, 195–96
increased arterial pCO₂, 197
titratable acid excretion, 194–95
Hydronephrosis, prenatal, algorithm
for evaluation of, 447
Hyperadrenocorticoid states,
hypernatremia, 12
Hyperaldosteronism, potassium loss
and, 62–63
Hyperalimentation, nasogastric,
hypernatremia, 12
Hypercalcemia, 88t, 88–98, 204–5
bicarbonate reclamation, 193
causes, 88–95
clinical features, 88, 88t
diagnostic evaluation, 88t, 95–96
electrolyte abnormalities, surgical
patient, perioperative period, 345,
345t
fluid and electrolyte balance, 330–31,
331t
magnesium balance, 124
malignancies associated with, 88
treatment, 96t, 97–98
Hypercalciuria, 170–74, 171t
calcium stones and, 169–78
diet versus thiazide, 173–74, 174t
etiology, 170, *171*
follow-up, outcome, and prognosis,
174
low-calcium diet, 173, 174t
pathogenesis, 172, *172*, 172–73, *173*
thiazide diuretic agents, 170t, 173,
173
Hypercapnia
defined, 293
respiratory acidosis, 295
Hypercapnic encephalopathy, usage of
term, 295
Hypercoagulability treatment,
nephrotic syndrome, 414–15
Hypercystinuria, 672
Hyperkalemia, 65–66, 70
beta-adrenergic blocking drugs, 68
continuous ambulatory peritoneal
dialysis, 942
cyclosporine, 70
diagnosis, 65–71, *67*
excess intake, 67
real insufficiency, 66–67
digoxin, 68
diuretics, potassium-sparing, 69
drug-induced, 68
effects of, 66
electrocardiogram, *58*, 66
factitious, 66

familial hyperkalemic periodic
paralysis, 69
fluid and electrolyte balance, 329,
329t
heparin, 70
hypertonicity, 68
insulin deficiency, 67–68
mineralocorticoid-related impairment
of excretion, 71
pentamidine, 70
pseudohypoaldosteronism, 70
real failure, 69
renal tubular acidosis, 71, 272–73
symptoms, 66
therapy, 71–74
acute management, 71t, 71–74
sustained hyperkalemia, 73
tissue breakdown, 69, *69*
trimethaprim, 70
Hyperlipidemia
after transplant, 1144–46, 1178
cholestyramine, 1145
gemfibrozil, 1145
lovastatin, 1145
nicotinic acid, 1145–46
provastatin, 1145
in nephrotic syndrome, 414, 803–15
blood lipids, mechanism, acquired
disorders in, 805–7
dietary, 809–10
dislipidemia, 803–8
lipid disorders, deleterious role of,
803–5
lipid-lowering agents, 810
lipoprotein catabolism, decreased,
807–8
treatment, 808–10
renal insufficiency and, 769
Hypermagnesemia
causes of, 135
disorders of, 135–36
symptoms of, 135–36
Hypernatremia
acute renal failure, 12
in adults, 12
brain adaptation to, 11–12
causes of, 12
children, 12
clinical manifestations, 13
extremities, myoclonic jerking of,
13
food intake, decreased, 13
nystagmus, 13
respiratory failure, 13
seizures, 13
sensorium, depression of, 13
tachypnea, 13

weight loss, 13
diabetes insipidus, 12
fluid and electrolyte balance, 324t,
328–29
gastroenteritis, 12
hyperadrenocorticoid states, 12
liver disease and, 12
morbidity, 13
mortality, 13
nasogastric hyperalimentation, 12
nonketotic hyperosmolar coma, 12
patient evaluation, 11–12
renal tubular damage, 12
seawater ingestion, 12
Hypernatremic states, 11
Hypernephroma, usage of term, 695
Hyperosmolar coma, nonketotic,
hypernatremia, 12
Hyperosmolar nonketotic syndrome,
245, 245–48
clinical manifestations, 245–46, 246–
47t
diagnosis, 245–46, 246–47t
ketosis, absence of, 248
renal dysfunction and, 246–48, 247t
therapy, 239t, 242–44t, 248
Hyperosmolar states, treatment, 13–14,
14
Hyperoxaluria, 179–82
enteric hyperoxaluria, 179–81
dietary hyperoxaluria, 179–81, 181t
ileal resection or bypass, 181
oxalate, overproduction of, 181–82
ascorbic acid, 181
primary hyperoxaluria, 181
primary, transplant, 1160
Hyperparathyroidism
correction of, in renal failure, 885
primary, 178–79
clinical characteristics, 179, *180*, 180t
pathogenesis of stones, 178–79
treatment, 179
secondary, 771–72
renal insufficiency and, 771–72
tertiary, 95
Hyperphosphatemia, 155–59
causes of, 155t, 155–58
endogenous load, increased, 157–58
increased exogenous load, 156
urinary excretion, decreased, 156t,
156–57
consequences of, 158, 158t
treatment, 158t, 158–59
Hypertension
acute glomerulonephritis and, 388–
90, 389t
after transplant, 1177–78

autosomal dominant polycystic
kidney disease and, 645
essential hypertension, 1183–94
magnesium balance, 128–30
malignant, noninflammatory vascular
disease, 492–93t, 494–96, 495–96t
with metabolic alkalosis, 203
mineralocorticoid excess, 202–3, 203t
posttransplant, 1207–17
in pregnancy, 578–84, 581t
progression of renal disease and,
759–62
renal, 1195–1206
renal insufficiency and, 767–68
renovascular, 1195–1206
with systemic lupus erythematosus,
462, 462t
Hypertensive encephalopathy, with
acute glomerulonephritis, 389–90t,
390
Hyperthyroidism, potassium balance
and, 59–60
Hypertonicity, pathological features,
12–13
intracranial pressure, 12
venous sinuses, thrombosis, 12
Hyperuricemic nephropathy, 541–46
chronic urate nephropathy, 543–44
diagnosis, 542
dialysis, 543
hyperuricemia, renal disease and, 544
patients with cancer, 543
prevention, 542
therapy, 543
uric acid-associated acute renal
failure, 541–43
Hyperuricosuria, 169–78
allopurinol, 170t, 176–77, 177t
citrate, 178
complications, 177, 178t
diet, 176
versus drugs, 177
pathogenesis, 174–76, *175*, 176t, *177*
purine, 176
thiazide, 170t, 177
Hypoalbuminemia, with nephrotic
syndrome, 413
Hypoaldosteronism, hyporeninemic,
potassium and, 70
Hypocalcemia, 87, 87t, 98–107, 99t
biochemical findings, 101
causes, 99–105
clinical features, 99t, 99–100
diagnostic evaluation, 101t, 105
fluid and electrolyte balance, 330
of magnesium depletion, 130
neonatal, 130

with nephrotic syndrome, 101
treatment, 105–7
Hypocapnia, defined, 293
Hypokalemia, 57, 60–64
antibiotics, 62
barium intoxication, 60
Bartter's syndrome, 63–64
cancer therapy, 61
diabetes mellitus, 64
diagnostic approach, 57–58, *58*
diuretics, 59t, 61–62
drug-induced, 59
electrocardiogram, 57, *58*
fluid and electrolyte balance, 328t,
329
gastrointestinal losses, 61, 61t
hyperthyroidism, 59–60
infectious diarrhea, 61
leukemia, 64–65
magnesium depletion, 64
mineralocorticoid excess, 62, 63, 63t
periodic paralysis, 60
from potassium depletion, 60–65
primary hyperaldosteronism, 62
renal losses, *58*, 61–65
renal tubular acidosis, 64, 65t
secondary hyperaldosteronism, 62–63
stress/excessive catecholamine
release, 58
symptoms, 57
vomiting, 62
Hypomagnesemia
symptoms, 128–30, 129
treatment of, 131–33
Hyponatremia, 2, 857–58
adaptation to, 1
asymptomatic, 8
demeclocyline, 8
LeVeen shunt, 8
lithium, 8
vesopressinoic acid, 8
brain adaptation, 1, 2–3
causes, 327
cerebral demyelinating lesions, risk
factors, 10
clinical classification, treatment, 327
delayed diagnosis of, 7
diuretic-associated, 6
encephalopathy, *6*, 6–7, 7t
fluid and electrolyte balance, *327*,
327t, 327–28
intravenous fluid therapy,
postoperative, 5
oxytocin-associated, 5
with polydipsia, 5–6
postoperative, 4t, 4–5
with psychiatric disorders, 5–6

symptoms, 4t, 4–8
clinical settings, 4
therapy, 9
transurethral resection of prostate,
water balance, 5
treatment, 327
water balance, in postoperative
patients, 4
Hyponatremic encephalopathy, 6–8
differential diagnosis, 7t, 7–8
Hypoosmolar states, 1
Hypoparathyroidism, 204–5
biochemical findings in, 101
hypocalcemia and, 100–101, 101t
Hypophosphatemia, 147–55
causes of, 147, 147t
from decreased intestinal absorption,
147
from excess renal loss, 148–50
indication of treatment, 154
oncogenic hypophosphatemic
osteomalacia, defined, 148
oxygen dissociation curve, 152
from phosphate redistribution, 148–
49
treatment, 154–55
complications of, 155
modalities, 154–55, 155t
Hyporeninemic hypoaldosteronism,
potassium and, 70
Hypotension, vasopressin levels, 23
Hypotension thirst, 24
Hypotonic states
central pontine myelinolysis, 8
cerebral salt-wasting syndrome, 9
furosemide, 8
polydipsia, 10
therapy, 9
thiazide diuretics, 9
treatment of, 8–11, *9*, *10*, 10t
Hypovolemia, in obstructive jaundice,
bile salt, *551*, 551–52
Hypoxia, effects of, 3–4
Hysteroscopic endometrial ablation,
water balance, 5

I
IgA. *See* Immunoglobulin A
Ileostomy, losses of fluid and
electrolytes, 325
Iminoglycinuria, 671
Imipramine, voioding dysfunction, 1236
Immune response, immunosuppressive
agents, 1107–8, *1109*
Immunoglobulin A nephropathy
hematuria, 429–34

clinical course, 430–31
clinical features, 430
differential diagnosis, 431
epidemiology, 429
pathology, 429–30
mesangial, 422
post-streptococcal
 glomerulonephritis, distinguishing,
 431
Immunological impairment, renal
 insufficiency and, 773
Immunosuppressors, 1107–12, *1109*
 nephrotoxicity, 731–34
 cyclosporines, 731t, 731–34
 neuropsychiatric complications, 869
 rejection, 1107–37
 thrombotic microangiopathy, 520
 transplantation, 1107–37
Indacrinone, site of action of, 36
Indapamide
 for hypertension, 492
 site of action of, 36
Indwelling urethral catheters, 1222–24
Infections
 with acute renal failure, 375
 with autosomal dominant polycystic
 kidney disease, 643–45, 644t
 complications, from transplant, 1172–
 77
 kidney stones and, 168
 from neoplasms, 621–23
 opportunistic infection, renal, 621–23
 with systemic lupus erythematosus,
 462, 462t
 tumors, renal infection, 622–23
 urinary tract, 435–40
 bacteriuria, asymptomatic, 439
 candida, vulvovaginitis secondary to,
 437
 catheter-related, 438–39
 chlamydia, 437
 clinical presentation, 436
 complicated, 438
 cystitis, acute, 435–38
 diagnosis, 436
 differential diagnosis, 436–37
 E. coli, 435, 436
 neisseria, 437
 pathogenesis, 435–36
 pyelonephritis, acute, 435–38
 recurrent infections, 437–38
 Staphylococcus saprophyticus, 435
 treatment, 437
 trichomonas, 437
 vulvovaginitis secondary to, 437
 uncomplicated, 435–38
 urethritis, 436–37

Infectious diarrhea, gastrointestinal
 potassium loss, 61
Infective endocarditis, end-stage renal
 disease, 830–34
 Aspergillus species, therapy, 833
 clinical presentation, 830–31t, 830–32
 etiology, 830
 fungi candida species, therapy, 833
 management, 832–33t, 832–34
 Pseudomonas aeruginosa, therapy,
 833
 Staphylococcus aureus, therapy, 833
 Staphylococcus epidermidis, therapy,
 833
 Streptococcus, therapy, 833
Influenza A, transplant, 1176
Influenza B, transplant, 1176
Inherited renal disease
 genetic counseling, 690–93
 natural history, 690–91
 prenatal diagnosis, 692t, 692–93
 presymptomatic testing, 691–92
 risks, of pregnancy, 691
 genetic diagnosis, 685–90
 biochemical tests, 687
 clinical diagnosis, 685–87, 686t
 DNA testing, 688–90
 radiological diagnosis, 687–88, 687–
 88t
 renal pathology, 688
Insulin
 deficiency, hyperkalemia, 67–68
 potassium balance and, 53
 role of, 234
Intermittent catheterization, 1226–27,
 1239
Intermittent peritoneal dialysis, 922t,
 922–23
Intestinal absorption of, 143–44, *144*
Intra-abdominal pressure,
 complications from, continuous
 ambulatory peritoneal dialysis,
 944–45
Intracranial hemorrhage, dialysis and,
 863–64
Intracranial pressure, hypertonicity, 12
Intraglomerular pressure, diabetic renal
 disease, 605
Intraoperative fluid management, fluid
 and electrolytes, 337–38, 338t
 plasma and protein replacement,
 338
Intrarenal acute renal failure, 360t,
 360–61
Intravenous drug abuse, 619–21, 620t
Intravenous fluid therapy,
 postoperative, 5

IPD. *See* Intermittent peritoneal
 dialysis
Iron
 supplementation, in renal failure,
 883–85, *884*
 uremia, 794
Ischemic acute renal failure, 363–65
Isoniazid
 detecting hypersensitivity to
 antituberculous drugs, 455
 genitourinary tuberculosis
 chemotherapy, 452–53
 with renal insufficiency, 456
Israpidine for hypertension, 493

J
Jaundice, obstructive
 altered systemic hemodynamics in,
 549–51
 impaired cardiac performance in,
 553–54
 renal failure in, role of bile
 constituents, 552–53
 renal function, systemic
 hemodynamics, 548–49, 549t
Jaundiced heart, 553–54
Juvenile nephronopthisis, familial, 652–
 53

K
K-phos neutral tablets, for
 hypophosphatemia, 154
Ketoacidosis
 diabetic, 234–44, *235*
 cerebral edema, 244, 244t
 clinical manifestations, 235–36, 236t
 metabolic acidosis, 236–39
 phosphorus, 243–44
 potassium, 241–43
 sodium, 240–41
 metabolic acidosis from, 266t, 266–67
Ketoconazole, hypocalcemia and, 104
Ketosis, absence of, hyperosmolar
 nonketotic syndrome, 248
Kidney
 acute renal failure, 359–86
 catheters, 953–79, 1219–32
 cholemia, 547–59
 complications, of transplant, 1169–82
 continuous ambulatory peritoneal
 dialysis, 935–51
 cystic disease, 639–62
 diabetic ketoacidosis, and
 hyperosmolar nonketotic
 syndrome, 233–51

1256   *Index*

diabetic renal disease, 605–17
dialysate, 1005–28
dialysis, 989–1003, 1043–64
drugs usage, 1065–78
dialyzer, 1005–28
donor selection, transplant, 1079–
    1105
drug intoxications, 747–56
essential hypertension, 1183–94
fluid, electrolyte abnormalities
children, 319–34
surgical patient, 335–50
thermally injured, 351–57
genetic diagnosis, counseling,
    inherited renal disease, 685–94
glomerulonephritis, acute, 387–93
Goodpasture's syndrome, 401–11
hematologic disorders, renal failure,
    875–92
hematuria, immunoglobulin A
    nephropathy and, 429–34
hemofiltration, 1043–64
hepatitis, in renal patient, 893–914
HIV infection, 619–37
hyperlipidemia, nephrotic syndrome,
    803–15
hyperosmolar nonketotic syndrome,
    233–51
hyperuricemic nephropathy, 541–46
hypophosphatemia
consequences of, 151
effect on, 151
immunoglobulin nephropathy, 429–
    34
immunosuppression, in transplant,
    1107–37
inherited systemic, metabolic
    diseases, transplant, 1153–67
intravenous drug abuse, 619–37
jaundice, 547–59
lactic acidosis, 211–31
magnesium, 115–41
maturation of
fluid and electrolyte balance, 320
functional, anatomic, 320
membrane biocompatibility, 1029–
    42
metabolic acidosis, 253–74
metabolic alkalosis, 189–210
metabolic dysfunction, after
    transplant, 1139–52
mixed acid-base disorders, 307–18
multiple myeloma, with plasma cell
    dyscrasias, 529–39
nephrocalcinosis, 167–87
nephrolithiasis, 167–87
nephrotic syndrome, 413

neurological disorders, in renal
    disease, 855–73
noninflammatory vascular disease,
    489–503
nutritional management, uremic
    patient, 783–802
osteodystrophy, renal, 841–53
peritoneal dialysis, 915–33
peritonitis, 981–87
phosphate metabolism, 143–66
posttransplant hypertension, 1207–17
pregnancy, renal complications, 561–
    603
progression, renal disease,
    prevention, 757–66
psychiatric disorders, in renal
    diseases, 855–73
recipient selection, transplant, 1079–
    105
rejection, in transplant, 1107–37
renal failure, anesthesia, surgery,
    777–82
renal hypertension, 1195–206
renal insufficiency, 767–75
renal tubular acidosis, 275–91
renovascular hypertension, 1195–
    206
respiratory acid-base disorders, 293–
    305
sickle cell hemoglobinopathy, 663–70
stones. *See* Kidney stones
systemic lupus erythematosus, 459–
    78
thrombotic microangiopathy, 513–27
toxic nephropathy, 723–45
transplant. *See* Transplant
tuberculosis, 451–58
tubular dysfunction, following
    transplant, 1139–52
ultrafiltration, 1043–64
uremia
dialysis, cardiovascular
    complications, 817–39
drugs usage, 1065–78
vasculitic diseases, 479–88
Kidney stones
Aerobacter, 185
ammonium acid urate, 167
calcium, 167, 169t, 169–84
hypercalciuria, 169–78
diet *versus* thiazide, 173–74, 174t
etiology, 170, *171*
follow-up, outcome, and prognosis,
    174
idiopathic, 170–74, 171t
low-calcium diet, 173, 174t
pathogenesis, 172, *172*, 172–73, *173*

thiazide diuretic agents, 170t, 173,
    173
hyperoxaluria, 179–82
enteric hyperoxaluria, 179–81
dietary hyperoxaluria, 179–81, 181t
ileal resection or bypass, 181
overproduction of oxalate, 181–82
ascorbic acid, 181
primary hyperoxaluria, 181
hyperparathyroidism, primary, 178–
    79
clinical characteristics, 179, *180*, 180t
pathogenesis of stones, 178–79
treatment, 179
hyperuricosuria, 169–78
allopurinol, 170t, 176–77, 177t
citrate, 178
complications, 177, 178t
diet, 176
versus drug, 177
pathogenesis, 174–76, *175*, 176t, *177*
purine, 176
thiazide, 170t, 177
medullary sponge kidney, 178, *179*
natural history, 169, *169*, 170t
no metabolic disorder, 178
diet, 174t, 178
thiazide, 170t, 178
renal tubular acidosis, 182
pathogenesis of stones, 182
mechanism of hypercalciuria, 182
reason for low urine citrate, 182
cystine, 167
cystinuria, 184–85
Klebsiella, 185
management, 168–69
chronic pain, 168–69
colic, 168
infection, 168
obstruction, 168
obstruction, 167
pain, 167
people at risk, 167–68
Proteus, 185
Pseudomonas, 185
renal colic, 167
struvite stones, 167, 185
triampterine, 167
types of stones, 167, 168t
uric acid stones, 182–84
calcium-uric acid stones, 184, *184*
clinical stones disease, 183
dissolution, 184
gout, 183
ileostomy, 183
inflammatory ileocolitis, 183
Lesch-Nyhan syndrome, 183

pathogenesis of stones, 182–83
small bowel bypass, 183
treatment, 183–84
hyperuricosuria, *183*, 183–84
increased urine volume, 184
urine acidity, 183, *183*
tumor-lysis syndrome, 183
xanthine, 167
Klebsiella
kidney stones and, 185
peritonitis, 985
Kussmaul, Adolph, 233

L
L-lactic acidosis, metabolic acidosis
from, 267–69, 268t
Labetalol
for chronic hypertension, in
pregnancy, 577
dosage, side effects, 1197
for hypertensive emergency, 496
for severe hypertension, in
pregnancy, 581
Labor, epidural anesthesia in, 584
Lactation, magnesium balance, 126
Lactic acidosis, 211–31
Bifidobacterium, 227
classification, 212–14, 213t
diagnosis, *214*, 214–15
disorders associated with
catecholamine excess, 225–26
congenital defects, lactic acid
metabolism, 226
D-lactic acid, excessive production
of, 227
diabetes, 222–23
liver disease, 223
malignancy, 222
nutritional causes of, 226
obstructive pulmonary disease, 223
seizures, 225
toxins, acidosis due to, 223–25
Eubacterium, 227
Lactobacillus, 227
pathophysiology of, 211–12, *212*, 212t
phosphofructokinase, inhibition of,
211
physiology of, 211–12, *212*, 212t
therapy, *214*, 215–22
bicarbonate therapy, *212*, 218–20
calcium administration, 220
carbicarb, 220t, 220–21
dialysis, 222
dichloroacetate, 221, *221*
improve tissue oxygen delivery, 216–
18

Lactobacillus, lactic acidosis, 227
LDL, 803–5
renal insufficiency and, 767–75
Lead, nephtrotoxicity, 737
Leflunomide, 1116–17
rejection, 1116–17
Leukemia, potassium loss and, 64–65
Leukocyte function, in renal failure,
886–87
LeVeen shunt, hyponatremia, 8
Licorice ingestion, metabolic alkalosis,
202–3
Liddle's syndrome, 680
with metabolic alkalosis, 203
Light chain deposition disease
AL amyloididosis, combined, 532
follow-up and treatment, 532
heavy chain, multiple myeloma,
plasma cell dyscrasias, 532
multiple myeloma, plasma cell
dyscrasias, 531
clinical features, 531
Light chain proteinuria, asymptomatic,
multiple myeloma with plasma cell
dyscrasias, 532
Lipid-lowering agents, nephrotic
syndrome, 414, 810
Lisinopril for hypertension, 493
Lithium
hypercalcemia and, 94
hyponatremia, 8
nephrogenic diabetes insipidus and,
26
Liver disease
in alcoholism, hypernatremia and, 12
hypernatremia and, 12
hypocalcemia and, 101
with lactic acidosis, 223
Loading dose, drugs, 1065–68, 1066t
Loop blockers, onset and duration of
action, 38
Loop of Henle, diuretics acting on, *36*,
38t, 39
early distal loop
metolazone, 40
thiazides, *36*, 36t, 38t, 40
early distal tubule, 40
late distal loop, potassium-sparing
agents, *36*, 40
late distal tubule, *36*, 40
Lovastatin, nephrotic syndrome, 414
Low-density lipoprotein. *See* LDL
Lower airways obstruction
as cause of acute respiratory acidosis,
296
as cause of chronic respiratory
acidosis, 297

Lowe's syndrome, 678
Lpha-adrenergic catecholamines,
potassium balance and, 55
Lung cancer, hypercalcemia and, 88
Lupus erythematosus, 459–78
fetal and maternal morbidity and
mortality, 462–63
hypertension and atherosclerosis,
462, 462t
infection and immunization, 462, 462t
neonatal lupus, 463
nephritis-related complications, 460–
63
pregnancy and, 584
proteinuria, 461
renal insufficiency, 460–61, 461t
therapy, 463–71
Lupus glomerulonephritis, therapy,
465–71
Lymphatic complications, transplant,
1171–72, *1172*
Lymphoid irradiation, for murine lupus
nephritis, 463

M
Magnesium, 115–41
absorption, factors affecting, 117–18
acute magnesium overload,
management of, 136
asthma, 135
Bartter's syndrome, 124
body pool, *118*, 118–19
bone pool, 118
burns with dermal losses, 126
calcitriol administration for
depletion, 132
calcium, chemical differentiation, 115
cardiac arrhythmias, 134
concentration in foods, 116
cytomegalovirus, 124
depletion, 122
diagnosis, 126–27
intracellular, 127
retention following standardized
load, 127
serum, 126–27
urinary, 127
mechanisms of, 121–26, 122t
potassium loss and, 64
treatment, 131–33
diabetic complications, 130
dialysis patients, magnesium
metabolism in, 136
electrolyte abnormalities, 130–31
hypocalcemia of depletion, 130
hypocalcemia of pancreatitis, 131

neonatal hypocalcemia, 130
renal potassium wasting, 131
surgical patient, perioperative period,
    345–46, 346t
essential hypertension, 133
excess of, 135–36
extracellular pool, 118
gastrointestinal, 115–18, *116*, 116t,
    121
absorbed, 116
Gitelman's syndrome, 124
granulocyte-macrophage colony
    stimulating factor, 123
gut, sites of bsorption, 116
hormonal factors, renal magnesium
    reabsorption, 119
hypermagnesemia, 135–36
symptoms of, 135–36
hypertension, 128–30
hypomagnesemia, 121–26, 122t
causes of, 122
conditions associated with, 127–28
elderly patients, 128
electrolyte abnormalities, 127–28
intensive care unit, 128
mechanisms of, 121–26, 122t
in pregnancy, 130
symptoms of, 128–30
cardiac patients, 128
treatment, 131–33
intercompartmental shifts, 125
intracellular pool, 119–21, *120*
intravenous magnesium, 131
kidney pool, *118*, 118–19
lactation, 126
mechanisms of transport, 116–17
myocardial ischemia, 134, 134t
nephrolithiasis, 135
normal homeostasis, 115–21, *116*
gastrointestinal pool, 115–18, *116*,
    116t
oral magnesium replacement
    therapy, 131–32, 132t
potassium-sparing diuretics, 132–33
preeclampsia, 133–34
reabsorption, nonhormonal factors
    affecting, 119
renal failure, magnesium metabolism
    in, 136
renal handling of, drugs affecting,
    121–24, 122t
renal losses, 121
depletion from mixed causes, 125–26
drugs affecting
aminoglycoside antibiotics, 122–23
cyclosporine, 123
diuretics, 121–22

hypomagnesemia, 122
intercompartmental shifts, 125
secreted, 116
status asthmaticus, 135
sweating, 126
urinary, factors altering, 119, 119t
vitamin D, 117–18
Magnesium balance disorders, 331–32,
    331–32t
Magnesium carbonate, treatment of
    hyperphosphatemia, 158
Magnesium hydroxide, treatment of
    hyperphosphatemia, 158
Magnesium metabolism, after
    transplant, 1142–43
Magnesium salts, treatment of
    hyperphosphatemia, 158
Magnesium sulphate, to prevent
    eclampsia, 583
Magnesurias, 677
Maintenance dose, drugs, 1068–69
Maintenance fluids, usage of term, 320
Malignancy, with lactic acidosis, 222
Malignant disease, hypocalcemia
    associated with, 104
Malignant hypertension, 492–93t, 494–
    96, 495–96t
noninflammatory vascular disease,
    492–93t, 494–96, 495–96t
Malnutrition
causes of, continuous ambulatory
    peritoneal dialysis, 791
in maintenance dialysis, 788–90,
    789t
energy intake, 789–90
protein intake, 789–90
Mannitol
acute renal failure, 370–71
site of action of, 36
Maternal morbidity, mortality, with
    systemic lupus erythematosus, 462–
    63
Meat
magnesium concentration in, 116
phosphorus content in, 843
Medication. *See* Drug
Medulla, renal, cystic diseases of, 652–
    54
familial juvenile nephronopthisis,
    652–53
medullary cystic disease, 652–53
medullary sponge kidney, 653–54
Membrane biocompatibility,
    hemodialysis, 1029–42
amyloid disease, beta-microglobulin
    associated, 1036–37
anaphylactoid reactions, 1032–34

circuit components, 1029–30
dialysis-induced hypoxemia, 1034
incompatibility
impaired immunity, 1034–36
mechanisms of, 1030–31
middle-molecule clearance, reuse,
    1037
mortality rates, different dialysis
    membranes, 1037
protein catabolism, 1037
renal function, dialysis membranes
    affecting, 1036
thrombosis in dialysis circuit, 1031–
    32
Membrane failure, continuous
    ambulatory peritoneal dialysis,
    945–46
Membranoproliferative
    glomerulonephritis, *421*, 421–22
Membranous nephropathy, 419–21,
    420t
Mesangial nephritis, immunoglobulin
    A, 422
Metabolic abnormalities, in uremia,
    nutrition, 792
Metabolic acid-base disorders, 332–33
fluid and electrolyte balance
metabolic acidosis, 332, 332t
metabolic alkalosis, 332–33, 333t
Metabolic acidosis, 253–74, 858
added acids, 253–55, 254t
D-lactic acidosis, 271–72
ethylene glycol poisoning, 270
fluid and electrolyte balance, 332,
    332t
from gastrointestinal tract, 271–72
glue-sniffing, *254*, 271
hyperkalemia, renal tubular acidosis
    with, 272–73
ketoacidosis, 266t, 266–67
L-lactic acidosis, 267–69, 268t
management, 262–66
$NaHCO_3$, use of, 262–65
maximal acid-excretion during, renal
    tubular acidosis, 284–86, *287*
methanol poisoning, 269–70
$NaHCO_3$, loss of, *255*, 255–56
partial pressure of carbon dioxide,
    alteration of, in tissues, 265–66
patient assessment, 256–62
basis of disorder, determination of,
    256–57
renal response to, 260–62
threat to life, 257–60, 258t
potassium status, management of,
    266, 266t
renal acidosis, 254t, 272–73

salicylate intoxication, 270–71
specific causes of, 266–73
subgroups of, 253–56, 254t
Metabolic alkalosis, 189–210
effects of, 205
excessive bicarbonate loads, 204
extrarenal acid buffering, 198
fluid and electrolyte balance, 332–33,
333t
gastric alkalosis, 198t, 201–2, 201–2t
pathogenesis of, 201
hydrogen, renal secretion of, 189–98
bicarbonate reclamation, 189–94, *190*,
191t
arterial pCO_2, acidity and, 192
carbonic anhydrase, *190*, 192–93
glucose loading, 191t, 194
hypercalcemia, 193
parathyroid hormone, 193
phosphate depletion, 193
bicarbonate regeneration, 189
renal acid excretion, 194–98
ammonium excretion, 195
distal acidification, 195–98
aldosterone excess, 196–97
buffer content, 191t, 197–98, 198t
decreased arterial pH, 197
distal sodium delivery, *194*, 195–96
increased arterial pCO_2, 197
titratable acid excretion, 194–95
hypercalcemia, 204–5
maintenance of, 200t, 200–201
mineralocorticoid excess, 202–4
Bartter's syndrome, 203–4
congenital chloride-losing diarrhea,
204
diuretic administration, 203
hypertensive disorders, 202–3, 203t
posthypercapnic metabolic alkalosis,
204
pathophysiologic states associated
with, 201–5
postfasting metabolic alkalosis, 204
respiratory compensation, 205
therapy, 205–6
Metabolic bone disease, after
transplant, 1140–42
Metabolites, active, drugs, 1074–75,
1075t
Methanol poisoning, metabolic acidosis
from, 269–70
Methyldopa
for chronic hypertension in
pregnancy, 577
dosage, side effects, 1197
with hydralazine, for hypertension in
pregnancy, 579

for hypertension, 492
in pregnancy, 578
for hypertensive emergency, 496
Metolazone
edema, 40
for hypertension, 492
loop of Henle, early distal loop, 40
onset and duration of action, 38
site of action of, 36
Metoprolol for hypertension, 492
Microalbuminuria, diabetic renal
disease, 613
Microangiopathy, thrombotic, 513–27
clinical features, 516–18
endothelial cell dysfunction, 514–15
etiology, 513–14
hemolytic uremic syndrome
cancer-associated, 517–18
cyclosporine-associated, 518
epidemic, 516
hereditary, hemolytic uremic
syndrome, 518
postpartum, 517
pregnancy-associated, 517
sporadic, 516–17
thrombotic thrombocytopenic
purpura, 518
acute, 518
chronic, 518
relapsing, 518
pathology, 515–16
treatment, 518–21, 519t
antioxidants, 521
antiplatelet agents, 520
antithrombotic treatment, 520–21
glucocorticoids, 520
heparin, 521
immunosuppressive treatment, and
splenectomy, 520
plasma manipulation, 519–20
renal failure, 521
splenectomy, 520
vitamin E, 521
Milk, phosphorus content, 843
Milk-alkali syndrome, 94
Mineral metabolism, continuous
ambulatory peritoneal dialysis,
937, 942–43
Mineralocorticoids
adrenogenital syndromes, 202
with metabolic alkalosis, 203
Bartter's syndrome, 203–4
with metabolic alkalosis, 203
congenital chloride-losing diarrhea,
204
with metabolic alkalosis, 203
deficiency, potassium and, 70–71

diuretics, 203
with metabolic alkalosis, 203
excess, 202–4
hemangiopericytoma with metabolic
alkalosis, 203
hypertension with metabolic
alkalosis, 203
hypertensive disorders, 202–3, 203t
licorice ingestion, 202–3
Liddle's syndrome with metabolic
alkalosis, 203
posthypercapnic, 203–4
potassium loss and, 62, 63, 63t
primary aldosteronism, 202
with metabolic alkalosis, 203
renal artery stenosis, 202
with metabolic alkalosis, 203
surgical patient, fluid and electrolyte
disorders, 335–36
vomiting with metabolic alkalosis,
203
Minimal-change nephropathy, 415–17
Minkowsky, Oskar, 233
Minoxidil, 492
dosage, side effects, 1197
Mithramycin, hypercalcemia and, 98
Mixed acid-base disorders, 307–18
coexistence of different simple
disturbances, 307–10
additive combination, two simple
disorders, 307–9
counterbalancing combination, two
simple disorders, 309–10
more than two simple disorders,
combinations of, 308t, 310
coexistence of disturbances, entities
of single simple disturbance, 308t,
311–17
clinical manifestations, 311
diagnosis, 311–16, 312t, *313*
therapeutic principles, 316–17
coexistence of entities of single,
simple disturbance, different
pathogenesis, time course, 308t,
310–11
Mizoribine, 1112
rejection, 1112
Monoclonal antibodies, 1111–12
experimental studies, 1117–18
anti-CD4 monoclonal antibodies,
1118
anti-interleukin-2 monoclonal
antibodies, 1118
ICAM-1/CD54, 1118
LFA-1, 1118
MNA 031, 1117–18
rejection, 1117–18

anti-CD4 monoclonal antibodies,
    1118
anti-interleukin-2 monoclonal
    antibodies, 1118
ICAM-1/CD54, 1118
LFA-1, 1118
MNA 031, 1117–18
T10B9.1A-31, 1118
    for murine lupus nephritis, 463
Monoclonal gammapathies, transplant,
    1155–56
Morbid obesity, focal segmental
    glomerular sclerosis, 417
Mucous membranes, examination
    evidence of dehydration, 323
Multiple myeloma with plasma cell
    dyscrasias, 529–39
    AL amyloidosis, 529–31
        clinical features, 530
        treatment, 530–31
    cast nephropathy, 532–34, *533*, 533t
    Fanconi syndrome, 532
    light, heavy chain deposition disease,
        532
    light chain deposition disease, 531
    and AL amyloididosis, combined,
        532
    follow-up and treatment, 532
        clinical features, 531
    light-chain excretion, renal
        involvement related to, 532
    asymptomatic light-chain proteinuria,
        532
    distal tubular dysfunction, 532
    Fanconi syndrome, 532
    proximal, distal tubular dysfunction,
        combined, 532
    proximal tubular dysfunction, 532
    rapidly progressive renal failure,
        approach to, 536
    treatment, 534–37
        chemotherapy, 534–35, 535t
        renal insufficiency, 536–37
        symptomatic measures, 535–36
Musculoskeletal system,
    hypophosphatemia, consequences
    of, 151
Mycophenolate nofetil, 1112–13
    rejection, 1112–13
Myocardial ischemia, magnesium, 134,
    134t
Myopathy, after transplant, 1144

N
Na. *See* Sodium
Nadolol for hypertension, 492

NaHCO₃, metabolic acidosis, *255*, 255–
    56, 262–65
Nasogastric hyperalimentation,
    hypernatremia, 12
Nausea, release of vasopressin, 23
Necrotizing glomerulonephritis
    corticosteroids for, 483
    cyclophosphamide for, 483
Negative cultures, peritonitis, 985
Neisseria, 437
Neonatal lupus, 463
Neonatal severe hyperparathyroidism,
    92–93
Nephritis, hereditary, in pregnancy, 585
Nephrocalcinosis, 167–87
Nephrogenic diabetes insipidus, 25–27,
    26t
    causes of, 26
    polyuria, 25–27, 26t, 30–31
Nephrolithiasis, 167–87
    autosomal dominant polycystic
        kidney disease, 646, *647*
    magnesium, 135
Nephrology, hepatitis and, 903
Nephron
    diluting segment of, 2
    diuretic agent site of action, 36
Nephronopthisis, juvenile, familial,
    652–53
Nephropathy
    analgesic, 735–37
    cast, 532–34, *533*, 533t
    multiple myeloma with, 532–34, *533*,
        533t
    chemotherapeutic agent-induced,
        729–31
    cisplatin nephropathy, 729–30
    methotrexate nephropathy, 730
    contrast medium-associated, 728–29
    diabetic, 587, 612t, 612–13, 1147
    pregnancy and, 584
    gold, 739–40
    hyperuricemic, 541–46
    immunoglobulin, 429–34
    immunoglobulin A
        hematuria and, 429–34
    post-streptococcal
        glomerulonephritis, distinguishing,
        431
    membranous, 419–21, 420t
    minimal-change, 415–17
    reflux, 441–49, 443–44, 587
    focal segmental glomerular sclerosis,
        417
    pregnancy, 584, 587
    vesicourteral reflux and, 441–49
    sickle cell, 667–69

    hemoglobinopathy, 667–69
        outcome, 668
        treatment, 668–69
    toxic, 723–45
        acyclovir, 728
        amphotericin B, 727–28
        carbapenum, 727
        cephalosporin, 776–27
        penicillin, 726
        pentamidine, 728
        rifampin, 727
        sulfonamide, 727
        tetracycline, 727
        vancomycin, 727
Nephrostomy
    percutaneous, genitourinary
        tuberculosis, 452
    tubes, 1227
Nephrotic syndrome
    bezafibrate, 414
    clofibrate, 414
    edema and, 45–46
    focal segmental glomerular sclerosis,
        417–19, *418*
    gemfibrozil, 414
    hypercoagulability treatment, 414–15
    hyperlipidemia in, 414, 803–15
        dietary treatment, 809–10
        dislipidemia, 803–8
    lipid
        disorders of, deleterious role of, 803–
            5
        lowering agents, 810
        mechanism, acquired disorders in,
            805–7
        lipoprotein catabolism, decreased,
            807–8
        treatment, 808–10
    hypocalcemia and, 101
    immunoglobulin A mesangial
        nephritis, 422
    lipid-lowering drugs, 414
    lovastatin, 414
    membranoproliferative
        glomerulonephritis, *421*, 421–22
    membranous nephropathy, 419–21,
        420t
    minimal-change nephropathy, 415–17
    in pregnancy, 588–89, 589t
    symptomatic therapy, 413–15
        edema, 413
        hyperlipidemia, 414
        hypoalbuminemia, 413
        proteinuria, 413–14
        therapy, 415–22
Nephrotoxicity, 723–45
    from analgesic, 735–37

clinical presentation of AN, 735
epidemiology of AN, 735–37, 736t
from angiotensin-converting enzyme inhibitors, 738
antibiotic-induced, 725–28
acyclovir nephropathy, 728
aminoglycoside antibiotic nephrotoxicity, 725–26
amphotericin B nephropathy, 727–28
carbapenum nephropathy, 727
cephalosporin nephropathy, 726–27
foscarnet, 728
penicillin nephropathy, 726
pentamidine nephropathy, 728
rifampin nephropathy, 727
sulfonamide nephropathy, 727
tetracycline nephropathy, 727
vancomycin nephropathy, 727
from cadmium, 737–38
cellular mechanisms of injury, 724–25
cellular uptake, nephrotoxins, 724
intracellular sites, nephrotoxicity, 724–25
mechanisms, nephrotoxicity, 724–25
from chemotherapeutic agents, 729–31
cisplatin nephropathy, 729–30
methotrexate nephropathy, 730
nitrosoureas, 730
contrast medium-associated, 728–29
management, 729
prevention, 729
risk factors, 728–29
defined, 723–24
diagnosis, 723–24
from environmental toxicants, 740
glomerular filtration rate, 723
gold nephropathy, 739–40
from heavy metals, 740
illicit drug abuse, 739
from immunosuppressive drugs, 731–34
cyclosporines, 731t, 731–34
from lead, 737
from nonsteroidal anti-inflammatory drugs, 734t, 734–35
from penicillamine, 739
Tolypocladium inflatum gams, 731
Nervous system, hypophosphatemia consequences of, 151
effect on, 153
Neurogenic diabetes insipidus. *See* Central diabetes insipidus
Neurological complications of dialysis, 861–64
carpal tunnel syndrome, 863

dialysis disequilibrium syndrome, 861–62
dialytic encephalopathy, 862–63
intracranial hemorrhage, 863–64
Werniche's encephalopathy, 864
Neuromuscular impairment
as cause of acute respiratory acidosis, 296
as cause of chronic respiratory acidosis, 297
Neuropsychiatric complications, drug treatment in renal patients, 869
antimicrobials, 869
diuretics, 869
drugs, acting on central nervous system, 869
immunosuppressive drugs, 869
OKT3 monoclonal antibodies, 869
recombinant erythropoietin, 869
Neutral sodium phosphate, for hypophosphatemia, 154
Neutral sodium potassium phosphate, for hypophosphatemia, 154
Neutraphos capsules, for hypophosphatemia, 154
Neutraphos K capsules, for hypophosphatemia, 154
Nicardipine, 493
dosage, side effects, 1197
Nicotine
central diabetes insipidus and, 24
vasopressin levels, 23
Nifedipine
acute glomerulonephritis, 389–90
for chronic hypertension in pregnancy, 577
dosage, side effects, 1197
for hypertension, 493
for hypertensive emergency, 496
Nitrogen balance, nutrition and, 783–84
Nitroglycerin for hypertensive emergency, 496
Nitroprusside, acute glomerulonephritis, 390
Nocturnal peritoneal dialysis, 922t, 924
Noninflammatory vascular disease, 489–503
embolic disease of kidney, 500–502
embolization, 500–502
large-vessel, 500–501
small-vessel, 501–2
high blood pressure—primary hypertension, 489–94, *490*, 492–93t
malignant hypertension, 492–93t, 494–96, 495–96t
renal vascular hypertension, 496–98, 498t

renal vein thrombosis, 502–3
scleroderma-progressive systemic sclerosis, 495t, 499–500
Nonketotic hyperosmolar coma, hypernatremia, 12
Nonsteroidal anti-inflammatory drugs
nephrotoxicity, 734t, 734–35
potassium, effect, 70
Noodles, phosphorus content, 843
NPD. *See* Nocturnal peritoneal dialysis
Numetanide, onset and duration of action, 38
Nutrition
with acute renal failure, 374
continuous ambulatory peritoneal dialysis, 790–92
malnutrition
outcome of, 790–91
prevalence, 790–91
prevention, protein energy malnutrition, 791t, 791–92
with uremia, 783–802
acute renal failure, 792–93
metabolic abnormalities, 792
nutritional approach, 792–93
ascorbic acid, 795
biochemical measurements, 785
body composition, 784–85
catabolic factors, dialysis treatment, 787t, 787–88
chronic renal failure, nutritional status in, 783–85, 784t
during continuous ambulatory peritoneal dialysis, 790–92
causes of malnutrition, 791
malnutrition
outcome of, 790–91
prevalence, 790–91
prevention, protein energy malnutrition, 791t, 791–92
copper, 795
cyanocobalamin, 795
dietary compliance, assessment of, 783
dietary intake, assessment of, 783
iron, 794
malnutrition, in maintenance dialysis, 788–90, 789t
drug intervention, 790
energy intake, 789–90
growth hormone, 790
intradialytic parenteral nutrition, 790
protein intake, 789–90
treatment, 789t, 789–90
nitrogen balance, 783–84
pre dialysis stage, chronic renal failure, 785–86

conventional low-protein diet, 786
energy requirements, 786
very low-protein diet, amino acid
    supplement, 786
very-low-protein diet, keto acid
    supplement, 786
protein intake, patient compliance,
    783–85, 784t
pyridoxine, 795, 795t
selenium, 794
tocopherol, 795
transplant, 793–94
vitamins, 794–96
vitamin A, 796
wasting, in chronic renal failure, 786
endocrine disorders, 787
metabolic disorders, 787
poor protein energy intake, 787
zinc, 794–95
Nuts, magnesium concentration in, 116
Nystagmus, with hypernatremia, 13

O
Oasthouse syndrome, 672
Oatmeal, phosphorus content, 843
Obesity
morbid, focal segmental glomerular
    sclerosis, 417
transplant, 1154–55
Obstructive jaundice
altered systemic hemodynamics in,
    549–51
hypovolemia, bile salt, *551*, 551–52
impaired cardiac performance in,
    553–54
renal failure in, role of bile
    constituents, 552–53
renal function, systemic
    hemodynamics, 548–49, 549t
Obstructive pulmonary disease, with
    lactic acidosis, 223
OKT3
metabolic side effects of, 1148–49
monoclonal antibodies,
    neuropsychiatric complications,
    869
Oligonephronia, focal segmental
    glomerular sclerosis, 417
Opiates, vasopressin levels, 23
Oral calcium preparations, 101
Osmolality, extracellular fluid, 1–19
Osmotic diuretics, nephrogenic
    diabetes insipidus and, 26
Osteitis fibrosa, 843–46
hyperphosphatemia
    management of, 843t, 843–44

prevention, 843t, 843–44
phosphorus retention, 843
Osteodystrophy, renal, 841–53
beta-2-microglobulin amyloidosis,
    848–49, 849
defined, 841
osteitis fibrosa, 843–46
calcitrol deficiency, 844, *844*
calcium supplementation, 845
hyperphosphatemia
management of, 843t, 843–44
prevention, 843t, 843–44
parathyroidectomy, 845–46, 846t
phosphorus retention, 843
vitamin D metabolite
    supplementation, 844–55
osteomalacia, *842*, 846–48
adynamic bone disease, ideopathic,
    848
aluminum-related bone disease, 847–
    48
therapeutic strategies, integration of,
    849t, 849–50
Osteomalacia, *842*, 846–48
adynamic bone disease, ideopathic,
    848
aluminum-related bone disease, 847–
    48
Outflow resistance, decreasing, 1237
Overhydration, fluid and electrolyte
    balance, 326t, 326–27

P
Pain
with autosomal dominant polycystic
    kidney disease, 641–42
with kidney stones, 168–69
release of vasopressin, 23
Pamidronate, 96, 97
Pancreatic juice, losses of fluid and
    electrolytes, 325
Pancreatitis
hypocalcemia of, 131
magnesium balance, 125
Papillary necrosis, with sickle cell
    hemoglobinopathy, 666–67
Papilloma, transplant, 1176
Parainfluenza, transplant, 1176
Paralysis, familial hyperkalemic
    periodic, 69
Paraproteinemias, transplant, 1155–56
Parasomnias, hypomagnesemia and,
    129
Parathesias, hypomagnesemia and,
    129
Parathyroid hormone

bicarbonate reclamation, 193
protein, hypercalcemia and, 89
Parathyroidectomy
osteitis fibrosa, 845–46, 846t
transplantation and, 1088
Parenchymal renal disease, unilateral,
    1200–1201
Parenteral phosphate preparations, for
    hypophosphatemia, 154
Parkinson-dementia complex of Guam,
    hypomagnesemia and, 129
Partial pressure of carbon dioxide,
    alteration of, in tissues, with
    metabolic acidosis, 265–66
Pasta, phosphorus content, 843
PCO_2. *See* Partial pressure of carbon
    dioxide
Peanuts, phosphorus content, 843
Pelvis, renal, neoplasms of, *701*, 702–2
Penethazine, vasopressin levels, 23
Penicillamine, nephrtotoxicity, 739
Pentamidine
for AIDS, 622
hypocalcemia and, 104
magnesium balance, 123
potassium and, 70
Periarteritis nodosa, pregnancy, 584,
    586–87
Pericardial tamponade, acute,
    pericarditis, 822
Pericarditis, 818–22
acute pericardial tamponade, 822
clinical presentation, 819–20, 820t
complications, 820–21, *821*, 821t
end-stage renal disease, therapy, 821
incidence, 818
management, 821–22
pathogenesis, 818–19, 819t
pathology, 818–19, 819t
uremic, renal insufficiency and, 773
Peritoneal catheters, 953–79
break-in, 966–68
care of, 966–68
exit, 966–68
immediate intraperitoneal segment
    care, 966
long-term results, 974–76
National CAPD Registry survey,
    974–75
swan-neck catheters, 975
United States Renal Data System
    Report, 975–76
peritoneal dialysis, 966
removal, 973–74
functioning catheter, with
    complication, 973–74
malfunction, 973

nonfunctioning catheter, 974
rigid catheters, 953–55
complications, 954t, 954–55
insertion, 953–54
preinsertion, patient assessment, 953
soft catheters, 955t, 955–58
complications, 968–73
early, 968–69
late, 969–73
implantation of, 958–66
catheter preparation, 959
flange, anchoring, 962
implantation method, 959–66
patient preparation, 958–59
straight, coiled Tenckhoff catheters, 956, *956*
swan-neck catheters, *956*, 956t, 956–58
Peritoneal dialysis, 915–33
access, 1001–3
acute peritoneal dialysis, 915–21
access, 916–17
complications, 918t, 918–21
contraindications, 905–6
indications, 905–6
schedules, 917–18
solutions, 917, 917t
technique, 917–18
ambulatory, with pregnancy, 591
chronic peritoneal dialysis, 921–29
access, 921
complications, 925t, 925–29
continuous cyclic, 922t, 923–24
delivery systems, 921–22
intermittent, 922t, 922–23
nocturnal, 922t, 924
tidal, 924–25
continuous ambulatory, 935–51, 981
complications, 944–47
catheter-related, 944, 944t
from intra-abdominal pressure, 944–45
membrane failure, 945–46
metabolic, 946–47
peritonitis, 944, 944t
edema, 44
individualized dialysis, 937–44
acid-base balance, 942
adequacy, *937*, 937–40
blood pressure, 941–42
dietary requirements, 943t, 943–44
hyperkalemia, 942
mineral metabolism, *937*, 942–43
sodium balance, 941–42
nutrition, 790–92
causes of malnutrition, 791
malnutrition

outcome of, 790–91
prevalence, 790–91
prevention, protein energy malnutrition, 791t, 791–92
patient selection, 935–36
advantages of, 935–36, 936t
contraindications, 936, 936t
indications, 936, 936t
patient training, 937
peritoneal access, 936
continuous cyclic, 922t, 923–24
operative technique, 1001–2, *1002*
peritonitis, 981–87
Peritonitis, 981–87
antibiotic selection, initial, 984–85
gram-negative organisms, 985
gram-positive organisms, 984–85
yeast, gram stain, 985
cellular factors, 982–84
clinical course, 983–84t, 984
clinical presentation, initial assessment, 984
continuous ambulatory peritoneal dialysis, 944, 944t
E. coli, 985
gram-negative microorganisms, 985–86
gram-positive microorganisms, 985
host defense mechanisms, 981–82, *982*
humoral factors, 982
incidence, 981
Klebsiella, 985
negative cultures, 985
pathogenesis, 981, 982t
prophylactic therapies, 986
Proteus, 985
Pseudomonas, 985–86
treatment, 983–84t, 984–86
tunnel infections, 986
Xanthomonas, 985–86
Permanent dialysis access, 991–1001
Phenobarbital, hypocalcemia and, 104
Phophaturias, 674–77
hypophosphatemic nonrachitic bone disease, 676
hypophosphatemic rickets, with hypercalcemia, 676
oncogenous rickets, with phosphaturia, 676
osteomalacia, adult, sporadic, 676–77, 677t
X-linked hypophosphatemic rickets, 675, 675t
Phosphate, oral, for hypercalcemia, 96
Phosphate depletion, magnesium and, 124

Phosphate metabolism, 143–66
after transplant, 1142
hyperphosphatemia, 155–59
causes of, 155t, 155–58
endogenous load, increased, 157–58
increased exogenous load, 156
urinary excretion, decreased, 156t, 156–57
consequences of, 158, 158t
treatment, 158t, 158–59
hypophosphatemia, 147–55
in alcoholism, 150, *150*
causes of, 147, 147t
clinical manifestations, 150–53, 151t
consequences of, 150–53, 151t
from decreased intestinal absorption, 147
diabetic ketoacidosis, 149–50, *150*
from excess renal loss, 148–50
indication of treatment, 154
oncogenic hypophosphatemic osteomalacia, defined, 148
from phosphate redistribution, 148–49
postrenal transplantation, 150
treatment, 154–55, 155t
complications of, 155
intestinal absorption of, 143–44, *144*
plasma, phosphate composition in, 143
renal excretion of, 144–47
glomerular filtration, 144
regulation, 145, 145t, 145–47
tubular reabsorption, 144–45
Phosphate preparations, for hypophosphatemia, 154
Phosphate restriction, renal insufficiency and, 768
Phosphofructokinase, inhibition of, lactic acidosis and, 211
Phosphorus
diabetic ketoacidosis, 243–44
electrolyte abnormalities, surgical patient, perioperative period, 346–47
Physical activity, autosomal dominant polycystic kidney disease and, 641
Pindolol, 492
dosage, side effects, 1197
PKD. *See* Polycystic kidney disease
Plasma
exchange, for hypertension in pregnancy, 581
manipulation, thrombotic microangiopathy, 519–20
phosphate composition in, 143

replacement, intraoperative, fluid and electrolytes and, 338
separation, hemodialysis, 1050t, 1050–51
tonicity, brain adaption, 2
Plasma cell dyscrasias, multiple myeloma with, 529–39
AL amyloidosis, 529–31
clinical features, 530
treatment, 530–31
cast nephropathy, 532–34, *533*, 533t
light, heavy chain deposition disease, 532
light chain deposition disease, 531
and AL amyloididosis, combined, 532
follow-up and treatment, 532
clinical features, 531
light-chain excretion, renal involvement related to, 532
asymptomatic light-chain proteinuria, 532
distal tubular dysfunction, 532
Fanconi syndrome, 532
proximal, distal tubular dysfunction, combined, 532
proximal tubular dysfunction, 532
rapidly progressive renal failure, approach to, 536
treatment, 534–37
chemotherapy, 534–35, 535t
renal insufficiency, 536–37
symptomatic measures, 535–36
Plasmapheresis, for poisoning, 753–54, 754t
Plicamycin
hypercalcemia and, 98
hypocalcemia and, 104
Plicamycin for hypercalcemia, 96
Poisoning
diagnosis, 747–48, *748*, 748t
dialysis, 754
drug elimination techniques, 749–54
dialysis, 753
criteria for, 754, 754t
techniques, 750–51t, 751–52
diuresis, forced, 749–51
exchange blood transfusion, 753–54, 754t
hemoperfusion, 753
criteria for, 754, 754t
plasmapheresis, 753–54, 754t
sorbent hemoperfusion, 752–53, 752–53t
treatment, 748–49
future trends, 754
Polyangitis

corticosteroids for, 483
microscopic
corticosteroids for, 483
cyclophosphamide for, 483
treatment, 482–84
vasculitic disease, 480
Polyarteritis nodosa
treatment, 481–82
vasculitic disease, 480
Polyclonal antilymphocyte agents, 1110–11
Polycystic kidney disease
pregnancy, 584, 588
transplant, 1158–59
Polycythemia, in renal failure, 886
Polydipsia, 10
Polyneuropathy, uremic, 858–60
clinical features, 859
electrophysiological findings, 859
morphology, 859
pathophysiology, 859
treatment, 859–60
Polyoma, transplant, 1176
Polyuric syndrome, 21–33
arginine vasopressin, 21
defined, 21
dehydration tests, interpretation, 28
diagnosis, 29
polyuria
defined, 21
disorders of, 24–27, *25*
type I polyuric disorders, 24–27
central diabetes insipidus, 24t, 24–25
causes of, 24
nephrogenic diabetes insipidus, 25–27, 26t
causes of, 26
type II polyuric disorders, 27
treatment, 27–29, 28t, *29*, 30–31
central diabetes insipidus, 30
nephrogenic diabetes insipidus, 30–31
type II disorders, 31
type I polyuric disorders, 24–27
type II disorders, 31
type II polyuric disorders, 27
water balance, normal, 21–24
thirst, *22*, 23–24
vasopressin, 21–23, *22*
Pontine myelinolysis, 8
Post-streptococcal glomerulonephritis, immunoglobulin A nephropathy, distinguishing, 431
Postfasting metabolic alkalosis, 204
Posthypercapnic metabolic alkalosis, 204
Postoperative patient

hyponatremia, 4t, 4–5
water balance in, 4
Postpartum hemolytic uremic syndrome, 517
Postrenal acute renal failure, 360, 360t
Poststreptococcal glomerulonephritis, prevention of, 392
Posttransplant hypertension, 1207–17
causes of, 1207–12
therapy, 1212–13
Potassium, 53–83
bicarbonate reclamation, 191–92, *192*
diabetic ketoacidosis and, 241–43
dietary sources, 73
disorders, 858
after transplant, 1139–40
of homeostasis, 57–74
electrolyte abnormalities, surgical patient, perioperative period, 341–44
hyperkalemia, 70
beta-adrenergic blocking drugs, 68
cyclosporine, 70
diagnosis, 65–71, *67*
excess intake, 67
real insufficiency, 66–67
digoxin, 68
diuretics, potassium-sparing, 69
drug-induced, 68
effects of, 66
electrocardiogram, *58*, 66
factitious, 66
familial hyperkalemic periodic paralysis, 69
heparin, 70
hypertonicity, 68
insulin deficiency, 67–68
mineralocorticoid-related impairment of excretion, 71
pentamidine, 70
pseudohypoaldosteronism, 70
real failure, 69
symptoms, 66
therapy, 71–74
acute management, 71t, 71–74
sustained hyperkalemia, 73
tissue breakdown, 69, *69*
trimethaprim, 70
hypokalemia, 57, 60–64
antibiotics, 62
barium intoxication, 60
Bartter's syndrome, 63–64
cancer therapy, 61
diabetes mellitus, 64
diagnostic approach, 57–58, *58*
diuretics, 59t, 61–62
drug-induced, 59

electrocardiogram, 57, *58*
gastrointestinal losses, 61, 61t
hyperthyroidism, 59–60
infectious diarrhea, 61
leukemia, 64–65
magnesium depletion, 64
mineralocorticoid excess, 62, 63, 63t
periodic paralysis, 60
from potassium depletion, 60–65
primary hyperaldosteronism, 62
renal losses, *58*, 61–65
renal tubular acidosis, 64, 65t
secondary hyperaldosteronism, 62–63
signs and symptoms, 57
stress/excessive catecholamine
    release, *58*
vomiting, 62
normal homeostasis, 53–57, *54*
acid-base perturbations, 55–56, *56*
aldosterone, *54*, 55
alpha-adrenergic catecholamines, 55
beta adrenergic catecholamines, 53
excretion, regulation of, 56–57
influences, 55–56
insulin, 53
intracellular calcium, 55
potassium depletion, 55
thyroid hormone, 55
transcellular balance, 53–55
phosphate, for hypophosphatemia,
    154
renal handling, sickle cell
    hemoglobinopathy, 665
replacement therapy, 65, 65t
Potassium-sparing agents, loop of
    Henle, diuretics acting on, *36*, 40
Potassium status, management of, with
    metabolic acidosis, 266, 266t
Prazosin, 492, 577
dosage, side effects, 1197
Preeclampsia
edema and, 49
magnesium, 133–34
Pregnancy
acute cystitis, 565
acute fatty liver of pregnancy, 570–
    71
acute pyelonephritis, 565, 565t
acute renal failure, 567–68
and preeclampsia/eclampsia, 570
and pyelonephritis, 570
acute symptomatic urinary tract
    infection, 565
ambulatory peritoneal dialysis, 591
anatomic changes, 561
antenatal care, 574
antihypertensive therapy, 578

assessment of renal function during
    pregnancy, *562, 573,* 575–76
asymptomatic bacteriuria, 562–65
autosomal dominant polycystic
    kidney disease and, 649
clinical implications, 563–64
cortical necrosis in pregnancy, 571–
    72
counseling
renal disease, 590, 591t, 591–92
delivery, 576
diabetic nephropathy, 587
diagnosis, 562–63, 567
dialysis, 567–68
chronic, patients undergoing, 590–91
eclampsia
magnesium sulphate to prevent, 583
sedation to prevent, 583–84
epidural anesthesia in labor, 584
evaluation during pregnancy, 574
forms of acute renal failure found in
    pregnancy, 568–72
functional changes, 561–62
general management plan for renal
    disease in pregnancy, 574–78
GFR. *See* Glomerular filtration rate
glomerulonephritis
acute, 584
chronic, 585
hereditary nephritis, 585
hypertension, 576–78
anticoagulant therapy, 580
bed rest, 578
beta-adrenoceptor blocking agents,
    579
alpha-, combined, 579
calcium channel blockers, 579
diet, 578
diuretics, 579–80
hydralazine, 579
low-dose aspirin, 581–82
management regimes, 578–84
methyldopa, 578
with hydralazine, 579
plasma exchange, 581
prostaglandin therapy, 581–82
sedation, 578
severe, 581t, 582
volume-expansion therapy, 580–81
hypertensive emergencies, blood
    transfusion policy, 584
hypomagnesemia in, 130
idiopathic postpartum renal failure
    or hemolytic uremic syndrome,
    571
inherited renal disease, risks, 691
kidney in normal pregnancy, 561–62

lupus erythythematosus and, 584
magnesium balance, 125–26
management, 564–67
nephrotic syndrome, 588–89, 589t
nontraumatic rupture of urinary
    tract, 566, 566t
obstetric renal failure, 572
obstructive uropathy, 572
periarteritis nodosa, 586–87
perspective, 565, 567
polycystic kidney disease, 588
pregnancy assessment, early, 590
preserved/mildly impaired renal
    function, *573,* 573–74
pyelonephritis, 587
reflux nephropathy, 587
renal biopsy, in antenatal
    management, 574–75
renal complications, 561–603
renal failure in septic abortion or
    septic shock, 568
renal insufficiency and, 770
severe renal insufficiency, 573t, 574
site of infection, 563
solitary kidney, 588
systemic lupus erythematosus, 585–86
systemic sclerosis, 586
transplant patients, 591–96, 1149
delivery, 594–95
pediatric management, 595
postnatal assessment, 595
pregnancy counseling, 591t, 591–92
pregnancy management, 592–94
urinary tract surgery, previous, 588
urolithiasis, 587–88
Wegener's granulomatosis, 588
Pregnancy assessment, with renal
    disease, 590
Pregnancy-associated hemolytic uremic
    syndrome, 517
Premenstrual syndrome, edema and,
    49
Prenatal diagnosis, with inherited renal
    disease, 692t, 692–93
Prerenal acute renal failure, 359, 360t
Pretransplant evaluation, potential
    recipient, transplantation, 1084–87,
    1085t
laboratory tests, 1086
patient history, 1085
physical examination, 1085–86
radiographic studies, 1086
selected studies, 1086–87
urologic studies, 1086
Previous urinary tract surgery,
    pregnancy and, 584
Primary aldosteronism

with metabllic alkalosis, 202
with metabolic alkalosis, 203
Primary hyperparathyroidism,
    hypercalcemia and, *86*, 88t, 90–92
Progression of renal disease
    control, 767–69
    diet, 768
    hypertension, 767–68
    phosphate restriction, 768
    proteinuria, reduction of, 768–69
    prevention, 757–66
    assessing progression, 757–58
    creatinine clearance, 757
    serum creatinine, 757–58
    reciprocal of, 758
    urea, 758
    intercurrent events affecting, 764t,
        764–65
    risk factors, 759
    dietary protein, 762–64
    hypertension, systemic, 759–62
Promethazine, central diabetes
    insipidus and, 24
Prophylactic therapies, peritonitis, 986
Propoxyphene, nephrogenic diabetes
    insipidus and, 26
Propranolol, 492, 496
    dosage, side effects, 1197
Prostaglandins
    for hypertension in pregnancy, 581–
        82
    for murine lupus nephritis, 463
    vasopressin-mediated water
        permeability, 23
Prostate, transurethral resection, water
    balance, 5
Prostate cancer, 712–17
    diagnosis, 714–15
    early, 712–14, 713t, *714*
    hypercalcemia and, 88
    pathology, 712
    staging, 714–15
    treatment, *715–16*, 715–17
Prostatic hyperplasia, benign, 1237–39
Protein
    dietary, renal disease, risk factors,
        762–64
    intake
        diabetic renal disease, 606
        in uremia, patient compliance, 783–
            85, 784t
    replacement, intraoperative, fluid
        and electrolytes and, 338
Proteinuria
    autosomal dominant polycystic
        kidney disease, 645
    with nephrotic syndrome, 413–14

reduction of, renal insufficiency and,
    768–69
with systemic lupus erythematosus,
    461
Proteus
    kidney stones, 185
    peritonitis, 985
Protozoal infection, transplant, 1177
Proximal renal tubular acidosis, 275–77
    clinical features, 275–76, *276*, 276–77t
    diagnosis, *276*, 277
    pathophysiology, 275–76, *276*, 276–
        77t
    therapy, 277
Pruritus, renal insufficiency and, 774
Pseudohyperparathyroidism,
    hypercalcemia and, 89
Pseudohypo-parathyroidism,
    biochemical findings in, 101
Pseudohypoaldosteronism, potassium
    and, 70
Pseudohyponatremia, 1–2
Pseudohypoparathyroidism, 101–2
    defined, 101
Pseudomonas
    kidney stones, 185
    peritonitis, 985
Pseudomonas aeruginosa
    peritonitis, 985–86
    therapy, infective endocarditis, end-
        stage renal disease, 833
Pseudopseudohypoparathyroidism, 102
Psychiatric disorders
    hyponatremia and, 5–6
    renal diseases, 855–73
Psychosis, hypomagnesemia and, 129
Pulmonary alveoli, occupation, as cause
    of respiratory acidosis, 296
Pulmonary edema, 44–45, 45t
Pulmonary infection, transplant, 1173–
    74
Pulmonary perfusion defect, as cause of
    acute respiratory acidosis, 296
Pyelography, retrograde, genitourinary
    tuberculosis, 452
Pyelonephritis
    acute, 435–38
    pregnancy, 584, 587
Pyrazinamide
    detecting hypersensitivity to
        antituberculous drugs, 455
    genitourinary tuberculosis, 453, 454
    with renal insufficiency, 456
Pyridoxine, uremia, 795, 795t
Pyrogenic reactions, dialysis water
    treatment, during dialysis, 1018–19,
    1019t

Q
Quinapril for hypertension, 493

R
R-HuEPO, in renal failure, 881
Ramipril for hypertension, 493
Rapamycin, rejection, 1116
Recipient selection, transplantation,
    1079–1105
Recombinant erythropoietin,
    neuropsychiatric complications,
    869
Reflux nephropathy, 441–49
    focal segmental glomerular sclerosis,
        417
    medical therapy, 441–43
    vs. surgical therapy, 443–44
    treatment of urinary tract infection,
        443
    pregnancy, 584, 587
    prenatal hydronephrosis, algorithm
        for evaluation of, 447
    prevention, 446
    surgical therapy, 443
    therapy, 446–47, *447*
Refractory arrhythmias,
    hypomagnesemia and, 129
Regional anesthesia, 780–81
Removal, peritoneal catheters, 973–74
    functioning catheter, with
        complication, 973–74
    malfunction, 973
    nonfunctioning catheter, 974
Renal acid excretion
    distal acidification, 195–98
    aldosterone excess, 196–97
    buffer content, 191t, 197–98, 198t
    decreased arterial pH, 197
    distal sodium delivery, *194*, 195–96
    increased arterial pCO_2, 197
    titratable acid excretion, 194–95
Renal artery stenosis
    with metabolic alkalosis, 203
    pregnancy and, 584
Renal cancer, hypercalcemia and, 88
Renal colic, kidney stones and, 167
Renal cystic disease, 639–62
    acquired renal cystic disease, 654–
        55
    management, 654–55, 655t
    autosomal dominant polycystic
        kidney disease, 639–50
    African-Americans, 649
    cardiovascular system, 645–46
    in childhood, 649–50
    counseling, 648–49

fluid and electrolyte management, 640–41
gastrointestinal abnormalities, 646–48, *648*
genetic counseling, 648–49
hematuria, 642–43
hypertension, 645
infection, 643–45, 644t
lifestyle, 641
nephrolithiasis, 646, *647*
pain, 641–42
physical activity, 641
pregnancy, 649
prognosis, 650
proteinuria, 645
renal replacement therapy, 650
autosomal recessive polycystic kidney disease, 650–52
management, 651–52
cystic diseases of renal medulla, 652–54
familial juvenile nephronopthisis, 652–53
medullary cystic disease, 652–53
medullary sponge kidney, 653–54
simple cysts, 655–56
Renal excretion, phosphate, 144–47
glomerular filtration, 144
regulation, 145t, 145–47
tubular reabsorption, 144–45
Renal failure
acute, 359–86
complications, 375–76
bleeding, 375–76
cardiopulmonary complications, 375
infections, 375
diagnosis, 361–63
chart review, 361
medical history, 361–62
physical examination, 361–62
urinalysis, 362
urinary indices, 362–63, 363t
urine output pattern, 360t, 362
edama and, 47
etiology of acute renal failure, 359–61
hypernatremia, 12
intrarenal acute renal failure, 360t, 360–61
outcome, 376–78
recovery, 377–78
survival, factors influencing, 376–77
pathogenesis, 363–69
drug-induced, 366–69
heme-pigment-associated, 365
ischemic acute renal failure, 363–65
pathophysiology, 363–69

postrenal acute renal failure, 360, 360t
prerenal acute renal failure, 359, 360t
prevention, 369–71
mannitol, 370–71
overview, 369t, 369–70
treatment, 371–74
conservative management, 371–73
nutrition, 374
renal replacement therapies, 373–74
hypercalcemia, 95
hypocalcemia and, 101
with thrombotic microangiopathy, 521
Renal hypertension, 1195–1206
accelerated, 1198–1200, 1199t
Renal insufficiency, 767–75. *See also* Renal failure
atheroembolic renal disease, 770
cardiac dysfunction, 773
contrast agents, 770
drugs, 769–70
endocrine disorders, 772
fluid and electrolyte disorders, 771
gastrointestinal complications, 773
hematologic abnormalities, 772–73, 773t
hyperlipidemia and, 769
hyperparathyroidism, secondary, 771–72
immunological impairment, 773
neurological disorders, 773
pregnancy, 770
progression, controlling, 767–69
diet, 768
experimental therapies, 769
hyperlipidemia, 769
hypertension, 767–68
LDL, 767–75
phosphate restriction, 768
proteinuria, reduction of, 768–69
pruritus, 774
renal replacement therapy, patient preparation, 774, 774t
reproductive dysfunction, 772
sexual dysfunction, 772
with systemic lupus erythematosus, 460–61, 461t
uremia, management of, 770–74
uremic pericarditis, 773
Renal medulla, cystic diseases of, 652–54
familial juvenile nephronopthisis, 652–53
medullary cystic disease, 652–53
medullary sponge kidney, 653–54
Renal osteodystrophy, 841–53

defined, 841
osteitis fibrosa
calcium supplementation, 845
parathyroidectomy, 845–46, 846t
vitamin D metabolite supplementation, 844–55
therapeutic strategies, integration of, 849t, 849–50
Renal parenchymal diseases, dialysis and, 1195–98
Renal pelvis, neoplasms of, *701*, 702–2
Renal potassium
losses, *58*, 61–65
wasting, magnesium balance and, 131
Renal replacement therapy, 373–74
autosomal dominant polycystic kidney disease, 650
patient preparation, 774, 774t
Renal transplant. *See* Transplant
Renal transport, familial disorders of, magnesium balance, 124–25
Renal tubular acidosis, 64, 65t, *255*, 256, 256t, 275–91, 672–74, 673t
calcium stone, 182
pathogenesis of stones, 182
mechanism of hypercalciuria, 182
reason for low urine citrate, 182
diagnostic tests, 283–89, *284–85*, 286t
amiloride test, 288–89
bumetanide test, 288
furosemide test, 288
immunocytochemical analysis, 289, *289*
metabolic acidosis, maximal acid-excretion during, 284–86, *287*
minimal urine acidity, 284–86, *287*
sodium sulfate infusion, 288
urinary anion gap, 284, *286–87*
urinary electrolytes, 284, *286–87*
urinary pCO_2, index of distal acidification, 286–88
distal, 277–83, *278*, 278t
classic, 278–80
hyperkalemic types of, 280–83
incomplete, 280
pseudohypoaldosteronism, 283
hyperkalemia, 71, 673, 674t
hypoaldosteronism, hyporeninemic, 674
proximal, 275–77
clinical features, 275–76, *276*, 276–77t
diagnosis, *276*, 277
pathophysiology, 275–76, *276*, 276–77t
therapy, 277
pseudohypoaldosteronism, 673–74

type I, 278–80, 672–73
type II, 275–77, 673
Renal tubular damage, hypernatremia, 12
Renal vascular hypertension, 496–98, 498t
Renin-secreting tumors, 1203–4
Renovascular disease, overview, 1201–3
Renovascular hypertension, 1195–206
Reproductive dysfunction, renal insufficiency and, 772
Reserpine, 492, 496
Respiratory acid-base disorders, 293–305
  hypercapnia, defined, 293
  hypocapnia, defined, 293
  respiratory acidosis, 294–301
  respiratory alkalosis, 301–4
Respiratory acidosis, 294–301
  acute, treatment of, 298–99
  chronic, treatment of, 297t, 299–301
  clinical manifestations, 295–96
  diagnosis, 297–98
  etiology, 295, 296–97t
  factors influencing development of, 294–95
  hypercapnia, 295
  plasma electrolyte composition, 295
Respiratory alkalosis, 301–4
  clinical manifestations, 303
  diagnosis, 303–4
  etiology, 302t, 302–3
  plasma electrolyte composition, 301–2
  treatment, 304
Respiratory failure, with hypernatremia, 13
Respiratory insufficiency, brain adaptation, 3
Retrograde pyelography, genitourinary tuberculosis, 452
Ribavirin, for murine lupus nephritis, 463
Rice, magnesium concentration in, 116
Rickets
  hypocalcemia and, 101
  hypophosphatemic, with hypercalcemia, 676
  oncogenous, with phosphaturia, 676
  with phosphaturia, oncogenous, 676
  X-linked hypophosphatemic, 675, 675t
Rifampicin
  detecting hypersensitivity to antituberculous drugs, 455
  genitourinary tuberculosis, 454

toxicity, 455
genitourinary tuberculosis
  chemotherapy, 452
  with renal insufficiency, 456
Rigid peritoneal catheters, 953–55
  complications, 954t, 954–55
  insertion, 953–54
  preinsertion, patient assessment, 953
Root beer, phosphorus content, 843
RRT. *See* Renal replacement therapy
RS-61443, rejection, 1112–13
RTA. *See* Renal tubular acidosis

S
Salicylate intoxication, metabolic acidosis from, 270–71
Salt, bile, diuretic, natriuretic effect of, 551, 551–52
Salt-wasting syndrome, cerebral, 9
Sandimmune, 1147–48
Scleroderma, pregnancy and, 584
Scleroderma-progressive systemic sclerosis, 495t, 499–500
Sclerosis, systemic, in pregnancy, 586
Seawater ingestion, hypernatremia, 12
Sedation
  for hypertension in pregnancy, 578
  to prevent eclampsia, 583–84
Seizures
  hypernatremia, 13
  hypomagnesemia, 129
  lactic acidosis, 225
Selenium, uremia, 794
Sensorium, depression of, with hypernatremia, 13
Septicemia, transplant, 1175
Sequential ultrafiltration, hemodialysis, 1047
Serum creatinine
  progression of renal disease and, 757–58
  reciprocal of, progression of renal disease and, 758
Sexual dysfunction, 772
  renal insufficiency and, 772
Shellfish, magnesium concentration in, 116
Sickle cell hemoglobinopathy, 663–70
  acute renal failure, 667
  blood pressure, 666
  chronic renal failure, 667–69
  hematuria, 666
  renal function abnormalities, 663–66
  acid-base homeostasis, renal acidification and, 665
  potassium, renal handling of, 665

renal concentrating defect, 665
renal hemodynamics, 663–65
renal papillary necrosis, 666–67
sickle cell nephropathy, 667–69
  outcome, 668
  treatment, 668–69
  urinary tract infection, 667
Sirolimus, 1116
Skeletal muscle, hypophosphatemia, 152–53
SKF-105685, 1117
Skin elasticity, examination evidence of dehydration, 323
Sleep disorders in uremia, 864
Small bowel, losses of fluid and electrolytes, 325
Sodium
  balance, continuous ambulatory peritoneal dialysis, 941–42
  diabetic ketoacidosis and, 240–41
  dietary restriction, for edema, 36–37, 37t
  electrolyte abnormalities and, perioperative period, 339–41
  nitroprusside for hypertensive emergency, 496
  phosphate, for hypophosphatemia, 154
Sodium-restricted diets, foe edema, 37
Sodium sulfate infusion, renal tubular acidosis, 288
Soft peritoneal catheters, 955t, 955–58
  complications, 968–73
  early, 968–69
  late, 969–73
  implantation of, 958–66
  catheter preparation, 959
  flange, anchoring, 962
  implantation method, 959–66
  patient preparation, 958–59
  straight, coiled Tenckhoff catheters, 956, 956
  swan-neck catheters, 956, 956t, 956–58
Solitary kidney, pregnancy, 584, 588
Solutes
  acute peritoneal dialysis, 917, 917t
  arginine vasopressin, 2
  cell content, steady state, 1
  diluting segment of nephron, 2
  hyponatremia, 2
  pseudohyponatremia, 1–2
Sorbent hemoperfusion, for poisoning, 752–53, 752–53t
Spasticity, hypomagnesemia and, 129
Spironolactone
  for hypertension, 492

onset and duration of action, 38
  site of action of, 36
Splenectomy, thrombotic
  microangiopathy, 520
Sponge kidney, medullary, 653–54
Staphylococcus aureus
  bacterial endocarditis,
    glomerulonephritis in, 395–400
  therapy, infective endocarditis, end-
    stage renal disease, 833
Staphylococcus epidermidis, therapy,
    infective endocarditis, end-stage
    renal disease, 833
Staphylococcus saprophyticus, urinary
    tract infection, 435
Status asthmaticus, magnesium balance,
    135
Steroids
  genitourinary tuberculosis
    chemotherapy, 454
  supplementation, after transplant,
    1147
Streptococcus, therapy, infective
    endocarditis, end-stage renal
    disease, 833
Streptomycin
  detecting hypersensitivity to
    antituberculous drugs, 455
  genitourinary tuberculosis
    chemotherapy, 453
  with renal insufficiency, 456
Stroke, hypomagnesemia and, 129
Struvite stones, 167, 185
Sulfadiazine, for AIDS, 622
Sunflower seeds, phosphorus content,
    843
Suprapubic catheters, 1229
Surgical patient, fluid and electrolyte
    disorders, 335–50
Swan-neck catheters, 975
Sweating, magnesium balance, 126
Symptomatic hyponatremia, 4t, 4–8
  delayed diagnosis of, 7
Systemic lupus erythematosus, 459–
    78
  fetal and maternal morbidity and
    mortality, 462–63
  hypertension and atherosclerosis,
    462, 462t
  infection and immunization, 462,
    462t
  neonatal lupus, 463
  nephritis-related complications, 460–
    63
  in pregnancy, 585–86
  proteinuria, 461
  renal insufficiency, 460–61, 461t

therapy, 463–71
  transplant, 1156
Systemic sclerosis, in pregnancy, 586

T
Tachypnea, with hypernatremia, 13
Tacrolimus, 1115–16
  rejection, 1115–16
Tears, examination evidence of
    dehydration, 323
Temporary dialysis access, 989–91
Terazosin, dosage, side effects, 1197
Tetany, hypomagnesemia and, 129
Theophylline-induced hypercalcemia,
    94
Thermally injured, fluid and electrolyte
    disorders in, 351–57
  burn shock, 351–54, *352*
  adrenal failure, 353
  concomitant injury, 353
  elderly patients, 353
  pediatric patients, 353
  vasoconstrictor shock, 352
  young adults, 352–53, *352–53*
  later postburn period, 354
  electrical burns, 354
  preexisting diseases, 354
  postresuscitation period, immediate,
    354–56, *355*
Thiazide, 9
  for chronic hypertension in
    pregnancy, 577
  edema, *36*, 36t, 38t, 40
  hypercalcemia and, 94
  kidney stones and, 170t, 178
  loop of Henle, early distal loop, *36*,
    36t, 38t, 40
Thirst
  center, hypothalamic subfornical
    region, 24
  polyuric syndromes and, *22*, 23–24
Thrombocyte function, in renal failure,
    887
Thrombosis
  renal vein, 502–3
  venous sinuses, hypertonicity, 12
Thrombotic complications, in renal
    failure, 887
Thrombotic microangiopathy, 513–27
  clinical features, 516–18
  endothelial cell dysfunction, 514–15
  etiology, 513–14
  hemolytic uremic syndrome
    cancer-associated, 517–18
    cyclosporine-associated, 518
    epidemic, 516

hereditary, hemolytic uremic
    syndrome, 518
  postpartum, 517
  pregnancy-associated, 517
  sporadic, 516–17
  thrombotic thrombocytopenic
    purpura, 518
    acute, 518
    chronic, 518
    relapsing, 518
  pathology, 515–16
  treatment, 518–21, 519t
    antioxidants, 521
    antiplatelet agents, 520
    antithrombotic treatment, 520–21
    glucocorticoids, 520
    heparin, 521
    immunosuppressive treatment, and
      splenectomy, 520
    plasma manipulation, 519–20
    renal failure, 521
    splenectomy, 520
    vitamin E, 521
Thrombotic thrombocytopenic purpura,
    868
  acute, hemolytic uremic syndrome,
    518
  chronic, hemolytic uremic syndrome,
    518
  hemolytic uremic syndrome, 518
  relapsing, 518
Thyroid hormone, potassium balance
    and, 55
Tidal peritoneal dialysis, 924–25
Timolol for hypertension, 492
Tissue oxygen delivery, improvement
    of, for lactic acidosis, 216–18
Tobacco smoking, bladder carcinoma
    and, 705
Tocopherol, uremia, 795
Tolazamide, nephrogenic diabetes
    insipidus and, 26
Tolypocladium inflatum gams,
    nephrotoxicity, 731
Torasemide
  onset, duration of action, 38
  site of action of, 36
Torsades des pointes treatment,
    hypomagnesemia and, 129
Toxic nephropathy, 723–45
  from analgesic, 735–37
  clinical presentation of AN, 735
  epidemiology of AN, 735–37, 736t
  from angiotensin-converting enzyme
    inhibitors, 738
  antibiotic-induced, 725–28
  acyclovir, 728

aminoglycoside antibiotic
   nephrotoxicity, 725–26
amphotericin B, 727–28
carbapenum, 727
cephalosporin, 726–27
foscarnet, 728
penicillin, 726
pentamidine, 728
rifampin, 727
sulfonamide, 727
tetracycline, 727
vancomycin, 727
from cadmium, 737–38
cellular mechanisms of injury, 724–25
cellular uptake, nephrotoxins, 724
intracellular sites, nephrotoxicity,
   724–25
mechanisms, nephrotoxicity, 724–25
from chemotherapeutic agents, 729–
   31
cisplatin, 729–30
methotrexate, 730
nitrosoureas, 730
contrast medium-associated, 728–29
management, 729
prevention, 729
risk factors, 728–29
defined, 723–24
diagnosis, 723–24
from environmental toxicants, 740
glomerular filtration rate, 723
gold nephropathy, 739–40
from heavy metals, 740
illicit drug abuse, 739
from immunosuppressive drugs, 731–
   34
cyclosporines, 731t, 731–34
from lead, 737
from nonsteroidal anti-inflammatory
   drugs, 734t, 734–35
from penicillamine, 739
Tolypocladium inflatum gams, 731
Toxins. *See under* specific toxin
TPD. *See* Tidal peritoneal dialysis
Transferred cancer, after transplant,
   1179
Transfusion. *See* Blood transfusion
Transplantation
acid-base disorders, 1139–40
amyloidosis, 1143
dialysis amyloidosis, 1143
in familial mediterranean fever, 1143
recurrent, renal allograft, 1143
complications of, 1169–82
technical, 1169–72
contraindications, 1081–83
cyclosporin, 1146

cytomegalovirus, 1098
diabetes mellitus, posttransplant,
   1146–47
diabetic nephropathy, 1147
donor selection, 1079–105
cadaver donors, 1093–94
HLA antigens, 1096–98
living related donors, 1089–92, *1090*
living unrelated donors, 1092t, 1092–
   93
pretransplant evaluation of potential
   living donor, 1092t, 1093
drugs used for immunosuppression,
   adverse effects, 1147–48, 1148t
azathioprine, 1148
cyclosporine, 1147–48
glycocorticoids, 1148
elderly patients, 1149
end-stage renal disease, leading to
   transplant, causes, 1083t, 1083–84
Epstein-Barr vizoster virus, 1098
erythrocytosis
after, 1147
posttransplant, 1147
extrarenal complications, 1146–47
gout, 1143–44
growth hormone after transplant,
   1149
hepatitis and, 907–8
hyperlipidemia, 1144–46
cholestyramine, 1145
gemfibrozil, 1145
lovastatin, 1145
nicotinic acid, 1145–46
provastatin, 1145
hyperuricemia, 1143–44
immunosuppression, 1107–37
rejection, 1107–37
indications for, 1079–81, *1080–81*
in inherited systemic disease, 1153–
   67
magnesium metabolism, 1142–43
metabolic bone disease, 1140–42
in metabolic diseases, 1153–67
metabolic dysfunction following,
   1139–52
metabolic status of myocardium
   following, 1144
myopathy after, 1144
nephrectomy, 1087–89
blood transfusion, *1088*, 1089
gastrointestinal disease, 1088
lower urinary tract dysfunction,
   1087
parathyroidectomy, 1088
splenectomy, 1087–88
nutrition and, 793–94

obesity, 1146
OKT3, metabolic side effects of,
   1148–49
phosphate metabolism, 1142
potassium disorders, 1139–40
pregnancy, 591–96, 1149
counseling, 591t, 591–92
delivery, 594–95
management, 592–94
pediatric management, 595
postnatal assessment, 595
pretransplant evaluation, potential
   recipient, 1084–87, 1085t
laboratory tests, 1086
patient history, 1085
physical examination, 1085–86
radiographic studies, 1086
urologic studies, 1086
recipient selection, 1079–105
rejection, 1107–37
steroids, 1146
supplementation with, 1147
surgical preparation, 1087
tubular dysfunction following, 1139–
   52
viral infections, 1098–99
Transurethral resection of prostate,
   water balance, postoperative, 5
Tremors, hypomagnesemia and, 129
Triamethaphan camsylate for
   hypertensive emergency, 496
Triampterine, kidney stones, 167
Triamterene
for hypertension, 492
onset and duration of action, 38
site of action of, 36
Trichlomethiazide, for hypertension,
   492
Trichomonas, 437
vulvovaginitis secondary to, 437
Trimethaprim, potassium and, 70
Trimethroprim-sulfamethoxazole, for
   AIDS, 622
TTP. *See* Thrombotic
   thrombocytopenic purpura
Tuberculosis, genitourinary, 451–58
algorithm for, 457
chemotherapy, 452–54, 453t
ethambutol, *453*, 453–54, 454t
isoniazid, 452–53
pyrazinamide, 453
rifampicin, 452
steroids, 454
streptomycin, 453
HIV, 455–56
investigations, 451–52
arteriography, 452

endoscopy, 452
intravenous urogram, 451–52
percutaneous nephrostomy, 452
radiography, 451
retrograde pyelography, 452
management, 452
pyrazinamide, 454
rifampicin, 454
streptomycin, 454
surgery, 456–58
diseased tissue, removal of, 456
follow-up, *457*, 458
reconstructive surgery, 456–58
toxicity, 454–55
antituberculous drugs, renal failure, 455, 456t
contraceptive pill, 455
hepatotoxicity, 455
hypersensitivity, 454–55
rifampicin, 455
Tubular disorders, inherited, 671–80
acidosis, 672–74, 673t
classical pseudohypoaldosteronism, 673–74
hyperkalemic, 673, 674t
hyporeninemic hypoaldosteronism, 674
proximal, 673
pseudohypoaldosteronism, 673–74
type I, 672–73
type II, 673
aminoaciduria, 671–72
Bartter's syndrome, 679–80
chloride shunt syndrome, 680
dicarboxylic aminoaciduria, 671
Fanconi syndrome, 677–79, 678t
Gitelman's syndrome, 679
glycinuria, 672
glycosuria, 672
Hartnup disease, 671
hereditary fructose intolerance, 678
histidinuria, 672
hypercystinuria, 672
iminoglycinuria, 671
Liddle's syndrome, 680
Lowe's syndrome, 678
magnesurias, 677
Oasthouse syndrome, 672
phophaturias, 674–77
adult sporadic osteomalacia, 676–77, 677t
hereditary hypophosphatemic rickets with hypercalcemia, 676
hypophosphatemic nonrachitic bone disease, 676
hypophosphatemic rickets, with hypercalcemia, 676

osteomalacia, adult, sporadic, 676–77, 677t
primary or X-linked hypophosphatemic rickets, 675, 675t
rickets, oncogenous, with phosphaturia, 676
X-linked hypophosphatemic rickets, 675, 675t
tyrosinosis, 678
untyped glycogen storage disease, 679
vitamin D deficiency, 679
Wilson's disease, 679
Tubular dysfunction, after transplant, 1139–52
Tubulointerstitial disease, in pregnancy, 587
Tumors of kidney, malignant, 695–701
diagnosis, *696–97*, 699–700, 699–700t
metastases, 701
pathology, 696–99
staging, *696–97*, 699–700, 699–700t
treatment, *698*, 700t, 700–701
Tunnel infections, peritonitis, 986
TURP. *See* Transurethral resection of prostate
Tyrosinosis, 678

U
United States Renal Data System Report, catheter evaluation, 975–76
Upper airways obstruction
as cause of acute respiratory acidosis, 296
as cause of chronic respiratory acidosis, 297
Urea, progression of renal disease and, 758
Uremia
autonomic nervous system dysfunction, 861
cardiovascular complications, 817–39
drugs, 1065–78
nutritional management, 783–802
acute renal failure, 792–93
metabolic abnormalities, 792
nutritional approach, 792–93
ascorbic acid, 795
biochemical measurements, 785
body composition, 784–85
catabolic factors, dialysis treatment, 787t, 787–88
chronic renal failure, nutritional status in, 783–85, 784t

during continuous ambulatory peritoneal dialysis, 790–92
causes of malnutrition, 791
malnutrition
outcome of, 790–91
prevalence, 790–91
prevention, protein energy malnutrition, 791t, 791–92
copper, 795
cyanocobalamin, 795
dietary compliance, assessment of, 783
dietary intake, assessment of, 783
iron, 794
malnutrition, in maintenance dialysis, 788–90, 789t
drug intervention, 790
energy intake, 789–90
growth hormone, 790
intradialytic parenteral nutrition, 790
protein intake, 789–90
treatment, 789t, 789–90
nitrogen balance, 783–84
pre dialysis stage, chronic renal failure, 785–86
conventional low-protein diet, 786
energy requirements, 786
very low-protein diet
amino acid supplement, 786
keto acid supplement, 786
protein intake, patient compliance, 783–85, 784t
pyridoxine, 795, 795t
selenium, 794
tocopherol, 795
transplant, 793–94
vitamins, 794–96
vitamin A, 796
wasting, in chronic renal failure, 786
endocrine disorders, 787
metabolic disorders, 787
poor protein energy intake, 787
zinc, 794–95
renal insufficiency and, 770–74
sleep disorders in, 864
Uremiahemolytic-uremic syndrome, autonomic nervous system dysfunction in, 868
Uremic cardiomyopathy, heart failure, 822–27, *823*
etiology, 823–24
incidence, 822–23
left ventricular morphology, 824, *825*
management, 824–27, 826t
Uremic encephalopathy, 855–57
acidosis, encephalopathy due to, 857–58

clinical features, 855
electrophysiological findings, 855–56
maintenance dialysis, 856
morphology, 856
pathophysiology, 856
treatment, 856–57
Uremic pericarditis, 773
Uremic polyneuropathy, 858–60
clinical features, 859
electrophysiological findings, 859
morphology, 859
pathophysiology, 859
treatment, 859–60
Ureter, neoplasms of, *701*, 702–2
Ureteral stents, 1227–28, 1228t
Urethra, anatomy, 1234
Urethritis, 436–37
Uric acid stones, 167, 182–84
calcium-uric acid stones, 184, *184*
dissolution, 184
gout, 183
ileostomy, 183
inflammatory ileocolitis, 183
Lesch-Nyhan syndrome, 183
pathogenesis, 182–83
small bowel bypass, 183
treatment, 183–84
hyperuricosuria, *183*, 183–84
increased urine volume, 184
urine acidity, 183, *183*
tumor-lysis syndrome, 183
Urinalysis, acute renal failure diagnosis, 362
Urinary anion gap, renal tubular acidosis, 284, *286–87*
Urinary electrolytes, renal tubular acidosis and, 284, *286–87*
Urinary pCO_2, index of distal acidification, renal tubular acidosis, 286–88
Urinary tract infections, 435–40
bacteriuria, asymptomatic, 439
candida, vulvovaginitis secondary to, 437
catheter-related, 438–39
chlamydia, 437
clinical presentation, 436
complicated, 438
cystitis, acute, 435–38
diagnosis, 436
differential diagnosis, 436–37
E. coli, 435–36
neisseria, 437
pathogenesis, 435–36
pyelonephritis, acute, 435–38
recurrent infections, 437–38

with sickle cell hemoglobinopathy, 667
Staphylococcus saprophyticus, 435
transplant, 1174–75
treatment, 437
trichomonas, 437
vulvovaginitis secondary to, 437
uncomplicated, 435–38
urethritis, 436–37
Urinary tract surgery, in pregnancy, previous, 588
Urine acidity, renal tubular acidosis, 284–86, *287*
Urine output
examination evidence of dehydration, 323
pattern of, acute renal failure diagnosis, 360t, 362
Urogram, intravenous, genitourinary tuberculosis, 451–52
Urolithiasis, in pregnancy, 584, 587–88
Urologic complications, transplant, 1170–71
UTI. *See* Urinary tract infection

V

Vascular complications, in transplantation, 1169–70, *1171*
Vasculitic disease, 479–88
clinical features, 480–81
Henoch-Schonlein nephritis, 484–85
prognostic considerations, 485
renal involvement, 484–85
therapeutic approaches, 485
natural history of, 480–81
necrotizing-crescentic glomerulonephritis, 480–81
polyangitis, microscopic, 480
polyarteritis nodosa, 480
treatment, 481–84
cytotoxic drugs, complications of, 484
necrotizing-crescentic glomerulonephritis, 482–84
polyangitis, microscopic, 482–84
polyarteritis nodosa, 481–82
Wegener's granulomatosis, and necrotizing-crescentic glomerulonephritis, 482–84
vasculitic syndrome, 479–88
antineutrophil cytoplasmic antibodies, 479
classification, 479, 480t
Wegener's granulomatosis, 480
Vasculitides, transplant, 1157–58
Vasoconstrictor shock, in thermally injured, 352

Vasopressin, 2–3
cerebral effects of, 3
hypotension, 23
polyuria, 21–23, *22*
Vasopressin-mediated water permeability
atrial natriuretic peptide, 23
polyuria, 23
Vegetables, phosphorus content, 843
Venous sinuses, thrombosis, hypertonicity, 12
Ventilatory restriction
as cause of acute respiratory acidosis, 296
as cause of chronic respiratory acidosis, 297
Verapramil for hypertension, 493
Verney, E.B., 21–22
Vesicourethral dysfunction, nonsurgical management, 1233–40
anatomy, 1234
bladder, 1234
urethra, 1234
benign prostatic hyperplasia, 1237–39
medical treatment, 1238–39
intermittent catheterization, 1239
neurophysiology, 1233–34
autonomic nervous system, 1233–34
somatic nervous system, 1234
outflow resistance, decreasing, 1237
treatment, voiding dysfunction, 1235–37
bladder emptying, failure of, 1236–37
bladder storage, failure of, 1235–36
imipramine, lower urinary tract, 1236
Vesicourteral reflux
complications, 444–46
hypertension, 445
renal scarring, 444–45
voiding dysfunction, 445–46
endoscopic treatment, 444
medical therapy, 441–43
vs. surgical therapy, 443–44
treatment of urinary tract infection, 443
prenatal hydronephrosis, algorithm for evaluation of, 447
reflux nephropathy and, 441–49
reflux, 443–44
surgical therapy, 443
therapy, 446–47, *447*
Vesopressinoic acid, hyponatremia, 8
Vinblastine, nephrogenic diabetes insipidus and, 26

Viral infection. *See also under* specific virus
    transplantation and, 1098–99, 1175
Vitamins
    uremia and, 794–96
    vitamin A, 94, 796
    vitamin D deficiency, 101, 679
    vitamin D intoxication, hypercalcemia and, 94
    vitamin D metabolite supplementation, osteitis fibrosa, 844–55
    vitamin E, thrombotic microangiopathy, 521
Voiding dysfunction
    bladder
        emptying, failure of, 1236–37
        storage, failure of, 1235–36
        imipramine, lower urinary tract, 1236
        treatment, 1235–37
Volume, of cell
    determination of, 1
    regulation of, 1, 2t
Volume disorders, in surgical patient, fluid and electrolytes, 336–37
    volume depletion, 336–37, 336–37t
    volume overload, 337

Volume-expansion therapy, for hypertension in pregnancy, 580–81
Vomiting
    with metabolic alkalosis, 203
    potassium loss and, 62

W
Waldenstrom's macroglobulinemia, 529
Water balance
    normal, 21–24
    in postoperative patients, 4
Water deprivation test, polyuria, 28–29
Water treatment, dialysis, 1015t, 1015–21
    Association for Advancement of Medical Instrumentation, standards, 1021–26, 1022t
    chemical contaminants in, 1015
    hazards associated with, 1015, 1016t
    microbiology, 1018, 1018t
    pathogenesis, pyrogenic reactions, 1020–21, 1020–21t, *1021*
    pyrogenic reactions, during dialysis, 1018–19, 1019t

purification, components of, 1016–18, *1017*
Wegener's granulomatosis, 480, 868
    corticosteroids for, 483
    cyclophosphamide for, 483
    in pregnancy, 588
Weight loss, with hypernatremia, 13
Werniche's encephalopathy, dialysis and, 864
White blood cells, in renal failure, 886–87
Whole wheat bread, phosphorus content, 843
Willis, Thomas, 233
Wilson's disease, 679
Wound, transplantation
    complications, 1172
    infection, 1175

X
Xanthine, kidney stones, 167

Z
Zinc, uremia and, 794–95